19th Edition

HARRISON'S™ PRINCIPLES OF INTERNAL MEDICINE

SELF-ASSESSMENT AND BOARD REVIEW

Editorial Board

19th Edition

HARRISON'S™ PRINCIPLES OF INTERNAL MEDICINE

SELF-ASSESSMENT AND BOARD REVIEW

For use with the 19th edition of HARRISON'S PRINCIPLES OF INTERNAL MEDICINE

EDITED BY

CHARLES M. WIENER, MD
Vice President of Academic Affairs
Johns Hopkins Medicine International
Professor of Medicine and Physiology
Johns Hopkins School of Medicine
Baltimore, Maryland

CYNTHIA D. BROWN, MD
Associate Professor of Clinical Medicine
Division of Pulmonary, Critical Care, Sleep and Occupational Medicine
Indiana University
Indianapolis, Indiana

BRIAN HOUSTON, MD
Assistant Professor of Medicine
Division of Cardiology
Medical University of South Carolina
Charleston, South Carolina

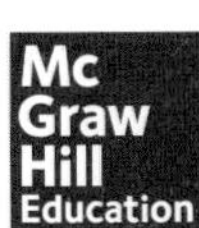

New York Chicago San Francisco Athens London Madrid Mexico City
Milan New Delhi Singapore Sydney Toronto

Harrison's®
PRINCIPLES OF INTERNAL MEDICINE, 19th Edition
Self-Assessment and Board Review

3 4 5 6 7 8 9 LWI 21 20 19 18

ISBN 978-1-259-64288-3
MHID 1-259-64288-7
ISSN 2167-7808

Notice

Medicine is an ever-changing science. As new research and clinical experience broaden our knowledge, changes in treatment and drug therapy are required. The authors and the publisher of this work have checked with sources believed to be reliable in their efforts to provide information that is complete and generally in accord with the standards accepted at the time of publication. However, in view of the possibility of human error or changes in medical sciences, neither the authors nor the publisher nor any other party who has been involved in the preparation or publication of this work warrants that the information contained herein is in every respect accurate or complete, and they disclaim all responsibility for any errors or omissions or for the results obtained from use of the information contained in this work. Readers are encouraged to confirm the information contained herein with other sources. For example and in particular, readers are advised to check the product information sheet included in the package of each drug they plan to administer to be certain that the information contained in this work is accurate and that changes have not been made in the recommended dose or in the contraindications for administration. This recommendation is of particular importance in connection with new or infrequently used drugs.

This book was set in Minion Pro by Cenveo® Publisher Services.
The editors were James F. Shanahan and Kim J. Davis.
The production supervisor was Catherine H. Saggese.
Project management was provided by Surbhi Mittal, Cenveo Publisher Services.
Cover image: animate4.com ltd. / Science Source.

This book is printed on acid-free paper.

International Edition ISBN 978-1-259-92138-4; MHID 1-259-92138-7. Copyright © 2017. Exclusive rights by McGraw-Hill Education, for manufacture and export. This book cannot be re-exported from the country to which it is consigned by McGraw-Hill. The International Edition is not available in North America.

CONTENTS

PREFACE

This is the fourth edition of *Harrison's Self-Assessment and Board Review* that we have had the honor of working on. We thank the editors of the 19th edition of *Harrison's Principles of Internal Medicine* for their continued confidence in our ability to produce a worthwhile companion to their exceptional textbook. It is truly inspirational to remind ourselves why we love medicine broadly, and internal medicine specifically.

The care of patients is a privilege. As physicians, we owe it to our patients to be intelligent, contemporary, and curious. Continuing education takes many forms; many of us enjoy the intellectual stimulation and active learning challenge of the question-and-answer format. It is in that spirit that we offer the 19th edition of the *Self-Assessment and Board Review* to students, housestaff, and practitioners. We hope that from it you will learn, read, investigate, and question. The questions and answers are particularly conducive to collaboration and discussion with colleagues.

This edition contains over 1100 questions and comprehensive explanations. The questions, whenever possible, use realistic patient scenarios, including radiographic or pathologic images. Our answers attempt to explain the correct or best choice, often supported with figures from the 19th edition of *Harrison's Principles of Internal Medicine* to stimulate learning.

Readers will note important changes in this new edition. We have replaced more than 60% of questions from the prior edition, thus hundreds of brand new questions and explanations are included herein. The format of the book has also changed, allowing for the more effective use of color images throughout. Readers will appreciate the convenience of having color images next to their citations in the text. This new edition is tied directly to all the great and updated content in the 19th edition of *Harrison's Principles of Internal Medicine,* assuring readers that the content of the *Self Assessment and Board Review* reflects the latest knowledge and developments in the field.

The content of this book is available in a variety of delivery formats. In addition to the print edition, an "app" will be available that offers adaptive learning features so that users can focus their studies on areas of greatest need. Several eBook formats are available, and as before the content is available on the widely used www.accessmedicine.com resource, where users can easily toggle over the *Harrison's* content for greater explanation and context of all the Q&A in this book.

Even though two of the authors (C.D.B., B.H.) have physically left the Osler Medical Service at Johns Hopkins Hospital, they will never leave spiritually. Our experiences with colleagues and patients at Johns Hopkins have defined our professional lives. In the words of William Osler, "We are here to add what we can to life, not to get what we can from life." We hope this addition to your life stimulates your mind, challenges your thinking, and translates benefit to your patients.

SECTION I

General Considerations in Clinical Medicine

QUESTIONS

DIRECTIONS: Choose the one best response to each question.

I-1. All of the following statements regarding practice guidelines set forth by governing agencies and professional organizations are true EXCEPT:

A. Clinical practice guidelines protect caregivers against inappropriate charges of malpractice, yet do not provide protection for patients from receiving substandard care.
B. Practice guidelines have largely reached a stage of nuance allowing them to address every unique illness and patient presented to the modern physician.
C. Practice guidelines provide a legal constraint to physicians, and deviation from guideline-based care invariably leaves physicians vulnerable to legal action.
D. Where different organizations disagree regarding practice guidelines, a third-party agency has been appointed to mitigate these disagreements such that now all major organizations' guidelines are consistent.
E. All of the above statements are not true.

I-2. Regarding molecular medicine, which of the following statements represents an INACCURATE example of the listed area of study:

A. Exposomics: An endocrinologist studies sunlight exposure and population risk of hip fracture.
B. Metabolomics: A biochemist studies the rate of flux through the creatine kinase pathway during the cardiac cycle.
C. Metagenomics: A biologist studies the genomic alterations in molds commonly found in human dwellings.
D. Microbiomics: A microbiologist studies the genomic variation in thermophiles, bacteria that can survive extreme heat near deep ocean vents.
E. Proteomics: A cardiologist studies desmosomal proteins and their posttranslational modifications in studying arrhythmogenic right ventricular dysplasia.

I-3. Which of the following is the best definition of evidence-based medicine?

A. A summary of existing data from existing clinical trials with a critical methodologic review and statistical analysis of summative data
B. A type of research that compares the results of one approach to treating disease with another approach to treating the same disease
C. Clinical decision-making support tools developed by professional organizations that include expert opinions and data from clinical trials
D. Clinical decision making supported by data, preferably randomized controlled clinical trials
E. One physician's clinical experience in caring for multiple patients with a specific disorder over many years

I-4. Which of the following is the standard measure for determining the impact of a health condition on a population?

A. Disability-adjusted life-years
B. Infant mortality
C. Life expectancy
D. Standardized mortality ratio
E. Years of life lost

I-5. Which of the following statements regarding disease patterns worldwide is true?

A. Childhood undernutrition is the leading risk factor for global disease burden.
B. In a 2006 publication, the World Health Organization (WHO) estimated that 10% of the total global burden of disease was due to modifiable environmental risk factors.
C. In 2010, ischemic heart disease was the leading cause of death among adults.
D. In the last two decades, mortality attributed to communicable diseases, maternal and perinatal conditions, and nutritional deficiencies has remained fairly stable, with the majority (76%) of mortality from these causes occurring in sub-Saharan Africa and southern Asia.
E. While poverty status has been shown to be linked to health status on the individual level, the same relationship does not hold true when studying the link between national health indicators and gross domestic product per capita among nations.

I-6. You are appointed to a governmental healthcare advisory subcommittee concerned with addressing problems facing the global health community. Your task is to draw general conclusions from the global fight against tuberculosis (TB) and human immunodeficiency virus (HIV)/acquired immunodeficiency syndrome (AIDS) that may be applied in combatting other diseases, including noncommunicable diseases. Which of the following conclusions is reasonable when considering HIV/AIDS and TB as chronic diseases?

A. Barriers to adequate healthcare and patient adherence imposed by extreme poverty must be concomitantly addressed to adequately treat and prevent chronic disease in developing nations.
B. Charging small fees for health services (e.g., AIDS prevention and care) supplies the patient with a sense of the treatment's value and increases compliance and overall public health.
C. Despite adequate available tools to practice their trade locally in developing nations, many physicians and nurses emigrate to developed nations to practice their respective trades, a phenomenon called "brain drain."
D. In developed nations where physicians are abundant, community health worker supervision of the care of chronically ill patients is not effective.
E. In the case of chronic infectious diseases, switching from one drug to another through a prolonged course of treatment provides the highest cure rate by obviating the infectious agent's ability to develop resistance to any single drug.

I-7. Mrs. Jones, a 22-year-old African American woman, presents to Dr. Smith, an internal medicine specialist, with a facial rash. Mrs. Jones states that the rash began after spending a day at the beach with her family. She also notes that her metacarpophalangeal and proximal interphalangeal joints have been painful and swollen for the preceding 2 weeks. On examination, the joints are swollen and tender. Laboratory analysis discloses reduced creatinine clearance, proteinuria, and hemolytic anemia. Antinuclear antibodies (a test with a high negative predictive value for systemic lupus erythematosus) are detected at significant titer, and ultimately, the diagnosis of systemic lupus erythematosus is made.

Two weeks later, Mrs. Johnson, a 24-year-old African American woman, presents with a facial rash and elbow pain to Dr. Smith. After a cursory interview and brief physical exam, Dr. Smith sends blood work only testing for antinuclear antibodies. When the test returns negative (no antibodies detected), Dr. Smith presumes this to be a false-negative result and starts Mrs. Johnson on hydroxychloroquine and prednisone for treatment of systemic lupus erythematosus. Which heuristic(s) did Dr. Smith likely employ in diagnosing Mrs. Johnson with systemic lupus erythematosus?

A. Availability heuristic
B. Anchoring heuristic
C. Bayes' rule
D. Confirmation bias
E. A and B

I-8. You have invented a blood test, which you name "veritangin," to determine if patients are having a myocardial infarction. You devise an experiment to determine the performance of your veritangin assay by testing it versus the troponin assay, the currently accepted gold standard for determining myocardial infarction, in 100 random emergency department patients with chest pain. You choose a veritangin result >1 ng/dL as positive for myocardial infarction. Your results are listed in the table below.

	Troponin Status	
Veritangin Status	Troponin Positive	Troponin Negative
Veritangin Positive	15	5
Veritangin Negative	10	70

Which of the following statements regarding the characteristics of the veritangin assay in this trial is true?

A. The posttest probability of the veritangin test does not depend on the population studied.
B. The sensitivity of the veritangin assay depends on the population studied and the disease prevalence in that population.
C. The sensitivity of the veritangin assay will decrease by 50% if you reduce the threshold for a positive result to >0.5 ng/dL.
D. The sensitivity of the veritangin test cannot be calculated based on the above data.
E. The specificity of the veritangin assay is 0.93 (70/75).

I-9. You are designing a clinical trial to test the use of a novel anticoagulant, clotbegone, in the treatment of deep vein thrombosis. Which of the following statements regarding the design of the trial is true?

A. An optimal study design would assign many patients to clotbegone and compare their outcomes to the outcomes of prior (historical) patients not taking clotbegone. This would allow faster trial completion.
B. If the trial returns a positive result (clotbegone is superior to placebo), that means that any patient with a clot would benefit from clotbegone therapy.
C. Observing the outcomes of patients already taking clotbegone versus patients who are not is preferable to assigning patients to clotbegone or placebo in a blinded fashion. The observational strategy is more "real world," applicable to the general population, and free of bias.
D. Population selection for the trial enrollment is not important as long as careful attention to randomization and blinding is observed.
E. The advantage of performing a randomized clinical trial of clotbegone over a prospective observational study of clotbegone is the avoidance of treatment selection bias.

I-10. A receiver operating characteristic (ROC) curve is constructed for a new test developed to diagnose disease X. All of the following statements regarding the ROC curve are true EXCEPT:

A. One criticism of the ROC curve is that it is developed for testing only one test or clinical parameter with exclusion of other potentially relevant data.
B. ROC curve allows the selection of a threshold value for a test that yields the best sensitivity with the fewest false-positive tests.
C. The axes of the ROC curve are sensitivity versus 1 – specificity.
D. The ideal ROC curve will have a value of 0.5.
E. The value of the ROC curve is calculated as the area under the curve generated from the true-positive rate versus the false-positive rate.

I-11. When considering a potential screening test, what end points should be considered to assess the potential gain from a proposed intervention?

A. Absolute and relative impact of screening on the disease outcome
B. Cost per life-year saved
C. Increase in the average life expectancy for the entire population
D. Number of subjects screened to alter the outcome in one individual
E. All of the above

I-12. You are appointed to an advisory committee in the WHO tasked with making recommendations regarding breast cancer screening and prevention. In regard to screening and preventing breast cancer in women, which of the following potential recommendations from your committee would be valid?

A. Any breast cancer detected by screening mammography and adequately treated represents a reduction in breast cancer mortality.
B. Screening is most effective when applied to relatively common diseases. Breast cancer, with a lifetime risk of 10% in women, meets this criterion.
C. The presence of a latent (asymptomatic) stage of breast cancer renders it a less ideal disease candidate for screening at the population level.
D. When studying the effectiveness of breast cancer screening with mammography in a population, length of disease survival is the most important outcome to consider.
E. Women in the general population should undergo just as rigorous screening and prevention measures for breast cancer as women with the *BRCA1* or *BRCA2* mutations.

I-13. You are seeing Mr. Brown today in the primary care clinic. He has a long history of tobacco abuse, and you notice on his intake form that he wishes to discuss lung cancer screening today. Which of the following statements regarding lung cancer screening can you truthfully make to Mr. Brown?

A. "Recently, a large National Heart, Lung, and Blood Institute study demonstrated a significant reduction in mortality by employing low-dose chest computed tomography as a screening tool in patients with a significant smoking history."
B. "Screening for lung cancer has a long history of successful implementation given the ease of obtaining a chest x-ray and the fact that most lung cancers are curable at the time of screening detection."
C. "Screening for lung cancer is a 'no-brainer'; there is really no harm in a false-positive test. The only real worry is always that you might have a cancer that we don't know about."
D. "Because the sensitivity and specificity of any screening test do not depend on the population studied, your odds of having lung cancer after a positive chest x-ray do not depend on his smoking history."
E. "There is really no evidence of benefit for lung cancer screening by any modality."

I-14. Which preventative intervention leads to the largest average increase in life expectancy for a target population?

A. A regular exercise program for a 40-year-old man
B. Getting a 35-year-old smoker to quit smoking
C. Mammography in women age 50–70
D. Pap smears in women age 18–65
E. Prostate-specific antigen (PSA) and digital rectal examination for a man >50 years old

I-15. The U.S. Preventive Services Task Force (USPSTF) recommends which of the following screening tests for the listed patients?

A. 16-year-old male: immunoassay for HIV if not performed before
B. 32-year-old sexually active woman: nucleic acid amplification on a cervical swab for chlamydia
C. 50-year-old woman with a smoking history: dual-energy x-ray absorptiometry (DEXA) scan for osteoporosis
D. 58-year-old prior smoker: ultrasound for abdominal aortic aneurysm
E. 80-year-old man: anti–hepatitis C virus (HCV) antibody for hepatitis C

I-16. Patients taking which of the following drugs should be advised to avoid drinking grapefruit juice?

A. Amoxicillin
B. Aspirin
C. Atorvastatin
D. Prevacid
E. Sildenafil

I-17. A 26-year-old woman received an allogeneic bone marrow transplantation 9 months ago for acute myelogenous leukemia. Her transplant course is complicated by graft-versus-host disease with diarrhea, weight loss, and skin rash. She is immunosuppressed with tacrolimus 1 mg twice a day (bid) and prednisone 7.5 mg daily. She recently was admitted to the hospital with shortness of breath and fevers to 101.5°F. She has a chest computed tomography (CT) showing nodular pneumonia, and fungal organisms are seen on a transbronchial lung biopsy. The culture demonstrates *Aspergillus fumigatus*, and a serum galactomannan level is elevated. She is initiated on therapy with voriconazole 6 mg/kg IV every 12 hours for 1 day, decreasing to 4 mg/kg IV every 12 hours beginning on day 2. Two days after starting voriconazole, she is no longer febrile but is complaining of headaches and tremors. Her blood pressure is 150/92 mmHg, up from 108/60 mmHg on admission. On examination, she has developed 1+ pitting edema in the lower extremities. Her creatinine has risen to 1.7 mg/dL from 0.8 mg/dL on admission. What is the most likely cause of the patient's current clinical picture?

A. *Aspergillus* meningitis
B. Congestive heart failure
C. Recurrent graft-versus-host disease
D. Tacrolimus toxicity
E. Thrombotic thrombocytopenic purpura caused by voriconazole

I-18. A 43-year-old woman is diagnosed with pulmonary blastomycosis and is initiated on therapy with oral itraconazole therapy. All of the following could affect the bioavailability of this drug EXCEPT:

A. Coadministration with a cola beverage
B. Coadministration with oral contraceptive pills
C. Formulation of the drug (liquid vs. capsule)
D. pH of the stomach
E. Presence of food in the stomach

I-19. Mr. Jonas is a 47-year-old truck driver with a history of HIV, hypertension, coronary artery disease, atrial fibrillation, and ischemic cardiomyopathy. He is on antiretroviral therapy. He presents today complaining of a new rash on his chest and axilla, which you astutely diagnose as tinea corporis. You would like to prescribe a course of oral ketoconazole for therapy. You should consider dose adjustment for all of the following medicines that he is already taking EXCEPT:

A. Carvedilol
B. Lovastatin
C. Mexiletine
D. Ritonavir
E. Saquinavir

I-20. Which of the following pharmacokinetic concepts is accurate?

A. After four half-lives of a zero-order drug, 93.75% of drug elimination is achieved.
B. Elimination half-life is the sole determinant of the time required for steady-state plasma concentrations to be achieved after any change in drug dosing.
C. First-order elimination refers to the priority a drug has for its elimination enzyme versus drugs of alternative orders. For example, a first-order drug will have a higher affinity for the enzyme than a second-order drug.
D. Steady state describes the situation during chronic drug dosing when the plasma concentration of drug is identical from minute to minute. One can only truly achieve steady state with continuous intravenous infusion.
E. The only method by which a drug can be removed from the central compartment is by elimination.

I-21. Mr. Brooks has been seeing you in the primary care clinic for over 20 years. Recently, he was diagnosed with amyotrophic lateral sclerosis (ALS), an almost universally fatal degenerative neurologic condition. In consultation with his neurologist, you have started him on a high dose of a new medication, Drug X, to alleviate muscle spasms. However, although Mr. Brooks's muscle spasms have improved drastically, he is experiencing dry mouth and dry eyes, side effects that were not described in very large clinical trials of Drug X. A recent postmarketing study of Drug X was released showing that patients with ALS taking it live, on average, 14 days less than patients not taking it. As you discuss the plan regarding Drug X with Mr. Brooks, which statement would be valid?

A. "A recent study shows that patients taking Drug X die sooner, on average, than those not taking it. I want to discuss your thoughts on continuing Drug X, perhaps at a lower dose, versus stopping it."
B. "A recent study shows that patients taking Drug X die sooner, on average, than those not taking it. I recommend stopping it, and I anticipate the drug will be discontinued soon."
C. "If you're having side effects at the high dose, it's certain that you'll have the same side effects at a lower dose."
D. No discussion is needed given the postmarketing data. You should stop Drug X and report the new side effect to the U.S. Food and Drug Administration (FDA).
E. "These side effects you describe were not described in clinical trials enrolling hundreds of patients with ALS. They cannot be from Drug X. Let's figure out what other medication might be causing them."

I-22. The graph below represents a plasma time-concentration curve after a single dose of Drug A. Which of the following statements regarding Figure I-22A is true?

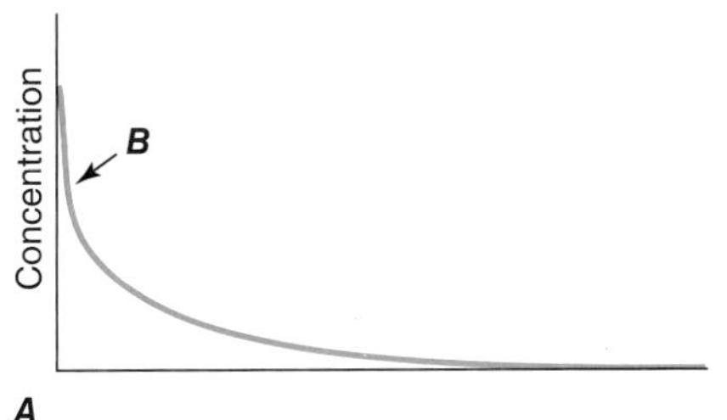

FIGURE I-22A

A. This drug was likely administered orally.
B. This drug demonstrates zero-order kinetics.
C. The shift in rapid reduction in plasma concentration to a more gradual reduction (point B) likely represents a saturation of the eliminating enzyme.
D. Point B represents the time when drug is distributed both to and from a peripheral compartment and eliminated from the central compartment.
E. This drug does not have a half-life given the curvilinear shape of its elimination curve.

I-23. All of the following patients are correctly matched to the drug and dose adjustment that should be considered given their concomitant listed comorbidity EXCEPT:

A. A 57-year-old man with cirrhosis: reduced dose of sotalol
B. A 35-year-old man with renal disease: reduced dose of meperidine
C. A 97-year-old man with normal creatinine and bilirubin: reduced dose of diazepam
D. A 42-year-old man with cirrhosis: reduced dose of meperidine
E. A 35-year-old woman with a known loss-of-function allele in CYP2C9: reduced initial dose of warfarin

I-24. Which of the following sets of drug–drug interaction and mechanism is accurately described?

A. Ibuprofen and warfarin: increased risk of GI bleeding; ibuprofen inhibition of CYP2C9
B. Sotalol and furosemide: increased risk of QT prolongation and torsades de pointes; furosemide-induced inhibition of CYP3A4
C. Sildenafil and sublingual nitroglycerin: increased risk of hypotension; sildenafil inhibition of the phosphodiesterase type 5 isoform that inactivates cyclic guanosine monophosphate
D. Ritonavir and lovastatin: increased risk of myotoxicity; ritonavir inhibition of CYP2C19
E. Allopurinol and azathioprine: increased risk of blood dyscrasias; allopurinol inhibition of P-glycoprotein

I-25. Which of the following statements regarding coronary heart disease (CHD) in women when compared to men is true?

A. Angina is a rare symptom in women with CHD.
B. At the time of diagnosis of CHD, women typically have fewer comorbidities when compared to men.
C. Physicians are less likely to consider CHD in women and are also less likely to recommend both diagnostic and therapeutic procedures in women.
D. Women and men present with CHD at similar ages.
E. Women are more likely to present with ventricular tachycardia, whereas men more commonly have cardiac arrest or cardiogenic shock.

I-26. All of the following diseases are more common in women than men EXCEPT:

A. Depression
B. Hypertension
C. Obesity
D. Rheumatoid arthritis
E. Type 1 diabetes mellitus

I-27. Which of the following statements regarding sex differences in the United States is true?

A. Due to extensive public awareness campaigns, the majority of physicians are counseling their female patients about their risk for cardiovascular disease.
B. The leading causes of death are the same for women and men.
C. Women's bone density and their risk for cardiovascular disease decline after menopause.
D. Women have a longer average life expectancy than men, and this difference has been unchanged for decades.
E. Women younger than age 65 correctly believe that breast cancer is their leading health risk.

I-28. You are seeing Mrs. Robin today, a 58-year-old woman with a history of tobacco use, treated hypertension, and moderate obesity. She is recently menopausal. You note on her intake form that she has questions about hormone replacement therapy to reduce her risk of coronary heart disease and stroke. Which of the following statements to Mrs. Robin would be true?

A. "Most studies suggest that combined continuous equine estrogen combined with medroxyprogesterone acetate is superior to combined continuous equine estrogen alone in regard to risk for stroke or heart attack."
B. "Studies suggest that initiating hormone therapy can reduce the incidence of hot flashes, night sweats, mood, sexual function, and bone density, but there is no change in risk for stroke, myocardial infarction, or venous thromboembolism."
C. "The largest trial done on hormone therapy demonstrated a benefit for hormone therapy in reducing the risk for heart attack and stroke."
D. "What is truly important for hormone therapy is the timing of initiation. Since you are recently menopausal, we know that starting hormone therapy now will reduce your risk of future heart attack."
E. "You should definitely take low-dose aspirin daily. It has been shown to reduce the risk of coronary heart disease in women more than men."

I-29. Which of the following statements is true regarding sex differences in disease?

A. Most autoimmune diseases are more prevalent in women than men. This is attributed to stimulatory actions of estrogens and the inhibitory actions of androgens on the cellular mediators of immunity, and hormone therapy with oral contraceptives increases the risk of autoimmune disease.
B. Obesity decreases the risk of endometrial cancer in women.
C. Testosterone administered to hypogonadal men will increase the incidence or severity of obstructive sleep apnea. This does not occur with testosterone administered to hypogonadal women.
D. Women are more sensitive to insulin than are men, and thus, women's risk for type 2 diabetes mellitus is lower.
E. Women have a longer QT interval on average than men and are at higher risk for drug-induced torsades de pointes.

I-30. A 67-year-old man with hypertension and sleep apnea presents to your clinic for routine follow-up. As you open your discussion with him, he says that he has seen some commercials advising him to ask his doctor about "low T" (low testosterone). He is interested in getting tested. Which of the following statements to this patient is valid?

A. "If you are found to be testosterone deficient, therapy with exogenous testosterone may worsen your sleep apnea."
B. "It is recommended that every man above the age of 60 be tested for low total and bioavailable testosterone."
C. "Most studies show that testosterone concentration does not, on average, decline with advancing age. Instead, the endogenous testosterone made is less potent."
D. "Testosterone levels are associated with a risk for dementia in men."
E. "While exogenous testosterone therapy can increase lean muscle mass, it also increases visceral fat mass."

I-31. A 29-year-old former competitive power-lifter who stopped competing 6 months earlier due to a deltoid muscle tear confides that he and his wife have been unable to conceive despite over a year of sexual intercourse without contraception. He wonders if there is a "shot or something that can, you know, help me out." You suspect that the patient may be using anabolic-androgenic steroids (AAS). Which of the following statements is true regarding AAS use?

A. AAS users have the same mortality as the general population.
B. An elevated hematocrit should increase suspicion for AAS abuse.
C. Elevated luteinizing hormone levels and suppressed follicle-stimulating hormone levels are clues suggesting AAS abuse.
D. Increased testicular volume is a clue for AAS abuse.
E. Several prolonged clinical trials of AAS abuse have provided the medical community with a sophisticated understanding of the adverse effects of AAS abuse.

I-32. Mr. Brooks returns to clinic in August for his yearly follow-up. He is a 78-year-old former long-haul trucker who enjoys fishing and traveling. During the spring and summer months, he takes diphenhydramine daily for seasonal allergies. He has been generally feeling well, but has recently noticed some urinary urgency, straining to void, and even urinary incontinence. You perform a complete physical examination including a digital prostate exam and confirm benign prostatic hypertrophy. The International Prostate Symptom Score indicates that Mr. Brooks's symptoms are moderate. Which of the following statements to Mr. Brooks would be appropriate?

A. "I recommend primary therapy with tolterodine, an anticholinergic agent targeted at treated overactive bladder symptoms."
B. "Therapy with finasteride can reduce progression to acute urinary retention and need for prostate surgery."
C. "Urodynamic studies are warranted; I'll refer you now."
D. "We should go straight to surgery. Given the severity of your symptoms, medical therapy is unlikely to help much."
E. "Your use of diphenhydramine is probably working to improve your lower urinary tract symptoms given its anticholinergic properties."

I-33. A 24-year-old woman comes to clinic for a routine visit. She is 28 weeks pregnant with her first child. To date, her pregnancy has been unremarkable and she has no family history of complicated pregnancies. Her past medical history is unremarkable except for a history of mitral valve prolapse. A blood pressure greater than which of the following would be considered potentially abnormally elevated?

A. 110/80 mmHg in the standing position
B. 120/80 mmHg in the standing position 2 minutes after rising from the supine position
C. 130/85 mmHg in the left lateral recumbent position
D. 130/85 mmHg in the seated position
E. 140/90 mmHg in the seated position

I-34. A 36-year-old nulliparous woman is found to have a blood pressure of 150/95 mmHg on a routine prenatal screening examination at 25 weeks' gestation. Prior to this visit, her blood pressure was typically 125/80 mmHg. She has a history of well-controlled diabetes and hyperlipidemia. Her exam is notable for a body mass index (BMI) of 28, 2+ pretibial edema, and a 3/6 systolic flow murmur. Laboratories are notable for normal electrolytes, serum creatinine of 1.0 mg/dL, and a urine protein/creatinine ratio of 0.4. Which of the following findings in this patient is necessary to confirm the diagnosis of preeclampsia?

A. Diabetes
B. Hyperlipidemia
C. Obesity
D. Pedal edema
E. Protein/creatine ratio

I-35. A 29-year-old woman who is 35 weeks pregnant has been managed with aspirin and labetalol for preeclampsia after she was found to have elevated blood pressure and proteinuria. All of the following findings characterize preeclampsia with severe features EXCEPT:

A. Asthma
B. Hemolysis
C. Hepatocellular injury
D. Seizure
E. Thrombocytopenia

I-36. A 33-year-old woman with diabetes mellitus, renal insufficiency, and hypertension presents to the hospital with seizures during week 38 of her pregnancy. Her blood pressure is 165/95 mmHg. She has 4+ proteinuria. Management should include all of the following EXCEPT:

A. Emergent delivery
B. Intravenous labetalol
C. Intravenous magnesium sulfate
D. Intravenous phenytoin

I-37. All of the following statements regarding a patient with type 1 diabetes who becomes pregnant are true EXCEPT:

A. Early delivery should be avoided and undertaken only for obstetric or fetal indications.
B. Fasting blood glucose should be maintained 140–180 mg/dL to avoid fetal hypoglycemia.
C. Prenatal folate supplementation will decrease the risk of a fetal neural tube defect.
D. She and her child are at higher perinatal mortality risk than a patient without diabetes.
E. The child is at higher risk of macrosomia than a child from a mother without diabetes.

I-38. Which of the following thyroid function tests will likely be altered due to pregnancy?

A. Free T_3
B. Free T_4
C. Total T_3
D. Thyroid-stimulating hormone (TSH)

I-39. Which of the following cardiovascular conditions is a contraindication to pregnancy?

A. Atrial septal defect without Eisenmenger syndrome
B. Idiopathic pulmonary arterial hypertension
C. Marfan syndrome
D. Mitral regurgitation
E. Prior peripartum cardiomyopathy with a current ejection fraction of 65%

I-40. All of the following are changes in the cardiovascular system seen in pregnancy EXCEPT:

A. Decreased blood pressure
B. Increased cardiac output
C. Increased heart rate
D. Increased plasma volume
E. Increased systemic vascular resistance

I-41. A 27-year-old woman develops left leg swelling during week 20 of her pregnancy. Left lower extremity ultrasound reveals a left iliac vein deep vein thrombosis (DVT). Proper management includes:

A. Bedrest
B. Catheter-directed thrombolysis
C. Enoxaparin
D. Inferior vena cava filter placement
E. Warfarin

I-42. In addition to a history and physical examination, which of the following should be performed preoperatively to identify intermediate- or high-risk patients who may benefit from a more detailed clinical evaluation?

A. Chest radiograph
B. Electrocardiogram
C. Liver function tests
D. Serum creatinine
E. Serum electrolytes (sodium, potassium, chloride, bicarbonate)

I-43. Which of the following patients should receive a cardiac catheterization prior to the proposed surgery?

A. A 38-year-old man for elective bariatric surgery. He has a history of medically controlled familial hyperlipidemia but no history of chest pain and a normal electrocardiogram (ECG). He has a normal cardiac and pulmonary examination and can easily climb more than two flights of stairs without stopping.
B. A 45-year-old man with a history of coronary artery bypass graft surgery 8 years ago who has sustained a motor vehicle accident and has findings in the emergency department of abdominal visceral bleeding.
C. A 54-year-old woman for elective cholecystectomy. She was evaluated for chest pain in the emergency department and found to have no coronary artery calcifications on cardiac CT.
D. A 58-year-old man for elective pulmonary lobectomy to resect a malignant nodule. The patient had an executive physical examination where the nodule was found on a chest CT; he also had an abnormal exercise stress test.
E. A 68-year-old man for an elective radical prostatectomy. He had a coronary artery bypass graft 2 years ago and has no symptoms of heart failure or angina.

I-44. All of the following risk factors are components of the Revised Cardiac Risk Index (RCRI) that is used to assess the risk of perioperative major cardiac events EXCEPT:

A. Congestive heart failure
B. High-risk surgery
C. Ischemic heart disease
D. Renal dysfunction
E. Thrombocytopenia

I-45. A 74-year-old man is scheduled to undergo total colectomy for recurrent life-threatening diverticular bleeding. He has a history of idiopathic cardiomyopathy, renal insufficiency, hypercholesterolemia, and chronic obstructive pulmonary disease (COPD). His current medications include metoprolol, atorvastatin, enalapril, metformin, and albuterol/ipratropium inhaler. His symptoms are well controlled, and he has had no emergency department visits in the past year for exacerbations of his cardiomyopathy or COPD. His blood pressure is 128/86 mmHg. His physical examination is normal. His most recent hemoglobin A1C was 6.3%, and his creatinine is 1.5 mg/dL. Which of his medications should be discontinued before surgery?

A. Albuterol/ipratropium inhaler
B. Atorvastatin
C. Enalapril
D. Metoprolol

I-46. A 73-year-old man with a history of COPD and an forced expiratory volume in 1 second (FEV_1) of 1.3 L (40% predicted) is undergoing an elective cholecystectomy. In the postoperative period, which of the following interventions has been shown to decrease the likelihood of pulmonary complications?

A. Eliminating administration of narcotics
B. Incentive spirometry
C. Pulmonary artery catheterization
D. Total enteral nutrition
E. Total parenteral nutrition

I-47. Which of the following surgeries would be considered to have the greatest risk for postsurgical complications?

A. Carotid endarterectomy
B. Nonemergent repair of a thoracic aortic aneurysm
C. Resection of a 5-cm lung cancer
D. Total colectomy for colon cancer
E. Total hip replacement

I-48. All of the following are risk factors for postoperative pulmonary complications EXCEPT:

A. Age >60 years
B. Asthma with a peak expiratory flow rate of 220 L/min
C. Chronic obstructive pulmonary disease
D. Congestive heart failure
E. FEV_1 of 1.5 L

I-49. You are caring for a 56-year-old woman who was admitted to the hospital with a change in mental status. She underwent a right-sided mastectomy and axillary lymph node dissection 3 years previously for stage IIIB ductal carcinoma. Serum calcium is elevated at 15.3 mg/dL. A chest radiograph demonstrates innumerable pulmonary nodules, and a head CT shows a brain mass in the right frontal lobe with surrounding edema. Despite correcting her calcium and treating cerebral edema, the patient remains confused. You approach the family to discuss the diagnosis of widely metastatic disease and the patient's poor prognosis. All of the following are components of the seven elements for communicating bad news (P-SPIKES approach) EXCEPT:

A. Assess the family's perception of her current illness and the status of her underlying cancer diagnosis
B. Empathize with the family's feelings and provide emotional support
C. Prepare mentally for the discussion
D. Provide an appropriate setting for discussion
E. Schedule a follow-up meeting in 1 day to reassess whether there are additional informational and emotional needs

I-50. All of the following statements regarding end-of-life epidemiology in the United States are true EXCEPT:

A. More than 70% of deaths occur in people over 65 years old.
B. Approximately 30% of patients die as hospital inpatients.
C. Approximately 70% of deaths are preceded by a known illness.
D. Cardiovascular disease and cancer are the most common causes of death.
E. HIV/AIDS is one of the top 10 causes of death.

I-51. All of the following are components of a living will EXCEPT:

A. Delineation of specific interventions that would be acceptable to the patient under certain conditions
B. Description of values that should guide discussions regarding terminal care
C. Designation of a healthcare proxy
D. General statements regarding whether the patient desires receipt of life-sustaining interventions such as mechanical ventilation

I-52. A 72-year-old woman has stage IV ovarian cancer with diffuse peritoneal studding. She is developing increasing pain in her abdomen and is admitted to the hospital for pain control. She previously was treated with oxycodone 10 mg orally every 6 hours as needed. Upon admission, she is initiated on morphine intravenously via patient-controlled analgesia. During the first 48 hours of her hospitalization, she received an average daily dose of morphine of 90 mg and reports adequate pain control unless she is walking. What is the most appropriate opioid regimen for transitioning this patient to oral pain medication?

	Sustained-Release Morphine	Immediate-Release Morphine
A.	None	15 mg every 4 hours as needed
B.	45 mg twice daily	5 mg every 4 hours as needed
C.	45 mg twice daily	15 mg every 4 hours as needed
D.	90 mg twice daily	15 mg every 4 hours as needed
E.	90 mg three time daily	15 mg every 4 hours as needed

I-53. You are asked to consult on 62-year-old man who was recently found to have newly metastatic disease. He was originally diagnosed with cancer of the prostate 5 years previously and presented to the hospital with back pain and weakness. Magnetic resonance imaging (MRI) demonstrated bony metastases to his L2 and L5 vertebrae with cord compression at the L2 level only. On bone scan images, there was evidence of widespread bony metastases. He has been started on radiation and hormonal therapy, and his disease has shown some response. However, he has become quite depressed since the metastatic disease was found. His family reports that he is sleeping for 18 or more hours daily and has stopped eating. His weight is down 12 lb over 4 weeks. He expresses profound fatigue, hopelessness, and a feeling of sadness. He claims to have no interest in his usual activities and no longer interacts with his grandchildren. What is the best approach to treating this patient's depression?

A. Do not initiate pharmacologic therapy because the patient is experiencing an appropriate reaction to his newly diagnosed metastatic disease.
B. Initiate therapy with doxepin 75 mg nightly.
C. Initiate therapy with fluoxetine 10 mg daily.
D. Initiate therapy with fluoxetine 10 mg daily and methylphenidate 2.5 mg twice daily in the morning and at noon.
E. Initiate therapy with methylphenidate 2.5 mg twice daily in the morning and at noon.

I-54. You are treating a 76-year-old woman with Alzheimer disease admitted to the intensive care unit for aspiration pneumonia. After 7 days of mechanical ventilation, her family requests that care be withdrawn. The patient is palliated with fentanyl intravenously at a rate of 25 μg/hr and midazolam intravenously at 2 mg/hr. You are urgently called to the bedside 15 minutes after the patient is extubated because the patient's daughter is distraught. She states that you are "drowning" her mother and is upset because her mother appears to be struggling to breathe. When you enter the room, you hear a gurgling noise that is coming from accumulated secretions in the oropharynx. You suction the patient for liberal amounts of thin salivary secretions and reassure the daughter that you will make her mother as comfortable as possible. Which of the following interventions may help with the treatment of the patient's oral secretions?

A. Increased infusion rate of fentanyl
B. *N*-Acetylcysteine nebulized
C. Pilocarpine drops
D. Placement of a nasal trumpet and oral airway to allow easier access for aggressive suctioning
E. Scopolamine patches

I-55. You are caring for a 68-year-old man with end-stage idiopathic pulmonary fibrosis. His performance status is currently 0; he is bed-bound and starting home hospice care. He is chronically on nasal oxygen at 4 L/min with SaO_2 of 94%. The patient reports relentless and severe dyspnea that has worsened over the last 1–2 months. It is now his most notable complaint. Physical examination is notable for normal vital signs other than a respiratory rate of 25/min. There is no evidence of ongoing infection or other acute pulmonary process. Which of the following interventions would be a reasonable first step to improve comfort for this patient?

A. Albuterol
B. Codeine
C. Increase nasal oxygen to 8 L/min
D. Lorazepam
E. Nebulized morphine

I-56. All of the following statements regarding euthanasia or physician-assisted suicide are true EXCEPT:

A. Over 70% of patients with terminal disease consider euthanasia or physician-assisted suicide for themselves.
B. Over 75% of patients who seek physician-assisted suicide identify loss of autonomy or dignity and inability to engage in enjoyable activities as their main reason.
C. Patients with cancer are the most common to consider euthanasia or physician-assisted suicide for themselves.
D. Physician-assisted suicide is legal in some states in the United States.
E. Voluntary active euthanasia is not legal in the United States.

I-57. Which continent has the highest median population age?

A. Africa
B. Asia
C. Australia
D. Europe
E. North America

I-58. The systemic effects of aging cluster into four domains: body composition, discrepancy between energy demand and utilization, homeostatic dysregulation, and neurodegeneration. All of the following statements regarding these effects are true EXCEPT:

A. Lean muscle mass decreases after the third decade of life, whereas fat mass increases progressively after middle age.
B. Most older individuals, even those who are healthy, develop mild increases in markers of inflammation such as C-reactive protein and interleukin-6 when compared to younger individuals.
C. Peak oxygen consumption declines progressively with age.
D. The regions of the brain most likely to be atrophied with mild cognitive impairment are the lateral prefrontal cortex and hippocampus.

I-59. Which of the following age groups is the fastest growing worldwide?

A. 1–20 years old
B. 21–40 years old
C. 41–60 years old
D. 61–79 years old
E. >80 years old

I-60. Which of the following is the most common type of preventable adverse event in hospitalized patients?

A. Adverse drug events
B. Diagnostic failures
C. Falls
D. Technical complications of procedures
E. Wound infections

I-61. All of the following are steps in a cycle to rapidly improve a specific process EXCEPT:

A. Act
B. Check
C. Do
D. Plan
E. Reevaluate

I-62. Which of the following is projected to cause the most deaths in low- and middle-income countries in 2030?

A. Cancer
B. Cardiovascular disease
C. HIV/AIDS, TB, malaria, and other infectious diseases
D. Intentional injuries
E. Road traffic accidents

I-63. The 2008 WHO World Health Report describes how a primary healthcare approach is necessary "now more than ever" to address global health priorities. All of the following areas of reform were highlighted in the report, EXCEPT:

A. Drug development
B. Leadership
C. Public policy
D. Service delivery
E. Universal health coverage

I-64. Which of the following statements regarding the Dietary Supplements Health and Education Act (DSHEA), passed in 1994, is true?

A. Dietary supplement vendors can claim that dietary supplements maintain normal structure and function of body systems.
B. Dietary supplement vendors can claim that dietary supplements prevent or treat diseases.
C. The FDA is given the authority to regulate advertising and marketing claims related to dietary supplements.
D. The FDA is given the authority to regulate homeopathic products.

I-65. Which of the following descriptions best describes the term *moral hazard* as currently used in the health insurance context?

A. A condition in which some individuals can be made better off without making anyone else worse off
B. A situation in which physicians are reimbursed a fixed amount per patient and will have a financial incentive to avoid sick patients
C. The branch of economics that seeks to explain actual phenomena without making a judgment about the desirability of these phenomena
D. The incentives for better-insured individuals to use more medical services
E. The system in which the price of a good or service is dictated by a governmental or other governing agency rather than by market forces

I-66. Independent of insurance status, income, age, and comorbid conditions, disparities exist between the care received by black and white patients for which of the following scenarios?

A. Prescription of analgesics for pain control
B. Referral to renal transplantation
C. Surgical treatment for lung cancer
D. Referral for cardiac catheterization and bypass grafting
E. All of the above

I-67. All of the following are legally relevant criteria for a physician establishing decision-making capacity in a patient EXCEPT:

A. The ability to answer basic orientation questions such as name, year, and home address
B. The ability to appreciate the situation and its consequences
C. The ability to communicate a choice
D. The ability to reason about treatment options
E. The ability to understand the relevant information

I-68. In which of the following conditions has stem cell therapy been shown to have in vivo benefit?

A. Cirrhosis
B. Ischemic heart disease
C. Parkinson disease
D. Spinal cord injury
E. Type 1 diabetes mellitus

I-69. The greatest source of nutrients and calories in an individual's diet should come from which source?

A. Alcohol
B. Carbohydrates
C. Fat
D. Protein

I-70. You are evaluating the vitamin D intake for a 32-year-old woman who is not pregnant or lactating. It is found to be below the recommended dietary allowance (RDA), although a serum level of vitamin D has been measured previously as within normal limits. Which statement is true with regard to this scenario?

A. Dietary reference intakes (DRI) would have been a better tool to determine if her nutrient intake was adequate.
B. Given the normal serum level of vitamin D, there is no reason to increase her intake of vitamin D.
C. RDA is not the best measure for evaluating the nutrient requirements of this individual.
D. All of the above statements are true with regard to this scenario.

I-71. A 56-year-old man was admitted to the surgical service for care due to exposure injury and frostbite in his distal extremities. He has a longstanding history of alcoholism, drinking about 1 L of vodka on a daily basis. You are asked to consult due to concerns of bizarre behaviors exhibited by the patient. He is expressing a belief that his wounds were the result of burns that were inflicted upon him by "torturers" in the government because he "knows too much" about government surveillance plans. The surgical team reports it is difficult to keep the patient in his bed, and he seems unsteady on his feet at times. He has been medicated throughout his stay for prevention of alcohol withdrawal via a symptom-triggered approach and last received lorazepam 2 mg orally about 2 hours ago. At that time, the patient was noted to be tremulous, tachycardic, and hypertensive. The delusional thoughts are not responsive to treatment of alcohol withdrawal symptoms. When you see the patient, he is sleeping quietly. Vital signs are blood pressure 110/82, heart rate 94, respiratory rate 16, temperature 37.1°C, and SaO_2 97% on room air. He awakens easily and has a minimal resting tremor. On neurologic examination, he exhibits past pointing, difficulty with rapid alternating movements, horizontal nystagmus, and decreased sensation to light touch and pinprick in the lower extremities below the mid-tibia. His gait is wide based and ataxic. He no longer expresses his prior delusional beliefs, but he is disoriented and thinks he is in jail. He states he was brought to "this gulag" so that the government could experiment on him. He has 5% dextrose in half-normal saline infusing at 100 mL/hr and is also receiving nafcillin 2 g IV every 4 hours for cellulitis. What do you suspect is the cause of the patient's altered mental state?

A. Hypoglycemia
B. Hyponatremia
C. Niacin deficiency
D. Thiamine deficiency
E. Undertreated alcohol withdrawal

I-72. A 30-year-old woman expresses the desire to maintain a healthy lifestyle and has a focus on preventative health. She believes that she can prevent illness and cancer through ingesting supplements and antioxidants. When reviewing her current intake, you determine she is taking vitamin A 20,000 IU daily and has been for the past 12 months. What advice can you give her regarding this dose?

A. Chronic ingestion of this dose could be associated with an increased risk of lung cancer even in nonsmokers.
B. Chronic ingestion of this dose is associated with yellowing of the skin but not the sclerae.
C. She should discontinue this dose prior to attempting a pregnancy as this dose could lead to an increased risk of spontaneous abortions and congenital malformations, including craniofacial abnormalities and valvular heart disease.
D. This dose is the highest daily recommended dose that is proven to be safe without toxicity.

I-73. A 48-year-old man is diagnosed with carcinoid syndrome after presenting with diarrhea, flushing, and hypotension. With appropriate treatment, he experiences an appropriate response biochemically, and his flushing and blood pressure are markedly improved. However, he continues to have some mild diarrhea and also has mouth soreness. He remains fatigued with a loss of appetite and irritability. On examination, you notice his tongue is bright red and somewhat enlarged. It is tender to touch. In addition, he has a pigmented and scaling rash that is most prominent around his neckline. What is the most likely vitamin or mineral deficiency in this patient?

A. Copper
B. Niacin
C. Riboflavin
D. Vitamin C
E. Zinc

I-74. Vitamin A deficiency is associated with an increased risk of which of the following:

A. Blindness
B. Maternal infection and death
C. Mortality from dysentery
D. Mortality from malaria
E. All of the above

I-75. A 51-year-old alcoholic man presents to the emergency department complaining of vomiting blood. Upon further evaluation including gastric lavage, you determine that he is not experiencing an upper gastrointestinal (GI) bleed, but rather is having significant gingival bleeding. He is intoxicated and complains of fatigue. Reviewing his chart, you find that he had a hemarthrosis evacuated 6 months ago and has been lost to follow-up since then. He takes no medications. Laboratory data show platelets of 250,000 and international normalized ratio (INR) of 0.9. He has a diffuse hemorrhagic eruption on his legs that is centered around hair follicles. What is the recommended treatment for this patient's underlying disorder?

A. Folate
B. Niacin
C. Thiamine
D. Vitamin C
E. Vitamin K

I-76. A 21-year-old woman is admitted to the cardiac care unit after collapsing in her college dormitory. When emergency personnel arrived at her home, she was found to be in a torsades de pointes arrhythmia and was pulseless. She received cardiopulmonary resuscitation, defibrillation, and magnesium en route to the hospital. Upon arrival, her initial potassium is 1.2 mEq/L. Her physical examination is remarkable for an excessively thin appearance with lanugo hair on arms and chest. Her BMI is 14.6 kg/m^2. Which of the following statements is true regarding this patient's nutritional state?

A. Mortality in the disease is most commonly due to complications of malnutrition.
B. Poor wound healing and frequent skin infections are common complications.
C. Systemic inflammation is a predominant finding on laboratory examination.
D. The serum albumin is typically less than 2.8 g/dL.
E. Triceps skinfold <3 mm and mid-arm muscle circumference <15 cm are useful diagnostic criteria.

I-77. A 74-year-old woman is hospitalized in the surgical intensive care unit after undergoing an emergent colectomy for ischemic colitis related to vascular disease. At the time of surgery, she had experienced a bowel perforation. She is currently postoperative day 10 and remains intubated and sedated with evidence of ongoing multiorgan system failure. She requires norepinephrine infusion continuously at a rate of 10 μg/min. She has acute renal failure and is on continuous venovenous hemodialysis. Her blood cultures were positive for *Escherichia coli*, and she is being treated with cefepime 2 g IV every 8 hours and metronidazole 500 mg every 8 hours. She has a colostomy in her right lower quadrant, but the surgeons were unable to primarily close her abdomen due to the bowel perforation. She has returned to the operating room for reexploration and wash out of the peritoneum. Since admission, her fluid balance is positive more than 30 L. She has marked anasarca and has not been fed since admission, although the team plans to initiate total parenteral nutrition today. Which statement is most likely true regarding her nutritional state?

A. Aggressive nutritional support should be avoided.
B. Immune function is not affected.
C. The albumin is less than 2.8 g/dL.
D. The body mass index will be less than 18.5 kg/m^2.
E. The nutritional state does not confer any increased mortality risk for this patient.

I-78. Which of the following patients would be LEAST likely to be at high risk of nutritional depletion?

A. A 21-year-old woman with a history of anorexia nervosa in remission for 2 months with a BMI of 19.1 kg/m^2 admitted to the hospital with an asthma exacerbation
B. A previously healthy 28-year-old man admitted to the intensive care unit with third-degree burns covering 85% of his body surface area
C. A 32-year-old man with alcoholism admitted with acute pancreatitis who has been NPO for 6 days
D. A 41-year-old woman with short gut syndrome following resection of small bowel for a gastrointestinal stromal tumor admitted to the hospital with dehydration
E. A 55-year-old woman admitted to the hospital for right mastectomy for breast cancer who has recently lost 25 lb (from 200 to 175 lb) unintentionally

I-79. You are caring for a 54-year-old woman in the intensive care unit who was admitted for treatment of severe sepsis and pneumonia. You would like to initiate enteral nutrition and plan to calculate basal energy expenditure for the patient. All of the following factors are used to determine the patient's caloric needs EXCEPT:

A. Age
B. Albumin
C. Gender
D. Height
E. Weight

I-80. A 65-year-old man is admitted for colectomy for stage III colon cancer. On the second postoperative day, he requires repeat exploratory laparotomy due to bleeding complications. It is now postoperative day 7 from his original resection, and the patient has had no nutrition since before surgery. His BMI before surgery was 28.7 kg/m^2, and he was felt to have normal nutritional status. He is currently clinically stable, but delirious and at high aspiration risk. He has bowel sounds present, and ileostomy output is good. What would be recommended at the present time for this patient?

A. Continued NPO status because 5–7 days without nutritional support is acceptable for this patient
B. Initiate a clear liquid diet and supplement with intravenous fluids with dextrose to maintain adequate intake
C. Placement of a central venous catheter and initiation of total parenteral nutrition
D. Placement of a nasogastric tube and initiation of enteral nutrition
E. Placement of a nasojejunal tube and initiation of enteral nutrition

I-81. All of the following statements support the use of enteral feeding for critically ill patients EXCEPT:

A. Enteral feeding increases splanchnic blood flow.
B. Enteral feeding stimulates secretion of gastrointestinal hormones to promote trophic gut activity.
C. Immunoglobulin (Ig) A antibody release is stimulated by enteral feeding.
D. Neuronal activity to the gut is decreased by enteral feeding.
E. Seventy percent of nutrients used by the gut are directly derived from food within the lumen of the gut.

I-82. What body mass index is likely to be lethal in males?

A. <10 kg/m^2
B. 11 kg/m^2
C. 13 kg/m^2
D. 16 kg/m^2
E. 18.5 kg/m^2

I-83. A 43-year-old woman develops hemorrhagic pancreatitis with severe systemic inflammation response syndrome. She is intubated and sedated in the medical intensive care unit with acute respiratory distress syndrome, hypotension, and renal dysfunction. She has ongoing daily fevers to as high as 104.5°F (40.3°C). She is initiated on parenteral nutrition (PN) and develops hyperglycemia as high as 500 g/dL. She is also noted to have an increasingly positive fluid balance of more than 2 L daily. What is the most appropriate approach to management of PN in the context of her hyperglycemia and fluid retention?

A. Addition of regular insulin to the total PN formula
B. Limiting sodium to less than 40 mEq/d
C. Limiting glucose to less than 200 g/d
D. Providing both glucose and fat to the total PN mixture
E. All of the above

I-84. Microbial agents have been used as bioweapons since ancient times. All of the following are key features of microbial agents that are used as bioweapons EXCEPT:

A. Environmental stability
B. High morbidity and mortality rates
C. Lack of rapid diagnostic capability
D. Lack of readily available antibiotic treatment
E. Lack of universally available and effective vaccine

I-85. Ten individuals in Arizona are hospitalized over a 4-week period with fever and rapidly enlarging and painful lymph nodes. Seven of these individuals experience severe sepsis and three die. While reviewing the epidemiologic characteristics of these individuals, you note that they are all illegal immigrants and have recently stayed in the same immigrant camp. Blood cultures are growing gram-negative rods that are identified as *Yersinia pestis*. You notify local public health officials and the Centers for Disease Control and Prevention. Which of the following factors indicates that this is NOT likely to be an act of bioterrorism?

A. The area affected was limited to a small immigrant camp.
B. The individuals presented with symptoms of bubonic plague rather than pneumonic plague.
C. The individuals were in close contact with one another, suggesting possible person-to-person transmission.
D. The mortality rate was less than 50%.
E. *Y pestis* is not environmentally stable for longer than 1 hour.

I-86. Which of the following routes of dispersal is/are likely for botulinum toxin used as a bioweapon?

A. Aerosol
B. Contamination of the food supply
C. Contamination of the water supply
D. A and B
E. All of the above

I-87. Anthrax spores can remain dormant in the respiratory tract for how long?

A. 1 week
B. 6 weeks
C. 6 months
D. 1 year
E. 3 years

I-88. Twenty recent attendees at a National Football League game arrive at the emergency department complaining of shortness of breath, fever, and malaise. Chest roentgenograms show mediastinal widening on several of these patients, prompting a concern for inhalational anthrax as a result of a bioterror attack. Antibiotics are initiated and the Centers for Disease Control and Prevention is notified. What form of isolation should be instituted for these patients in the hospital?

A. Airborne
B. Contact
C. Droplet
D. None

I-89. The Centers for Disease Control and Prevention has designated several biologic agents as category A in their ability to be used as bioweapons. Category A agents include agents that can be easily disseminated or transmitted, result in high mortality, can cause public panic, and require special action for public health preparedness. All the following agents are considered category A EXCEPT:

A. *Bacillus anthracis*
B. *Francisella tularensis*
C. Ricin toxin from *Ricinus communis*
D. Smallpox virus
E. *Y pestis*

I-90. In September 2001, the U.S. public was exposed to a bioweapon agent delivered through the U.S. Postal Service. Characteristic lesions of this infectious agent are shown in Figure I-90, Parts A and B, below.

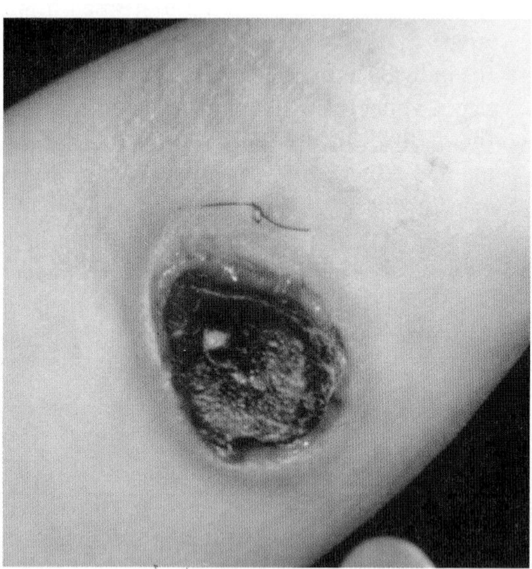

A

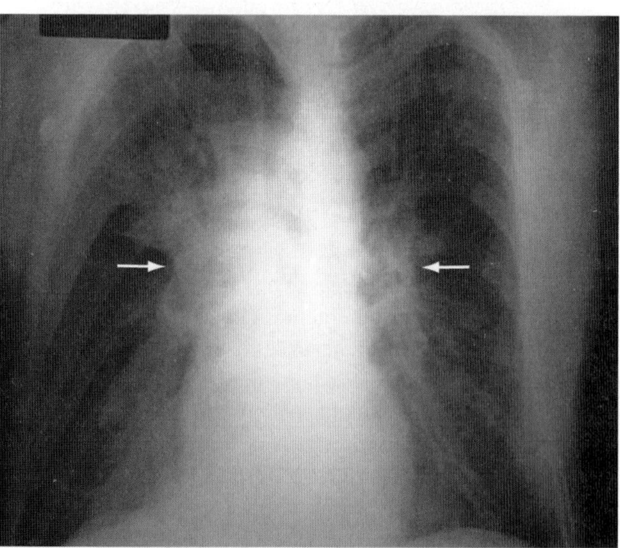

B

FIGURE I-90

Which of the following was the agent responsible for this event?

A. *B anthracis*
B. Botulinum toxin
C. Ebola virus
D. Variola major
E. *Y pestis*

I-91. All of the following chemical agents of bioterrorism are correctly identified by their mechanism of injury EXCEPT:

A. Arsine—asphyxiant
B. Chlorine gas—pulmonary damage
C. Cyanogen chloride—nerve agent
D. Mustard gas—vesicant
E. Sarin—nerve agent

I-92. Over the course of 12 hours, 24 individuals present to a single emergency department complaining of a sunburn-like reaction with development of large blisters. Most of these individuals are also experiencing irritation of the eyes, nose, and pharynx. Two individuals developed progressive dyspnea, severe cough, and stridor requiring endotracheal intubation. On physical examination, all of the patients exhibited conjunctivitis and nasal congestion. Erythema of the skin was greatest in the axillae, neck, and antecubital fossae. Many of the affected individuals had large, thin-walled bullae on the extremities that were filled with a clear or straw-colored fluid. On further questioning, all of the affected individuals had been shopping at a local mall within the past 24-hours and ate at the food court. Many commented on a strong odor of burning garlic in the food court at that time. You suspect a bioterrorism act. Which of the following statements is true with regard to the likely agent causing the patients' symptoms?

A. 2-Pralidoxime should be administered to all affected individuals.
B. The associated mortality of this agent is more than 50%.
C. The cause of respiratory distress in affected individuals is related to direct alveolar injury and adult respiratory distress syndrome.
D. The erythema that occurs can be delayed as long as 2 days following exposure and depends upon several factors including ambient temperature and humidity.
E. The fluid within the bullae should be treated as a hazardous substance that can lead to local reactions and blistering with exposure.

I-93. A 24-year-old man is evaluated immediately following exposure to chlorine gas as an act of chemical terrorism. He currently denies dyspnea. His respiratory rate is 16/min, and oxygen saturation is 97% on room air. All of the following should be included in the immediate treatment of this individual EXCEPT:

A. Aggressive bathing of all exposed skin areas
B. Flushing of the eyes with water or normal saline
C. Forced rest and fresh air
D. Immediate removal of clothing if no frostbite
E. Maintenance of a semi-upright position

I-94. You are a physician working in an urban emergency department when several patients are brought in after the release of an unknown gas at the performance of a symphony. You are evaluating a 52-year-old female who is not able to talk clearly because of excessive salivation and rhinorrhea, although she is able to tell you that she feels as if she lost her sight immediately upon exposure. At present, she also has nausea, vomiting, diarrhea, and muscle twitching. On physical examination, the patient has a blood pressure of 156/92 mmHg, a heart rate of 92, a respiratory rate of 30, and a temperature of 37.4°C (99.3°F). She has pinpoint pupils with profuse rhinorrhea and salivation. She is also coughing profusely, with production of copious amounts of clear secretions. A lung examination reveals wheezing on expiration in bilateral lung fields. The patient has a regular rate and rhythm with normal heart sounds. Bowel sounds are hyperactive, but the abdomen is not tender. She is having diffuse fasciculations. At the end of your examination, the patient abruptly develops tonic-clonic seizures. Which of the following agents most likely caused this patient's symptoms?

A. Arsine
B. Cyanogen chloride
C. Nitrogen mustard
D. Sarin
E. VX

I-95. All the following should be used in the treatment of the patient in the previous question EXCEPT:

A. Atropine
B. Decontamination
C. Diazepam
D. Phenytoin
E. 2-Pralidoxime chloride

I-96. All of the following statements regarding the results of detonation of a low-yield nuclear device by a terror group are true EXCEPT:

A. After recovery of initial exposure symptoms, the patient remains at risk of systemic illness for up to 6 weeks.
B. Appropriate medical therapy can change the median lethal dose from approximately 4 Gy to 8 Gy.
C. Initial mortality is mostly due to shock blast and thermal damage.
D. Most of the total mortality is related to release of alpha and beta particles.
E. The hematopoietic, gastrointestinal, and neurologic systems are most likely involved in acute radiation syndrome.

I-97. A "dirty" bomb is detonated in downtown Boston. The bomb was composed of cesium-137 with trinitrotoluene. In the immediate aftermath, an estimated 30 people were killed due to the power of the blast. The fallout area was about 0.5 mile, with radiation exposure of approximately 1.8 Gy. An estimated 5000 people have been potentially exposed to beta and gamma radiation. Most of these individuals show no sign of any injury, but about 60 people have evidence of thermal injury. What is the most appropriate approach to treating the injured victims?

A. All individuals who have been exposed should be treated with potassium iodide.
B. All individuals who have been exposed should be treated with Prussian blue.
C. All individuals should be decontaminated prior to transportation to the nearest medical center for emergency care to prevent exposure of healthcare workers.
D. Severely injured individuals should be transported to the hospital for emergency care after removing the victims' clothes, because the risk of exposure to healthcare workers is low.
E. With this degree of radiation exposure, no further testing and treatment are needed.

I-98. A 38-year-old man was hiking in a national forest near Tallahassee, Florida, when he was bitten on his lower right leg by a snake that his hiking companion identified as a rattlesnake. The man was wearing shorts and hiking boots. There are two clear puncture wounds that are oozing blood just above the sock line of his right boot, and the man is beginning to complain of increasing pain in the right leg. The man and his companion are about 15 minutes away from the trailhead and do not have a cell phone. What should be done immediately in the care of this patient?

A. Apply a splint if available to support the limb and decrease pain and seek immediate medical care
B. Apply a tourniquet superior to the bite to limit circulation of the venom
C. Incise or apply suction to the site of the bite immediately to attempt to remove injected venom
D. When possible, elevate the limb to heart level
E. A and D only
F. All of the above

I-99. The companion of the patient in Question I-98 assists him to the trailhead and activates emergency medical services. Upon arrival to the emergency department, the patient is noted to have increasing swelling and pain in the right lower extremity. The vital signs are blood pressure 98/52 mmHg, heart rate 132 bpm, respiratory rate 24/min, SaO_2 96% on room air, and temperature 37.0°C. The limb is positioned at the level of the heart. The maximum level and progression of swelling is marked. Two large-bore IV's are placed, and aggressive fluid resuscitation is begun. Which of the following is an indication for administration of antivenom?

A. Coagulopathy
B. Hypotension unresponsive to fluid administration
C. Swelling in the right lower leg that crosses the ankle
D. Swelling in the right lower leg that involves more than half of the leg
E. All of the above would be indications for antivenom administration

I-100. Four individuals from the same family present to the emergency department with symptoms of abdominal pain, nausea, vomiting, and diarrhea. Two of the family members are also reporting strange tingling sensations around their lips, and one person says he feels like he is swallowing bubbles. The family is vacationing in Florida and have been deep sea fishing all day. For dinner, they ate some of the fish they had caught, including some small barracuda. Emergency department evaluation is unrevealing, and they are discharged with only symptomatic nausea treatment. Over the next 24 hours, their GI symptoms peak and then resolve within 3 days. The two individuals with mild paresthesias also resolve over 3 days. However, one individual develops reversal of hot and cold perception after 3 days. This symptom continued to persist after 6 weeks. What was the likely cause of the patients' illness?

A. Ciguatera poisoning
B. Diarrhetic shellfish poisoning
C. Domoic acid intoxication
D. Scombroid poisoning
E. Tetrodotoxin poisoning

I-101. A 42-year-old woman and her 6-year-old daughter have each been treated for head lice with two applications of over-the-counter 1% permethrin separated by 10 days. Mechanical removal of lice and their eggs was performed after each application. Environmental measures have included washing all bedding in hot water and drying at >55°C. The father's head is shaved. Despite this, the daughter is again found to have live lice on her scalp. What measures would you recommend at this time?

A. Apply topical treatments such as petrolatum to avoid further exposure to pesticide
B. Complete an additional treatment with 1% permethrin
C. Perform a more thorough environmental investigation for possible fomite transmission
D. Refrain from all participation in school until the child is determined to be free of all nits (lice eggs)
E. Treat with topical spinosad due to permethrin resistance

I-102. A 56-year-old man seeks evaluation due to a spider bite. He was dressing this morning and pulled a sweatshirt over his head. He felt a sharp sting on his upper arm and found a brown recluse spider in his clothing. He has noticed some redness in this area. On examination, you see a 3 × 2 cm lesion on the inner area of his upper arm. In the center, it is somewhat pale and indurated, but the surrounding area is erythematous and painful to touch. What is the best treatment for this patient?

A. Administer antivenom
B. Advise the patient that most patients develop ischemic necrosis that requires prolonged healing
C. Apply RICE (rest, ice, compression, and elevation) and observe closely for signs of ischemia
D. Prescribe clindamycin 600 mg qid for cellulitis
E. Refer to the emergency department for further evaluation and possible debridement

I-103. One of your patients is contemplating a trekking trip to Nepal at elevations between 2500 and 3000 meters. Five years ago, while skiing at Telluride (altitude 2650 meters), she recalls having headache, nausea, and fatigue within a day of arriving that lasted about 2–3 days. All of the following statements are true regarding the development of acute mountain sickness in this patient EXCEPT:

A. Acetazolamide starting 1 day before ascent is effective in decreasing the risk.
B. *Ginkgo biloba* is not effective in decreasing the risk.
C. Gradual ascent is protective.
D. Her prior episode increases her risk for this trip.
E. Improved physical conditioning before the trip decreases the risk.

I-104. A 36-year-old man develops shortness of breath, dyspnea, and dry cough 3 days after arriving for helicopter snowboarding in the Bugaboo mountain range in British Columbia (elevation 3000 meters). Over the next 12 hours, he becomes more short of breath and produces pink frothy sputum. An emergency medical technician (EMT)–trained guide hears crackles on chest examination. All of the following statements are true regarding his illness EXCEPT:

A. Descent and oxygen are most therapeutic.
B. Exercise increased his risk.
C. Fever and leukocytosis may occur.
D. He should never risk return to high altitude after recovery.
E. Pretreatment with nifedipine or tadalafil would have lowered his risk.

I-105. Which of the following is considered an absolute contraindication to hyperbaric oxygen therapy?

A. Carbon monoxide poisoning
B. History of COPD
C. History of high-altitude pulmonary edema
D. Radiation proctitis
E. Untreated pneumothorax

I-106. A 35-year-old woman is scuba diving while vacationing in Malaysia. During her last dive of the day, her regulator malfunctioned, requiring her to ascend from 20 meters to the surface rapidly. Upon returning to the boat she felt well. However, about 6 hours after returning to shore, she develops diffuse itching and muscle aches, leg pain, blurred vision, slurred speech, and nausea. Which of the following statements regarding her condition is true?

A. Decompression illness is unlikely at 20-meter water depth.
B. Inhalation of 100% oxygen is contraindicated.
C. She can never again scuba dive to a depth greater than 6 meters.
D. She should receive recompression and hyperbaric oxygen therapy.
E. She should remain upright as much as possible.

I-107. A 48-year-old man is brought to the emergency department in January after being found unresponsive in a city park. He suffers from alcoholism and was last seen by his daughter about 12 hours before being brought to the emergency department. At that time, he left their home intoxicated and agitated. He left seeking additional alcohol as his daughter had poured out his last bottle of vodka hoping that he would seek treatment. On presentation, he has a core body temperature of 88.5°F (31.4°C), heart rate of 48 bpm, respiratory rate of 28/min, and blood pressure of 88/44 mmHg; oxygen saturation is unable to be obtained. The arterial blood gas demonstrates a pH of 7.05, $PaCO_2$ of 32 mmHg, and PaO_2 of 56 mmHg. Initial blood chemistries demonstrate a sodium of 132 mEq/L, potassium of 5.2 mEq/L, chloride of 94 mEq/L, bicarbonate of 10 mEq/L, blood urea nitrogen (BUN) of 56 mg/dL, and creatinine of 1.8 mg/dL. Serum glucose is 63 mg/dL. The serum ethanol level is 65 mg/dL. The measured osmolality is 328 mOsm/kg. ECG demonstrates sinus bradycardia with a long first-degree atrioventricular block and J waves. In addition to initiating a rewarming protocol, what additional tests should be performed in this patient?

A. Endotracheal intubation with hyperventilation to a goal $PaCO_2$ of less than 20 mmHg
B. Intravenous hydration with a 1- to 2-L bolus of warmed lactated Ringer's solution
C. No other measures necessary because interpretation of the acid-base status is unreliable with this degree of hypothermia
D. Measure levels of ethylene glycol and methanol
E. Placement of a transvenous cardiac pacemaker

I-108. A homeless male is evaluated in the emergency department. He has noted that after he slept outside during a particularly cold night his left foot has become clumsy and feels "dead." On examination, the foot has hemorrhagic vesicles distributed throughout the foot distal to the ankle. The foot is cool and has no sensation to pain or temperature. The right foot is hyperemic but does not have vesicles and has normal sensation. The remainder of the physical examination is normal. Which of the following statements regarding the management of this disorder is true?

A. Active foot rewarming should not be attempted.
B. During the period of rewarming, intense pain can be anticipated.
C. Heparin has been shown to improve outcomes in this disorder.
D. Immediate amputation is indicated.
E. Normal sensation is likely to return with rewarming.

I-109. Which of the following is the major source of heat loss in normal adults?

A. Kidney/urine
B. Skin
C. Stomach/bowel
D. Upper/lower respiratory system

I-110. A 74-year-old man is brought to the emergency department by ambulance after being found in his yard confused and somnolent. He was outside trimming hedges with an electric cutter during a hot summer day for about 2–3 hours prior to being found by his wife. He has a history of mild-moderate systolic heart failure, and his medications include atorvastatin, metoprolol, and losartan. He lives with his wife and works as a TSA officer in the airport. On examination, he is difficult to arouse and confused, with a heart rate of 120 bpm, blood pressure of 100/50 mmHg, respiratory rate of 26 breaths/min, oxygen saturation of 97% on room air, and temperature of 41°C. His skin is dry and warm with the rest of the physical examination unremarkable. His laboratory studies are notable for a sodium of 146 mEq/L, potassium of 3.8 mEq/L, creatine kinase of 250 U/L (reference 25–200 U/L), glucose of 120 mg/dL, BUN of 35 mg/dL, and creatinine of 1.2 mg/dL. Which of the following is the most likely diagnosis?

A. Cerebral hemorrhage
B. Classic heat stroke
C. Exertional heat stroke
D. Neuroleptic malignant syndrome
E. Statin-induced rhabdomyolysis

I-111. In the patient described in Question I-110, which is the most appropriate therapy?

A. Cold water bladder irrigation
B. Cooling blankets
C. Evaporative cooling
D. Immersion cooling
E. Phenylephrine

ANSWERS

I-1. **The answer is E.** *(Chap. 1)* Practice guidelines have been developed by many professional organizations and agencies as a decision-making aid to caregivers. Most organizations attempt to incorporate the most recent available evidence and concerns of cost-effectiveness into their guideline formulations. Despite increasing levels of nuance in current guidelines, they cannot be expected to account for the uniqueness of each individual and his or her illness. Furthermore, many discrepancies exist in guidelines from major organizations. By setting a standard of reasonable care in most cases, clinical guidelines provide protection to both clinicians (from inappropriate charges of malpractice) and to patients, particularly those with inadequate healthcare resources. Even though guidelines do provide this protection, they do not provide a rigid legal constraint for the conscientious physician. The physician's challenge is to incorporate the useful recommendations provided by the experts in guidelines and incorporate them into the care of each individual patient.

I-2. **The answer is D.** *(Chap. 1)* The field of molecular medicine is seeing rapid progress in fields other than genetics, bringing a new era of "-omics." *Metagenomics* is the genomic study of environmental species that have the potential to influence human biology directly or indirectly. *Metabolomics* is the study of the range of metabolites in cells or organs and ways in which they are altered in disease states. *Microbiomics* is the study of the resident microbes in humans and other mammals. Thermophiles do not reside in humans or other mammals by definition, and thus, their study would not be included in the field of microbiomics. This field has proven particularly rich; the microbes residing on and in the human body comprise over 3–4 million genes (vs. the 20,000 genes in the human haploid genome). *Proteomics* is the study of the library of proteins made in a cell or organ (including posttranslational modifications) and its complex relationship to disease. *Exposomics* is the study cataloguing environmental exposures and their impact on health and disease.

I-3. **The answer is D.** *(Chap. 1)* Evidence-based medicine (EBM) is an important cornerstone to the effective and efficient practice of medicine. EBM refers to the concept that clinical decisions should be supported by data with the strongest evidence gleaned from randomized controlled clinical trials. In many situations, data from observational studies such as cohort or case-control studies supply important information and contribute to the evidence used in clinical decisions in EBM. EBM is used by professional organizations and other agencies to formulate clinical practice guidelines, which are support tools to aid clinical decision making (option C). Systematic reviews summarize the accumulated data from all existing clinical trials (option A). Comparative effectiveness research (option B) compares different approaches to treating disease to determine effectiveness from a clinical and cost-effectiveness standpoint. Anecdotal evidence (option E) is the weakest type of evidence, represents one individual's clinical experience, and is subject to the bias inherent in one practitioner's personal experience.

I-4. **The answer is A.** *(Chap. 2)* The disability-adjusted life-year (DALY) is the standard measure for determining global burden of disease by the World Health Organization. This measure takes into account both absolute years of life lost due to disease (premature death) as well as productive years lost due to disability. DALY is felt to more accurately reflect the true effects of disease within a population because individuals who become disabled cannot contribute fully to society. Life expectancy, years of life lost due to disease, standardized mortality ratios, and infant mortality do provide important information about the general health of a population but do not capture the true burden of disease.

I-5. **The answer is C.** *(Chap. 2)* Although 24.6% of deaths worldwide were due to communicable diseases, maternal and perinatal conditions, and nutritional deficiencies in 2010, this represented a striking decrease with figures from 1990, when these conditions accounted for 34% of worldwide mortality (option A). The majority of mortality from these causes occurs in sub-Saharan Africa or southern Asia (76%). Poverty status and health are strongly linked both at the individual and national levels (option C). In 1990, childhood undernutrition was the leading risk factor for global disease burden. However, in 2010, the three leading risk factors for global disease burden were high blood pressure, tobacco smoking (including secondhand smoke), and alcohol use (option D). Childhood undernutrition ranked eighth in 2010, which remains vexing given the rise of obesity as a global risk factor for disease. The WHO in 2006 estimated that a full 25% of total global burden of disease was due to modifiable risk factors. This includes remarkable estimates that 80% of cardiovascular disease and type 2 diabetes and 40% of all cancers can be prevented through healthier diets, increased physical activity, and avoidance of tobacco.

I-6. **The answer is A.** *(Chap. 2)* Examining AIDS and TB as chronic diseases—instead of simply communicable diseases—makes it possible to draw a number of conclusions, many of them pertinent to global health in general. One of the most striking lessons is that these chronic infections are best treated with multidrug regimens to which the infecting strains are susceptible. This involves the concomitant administration of several drugs, instead of a switching from one drug to another throughout the course of treatment (option E), a strategy more likely to lead to multidrug resistance in chronic infections. For people living in poverty, even small fees (option A) for health services often pose insurmountable problems and obviates these people's ability to obtain important healthcare. Such services might best be seen as a public good promoting public health. Many physicians and nurses do indeed emigrate from their homes in resource-poor settings to practice their trades elsewhere (option C). However, a lack of tools necessary for their practice in their home nations is the primary reason cited for their emigration. Even in areas where physicians are abundant, community-based supervision represents the highest standard of care for chronic disease (option D). Option B is correct;– barriers to adequate healthcare and adherence imposed by extreme poverty (e.g., food supplements for the hungry, child care, housing) must be addressed when treating and preventing chronic diseases in developing nations.

I-7. **The answer is E.** *(Chap. 3)* Dr. Smith likely employed both the availability heuristic and anchoring heuristic in diagnosing Mrs. Johnson with systemic lupus erythematosus (SLE). Heuristics are decision-making "shortcuts" or "rules of thumb" that clinicians employ to simplify decision strategies. The availability heuristic involves judgments based on how easily the current case brings to mind prior cases. Mrs. Johnson likely reminded Dr. Smith of Mrs. Jones, a recent young African American woman with facial rash and joint pain who turned out to have SLE. After the negative test for antinuclear antibodies, Dr. Smith failed to adjust her posttest probability appropriately, settling on the diagnosis of SLE regardless of the negative test result. This represents the anchoring heuristic, whereby a clinician insufficiently adjusts the probability up or down based on a test result; –in effect, they are stuck or "anchored" to their pretest diagnosis. The anchoring heuristic often represents a failure of the clinician to properly employ Bayes' rule. This rule states that a posttest probability of diagnosis depends on three parameters: the pretest probability of disease, the test sensitivity, and the test specificity. Mathematically, it is expressed as follows for a positive test:

$$\text{Posttest probability} = (\text{Pretest probability} \times \text{Sensitivity})/[\text{Pretest probability} \times \text{Sensitivity} + (1 - \text{Pretest probability}) \times \text{False-positive rate}]$$

Confirmation bias is defined as the tendency to look for confirming evidence to support a diagnosis rather than look for discomfirming evidence to refute it (despite the latter often being more persuasive and definitive). In this case, the antinuclear antibody test has a high specificity and high negative predictive value for SLE. Thus, despite Dr. Smith's high pretest probability, a negative test for antinuclear antibodies provides a very low posttest probability that Mrs. Johnson has SLE. Dr. Smith fails to take this into account, "anchoring" instead on the diagnosis of SLE to the point of starting treatment.

I-8. **The answer is E.** *(Chap. 3)* Specificity is the number of true negatives of the test studied divided by the number of subjects in the population without the disease (true negatives + false positives). In this case, 70 subjects with a negative troponin assay had a negative veritangin assay, and 5 patients with a negative troponin assay has a positive veritangin assay (false positive). Thus, the specificity of veritangin is 0.93 (70/75). Sensitivity and specificity of a test do not depend on the disease prevalence in a population (option B). However, posttest probability depends heavily on pretest probability by Bayes' rule (option A). For example, if you chose a population where every patient had a positive troponin (the gold standard blood test for myocardial infarction), your pre- and posttest probability for myocardial infarction would be 1.0 regardless of any other test performed. By decreasing the cut point of the studied assay, the sensitivity will increase by reducing the number of false-negative tests (option C). Without other data, it is unknown by how much the sensitivity would increase. The sensitivity of a test is calculated by the number of true positives divided by the total number of patients with the disease by gold standard testing (true positives + false negatives). In this case, 25 patients had myocardial infarctions by troponin assay, 10 of whom had a positive veritangin assay (true positive). Thus, the sensitivity is 10/25, or 0.4 (option D).

I-9. **The answer is E.** *(Chap. 3)* In prospective observational studies, the investigator does not control patient care. Thus, any intervention studied is subject to treatment selection bias (–i.e., clinical practice in selecting patients in the population for the treatment may not be random). Although certain statistical models may be employed to attempt to adjust for treatment selection bias in observational studies, randomized controlled trials obviate treatment selection bias by their prospective random assignment of patients to treatment or placebo arms of the trial. While observational trials can be very useful and provide immense insight, randomized controlled trials are generally deemed superior if feasible (option A). Likewise, the use of concurrent controls is superior to historical controls (option C). The use of historical controls can be misleading because it may not account for advances in clinical medicine that have occurred between the treatment of the control and intervention arms of the trial. Population selection of any randomized trial is crucial to determining the external validity (generalizability) of the results to practicing clinicians (option D). The savvy physician will read randomized controlled trials published in high-impact journals to determine if their patients fit the population studied. A "positive" trial does not mean that any patient with clotbegone would benefit from therapy. For example, if the trial did not enroll women, the results could not be generalized to that population (option B).

I-10. **The answer is D.** *(Chap. 3)* A receiver operating characteristic (ROC) curve plots sensitivity (or true-positive rate) on the y-axis and 1 – specificity (or false-positive rate) on the x-axis. Each point on the curve represents a cutoff point of sensitivity and 1 – specificity, and these cutoff points are used to select the threshold value for a diagnostic test that yields the best trade-off between true-positive and false-positive tests. The area under the curve can be used as a quantitative measure of the information content of a test. Values range from 0.5 (a 45 degree line), representing no diagnostic information, to 1.0 for an ideal test. In the medical literature, ROC curves are often used to compare alternative diagnostic tests, but the interpretation of a specific test and ROC curve is not as simple in clinical practice. One criticism of the ROC curve is that it evaluates only one test parameter with exclusion of other potentially relevant clinical data. Also, one must consider the underlying population in which the ROC curve was validated and how generalizable this is to the entire population with disease.

I-11. **The answer is E.** *(Chap. 4)* Within a population, it is certainly impractical to perform all possible screening procedures for the variety of diseases that exist in that population. This approach would be overwhelming to the medical community and would not be cost-effective. Indeed, the amount of monetary and psychological stress that would occur from pursuing false-positive test results would add an additional burden on the population. When determining which procedures should be considered as screening tests, a variety of end points can be used. One of these is to determine how many individuals would need to be screened in the population to prevent or alter the outcome in one individual with disease. While this can be statistically determined, there are no recommendations for what the threshold value should be, and may change based on the invasiveness or cost of the test and the potential outcome avoided. Additionally, one should consider both the absolute and relative impact of screening on disease outcome. Another measure used in considering the utility of screening tests is the cost per life-year saved. Most measures are considered cost-effective if they cost <$30,000–$50,000 per year of life saved. This measure is also sometimes adjusted for the quality of life as well and presented as quality-adjusted life-years saved. A final measure that is used in determining the effectiveness of a screening test is the effect of the screening test on life expectancy of the entire population. When applying the test across the entire population, this number is surprisingly small, and a goal of about 1 month is desirable for a population-based screening strategy.

I-12. **The answer is B.** *(Chap. 4)* Screening is indeed most effective when applied to relatively common diseases within the population. Because no test is perfect and posttest probability depends heavily on the disease prevalence within the population studied (pretest probability) by Bayes' rule, any screening test will perform poorly if employed in the wrong population. To use an extreme example, screening for prostate cancer in women with prostate-specific antigen testing can only lead to an unacceptable level of false-positive results. On the other hand, populations with very high risk of the disease should undergo more rigorous screening and prevention measures. Patients with the *BRCA1* or *BRCA2* mutations have a very high lifetime risk of breast cancer. Thus, their chance of experiencing a false-negative result with traditional screening methods is unacceptable. It is recommended that these patients undergo breast magnetic resonance imaging for screening (option E). This is not necessary in the general population, as their baseline risk of breast cancer is lower. In general, the presence of a latent period (asymptomatic presence of the disease) is a necessity for successful screening. If a disease has no latent period, screening becomes less effective as early treatment and prevention are obviated (option C). When considering the effectiveness of any screening method, disease incidence and overall mortality are the most important outcomes (option D). Comparing length of disease survival will be susceptible to lead and length time biases. Lead time bias occurs because screening identifies a case before it would have presented clinically, thereby creating the perception that a patient lived longer after diagnosis simply by moving the date of diagnosis earlier rather than the date of death later. Length time bias occurs because screening is more likely to identify slowly progressive disease than rapidly progressive disease. Thus, within a fixed period of time, a screened population will have a greater proportion of these slowly progressive cases and will appear to have better disease survival than an unscreened population. It is also important to remember that every detected and treated disease by any screening mechanism does not necessarily represent a reduction in mortality (option A). Certain diseases have a long enough latent period that many patients die *with* the disease and not *from* the disease. In fact, recent estimates suggest that as many as 15%–25% of breast cancers identified by mammography screening would never have presented clinically.

I-13. **The answer is A.** *(Chap. 4)* Recently, the National Heart, Lung, and Blood Institute found that low-dose chest CT scanning can detect tumors earlier, and CT was recently demonstrated to reduce lung cancer mortality by 20% in individuals who had at least a 30-pack-year history of smoking (option E). This represented somewhat of a paradigm shift in how lung cancer screening was viewed. Historically, lung cancer screening in even high-risk populations had proven largely unsuccessful as many detected cancers were incurable at the time of detection by screening (option B). A screening test is hardly ever a "no-brainer." In the case of lung cancer screening, several risks need to be discussed with the patient prior to referral for low-dose CT scanning. First, there is the risk of detection of an incurable cancer as discussed above. Second, even low-dose CT scanning exposes the patient to radiation and may increase their risk for subsequent neoplasm. Finally, every screening test carries a risk of a false positive. In the case of lung cancer screening, false-positive results may lead to invasive biopsies and even drastic surgeries such as pneumonectomy (option C). Finally, although the sensitivity and specificity of a test do not depend on the population risk (a patient's pretest probability), the posttest probability of disease provided by a positive or negative test does strongly depend on the pretest probability (option D). This is the reason why carefully choosing the appropriate risk patient for each screening test is important.

I-14. **The answer is B.** *(Chap. 4)* Predicted increases in life expectancy are average numbers that apply to populations, not individuals. Because we often do not understand the true nature of risk of disease, screening and lifestyle interventions usually benefit a small proportion of the total population. For screening tests, false positives may also increase the risk of diagnostic tests. While Pap smears increase life expectancy overall by only 2–3 months, for the individual at risk of cervical cancer, Pap smear screening may add many years to life. The average life expectancy increases resulting from mammography (1 month), PSA (2 weeks), or exercise (1–2 years) are less than from quitting smoking (3–5 years).

I-15. **The answer is C.** *(Chap. 4)* The U.S. Preventive Services Task Force (USPSTF) is an independent panel of experts selected by the federal government to provide evidence-based guidelines for prevention and screening for disease. The panel typically consists of primary care providers from internal medicine, family medicine, pediatrics, and obstetrics and gynecology. The USPSTF recommends screening all patients age 15–65 once for HIV. Ultrasound for abdominal aortic aneurysm should be performed in men age 65–75 who have smoked (option D). Screening for chlamydia and gonorrhea should be performed in sexually active women <25 years old (option B). Hepatitis C screening is recommended for adults born between 1945 and 1965 (option E). DEXA scanning for osteoporosis screening is recommended for woman >65 or >60 years old with risk factors (option C).

I-16. **The answer is C.** *(Chap. 5)* Grapefruit juice inhibits CYP3A4 in the liver, particularly at high doses. This can cause decreased drug elimination via hepatic metabolism and can increase potential drug toxicities. Atorvastatin is metabolized via this pathway. Drugs that may enhance atorvastatin toxicity via this mechanism include phenytoin, ritonavir, clarithromycin, and azole antifungals. Aspirin is cleared via renal mechanisms. Prevacid can cause impaired absorption of other drugs via its effect on gastric pH. Sildenafil is a phosphodiesterase inhibitor that may enhance the effect of nitrate medications and cause hypotension.

I-17. **The answer is D.** *(Chap. 5)* Calcineurin inhibitors such as tacrolimus and cyclosporine are immunosuppressive agents that are used following solid organ transplantations as well as for treatment of graft-versus-host disease in bone marrow transplant patients. These drugs are primarily metabolized via the cytochrome P450 pathway and excreted into bile. Many drugs and foods can be inhibitors or inducers of this pathway, and thoughtful consideration of possible drug interactions must be considered when starting any patient on a new medication while on tacrolimus or cyclosporine. In this case, voriconazole inhibits metabolism of tacrolimus, leading to increased serum concentrations of the drug. The clinical signs and symptoms of tacrolimus toxicity include hypertension, edema, headaches, insomnia, and tremor. In addition, elevated levels of tacrolimus can lead to worsening renal function and electrolyte abnormalities including hyperkalemia, hypomagnesemia, hypophosphatemia, and hyperglycemia. It is recommended that the tacrolimus dose be decreased to one-third of the original dose when it is necessary to coadminister tacrolimus and voriconazole. Aspergillus meningitis is a rare infection that typically results from direct invasion from a rhinosinusitis. Congestive heart failure is unlikely in the clinical scenario as this is a young woman with no known heart disease and the neurologic symptoms are not consistent with that diagnosis. Graft-versus-host disease (GVHD) occurs when transplanted immune cells recognize the host cells as foreign and initiate an immune response. GVHD occurs following allogeneic hematopoietic stem cell transplantations, and there is increased risk of GVHD in those with a greater disparity of human leukocyte antigens (HLAs) between the graft and the host. GVHD presents acutely with a diffuse maculopapular rash, fever, elevations in bilirubin and alkaline phosphatase, and diarrhea with abdominal cramping. There are case reports of nephritic syndrome related to GVHD, but renal involvement is not common. Also unlikely are neurologic symptoms, headache, hypertension, and tremor. Thrombotic thrombocytopenic purpura (TTP) could be considered in an individual with renal disease, altered mental status, and hypertension if there was concurrent evidence of an intravascular hemolytic process. However, TTP has not been associated with administration of voriconazole.

I-18. **The answer is B.** *(Chap. 5)* Bioavailability refers to the amount of the drug that is available to the systemic circulation when administered by routes other than the intravenous route.

In this setting, bioavailability may be much less than 100%. The primary factors affecting bioavailability are the amount of drug that is absorbed and metabolism of the drug prior to entering the systemic circulation (the first-pass effect). Oral itraconazole is the recommended treatment for mild blastomycosis, but a problem with use of this drug is its bioavailability which is estimated at about 55%. While oral itraconazole does not experience a significant first-pass effect, its absorption from the stomach can be quite variable under different conditions. A first important consideration is the drug preparation. The liquid formulation should be taken on an empty stomach, whereas the capsule should be taken after a meal. Furthermore, having an acid pH improves bioavailability, and use of gastric acid suppressors such as H2 blockers or proton pump inhibitors should be avoided with itraconazole use. When acid suppressors cannot be withheld, it is recommended to co-administer itraconazole with a cola beverage, which has been shown to enhance absorption in some clinical trials. Oral contraceptive pills will not affect the bioavailability of itraconazole; however, azole antifungals (including itraconazole) inhibit CYP450 3A4 and may increase the serum levels of estrogens and progestins.

I-19. **The answer is A.** *(Chap. 5)* Mexiletine, lovastatin, ritonavir, and saquinavir are all substrates of the cytochrome P450 enzyme CYP3A4. As one of the most ubiquitous drug clearance enzymes, CYP3A4 metabolism is often a culprit in adverse drug–drug interactions, and the savvy clinician will be wary of co-prescribing drugs metabolized by this enzyme. Ketoconazole is a powerful inhibitor of CYP3A4, and co-administration of ketoconazole with lovastatin, mexiletine, ritonavir, and saquinavir may lead to impressive increases in the plasma level of these medications, resulting in potential toxicity. In fact, the CYP3A4-inhibition qualities of ketoconazole are sometimes leveraged to increase drug levels of medications like tacrolimus in the posttransplant patient when stable and elevated tacrolimus levels are required to prevent organ rejection. Carvedilol is metabolized by CYP2C19 and would not be affected by concomitant ketoconazole dosing.

I-20. **The answer is B.** *(Chap. 5)* Elimination half-life refers to the time required to metabolize half of the available drug in a first-order elimination system. After four half-lives of a first-order drug, 93.75% of drug elimination is achieved. However, in a zero-order elimination system, the drug is completely eliminated after two half-lives because it's elimination is not dependent on the amount of drug available. Drug can be removed from the central compartment by elimination or by distribution to another compartment. Steady state is the situation of chronic drug administration when the amount of drug administered per unit of time equals drug eliminated per unit of time. With a continuous intravenous infusion, plasma concentrations at steady state are stable, whereas with chronic oral drug administration, plasma concentrations vary during the dosing interval but the time-concentration profile between dosing intervals is stable. Most pharmacokinetic processes, such as elimination, are first order; that is, the rate of the process depends on the amount of drug present. This does not refer to the relative priority of a drug for its elimination enzyme.

I-21. **The answer is A.** *(Chap. 5)* Mr. Brooks, unfortunately, has a serious and highly symptomatic disease. In these cases, it is appropriate to consider the use of medications that alleviate symptoms but may shorten life. As with every intervention or test, a frank discussion of the known risks and benefits of the medication should be had with the patient. Many patients will consider therapies that reduce life-altering symptoms at the cost of an increased mortality, particularly those with serious diagnoses such as cancer, ALS, and heart failure (options B and E). Often, side effects occur when the dose of a medication exceeds its therapeutic window. This is described as the margin between the doses required to produce a therapeutic effect and those producing toxicity. Lowering Mr. Brooks's dose of Drug X may reduce the side effects while still producing the desired therapeutic effects (option C). Experienced clinicians know that individual patients may display responses that are not expected from large population studies and often have comorbidities that typically exclude them from large clinical trials. Simply because a side effect was not reported in the initial clinical trial does not mean it cannot be attributed to the medication in every individual patient (option E).

I-22. The answer is D. *(Chap. 5)* After point B, this drug demonstrates typical first-order kinetics, where the elimination rate of the medication depends on the current plasma concentration. Drugs with zero-order kinetics demonstrate a straight time-concentration curve as their rate of elimination is constant and does not depend on drug concentration (option B). However, prior to point B, the drug concentration rapidly declines from the central compartment (plasma). This rapid initial decline of concentration reflects not drug elimination but distribution to a peripheral compartment (option D). If a drug saturates its eliminating enzyme, it will shift from first-order to zero-order kinetics, where the elimination rate is constant regardless of the drug concentration (option C). All drugs with first-order kinetics have a half-life (option E). It is most likely that this drug was administered intravenously given the initial maximal plasma concentration and the rapid decline in concentration from the central compartment. Due to incomplete absorption and bioavailability, orally administered drug time-concentration curves do not start out with maximal concentration (option A). This is demonstrated in Figure I-22B which shows differences in typical time-concentration curves for intravenous (IV) versus orally administered drugs.

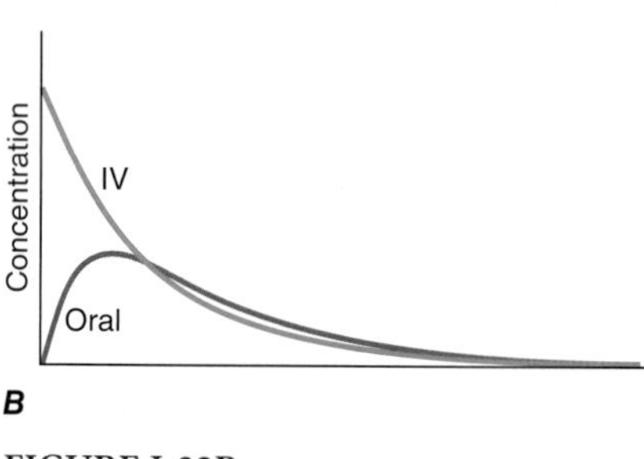

FIGURE I-22B

I-23. The answer is A. *(Chap. 5)* Sotalol is almost exclusively renally cleared, and dose reduction should be considered in patients with renal disease. Meperidine undergoes extensive hepatic metabolism, so that renal failure has little effect on its plasma concentration. However, its metabolite, normeperidine, does undergo renal excretion, accumulates in renal failure, and probably accounts for the signs of central nervous system (CNS) excitation, such as irritability, twitching, and seizures, that appear when multiple doses of meperidine are administered to patients with renal disease (options B and D). Adverse drug reactions are especially common in the elderly because of altered pharmacokinetics and pharmacodynamics, the frequent use of multidrug regimens, and concomitant disease. For example, use of long half-life benzodiazepines is linked to the occurrence of hip fractures in elderly patients (option C). Individuals with loss-of-function alleles in CYP2C9, responsible for metabolism of the active *S*-enantiomer of warfarin, appear to be at increased risk for bleeding (option E).

I-24. The answer is C. *(Chap. 5)* Sildenafil and nitroglycerin should not be co-prescribed. The pharmacologic effects of sildenafil result from inhibition of the phosphodiesterase type 5 isoform that inactivates cyclic guanosine monophosphate (GMP) in the vasculature. Nitroglycerin and related nitrates used to treat angina produce vasodilation by elevating cyclic GMP. Thus, co-administration of these nitrates with sildenafil can cause profound hypotension, which can be catastrophic in patients with coronary disease. Nonsteroidal anti-inflammatory drugs (NSAIDs) cause gastric ulcers, and in patients treated with warfarin, the risk of upper gastrointestinal bleeding is increased almost threefold by concomitant use of an NSAID such as ibuprofen. This is not mediated by inhibition of a cytochrome P450 enzyme (option A). Torsades de pointes ventricular tachycardia during administration of QT-prolonging antiarrhythmics (quinidine, sotalol, dofetilide) occurs much more frequently in patients receiving diuretics, probably reflecting hypokalemia instead of inhibition of any cytochrome P450 enzyme (option B). Ritonavir is a powerful inhibitor of CYP3A4 (not 2C19) (option D) and should not be co-prescribed with lovastatin. Allopurinol does increase the risk of blood dyscrasias when co-administered with azathioprine, although this is mediated by xanthine oxidase inhibition (option E).

I-25. **The answer is C.** *(Chap. 6e)* Coronary heart disease (CHD) is the most common cause of death in men and women, but important sex differences exist in the presentation and treatment of CHD. At the time of presentation of CHD, women are typically about 10–15 years older than men with CHD. In addition, women have a greater number of medical comorbidities at the time of diagnosis, including hypertension, heart failure, and diabetes mellitus. Angina is the most common presenting symptom of CHD in women and may have atypical features including nausea, indigestion, and upper back pain. Women who present with a myocardial infarction (MI) more often present with cardiogenic shock or cardiac arrest, whereas men have a greater risk of ventricular tachycardia on presentation with MI. In the past, women had a greater risk of death due to MI when presenting at younger ages, but this gap has decreased in recent years. However, women are still referred less often by physicians for diagnostic and therapeutic cardiovascular procedures, and there are more false-positive and false-negative diagnostic tests in women. Women are also less likely than men to receive angioplasty, thrombolysis, coronary artery bypass grafting, aspirin, and β-blockers. Despite this, the 5- and 10-year survival rates following coronary artery bypass grafting are the same between the sexes.

I-26. **The answer is E.** *(Chap. 6e)* Sex differences exist in the prevalence of many common diseases. Hypertension is more common in women, particularly in those older than 60 years. In addition, most autoimmune diseases are more common in women, including rheumatoid arthritis, systemic lupus erythematosus, and autoimmune thyroid disease. Major depression is twice as common in women compared to men, and this is true even in developing countries. Other psychological disorders that are more common in women are eating disorders and anxiety. Endocrine disorders including obesity and osteoporosis are more common in women, and 80% of patients referred for bariatric surgery are women. However, the prevalence of both type 1 and type 2 diabetes mellitus is the same between men and women.

I-27. **The answer is B.** *(Chap. 6e)* Although many patients and physicians have a different perception, the leading causes of death are indeed the same for men and women: (1) heart disease and (2) cancer. In fact, the leading cause of cancer death, lung cancer, is the same in both sexes. After menopause, many biologic changes occur in women, and disease incidence changes. Although bone density does decline after menopause, the risk of cardiovascular disease increases (option C). In the United States, women currently live about 5 years longer than men on average. However, this difference has been slowly diminishing. If it continues to decline at the current rate, women and men will have identical average longevity by the year 2054 (option D). While it is true that women younger than 65 believe that breast cancer is their leading health risk, this is not correct (option E). Although a woman's lifetime risk of developing breast cancer if she lives past 85 years is about 1 in 9, it is much more likely that she will die from cardiovascular disease than from breast cancer. In other words, many elderly women have breast cancer but die from other causes. Despite extensive public awareness campaigns, in 2012, only 21% of U.S. women surveyed reported that their physicians had counseled them about their risk for heart disease (option A).

I-28. **The answer is B.** *(Chap. 6e)* The most recent trial of hormone therapy (HT) for women, the Kronos Early Estrogen Prevention Study (KEEPS), found no difference in risk for stroke, myocardial infarction, or venous thromboembolism. However, there was a reduction in the incidence of hot flashes, night sweats, mood, sexual function, and bone density. KEEPS used combined continuous equine estrogen (CEE) alone without medroxyprogesterone acetate (MPA). In contrast, the Women's Health Initiative study (WHI) studied women treated with CEE plus MPA and CEE alone. The WHI found that CEE plus MPA was associated with an increased risk for coronary heart disease (CHD), particularly in the first year of therapy, whereas CEE alone neither increased nor decreased CHD risk. Both CEE plus MPA and CEE alone were associated with an increased risk for ischemic stroke. The WHI is the largest trial done to date on HT and did not demonstrate a benefit for HT in reducing the risk for heart attack and stroke. Although the WHI substudies showed a suggestion of a reduction in CHD risk in women who initiated HT closer to menopause, the KEEPS study (performed in this specific population) showed no difference in risk for stroke, myocardial infarction, or venous thromboembolism. Aspirin has curiously shown no benefit in women for the primary prevention of myocardial infarction, although it does reduce the risk of stroke in women with elevated risk.

I-29. The answer is E. *(Chap. 6e)* Women do have a longer and more vulnerable QT interval on average. Two-thirds of cases of drug-induced torsades de pointes, a rare, life-threatening ventricular arrhythmia, occur in women. Testosterone administered to women or men increases the incidence or severity of obstructive sleep apnea. Women are more sensitive to insulin than men. Despite this, the prevalence of type 2 diabetes is similar in men and women. There is a sex difference in the relationship between endogenous androgen levels and diabetes risk. Higher bioavailable testosterone levels are associated with increased risk in women, whereas lower bioavailable testosterone levels are associated with increased risk in men. Obesity has been shown to increase the risk for endometrial cancer in women. This is likely due to the increased extragonadal source of estrogen produced by adipose tissue. Although most autoimmune diseases are more common in women (with type 1 diabetes and ankylosing spondylitis as exceptions), the use of oral contraceptives and hormone therapy in women does not increase the risk of autoimmune diseases.

I-30. The answer is A. *(Chap. 7e)* Testosterone therapy can worsen existing obstructive sleep apnea (OSA) or lead to the development of OSA. In patients with severe OSA, testosterone therapy should be employed with caution and careful monitoring. Most studies show that, on average, male testosterone levels decline with age. The Framingham Heart Study (FHS), the European Male Aging Study (EMAS), and the Osteoporotic Fractures in Men Study (MrOS) all confirmed this finding. Only men with symptoms or signs attributable to androgen deficiency should be tested for testosterone deficiency. Testosterone therapy increases lean muscle mass and *decreases* visceral fat mass. A summary of the effects of testosterone therapy on body composition, muscle strength, bone mineral density, and sexual function in intervention trials is shown in Figure I-30. Testosterone levels are not associated with a risk for dementia.

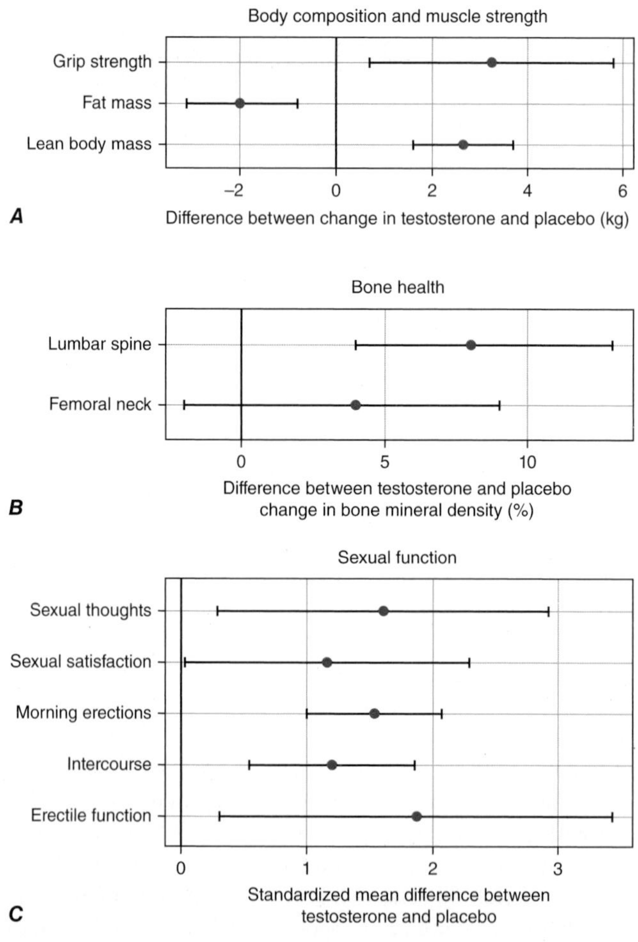

FIGURE I-30

I-31. **The answer is B.** *(Chap. 7e)* AAS use can cause increased erythropoiesis, and elevated hemoglobin and hematocrit can be clues to AAS. AAS abuse causes suppression of both luteinizing hormone (LH) and follicle-stimulating hormone (FSH) and subsequent testicular atrophy with reduction in testicular volumes. Observational studies inform us that AAS users have an increased mortality and morbidity when compared to the general population. However, the adverse effects of long-term AAS abuse remain poorly understood. Most of the information about the adverse effects of AAS has emerged from case reports, uncontrolled studies, or clinical trials that used replacement doses of testosterone. Of note, AAS users may administer 10–100 times the replacement doses of testosterone over many years, making it unjustifiable to extrapolate from trials using replacement doses. It is unclear what risk isolated AAS abuse carries. A substantial fraction of AAS users also use other drugs that are perceived to be muscle building or performance enhancing, such as growth hormone; erythropoiesis-stimulating agents; insulin; stimulants such as amphetamine, clenbuterol, cocaine, ephedrine, and thyroxine; and drugs perceived to reduce adverse effects such as human chorionic gonadotropin, aromatase inhibitors, or estrogen antagonists. The men who abuse AAS are more likely to engage in other high-risk behaviors than nonusers. The adverse events associated with AAS use may be due to AAS themselves, concomitant use of other drugs, high-risk behaviors, and host characteristics that may render these individuals more susceptible to AAS use or to other high-risk behaviors.

I-32. **The answer is B.** *(Chap. 7e)* Finasteride is a 5α-reductase inhibitor. These medications (which include finasteride and dutasteride) have been shown to reduce the progression of lower urinary tract symptoms (LUTS) and reduce the need for surgery due to acute urinary retention. Therapy with selective α-adrenergic antagonists (prazosin, doxazosin) is typically first line in men with mild symptoms. Combined administration of a steroid 5α-reductase inhibitor and α_1-adrenergic blocker can both rapidly improve urinary symptoms and reduce the relative risk of acute urinary retention and surgery. Medications with antihistaminergic properties (such as diphenhydramine) can worsen urinary retention and LUTS. Surgery is not warranted for patients with moderate LUTS who have not tried medical therapy. Urodynamic studies are not required in most patients but are recommended when invasive surgical therapies are being considered, which is not the case for this patient. Although tolterodine and other similar anticholinergic agents are useful for treating LUTS due to overactive bladder, this patient has LUTS due to benign prostatic hyperplasia.

I-33. **The answer is E.** *(Chap. 8)* In pregnancy, cardiac output increases by 40%, with most of the increase due to an increase in stroke volume. Heart rate increases by ~10 bpm during the third trimester. In the second trimester, systemic vascular resistance decreases, and this decline is associated with a fall in blood pressure. During pregnancy, a blood pressure of 140/90 mmHg is considered to be abnormally elevated and is associated with an increase in perinatal morbidity and mortality. In all pregnant women, the measurement of blood pressure should be performed in the sitting position, because the lateral recumbent position may result in a blood pressure lower than that recorded in the sitting position. The diagnosis of pregnancy-associated hypertension requires the measurement of two elevated blood pressures at least 6 hours apart. Hypertension during pregnancy is usually caused by preeclampsia, chronic hypertension, gestational hypertension, or renal disease.

I-34. **The answer is E.** *(Chap. 8 and Obstet Gynecol 2013;122(5):1122–1131)* Approximately 5%–7% of all pregnant women develop preeclampsia, new onset of hypertension (blood pressure >140/90 mmHg), and typically proteinuria (either a 24-hour urinary protein >300 mg/24 hr, or a protein/creatinine ratio >0.3) after 20 weeks of gestation. The recent American Congress of Obstetricians and Gynecologists (ACOG) Task Force on Hypertension in Pregnancy recommended removing the absolute necessity for proteinuria for the diagnosis of preeclampsia. In the absence of proteinuria, preeclampsia can be diagnosed in a patient with hypertension and thrombocytopenia, liver dysfunction, new or worsening renal insufficiency, pulmonary edema, or CNS symptoms. Recent studies suggest the pathophysiology of preeclampsia may involve placental production of antagonists to vascular epithelial growth factor (VEGF) and transforming growth factor β (TGF-β) altering endothelial and glomerular function. Pedal edema is a characteristic finding in preeclampsia but does not confirm the diagnosis. Diabetes, obesity, and renal insufficiency are risk factors for preeclampsia, as are nulliparity, chronic hypertension, prior history of preeclampsia, extremes of maternal age (>35 years or <15 years), antiphospholipid antibody syndrome, and multiple gestation. Low-dose aspirin (81 mg daily, initiated at the end of the first trimester) may reduce the risk of preeclampsia in pregnant women at high risk of developing the disease.

I-35. **The answer is A.** *(Chap. 8 and Obstet Gynecol 2013;122(5):1122–1131)* The recent ACOG task force report on hypertension in pregnancy replaced the terms mild and severe preeclampsia with the new characterization of preeclampsia either with or without severe features. Preeclampsia with severe features is the presence of new-onset hypertension and proteinuria accompanied by end-organ damage. Features may include severe elevation of blood pressure (>160/110 mmHg), evidence of CNS dysfunction (headaches, blurred vision, seizures, coma), renal dysfunction (oliguria or creatinine >1.5 mg/dL), pulmonary edema, hepatocellular injury (serum alanine aminotransferase level more than twofold the upper limit of normal), hematologic dysfunction (platelet count <100,000/L or disseminated intravascular coagulation [DIC]). The HELLP syndrome (*h*emolysis, *e*levated *l*iver enzymes, *l*ow *p*latelets) is a special subtype of severe preeclampsia and is a major cause of morbidity and mortality in this disease. Platelet dysfunction and coagulation disorders further increase the risk of stroke.

I-36. **The answer is D.** *(Chap. 8)* This patient has preeclampsia with severe features, and delivery should be performed as rapidly as possible. In mothers at <34 weeks of gestation, corticosteroids should be administered for fetal benefit and delivery delayed 24–48 hours if possible . Aggressive management of blood pressure, usually with labetalol or hydralazine intravenously, decreases maternal risk of stroke. However, like any hypertensive crisis, the decrease in blood pressure should be achieved slowly to avoid hypotension and risk of decreased blood flow to the fetus. Eclamptic seizures should be controlled with magnesium sulfate, which has been shown to be superior to phenytoin and diazepam in large randomized clinical trials. Women who have had preeclampsia appear to be at increased risk of cardiovascular and renal disease later in life.

I-37. **The answer is B.** *(Chap. 8)* Diabetic patients who become pregnant have a higher maternal morbidity and mortality, as do their fetuses/infants. This knowledge and prenatal counseling are vital to reducing maternal and fetal complications. Folate supplementation reduces the incidence of fetal neural tube defects, which occur with greater frequency in fetuses of diabetic mothers. Once pregnancy is established, glucose control should be managed more aggressively than in the nonpregnant state. Fasting blood glucose should be maintained at <105 mg/dL, and nonfasting levels should be maintained <140 mg/dL. Often conversion to an insulin pump is recommended. Pregnant diabetic patients without vascular disease are at greater risk for delivering a macrosomic fetus, and attention to fetal growth via clinical and ultrasound examination is important. Fetal macrosomia is associated with an increased risk of maternal and fetal birth trauma, including permanent newborn Erb palsy. Pregnant women with diabetes have an increased risk of developing preeclampsia, and those with vascular disease are at greater risk for developing intrauterine growth restriction, which is associated with an increased risk of fetal and neonatal death.

I-38. **The answer is C.** *(Chap. 8)* In pregnancy, elevated estrogen causes an increase thyroid-binding globulin. Thus, total T_3 and total T_4 will be elevated because they are protein bound. Free T_3, free T_4, and TSH will be unaffected by the increase in thyroid-binding globulin. TSH may be used to screen for hypothyroidism. Children born to women with an elevated serum TSH (and a normal total T_4) during pregnancy may have impaired performance on neuropsychological tests. Hyperthyroidism in pregnancy is usually caused by Graves disease.

I-39. **The answer is B.** *(Chaps. 8 and 304)* Most cardiovascular conditions can be managed safely in pregnancy, although these pregnancies are often considered high risk. The conditions that are considered to be contraindications to pregnancy are idiopathic pulmonary arterial hypertension and Eisenmenger syndrome (congenital heart disease resulting in pulmonary hypertension with right-to-left shunting). In these cases, it is typically recommended to terminate the pregnancy because there is a high risk of maternal and fetal death. Peripartum cardiomyopathy can recur in subsequent pregnancies, and it is recommended that individuals with an abnormal ejection fraction avoid further pregnancies. Approximately 15% of individuals with Marfan syndrome will have a major cardiovascular complication in pregnancy, although the condition is not considered a contraindication to pregnancy. An aortic root diameter of less than 40 mm is generally associated with the best outcomes in pregnancy. The valvular heart disease with the greatest risk in pregnancy is mitral stenosis. There is an increased risk of pulmonary edema, and pulmonary hypertension is a common long-term consequence of mitral stenosis. However, aortic stenosis, aortic regurgitation, and mitral regurgitation are typically well tolerated. Congenital heart disease in the mother is associated with an increased risk of congenital heart disease in the offspring, but atrial and ventricular septal defects are usually well tolerated in pregnancy as long as there is no evidence of Eisenmenger syndrome.

I-40. **The answer is E.** *(Chap. 8)* The cardiovascular system undergoes many changes in the pregnant woman to accommodate the needs of the developing fetus. Plasma volume begins to expand early in pregnancy and ultimately is increased by about 40%–50% at term. Coincident with the increased plasma volume, cardiac output increases as well by about 40%. Although this is primarily due to increases in stroke volume, heart rate also increases in pregnancy by ~10 bpm. In the second trimester, systemic vascular resistance falls, and subsequently blood pressure decreases as well. Thus, a blood pressure greater than 140/90 mmHg is considered abnormal and is associated with increased maternal and fetal morbidity and mortality.

I-41. **The answer is C.** *(Chap. 8)* Pregnancy causes a hypercoagulable state, and deep vein thrombosis (DVT) occurs in about 1 in 2000 pregnancies. DVT occurs more commonly in the left leg than the right leg during pregnancy due to compression of the left iliac vein by the gravid uterus. In addition, pregnancy represents a procoagulant states with increases in factors V and VII and decreases in proteins C and S. Approximately 25% of pregnant women with DVT have a factor V Leiden mutation, which also predisposes to preeclampsia. Warfarin is strictly contraindicated due to risk of fetal abnormality. Low-molecular-weight heparin is appropriate therapy at this point in pregnancy but is typically switched to unfractionated heparin 4 weeks prior to anticipated delivery because low-molecular-weight heparins may be associated with an increased risk of epidural hematoma. Ambulation, rather than bedrest, should be encouraged as with all DVTs. There is no proven role for local thrombolytics or an inferior vena cava filter in pregnancy. The latter would be considered only in scenarios where anticoagulation is not possible. When DVT occurs in the postpartum period, low-molecular-weight heparin therapy for 7–10 days may be followed by warfarin therapy for 3–6 months. Warfarin is not contraindicated in breast-feeding women.

I-42. **The answer is B.** *(Chap. 9)* Evaluation of such patients for surgery should always begin with a thorough history and physical examination and with a 12-lead resting electrocardiogram (ECG), in accordance with the American College of Cardiology/American Heart Association (ACC/AHA) guidelines. The history should focus on symptoms of occult cardiac or pulmonary disease. The urgency of the surgery should be determined, because true emergency procedures are associated with unavoidably higher morbidity and mortality risk. Preoperative laboratory testing should be carried out only for specific clinical conditions, as noted during clinical examination. Thus, healthy patients of any age who are undergoing elective surgical procedures without coexisting medical conditions should not require any testing unless the degree of surgical stress may result in unusual changes from the baseline state.

I-43. **The answer is D.** *(Chap. 9)* A patient with a recent history of abnormal exercise stress test should be considered for cardiac revascularization prior to elective surgery. Cardiac catheterization is not necessary prior to emergent surgery (patient B); in an asymptomatic patient with a normal ECG, normal physical examination, and >4 metabolic equivalent

(MET) exercise tolerance (patient A); in a patient with a recent negative coronary evaluation (patient C); or in a patient who had coronary revascularization within 5 years and has no recurrent symptoms.

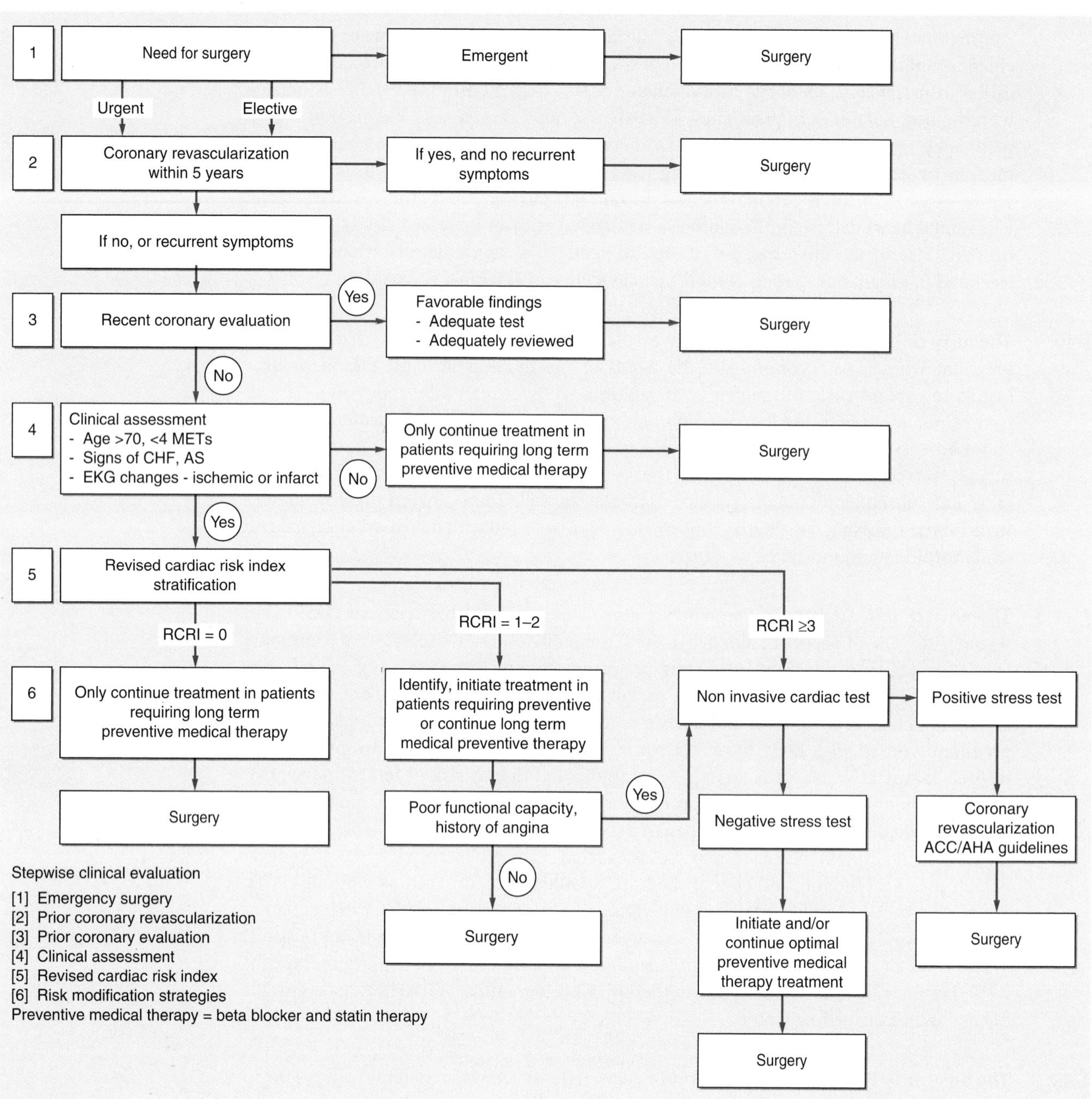

FIGURE I-43

I-44. **The answer is E.** *(Chap. 9)* The RCRI is favored over the American Society of Anesthesiologists system of assigning risk of perioperative major cardiac events (myocardial infarction, pulmonary edema, ventricular fibrillation or primary cardiac arrest, and complete heart block) due to its simplicity and accuracy. The RCRI relies on the presence or absence of six identifiable predictive factors: high-risk surgery, ischemic heart disease, congestive heart failure, cerebrovascular disease, diabetes mellitus, and renal dysfunction. Each of these predictors is assigned one point. An RCRI score of 0 signifies a 0.4%–0.5% risk of cardiac events; RCRI 1, 0.9%–1.3%; RCRI 2, 4%–7%; and RCRI ≥3, 9%–11%. The clinical utility of the RCRI is to identify patients with three or more predictors who are at very high risk (≥11%) for cardiac complications and who may benefit from further risk stratification with noninvasive cardiac testing or initiation of preoperative preventive medical management (Table I-44).

TABLE I-44 Clinical Markers Included in the Revised Cardiac Risk Index

High-Risk Surgical Procedures
Vascular surgery
Major intraperitoneal or intrathoracic procedures
Ischemic Heart Disease
History of myocardial infarction
Current angina considered to be ischemic
Requirement for sublingual nitroglycerin
Positive exercise test
Pathologic Q waves on ECG
History of PCI and/or CABG with current angina considered to be ischemic
Congestive Heart Failure
Left ventricular failure by physical examination
History of paroxysmal nocturnal dyspnea
History of pulmonary edema
S_3 gallop on cardiac auscultation
Bilateral rales on pulmonary auscultation
Pulmonary edema on chest x-ray
Cerebrovascular Disease
History of transient ischemic attack
History of cerebrovascular accident
Diabetes Mellitus
Treatment with insulin
Chronic Renal Insufficiency
Serum creatinine >2 mg/dL

Abbreviations: CABG, coronary artery bypass grafting; ECG, electrocardiogram; PCI, percutaneous coronary interventions.
Source: Adapted from TH Lee et al: *Circulation* 100:1043, 1999.

I-45. **The answer is C.** *(Chap. 9)* This patient has an RCRI of 3 (high-risk surgery, cardiomyopathy, and renal insufficiency) and therefore is at high risk of a perioperative cardiac event. The results from the Perioperative Ischemic Evaluation (POISE) trial showed that, although cardiac death, nonfatal myocardial infarction, or cardiac arrest was reduced among patients who received metoprolol rather than placebo, there was an increased incidence of death and stroke among metoprolol recipients because of a high and rapidly loading dose of this drug. The ACC/AHA guidelines recommend the following: (1) β-blockers *should be continued* in patients with active cardiac conditions who are undergoing surgery and are receiving β-blockers. (2) β-Blockers titrated to heart rate and blood pressure are *probably recommended* for patients undergoing vascular surgery who are at high cardiac risk defined by coronary artery disease (CAD) or cardiac ischemia on preoperative testing. (3) β-Blockers are *reasonable* for high-risk patients (RCRI ≥2) who undergo vascular surgery. (4) β-Blockers are *reasonable* for patients with known CAD or at high risk (RCRI ≥2) who undergo intermediate-risk surgery. (5) Nondiscriminant administration of high-dose β-blockers without dose titration to effectiveness is *contraindicated* for patients who have never been treated with a β-blocker. A number of prospective and retrospective studies support the perioperative prophylactic use of statins for reduction of cardiac complications in patients with established atherosclerosis. The ACC/AHA guidelines support the protective efficacy of perioperative statins on cardiac complications in intermediate-risk patients undergoing major noncardiac surgery. For patients undergoing noncardiac surgery and currently taking statins, statin therapy *should be continued* to reduce perioperative cardiac risk. Statins are *reasonable* for patients undergoing vascular surgery with or without clinical risk factors (RCRI ≥1). Several prospective and retrospective meta-analyses of perioperative α_2-agonists (clonidine and mivazerol) demonstrated a reduction of cardiac death rates among patients with known CAD who underwent noncardiac surgery. α_2-Agonists thus *may be considered* for perioperative control of hypertension in patients with known coronary artery disease or an RCRI score ≥2. Administration of bronchodilators should be continued to reduce the risk of respiratory complications. Oral hypoglycemic agents should not be administered on the day of surgery. Evidence supports the discontinuation of angiotensin-converting enzyme inhibitors and angiotensin receptor blockers for 24 hours prior to noncardiac surgery due to adverse circulatory effects after induction of anesthesia.

I-46. **The answer is B.** *(Chap. 9)* Perioperative pulmonary complications are common, particularly after upper abdominal surgery; emergency or prolonged (3- to 4-hour) surgery; aortic aneurysm repair; vascular surgery; or major abdominal, thoracic, neurologic, head, or neck surgery; and with general anesthesia. Patients at higher risk of pulmonary complications should undergo incentive spirometry, deep-breathing exercises, cough encouragement, postural drainage, percussion and vibration, suctioning and ambulation, intermittent positive-pressure breathing, continuous positive airway pressure, and selective use of a nasogastric tube for postoperative nausea, vomiting, or symptomatic abdominal distention to reduce postoperative risk. Pain control is also important for promoting respiratory clearance, and narcotics may be used appropriately. Pulmonary artery catheterization, total parenteral nutrition, and total enteral nutrition have not been shown to reduce perioperative respiratory complications.

I-47. **The answer is B.** *(Chap. 9)* Medical providers are often asked to provide guidance regarding the postoperative risk of complications following a variety of noncardiac surgical procedures. When evaluating risk of complications, it is useful to categorize the surgical procedures into a low-, intermediate-, or high-risk category. Individuals who are at the highest risk of complications include those undergoing an emergent major operation, especially in the elderly. Other higher risk procedures include aortic and other noncarotid major vascular surgeries and surgeries with a prolonged operative time and large anticipated blood loss or fluid shifts (i.e., pancreaticoduodenectomy or Whipple procedure). Surgeries that are felt to be intermediate risk include major thoracic surgery, major abdominal surgery, carotid endarterectomy, head and neck surgery, orthopedic surgery, and prostate surgery. Lower risk procedures include eye, skin, and superficial surgery as well as endoscopy.

I-48. **The answer is B.** *(Chap. 9)* Pulmonary and cardiovascular complications are a major source of morbidity and mortality following surgery. Primary care physicians are often asked to determine a patient's postoperative risk of pulmonary complications. Factors identified by the American College of Physicians as conferring an increased risk of pulmonary complications are shown in Table I-48. While many of these factors are directly related to pulmonary function, some of these are not. Notably, the presence of congestive heart failure and a serum albumin level of less than 3.5 g/dL predict postoperative pulmonary complications. Asthma is

TABLE I-48 Risk Modification to Reduce Perioperative Pulmonary Complications

Preoperatively
• Cessation of smoking for at least 8 weeks before and until at least 10 days after surgery
• Training in proper lung expansion techniques
• Inhalation bronchodilator and/or steroid therapy, when indicated
• Control of infection and secretion, when indicated
• Weight reduction, when appropriate
Intraoperatively
• Limited duration of anesthesia
• Avoidance of long-acting neuromuscular-blocking drugs, when indicated
• Prevention of aspiration and maintenance of optimal bronchodilation
Postoperatively
• Optimization of inspiratory capacity maneuvers, with attention to:
Mobilization of secretions
Early ambulation
Encouragement of coughing
Selective use of a nasogastric tube
Adequate pain control without excessive narcotics

Source: From VA Lawrence et al: *Ann Intern Med* 144:596, 2006, and WF Dunn, PD Scanlon: *Mayo Clin Proc* 68:371, 1993.

not a predictor of pulmonary complications as long as the disease is under sufficient control. Factors listed in the table that are useful determinants of asthma control include peak expiratory flow rate >100 L or 50% predicted and forced expiratory volume in 1 second of <2 L.

I-49. **The answer is E.** *(Chap. 10)* Communication of bad news is an inherent component of the physician–patient relationship, and these conversations often occur in a hospital setting where the treating provider is not the primary care provider for the patient. Many physicians struggle with providing clear and effective communication to patients who are seriously ill and their family members. In the scenario presented in this case, it is necessary to have a discussion about the patient's poor prognosis and determine goals of care without the input of the patient as her mental status remains altered. Failure to provide clear communication in the appropriate environment can lead to tension in the relationship between the physician and patient and may lead to overly aggressive treatment. The P-SPIKES approach (Table I-49) has been advocated as a simple framework to assist physicians in effectively communicating bad news to patients. The components of this communication tool are:

- Preparation—Review what information needs to be communicated and plan how emotional support will be provided.
- Setting of interaction—This step is often the most neglected. Ensure a quiet and private environment and attempt to minimize any interruptions.
- Patient (or family) perceptions and preparation—Assess what the patient and family know about the current condition. Use open-ended questions.
- Invitation and information needs—Ask the patient or family what they would like to know and also what limits they want regarding bad information.
- Knowledge of the condition—Provide the patient and family with the bad news and assess understanding.
- Empathy and exploration—Empathize with the patient's and family's feelings and offer emotional support. Allow plenty of time for questions and exploration of feelings.
- Summary and planning—Outline the next steps for the patient and family. Recommend a timeline to achieve the goals of care.

Setting a follow-up meeting is not a primary component of the P-SPIKES framework but may be necessary when a family or patient is not emotionally ready to discuss the next steps in the care plan.

TABLE I-49 Elements of Communicating Bad News: —The P-SPIKES Approach

Acronym	Steps	Aim of the Interaction	Preparations, Questions, or Phrases
P	Preparation	Mentally prepare for the interaction with the patient and/or family.	Review what information needs to be communicated. Plan how you will provide emotional support. Rehearse key steps and phrases in the interaction.
S	Setting of the interaction	Ensure the appropriate setting for a serious and potentially emotionally charged discussion.	Ensure that patient, family, and appropriate social supports are present. Devote sufficient time. Ensure privacy and prevent interruptions by people or beeper. Bring a box of tissues.
P	Patient's perception and preparation	Begin the discussion by establishing the baseline and whether the patient and family can grasp the information. Ease tension by having the patient and family contribute.	Start with open-ended questions to encourage participation. Possible phrases to use: *What do you understand about your illness?* *When you first had symptom X, what did you think it might be?* *What did Dr. X tell you when he or she sent you here?* *What do you think is going to happen?*

(continued)

TABLE I-49 Elements of Communicating Bad News: —The P-SPIKES Approach (*Continued*)

Acronym	Steps	Aim of the Interaction	Preparations, Questions, or Phrases
I	Invitation and information needs	Discover what information needs the patient and/or family have and what limits they want regarding the bad information.	Possible phrases to use: *If this condition turns out to be something serious, do you want to know?* *Would you like me to tell you all the details of your condition? If not, who would you like me to talk to?*
K	Knowledge of the condition	Provide the bad news or other information to the patient and/or family sensitively.	Do not just dump the information on the patient and family. Check for patient and family understanding. Possible phrases to use: *I feel badly to have to tell you this, but ...* *Unfortunately, the tests showed ...* *I'm afraid the news is not good ...*
E	Empathy and exploration	Identify the cause of the emotions—e.g., poor prognosis. Empathize with the patient and/or family's feelings. Explore by asking open-ended questions.	Strong feelings in reaction to bad news are normal. Acknowledge what the patient and family are feeling. Remind them such feelings are normal, even if frightening. Give them time to respond. Remind patient and family you won't abandon them. Possible phrases to use: *I imagine this is very hard for you to hear.* *You look very upset. Tell me how you are feeling.* *I wish the news were different.* *We'll do whatever we can to help you.*
S	Summary and planning	Delineate for the patient and the family the next steps, including additional tests or interventions.	It is the unknown and uncertain that can increase anxiety. Recommend a schedule with goals and landmarks. Provide your rationale for the patient and/or family to accept (or reject). If the patient and/or family are not ready to discuss the next steps, schedule a follow-up visit.

Source: Adapted from R Buckman: *How to Break Bad News: A Guide for Health Care Professionals.* Baltimore: Johns Hopkins University Press, 1992.

I-50. **The answer is E.** *(Chap. 10)* Approximately 73% of all deaths occur in those >65 years old. The epidemiology of mortality is similar in most developed countries; cardiovascular diseases and cancer are the predominant causes of death, a marked change since 1900, when heart disease caused ~8% of all deaths and cancer accounted for <4% of all deaths. In 2010, the year with the most recent available data, AIDS did not rank among the top 15 causes of death, causing just 8369 deaths. Even among people age 35–44, heart disease, cancer, chronic liver disease, and accidents all cause more deaths than AIDS. It is estimated that in developed countries ~70% of all deaths are preceded by a disease or condition, making it reasonable to plan for dying in the foreseeable future. Over the last few decades in the United States, a significant change in the site of death has occurred that coincides with patient and family preferences. Nearly 60% of Americans died as inpatients in hospitals in 1980. By 2000, the trend was reversing, with ~31% of Americans dying as hospital inpatients. This shift has been most dramatic for those dying from cancer and COPD and for younger and very old individuals. In the last decade, it has been associated with the increased use of hospice care; in 2008, approximately 39% of all decedents in the United States received such care.

I-51. **The answer is C.** *(Chap. 10)* Advance care planning documentation is an increasing component of medical practice. As of 2006, 48 states and the District of Columbia had enacted legislation regarding advance care planning. There are two broad types of advance care planning documentation: living wills and designation of a healthcare proxy (option C).

While these two documents are often combined into a single document, designation of a health care proxy is not one of the primary components of a living will. The living will (or instructional directive) delineates the patient's preferences (option A) regarding treatment under different scenarios (e.g., whether condition is perceived as terminal). These documents can be very specific to a condition such as cancer, but may also be very broad in the case of elderly individuals who are not currently suffering from a terminal condition but want to outline their wishes for care in the event of an unexpected health crisis. Examples of what this might include general statements regarding the receipt of life-sustaining therapies (option D) and the values that should guide the decisions regarding terminal care (option B).

I-52. **The answer is C.** *(Chap. 10)* A primary goal of palliative care medicine is to control pain in patients who are terminally ill. Surveys have found that 36%–90% of individuals with advanced cancer have substantial pain, and an individualized treatment plan is necessary for each patient. For individuals with continuous pain, opioid analgesics should be administered on a scheduled basis around the clock at an interval based on the half-life of the medication chosen. Extended- release preparations are frequently used due to their longer half-lives. However, it is inappropriate to start immediately with an extended-release preparation. In this scenario, the patient was treated with a continuous intravenous infusion via patient-controlled analgesia for 48 hours to determine her baseline opioid needs. The average daily dose of morphine required was 90 mg. This total dose should be administered in divided doses two or three times daily (either 45 mg twice daily or 30 mg three times daily). In addition, an immediate-release preparation should be available for administration for breakthrough pain. The recommended dose of the immediate release preparation is 20% of the baseline dose. In this case, the dose would be 18 mg and could be given as either 15 or 20 mg four times daily as needed.

I-53. **The answer is D.** *(Chap. 10)* Depression is difficult to diagnose in individuals with terminal illness and is often an overlooked symptom by physicians as many individual believe it a normal component of terminal illness. Furthermore, symptoms commonly associated with depression such as insomnia and anorexia are also frequently seen in serious illness or occur as a side effect of treatment. Although about 75% of terminally ill patients express some depressive symptoms, only 25% or less have major depression. When assessing depression in terminally ill individuals, one should focus on symptoms pertaining to the dysphoric mood, including helplessness, hopelessness, and anhedonia. It is inappropriate to do nothing in the situation where one believes major depression is occurring (option A). The approach to treatment should include nonpharmacologic and pharmacologic therapies. The pharmacologic approach to depression should be the same in terminally ill individuals as in non–terminally ill individuals. If an individual has a prognosis of several months or longer, selective serotonin reuptake inhibitors (fluoxetine, paroxetine) or serotonin-noradrenaline reuptake inhibitors (venlafaxine) are the preferred treatment due to their efficacy and side effect profile. However, these medications take several weeks to become effective. Thus, starting fluoxetine alone (option C) is not preferred. In patients with major depression and fatigue or opioid-induced somnolence, combining a traditional antidepressant with a psychostimulant is appropriate (option D). Psychostimulants are also indicated in individuals with a poor prognosis who are not expected to live long enough to experience the benefits of treatment with a traditional antidepressant. A variety of psychostimulant medications are available including methylphenidate, modafinil, dextroamphetamine, or pemoline. Because this patient has a prognosis of several months or longer, methylphenidate alone is not recommended (option E). Because of their side effect profile, tricyclic antidepressants (option A) are not used in the treatment of depression in the terminally ill unless they are utilized as adjunctive treatment for chronic pain.

I-54. **The answer is E.** *(Chap. 10)* Withdrawal of care is a common occurrence in intensive care units. More than 90% of Americans die without performance of cardiopulmonary resuscitation. When a family decides to withdraw care, the treating care team of doctors, nurses, and respiratory therapists must work together to ensure that the dying process will be comfortable for both the patient and the family. Commonly, patients receive a combination of anxiolytics and opioid analgesics. These medications also provide relief of dyspnea in the dying patient. However, they have little effect on oropharyngeal secretions (option A). The accumulation of secretions in the oropharynx can produce agitation, labored breathing, and noisy breathing that has been labeled the "death rattle." This can be quite distressing to the family. Treatments for excessive oropharyngeal secretions are primarily anticholinergic medications including scopolamine delivered transdermally (option E) or intravenously, atropine, and glycopyrrolate. While placement of a nasal trumpet or oral airway (option D) may allow better access for suctioning of secretions, these can be uncomfortable or even painful interventions that are typically discouraged in a palliative care situation. *N*-Acetylcysteine (option B) can be used as a mucolytic agent to thin lower respiratory secretions. Pilocarpine (option C) is a cholinergic stimulant and increases salivary production.

I-55. **The answer is B.** *(Chap. 10)* It is common for patients with end-stage lung or heart disease to develop debilitating dyspnea. It is an extremely distressing symptom, possibly worse than pain for many patients. The symptom may not correlate with objective parameters like SaO_2 or $PaCO^2$. Potentially reversible or treatable causes of dyspnea include infection, pleural effusions, pulmonary emboli, pulmonary edema, asthma, and tumor encroachment on the airway. Depending on the diagnosis and the overall prognosis, specific therapy may be indicated in some cases. Opioids reduce the sensitivity of the central respiratory drive center and often reduce the sensation of dyspnea. In patients not already on an opioid, codeine is often a useful first intervention. In patients already on some opioids, morphine or another strong opioid may be used. There are no data supporting the use of nebulized morphine for dyspnea at the end of life. In the absence of bronchospasm, albuterol could worsen dyspnea as a respiratory stimulant. Benzodiazepines may help if there is concurrent anxiety but should not be used as the sole therapy for dyspnea. The use of oxygen is controversial in nonhypoxic patients. In this patient whose SaO_2 is already greater than 90% on current therapy, there is no role for increasing the FiO_2.

I-56. **The answer is A.** *(Chap. 10)* Voluntary active euthanasia is defined as intentionally administering medications or other interventions to cause the patient's death with the patient's informed consent. It is legal in Belgium and the Netherlands, but not the United States. Physician-assisted suicide is defined as a physician providing medications or other interventions to a patient with the understanding that the patient can use them to commit suicide. This practice is legal in Montana, Oregon, Vermont, and Washington State. Fewer than 10%–20% of terminally ill patients actually consider euthanasia and/or physician-assisted suicide for themselves. In the Netherlands and Oregon, >70% of patients using these interventions are dying of cancer; in Oregon, in 2013, just 1.2% of physician-assisted suicide cases involved patients with HIV/AIDS and 7.2% involved patients with amyotrophic lateral sclerosis. Pain is not a primary motivator for patients' requests for or interest in euthanasia and/or physician-assisted suicide. Fewer than 25% of all patients in Oregon cite inadequate pain control as the reason for desiring physician-assisted suicide. Depression, hopelessness, and, more profoundly, concerns about loss of dignity or autonomy or being a burden on family members appear to be primary factors motivating a desire for euthanasia or physician-assisted suicide. Over 75% cite loss of autonomy or dignity and inability to engage in enjoyable activities as the reason for wanting physician-assisted suicide. About 40% cite being a burden on family.

I-57. **The answer is D.** *(Chap. 11)* Figure I-57 demonstrates the median population age over time across the populated continents. Individuals in Europe experience the highest median population age currently, with Australia and North America falling closely behind. The populations of Asia and South America, however, are rapidly aging and are predicted to approach the median age of North American by the middle of the current century. The fastest-growing segment of the population is the "oldest old," those >80 years of age, and Japan and Italy are the two countries with the greatest percentage of individuals in this category.

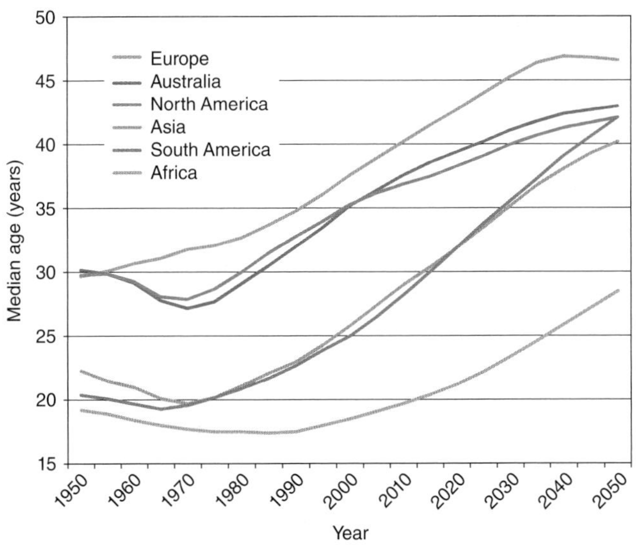

FIGURE I-57 From United Nations World Population Prospects: The 2008 Revision, http://www.un.org/esa/population/publications/wpp2008/wpp2008_highlights.pdf.

I-58. **The answer is A.** *(Chap. 11)* The systemic effects of aging are multidimensional and contribute overall to the concept of frailty. Frailty is defined as a physiologic syndrome characterized by diminished reserve and decreased resistance to stressors. Frailty increases an individual's vulnerability to adverse outcomes and death. The four recognized domains are: body composition, discrepancy between energy demand and utilization, homeostatic dysregulation, and neurodegeneration. Body composition changes are marked by a progressive loss of lean muscle mass following the third decade of life. The loss of muscle mass is greater in fast-twitch than in slow-twitch fibers and is associated with a loss in muscle strength. The reason behind the loss is unknown, but some research suggests this is due to loss of motor neurons. Coincident with the loss of muscle mass is an increase of fat mass that begins in middle age. However, late in life, fat mass begins to decrease again (option A). This mirrors changes in weight, which tends to increase until about 65 to 70 years in men and somewhat later in women before declining later in life. Waist circumference does increase throughout the life span, indicating ongoing fat deposition in the viscera. The effects of aging on the balance between energy demand and utilization are reflected by decreases in the maximal oxygen consumption (option C) as well as progressive decreases in the resting metabolic rate (RMR). Although the RMR does decline with aging, one should have caution in the setting of acute illness when the RMR may rise substantially. The high RMR in the setting of acute illness is associated with higher mortality. Homeostasis is generally measured by evaluating signaling pathways that involve hormones, inflammatory mediators, and antioxidants. Testosterone and estrogens decrease with aging, whereas inflammatory cytokines, including C-reactive protein and interleukin-6 (option B), rise. In addition, there is also evidence of oxidative stress and production of reactive oxygen species with aging. Neurodegeneration begins to become more evident after the age of 60 and is more apparent is some areas of the brain than others. The lateral prefrontal cortex and hippocampus (option D) are most likely to show evidence of atrophy in individuals with mild cognitive impairment, whereas the primary visual cortex is relatively preserved. In addition, functional imaging studies may show impaired coordination between brain areas responsible for higher order functioning with more diffuse activation rather than highly localized activity that is seen in younger individuals.

I-59. **The answer is E.** *(Chap. 11)* Population aging occurs at different rates in varying geographic regions of the world. Over the past century, Europe, Australia, and North America have had the populations with the greatest proportions of older persons, but the populations of Asia and South America are aging rapidly, and the population structure on these continents will resemble that of "older" countries by around 2050. Among older persons, the oldest old (those >80 years of age) are the fastest-growing segment, and the pace of population aging is projected to accelerate in most countries over the next 50 years. There is no evidence that the rate of population aging is decreasing. As shown in Figure I-59, it is projected that by 2050 over 15% of Japan's population will be over 80 years age.

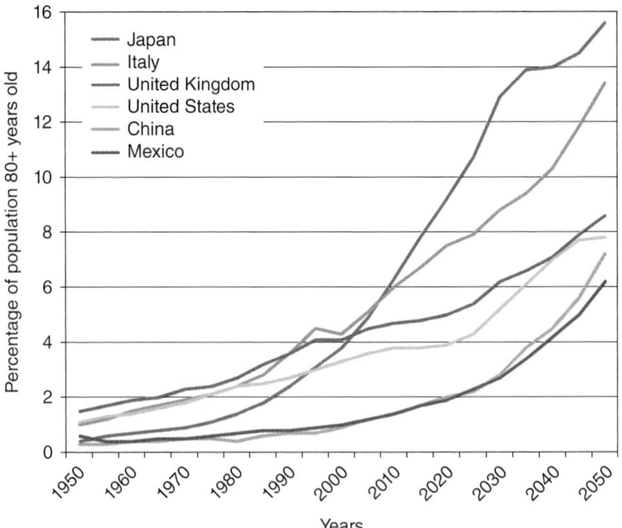

FIGURE I-59 From United Nations World Population Prospects: The 2008 Revision. http://www.un.org/esa/population/publications/wpp2008/wpp2008_highlights.pdf.

I-60. **The answer is A.** *(Chap. 12e)* In recent years, there has been increasing focus on both the safety and quality of healthcare provided throughout the world. The Institute of Medicine has suggested that safety is the first part of quality and that the healthcare system must guarantee that it will deliver safe care. Improving safety and quality in healthcare relies on understanding the frequency and type of adverse events that are occurring in the healthcare system. An adverse event is defined as an injury caused by medical management rather than the underlying disease of the patient. One of the largest studies that attempted to quantify adverse events in hospitalized patients was the Harvard Medical Practice Study. In this study, the most common adverse events were adverse drug events, which occurred in 19% of hospitalizations. Other common adverse events included wound infections (14%) and technical complications of a procedure (13%). Among nonoperative events, 37% were adverse drug events, 15% were diagnostic mishaps, 14% were therapeutic mishaps, and 5% were falls.

I-61. **The answer is E.** *(Chap. 12e)* Avedis Donabedian, founder of the study of quality of healthcare in America, suggested that quality of care can be studied by examining structures, processes, and outcomes. The theory of continuous quality improvement suggests that organizations should be evaluating the care they deliver on an ongoing basis and continually making small changes to improve individual processes. One of most important and widely adopted tools to help improve process performance is the Plan–Do–Check–Act cycle. First, planning is undertaken, and several potential improvement strategies are identified. Next, these strategies are evaluated in small "tests of change." "Checking" entails measuring whether the strategies have appeared to make a difference, and the results are then acted upon.

I-62. **The answer is B.** *(Chap. 13e)* The current average life expectancy at birth in high-income countries is 74 years, but it is only 68 years in middle-income countries and 58 years in low-income countries. Initially this difference was largely attributed to high fertility and high infant, child, and maternal mortality rates as well as infectious and tropical diseases in largely rural populations. However, low- and middle-income countries now have growing adult and elderly populations and changing lifestyles linked to global forces of urbanization. Thus, these countries are facing a new set of health challenges characterized by chronic disease and environmental overcrowding. The majority of tobacco-related deaths globally now occur in low- and middle-income countries, and the risk of a child's dying from a road traffic injury in Africa is more than twice that of Europe. Thus, road traffic accidents, cancers, cardiovascular diseases, and intentional injuries are all projected to cause increased disease burdens in low- and middle-income countries between 2004 and 2030, with only infectious disease mortality declining. Of these categories, cardiovascular disease is projected to cause the majority of deaths in the year 2030.

I-63. The answer is A. *(Chap. 13e)* The WHO noted that these four groups reflect: the evidence of what is needed for an effective response to today's healthcare challenges; the values of equity, solidarity, and social justice; and the growing expectations of the population in modernizing societies. Universal coverage reforms ensure that health systems contribute to health equity and the end of exclusion by moving toward universal access and social health protection. Service delivery reforms aim to make health systems more people centered. Leadership reforms aim to make health authorities more reliable. Public policy reforms aim to promote the health of communities. Drug development was not highlighted in this report as an area for reform.

I-64. The answer is A. *(Chap. 14e)* Multiple studies have shown that nearly 40% of Americans utilize at least one form of complementary and alternative medicine (CAM). According to the National Health Interview Survey, nonmineral, nonvitamin dietary supplements are the most prevalent form of CAM used, by 18% of Americans. In 1994, the DSHEA gave the FDA authority to regulate dietary supplements; homeopathic medications predated these regulations and are sold with no requirement that they are proved effective. Purveyors of dietary supplements may not claim that they can prevent or treat diseases without evidence, but can claim that they can maintain normal structure and function of body systems. The Federal Trade Commission, not the FDA, has the authority to regulate advertising and marketing claims related to dietary supplements. DSHEA regulations have led, for example, to the banning of ephedra-containing products such as ma huang.

I-65. The answer is D. *(Chap. 15e)* The term *moral hazard* comes from the actuarial literature and originally referred to the weaker incentives of an insured individual to prevent the loss against which he or she is insured. In the context of health insurance, *moral hazard* classically referred to potentially reduced incentives to prevent illness, but this is generally not considered a major issue (people have other incentives to remain healthy and disease free). *Moral hazard* typically refers to the incentives for better-insured individuals to use more medical services. In the RAND Health Insurance Experiment, families were randomized to various amounts of co-pays/co-insurance, and families who had complete coverage used 40% more services in a year than those with catastrophic insurance. However, there was no difference in outcomes between the groups. Option A is the definition of *market failure*; option B is the definition of *capitation*; option C is the definition of *positive economics*; option E is the definition of *administered pricing.*

I-66. The answer is E. *(Chap. 16e)* Minority patients have poorer health outcomes from many preventable and treatable conditions such as cardiovascular disease, asthma, diabetes, cancer, and HIV/AIDS. The causes of these differences are multifactorial and include social determinants (such as lower socioeconomic status, inadequate housing, and racism) and access to care (which often leads to more serious illness before seeking care). However, there are also clearly described racial differences in quality of care once patients enter the healthcare system. Eliminating these differences will require systematic changes in health system factors, provider-level factors, and patient-level factors.

I-67. The answer is A. *(Chap. 17e)* Ethical principles can serve as general guidelines to help physicians determine the right thing to do. Respecting patients and acting justly are two key ethical principles. Tenets of respecting patients include obtaining informed consent, avoiding deception, maintaining confidentiality, caring for patients who lack decision-making capacity, and acting in the best interests of patients. Determining whether a patient has decision-making capacity can be a challenge for physicians. Legal standards vary across jurisdictions, but generally encompass the four criteria listed in options B,

C, D, and E as originally elucidated by Grisso and Appelbaum in the *New England Journal of Medicine*. A patient simply being oriented to person, place, and time is not adequate to establish decision-making capacity.

I-68. **The answer is B.** *(Chap. 90e)* There is great excitement for the future of stem cells to reverse organ disease, repair injury, or replace dysfunctional cells. However, to date, few clinical studies have demonstrated benefit, and of the options listed, benefit has only been shown in ischemic heart disease. Recent studies have demonstrated that the heart has the capacity for low levels of cardiomyocyte regeneration. This regeneration appears to be accomplished by cardiac stem cells resident in the heart and possibly also by cells originating in the bone marrow. Early studies suggested that stem cells might have the potential to engraft and generate cardiomyocytes. However, most investigators have found that the generation of new cardiomyocytes by these cells is at best a rare event and that graft survival over long periods is poor. The preponderance of evidence suggests that the observed beneficial effects of most experimental therapies were not derived from direct stem cell generation of cardiomyocytes but rather from indirect effects of the stem cells on resident cells. It is not clear whether these effects reflect the release of soluble trophic factors, the induction of angiogenesis, the release of anti-inflammatory cytokines, or another mechanism. A number of studies utilizing stem cells have shown a small but measurable improvement in cardiac function and, in some cases, reduction in infarct size. Mesenchymal stem cells (MSCs) and neural stem cells both reportedly have the capacity to generate insulin-producing cells, but there is no convincing evidence that either cell type will be clinically useful in type 1 or type 2 diabetes; however, clinical trials are ongoing. For Parkinson disease, two clinical trials of fetal nigral transplantation failed to meet their primary end point and were complicated by the development of dyskinesia. Embryonic stem (ES) cells and MSCs can facilitate remyelination after experimental spinal cord injury (SCI). Clinical trials of MSCs in this disorder have commenced in a number of countries, and SCI was the first disorder targeted for the clinical use of ES cells. However, the ES cell trial in SCI was terminated early for nonmedical reasons. At present, no population of transplanted stem cells has been shown to have the capacity to generate neurons that extend axons over long distances to form synaptic connections (as would be necessary for replacement of upper motor neurons in ALS, stroke, or other disorders). Although a series of studies in humans as well as animals suggested that transplanted stem cells can generate hepatocytes, fusion of the transplanted cells with endogenous liver cells, giving the erroneous appearance of new hepatocytes, appears to be the underlying event in most circumstances. Clinical trials of stem cells in cirrhosis are ongoing.

I-69. **The answer is B.** *(Chap. 95e)* Carbohydrates, proteins, and fats contribute the primary sources of nutrients in the diet. The largest source of calories and nutrients in the diet is carbohydrates. At least 45%–55% of a person's total calories are derived from carbohydrates. The second biggest source of calories in the diet is fats. Although it is recommended that no more than 30% of one's calories come from fats, a typical American diet consists of about 34% fat. Proteins contribute 10%–15% of daily caloric intake. Finally, although alcohol can contribute calories to one's diet, it does not contribute any nutrients.

I-70. **The answer is D.** *(Chap. 95e)* This individual has a normal measured level of vitamin D and thus is unlikely to have inadequate oral intake. Since the early 1990s, the best reference values for estimating the appropriate intake of nutrients are the dietary reference intakes (DRIs). The DRIs include the estimated average requirement, adequate intake, recommended dietary allowance (RDA), and tolerable upper level rather than a single measure of intake such as the RDA. The RDA underperforms as a criterion for determining nutritional adequacy for any single individual. By definition, the RDA is meant to identify individuals who would require intake of a nutrient that statistically would be greater than two standard deviations above the estimated average intake. So clearly, most individuals whose intake falls below the RDA are obtaining adequate nutritional intake.

I-71. **The answer is D.** *(Chap. 96e)* This patient is manifesting symptoms of thiamine deficiency. The most common causes of thiamine deficiency in developed countries are alcoholism and chronic illnesses such as cancer. Alcohol interferes with the absorption of thiamine as well as the synthesis of thiamin pyrophosphate. In addition, alcohol increases the excretion of thiamine in the urine. Moreover, most chronic alcoholics have low dietary intake of thiamine. Chronic thiamine deficiency manifests as beriberi, which is classically described as "wet" or "dry," depending on whether significant heart failure symptoms are present. However, there is often overlap between the syndromes of "wet" and "dry" beriberi. Both forms of the disease often exhibit paresthesias and neuropathic pain. Wet beriberi symptoms include those of high-output heart failure with tachycardia, cardiomegaly, and peripheral edema. Dry beriberi symptoms more commonly are those of both a motor and sensory neuropathy, predominantly affecting the legs. Alcoholic patients also demonstrate central nervous system effects. Acutely, this can consist of horizontal nystagmus, ophthalmoplegia, cerebellar ataxia, and mental impairment. This constellation of findings is called Wernicke encephalopathy. When there is additional loss of memory with confabulatory psychosis, as this individual is exhibiting, the syndrome is called Wernicke-Korsakoff syndrome. Rehydration with glucose-containing solutions without thiamine repletion can precipitate acute worsening of thiamine deficiency with lactic acidosis and coma and should be studiously avoided. In this case, the IV fluids with glucose should be held until thiamine repletion has begun. Thiamine should be repleted intravenously at a dose of 200 mg IV three times daily until there is no further improvement in acute symptoms, and then long-term oral thiamine at a dose of 10 mg daily should be continued until recovery is complete. In cases of Wernicke-Korsakoff syndrome, long-term memory loss is common.

I-72. **The answer is C.** *(Chap. 96e)* Vitamin A toxicity can occur acutely with large ingestions of vitamin A supplements and was noted historically in Arctic explorers who ingested polar bear liver. Acute toxicity manifests as increased intracranial pressure, diplopia, vertigo, seizures, and exfoliative dermatitis. Death can occur. Chronic ingestion of doses higher than the recommended daily doses (15 mg/d in adults or 6 mg/d in children) can lead to symptoms of chronic intoxication. More commonly, vitamin A is labelled in international units, or IU. The highest daily recommended IU for adults is 10,000 IU daily. Symptoms of chronic vitamin A toxicity can be varied and include dry skin, cheilosis, glossitis, vomiting, alopecia, bone demineralization and pain, hypercalcemia, lymph node enlargement, hyperlipidemia, amenorrhea, and increased intracranial pressure with pseudotumor cerebri. Liver fibrosis with portal hypertension may also occur. Excess vitamin A in pregnancy can result in spontaneous abortion and congenital malformations including craniofacial abnormalities and valvular heart disease. High doses of carotenoids were given in a chemoprevention trial to smokers, and those who were given the carotenoids were found to have a higher incidence of lung cancer. However, vitamin A has not been demonstrated to cause lung cancer in nonsmokers. Carotenemia is a condition that is associated with yellowing of the skin but not the sclerae. This condition is associated with the ingestion of >30 mg of β-carotene on a daily basis for a prolonged period. β-Carotene is an organic compound found in plants and fruits and is a precursor to vitamin A. It should not be found in the individual's supplement, and therefore, the individual is not at risk of carotenemia from her excessive use of vitamin A supplements.

I-73. **The answer is B.** *(Chap. 96e)* Niacin (vitamin B_3) has high bioavailability from beans, milk, meat, and eggs. While the bioavailability from grains is lower, most flour is enriched with "free" niacin; thus, deficiency of niacin is rare in Western diets. Niacin deficiency can be found in individuals with corn-based diets in some parts of China, Africa, and India; individuals with alcoholism; and individuals with genetic defects limiting absorption of tryptophan. In addition, individuals with carcinoid syndrome are at increased risk of niacin deficiency because of increased conversion of tryptophan to serotonin. Clinically, the syndrome of niacin deficiency is known as pellagra. Early symptoms of niacin deficiency are loss of appetite, generalized weakness, abdominal pain, and vomiting. Glossitis is characteristic of pellagra with a beefy red tongue. Pellagra also has many dermatologic manifestations including a characteristic skin rash appearing on sun-exposed area. The rash is scaling and erythematous. Often, the rash forms a ring around the neck, known as Casal's necklace. The four *d's* of niacin deficiency—diarrhea, dermatitis, dementia, and death—are seen only in the most severe cases.

I-74. The answer is E. *(Chap. 96e)* Vitamin A, also known as retinol, is a fat-soluble vitamin that has biologically active metabolites retinaldehyde and retinoic acid that are all important for good health. Collectively, these molecules are known as retinoids and are important for normal vision, cell growth and differentiation, and immunity. Vitamin A is found in its preformed state in liver, fish, and eggs, and it is often consumed as carotenoids from dark green and deeply colored fruits and vegetables. In developing countries, chronic vitamin A deficiency is endemic in many areas and is the most common cause of preventable blindness. In milder stages, vitamin A deficiency causes night blindness and conjunctival xerosis. This can progress to keratomalacia and blindness. Given the broad biologic functions of vitamin A, however, deficiency at any stage increases the risk of mortality from diarrhea, dysentery, measles, malaria, and respiratory disease. Vitamin A supplementation has been demonstrated to decrease childhood mortality by 23%–34%. About 10% of pregnant women in undernourished settings develop night blindness in the later trimesters of pregnancy, and vitamin A deficiency in pregnancy is associated with an increased risk of maternal infection and death.

I-75. The answer is D. *(Chap. 96e)* This patient presents with gingival bleeding and has the classic perifollicular hemorrhagic rash of scurvy (vitamin C deficiency). In the United States, scurvy is primarily a disease of alcoholics and the elderly who consume <10 mg/d of vitamin C. Other individuals who are at risk of the disease are the poor and those who consume macrobiotic diets that are high in grains and seafood but avoid citrus fruits. In addition to nonspecific symptoms of fatigue, these patients also have impaired ability to form mature connective tissue and can bleed into various sites, including the joints, skin and gingiva. A normal INR excludes symptomatic vitamin K deficiency. Thiamine, niacin, and folate deficiencies are also seen in patients with alcoholism. Thiamine deficiency may cause a peripheral neuropathy (beriberi), high-output heart failure, ataxia, and memory impairment. Folate deficiency causes macrocytic anemia and thrombocytopenia. Niacin deficiency causes pellagra, which is characterized by glossitis and a pigmented, scaling rash that may be particularly noticeable in sun-exposed areas.

I-76. The answer is E. *(Chap. 97)* The patient in this scenario has evidence of chronic starvation-related malnutrition, most likely related to anorexia nervosa. Starvation-related malnutrition that occurs without evidence of systemic inflammation is also known as marasmus and develops over months or years due to prolonged decreases in energy and protein intake. The patient exhibits a starved appearance with a low body mass index ($<18.5\ kg/m^2$). The diagnosis is based on diminished skinfold thickness, which reflects loss of fat stores and reduced arm circumference and demonstrates muscle wasting. In addition, temporal and interosseous muscle wasting is also commonly seen. Routine laboratory testing is not remarkably abnormal. Albumin may be low, but is typically not less than 2.8 g/dL. However, despite a morbid appearance, immunocompetence and wound healing are preserved. Because the process is a chronic and fairly well-adapted process, treatment should be planned in concert with a dietitian to slowly allow a return to normal body weight. Overly aggressive nutritional support can lead to life-threatening metabolic imbalances. When mortality occurs in anorexia nervosa, it is most commonly related to complications of the disease and rarely due to malnutrition itself. Indeed, suicide is a more common cause of death in the disease than malnutrition. In certain processes such as cancer or chronic obstructive pulmonary disease, a similar loss of fat and protein can occur in the setting of systemic inflammation resulting in a wasted appearance. This process is known as cachexia. The diagnostic criteria are similar with regard to skinfold thickness and arm circumference. However, due to the concomitant systemic inflammation, individuals with cachexia are more likely to have lower albumin levels and can be immunocompromised.

I-77. The answer is C. *(Chap. 97)* Kwashiorkor is the term that describes acute disease- or injury-related malnutrition. In developed countries, the most common causes of kwashiorkor are trauma and sepsis. Pathophysiologically, the body has increased protein and energy requirements in these settings. However, intake is often reduced or absent for prolonged periods of time. Signs of kwashiorkor can develop within a period as short as 2 weeks. Body mass index is a poor predictor and is often normal. Acute weight loss is often masked by the development of edema. Easy hair pluckability, skin breakdown, and wound healing are common signs. On laboratory examination, there are marked decreases in serum proteins, including albumin <2.8 g/dL, transferrin <150 mg/dL, and total iron-binding capacity <200 μg/dL. Cellular immunity is impaired, with low lymphocyte counts and presence of anergy. Presence of kwashiorkor portends a poor prognosis and high mortality from the underlying medical condition. Surgical wounds exhibit poor healing and often dehisce. There is an increased risk of development of decubitus ulcers. Aggressive nutritional support is indicated. Use of enteral feeding in general can be difficult and may be contraindicated in this patient due to her surgical issues. Patients with kwashiorkor frequently exhibit gastroparesis with enteral feedings and also have an increased risk of gastrointestinal bleeding from stress ulcers.

I-78. **The answer is A.** *(Chap. 97)* Several factors can help identify an individual who is at high risk of nutritional depletion upon hospital admission. The first factor to consider is the body mass index (BMI) and recent weight loss. If a patient is underweight (BMI <18.5 kg/m^2) or has recently lost more than 10% of body weight, this would confer increased nutritional risk. Other general categories that increase nutritional risk include poor intake, excessive nutrient losses, hypermetabolic states, alcoholism, or medications that increase metabolic requirements. Poor oral intake can be related to current anorexia, food avoidance, or NPO status for more than 5 days among others. Examples of excessive nutrient loss include malabsorption syndromes, enteric fistulae, draining wounds, or renal dialysis. Common hypermetabolic states are trauma, burns, sepsis, and prolonged febrile illness. The patient with anorexia in remission and a normal BMI would be least likely among these patients to have excessive nutritional risk.

I-79. **The answer is B.** *(Chap. 97)* A patient's basal energy expenditure (BEE) can be calculated by the Harris-Benedict equation. The factors that are used for determining BEE are age, gender, height, and weight. The BEE for hospitalized patients is then adjusted by a factor of 1.1–1.4 depending on the severity of illness, with the highest values used for patients admitted with marked stress such as trauma or severe sepsis. The BEE serves as an estimate only. If it is important to have an exact calculation of energy expenditure, indirect calorimetry can be performed. Protein needs can also be calculated more definitively by the use of urine urea nitrogen (UUN) as an estimate of protein catabolism.

I-80. **The answer is E.** *(Chap. 98e)* This patient would have at least a moderate systemic response to inflammation as would be expected in the postoperative period. In such a situation, an individual benefits from adequate feeding by day 5–7. Picking the appropriate nutritional support should take into account his overall clinical course. Generally, the enteral route is preferred to promote the ongoing health and immunologic barrier function of the gut as long as there are no contraindications. Parenteral nutrition alone is generally only indicated for prolonged ileus, obstruction, or hemorrhagic pancreatitis. Because this patient has bowel sounds and evidence of ileostomy output, he is not exhibiting ileus at the present time. Thus, enteral nutrition would be used. Given his delirium and aspiration risk, he should not be initiated on an oral diet, and nasogastric feeding is also associated with a higher aspiration risk. The preferred feeding method would be use of a nasojejunal feeding tube placed post ligament of Treitz.

I-81. **The answer is D.** *(Chap. 98e)* When possible, at least a portion of the nutritional support given to a critically ill patient should be in the form of enteral nutrition. Use of the enteral route is particularly important for maintaining overall health of the gastrointestinal tract. Seventy percent of the nutrients utilized by the bowel and its associated digestive organs are directly derived from food within the bowel lumen. Moreover, enteral feedings are important for maintaining the immunologic function of the gut as they stimulate secretion of IgA and hormones to promote trophic activity of the gut. In addition, enteral feedings improve splanchnic blood flow and stimulate neuronal activity to prevent ischemia and ileus.

I-82. **The answer is C.** *(Chap. 98e)* It is important to understand the thresholds of body mass index (BMI) that indicate malnutrition. Normal BMI ranges between 20 and 25 kg/m^2, and a patient is considered underweight with likely moderate malnutrition at a BMI of

18.5 kg/m^2. Severe malnutrition is expected with a BMI of <16 kg/m^2. In men, a BMI of <13 kg/m^2 is lethal, whereas in women, the lethal BMI is <11 kg/m^2.

I-83. **The answer is E.** *(Chap. 98e)* The two most common problems with use of parenteral nutrition (PN) are fluid retention and hyperglycemia. The fluid retention is greater than would be expected by the volume of PN and is linked to the hyperglycemia. The dextrose provided by PN is hypertonic and stimulates greater insulin secretion than is generated by meal feeding. Insulin itself has antinatriuretic and antidiuretic properties that exacerbate fluid and sodium retention. Strategies to minimize fluid and sodium retention include providing both glucose and fat as energy source and limiting sodium intake to less than 40 mEq daily. In addition, glucose should be provided initially at a dose of 200 g daily or less, and regular insulin should be added to the PN formula. In addition to providing insulin with the PN formula, additional subcutaneous insulin should be given based on a sliding scale every 6 hours with about two-thirds of the total dose given during a 24-hour period added to the PN formula the next day. In more severe cases, intensive insulin support with a separate infusion of insulin should be used. If a patient has known insulin-dependent diabetes mellitus, the dose of insulin required is usually twice the home dosage.

I-84. **The answer is D.** *(Chap. 261e)* Microbial agents have been used as bioweapons as far back as the sixth century B.C. when water supplies were poisoned with *Claviceps purpurea* by the Assyrians. In modern times, science that has been often sponsored by governmental agencies has led to new ways to enhance and spread microbial bioweapons. Bioterrorism should be delineated from biowarfare. Although bioterrorism has the potential to lead to thousands of deaths if employed in a large-scale manner, the primary impact is the fear and terror generated by the attack. However, biowarfare specifically targets mass casualties and seeks to weaken the enemy. The Working Group for Civilian Biodefense has outlined key features that characterize agents that are the most effective bioweapons. These 10 features are:

1. High morbidity and mortality rates
2. Potential for person-to-person spread
3. Low infective dose and highly infectious by the aerosol route
4. Lack of rapid diagnostic capability
5. Lack of universally available effective vaccine
6. Potential to cause anxiety
7. Availability of pathogen and feasibility of production
8. Environmental stability
9. Database of prior research and development
10. Potential to be weaponized

A lack of effective and available treatment is not one of the characteristics of an effective bioweapon. *Bacillus anthracis* is the causative organism of anthrax, one of the most prototypical microbial bioweapons, but many antibiotics have efficacy against anthrax and can be life-saving if initiated early.

I-85. **The answer is B.** *(Chap. 261e) Yersinia pestis* is a gram-negative rod that causes the plague and has been one of the most widely used bioweapons over the centuries. Although *Y pestis* lacks environmental stability, it is highly contagious and has a high mortality rate, making it an effective agent of bioterrorism. There are two major syndromes caused by *Y pestis* that reflect the mode of infection. These patients presented with symptoms typical of bubonic plague, which still exists widely in nature. In the United States, the area with the greatest number of naturally occurring cases of bubonic plague is in the southwest with transmission occurring via contact with infected animals or fleas. In this case, infected animals or fleas were present in the concentrated population of an immigrant camp that had poor sanitation. Once an individual is bitten by an infected vector, the bacteria travel through the lymphatics to regional lymph nodes where they are phagocytized but not destroyed. The organisms can then multiply with the cells, leading to inflammation, painful and markedly enlarged lymph nodes, and fever. The affected lymph nodes can develop necrosis and are characteristically called buboes. Infection can progress to severe sepsis and death. The mortality rate for treated bubonic plague is 1%–15% and 40%–60% in untreated cases. If *Y pestis* was used as an agent of bioterrorism, it would aerosolize to a large area, and the affected cases would present primarily with pneumonic plague. Pneumonic plague presents with fever, cough, hemoptysis, and gastrointestinal symptoms that occur 1–6 days following exposure. Without treatment, pneumonic plague has an 85% morality rate with death occurring rapidly within 2–6 days. The treatment for *Y pestis* could include aminoglycosides or doxycycline.

I-86. **The answer is D.** *(Chap. 261e)* In the event of a bioterrorism attack, botulinum toxin would be most likely delivered by either aerosol or contamination of the food supply. Contamination of the water supply is possible, but it is not an optimal route for bioterrorism. Botulinum toxin is inactivated by chlorine, which is used in many water supplies for purification. In addition, heating any food or water to >85°C for longer than 5 minutes will inactivate the toxin. Finally, there is an environmental decay rate of 1% per minute. So the time interval between release and ingestion would need to be very short, which would be difficult with an entire city water supply.

I-87. **The answer is B.** *(Chap. 261e)* Anthrax is caused by the gram-positive spore-forming rod *Bacillus anthracis*. Anthrax spores may be the prototypical disease of bioterrorism. Although not spread person to person, inhalational anthrax has a high mortality, has a low infective dose (five spores), and may be spread widely with aerosols after bioengineering. It is well documented that anthrax spores were produced and stored as potential bioweapons. In 2001, the United States was exposed to anthrax spores delivered as a powder in letters. Of 11 patients with inhalational anthrax, 5 died. All 11 patients with cutaneous anthrax survived. Because anthrax spores can remain dormant in the respiratory tract for 6 weeks, the incubation period can be quite long, and postexposure antibiotics are recommended for 60 days. Trials of a recombinant vaccine are under way.

I-88. **The answer is D.** *(Chap. 261e)* The three major clinical forms of anthrax are gastrointestinal (GI), cutaneous, and inhalational. GI anthrax results from eating contaminated meat and is an unlikely bioweapon. Cutaneous anthrax results from contact with the spores and results in a black eschar lesion. Cutaneous anthrax had a 20% mortality before antibiotics became available. Inhalational anthrax typically presents with the most deadly form and is the most likely bioweapon. The spores are phagocytosed by alveolar macrophages and transported to the mediastinum. Subsequent germination, toxin elaboration, and hematogenous spread cause septic shock. A characteristic radiographic finding is mediastinal widening and pleural effusion. Prompt initiation of antibiotics is essential because mortality is likely 100% without specific treatment. Inhalational anthrax is not known to be contagious. Provided that there is no concern for release of another highly infectious agent such as smallpox, only routine precautions are warranted.

I-89. **The answer is C.** *(Chap. 261e)* Using the characteristics listed in the question, the Centers for Disease Control and Prevention (CDC) developed classifications of biologic agents that are based on their potential to be used as bioweapons. Six types of agents have been designated as category A: *Bacillus anthracis*, botulinum toxin, *Y pestis*, smallpox, tularemia, and the many viruses that cause viral hemorrhagic fever. Those viruses include Lassa virus, Rift Valley fever virus, Ebola virus, and yellow fever virus.

I-90. **The answer is A.** *(Chap. 291e)* In September 2001, the American public was exposed to anthrax spores as a bioweapon delivered through the U.S. Postal Service by an employee of the U.S. Army Medical Research Institute for Infectious Diseases (USAMRIID) who had access to such materials and who committed suicide prior to being indicted for this crime. The CDC identified 22 confirmed or suspected cases of anthrax as a consequence of this attack. These included 11 patients with inhalational anthrax, 5 of whom died, and 11 patients with cutaneous anthrax (7 confirmed), all of whom survived. Cases occurred in individuals who opened contaminated letters as well as in postal workers involved in the processing of mail. The arm lesion is typical of *cutaneous anthrax* and typically starts as a papule at the site of bacterial entry and progresses to a coal-black eschar. The chest radiograph shows the mediastinal widening typical of *inhalational anthrax*. The other listed agents are Category A bioweapon agents, and their typical clinical syndrome, incubation period, diagnostic method, treatment, and prophylaxis are listed in Table I-90.

SECTION I General Considerations in Clinical Medicine

TABLE I-90 Clinical Syndromes, Prevention, and Treatment Strategies for Diseases Caused by Category A Agents

Agent	Clinical Syndrome	Incubation Period	Diagnosis	Treatment	Prophylaxis
Bacillus anthracis (anthrax)	Cutaneous lesion: Papule to eschar Inhalational disease: Fever, malaise, chest and abdominal discomfort, pleural effusion, widened mediastinum on chest x-ray	Cutaneous: 1–12 d Inhalational: 1–60 d	Culture, Gram stain, PCR, Wright stain of peripheral smear	Postexposure: Ciprofloxacin, 500 mg PO bid × 60 d *or* Doxycycline, 100 mg PO bid × 60 d *or* Amoxicillin, 500 mg PO q8h × 60 d, likely to be effective if strain is penicillin sensitive Active disease: Ciprofloxacin, 400 mg IV q12h *or* doxycycline, 100 mg IV q12h *plus* Clindamycin, 900 mg IV q8h and/or rifampin, 300 mg IV q12h; switch to PO when stable × 60 d total *plus* Antitoxin Raxibacumab, 40 mg/kg IV over 2.25 h; diphenhydramine to reduce reaction	Anthrax vaccine adsorbed Recombinant protective antigen vaccines are under study Raxibacumab when alternative therapies are not available or appropriate
Yersinia pestis (pneumonic plague)	Fever, cough, dyspnea, hemoptysis Infiltrates and consolidation on chest x-ray	1–6 d	Culture, Gram stain, direct fluorescent antibody, PCR	Gentamicin 2.0 mg/kg IV loading then 1.7 mg/kg q8h IV *or* Streptomycin 1.0 g q12h IM or IV Alternatives include doxycycline 100 mg bid PO or IV; chloramphenicol 500 mg qid PO or IV	Doxycycline, 100 mg PO bid *or* Levofloxacin, 500 mg PO daily Formalin-fixed vaccine (FDA licensed; not available)
Variola major (smallpox)	Fever, malaise, headache, backache, emesis Maculopapular to vesicular to pustular skin lesions	7–17 d	Culture, PCR, electron microscopy	Supportive measures; consideration for cidofovir, tecovirimat, antivaccinia immunoglobulin	Vaccinia immunization
Francisella tularensis (tularemia)	Fever, chills, malaise, myalgia, chest discomfort, dyspnea, headache, skin rash, pharyngitis, conjunctivitis Hilar adenopathy on chest x-ray	1–14 d	Gram stain, culture, immunohistochemistry, PCR	Streptomycin 1 g IM bid *or* Gentamicin 5 mg/kg/d divided q8h IV for 14 d *or* Doxycycline 100 mg IV bid *or* Chloramphenicol 15 mg/kg up to 1 g IV qid *or* Ciprofloxacin 400 mg IV bid	Doxycycline 100 mg PO bid × 14 d *or* Ciprofloxacin 500 mg PO bid × 14 d
Viral hemorrhagic fevers	Fever, myalgia, rash, encephalitis, prostration	2–21 d	RT-PCR, serologic testing for antigen or antibody Viral isolation by CDC or U.S. Army Medical Research Institute of Infectious Diseases (USAMRIID)	Supportive measures Ribavirin 30 mg/kg up to 2 g × 1, followed by 16 mg/kg IV up to 1 g q6h for 4 d, followed by 8 mg/kg IV up to 0.5 g q8h × 6 d	No known chemoprophylaxis Consideration for ribavirin or monoclonal antibodies in high-risk situations
Botulinum toxin (*Clostridium botulinum*)	Dry mouth, blurred vision, ptosis, weakness, dysarthria, dysphagia, dizziness, respiratory failure, progressive paralysis, dilated pupils	12–72 hr	Mouse bioassay, toxin immunoassay	Supportive measures including ventilation, HBAT equine antitoxin from the CDC Emergency Operations Center, 770-488-7100	Administration of antitoxin

Abbreviations: CDC, U.S. Centers for Disease Control and Prevention; FDA, U.S. Food and Drug Administration; HBAT, heptavalent botulinum antitoxin; IM, intramuscular; IV, intravenous; PCR, polymerase chain reaction; PO, oral; RT-PCR, reverse transcriptase polymerase chain reaction.

I-91. **The answer is C.** *(Chap. 262e)* Chemical agents were first used in modern warfare during World War I when 1.3 million people died as a result of chemical agents. Since then, chemical agents have been used during warfare and bioterrorism, but most agents have a fairly low associated mortality. The chemical agents generally fall into one of five categories: nerve agents, asphyxiants, pulmonary damaging, vesicants, and behavior altering/incapacitating. Nerve agents include cyclohexyl sarin, sarin, soman, tabun, and VX and largely exert their effects through acetylcholinesterase inhibition. The most common asphyxiant is cyanide, which is liberated through cyanogen chloride or hydrogen cyanide. Chlorine gas, hydrogen chloride, nitrogen oxide, and phosgene are common agents that primarily cause pulmonary damage and adult respiratory distress syndrome. Vesicants include mustard gas and phosgene oxime, and agent 15/BZ is the primary chemical causing alterations in behavior or incapacitation.

I-92. **The answer is D.** *(Chap. 262e)* Sulfur mustard was first used as a chemical warfare agent in World War I. This agent is considered a vesicant and has a characteristic odor of burning garlic or horseradish. It is a threat to all exposed epithelial surfaces, and the most commonly affected organs are the eyes, skin, and airways. Large exposures can lead to bone marrow suppression. Erythema resembling a sunburn is one of the earliest manifestations of sulfur mustard exposure and begins within 2 hours to 2 days of exposure. The timing of exposure can be delayed as long as 2 days depending on the severity of exposure, ambient temperature, and humidity. The most sensitive body areas are warm, moist locations including the axillae, perineum, external genitalia, neck, and antecubital fossae. Blistering of the skin is frequent and may be anything from small vesicles to large bullae. The bullae are dome-shaped and flaccid. Filled with clear or straw-colored fluid, these bullae are not hazardous because the fluid does not contain any vesicant substances. The respiratory passages are also affected. With mild exposure, the only manifestation may be a complaint of irritation and congestion. Laryngospasm may occur. In severe cases, there is necrosis of the airways with pseudomembrane formation. The damage that occurs following sulfur mustard exposure is airway predominant, and alveolar damage is very rare. The eyes are particularly sensitive to sulfur mustard, and eye injury has a shorter latency period than the skin injury. Almost all exposed individuals develop redness of the eyes. With higher exposure, there is a greater severity of conjunctivitis and corneal damage. The cause of death following mustard gas exposure is sepsis or respiratory failure, but the mortality rate is typically low. Even during World War I, when antibiotics and endotracheal intubation were not available, the mortality rate was only 1.9%. There is no antidote to sulfur mustard. Complete decontamination in 2 minutes stops clinical injury, and decontamination within 5 minutes can decrease skin injury by half. Treatment is largely supportive.

I-93. **The answer is A.** *(Chap. 262e)* Chlorine gas exposure primarily causes pulmonary damage and edema with respiratory distress syndrome. The initial decontamination of a victim exposed to chlorine gas should include removal of all clothing if no frostbite is present. The victim should gently wash the skin with soap and water with care to avoid aggressive bathing that may lead to serious abrasion of the skin. The eyes are flushed with water or normal saline. Supportive care should include forced rest, fresh air, and maintenance of a semi-upright position. Oxygen is not required because the patient is not hypoxemic or in any respiratory distress. Delayed pulmonary edema can occur even if the patient is initially asymptomatic. Thus, observation for a period of time following exposure is required.

I-94 and I-95. **The answers are D and D, respectively.** *(Chap. 262e)* This patient has symptoms of an acute cholinergic crisis as seen in cases of organophosphate poisoning. Organophosphates are the "classic" nerve agents, and several different compounds may act in this manner, including sarin, tabun, soman, and cyclosarin. Except for agent VX, all the organophosphates are liquid at standard room temperature and pressure and are highly volatile, with the onset of symptoms occurring within minutes to hours after exposure. VX is an oily liquid with a low vapor pressure; therefore, it does not acutely cause symptoms. However, it is an environmental hazard because it can persist in the environment for a longer period. Organophosphates act by inhibiting tissue synaptic acetylcholinesterase. Symptoms differ between vapor exposure and liquid exposure because the organophosphate acts in the tissue upon contact. The first organ exposed with vapor exposure is the eyes, causing rapid and persistent pupillary constriction. After the sarin gas attacks in the Tokyo subway in 1994 and 1995, survivors frequently complained that their "world went black" as the first symptom of exposure. This is rapidly followed by rhinorrhea, excessive salivation, and lacrimation. In the airways, organophosphates cause bronchorrhea and bronchospasm. It is in the alveoli that organophosphates gain the greatest extent of entry into the blood. As organophosphates circulate, other symptoms appear, including nausea, vomiting, diarrhea, and muscle fasciculations. Death occurs with central nervous system penetration causing central apnea and status epilepticus. The effects on the heart rate and blood pressure are unpredictable. Treatment requires a multifocal approach. Initially, decontamination of clothing and wounds is important for both the patient and the caregiver. Clothing should be removed before contact with the healthcare provider. In Tokyo, 10% of emergency personnel developed miosis related to contact with patients' clothing. Three classes of medication are important in treating organophosphate poisoning: anticholinergics, oximes, and anticonvulsant agents. Initially, atropine at doses of 2 to 6 mg should be given intravenously or intramuscularly to reverse the effects of organophosphates at muscarinic receptors; it has no effect on nicotinic receptors. Thus, atropine rapidly treats life-threatening respiratory depression but does not affect neuromuscular or sympathetic effects. This should be followed by the administration of an oxime, which is a nucleophile compound that reactivates the cholinesterase whose active site has been bound to a nerve agent. Depending on the nerve agent used, oxime may not be helpful because it is unable to bind to "aged" complexes that have undergone degradation of a side chain of the nerve agent, making it negatively charged. Soman undergoes aging within 2 minutes, thus rendering oxime therapy useless. The currently approved oxime in the United States is 2-pralidoxime. Finally, the only anticonvulsant class of drugs that is effective in seizures caused by organophosphate poisoning is benzodiazepines. The dose required is frequently higher than that used for epileptic seizures, requiring the equivalent of 40 mg of diazepam given in frequent doses. All other classes of anticonvulsant medications, including phenytoin, barbiturates, carbamazepine, and valproic acid, will not improve seizures related to organophosphate poisoning.

I-96. **The answer is D.** *(Chap. 263e)* Detonation of a nuclear device is the most likely scenario of radiation bioterror. The initial blast will cause acute mortality due to the shock wave and thermal damage. Subsequent mortality would be due to acute radiation exposure and fallout to more distant populations that largely depend on weather patterns. The initial detonation releases mostly highly damaging gamma particles and neutrons. Alpha and beta particles are not highly toxic in this situation. Alpha particles are large, have limiting penetrating power, and are stopped by cloth and human skin. Beta particles, while small, travel only a short distance (a few millimeters) in tissue and cause mostly burn-type injuries. Radioactive iodine is a beta particle emitter. Acute radiation syndrome causes death by hematopoietic bone marrow suppression and aplasia, gastrointestinal (GI) tract damage with malabsorption and translocation of bacteria, and in severe cases, neurologic damage. Appropriate medical supportive therapy can reduce mortality and allow patients with more severe exposure to survive. Radiation causes dose-dependent bone marrow suppression that at high doses is irreversible. Bone marrow transplantation is controversial in cases of nonrecovery of bone marrow. The acute exposure symptoms, predominantly thermal injury, respiratory distress, and GI symptoms, may resolve within days. However, subsequent bone marrow dysfunction typically develops within 2 weeks but may take as long as 6 weeks to manifest.

I-97. **The answer is D.** *(Chap. 263e)* Much of the initial damage related to a "dirty" bomb is related to the power of the blast rather than the radiation. Following a terrorist attack, it is important to identify all individuals who might have been exposed to radiation. The initial treatment of these individuals should be to stabilize and treat the most severely injured. Those with severe injuries should have contaminated clothing removed prior to transportation to the emergency department, but further care should not be withheld for additional decontamination because the risk of exposure to healthcare workers is low. Individuals with minor injuries who can be safely decontaminated without increasing the risk of medical complications should be transported to a centralized area for decontamination. A further consideration regarding treatment following radiation exposure is the total dose of radiation that an individual was exposed to. At a dose <2 Gy, there are usually no significant adverse outcomes, and no specific treatment is recommended unless symptoms develop. Many individuals will develop flulike symptoms. However, a complete blood count should be obtained every 6 hours for the first 24 hours because bone marrow suppression can develop with radiation exposure as low as 0.7 Gy. The earliest sign of this is a fall in the lymphocyte count of >50%. Potential treatments of radiation exposure include use of colony-stimulating factors and supportive transfusions. Stem cell transfusion and bone marrow transplantation can be considered in the case of severe pancytopenia that does not recover. However, this is controversial, given the lack of experience with the procedure for this indication. Following the Chernobyl nuclear reactor accident, none of the bone marrow transplants were successful.

I-98 and I-99. The answers are E and E, respectively. *(Chap. 474)* Most snakebites that occur are due to nonvenomous snakes. However, about 7000–8000 individuals in the United States are bitten by venomous snakes each year, and of these, 5 will die (www.cdc.gov). In the developing countries with temperate and tropical climates, snakebites are a more serious problem because access to healthcare resources may be quite sparse, and it is estimated at 20,000–94,000 individuals die worldwide from snakebites yearly. Venomous snakes belong to the families Viperidae (pit vipers including rattlesnakes, copperheads, and cottonmouth water moccasins), Elapidae (including cobras and coral snakes), Lamprophiidae (asps), and Colubridae, which are largely nonvenomous but have a few toxic species. Most snakes have venom glands situated below and behind the eyes that are connected by ducts to hollow maxillary fangs. The fangs are retractable in most pit vipers and brought into an upright position for striking. It is notable when evaluating a snake bite to know that about 20% of pit viper bites and higher percentages of other snakebites bites contain no venom. Significant envenomation occurs in only about 50% of all snakebites. Snake venoms are complex mixtures of enzymes, glycoproteins, and low-molecular-weight polypeptides, among other constituents, that lead to tissue hemorrhage, vascular leak, and proteolysis with tissue necrolysis. Some snake venoms have myocardial depressant factors and neurotoxins as well. The time from the bite to symptom onset is variable and depends on the species of snake, amount of envenomation, and site of the bite. Progressive local pain, swelling, and ecchymosis are common with development of hemorrhagic or serum-filled bullae. Systemic findings are quite variable and may include tachycardia or bradycardia, hypotension, weakness, coagulopathy, renal dysfunction, and neurologic dysfunction. If a patient has suffered a venomous snakebite, the most important aspect of prehospital care is supportive care with rapid transport to a medical facility where antivenom therapy is available. It is notable that most of the first-aid measures recommended in the past are of little benefit and may actually worsen local tissue damage. For supportive care, a splint may be applied to decrease pain and lessen bleeding. If possible, the injured limb should be elevated to the level of the heart. Attempting to capture the offending snake alive or dead is not recommended and could only lead to more injury in others. Digital photographs taken from a safe distance away will suffice to allow identification of the snake. There is no role for incising or applying suction to the wound. This will not allow the venom to be removed and may introduce additional bacterial contamination. Applying a tight tourniquet also does not limit spread of venom and may endanger the affected limb by limiting blood flow. The only role for pressure-immobilization is in Elapid venoms (cobra), which are neurotoxic. This technique requires specific training to effectively apply to an entire limb and to a precise pressure. After application, the victim must be carried from the field and remain immobile in order to prevent spread of the neurotoxin. Upon arrival at the hospital, victims of snakebite should be carefully monitored for signs of significant envenomation that would require antivenom therapy. The patient should be monitored on telemetry with frequent vital signs. The area of snakebite should be cleaned and clearly marked. Limb circumference should be measured every 15 minutes. The extremity should remain at the level of the heart. Volume resuscitation should ensue, and large-bore IV access should be maintained. Indications for the use of antivenom therapy include significant local progression including soft tissue swelling that crosses a joint or involves more than half of the bitten limb. In addition, any evidence of systemic involvement should prompt the use of antivenom therapy. Signs of systemic involvement could include hypotension, altered mental status, coagulopathy, renal dysfunction, rhabdomyolysis, hepatic dysfunction, or neurologic dysfunction. It is important to know the type of snake when administering antivenom therapy because it is specific to the type of snake. Prompt and serious allergy reaction can occur including anaphylaxis. Use of IV antihistamines is typical as a pretreatment. Posttreatment serum sickness reactions may occur.

I-100. The answer is A. *(Chap. 474)* Ciguatera poisoning is the most common nonbacterial food poisoning associated with fish consumption in the United States, occurring primarily in Hawaii and Florida. However, it is seen more commonly in other areas because imported fish are being transported nationwide. Ciguatera poisoning is caused by a toxin produced by warm water ocean reef microalgae that are then consumed by fish that feed at the reef. The toxin can then accumulate in these fish and enter the food chain. Specific fish that are susceptible to ciguatera toxin are barracuda, snapper, jack, and grouper. Most ciguatoxins are unaffected by freeze-drying, heat, cold, and gastric acid, and the toxins do not alter the taste, odor, or color of the fish. The onset of symptoms after ingesting affected fish may be within 15–30 minutes and typically is within 2–6 hours. Peak symptoms occur within the first 4–6 hours after onset of symptoms. Myriad symptoms have been attributed to ciguatera poisoning, but the typical initial symptoms are diarrhea, vomiting, and abdominal pain. These symptoms may persist up to 48 hours. Neurologic symptoms are also common and include paresthesias, pruritus, tongue and throat numbness, sensation of "carbonation" during swallowing, tremor, fasciculations, seizures, and coma. A pathognomonic symptom of ciguatera poisoning is reversal of hot and cold tactile perception. This symptom develops in some affected individuals after 3–5 days and may last for months. More severe symptoms tend to occur in individuals previously affected by an ingestion. Therapy is supportive and directed at symptom management. In severe cases where systemic symptoms including hypotension or bradycardia are present, volume resuscitation with use of atropine may be required. Amitriptyline may also alleviate some of the pruritus and dysesthesia through its anticholinergic actions. During recovery, care should be taken to avoid reexposure to ciguatoxin. An affected individual should avoid all fish consumption (fresh or preserved), fish sauce, and shellfish, as well as alcoholic beverages, nuts, and nut oils, for 6 months. Diarrhetic shellfish poisoning occurs after consuming shellfish that have been contaminated with the toxins okadaic acid and *Dinophysis* toxin acquired from feeding on dinoflagellates. Symptoms include diarrhea, nausea, vomiting, abdominal pain, and chills that occur within 30 minutes to 12 hours after eating shellfish. Domoic acid intoxication is also known as amnestic shellfish poisoning. This rare illness has been described in outbreaks in the United States, United Kingdom, Canada, and Spain and is caused by domoic acid–contaminated mussels. Symptoms begin within 24 hours and include confusion, disorientation, memory loss, severe headache, nausea, vomiting, and diarrhea. The symptoms may progress to seizures and coma. Scombroid poisoning occurs commonly worldwide and may be the most common seafood poisoning. Affected fish include tuna, mackerel, mahi-mahi, sardine, marlin, anchovy, herring, and wahoo, among many others. If fish are not preserved properly, the fish will undergo decomposition by *Proteus morganii* and *Klebsiella pneumoniae* with consequent decarboxylation of the amino acid L-histidine to histamine, histamine phosphate, and histamine hydrochloride. Buildup of these histaminic compounds in the fish leads to symptoms of mouth and lip tingling upon ingestion and nausea. More severe symptoms may include flushing, pruritus, urticaria, and bronchospasm. Tetrodotoxin poisoning can occur after ingestion of the puffer fish. This dangerous neurotoxin can result in death with as little as 1–2 mg of ingestion with a rapid ascending paralysis and cardiac depression with bradycardia.

I-101. The answer is E. *(Chap. 475)* Head lice (*Pediculus capitis*) is a common problem among school-aged children, affecting about 1% of elementary-aged children. Nymphs and adult lice feed exclusively on human blood and need to feed at least once daily. The saliva of the lice is an irritant and produces a morbilliform rash. In some individuals, it can be urticarial. The female louse cements her eggs, called nits, firmly onto the shaft of the hair. The eggs will hatch after about 10 days. However, unless manually removed, the nit can remain attached to the hair for months afterward. Contrary to popular belief, fomite transmission of head lice is rare. Most head lice are transmitted by direct head-to-head contact. The primary symptom of an infestation is a mild pruritus. To confirm an infestation requires discovery of a live louse as finding nits only demonstrates a prior infestation but cannot confirm if it is currently active. Once confirmed, the first-line treatment is a topical application of 1% permethrin, which kills both the adult louse and the unhatched eggs. A second application should be applied after 7–10 days. However, if lice persist after this treatment, permethrin resistance may be present, and an alternative treatment should be considered. Options include lindane, malathion, benzyl alcohol, spinosad, and ivermectin. Resistance to lindane and malathion has also been reported. Lindane cannot be used in children under 110 lb. A variety of alternative treatments have been used in communities over the years including covering the scalp in mayonnaise or petrolatum jelly to suffocate the lice. These have not been demonstrated to have any efficacy. Finally, schools will determine their own policies about participation if live lice are present. However, it is unnecessary to refrain from being in school until all nits are eliminated as nits are not evidence of active infection.

I-102. The answer is C. *(Chap. 475)* Brown recluse spiders live mainly in southern and central United States and have similar relative species in Central and South America, Africa, and the Middle East. These spiders are not aggressive toward humans and tend to hide under rocks or in caves. They will invade homes seeking dark and undisturbed hiding spots, such as closets, under furniture, and in storage rooms, attics, or garages. Despite the fact that these spiders are common, bites from the brown recluse are rare and usually minor with local edema and erythema only. However, envenomation can cause more severe tissue injury with necrosis of the skin and subcutaneous tissue and even more rarely systemic hemolysis. There is no effective antivenom specific to these spider bites. Bites tend to occur when an individual is dressing and typically occur on the hands, arms, neck, and lower abdomen. The bite can initially be painless or accompanied by a mild stinging sensation. Over a few hours, the site becomes painful and pruritic with an area of central induration. There is a pale ischemic zone surrounded by erythema. Initial management at this stage includes RICE (rest, ice, compression, and elevation). Analgesics, antihistamines, antibiotics, and tetanus prophylaxis can be considered if there are medical indications. The lesion needs to monitored for development of more severe ischemia. However, most lesions resolve over a few days without treatment. In more severe cases of envenomation, the center of the lesion will develop significant ischemia, leading to development of central necrosis. A black eschar or bulla may form prior to development of a craterous ulcer. Early debridement or surgical excision without closure may delay healing. Healing typically takes less than 6 months, but if the wound extends deeply into the fatty tissue, healing may be quite prolonged.

I-103. The answer is E. *(Chap. 476e)* Acute mountain sickness (AMS) is the benign form of altitude illness, whereas high-altitude cerebral edema (HACE) and high-altitude pulmonary edema (HAPE) are life threatening. Altitude illness is likely to occur above 2500 meters but has been documented even at 1500–2500 meters. The acclimation to altitude includes hyperventilation in response to the reduced inspired PO_2 initially, followed by increased erythropoietin and 2,3-bisphosphoglycerate. AMS is characterized by nonspecific symptoms (headache, nausea, fatigue, and dizziness) with a paucity of physical findings developing 6–12 hours after ascent to a high altitude. AMS must be distinguished from exhaustion, dehydration, hypothermia, alcoholic hangover, and hyponatremia. The most important risk factors for the development of altitude illness are the rate of ascent and a history of high-altitude illness. Exertion is a risk factor, but lack of physical fitness is not. One protective factor in AMS is high-altitude exposure during the preceding 2 months. Children and adults seem to be equally affected, but people >50 years of age may be less likely to develop AMS than younger people. Most studies reveal no gender difference in AMS incidence. Sleep desaturation—a common phenomenon at high altitude—is associated with AMS. Gradual ascent is the best approach to prevent AMS. Acetazolamide or dexamethasone beginning 1 day prior to ascent and continuing for 2–3 days is effective if rapid ascent is necessary. A double-blind placebo-controlled trial demonstrated no benefit on AMS from *Ginkgo biloba*. Mild cases of AMS can be treated with rest, whereas more serious cases are treated with acetazolamide and oxygen. Descent is therapeutic in all serious cases, including HACE or HAPE. Patients who have recovered from mild cases of AMS may reascend carefully after recovery. Patients with HACE should not.

I-104. **The answer is D.** *(Chap. 476e)* High-altitude pulmonary edema (HAPE) is related to an enhanced or atypical pulmonary vascular response to hypoxia. It is not necessarily preceded by acute mountain sickness. HAPE develops within 2–4 days after arrival at high altitude; it rarely occurs after more than 4 or 5 days at the same altitude. A rapid rate of ascent, exercise, a history of prior HAPE, respiratory tract infections, and cold environmental temperatures are risk factors. Men are more susceptible than women. People with abnormalities of the cardiopulmonary circulation leading to pulmonary hypertension (—e.g., patent foramen ovale, mitral stenosis, primary pulmonary hypertension, or unilateral absence of the pulmonary artery) —are at increased risk of HAPE, even at moderate altitudes. Echocardiography is recommended when HAPE develops at relatively low altitudes (<3000 meters) and whenever cardiopulmonary abnormalities predisposing to HAPE are suspected. The initial manifestation of HAPE may be a reduction in exercise tolerance greater than that expected at the given altitude. A dry, persistent cough may presage HAPE and may be followed by the production of blood-tinged sputum. Tachypnea and tachycardia, even at rest, are important markers as illness progresses. Crackles may be heard on auscultation but are not diagnostic. Fever and leukocytosis may occur. Descent and oxygen (to raise SaO_2 >90%) are the mainstays of therapy for HAPE. Nifedipine can be used as adjunctive therapy. Inhaled β-agonists, which are safe and convenient to carry, are useful in the prevention of HAPE and may be effective in its treatment, although no trials have yet been carried out. Inhaled nitric oxide and expiratory positive airway pressure may also be useful therapeutic measures but may not be available in high-altitude settings. No studies have investigated phosphodiesterase-5 inhibitors in the treatment of HAPE, but reports have described their use in clinical practice. Patients with HAPE who have recovered may be able to reascend. In high-altitude cerebral edema, reascent after a few days is not advisable.

I-105. **The answer is E.** *(Chap. 477e)* Untreated pneumothorax has the risk of rapidly expanding and potentially causing tension upon decompression. Patients with extensive bullae should be considered carefully since they may incur a similar risk. The effect of hyperbaric oxygen in patients with chronic carbon dioxide retention is not studied. The other commonly quoted contraindication to hyperbaric oxygen therapy is a history of receiving bleomycin chemotherapy. Bleomycin is associated with a dose-dependent risk of pneumonitis, and this risk may be enhanced with hyperbaric oxygen exposure. There are reports of patients developing pneumonitis with high FiO_2 or hyperbaric therapy even years after receiving bleomycin. Radiation proctitis and carbon monoxide poisoning are clinical conditions where hyperbaric oxygen therapy may be warranted. The indications for hyperbaric oxygen therapy are evolving with some advocating therapy for delayed radiation injury, wound therapy, myonecrosis, thermal injuries, and other conditions where local hypoxia may occur or where impaired oxygen delivery may be present.

I-106. **The answer is D.** *(Chap. 477e)* Because for every 10.1-meter increase in depth of seawater, the ambient pressure (P_{amb}) increases by 1 standard atmosphere (atm), at a depth of 20 meters, a person is exposed to a P_{amb} of approximately 3 atm absolute. Decompression sickness (DCS) is caused by the formation of bubbles from dissolved inert gas (usually nitrogen) during or after ascent (decompression) from a compressed gas dive. Deeper and longer dives increase the amount of dissolved inert gas, and more rapid ascent increases the potential for bubbles to form and affect end organs. Although variable, DCS usually does not occur unless dive depth exceeds 7 meters (1.7 atm absolute). DCS usually develops within 8–12 hours of ascent. The majority of cases present with mild symptoms including musculoskeletal pain, fatigue, and minor neurologic manifestations, such as patchy paresthesias. A feared complication is cerebral arterial gas embolism (CAGE). To lessen the chance of gas bubbles entering the cerebral circulation, patients with DCS should remain in a horizontal posture. Initial first aid should include 100% oxygen to accelerate inert gas washout and resolution of bubbles. For patients with symptoms beyond mild DCS, recompression and hyperbaric oxygen therapy are generally recommended. If evacuated by air, the patient should be transported at low altitude by helicopter. After full recovery, diving can be restarted after at least 1 month.

I-107. **The answer is D.** *(Chap. 478e)* When evaluating a patient with hypothermia, it is important to consider all the possible factors that could contribute to hypothermia because treatment of hypothermia alone without treating the underlying cause could lead to delayed diagnosis and poor outcomes. In some instances, it is clear that the cause of hypothermia is simply prolonged exposure to cold without proper clothing. However, in patients such as this one, the clinician will need to look for findings that would be unexpected in a hypothermic patient. This patient has a moderate degree of hypothermia (between 28.0°C and 32.2°C). At this range of hypothermia, the expected clinical presentation would be one of a global slowing of metabolism. Clinically, this would include a depressed level of consciousness with papillary dilatation. Often these individuals experience a paradoxical instinct to take off their clothes. In addition, the heart rate, blood pressure, and respiratory rate would be expected to decrease. Carbon dioxide production by tissues typically decreases by 50% for each 8°C drop in body temperature. A common error in the treatment of hypothermic individuals is overly aggressive hyperventilation in the face of this known decrease in carbon dioxide production. In this patient, despite the hypothermia, there is an increased respiratory rate in the setting of a metabolic acidosis. This finding would suggest a lesion in the central nervous system or ingestion of an alcohol that would lead to a metabolic acidosis. Ingestion is confirmed by the presence of a very high anion gap (28) as well as an osmolar gap. The osmolar gap can be calculated as: (sodium × 2) + (BUN/2.8) + (glucose/18) + (ethanol/4.6). In this patient, the calculated osmolarity would be 301.6. Thus, the osmolar gap is 26, indicating the presence of some other osmotically active compound. In this case, it is prudent to measure toxic alcohol levels such as methanol and ethylene glycol. In the management of the patient's hypothermia, warmed intravenous fluids may be indicated. However, the lactated Ringer's solution should be avoided as the liver may be unable to metabolize lactate, which could lead to worsening metabolic acidosis. The cardiac complications of hypothermia may lead to bradyarrhythmias, but cardiac pacing is rarely indicated. If required, the transthoracic route is preferred because placement of any leads into the heart may lead to refractory ventricular arrhythmias.

I-108. **The answer is B.** *(Chap. 478e)* This patient presents with frostbite of the left foot. The most common presenting symptom of this disorder is sensory changes that affect pain and temperature. Physical examination can have a multitude of findings, depending on the degree of tissue damage. Mild frostbite will show erythema and anesthesia. With more extensive damage, bullae and vesicles will develop. Hemorrhagic vesicles are due to injury to the microvasculature. The prognosis is most favorable when the presenting area is warm and has a normal color. Treatment is with rapid rewarming, which usually is accomplished with a 37–40°C (98.6–104°F) water bath. The period of rewarming can be intensely painful for the patient, and often narcotic analgesia is warranted. If the pain is intolerable, the temperature of the water bath can be dropped slightly. Compartment syndrome can develop with rewarming and should be investigated if cyanosis persists after rewarming. No medications have been shown to improve outcomes, including heparin, steroids, calcium channel blockers, and hyperbaric oxygen. In the absence of wet gangrene or another emergent surgical indication, decisions about the need for amputation or debridement should be deferred until the boundaries of the tissue injury are well demarcated. After recovery from the initial insult, these patients often have neuronal injury with abnormal sympathetic tone in the extremity. Other remote complications include cutaneous carcinomas, nail deformities, and, in children, epiphyseal damage.

I-109. **The answer is B.** *(Chap. 479e)* Normally, the body dissipates heat into the environment via four mechanisms. The evaporation of skin moisture is the single most efficient mechanism of heat loss but becomes progressively ineffective as the relative humidity rises to >70%. The radiation of infrared electromagnetic energy directly into the surrounding environment occurs continuously. (Conversely, radiation is a major source of heat gain in hot climates.) Conduction—the direct transfer of heat to a cooler object—and convection—the loss of heat to air currents—become ineffective when the environmental temperature exceeds the skin temperature. Factors that interfere with the evaporation of diaphoresis significantly increase the risk of heat illness. Examples include dripping of sweat off the skin, constrictive or occlusive clothing, dehydration, and excessive humidity. The regulation of heat load is complex and involves the central nervous system (CNS), thermosensors, and thermoregulatory effectors. The central thermostat activates the effectors that produce peripheral vasodilation and sweating. The skin surface is in effect the radiator and the principal location of heat loss, since skin blood flow can increase 25–30 times over the basal rate. This dramatic increase in skin blood flow, coupled with the maintenance of peripheral vasodilation, efficiently radiates heat. At the same time, there is a compensatory vasoconstriction of the splanchnic and renal beds. Acclimatization to heat reflects a constellation of physiologic adaptations that permit the body to lose heat more efficiently. This process often requires 1 to several weeks of exposure and work in a hot environment. During acclimatization, the thermoregulatory set point is altered, and this alteration affects the onset, volume, and content of diaphoresis. The threshold for the initiation of sweating is lowered, and the amount of sweat increases, with a lowered salt concentration. Sweating rates can be 1–2 L/hr in acclimated individuals during heat stress. Plasma volume expansion also occurs and improves cutaneous vascular flow.

I-110. The answer is B. *(Chap. 479e)* The clinical manifestations of heat stroke reflect a total loss of thermoregulatory function. Typical vital sign abnormalities include tachypnea, various tachycardias, hypotension, and a widened pulse pressure. Although there is no single specific diagnostic test, the historical and physical triad of exposure to a heat stress, CNS dysfunction, and a core temperature >40.5°C helps establish the preliminary diagnosis. Heat exhaustion is distinguished from heat stroke by the loss of thermoregulatory control, typically manifest by a core temperature >40.5°C. The physiologic precipitants of heat exhaustion, which may progress to heat stroke, are water and sodium depletion. There are two forms of heat stroke with different manifestations (Table 1-110). Classic heat stroke (CHS) usually occurs in older adults during long periods of exposure to elevated ambient temperature and humidity. Patients with CHS commonly have chronic diseases that predispose to heat-related illness, and they may have limited access to oral fluids. Heat dissipation mechanisms are overwhelmed by both endogenous heat production and exogenous heat stress. Patients with CHS are often compliant with prescribed medications that can impair tolerance to a heat stress. In many of these dehydrated CHS patients, sweating has ceased and the skin is hot and dry. Exertional heat stroke typically occurs in younger adults with an identifiable cause. In this case, the clinical history is typical for CHS. The absence of focal neurologic findings, elevated creatine kinase, and precipitating medications makes the other diagnoses less likely.

TABLE I-110 Typical Manifestations of Heat Stroke

Classic	Exertional
Older patient	Younger patient
Predisposing health factors/medications	Healthy condition
Epidemiology (heat waves)	Sporadic cases
Sedentary	Exercising
Anhidrosis (possible)	Diaphoresis (common)
Central nervous system dysfunction	Myocardial/hepatic injury
Oliguria	Acute renal failure
Coagulopathy (mild)	Disseminated intravascular coagulation
Mild lactic acidosis	Marked lactic acidosis
Mild creatine kinase elevation	Rhabdomyolysis
Normoglycemia/calcemia	Hypoglycemia/calcemia
Normokalemia	Hyperkalemia

I-111. The answer is C. *(Chap. 479e)* Before cooling is initiated, patients should be evaluated for the ability to protect their airway, acid-base status, and volume status. Central venous pressure determination and continuous core temperature monitoring should be considered. Hypoglycemia is a frequent finding and should be addressed by glucose infusion. Because peripheral vasoconstriction delays heat dissipation, repeated administration of discrete boluses of isotonic crystalloid for hypotension is preferable to the administration of α-adrenergic agonists. Phenylephrine is relatively contraindicated because it inhibits peripheral vasodilation necessary for heat dissipation. Evaporative cooling is usually the most practical and effective technique. Rapid cooling is essential in both classic heat stroke (CHS) and exertional heat stroke (EHS). Cool water (15°C [60°F]) is sprayed on the exposed skin while fans direct continuous airflow over the moistened skin. Cold packs applied to the axillae and groin are a useful cooling adjunct. To avoid "overshoot hypothermia," active cooling should be terminated at ~38–39°C (100.4–102.2°F). Immersion cooling in cold water is an alternative option in EHS but induces peripheral vasoconstriction and intense shivering. This technique presents significant monitoring and resuscitation challenges in most clinical settings. The safety of immersion cooling is best established for young, previously healthy patients with EHS (but not for those with CHS). Cooling with commercially available cooling blankets should not be the sole technique used, since the rate of cooling is far too slow. Other methods are less efficacious and rarely indicated, such as IV infusion of cold fluids and cold irrigation of the bladder or gastrointestinal tract. Cold thoracic lavage and peritoneal lavage are efficient maneuvers but are invasive and rarely necessary.

SECTION II

Cardinal Manifestations and Presentation of Diseases

QUESTIONS

DIRECTIONS: Choose the one best response to each question.

II-1. When repeated intense stimuli are applied to damaged or inflamed tissue, which of the following responses occurs?

A. The threshold for activating primary afferent nociceptors is lowered, and the frequency of firing is higher for all stimulus intensities.
B. The threshold for activating primary afferent nociceptors is lowered, and the frequency of firing is lowered for all stimulus intensities.
C. The threshold for activating primary afferent nociceptors is raised and the frequency of firing is higher for all stimulus intensities.
D. The threshold for activating primary afferent nociceptors is raised and the frequency of firing is lower for all stimulus intensities.

II-2. Substance P, which is released from primary afferent nociceptors, has all of the following biologic activities EXCEPT:

A. Chemoattractant for leukocytes
B. Degranulation of mast cells
C. Increase intracellular concentration of cyclic guanosine monophosphate (GMP)
D. Increase the production and release of inflammatory mediators
E. Vasodilation

II-3. A 45-year-man with longstanding type 1 diabetes mellitus complains of pain in his feet and ankles that has been present for over a year. All of the following are consistent with neuropathic pain due to diabetes EXCEPT:

A. Burning pain
B. Electric shock quality
C. Exacerbated by light touch
D. Pain referred to scrotum
E. Tingling

II-4. A 28-year-old woman (shown in Figure II-4) has had pain and redness in her left hand for the last 3 months since falling and stopping the fall with that hand. Immediate radiographs showed no fracture. Over the last few days, she has developed forearm burning and edema. Range of motion is limited at her left shoulder and left wrist. In the picture below, she is trying to close her left hand. She also reports allodynia to touch over the back of her left hand. Her rheumatologic and radiographic evaluation has been unrevealing. She has no past medical history, is not sexually active, takes no medications, and does not use tobacco, alcohol, or illicit drugs. Which of the following is the most likely diagnosis?

A. Acute gonococcal arthritis
B. Carpal tunnel syndrome
C. Complex regional pain syndrome
D. Gout
E. Systemic lupus erythematosus

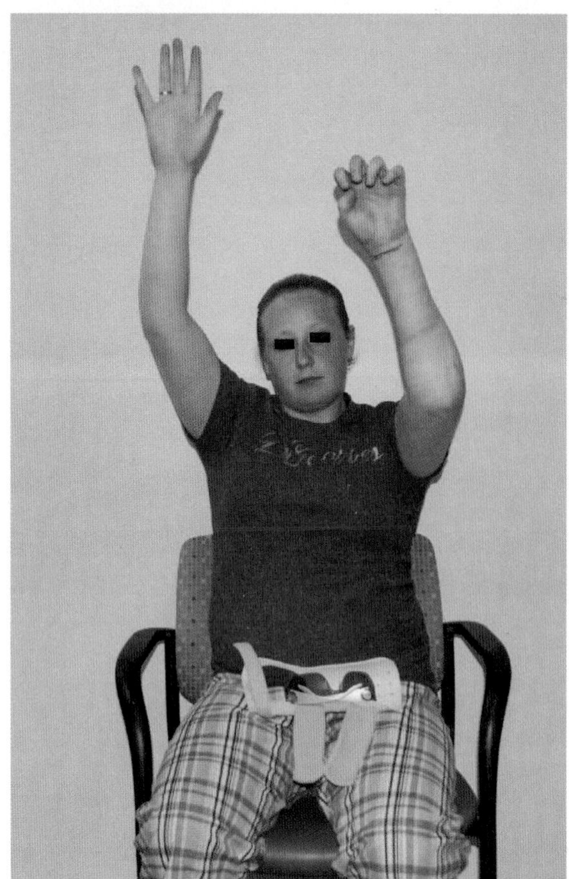

FIGURE II-4 From Imboden JB, Hellman DB, Stone JH: *Current Diagnosis & Treatment: Rheumatology*, 3rd ed. New York, NY: McGraw-Hill, 2013.

II-5. Which of the following statements regarding cyclooxygenase (COX) inhibitors is true?

A. Aspirin is a reversible inhibitor of COX-2.
B. COX-2–selective nonsteroidal anti-inflammatory drugs (NSAIDs) are contraindicated after surgery because they inhibit platelet aggregation.
C. COX-2–selective NSAID inhibitors have a lower risk of nephrotoxicity than nonselective NSAIDs.
D. Gastrointestinal (GI) irritation is the most common side effect of aspirin and NSAIDs.
E. NSAIDs may cause a decrease in blood pressure.

II-6. A 38-year-old woman is brought to the emergency department by her spouse because of decreased mental status. She had knee surgery 2 days ago and was prescribed oral oxycodone for pain. Her spouse notes that she finished the entire 7-day supply during that day. He denies any seizure activity. They have no other drugs or medications in the house. She is afebrile with blood pressure of 130/75 mmHg, heart rate of 70 bpm, respiratory rate of 4 breaths/min, and SaO_2 of 85% on room air. She barely responds to painful stimuli but moves all four extremities equally. Which of the following medications is most likely to improve her mental status?

A. Albuterol
B. Alvimopan
C. Flumazenil
D. *N*-Acetylcysteine
E. Naloxone

II-7. A 63-year-old man with a history of hypertension and hyperlipidemia comes to the emergency department complaining of 1 hour of chest pain that came on at rest. The pain is substernal and radiates to both shoulders. He describes the pain as "diffuse pressure, not sharp" and says he feels nauseated and sweaty. He also feels like the pain improves when he curls up on his left side. His physical examination is notable only for some mild diaphoresis and a heart rate of 105 bpm with blood pressure of 140/88 mmHg. All of the following aspects of his history increase the likelihood of acute coronary syndrome EXCEPT:

A. Associated with feeling sweaty
B. Associated with nausea
C. Improved when lying on left side
D. Pressure, not sharp pain
E. Radiation to both shoulders

II-8. Your mother calls you late at night saying that 63-year-old Uncle Albert went to the emergency department because of chest pain. She knows nothing more about the story or Uncle Albert's past medical history, but she's convinced he's going to die of a heart attack and wants to know what could happen. In addition to telling her to calm down, you tell your mother that:

A. Albert is more likely to have chest wall pain than ischemic cardiac disease.
B. Less than one-third of patients going to the emergency department with nontraumatic chest pain are found to have ischemic cardiac disease.
C. There is less than 25% chance he will be admitted to the hospital.
D. There is over a 60% chance the pain has a gastrointestinal source.
E. This is the most common reason patients go the emergency department.

II-9. A 28-year-old woman presents to the emergency department with 8 hours of worsening abdominal pain. She describes the pain as steady, aching, and located in the lower middle to right abdomen. Any movement worsens the pain. She denies any hematemesis, melena, or bright red blood in stools. She is sexually active with four to six partners over the last 6 months. Her only medication is an oral contraceptive. On physical examination, her temperature is 39.0°C, blood pressure is 110/75 mmHg, heart rate is 105 bpm, and respiratory rate is 18 breaths/min. Her abdominal examination is notable for tenderness below and to the right of the umbilicus with positive rebound. Any movement causes immediate worsening of the pain. Bowel sounds are diminished. Serum pregnancy test is negative. Which of the following is the most likely mechanism of her abdominal pain?

A. Abdominal wall disturbance
B. Distension of hollow viscus
C. Distension of visceral surface
D. Parietal peritoneal inflammation
E. Vascular disturbance

II-10. In the patient described in Question II-9, which of the following is the most likely diagnosis?

A. Acute cholecystitis
B. Pelvic inflammatory disease
C. Rectus sheath hematoma
D. Small bowel obstruction
E. Superior mesenteric artery embolism

II-11. In a patient complaining of headache, which of the following aspects of the history is worrisome and suggests further evaluation?

A. First severe headache
B. Onset after age 55
C. Pain associated with local tenderness
D. Subacute worsening over days or weeks
E. All of the above

II-12. A 42-year-old man seeks attention for acute-onset back pain that occurred while lifting heavy boxes. He reports the pain is localized to the right lower back, radiates to the buttocks and posterior thigh, and is worse with standing and improved with lying down. His medical history is only notable for hyperlipidemia for which he takes atorvastatin. His vital signs are normal, and the only positive examination finding is that raising his right leg straight while supine re-creates the pain exactly at approximately 30 degrees. There are no motor or sensory defects, and reflexes are normal. Which of the following lumbosacral nerve roots is likely involved in this process?

A. L1
B. L2
C. L3
D. L4
E. L5

II-13. For the patient described in Question II-12, all of the following treatments may be indicated EXCEPT:

A. Acetaminophen
B. Bedrest
C. Epidural glucocorticoid injection
D. Naproxen
E. Resumption of normal activities

II-14. A 68-year-old woman complains of worsening back, buttock, and bilateral upper leg pain over the last 6–9 months. She reports the pain is worst when she is standing for more than 10–15 minutes. The pain is also present during prolonged walking. In all cases, she feels better when she sits down. She denies any calf pain or swelling. Her medical history is notable for hypertension controlled with enalapril. Her only other medication is daily vitamin D. Her physical examination is unremarkable, with normal vital signs, no lower extremity swelling, and no vascular bruits. Which of the following is her most likely diagnosis?

A. Aortic dissection
B. Lumbar disk disease
C. Lumbar spinal stenosis
D. Takayasu arteritis
E. Vascular claudication

II-15. In the patient described in Question II-14, treatment may include all of the following EXCEPT:

A. Acetaminophen
B. Epidural corticosteroid injection
C. Exercise
D. NSAIDs
E. Surgery

II-16. A 38-year-old man seeks attention for new-onset lower back pain. It started after he played basketball with his teenage nephews and has not resolved in the past 5 days. His mobility is limited, and the pain improves with lying down. The pain is localized to the left lumbar region and does not radiate. He takes no medications. His physical examination is normal except for pain in the involved area. There are no sensory, motor, or reflex deficits, and his straight- and crossed-leg raise tests do not reproduce the pain. Which of the following is indicated at this time?

A. Acetaminophen
B. Computed tomography (CT) myelogram
C. Magnetic resonance imaging (MRI) of the spine
D. Plain films of the back
E. Protein electrophoresis

II-17. In the patient described in Question II-16, which of the following is considered evidence-based therapy at this time?

A. Cyclobenzaprine
B. Gabapentin
C. Ibuprofen
D. Prednisone
E. Tramadol

II-18. Hyperthermia is defined as:

A. A core temperature >40°C
B. A core temperature >41.5°C
C. An elevated temperature that normalizes with antipyretic therapy
D. An uncontrolled increase in body temperature despite a normal hypothalamic temperature setting
E. Temperature >40°C, rigidity, and autonomic dysregulation

II-19. Ms. Smith is a previously healthy 25-year-old woman. Two weeks prior, she had bacterial pharyngitis with 3 days of fever. She has symptomatically completely recovered now. She is working on her engineering degree and enjoys collecting and analyzing data. Thus, she has taken her temperature orally every hour for the past 2 weeks and brings in her temperature log to you. Which of the following statements regarding her expected body temperature pattern is true?

A. During the febrile illness, the normal diurnal variation in body temperature is absent.
B. Lowest body temperatures will occur at approximately noon.
C. Normal daily temperature variations are currently a bit higher than individuals in the normal population.
D. Oral temperature accurately reflects body core temperature.
E. Ovulation will not affect her body temperature.

II-20. A 32-year-old man with Crohn disease has been treated with infliximab for the past 6 months. He comes to your office in January and did not receive his influenza vaccine this year. Unfortunately, for the prior week, he has complained of a persistent cough and fever to 38.4°C. Which of the following statements regarding evaluation and treatment of his fever is true?

A. Even if the patient had a negative tuberculin skin test (TST) prior to initiating infliximab, active tuberculosis should be considered as a cause of his fever and cough.
B. Given the season, it would be reasonable to closely observe and symptomatically treat the patient's fever; it is most likely a viral upper respiratory infection.
C. It is very unusual for patients on anti–tumor necrosis factor (TNF) therapy to have a fever with infection.
D. Measurement of interleukin (IL)-1 would be useful in determining whether the fever is infectious in etiology.
E. One should avoid using antipyretics for the patient; there are convincing data that fever acts as an adjuvant to the immune system and antipyretics delay the resolution of viral and bacterial infections.

II-21. All of the following drugs exert an antipyretic effect through inhibition of cyclooxygenase EXCEPT:

A. Acetaminophen
B. Aspirin
C. Celecoxib
D. Ibuprofen
E. Prednisone

II-22. Which of the following patients is matched to an INCORRECT recommendation regarding treatment of fever?

A. A 6-year-old with pharyngitis and fever of 39.2°C—Treatment with aspirin
B. A 9-year-old with a prior history of febrile seizures, currently with rhinovirus and temperature of 39.2°C—Treatment with ibuprofen or acetaminophen.
C. A 46-year-old man with a temperature of 41°C and sepsis—Treatment with oral ibuprofen and cooling blankets
D. A 50-year-old man with an interventricular central nervous system (CNS) hemorrhage and fever to 41.2°C—Aggressive treatment to reduce core temperature including oral antipyretics, cooling blankets, and chilled saline infusion
E. A 66-year-old with severe chronic obstructive pulmonary disease (COPD) and fever to 39.2°C due to lower extremity cellulitis—Treatment with ibuprofen or acetaminophen

II-23. A recent 18-year-old immigrant from Kenya presents to a university clinic with fever, nasal congestion, severe fatigue, and a rash. The rash started with discrete lesions at the hairline that coalesced as the rash spread caudally. There is sparing of the palms and soles. Small white spots with a surrounding red halo are noted on examination of the palate. The patient is at risk for developing which of the following in the future?

A. Encephalitis
B. Epiglottitis
C. Opportunistic infections
D. Postherpetic neuralgia
E. Splenic rupture

II-24. A 23-year-old woman with a chronic lower extremity ulcer related to prior trauma presents with rash, hypotension, and fever. She has had no recent travel or outdoor exposure and is up to date on all of her vaccinations. She does not use intravenous (IV) drugs. On examination, the ulcer looks clean with a well-granulated base and no erythema, warmth, or pustular discharge. However, the patient does have diffuse erythema that is most prominent on her palms, conjunctiva, and oral mucosa. Other than profound hypotension and tachycardia, the remainder of the examination is nonfocal. Laboratory results are notable for a creatinine of 2.8 mg/dL, aspartate aminotransferase of 250 U/L, alanine aminotransferase of 328 U/L, total bilirubin of 3.2 mg/dL, direct bilirubin of 0.5 mg/dL, international normalized ratio (INR) of 1.5, activated partial thromboplastin time of 1.6× control, and platelet level of 94,000/μL. Ferritin is 1300 μg/mL. The patient is started on broad-spectrum antibiotics after appropriate blood cultures are drawn and is resuscitated with IV fluid and vasopressors. Her blood cultures are negative at 72 hours; at this point, her fingertips start to desquamate. What is the most likely diagnosis?

A. Juvenile rheumatoid arthritis (JRA)
B. Leptospirosis
C. Staphylococcal toxic shock syndrome
D. Streptococcal toxic shock syndrome
E. Typhoid fever

II-25. An 18-year-old man recently started his freshman year at a local university. He presents with a week of overwhelming malaise, fever, and sore throat. He says he finds it hard just to get out of bed in the morning. He was seen by your junior colleague 2 days ago who noted pharyngitis, and the patient was given a dose of intramuscular ampicillin for empiric treatment of streptococcal pharyngitis. The patient returns today with a lacy exanthematous rash and continued fever and malaise. You note striking cervical lymphadenopathy. He denies any recent travel outside of the United States. Which of the following is the likely etiology of his rash?

A. Chikungunya fever
B. Exanthematous drug eruption
C. Fifth disease
D. Rubella
E. Rubeola

II-26. A 47-year-old man from North Carolina with no known past medical history presents in August with a 2-day history of abdominal pain, diffuse myalgias, and debilitating headache. He has not traveled out of the state recently but does report that he spent a day 2 weeks ago clearing a nearby field in preparation for planting a garden and that 1 week ago he ate raw oysters. On examination, you note that the patient has blanchable macules on his wrists and ankles. You promptly admit him to the hospital for treatment, noting that his disease carries a mortality rate of approximately 40% if not treated appropriately. Which pathogen is likely responsible for this patient's disease?

A. *Borrelia burgdorferi*
B. *Rickettsia rickettsii*
C. *Spirillum minis*
D. *Salmonella typhi*
E. *Vibrio vulnificus*

II-27. A 42-year-old surveyor from Connecticut presents with a 2 day history of the rash seen in Figure II-27. Which of the following signs or symptoms is also likely to develop in this patient?

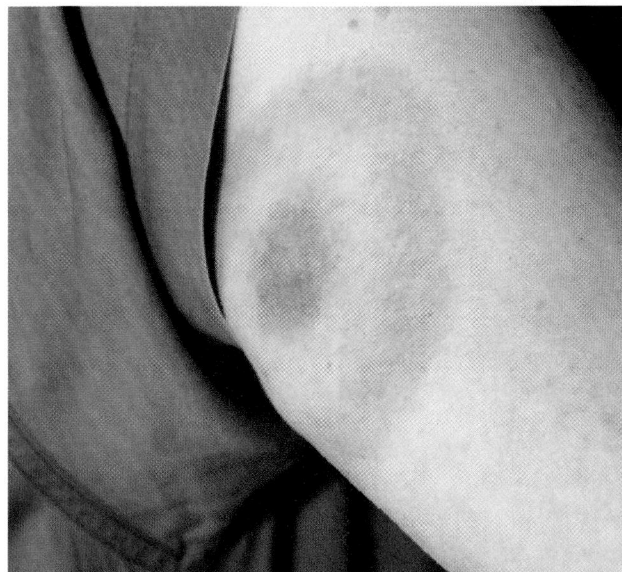

FIGURE II-27 Reprinted from KJ Knoop et al: *The Atlas of Emergency Medicine*, 4th ed. New York, McGraw-Hill, 2016. Photo contributor: James Gathany, Public Health Image Library, US Centers for Disease Control and Prevention.

A. A holosystolic murmur loudest at the cardiac apex and radiating to the axilla
B. A fissured lip, strawberry tongue, and coronary aneurysms
C. Bradycardia with an electrocardiogram finding of complete atrioventricular dissociation
D. Diffuse exanthematous rash with eventual desquamation of the hands and feet
E. White macular spots with an erythematous halo on the oral buccal mucosa

II-28. A 42-year-old man with a history of epilepsy presents to the emergency department after having a seizure. He is on maintenance levetiracetam for seizure prophylaxis at home and has been taking his medications as prescribed. In the emergency department, he has another generalized tonic-clonic seizure and is postictal after the event. He is given a dose of phenobarbital and admitted to the hospital. Over the ensuing 24 hours, skin eruption, depicted in Figure II-28, developed, which demonstrates early desquamation. He also developed hypotension requiring escalating vasopressor support, facial edema, generalized lymphadenopathy, abnormal liver function tests, and hepatomegaly. Differential on his complete blood count is below:

Neutrophils	72%
Lymphocytes	10%
Eosinophils	17%
Monocytes	1%
Basophils	None detected

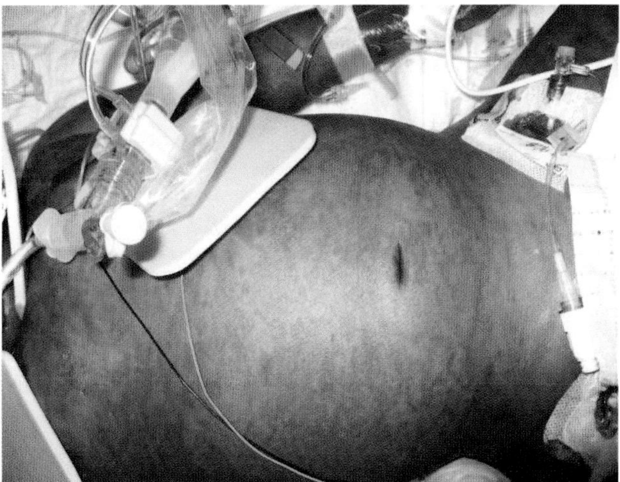

FIGURE II-28 Courtesy of Peter Lio, MD; with permission.

Which of the following is the most likely diagnosis?

A. Drug reaction with eosinophilia and systemic symptoms (DRESS)
B. Eosinophilic non-Hodgkin lymphoma with Sweet syndrome
C. Erythema multiforme
D. Staphylococcal toxic shock syndrome
E. Stevens-Johnson syndrome

II-29. A 27-year-old man presents for evaluation of the skin lesions pictured in Figure II-29. On examination, he has deep-seated, painful nodules and plaques in the areas seen in the figure. All of the following diseases are classically associated with this skin finding EXCEPT:

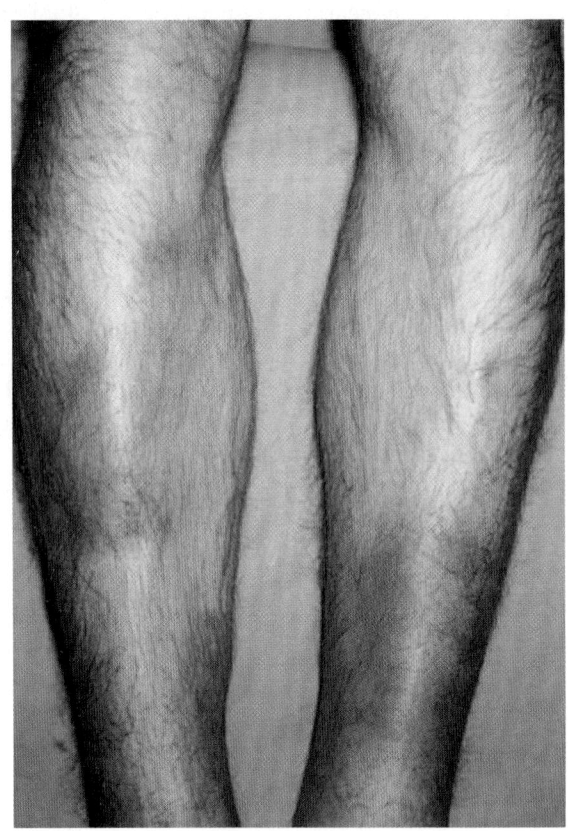

FIGURE II-29 Courtesy of Robert Swerlick, MD; with permission.

A. Drug exposure
B. Inflammatory bowel disease
C. Lung adenocarcinoma
D. Mycobacterial infection
E. Sarcoidosis

II-30. You review your upcoming daily clinic patients and note that you have quite a group this morning. Which of the following patients scheduled to see you today warrants the diagnosis of fever of unknown origin (FUO)?

A. A 29-year-old woman with nearly daily fever of 38.3°C for 3 weeks. She last saw you a week prior and complained of a facial rash, bilateral metacarpophalangeal arthralgias, and fatigue. Laboratory workup revealed proteinuria, anemia, and a positive test for antinuclear antibodies (ANA) at a titer of >1:640.
B. A 64-year-old man whom you saw 3 weeks ago. At that time, he had 1 week of twice-daily fever to 39.2°C, rigors, and a sore throat. He has since recovered and is asymptomatic now, but no cause was found despite extensive testing.
C. A 33-year-old man with subjective feeling of having a fever several times per week for 1 month. He also has rigors and an evanescent rash that has appeared on his legs, torso, and back.
D. A 45-year-old man with 4 weeks of nearly daily fevers to 38.5°C and crippling shin pain. You last saw him 1 week prior, and a comprehensive workup including erythrocyte sedimentation rate (ESR) and C-reactive protein (CRP) levels, complete blood count, electrolytes, lactate dehydrogenase, ferritin, ANA, rheumatoid factor, urinalysis, blood and urine cultures, chest x-ray, abdominal ultrasonography, and tuberculin skin test have all been unrevealing.
E. A 26-year-old woman on mycophenolate mofetil, tacrolimus, and prednisone after having undergone living unrelated donor kidney transplant 1 year prior. She has had fevers to >38.3°C for just over 3 weeks. Evaluation 2 weeks ago included unrevealing ESR and CRP levels, complete blood count, electrolytes, lactate dehydrogenase, ferritin, ANA, rheumatoid factor, urinalysis, blood and urine cultures, chest x-ray, abdominal ultrasonography, and tuberculin skin test.

II-31. Which of the following statements regarding the epidemiology and prognosis of FUO is true?

A. For patients with FUO, an etiologic diagnosis is more likely in elderly patients than in young patients.
B. FUO is usually caused by a very rare disease that escaped diagnosis during the initial obligatory workup.
C. In both Western countries and countries outside the West, infection accounts for over half of FUO cases.
D. In patients with an FUO, the ultimate inability to find an etiologic diagnosis portends a very poor prognosis.
E. In the West, the percentage of patients with FUO who remain undiagnosed has remained constant for decades despite advances in serologic and radiographic diagnostic techniques.

II.32 A 50-year-old man is evaluated for fevers and weight loss of uncertain etiology. He first developed symptoms 3 months ago. He reports daily fevers to as high as 39.4°C (103°F) with night sweats and fatigue. Over this same period, his appetite has decreased, and he has lost 50 lb when compared to his weight at his last annual examination. Fevers have been documented in his primary care physician's office to as high as 38.7°C (101.7°F). He has no exposures or ill contacts. His medical history is significant for diabetes mellitus, obesity, and obstructive sleep apnea. He is taking insulin glargine 50 U daily. He works in a warehouse driving a forklift. He has not traveled outside of his home area in a rural part of Virginia. He has never received a blood transfusion and is married with one female sexual partner for the past 25 years. On examination, no focal findings are identified. Multiple laboratory studies have been performed that have shown nonspecific findings only with exception of an elevated calcium at 11.2 g/dL. A complete blood count showed a white blood cell count of 15,700/μL with 80% polymorphonuclear cells, 15% lymphocytes, 3% eosinophils, and 2% monocytes. The peripheral smear is normal. The hematocrit is 34.7%. His ESR is elevated at 57 mm/hr. A rheumatologic panel is normal, and the ferritin is 521 ng/mL. Liver and kidney function are normal. The serum protein electrophoresis demonstrated polyclonal gammopathy. Human immunodeficiency virus (HIV), Epstein-Barr virus (EBV), and cytomegalovirus (CMV) testing are negative. Urine *Histoplasma* antigen is negative. Routine blood cultures for bacteria, chest radiograph, and purified protein derivative (PPD) testing are negative. A CT scan of the chest, abdomen, and pelvis shows borderline enlargement of lymph nodes in the abdomen and retroperitoneum to 1.2 cm. What would be the next best step in determining the etiology of fever in this patient?

A. Empiric treatment with corticosteroids
B. Empiric treatment for *Mycobacterium tuberculosis*
C. Needle biopsy of enlarged lymph nodes
D. Positron emission tomography (PET)-CT imaging
E. Serum angiotensin-converting enzyme levels

II-33. A 64-year-old woman complains of dizziness. Symptoms started suddenly approximately 12 hours ago and have persisted despite a good night's sleep. The dizziness is described as vertiginous, constant, and mild. There is no associated hearing loss, tinnitus, ear fullness, or rash. She has history of hypertension, diabetes mellitus, and dyslipidemia and smokes tobacco. No corrective saccade is noted bilaterally on the head impulse test. The Dix-Hallpike maneuver exacerbates her dizziness. No nystagmus is seen. What is the next most appropriate diagnostic or therapeutic step in her care?

A. Brain MRI
B. Caloric testing
C. Perform the Epley maneuver
D. Start meclizine
E. Start prednisone

II-34. A 42-year-old man presents to the emergency department complaining of severe vertiginous dizziness associated with nausea. Which of the following is most consistent with a peripheral cause of vertigo?

A. Downbeat nystagmus
B. Gaze-evoked nystagmus
C. Pure torsional nystagmus
D. Rebound nystagmus
E. Unidirectional horizontal nystagmus

II-35. A 62-year-old man presents to clinic complaining of frequent falls. He complains of feeling off balance. He denies vertigo or orthostatic symptoms, but complains that he feels unsteady, which is exacerbated in the dark or when his eyes are closed. He complains of increased difficulty focusing while moving because the world "jumps around," and is no longer able to read a book during his routine subway commute to work. He has no history of peripheral neuropathy or nutritional deficiency. He recently completed 6 weeks of antibiotic therapy for *Enterococcus faecalis* bacteremia with endocarditis. On examination, corrective saccades are noted bilaterally on the head impulse test. Which medication is most likely to have caused this patient's gait instability?

A. Ampicillin
B. Ceftriaxone
C. Gentamicin
D. Penicillin
E. Vancomycin

II-36. A 29-year-old woman presents for second opinion evaluation of chronic fatigue syndrome. She was well until 2 years ago when she developed insidious and recalcitrant weariness. She sleeps 10 hours a night but awakes feeling unrefreshed. She is unable to tolerate exercise, which only worsens her malaise, and she is no longer able to work. She has no significant past medical or psychiatric history. In addition to a detailed history and physical, which of the following is recommended as a reasonable approach to screening patients who complain of chronic fatigue?

A. Antinuclear antibody testing
B. Electromyography with nerve conduction studies
C. Epstein-Barr virus testing
D. Lyme serologies
E. Thyroid function testing

II-37. A 42-year-old man presents complaining of progressive weakness over a period of several months. He reports tripping over his toes while walking and has dropped a cup of hot coffee on one occasion because he felt too weak to continue to hold it. A disorder affecting lower motor neurons is suspected. All of the following findings would be found in an individual with a disease primarily affecting lower motor neurons EXCEPT:

A. Decreased muscle tone
B. Distal greater than proximal weakness
C. Fasciculations
D. Hyperactive tendon reflexes
E. Severe muscle atrophy

II-38 through II-40. Match the clinical presentation to the mostly likely origin of the weakness.

II-38. A 64-year-old man with marked hypothenar wasting and visible fasciculations.

II-39. A 55-year-old woman with atrial fibrillation, right leg weakness, hyperactive plantar reflex, and positive Babinski sign.

II-40. A 40-year-old woman who has difficulty arising from a chair and brushing her teeth. Patellar and biceps reflexes are normal. There is slight atrophy of her deltoids bilaterally.

A. Lower motor neuron
B. Myopathy
C. Psychogenic weakness
D. Upper motor neuron

II-41. All of the following sensations are mediated by unmyelinated and small myelinated afferent peripheral nerve fibers EXCEPT:

A. Cold temperature
B. Light touch
C. Pain
D. Vibration
E. Warm temperature

II-42. A 46-year-old tennis player presents with left neck pain. He has focal paresthesias and diminished sensation on the anterior and posterior lateral upper arm below the deltoid and above the elbow. Which of the following nerve roots is most likely involved in the injury?

A. C3
B. C4
C. C5
D. T1
E. T2

II-43. A 58-year-old sedentary man presents with acute lower back pain and diminished sensation on the anterior and posterior lateral right leg below the knee but extending to the dorsum of the foot. Which of the following nerve roots is most likely involved in the injury?

A. L2
B. L3
C. L4
D. L5
E. S1

II-44. A 78-year-old man is seen in clinic because of recent falls. He reports gait difficulties with a sensation of being off balance at times. One recent fall caused a shoulder injury requiring surgery to repair a torn rotation cuff. In epidemiologic cases series, what is the most common cause of gait disorders?

A. Cerebellar degeneration
B. Cerebrovascular disease with multiple infarcts
C. Cervical myelopathy
D. Parkinson disease
E. Sensory deficits

II-45. A 65-year-old man presents complaining of frequent falls and gait abnormalities. He first noticed the difficulty about 6 months ago. He has a history of hypertension, hypothyroidism, and hyperlipidemia. His current medications include amlodipine 10 mg daily, simvastatin 20 mg daily, and levothyroxine 75 μg daily. On neurologic examination, you observe his gait to be wide based with short shuffling steps. He has difficulty rising from his chair and initiating his gait. Upon turning, he takes multiple steps and appears unsteady. However, cerebellar testing is normal including heel to shin and Romberg testing. He has no evidence of sensory deficits in the lower extremities, and strength is 5/5 throughout all tested muscle groups. He shows no evidence of muscle spasticity on passive movement. His neurologic examination is consistent with which of the following causes?

A. Alcoholic cerebellar degeneration
B. Communicating hydrocephalus
C. Neurosyphilis
D. Multiple system atrophy
E. Lumbar myelopathy

II-46. A 67-year-old woman is admitted for management of sepsis of urinary source. You are called to evaluate a change in mental status. Her husband reports that she now appears withdrawn and apathetic, in contrast to her normally vivacious baseline. Her bedside nurse reports that her alertness has fluctuated throughout the day. On exam, she appears drowsy, although she easily arouses to verbal stimuli. According to the Confusion Assessment Method (CAM), which additional feature is necessary to diagnosis delirium?

A. Altered sleep-wake cycle
B. Disorientation
C. Inattention
D. Perceptual disturbances
E. Psychomotor agitation

II-47. A 76-year-old previously healthy man presents to the emergency department for evaluation of an acute change in mental status. He appears agitated and is pacing the room. He has difficulty focusing his attention and provides an incoherent history. His temperature is 98.4°F, blood pressure is 134/72 mmHg, pulse is 94 bpm, and room-air oxygen saturation is 99%. Laboratory investigations are unremarkable. His wife reports that he has been taking over-the-counter diphenhydramine for an itchy contact dermatitis for the past 2 days. Interference with which neurotransmitter most likely precipitated this change in mental status?

A. Acetylcholine
B. Dopamine
C. Histamine
D. Norepinephrine
E. Serotonin

II-48. An 82-year-old woman is admitted to the intensive care unit with severe sepsis due to pneumonia complicated by renal and respiratory failure. She is supportively treated with fluid resuscitation, vasopressors, broad-spectrum antibiotics, invasive mechanical ventilation, and chemical sedation. Although initially alert, calm, and cooperative, on morning rounds, the nurse reports the patient is now oriented only to person, appears withdrawn, has difficulty following a conversation, and is lethargic. Which of the following medications is most likely to have contributed to her acute cognitive dysfunction?

A. Cefepime
B. Dexmedetomidine
C. Lactated Ringer's solution
D. Midazolam
E. Norepinephrine

II-49. Which of the following tests is most appropriate in the initial evaluation of delirium?

A. Brain MRI with and without gadolinium
B. Electrolyte panel including calcium, magnesium, and phosphorus
C. Rapid plasmin reagin (RPR)
D. Serum ammonia
E. Serum vitamin B_{12}

II-50. Which of the following statements regarding Alzheimer disease is true?

A. Delusions are uncommon.
B. It accounts for over half of the cases of significant memory loss in patients over 70 years of age.
C. It typically presents with rapid (<6 months) significant memory loss.
D. Less than 5% of patients present with nonmemory complaints.
E. Pathologically, the most notable abnormalities are in the cerebellar regions.

II-51. All of the following medications have been shown to have potential efficacy in the treatment of Alzheimer disease EXCEPT:

A. Donepezil
B. Galantamine
C. Memantine
D. Oxybutynin
E. Rivastigmine

II-52. A 72-year-old right-handed male with a history of atrial fibrillation and chronic alcoholism is evaluated for dementia. His son gives a history of a stepwise decline in the patient's function over the last 5 years with the accumulation of mild focal neurologic deficits. On examination, he is found to have a pseudobulbar affect, mildly increased muscle tone, and brisk deep tendon reflexes in the right upper extremity and an extensor plantar response on the left. The history and examination are most consistent with which of the following?

A. Alzheimer disease
B. Binswanger disease
C. Creutzfeldt-Jakob disease
D. Multi-infarct dementia
E. Vitamin B_{12} deficiency

II-53. You are evaluating a previously healthy 73-year-old man with 3–4 months of cognitive decline as reported by his loving wife and daughter. They report that the patient was fully engaged in gardening and competitive board games; however, over the last 6 months, his garden has gone untended, and he expresses absolutely no interest in board games. He also has inappropriate outbursts of rage in social situations, such as in the mall. Over the last 2 months, he's gained about 15 pounds and always seems to be eating or snacking. His only medication is a atorvastatin, which he's been taking for 20 years. Based on this history, you are most concerned about which of the following diagnoses?

A. Alzheimer disease
B. Creutzfeldt-Jakob disease
C. Dementia with Lewy bodies
D. Frontotemporal dementia
E. Vascular dementia

II-54. Which of the following is the most common finding in aphasic patients?

A. Alexia
B. Anomia
C. Comprehension
D. Fluency
E. Repetition

II-55. A 65-year-old man experiences an ischemic cerebrovascular accident affecting the territory of the right anterior cerebral artery. Following the stroke, an assessment reveals the findings shown in Figure II-55.

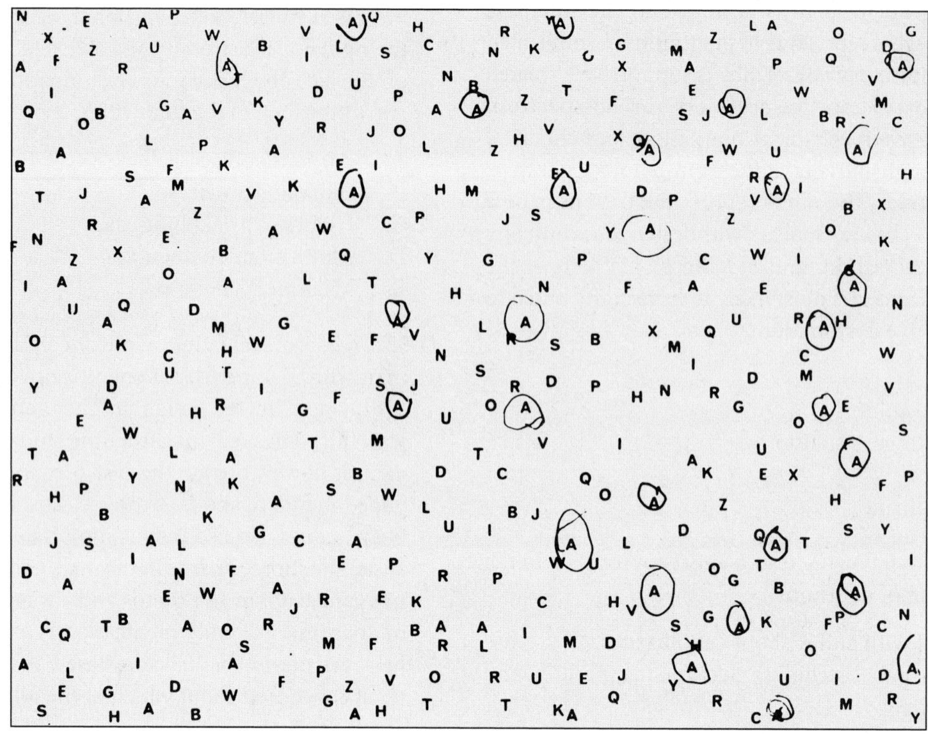

FIGURE II-55

What diagnosis does this figure suggest?

A. Construction apraxia
B. Hemianopia
C. Hemineglect
D. Object agnosia
E. Simultanagnosia

II-56. A 42-year-old man is evaluated for excessive sleepiness that is interfering with his ability to work. He works at a glass factory that requires him to work rotating shifts. He typically cycles across day (7 AM–3 PM), evening (3 PM–11 PM), and night (11 PM–7 AM) shifts over the course of 4 weeks. He notes the problem to be most severe when he is on the night shift. Twice he has fallen asleep on the job. While no accidents have occurred, he has been threatened with loss of his job if he falls asleep again. His preferred sleep schedule is 10 PM until 6 AM, but even when he is working day shifts, he typically only sleeps from about 10:30 PM until 5:30 AM. However, he feels fully functional at work on day and evening shifts. Following his night shifts, he states that he finds it difficult to sleep when he first gets home, frequently not falling asleep until 10 AM or later. He is up by about 3 PM when his children arrive home from school. He drinks about 2 cups of coffee daily, but tries to avoid drinking more than this. He does not snore and has a body mass index of 21.3 kg/m^2. All of the following are reasonable approaches to treatment in this gentleman EXCEPT:

A. Avoidance of bright light in the morning following his shifts
B. Exercise in the early evening before going to work
C. Melatonin 3 mg taken at bedtime on the morning following a night shift.
D. Modafinil 200 mg taken 30–60 minutes prior to starting a shift
E. Strategic napping of no more than 20 minutes during breaks at work

II-57. A 45-year-old woman presents for evaluation of abnormal sensations in her legs that keep her from sleeping at night. She first notices the symptoms around 8 PM when she is sitting quietly watching television. She describes the symptoms as "ants crawling in her veins." While the symptoms are not painful, they are very uncomfortable and worsen when she lies down at night. They interfere with her ability to fall asleep about four times weekly. If she gets out of bed to walk or rubs her legs, the symptoms disappear almost immediately only to recur as soon as she is still. She also sometimes takes a very hot bath to alleviate the symptoms. During sleep, her husband complains that she kicks him throughout the night. She has no history of neurologic or renal disease. She currently is perimenopausal and has been experiencing very heavy and prolonged menstrual cycles over the past several months. The physical examination, including thorough neurologic examination, is normal. Her hemoglobin is 9.8 g/dL and hematocrit is 30.1%. The mean corpuscular volume is 68 fL. Serum ferritin is 12 ng/mL. Which of the following is the most appropriate initial therapy for this patient?

A. Carbidopa/levodopa
B. Hormone replacement therapy
C. Iron supplementation
D. Oxycodone
E. Pramipexole

II-58. A 20-year-old man presents for evaluation of excessive daytime somnolence. He is finding it increasingly difficult to stay awake during his classes. Recently, his grades have fallen because whenever he tries to read he finds himself drifting off. He finds that his alertness is best after exercising or brief naps of 10–30 minutes. Because of this, he states that he takes 5 or 10 "catnaps" daily. The sleepiness persists despite averaging 9 hours of sleep nightly. In addition to excessive somnolence, he reports occasional hallucinations that occur as he is falling asleep. He describes these occurrences as a voice calling his name as he drifts off. Perhaps once weekly, he awakens from sleep but is unable to move for a period of about 30 seconds. He has never had apparent loss of consciousness but states that whenever he is laughing, he feels heaviness in his neck and arms. Once he had to lean against a wall to keep from falling down. He undergoes an overnight sleep study and multiple sleep latency test. There is no sleep apnea. His mean sleep latency on five naps is 2.3 minutes. In three of the five naps, rapid eye movement sleep is present. Which of the following findings in this patient is most specific for the diagnosis of narcolepsy?

A. Cataplexy
B. Excessive daytime somnolence
C. Hypnagogic hallucinations
D. Rapid eye movement sleep in more than two naps on a multiple sleep latency test
E. Sleep paralysis

II-59. Which of the following is the most common sleep disorder in the population?

A. Delayed sleep phase syndrome
B. Insomnia
C. Obstructive sleep apnea
D. Narcolepsy
E. Restless legs syndrome

II-60. From which stage of sleep are the parasomnias somnambulism and night terrors most likely to occur?

A. Stage 1
B. Stage 2
C. Slow-wave sleep
D. Rapid eye movement (REM) sleep

II-61. All of the following statements regarding the organization of a normal night's sleep in a healthy young adult are true EXCEPT:

A. REM sleep comprises 20%–25% of total sleep.
B. Sleep deprivation increases the amount of slow-wave sleep.
C. Sleep organization varies substantially from night to night.
D. Slow-wave (N3) non-REM (NREM) sleep progressively declines with age.
E. Slow-wave (N3) NREM sleep predominates in young adults.

II-62. A 44-year-old man is seen in the emergency department after a motor vehicle accident. The patient says, "I never saw that car coming from the right side." On physical examination, his pupils are equal and reactive to light. His visual acuity is normal; however, there are visual field defect in both eyes laterally (bitemporal hemianopia). Which of the following is most likely to be found on further evaluation?

A. Occipital lobe glioma
B. Optic nerve injury
C. Parietal lobe infarction
D. Pituitary adenoma
E. Retinal detachment

II-63. A 13-year-old girl with no past medical history has recently noticed that she is having trouble reading the board, particularly in her biology class where she sits near the back of the room. In her English literature class, where she sits in the front, she does not have nearly as much difficulty. After performing the standard tests for visual acuity, you determine that the young girl has a refractive error whereby her globe is too long, and light rays come to a focal point in front of the retina. Which term accurately describes this patient's ophthalmologic condition and is associated with the appropriate type of corrective lens?

A. Emmetropia – Diverging lens
B. Hyperopia – Diverging lens
C. Hyperopia – Converging lens
D. Myopia – Diverging lens
E. Presbyopia – Reading glasses

II-64. A 74-year-old man with a history of well-treated hypertension presents with painless blurry vision on one side. You perform the "swinging flashlight" test, shown in Figure II-64. Panel A shows the patient sitting in a dim room; panel B shows him with the flashlight shining in his right eye; and panel C shows the flashlight shining in his left eye. Which defect is present and is appropriately matched to a likely cause?

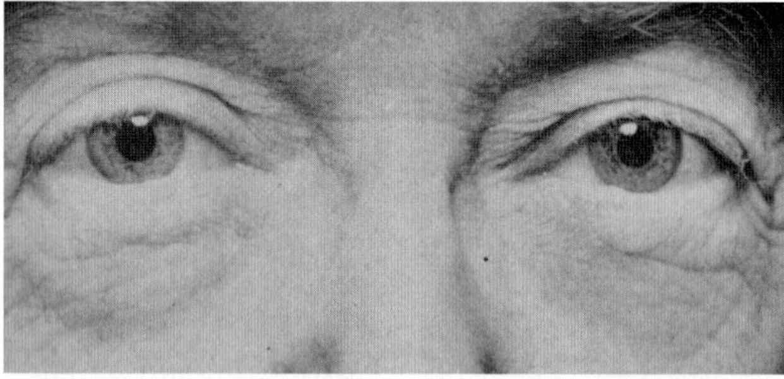

A

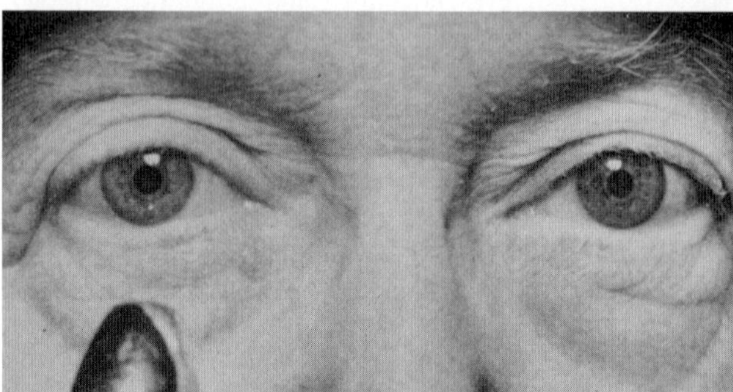

B

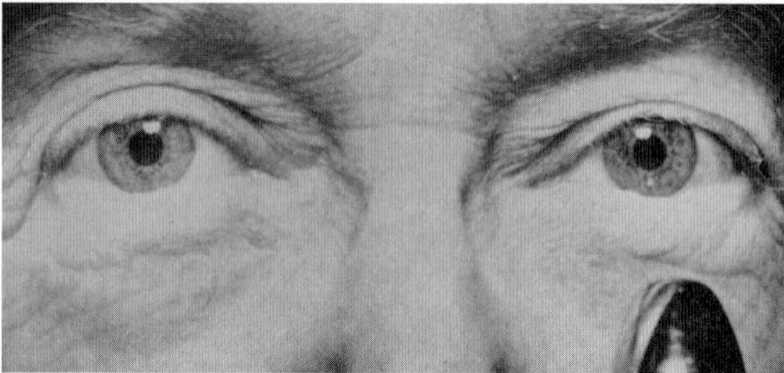

C

FIGURE II-64 From P Levatin: *Arch Ophthalmol* 62:768, 1959.

A. Homonymous hemianopsia – Optic chiasm lesion
B. Left Adie tonic pupil – Oculomotor nerve palsy
C. Left eye sympathetic paresis (Horner syndrome) – Left lung apical tumor
D. Left relative afferent pupillary defect – Left optic neuritis
E. Right afferent pupillary defect – Occipital stroke

II-65. You are seeing Mrs. Ruth today in clinic. For the preceding 6 weeks, she has noticed no symptoms other than occasionally running into doors and walls. You perform a complete physical examination and note abnormalities in her visual fields. Figure II-65A is a map of your visual field findings, with black representing areas where she cannot see in each eye, and white/gray representing areas she can see. You promptly refer Mrs. Ruth for brain MRI. Where do you anticipate finding a lesion?

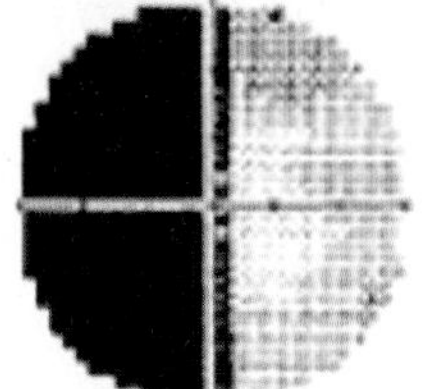

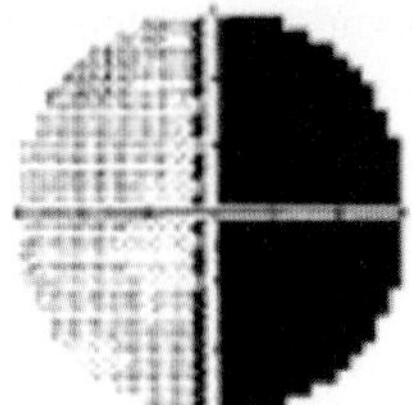

FIGURE II-65A

A. Left optic nerve
B. Left parietal lobe
C. Optic chiasm
D. Right occipital lobe
E. Right retina

II-66. Mrs. Tipover is a 72-year-old woman who enjoys kayaking on the nearby lake. She notes that over the preceding 2 months she has been progressively less able to kayak due to soreness in both shoulders and upper back. She feels tired all the time, and over the last few days reports near-persistent headache. She finally presents to your office today when she suddenly lost vision in her left eye. Ophthalmoscopy of her left eye is shown in Figure II-66. What is the next most reasonable step in the diagnosis and therapy of Mrs. Tipover's condition?

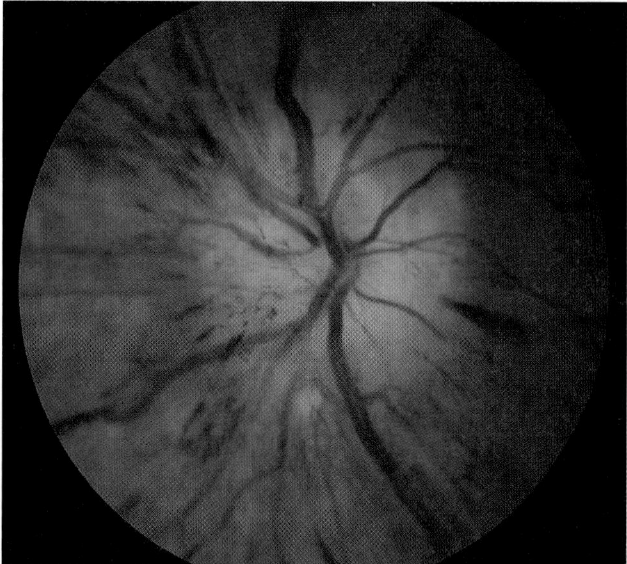

FIGURE II-66

A. Brain MRI to evaluate for demyelinating disease or tumor
B. Initiate high-dose glucocorticoid therapy and refer for temporal artery biopsy
C. Ocular massage for 2 minutes followed by repeat visual acuity testing
D. Topical β-blocker administration
E. Urgent temporal artery biopsy and admit to the hospital to await results

II-67. In what anatomic structural way is the olfaction system unique among the sensory systems?

A. Initial afferent projections bypass the thalamus and synapse directly with the primary olfactory cortex.
B. The olfactory system's primary sensory neurons uniquely are chemoreceptors.
C. Primary olfactory cortex is anatomically distant from the hippocampus and amygdala.
D. The primary sensory neuron synapses directly with the olfactory cortex
E. Thalamic damage enacts no olfactory deficit.

II-68. All of the cranial nerves below are matched correctly with their innervation territory in regard to the sense of taste EXCEPT:

A. VII – Anterior tongue
B. VII – Soft palate
C. IX – Posterior tongue
D. IX – Soft epiglottis
E. X – Larynx

II-69. Which of the following statements is true regarding presbyosmia and anosmia?

A. A majority of the population over the age of 80 years suffers from presbyosmia.
B. Anosmia is often a late feature of end-stage Parkinson disease.
C. Patients with trauma-related anosmia will not recover any olfactory function.
D. While irritating, presbyosmia confers no real health risk.
E. Women suffer from presbyosmia at a greater rate than men

II-70. Mr. McEvoy is a 42-year-old long-haul truck driver who comes to your clinic for an urgent care visit. Two days ago, he noticed that his face felt unusual. While checking the rearview mirror, he noticed that the left side of his face looked different from normal. He also noticed that he drooled some of his soda, and it tasted quite odd. These symptoms did not improve over the ensuing 2 days of his trip. He denies any tick exposures or any other neurologic symptoms. You explain to Mr. McEvoy that the most common cause of his facial paralysis and taste disturbance is viral involvement of which of the following cranial nerves (CN)?

A. CN V
B. CN VI
C. CN VII
D. CN IX
E. CN X

II-71. A 64-year-old man is evaluated for hearing loss that he thinks is worse in his left ear. His wife and children have told him for years that he doesn't listen to them. Recently, he has failed to hear the chime of the alarm on his digital watch, and he admits to focusing on the lips of individuals speaking to him as he sometimes has difficulties in word recognition. In addition, he reports a continuous buzzing that is louder in his left ear. He denies any sensation of vertigo, headaches, or balance difficulties. He has worked in a factory for many years that makes parts for airplanes, and the machinery that he works with sits to his left primarily. He has no family history of deafness, although his father had hearing loss as he aged. He has a medical history of hypertension, hyperlipidemia, and coronary artery disease. You suspect sensorineural hearing loss related to exposure to the intense noise in the factory for many decades. Which of the following findings would you expect on physical examination?

A. A deep tympanic retraction pocket seen above the pars flaccida on the tympanic membrane
B. Cerumen impaction in the external auditory canal
C. Hearing loss that is greater at lower frequencies on pure tone audiometry
D. Increased intensity of sound when a tuning fork is placed upon the mastoid process when compared to placement near the auditory canal
E. Increased intensity of sound in the right ear when a tuning fork is placed in the midline of the forehead

II-72. In the patient described in Question II-71, which of the following should be the next suggested diagnostic test?

A. Head CT scan
B. Brain MRI with gadolinium contrast
C. Pure tone and speech audiometry
D. Schirmer test
E. Tympanometry

II-73. A 19-year-old college student presents with 3 days of increasing left-sided pain below his ear with feeling feverish. He noted some nasal congestion over the last 2 weeks due to high pollen counts. The pain has worsened despite taking decongestants and acetaminophen. He has a history of allergic rhinitis and multiple episodes of otitis media. On examination, there is tenderness, some swelling at the left mastoid process, and fluid behind the left temporal membrane. Because of his history, a CT scan is obtained and is shown in Figure II-73.

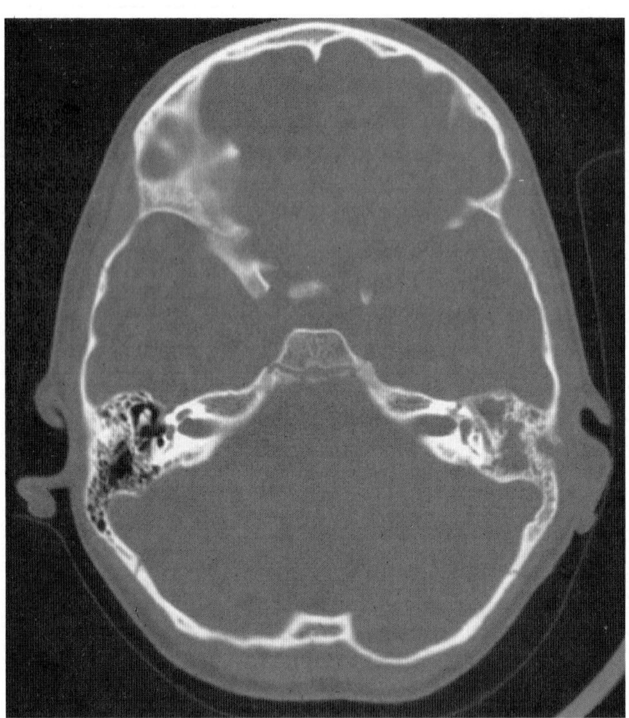

FIGURE II-73

Which of the following is the most likely diagnosis?

A. Acute mastoiditis
B. Otitis externa
C. Mucormycosis
D. Meningioma
E. Septic thrombosis

II-74. A 32-year-old woman presents to her primary care physician complaining of nasal congestion and drainage and headache. Her symptoms originally began about 7 days ago with rhinorrhea and sore throat. For the past 5 days, she has been having increasing feelings of fullness and pressure in the maxillary area that is causing her headaches. The pressure is worse when she bends over, and she also notices it while lying in bed at night. She is otherwise healthy and has not had fever. On physical examination, there is purulent nasal drainage and pain with palpation over bilateral maxillary sinuses. What is the best approach to ongoing management of this patient?

A. Initiate therapy with amoxicillin 500 mg three times daily for 10 days
B. Initiate therapy with levofloxacin 500 mg daily for 10 days
C. Perform a sinus aspirate for culture and sensitivities
D. Perform a sinus CT
E. Treat with oral decongestants and nasal saline lavage

II-75. A 28-year-old man seeks evaluation for sore throat for 2 days. He has not had a cough or rhinorrhea. He has no other medical conditions and works as a daycare provider. On examination, tonsillar hypertrophy with membranous exudate is present. What is the next step in the management of this patient?

A. Empiric treatment with amoxicillin 500 mg twice daily for 10 days
B. Rapid antigen detection test for *Streptococcus pyogenes* only
C. Rapid antigen detection test for *S pyogenes* plus throat culture if rapid test is negative
D. Rapid antigen detection test for *S pyogenes* plus throat culture regardless of result
E. Throat culture only

II-76. A 58-year-old man comes to clinic for a routine physical examination. He has a history of hyperlipidemia and hypertension controlled with atorvastatin and enalapril. Despite counseling, he smokes 1 pack of cigarettes per day. On physical examination, you notice some ulcerations in the mouth below the tongue (Figure II-76). The lesion is not painful, and the patient reports no recent mouth symptoms. Which of the following is the most likely diagnosis?

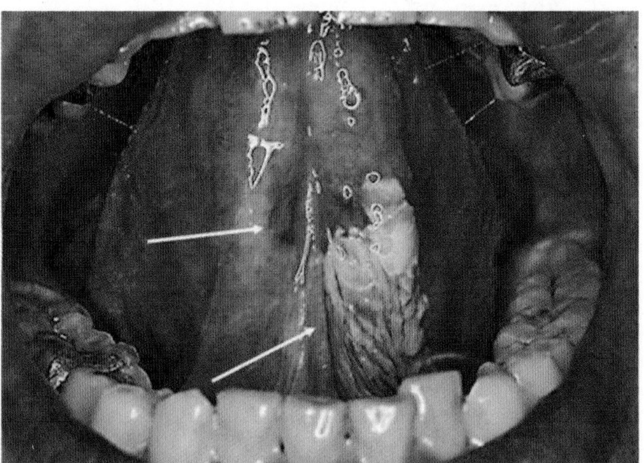

FIGURE II-76

A. Aphthous ulcer
B. Behcet disease
C. Herpes virus type 1 infection
D. HIV infection
E. Oral leukoplakia

II-77. The patient in Question II-76 is at greatest risk of which of the following disorders?

A. Celiac disease
B. Crohn disease
C. Oral candidiasis
D. Reactive arthritis
E. Squamous cell carcinoma

II-78. You are riding the bus home after a busy clinic one day. A man sits next you and, ignoring the easily seen signs, begins to smoke a cigarette. You feel a "tickle in your throat" and then proceed to cough. All of the following statements regarding the cough are true EXCEPT:

A. During a cough, rapid expiratory flows are generated but cannot exceed the normal envelop of maximum voluntary expiratory flow seen on a flow-volume curve assessment.
B. In initiating a cough, the vocal cords must first adduct.
C. In some patients, stimulation of the auricular branch of the vagus nerve in the external auditory meatus can stimulate a cough.
D. Pressures approaching 300 mmHg can be generated in the thorax during the cough reflex.
E. The velocity of expiratory airflow is crucial to dislodging mucus or other irritants from the airway walls.

II-79. Mrs. Jones is a 48-year-old woman with hypertension and obesity. She presents to your office for the second time today because of a cough. When you first saw her 2 weeks ago, she complained of a cough productive of scant sputum lasting for over 2 months. Physical examination, chest radiography, and laboratory examination were all unrevealing. She intermittently took some over-the-counter decongestants at night, but she now returns without any diminution in her cough. Regarding chronic cough, which of the following is true?

A. Angiotensin-converting enzyme (ACE) inhibitor–induced cough is believed to be due to decreased relative levels of bradykinin.
B. Cytologic examination of expectorated sputum is warranted in this case.
C. If a cough worsens when first lying down, this is an important clue to etiology.
D. In combination, postnasal drainage, gastroesophageal reflux, asthma, and ACE inhibitor use account for more than 90% of chronic cough.
E. Most etiologies of chronic cough are associated with improvement with exercise.

II-80. Mr. Boyle is a 19-year-old college student with cystic fibrosis. While studying for midterm exams, he suddenly begins coughing up large volumes of bright red blood. Emergency medical personnel are rapidly called and transfer him to the nearby university hospital emergency department, where you are working. Given his medical history, which blood vessel(s) do you suspect his bleeding is arising from?

A. Alveolar capillaries
B. Bronchial arteries
C. Gastric varices
D. Pulmonary artery
E. Pulmonary veins

II-81. The patient described in Question II-80 is coughing up large volumes of blood as he is wheeled into the sick bay in the emergency department. His blood pressure is 70/palp, heart rate is 145 bpm, oxygen saturation is 85% on room air, and he is breathing in excess of 40 times per minute. He is speaking in two- to three-word phrases only and appears pale and in distress. Auscultation reveals diminished breath sounds on the right. An emergent chest radiograph shows a dense opacity in the right lung. All of the following therapeutic steps are appropriate to consider for Mr. Boyle EXCEPT:

A. Bronchoscopic examination of the airways and consideration of bronchoscopically directed cauterization or laser therapy
B. Consultation with the interventional radiology team to evaluate for bronchial artery angiography and potential embolization
C. Endotracheal intubation with a dual-lumen endotracheal tube and mechanical ventilation
D. Placement of the patient in the left lateral decubitus position
E. Placement of two large-bore peripheral intravenous catheters and aggressive administration of intravenous crystalloids

II-82. A patient is evaluated in the emergency department for peripheral cyanosis. All of the following are potential etiologies EXCEPT?

A. Cold exposure
B. Deep venous thrombosis
C. Methemoglobinemia
D. Peripheral vascular disease
E. Raynaud phenomenon

II-83. You are reading a fascinating historical account of human experiments done in the mid-to-early 20th century to discover the physiologic effects of hypoxia. In these experiments, men reside in a large compression chamber for 1 month. The scientists then slowly reduce the oxygen content in the room's air by 0.5% per day until they reach a level where the men have a resting hemoglobin oxygen saturation of 87%. The men then reside in this state for 2 weeks. While you question the ethical considerations involved, you also think of the physiologic changes in the men residing in the compression chamber. You know that these men are likely to experience all of the following EXCEPT:

A. Elevated expression of hypoxia-inducible factor 1
B. Elevated production of erythrocytes
C. Reduced pulmonary arterial resistance
D. Reduced systemic arterial resistance
E. Upregulation of vascular endothelial growth factor

II-84. Each of the following five 50-year-old women has a PaO_2 (arterial oxygen partial pressure) of 60 mmHg. Which of them will have the highest arterial hemoglobin oxygen saturation?

A. A healthy woman standing on the top of a 3000-meter peak in the Peruvian Andes.
B. A woman with end-stage COPD from α_1-antitrypsin deficiency
C. A woman obtunded from an overdose of morphine
D. A woman found by paramedics after attempting suicide by placing a plastic bag over her head
E. A woman with severe neuromuscular weakness due to myasthenia gravis

II-85. Each of the following patients has the same skin tone, an identical cardiac output, and an identical arterial hemoglobin oxygen saturation of 80%. Which patient will likely appear most cyanotic?

A. A man with a gastrointestinal bleed from an esophageal varix and a hemoglobin of 8 g/dL
B. A normal, healthy man exultant after just having summited a 4000-meter peak in Tibet for the first time
C. A man with long-standing congenital heart disease due to uncorrected tetralogy of Fallot and a hemoglobin of 20 g/dL
D. A previously healthy man with bacterial pneumonia
E. A previously healthy man with a large pulmonary embolism

II-86. Which of the following changes in the lung microenvironment will result in a net overall movement of fluid volume from the intravascular space to the extravascular space leading to edema?

A. Decrease in pulmonary capillary hydrostatic pressure
B. Decrease in pulmonary capillary oncotic pressure
C. Increase in pulmonary interstitial hydrostatic pressure
D. Reduction in atmospheric pressure
E. None of the above

II-87. Mr. Johnson returns to your clinic for his second visit in 2 weeks. Last week, he presented for evaluation of lower extremity swelling. He felt like he had been gaining weight and that it was more difficult to put his shoes on in the morning. On examination, you note a laterally displaced cardiac point of maximal impulse, an S_3 gallop on auscultation, elevation of the jugular venous pulse, and pitting edema to his knees bilaterally. Transthoracic echocardiogram reveals a dilated left ventricle with a reduced ejection fraction of 20%–30%, confirming the diagnosis of cardiomyopathy. He is currently on no medications and has no other known medical conditions. All of the following are elevated or increased in Mr. Johnson EXCEPT:

A. Aldosterone
B. Brain natriuretic peptide
C. Effective arterial blood volume
D. Renal vascular resistance
E. Systemic capillary hydrostatic pressure

II-88. Mr. Carpentier presents to the emergency room with 2 weeks of fever and 30 minutes of acute, overwhelming shortness of breath. His heart rate on presentation is 120 bpm, blood pressure is 90/75 mmHg, and oxygen saturation is 84% on room air. Examination reveals diffuse pulmonary rales, and chest x-ray confirms pulmonary edema. After auscultation of his precordium, you suspect that he has acute mitral regurgitation. Compared to the murmur of chronic mitral regurgitation, the murmur you heard:

A. Is crescendo-decrescendo in pattern
B. Is holosystolic and proceeding to obscure S_2
C. Is likely louder and associated with a thrill
D. Is shorter, ending in early diastole and decrescendo in shape
E. Will likely be easily appreciated with the bell of the stethoscope off the chest

II-89. Mr. Johannson is a 76-year-old retired cricket coach with a history of hyperlipidemia. He presents to your office reporting escalating breathlessness on exertion. On auscultation, you note a systolic murmur and suspect severe aortic stenosis. All of the following are auscultatory clues that his aortic stenosis is severe EXCEPT:

A. A late-peaking systolic murmur
B. An apical S_4
C. An absent A_2
D. An early ejection sound that is high pitched, like a click along the left sternal border
E. Paradoxical splitting of S_2

II-90. Mr. Abraham is a 62-year-old former sea urchin collector with a history of right total knee replacement 10 years ago and prior tobacco abuse. He presents to your office complaining of chest pain with moderate exertion and some mild dyspnea with walking up hills. On examination, you note a mid-systolic murmur. After careful listening, you are unsure whether this is the murmur of aortic stenosis or of the obstructive form of hypertrophic cardiomyopathy. Which maneuver is appropriately matched to the clinical finding that would suggest that this murmur is due to obstructive hypertrophic cardiomyopathy as opposed to aortic valvular stenosis?

A. Handgrip maneuver – Diminished intensity of the murmur
B. Initiating milrinone intravenously – Augmentation of the systolic murmur
C. Palpation of the carotid impulse – A diminished, delayed carotid upstroke
D. Stand to squat – Augmentation of the intensity of the murmur
E. Valsalva maneuver – Augmentation of the intensity of the murmur

II-91. A 42-year-old man with known Marfan syndrome presents to your office for his yearly follow-up. His heart rate is 85 bpm, and blood pressure is 140/55 mmHg. His carotid pulses are bounding. On auscultation, you identify an early diastolic, blowing decrescendo murmur at the right second interspace, radiating to the right sternal border. Curiously, you also hear a lower pitched mid-to-late grade 2 diastolic murmur at the apex. While you are fairly certain the first murmur is from aortic regurgitation and are concerned about aortic root disease, you are not certain whether the latter murmur is due to the Austin Flint phenomenon (turbulence at the mitral inflow area from admixing of the regurgitant aortic flow and forward mitral flow) or from structural mitral valve stenosis. Unfortunately, your echocardiogram machine is broken. Which maneuver below is appropriately matched to the finding of the apical murmur that would convince you that this murmur is due to the Austin Flint phenomenon?

A. Hand grip – Increased murmur intensity
B. Amyl nitrate administration – Increased murmur intensity
C. Administration of phenylephrine – Decreased murmur intensity
D. Administration of immediate-release nifedipine – Increased murmur intensity
E. The murmur of valvular mitral stenosis and the Austin Flint murmur will respond identically to every maneuver.

II-92. Mrs. Edwards is a 37-year-old sushi chef, originally from the Izu Islands of Japan, with a history of rheumatic fever, continuous atrial fibrillation, and known mitral stenosis. She feels well at rest but is limited by dyspnea to mild exertional efforts only. She has stopped biking to the market to pick out the fresh fish daily, relegating these responsibilities to her son. On auscultation of Mrs. Edward's precordium, you expect to hear all of the following findings EXCEPT:

A. A mid-diastolic, low-pitched decrescendo murmur
B. An increase in the murmur just before systole
C. A loud S_1
D. A high-pitched sound occurring shortly after S_2
E. An augmentation of the murmur intensity with turning the patient in the left lateral decubitus position.

II-93. A 58-year-old former professional badminton champion presents to your clinic for evaluation of palpitations. Unfortunately, since his badminton career ended 25 years ago, he has not kept up his physical fitness. As his primary care provider, you have been trying to manage his hypertension, hyperlipidemia, tobacco abuse, and lack of physical exercise. Two weeks ago, he decided to take your advice and start jogging to increase his aerobic exercise. However, at your clinic visit with him today, he notes that every time he starts to jog, he senses palpitations, feels very short of breath, and feels like he is going to pass out. Once, he thinks he may have lost consciousness briefly after sitting at the side of the jogging track. These sensations last for several minutes after he stops to rest. What is the most appropriate response to this patient?

A. "I am going to refer you for an exercise treadmill electrocardiogram to see if we can capture any concerning arrhythmia or ischemic changes."
B. "Most patients with palpitations do not have serious arrhythmias or structural heart disease. Nothing to worry about. Keep up the good work with jogging!"
C. "Perhaps you should try swimming. Jogging is an intense orthostatic challenge for the physically unfit."
D. "Tobacco is a classic cause of palpitations. You should stop smoking, and I'll bet your palpitations will resolve completely."
E. "We should get a 48-hour Holter monitor. Do not jog again until I have had time to review the Holter report."

II-94. A 77-year-old woman seeks your opinion because she has lost weight over the last 9 months. She reports her weight has fallen from 165 to 140 lb without any effort on her part to lose weight. She had a hip fracture after a fall 3 months ago that was successfully surgically repaired. She reports that her mobility is good. There are no fevers or night sweats. Her review of systems is otherwise negative, and she reports an intact but not voracious appetite. Medications include warfarin with a well-controlled INR. She is a lifelong nonsmoker and has one glass of wine less than twice per week. All of the following should be ordered to evaluate her involuntary weight loss EXCEPT:

A. C-reactive protein
B. Complete blood count
C. Complete metabolic panel including renal and hepatic function
D. Low-dose CT of chest
E. Thyroid function tests

II-95. The normal small intestine contains about 200 mL of gas. Of the following, which of these gases is usually present in the normal small intestine and is *not* produced by bacteria living there?

A. Carbon dioxide
B. Carbon monoxide
C. Hydrogen
D. Methane
E. Nitrogen

II-96. Mr. Herlong presents with the complaint of abdominal swelling. For the past month, he has noticed that his abdomen has become increasingly large, and he has been forced to buy new pants with an increased waist size twice. He denies any change in bowel movements, but does now feel shortness of breath when walking and lying down. On physical examination, his abdomen is distended, but soft and nontender. His abdomen is dull to percussion, and you detect a fluid wave in his abdomen on physical examination. Curiously, you detect pulsations with light palpation over his liver. His lungs are clear to auscultation. Cardiac palpation reveals a systolic heave just to the left of the sternum, and a holosystolic murmur and loud P_2 are appreciated on auscultation. He has a positive Kussmaul sign. You insert (under sterile conditions) into his internal jugular vein a fluid-filled catheter connected to a pressure manometer located at the level of the patient's heart when supine. You advance the catheter into various venous spaces, occasionally inflating a balloon just proximal to the catheter tip to "wedge" it into the vein or artery. Which of the following locations will yield a normal pressure?

A. Internal jugular vein
B. Right ventricle
C. Unwedged hepatic vein
D. Wedged hepatic vein
E. None of the above

II-97. A 56-year-old man with an unknown past medical history presents to the hospital with abdominal swelling. Physical examination suggests ascites, and abdominal ultrasound confirms a large volume of intraperitoneal fluid, the absence of hepatic vein thrombus, and no identifiable liver masses. You perform a paracentesis, removing 4 L of serous fluid from the abdomen. Below are the laboratory results from the patient's serum and ascites studies.

Serum	
Sodium	132 mEq/dL
Creatinine	1.2 mg/dL
Albumin	3.6 g/dL
Bilirubin	4.2 mg/dL

Ascites	
Albumin	1.1 g/dL
Protein	0.9 g/dL

Which of the following is the mostly likely cause of this patient's ascites?

A. Acute Budd-Chiari syndrome
B. Cirrhosis
C. Heart failure (e.g., "cardiac ascites")
D. Intraperitoneal tumor
E. Tuberculosis

II-98. After paracentesis, you instruct the patient described in Question II-97 to comply with a sodium-restricted diet and initiate diuretic therapy with spironolactone and furosemide to prevent future ascites. Which of the following additional daily therapies is warranted?

A. Clonidine
B. Lactulose
C. Midodrine
D. Norfloxacin
E. Propranolol

II-99. Mr. Spearoti is a 47-year-old long-haul truck driver with a history of mild chronic kidney disease (baseline creatinine 1.4 mg/dL) and hypertension. Recently, he was complaining of some shoulder pain exacerbated by his work. Further, at his primary care appointment, his blood pressure was elevated at 150/95 mmHg. He was started on lisinopril 20 mg daily and advised to take naproxen 500 mg bid. Two weeks later, he presents to the emergency department with muscle cramps and is found to have a creatinine of 4.9 mg/dL. His blood pressure is 135/80 mmHg. Renal ultrasound reveals no hydronephrosis and normal-appearing kidneys. His urinalysis is bland, and urine microscopy reveals hyaline casts. Urinary sodium is undetectable. Which of the following is the likely cause of his acute renal failure?

A. Acute interstitial nephritis
B. Acute tubular necrosis
C. Glomerulonephritis
D. Glomerular vasomotor dysfunction
E. Obstructive uropathy

II-100. Mr. Fein is a 55-year-old South African movie star who presents with several months of fatigue. Physical examination is unrevealing, although extended review of systems reveals that he occasionally has noted very foamy urine. Urinary dipstick reveals a pH of 6.7, no hemoglobin or protein, and no cells or casts. Given his history, you send his urine for direct protein testing via sulfosalicylic acid, which returns very positive and is quantified as 2.5 g per 24 hours. What likely explains the discrepancy between the negative dipstick protein result and positive direct protein measurements?

A. The patient may have varying amounts of protein excretion at different times.
B. The protein in the patient's urine is likely albumin.
C. The protein in the patient's urine is likely not albumin.
D. The urinary pH caused a false negative on the dipstick test.
E. The urinary pH caused a false positive on the direct test.

II-101. As part of an experiment, you infuse a nonmetabolized osmotically active solute into a peripheral vein of a subject, measuring serum osmolality at a distant vein every 2 minutes. When osmolality reaches about 285 mOsm/kg, you know that several physiologic changes will occur. These include all of the following EXCEPT:

A. Aquaporin-2 water channels will be actively inserted in the luminal membrane of the glomerular collecting duct.
B. Neurons in the hypothalamus will release arginine vasopressin into the circulation via the posterior pituitary.
C. The patient will feel thirsty.
D. The renal medullary osmotic gradient will decrease.
E. Urinary osmolality will rise.

II-102. As you study for your upcoming high-stakes board examination, you start performing some arithmetic on sodium reabsorption in the kidney. You know that a normal glomerular filtration rate is about 180 L/d. At a serum sodium concentration of 140 mM, you calculate that the kidneys filter out about 1.5 kg of salt per day! Clearly, the majority of this salt must be reabsorbed by the nephron distal to the glomerulus. Which portion of the glomerulus is responsible for the bulk of sodium reabsorption?

A. Aldosterone-sensitive cells in the connecting tubule and collecting duct
B. Distal collecting tubule
C. Principal cells in the connecting tubule and collecting duct
D. Proximal tubule
E. Thick ascending limb of Henle

II-103. A patient presents to you with 2 days of frequent vomiting. On examination, he has dry mucous membranes and diminished skin turgor. While supine, blood pressure and heart rate are 110/75 mmHg and 90 bpm, respectively. When standing, blood pressure and heart rate are 85/55 mmHg and 110 bpm, respectively. Serum pH is 7.45 with a bicarbonate level of 32 mEq/dL. You obtain a urine sample for testing. Which of the following do you expect to be true?

A. Urine specific gravity will be <1.020
B. Urine chloride will be >25 mM
C. Urine osmolality will be <300 mOsm/kg
D. Urine sodium will be <20 mM
E. Urine sodium will be >20 mM

II-104. A 63-year-old woman presents to the emergency department with 4 days of diarrhea. On examination, she is mildly tachycardic with dry mucous membranes. Serum sodium is 132 mEq/dL, and urine sodium concentration is undetectably low. To correct her hyponatremia, you must do what?

A. Prescribe furosemide to allow free water loss
B. Prescribe hydrochlorothiazide to allow free water loss
C. Prescribe intravenous hydration to reduce antidiuretic hormone (ADH) levels and allow a free water diuresis
D. Prescribe tolvaptan therapy as an ADH antagonist
E. Provide extra sodium to correct her total body sodium deficiency

II-105. Which of the following conditions is associated with hyponatremia *and* suppression of circulating ADH levels?

A. Central diabetes insipidus
B. Cirrhosis
C. Dehydration
D. Heart failure
E. Psychogenic polydipsia

II-106. You are called in to consult on the curious case of Mr. Atah. He is a 21-year-old man who was admitted with mild pancreatitis. CT scan showed no gallstones, and he fervently denies any history of alcohol intake. Strangely, his serum sodium is measured by the core laboratory as between 117 and 121 mEq/dL on repeated tests, and prior reports faxed from his primary care clinic indicate that his serum sodium 1 year previously (in a state of normal health) was 121 mEq/dL. On examination, he has an arcus senilis and tendinous xanthomas. What is the likely cause of this patient's hyponatremia?

A. A mutation leading to a constitutively active V2 aquaporin protein in the nephron
B. Cirrhosis
C. Excess inappropriate activity of ADH
D. Polydipsia
E. Pseudohyponatremia

II-107. Mr. Jones, a previously healthy 45-year-old man, presents to the emergency department after he became acutely obtunded and suffered a seizure after completing a marathon race. After establishing an endotracheal airway and beginning mechanical ventilation, you send basic laboratory studies and obtain a head CT. You receive two back-to-back "panic value" calls. On the first, the laboratory informs you that the patient's sodium level is 115 mEq/dL. On the second, the radiologist informs you that the patient has diffuse cerebral edema with effacement of sulci without cerebral herniation. What therapy is most appropriate?

A. 1 L of normal saline bolus followed by 100 mL/hr
B. 180 mg of intravenous Lasix
C. Hypertonic (3%) saline targeted at increasing sodium 1–2 mM/hr
D. Initiation of desmopressin therapy and then administration of hypertonic saline
E. Stat infusion of intravenous conivaptan

II-108. Mr. Matherli is a 54-year-old man with nephrogenic diabetes insipidus (NDI) from lithium therapy. Usually, he is excellent about keeping up his free water intake to control his sodium level. However, he was involved in a car accident requiring operation at an outside hospital. There, they did not know about his NDI, and after being NPO for 48 hours, he was found to have a serum sodium of 160 mEq/dL. He is a 100-kg man. To correct his serum sodium over the next 24 hours, at what approximate rate should the physician run intravenous 5% dextrose in water (D5W; for free water)?

A. 50 mL/hr
B. 100 mL/hr
C. 150 mL/hr
D. 250 mL/hr
E. 350 mL/hr

II-109. A 66-year-old man presents to the urgent care center with vague complaints of nausea and decreased appetite over the last 4–6 weeks. Physical examination reveals normal vital signs and no abnormality other than a thin man with mild diffuse abdominal tenderness without guarding or rebound. The patient is found to have reduced serum calcium of 7.8 mg/dL. He denies any musculoskeletal symptoms. Additional laboratory studies are presented below:

Sodium	139 mEq/dL
Bicarbonate	26 mEq/dL
Creatinine	1.2 mg/dL
Glucose	109 mg/dL
Total protein	6.2 g/dL
Albumin	2.0 g/dL
Bilirubin	1.2 mg/dL
Potassium	3.8 mg/dL

For the patient's hypocalcemia, which of the following is the most appropriate response?

A. Administer calcium gluconate 1 g intravenously
B. Check magnesium levels and replete if deficient
C. Check vitamin D levels and replete if deficient
D. No further response necessary
E. Prescribe oral calcium bicarbonate daily

II-110. Mr. Wassim is a 45-year-old man with metastatic non–small-cell lung cancer undergoing chemotherapy. He presents to the hospital after his family noted that he was confused. Serum calcium is 11.5 mg/dL with a serum albumin of 2.5 g/dL. Vital signs are as follows: heart rate 132 bpm, blood pressure 90/55 mmHg, respiratory rate 18 breaths/min, temperature 37.2°C. What is the first appropriate therapeutic response for his hypercalcemia?

A. 80 mg of intravenous furosemide
B. Aggressive hydration with intravenous saline
C. Hydrocortisone 100 mg daily
D. No therapy is needed; the corrected serum calcium is normal
E. Zoledronic acid 4 mg intravenously

II-111. A 55-year-old man with a history of diabetes mellitus, hypertension, and prior narcotic abuse presents to the emergency department with altered mental status. On presentation, he is obtunded. Emergent laboratory values are shown below.

Arterial pH	7.21
$PaCO_2$	26
HCO_3^-	12
Sodium	145
Chloride	100
Glucose	280

What metabolic acid-base disorder does this patient have?

A. Combined metabolic acidosis and respiratory acidosis
B. Metabolic acidosis
C. Metabolic alkalosis
D. Respiratory acidosis
E. Respiratory alkalosis

II-112. All of the following clinical conditions may cause L-lactic acidosis EXCEPT:

A. Bowel ischemia
B. Carbon monoxide toxicity
C. Sepsis
D. Severe anemia
E. Short gut syndrome

II-113. Johns Rickerd is an 18-year-old man with a history of depression who presents to the emergency department after being found confused in his garage. He is noted to have a high anion gap metabolic acidosis, elevated creatinine, and rectangular coffin lid–appearing crystals in his urine on microscopic analysis. Ethylene glycol level is pending. Arterial pH is 7.33. Measured serum osmolality is 320 mmol; serum sodium is 140, blood urea nitrogen (BUN) is 28, and glucose is 180. What is the next appropriate step?

A. Administer fomepizole
B. Administer intravenous bicarbonate
C. Await ethylene glycol level before initiating therapy
D. Initiate emergent renal transplantation evaluation
E. Start intravenous antibiotics and obtain renal imaging to evaluate for staghorn calculi

II-114. All of the following statements regarding male sexual function are true EXCEPT:

A. Detumescence is mediated by the parasympathetic nervous system.
B. Ejaculation is stimulated by the sympathetic nervous system.
C. Nitric oxide enhances erection.
D. Sildenafil maintains erection by inhibiting the breakdown of cyclic GMP.
E. Testosterone enhances libido.

II-115. A 62-year-old man comes to clinic with his spouse complaining of erectile dysfunction. He has a 10-year history of moderately controlled diabetes mellitus and uses insulin. Over the last year, despite intact libido, he has been unable to attain or sustain an erection when attempting sexual intercourse with his wife. He reports that over this time he no longer awakes with an erection as he did previously. Serum chemistries are normal, hemoglobin A1C is 5.8%, and serum testosterone is normal for his age. Which class of drug is most likely to improve his ability to achieve and maintain erection?

A. 5α-Reductase inhibitor
B. Androgen
C. Corticosteroid
D. Phosphodiesterase-5 inhibitor
E. Selective serotonin reuptake inhibitor

II-116. A 54-year-old woman complains of difficulty having sex because of pain during intercourse. These symptoms began about 8 years ago but have worsened over the last year. She has one sexual partner and is on no medications. Which of the following is most likely to improve her symptoms?

A. Anastrozole
B. Estrogen cream
C. Paroxetine
D. Sildenafil
E. Tamoxifen

II-117. Ms. Chacco, a 19-year-old white woman, complains of worsening excess hairiness and is worried that she will be mocked as she starts college. She notes increasingly noticeable hair on her upper lip, chin, and arms. She takes no medications and reports a history of irregular menses. On examination, she has normal vital signs, and you note small to medium tufts of dark hair in the areas she mentioned plus in the midline above and below the umbilicus, along the inner thigh, and in the upper and lower back. All of the statements regarding her condition are true EXCEPT:

A. Further hormonal evaluation is likely necessary.
B. She likely has elevated androgen levels.
C. She meets the diagnostic criteria for hirsutism.
D. The most common cause of her condition is congenital adrenal hyperplasia.
E. This condition affects approximately 10% of women.

II-118. For the patient described in Question II-117, additional initial evaluation should include which of the following:

A. Abdominal/pelvic CT scan
B. Adrenocorticotropic hormone (ACTH) stimulation test
C. Dexamethasone suppression test
D. Measurement of serum prolactin
E. Measurement of serum testosterone

II-119. All of the following statements regarding menstrual function and dysfunction are true EXCEPT:

A. Pregnancy is the most common cause of secondary amenorrhea
B. Primary amenorrhea is defined as the absence of ever having a first menstrual flow.
C. Secondary amenorrhea is defined as absence of a menstrual flow for >3–6 months in a woman who previously menstruated.
D. The absence of menarche at age 17 years old in a normally developing woman warrants evaluation for primary amenorrhea.
E. There is no evidence that race or ethnicity affects the prevalence of amenorrhea.

II-120. A 28-year-old woman seeks evaluation for secondary amenorrhea. She had a normal menarche at age 14 with regular monthly periods lasting 5–6 days for the last 13 years. Over the last year, she's noticed greater irregularity and has had no menses for the last 6 months. She takes no medications and is sexually active with one partner using condoms as prophylaxis. Her physical examination is notable for normal vital signs, a body mass index (BMI) of 29 kg/m^2, normal breast development, and normal pelvic examination. Laboratory testing reveals a negative β-human chorionic gonadotropin (hCG), normal testosterone, normal dehydroepiandrosterone sulfate (DHEAS), elevated prolactin, and reduced follicle-stimulating hormone (FSH). Based on this information, what is the most likely diagnosis?

A. Androgen insensitivity syndrome
B. Neuroendocrine tumor
C. Polycystic ovary syndrome
D. Pregnancy
E. Premature menopause

II-121. You are evaluating a 23-year-old woman with heavy uterine bleeding. She reports menarche at age 13 with regular monthly 5–6 days menses until the age of 19. Starting at age 20, she began having three to four menses per year only lasting 3 days. For the last year, she has had four episodes of heavy uterine bleeding lasting 6–8 days. She has not had any menstruation for 9 months and is not sexually active. She has been diagnosed with type 2 diabetes and takes metformin. On examination, she is mildly hirsute, her blood pressure is 130/85 mmHg with heart rate of 85 bpm and respiratory rate of 14 breaths/min. Her BMI is 25 kg/m^2, and her SaO_2 on room air is 98%. Her β-gCG is negative, testosterone is elevated, and vaginal ultrasound reveals polycystic ovaries. Which of the following is the most effective treatment for her uterine bleeding?

A. Clomiphene
B. Letrozole
C. Prednisone
D. Progesterone
E. Testosterone

II-122. A 34-year-old woman seeks evaluation for a skin lesion. On examination, the lesion is present on the extensor surface of the right elbow. It measures 2.4 cm in diameter and is raised with a flat top and distinct edge. Overlying the lesion is an excess accumulation of stratum cornea. Further examination reveals several smaller lesions also located on extensor surfaces. Which term best characterizes the primary lesion for which the patient is seeking evaluation?

A. Macule with lichenification
B. Patch with a scale
C. Plaque with a crust
D. Plaque with a scale
E. Tumor

II-123. What term is used in dermatology to describe a coin-shaped lesion?

A. Herpetiform
B. Lichenoid
C. Morbilliform
D. Nummular
E. Polycyclic

II-124. A 5 year-old boy is brought in by his mother complaining of approximately 6 months of itching and scaling of the skin inside the elbows (Figure II-124). The area gets red occasionally and improves with over-the-counter topical steroid creams. There is no fever, chills, night sweats, or red streaks ascending the arm. The family has a pet cat and lives in a clean apartment. All of the following statements concerning this child are true EXCEPT:

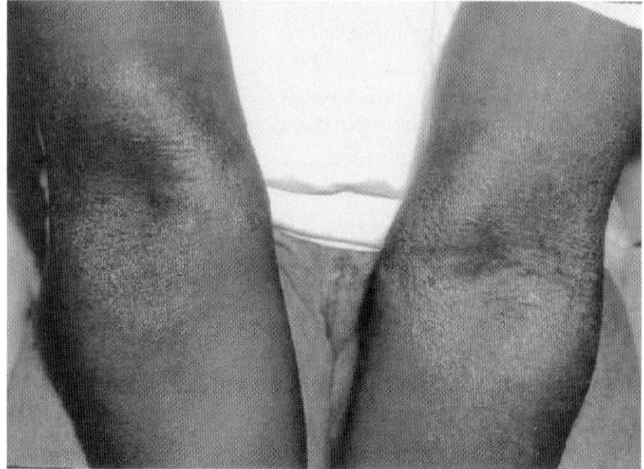

FIGURE II-124 Courtesy of Robert Swerlick, MD; with permission

A. Both of his parents have a history of atopic dermatitis.
B. He likely has a history of asthma or atopic rhinitis.
C. His serum immunoglobulin (Ig) E levels are elevated.
D. He has a greater than 70% chance of spontaneous resolution.
E. His lesions will likely respond to topical tacrolimus.

II-125. A 63-year-old woman has a 5-year history of psoriasis involving her elbows that has been controlled with topical glucocorticoids and a vitamin D analogue. However, in the past 9–12 months, her psoriasis has worsened, and she has developed new lesions involving her knees, gluteal regions, and scalp. She is increasingly uncomfortable and has noted swelling of her digits with pain and stiffness. She is up to date on all cancer screening and has no sign of systemic infection. Her physical examination is only notable for the psoriatic plaques that are red and scaling and swollen tender distal interphalangeal joints on both hands. All of the following therapies are indicated for worsening widespread systemic psoriatic disease EXCEPT:

A. Alefacept
B. Cyclosporine
C. Infliximab
D. Methotrexate
E. Prednisone

II-126. Ms. Magret brings her 73-year-old mother, Mrs. Lizz, to see you because she's worried about the skin of her mother's right foot and ankle (Figure II-126). Mrs. Lizz reports her skin has become progressively more abnormal over the last year. Her past medical history is notable for a history of right deep vein thrombosis (DVT) in her 50s after she hurt her leg snowboarding. She has no history of cardiac, liver, or renal disease. Her only medication is a vitamin D supplement. She is afebrile. There are a number of scaly, erythematous oozing patches with a number of 1- to 2-cm ulcers around the right ankle area. The patches and ulcers are neither tender nor inflamed. There are notable varicose veins in the calf and thigh. Which of the following is the indicated therapy for Mrs. Lizz?

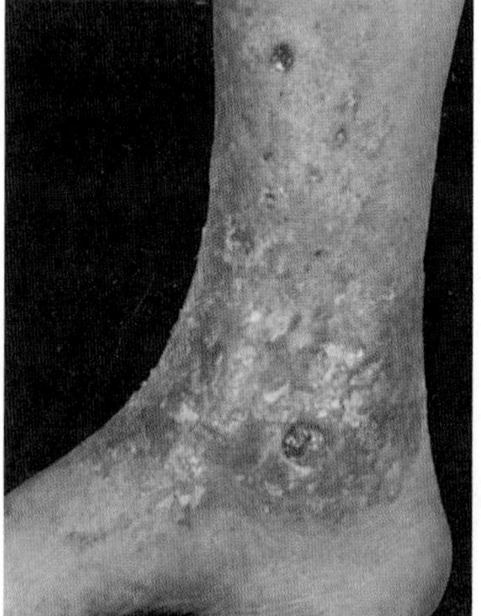

FIGURE II-126

A. Acyclovir
B. Augmentin
C. Compression stockings
D. Hemodialysis
E. Prednisone

II-127. A 45-year-old woman complains of hair loss. She states that whenever she brushes her hair she feels that there is excessive numbers of hairs that are shed, and she also notices the same phenomenon when she washes her hair. It has progressed to the point that she states her hair is noticeably thinner diffusely, and her hairdresser has commented on this as well. Approximately 5 months ago, she was hospitalized for acute gallstone pancreatitis with high fevers and underwent endoscopic retrograde cholangiopancreatography (ERCP). This was followed by laparoscopic cholecystectomy after 14 days. Overall, she was hospitalized for a total of 21 days. She has now returned to her baseline functional status. Her past medical history is significant for obesity, hyperlipidemia, and glucose intolerance. She is taking metformin 1000 mg daily and rosuvastatin 10 mg daily. On physical examination, she has only mild hair thinning. When a small area of the hair is pulled, more than 10 hairs are extracted at the root. There is no scaling or scarring on the scalp, and no broken hairs are seen. What treatment do you recommend?

A. Observation only
B. Oral terbinafine
C. Psychotherapy
D. Topical minoxidil
E. Topical anthralin

II-128. A 66-year-old man presents for evaluation of erythematous skin lesions on his lower extremities that have been present for the past 4 days. One week ago, he was seen by his primary care doctor for acute bronchitis and was prescribed cefuroxime 500 mg bid. His upper respiratory symptoms improved, but the rash developed. He is not having fever, chills, joint pains, myalgias, or hematuria. On physical examination, there are numerous nonblanching palpable erythematous lesions measuring 1–5 mm in diameter. What is the most likely diagnosis?

A. Capillaritis
B. Drug-induced thrombocytopenia
C. Ecthyma gangrenosum
D. Henoch-Schönlein purpura
E. Leukocytoclastic vasculitis

II-129. A 54-year-old man presents with oral lesions and blisters on his skin. He first noticed painful mouth sores about 2 months ago. He has now developed painful blisters on his trunk, neck, axillae, and groin. These blisters are fairly loose and quickly rupture, leaving behind erosions that heal without scarring. He had seen his dentist initially, who had given him topical steroids and chlorhexidine mouth rinses for presumed aphthous ulcers. These had not yielded any significant improvement in the oral lesions. He has a history of hypertension and hypercholesterolemia and is on treatment with candesartan 32 mg daily and atorvastatin 20 mg daily. On physical examination, there are three ill-defined erythematous oral erosions on bilateral buccal mucosal that are painful, with the largest measuring 4 mm in diameter. There are numerous erosions on the neck, trunk, axillae, and groin in various stages of healing. In some areas, flaccid blistering lesions on an erythematous base are seen, measuring up to 1 cm in diameter. However, most areas show denuded skin with crusted plaques in various stages of healing. When manual pressure is applied to the skin, some of the epidermis sloughs off. In healed areas, hyperpigmentation is present. Which of the following findings would be expected on immunopathology analysis of a skin biopsy?

A. Cell surface deposits of IgG on keratinocytes
B. Cell surface deposits of IgG and C3 on keratinocytes and possibly similar immunoreactants in epidermal basement membrane zone
C. Granular deposits of IgA in dermal papillae
D. Linear band of IgG, IgA, and/or C3 in epidermal basement membrane zone
E. Linear band of IgG and/or C3 in the epidermal basement membrane zone

II-130. A 73-year-old man develops pruritic blistering lesions on his lower abdomen, groin, and legs. The lesions begin with raised red itchy plaques and progress to tense bullae. After rupture, these lesions have largely healed without scarring except when excessively inflamed from excoriation. He has had no changes in his chronic medications for diabetes mellitus, gout, and benign prostatic hypertrophy. He was previously treated for renal cell carcinoma 15 years ago. An image of his rash is shown in Figure II-130. What is the most likely diagnosis?

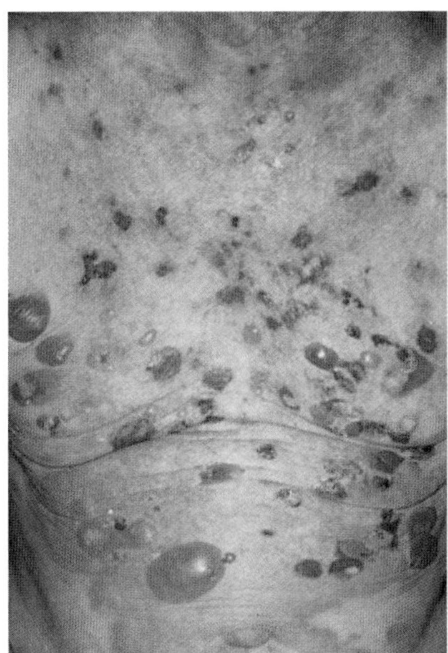

FIGURE II-130 Courtesy of the Yale Resident's Slide Collection; with permission.

A. Bullous pemphigoid
B. Epidermolysis bullosa acquisita
C. Paraneoplastic pemphigus
D. Pemphigus vulgaris
E. Urticarial vasculitis

II-131. A 24-year-old woman seeks evaluation for a rash that is present diffusely on her back, buttocks, elbows, and knees. The rash began abruptly, and the patient is complaining of severe pruritus and burning associated with the rash. A biopsy of the rash demonstrates neutrophilic dermatitis within the dermal papillae, and immunofluorescence highlights granular deposition of IgA in the papillary dermis and along the epidermal basement membrane zone. What treatment do you recommend for this patient?

A. Dapsone 100 mg daily
B. Gluten-free diet
C. Prednisone 40 mg daily
D. A and B
E. All of the above

II-132. Which of the following statements regarding sunburn is true?

A. At midday, ultraviolet (UV) B radiation predominates and contributes most of the effect to the development of sunburn at this time of day.
B. Individuals with red hair and fair skin typically have high activity of melanocortin-1 receptor and thus have high susceptibility to sunburn.
C. Tanning beds typically administer >90% UVB radiation.
D. The typical lag time from sun exposure to the development of visible redness is 1–2 hours.
E. UVB radiation is more efficient at provoking sunburn erythema than UVA radiation.

II-133. A 54-year-old woman is begun on glyburide 10 mg sustained release once daily for type 2 diabetes mellitus. After spending an afternoon in her garden, she develops an erythematous rash. Which of the following features would lead you to suspect a photoallergy over simple phototoxicity?

A. Intense pruritus
B. Involvement of mucous membranes
C. Persistent hypersensitivity to light after cessation of drug
D. Skin desquamation resembling a sunburn
E. A and C
F. All of the above

II-134. Which of the following statements regarding erythropoiesis is true?

A. Hypoxia-inducible factor-1α is downregulated in response to hypoxia and results in increased production of erythropoietin.
B. In response to erythropoietin, red blood cell production can increase to by a maximum factor of 2 over a 3–6 day period.
C. Normal red blood cell production results in replacement of approximately 1% of all circulating red blood cells each week.
D. The erythroid precursor, the pronormoblast, can produce 16–32 mature red blood cells.
E. With increased erythropoietin, each progenitor cell is stimulated to produce additional red blood cells.

II-135. A 36-year-old woman presents to your office complaining of easy fatigability. She is found to have anemia. On further questioning, she does report heavy menses and has been following a vegetarian diet. Her physical examination is normal with the exception of mildly pale conjunctiva. Her hemoglobin is 9.1 g/dL, and hematocrit is 27.6%. The mean corpuscular volume (MCV) is 65 fL, mean corpuscular hemoglobin (MCH) is 24 pg, and mean corpuscular hemoglobin concentration (MCHC) is 26%. The red cell distribution width is 16.7% The peripheral blood smear is shown in Figure II-135. Which of the following is present on the peripheral blood smear?

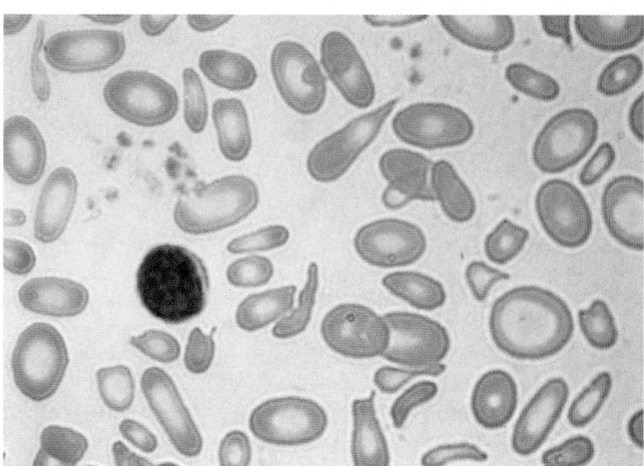

FIGURE II-135 From RS Hillman et al: *Hematology in Clinical Practice*, 5th ed. New York, McGraw-Hill, 2010.

A. Anisocytosis
B. Hypochromia
C. Poikilocytosis
D. A and B
E. All of the above

II-136. A 24-year-old woman is 12 weeks pregnant with her first child. She is referred for evaluation of an abnormal finding on complete blood count. She is asymptomatic and has had no complications thus far. She is of Turkish descent. She has no family members with significant anemias. Her hemoglobin is 12.2 g/dL and hematocrit is 37%. The MCV is 60 fL and MCH is 25 pg. Her ferritin is 50 μg/L and iron is 15 μmol/L. What is the characteristic finding expected on peripheral blood smear?

A. Burr cells
B. Howell-Jolly bodies
C. Schistocytes
D. Spherocytes
E. Target cells

II-137. You are asked to review the peripheral blood smear (Figure II-137) from a patient with anemia. Serum lactate dehydrogenase and total bilirubin are elevated, and there is hemoglobinuria. Which physical examination finding this patient is likely to have?

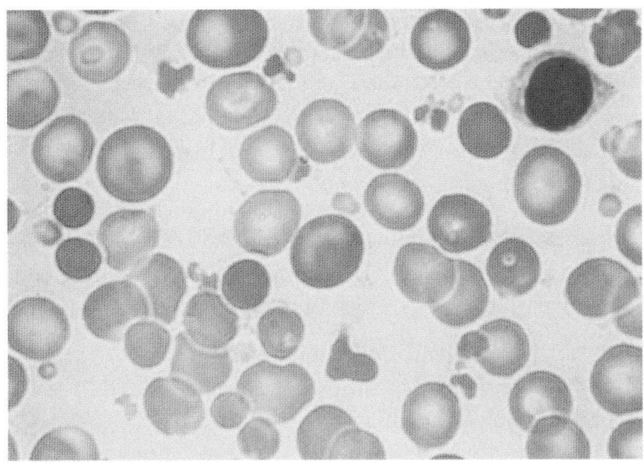

FIGURE II-137 From RS Hillman et al: *Hematology in Clinical Practice*, 5th ed. New York, McGraw-Hill, 2010.

A. Goiter
B. Heme-positive stools
C. Mechanical second heart sound
D. Splenomegaly
E. Thickened calvarium

II-138. You are seeing a patient in follow-up in whom you have begun an evaluation for an elevated hematocrit. You suspect polycythemia vera based on a history of aquagenic pruritus and splenomegaly. Which set of laboratory tests is consistent with the diagnosis of polycythemia vera?

A. Elevated red blood cell mass, high serum erythropoietin levels, normal oxygen saturation
B. Elevated red blood cell mass, low serum erythropoietin levels, normal oxygen saturation
C. Normal red blood cell mass, high serum erythropoietin levels, low arterial oxygen saturation
D. Normal red blood cell mass, low serum erythropoietin levels, low arterial oxygen saturation

II-139. Which protein is the primary mediating factor for platelet adhesion?

A. Collagen
B. Endothelin
C. Tissue factor
D. Thrombin
E. von Willebrand factor

II-140 through II-143. Match the following proteins involved in hemostasis with their definition.

II-140. Glycoprotein IIb/IIIa

II-141. Tissue factor

II-142. Plasmin

II-143. Protein S

A. A vitamin K–dependent cofactor that accelerates the anticoagulant action of protein C on factors V and VIII
B. The most abundant receptor on the surface of platelets that binds von Willebrand factor (vWF) and fibrinogen
C. The major protease enzyme of the fibrinolytic system
D. Primary trigger for activation of the coagulation system

II-144. You are consulted after an episode of postpartum hemorrhage in a 24-year-old woman. This was her first pregnancy, and she successfully delivered a healthy child at 39 weeks and 4 days. The child weighed 7 lb 12 oz, and the delivery was an uncomplicated spontaneous vaginal delivery. The uterine fundus contracted appropriately, but over the course of the next 12 hours, the patient had more than 1 L of bloody discharge. She has felt increasingly weak and has lightheadedness on standing. Her heart rate is 126 bpm, and blood pressure is 92/50 mmHg. She appears pale. Her pulses are thready. Cardiovascular examination shows regular tachycardia. Her hemoglobin prior to delivery was 9.2 g/dL. It is now 6.0 g/dL. Her prothrombin time (PT) is 12.0, INR is 1.1, and activated partial thromboplastin time (aPTT) is 42.5 seconds. Upon further questioning, the patient describes one other episode of prolonged oral bleeding in childhood at about age 7. At that time, she had a cap placed on a tooth and subsequently experienced significant bleeding. She bruises easily but has not had hemarthroses. She says she stopped playing soccer in grade school due to large bruises after minor injuries that were painful and embarrassing to her. She has had no other surgeries. She is taking iron supplements and prenatal vitamins. She has no allergies. She has a family history of excessive bleeding after a surgical procedure in her father from whom she is estranged. What do you suspect as the cause of the patient's illness?

A. Acquired inhibitor of coagulation
B. Factor VIII deficiency
C. Factor IX deficiency
D. Surreptitious ingestion of an anticoagulant
E. von Willebrand disease

II-145. A 68-year-old man is undergoing a total knee replacement for degenerative arthritis. His past medical history is significant for hypertension, diabetes mellitus, hyperlipidemia, gout, and obesity. His medication list includes metoprolol, sitagliptin, metformin, allopurinol, rosuvastatin, and aspirin daily. He is asked to stop his aspirin in preparation for surgery. Which of the following tests is/are indicated prior to surgery to ensure that the patient is not at increased risk of postoperative bleeding complications?

A. aPTT
B. Bleeding time
C. PT
D. A and C
E. A, B, and C

II-146. A 62-year-old woman is evaluated in a hematology clinic after a second episode of DVT. Her first episode occurred at age 34 following a pregnancy, and this episode occurred following an automobile accident that resulted in a femur fracture. She has no family history of DVT or pulmonary embolus. She is requesting a workup for hypercoagulability. Her automobile accident was 2 months ago. She remains casted and underwent surgical intervention on her fracture 4 weeks prior. She remains on low-molecular-weight heparin. What do you advise at the current time?

A. Do nothing. No further testing is indicated.
B. Send factor V Leiden and prothrombin 20210.
C. Send protein C and S levels.
D. Send antithrombin III levels.
E. Have the patient return in 3–6 months for further testing.

II-147. A 24-year-old woman seeks evaluation from her primary care provider for a "swollen gland" on the right side of her neck. She first noticed it about 2 weeks ago and has felt fatigued with a sore throat and low-grade fevers throughout this time. On examination, there is dominant 2-cm right posterior cervical lymph node that is rubbery and mobile. It is tender to palpation. In addition, there are also several 0.5–1 cm lymph nodes in the bilateral anterior and posterior cervical chains as well as the occipital area. All of the following findings favor a benign diagnosis EXCEPT:

A. Age <50
B. Multiple lymph node involvement
C. Presence of mobility on examination
D. Presence of tenderness to palpation
E. Size of dominant node ≥2 cm

II-148. A 58-year-old man presents with complaints of fatigue, dyspnea on exertion, and abdominal pain that is worst on the left side of his abdomen. He has a medical history of difficult-to-treat hypertension. His medical regimen includes lisinopril 40 mg daily, amlodipine 10 mg daily, hydrochlorothiazide 25 mg daily, and methyldopa 250 mg twice daily. He has been intolerant of β-blockers due to bradycardia. The most recent medication change was addition of the methyldopa approximately 6 months ago. His vital signs are as follows: heart rate 110 bpm, respiratory rate 18 breaths/min, temperature 37°C, blood pressure 148/84 mmHg, and SaO_2 95% on room air. He appears pale with mild jaundice. Scleral icterus is present. His chest examination is clear, and cardiovascular examination shows only a regular tachycardia. The liver is 10 cm to percussion and palpable 1 cm below the right costal margin. The spleen is palpable 10 cm below the left costal margin. There is no edema. On laboratory examination, the hemoglobin is 7.5 g/dL and hematocrit is 23.2%. The white blood cell count is 8,300/μL with a normal differential, and platelets are 123,000/μL. The peripheral smear shows spherocytes and anisocytosis. AST, ALT, and alkaline phosphatase are normal. The total bilirubin is 3.3 mg/dL, and the direct bilirubin is 0.4 mg/dL. What is the most likely cause of the patient's splenomegaly?

A. Autoimmune hemolytic anemia
B. Chronic myeloid leukemia
C. Hodgkin lymphoma
D. Myelofibrosis with myeloid metaplasia
E. Passive congestion due to portal hypertension

II-149. The presence of Howell-Jolly bodies, Heinz bodies, basophilic stippling, and nucleated red blood cells in a patient with hairy cell leukemia prior to any treatment intervention implies which of the following?

A. Diffuse splenic infiltration by tumor
B. Disseminated intravascular coagulation (DIC)
C. Hemolytic anemia
D. Pancytopenia
E. Transformation to acute leukemia

II-150. Which of the following is true regarding infection risk after elective splenectomy?

A. Patients are at no increased risk of viral infection after splenectomy.
B. Patients should be vaccinated 2 weeks after splenectomy.
C. Splenectomy patients over the age of 50 are at greatest risk for postsplenectomy sepsis.
D. *Staphylococcus aureus* is the most commonly implicated organism in postsplenectomy sepsis.
E. The risk of infection after splenectomy increases with time.

II-151. You are an internist at a community hospital and are asked to consult regarding an abnormality seen on a peripheral blood smear. A 64-year-old man was admitted to the orthopedic surgery service for a right total hip replacement surgery. His postoperative course was complicated by an aspiration event and subsequent pneumonia. His white blood cell count rose from 6.3/μL to 12.1/μL with 83% neutrophils and 10% bands. There was comment of an abnormal bilobed nucleus in a polymorphonuclear cell seen on the peripheral smear in the majority of granulocytes. The initial complete blood count (CBC) did not have a differential or peripheral smear performed. When you evaluate the smear, you see the following (Figure II-151). What is your recommendation?

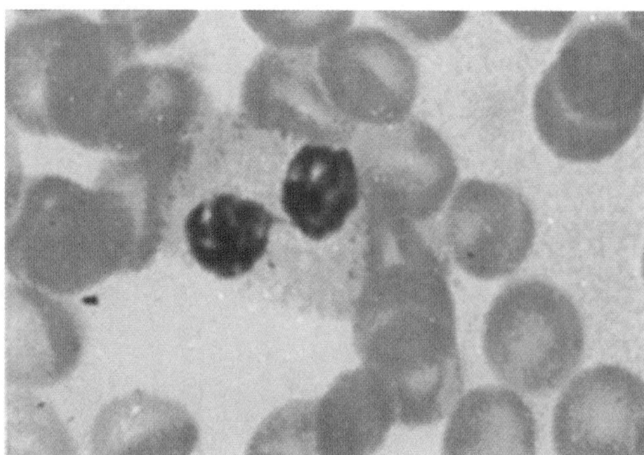

FIGURE II-151

A. A bone marrow biopsy should be performed.
B. A follow-up CBC with differential and peripheral smear should be evaluated in 4–6 weeks to ensure a return to normal.
C. No further follow-up is required. This is a benign inherited disorder.
D. No further follow-up is required. This is an expected reaction to the patient's infection.
E. Without a prior peripheral smear for comparison, the acuity of the change is unable to be determined. Either C or D could be correct.

II-152. An 18-year-old man presents with a gastric outlet obstruction. He has had frequent episodes of abdominal pain, diarrhea, and proctitis. A prior colonic biopsy has demonstrated sharply defined granulomas in the colon. In addition, he has had recurrent episodes of pneumonia. He has grown both *S aureus* and *Burkholderia cepacia* from his lungs. A dihydrorhodamine oxidation test shows no shift in fluorescence in response to neutrophil stimulation, confirming the suspected diagnosis of chronic granulomatous disease. All of the following would be potentially considered for initial treatment in this patient EXCEPT:

A. Glucocorticoids
B. Infliximab
C. Interferon-γ
D. Prophylactic itraconazole
E. Prophylactic trimethoprim-sulfamethoxazole

II-153. A patient with longstanding HIV infection, alcoholism, and asthma is seen in the emergency room for 1–2 days of severe wheezing. He has not been taking any medicines for months. He is admitted to the hospital and treated with nebulized therapy and systemic glucocorticoids. His CD4 count is 8 and viral load is >750,000. His total white blood cell (WBC) count is 5200 cells/μL with 90% neutrophils. He is accepted into an inpatient substance abuse rehabilitation program and before discharge is started on opportunistic infection prophylaxis, bronchodilators, a prednisone taper over 2 weeks, ranitidine, and highly active antiretroviral therapy. The rehabilitation center pages you 2 weeks later; a routine laboratory check reveals a total WBC count of 900 cells/μL with 5% neutrophils. Which of the following new drugs would most likely explain this patient's neutropenia?

A. Darunavir
B. Efavirenz
C. Ranitidine
D. Prednisone
E. Trimethoprim-sulfamethoxazole

Questions II-154 through II-158. For each patient below, choose the most likely peripheral blood smear.

II-154. A 22-year-old man with a hematocrit of 17%. He has sickle cell disease and is admitted with a vaso-occlusive crisis after an upper respiratory illness.

II-155. A 36-year-old woman with a hematocrit of 32%. She had a splenectomy 5 years ago after a motor vehicle accident.

II-156. A 55-year-old man with a hematocrit of 28%. He has advanced alcoholic liver disease with cirrhosis and is awaiting liver transplantation.

II-157. A 64-year-old woman with a hematocrit of 28%. She has heme-positive stool and a 2-cm adenomatous colonic polyp at colonoscopy.

II-158. A 72-year-old man a hematocrit of 33%. Four years ago, he received a mechanical prosthetic aortic valve because of aortic stenosis due to a congenital bicuspid valve.

A.

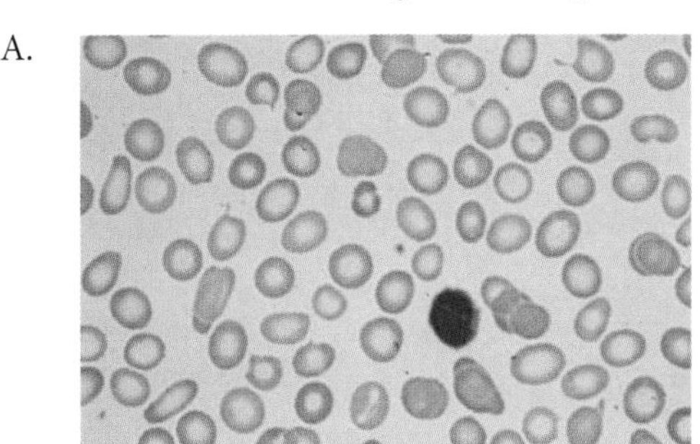

B.

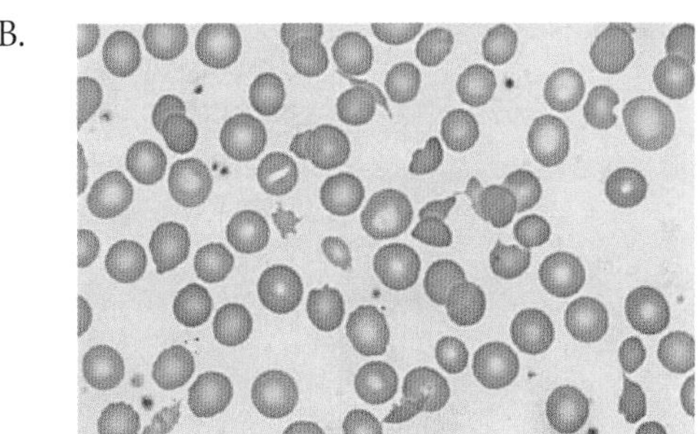

C.

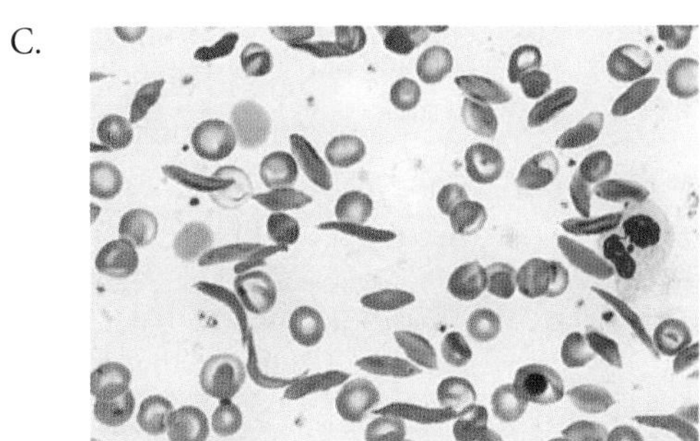

D.

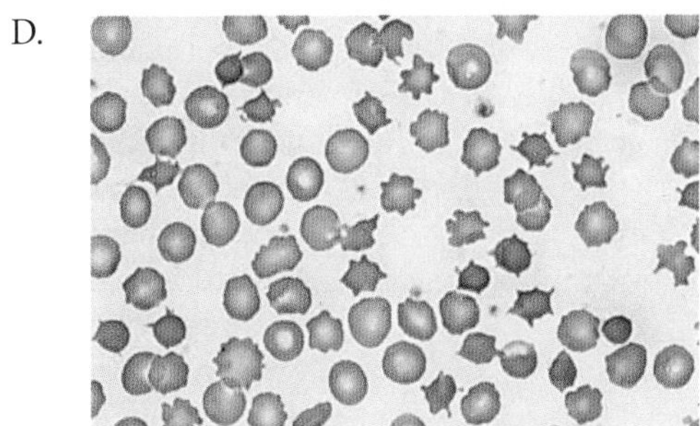

E.

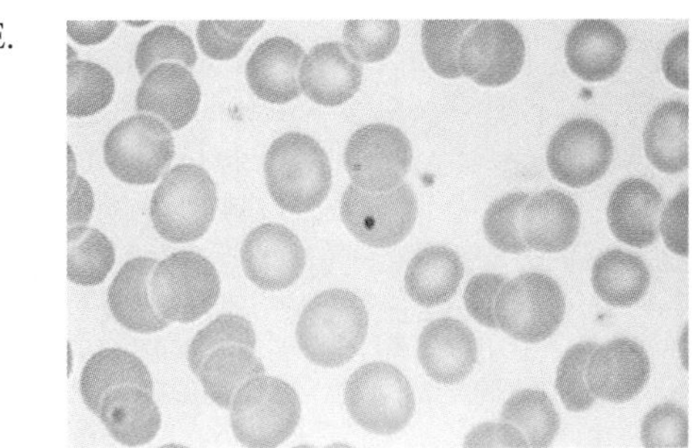

ANSWERS

II-1. **The answer is A.** *(Chap. 18)* When intense, repeated, or prolonged stimuli are applied to damaged or inflamed tissues, the threshold for activating primary afferent nociceptors (pain receptors) is lowered, and the frequency of firing is higher for all stimulus intensities. This process is called *sensitization*. Inflammatory mediators such as bradykinin, nerve-growth factor, some prostaglandins, and leukotrienes contribute to this process. Following injury and resultant sensitization, normally innocuous stimuli can produce pain (termed allodynia). Sensitization is a clinically important process that contributes to tenderness, soreness, and hyperalgesia (increased pain intensity in response to the same noxious stimulus; e.g., moderate pressure causes severe pain). A striking example of sensitization is the significant pain caused by minimal stimulus (light touch or shower) on sunburned skin. Sensitization is of particular importance for pain and tenderness in deep tissues. Viscera are normally relatively insensitive to noxious mechanical and thermal stimuli, although hollow viscera do generate significant discomfort when distended. In contrast, when affected by a disease process with an inflammatory component, deep structures such as joints or hollow viscera characteristically become exquisitely sensitive to mechanical stimulation.

II-2. **The answer is C.** *(Chap. 18)* Substance P is released from primary afferent nociceptors and has multiple biologic activities. It is a potent vasodilator, degranulates mast cells, is a chemoattractant for leukocytes, and increases the production and release of inflammatory mediators. Interestingly, depletion of substance P from joints reduces the severity of experimental arthritis. Phosphodiesterase inhibitors increase intracellular concentration of cyclic guanosine monophosphate (cGMP) or cyclic adenosine monophosphate (cAMP).

II-3. **The answer is D.** *(Chap. 18)* Peripheral neuropathic pain, which is typical in longstanding diabetes and postherpetic neuralgia, typically has an unusual burning, tingling, or electric shock–like quality and may be triggered by very light touch. These features are rare in other types of pain. Peripheral neuropathic pain will not radiate to other areas. On examination, a sensory deficit is characteristically present in the area of the patient's pain. Hyperpathia, a greatly exaggerated pain sensation to innocuous or mild nociceptive stimuli, is also characteristic of neuropathic pain; patients often complain that the very lightest moving stimulus evokes exquisite pain (allodynia). In this regard, it is of clinical interest that a topical preparation of 5% lidocaine in patch form is effective for patients with postherpetic neuralgia who have prominent allodynia.

II-4. **The answer is C.** *(Chap. 18)* This patient has complex regional pain syndrome. Patients with peripheral nerve injury occasionally develop spontaneous pain in the region innervated by the nerve. This pain is often described as having a burning quality. The pain typically begins after a delay of hours to days or even weeks and is accompanied by swelling of the extremity, periarticular bone loss, and arthritic changes in the distal joints. The pain may be relieved by a local anesthetic block of the sympathetic innervation to the affected extremity. Damaged primary afferent nociceptors acquire adrenergic sensitivity and can be activated by stimulation of the sympathetic outflow. This constellation of spontaneous pain and signs of sympathetic dysfunction following injury has been termed complex regional pain syndrome (CRPS). When this occurs after an identifiable nerve injury, it is termed CRPS type II (also known as posttraumatic neuralgia or, if severe, causalgia). When a similar clinical picture appears without obvious nerve injury, it is termed CRPS type I (also known as reflex sympathetic dystrophy). CRPS can be produced by a variety of injuries, including fractures of bone, soft tissue trauma, myocardial infarction, and stroke. CRPS type I typically resolves with symptomatic treatment; however, when it persists, detailed examination often reveals evidence of peripheral nerve injury. Although the pathophysiology of CRPS is poorly understood, the pain and the signs of inflammation, when acute, can be rapidly relieved by blocking the sympathetic nervous system. This implies that sympathetic activity can activate undamaged nociceptors when inflammation is present. Signs of sympathetic hyperactivity should be sought in patients with posttraumatic pain and inflammation and no other obvious explanation. Acute gonococcal arthritis and gout will have a focal joint fluid collection and inflammation. Systemic lupus can manifest in cryptic joint findings, but in this case, the focality and absence of systemic findings or serologic abnormalities make it less likely. Carpal tunnel syndrome, caused by injury to the median nerve, is not consistent with this presentation of the entire arm.

II-5. **The answer is D.** *(Chap. 18)* Nonsteroidal anti-inflammatory drugs (NSAIDs) and aspirin inhibit cyclooxygenase (COX) and have anti-inflammatory actions. They are particularly effective for mild to moderate headache and for pain of musculoskeletal origin. Because they are effective for these common types of pain and are available without prescription, COX inhibitors are by far the most commonly used analgesics. With chronic use, gastric irritation is a common side effect of aspirin and NSAIDs and is the problem that most frequently limits the dose that can be given. Gastric irritation is most severe with aspirin, which may cause erosion and ulceration of the gastric mucosa, leading to bleeding or perforation. Because aspirin irreversibly acetylates platelet cyclooxygenase and thereby interferes with coagulation of the blood, gastrointestinal bleeding is a particular risk. Older age and history of gastrointestinal disease increase the risks of aspirin and NSAIDs. In addition to the well-known gastrointestinal toxicity of NSAIDs, nephrotoxicity is a significant problem for patients using these drugs on a chronic basis. Patients at risk for renal insufficiency, particularly those with significant contraction of their intravascular volume as occurs with chronic diuretic use or acute hypovolemia, should be monitored closely. NSAIDs can also increase blood pressure in some individuals. Long-term treatment with NSAIDs requires regular blood pressure monitoring and treatment if necessary. There are two major classes of COX: COX-1 is constitutively expressed, and COX-2 is induced in the inflammatory state. COX-2–selective drugs have similar analgesic potency and produce less gastric irritation than the nonselective COX inhibitors. The use of COX-2–selective drugs does not appear to lower the risk of nephrotoxicity compared to nonselective NSAIDs. On the other hand, COX-2–selective drugs offer a significant benefit in the management of acute postoperative pain because they do not affect blood coagulation. Nonselective COX inhibitors are usually contraindicated postoperatively because they impair platelet-mediated blood clotting and are thus associated with increased bleeding at the operative site. COX-2 inhibitors, including celecoxib (Celebrex), are associated with increased cardiovascular risk. It appears that this is a class effect of NSAIDs, excluding aspirin. These drugs are contraindicated in patients in the immediate period after coronary artery bypass surgery and should be used with caution in elderly patients and those with a history of or significant risk factors for cardiovascular disease.

II-6. **The answer is E.** *(Chap. 18)* Opioids, such as oxycodone, work centrally and may cause significant respiratory depression and sedation. Because of the hypoventilation, hypoxemia is common although easily treated with supplemental oxygen. Naloxone is an opioid antagonist that may rapidly reverse the respiratory depression and sedation. Alvimopan is an oral opioid antagonist that is confined to the gut. It may be useful to counteract peripheral opioid side effects, such as constipation, but has no central actions. Albuterol is a β-agonist that may increase respiratory rate but will not reverse the opioid sedation. Flumazenil is a γ-aminobutyric acid (GABA) receptor antagonist that can be used for benzodiazepine overdose. *N*-Acetylcysteine is used for acetaminophen overdose. Many forms of oxycodone also include acetaminophen, so the clinician should be careful to elicit an accurate medication history because of the possibility of concurrent acetaminophen-induced liver toxicity.

II-7. **The answer is C.** *(Chap. 19)* The evaluation of nontraumatic chest discomfort relies heavily on the clinical history and physical examination to direct subsequent diagnostic testing. The evaluating clinician should assess the quality, location (including radiation), and pattern (including onset and duration) of the pain as well as any provoking or alleviating factors (Figure II-7). The presence of associated symptoms may also be useful in establishing a diagnosis. The quality of chest discomfort alone is never sufficient to establish a diagnosis. However, the characteristics of the pain are pivotal in formulating an initial clinical impression and assessing the likelihood of a serious cardiopulmonary process, including acute coronary syndrome in particular. Interestingly, radiation to the right arm

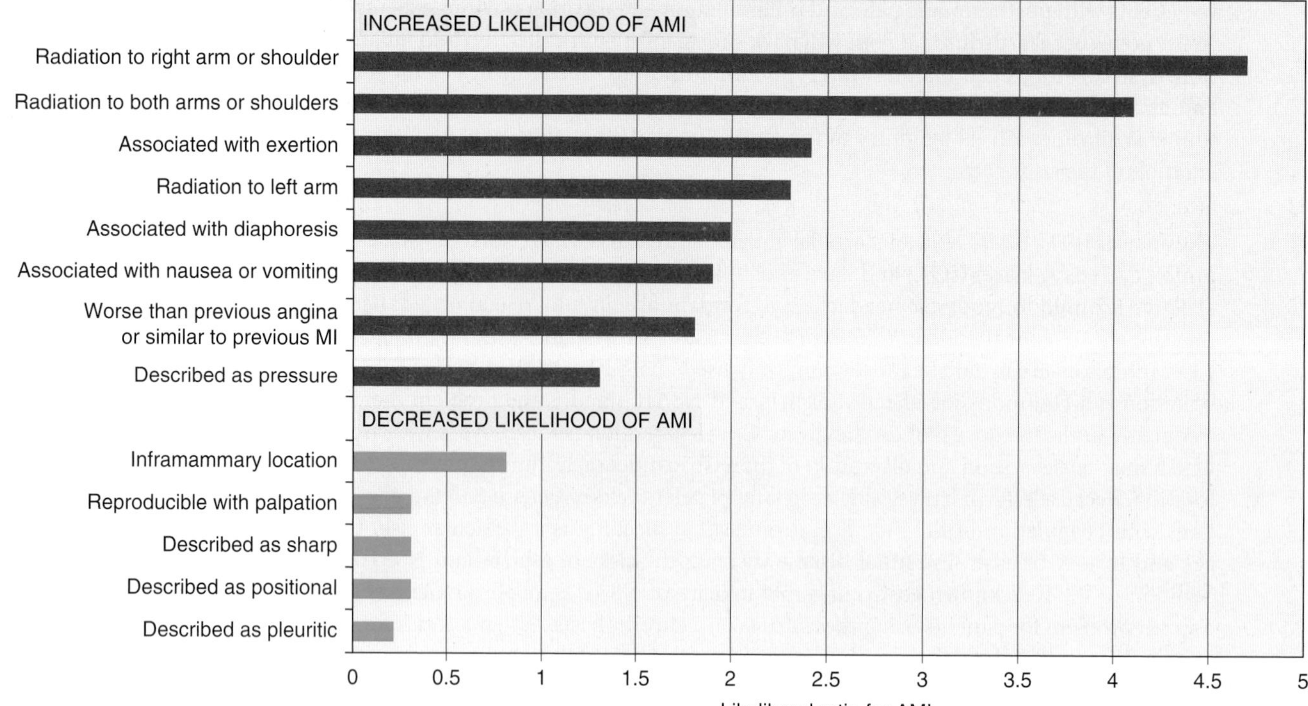

FIGURE II-7 Association of chest pain characteristics with the probability of acute myocardial infarction (AMI). MI, myocardial infarction. Figure prepared from data in CJ Swap, JT Nagurney: *JAMA* 294:2623, 2005.

has a greater likelihood of being related to acute coronary syndrome than radiation to the left arm. Of the factors listed, only positional quality of pain (which is often typical of pericardial inflammatory disease) lessens the likelihood of acute coronary syndrome. This patient has a high risk given his past medical history and acute complaints.

II-8. **The answer is B.** *(Chap. 19)* Chest discomfort is the third most common reason for visits to the emergency department (ED) in the United States, resulting in 6–7 million emergency visits each year. More than 60% of patients with this presentation are hospitalized for further testing, and the rest undergo additional investigation in the ED. Fewer than 25% of evaluated patients are eventually diagnosed with acute coronary syndrome (ACS), with rates of 5%–15% in most series of unselected populations. In the remainder, the most common diagnoses are gastrointestinal causes (Figure II-8), and fewer than 10% are other life-threatening cardiopulmonary conditions. In a large proportion of patients with transient

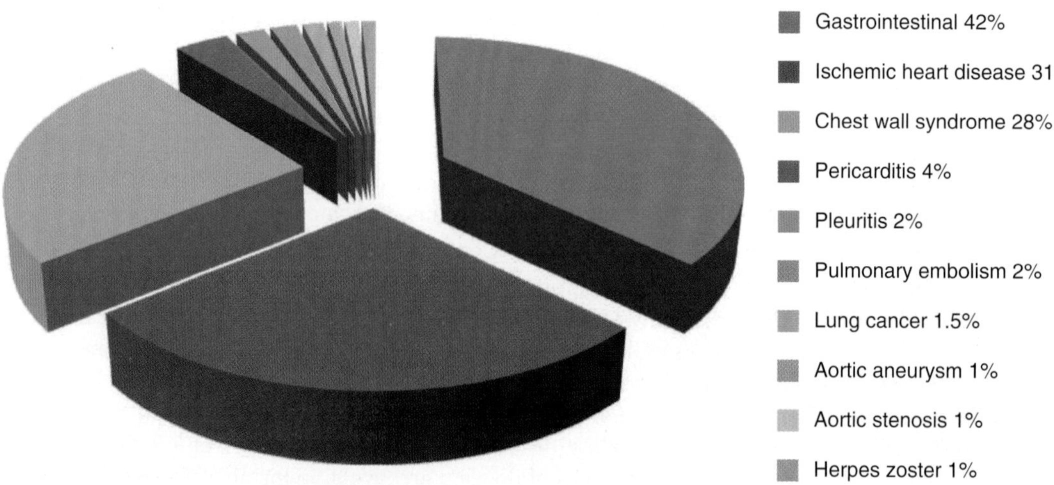

FIGURE II-8 Distribution of final discharge diagnoses in patients with nontraumatic acute chest pain. Figure prepared from data in P Fruergaard et al: *Eur Heart J* 17:1028, 1996.

acute chest discomfort, ACS or another acute cardiopulmonary cause is excluded but the cause is not determined. A disconcerting 2%–6% of patients with chest discomfort of presumed nonischemic etiology who are discharged from the ED are later deemed to have had a missed myocardial infarction (MI). Patients with a missed diagnosis of MI have a 30-day risk of death that is double that of their counterparts who are hospitalized.

II-9. **The answer is D.** *(Chap. 20)* The pain of parietal peritoneal inflammation is steady and aching in character and is located directly over the inflamed area, its exact reference being possible because it is transmitted by somatic nerves supplying the parietal peritoneum. The pain of peritoneal inflammation is invariably accentuated by pressure or changes in tension of the peritoneum, whether produced by palpation or by movement such as with coughing or sneezing. The patient with peritonitis characteristically lies quietly in bed, preferring to avoid motion, in contrast to the patient with colic, who may be thrashing in discomfort. Obstruction of hollow viscera classically elicits intermittent or colicky abdominal pain that is not as well localized as the pain of parietal peritoneal irritation. However, the absence of cramping discomfort should not be misleading because distention of a hollow viscus may also produce steady pain with only rare paroxysms. A frequent misconception is that pain due to intra-abdominal vascular disturbances is sudden and catastrophic in nature. Certain disease processes, such as embolism or thrombosis of the superior mesenteric artery or impending rupture of an abdominal aortic aneurysm, can certainly be associated with diffuse, severe pain. Yet, just as frequently, the patient with occlusion of the superior mesenteric artery only has mild continuous or cramping diffuse pain for 2 or 3 days before vascular collapse or findings of peritoneal inflammation appear. The early, seemingly insignificant discomfort is caused by hyperperistalsis rather than peritoneal inflammation. The absence of tenderness and rigidity in the presence of continuous, diffuse pain (e.g., "pain out of proportion to physical findings") in a patient likely to have vascular disease is quite characteristic of occlusion of the superior mesenteric artery. Pain arising from the abdominal wall is usually constant and aching. Movement, prolonged standing, and pressure accentuate the discomfort and associated muscle spasm. In the case of hematoma of the rectus sheath, now most frequently encountered in association with anticoagulant therapy, a mass may be present in the lower quadrants of the abdomen.

II-10. **The answer is B.** *(Chap. 20)* Of the causes listed, pelvic inflammatory disease causes pain due to parietal peritoneal inflammation, plus the patient is at risk with her sexual activity with multiple partners. Acute cholecystitis causes pain by distension of the gallbladder viscera. Sudden distention of the biliary tree produces a steady rather than colicky type of pain; hence, the term biliary colic is misleading. Acute distention of the gallbladder usually causes pain in the right upper quadrant with radiation to the right posterior region of the thorax or to the tip of the right scapula, but it is also not uncommonly found near the midline. Distention of the common bile duct often causes epigastric pain that may radiate to the upper lumbar region. Considerable variation is common, however, so that differentiation between these may be impossible. Rectus sheath hematoma causes pain related to abdominal wall distension. Small bowel obstruction often presents as poorly localized, intermittent periumbilical or supraumbilical pain. As the intestine progressively dilates and loses muscular tone, the colicky nature of the pain may diminish. With superimposed strangulating obstruction, pain may spread to the lower lumbar region if there is traction on the root of the mesentery.

II-11. **The answer is E.** *(Chap. 21)* The patient who presents with a new, severe headache has a differential diagnosis that is quite different from the patient with recurrent headaches over many years. In new-onset and severe headache, the probability of finding a potentially serious cause is considerably greater than in recurrent headache (Table II-11). Patients with recent onset of pain require prompt evaluation and appropriate treatment. Serious causes to be considered include meningitis, subarachnoid hemorrhage, epidural or subdural hematoma, glaucoma, tumor, and purulent sinusitis. When worrisome symptoms and signs are present, rapid diagnosis and management are critical. A careful neurologic examination is an essential first step in the evaluation. In most cases, patients with an abnormal examination or a history of recent-onset headache should be evaluated by a computed tomography (CT) or magnetic resonance imaging (MRI) study. As an initial screening procedure for intracranial pathology in this setting, CT and MRI methods

TABLE II-11 Headache Symptoms That Suggest a Serious Underlying Disorder

Sudden-onset headache
First severe headache
"Worst headache ever"
Vomiting that precedes headache
Subacute worsening over days or weeks
Pain induced by bending, lifting, cough
Pain that disturbs sleep or presents immediately upon awakening
Known systemic illness
Onset after age 55
Fever or unexplained systemic signs
Abnormal neurologic examination
Pain associated with local tenderness, e.g., region of temporal artery

appear to be equally sensitive. Brain tumor is a rare cause of headache and even less commonly a cause of severe pain. The vast majority of patients presenting with severe headache have a benign cause.

II-12. **The answer is E.** *(Chap. 22)* Radicular pain is typically sharp and radiates from the low back to a leg within the territory of a nerve root (Table II-12). Coughing, sneezing, or voluntary contraction of abdominal muscles (lifting heavy objects or straining at stool) may elicit the radiating pain. The pain may increase in postures that stretch the nerves and nerve roots. Sitting with the leg outstretched places traction on the sciatic nerve and L5 and S1 roots because the nerve passes posterior to the hip. The femoral nerve (L2, L3, and L4 roots) passes anterior to the hip and is not stretched by sitting. The straight-leg raising (SLR) maneuver is a simple bedside test for nerve root disease. With the patient supine, passive flexion of the extended leg at the hip stretches the L5 and S1 nerve roots and the sciatic nerve. Passive dorsiflexion of the foot during the maneuver adds to the stretch. In healthy individuals, flexion to at least 80 degrees is normally possible without

TABLE II-12 Lumbosacral Radiculopathy: Neurologic Features

	Examination Findings			
Lumbosacral Nerve Roots	Reflex	Sensory	Motor	Pain Distribution
L2[a]	—	Upper anterior thigh	Psoas (hip flexors)	Anterior thigh
L3[a]	—	Lower anterior thigh	Psoas (hip flexors)	Anterior thigh, knee
		Anterior knee	Quadriceps (knee extensors)	
			Thigh adductors	
L4[a]	Quadriceps (knee)	Medial calf	Quadriceps (knee extensors)[b]	Knee, medial calf
			Thigh adductors	Anterolateral thigh
L5[c]	—	Dorsal surface—foot	Peronei (foot evertors)[b]	Lateral calf, dorsal foot, posterolateral thigh, buttocks
		Lateral calf	Tibialis anterior (foot dorsiflexors)	
			Gluteus medius (hip abductors)	
			Toe dorsiflexors	
S1[c]	Gastrocnemius/soleus (ankle)	Plantar surface—foot	Gastrocnemius/soleus (foot plantar flexors)[b]	Bottom foot, posterior calf, posterior thigh, buttocks
		Lateral aspect—foot	Abductor hallucis (toe flexors)[b]	
			Gluteus maximus (hip extensors)	

[a]Reverse straight-leg raising sign present—see "Examination of the Back."
[b]These muscles receive the majority of innervation from this root.
[c]Straight-leg raising sign present.

causing pain, although a tight, stretching sensation in the hamstring muscles is common. The SLR test is positive if the maneuver reproduces the patient's usual back or limb pain. The patient may describe pain in the low back, buttocks, posterior thigh, or lower leg, but the key feature is reproduction of the patient's usual pain. The crossed SLR sign is present when flexion of one leg reproduces the usual pain in the opposite leg or buttocks. In disk herniation, the crossed SLR sign is less sensitive but more specific than the SLR sign. The reverse SLR sign is elicited by standing the patient next to the examination table and passively extending each leg with the knee fully extended. This maneuver, which stretches the L2–L4 nerve roots, lumbosacral plexus, and femoral nerve, is considered positive if the patient's usual back or limb pain is reproduced. For all of these tests, the nerve or nerve root lesion is always on the side of the pain.

II-13. The answer is B. *(Chap. 22)* The prognosis for acute low back and leg pain with radiculopathy due to disk herniation is generally favorable, with most patients showing substantial improvement over months. Serial imaging studies suggest spontaneous regression of the herniated portion of the disk in two-thirds of patients over 6 months. Nonetheless, there are several important treatment options to provide symptomatic relief while this natural healing process unfolds. Resumption of normal activity is recommended. Randomized trial evidence suggests that bed rest is ineffective for treating sciatica as well as back pain alone. Acetaminophen and NSAIDs are useful for pain relief, although severe pain may require short courses of opioid analgesics. Epidural glucocorticoid injections have a role in providing temporary symptom relief for sciatica due to a herniated disk. However, there does not appear to be a benefit in terms of reducing subsequent surgical interventions. Surgical intervention is indicated for patients who have progressive motor weakness due to nerve root injury demonstrated on clinical examination or electromyography (EMG).

II-14 and II-15. The answers are C and B, respectively. *(Chap. 22)* Lumbar spinal stenosis (LSS) describes a narrowed lumbar spinal canal and is frequently asymptomatic. Typical is neurogenic claudication, consisting of back and buttock or leg pain induced by walking or standing and relieved by sitting. Symptoms in the legs are usually bilateral. Unlike vascular claudication, symptoms are often provoked by standing without walking. Unlike lumbar disk disease, symptoms are usually relieved by sitting. Patients with neurogenic claudication can often walk much farther when leaning over a shopping cart and can pedal a stationary bike with ease while sitting. These flexed positions increase the anteroposterior spinal canal diameter and reduce intraspinal venous hypertension, resulting in pain relief. Focal weakness, sensory loss, or reflex changes may occur when spinal stenosis is associated with neural foraminal narrowing and radiculopathy. Severe neurologic deficits, including paralysis and urinary incontinence, occur only rarely. LSS by itself is frequently asymptomatic, and the correlation between the severity of symptoms and degree of stenosis of the spinal canal is variable. Conservative treatment of symptomatic LSS includes NSAIDs, acetaminophen, exercise programs, and symptomatic treatment of acute pain episodes. Surgical therapy is considered when medical therapy does not relieve symptoms sufficiently to allow for resumption of activities of daily living or when focal neurologic signs are present. Most patients with neurogenic claudication who are treated medically do not improve over time. Surgical management can produce significant relief of back and leg pain within 6 weeks, and pain relief persists for at least 2 years. However, up to one-quarter of patients develop recurrent stenosis at the same spinal level or an adjacent level 7–10 years after the initial surgery; recurrent symptoms usually respond to a second surgical decompression. There is insufficient evidence to support the routine use of epidural glucocorticoid injections.

II-16 and II-17. The answers are A and C, respectively. *(Chap. 22)* Surveys in the United States indicate that patients with back pain have reported progressively worse functional limitations in recent years, despite rapid increases in spine imaging, opioid prescribing, injections, and spine surgery. This suggests that more selective use of diagnostic and treatment modalities may be appropriate. Spine imaging often reveals abnormalities of dubious clinical relevance that may alarm clinicians and patients and prompt further testing and unnecessary therapy. Both randomized trials and observational studies have suggested a "cascade effect" of imaging, which may create a gateway to other unnecessary care. Based in part on such evidence, the American College of Physicians has made parsimonious spine imaging a high priority in its "Choosing Wisely" campaign, aimed at reducing unnecessary care. Successful efforts to reduce unnecessary imaging have included physician education by clinical leaders, computerized decision support to identify recent imaging tests and eliminate duplication, and requiring an approved indication to order an imaging test. Acute lumbar back pain (ALBP) is defined as pain of <3 months in duration without leg pain. Most patients have purely "mechanical" symptoms (i.e., pain that is aggravated by motion and relieved by rest). The initial assessment excludes serious causes of spine pathology that require urgent intervention including infection, cancer, or trauma (Table II-16). Laboratory and imaging studies are unnecessary if risk factors are absent. CT, MRI, and plain spine films are rarely indicated in the first month of symptoms unless a spine fracture, tumor, or infection is suspected. The prognosis is generally excellent. Many patients do not seek medical care and improve on their own. Even among those seen in primary care, two-thirds report being substantially improved after 7 weeks. This spontaneous improvement can mislead clinicians and researchers about the efficacy of treatment interventions unless subjected to rigorous prospective trials. Many treatments commonly used in the past but now known to be ineffective, including bed rest and lumbar traction, have been largely abandoned. Clinicians should reassure patients that improvement is very likely and instruct them in self-care. Education is an important part of treatment. Evidence-based guidelines recommend over-the-counter medicines such as acetaminophen and NSAIDs as first-line options for treatment of ALBP. Skeletal muscle relaxants, such as cyclobenzaprine or methocarbamol, may be useful, but sedation is a common side effect. Limiting the use of muscle relaxants to night time only may be an option for patients with back pain that interferes with sleep. There is no good evidence to support the use of opioid analgesics or tramadol as first-line therapy for ALBP. Their use is best reserved for patients who cannot tolerate acetaminophen or NSAIDs or for those with severe refractory pain. There is no evidence to support use of oral or injected glucocorticoids for ALBP without radiculopathy. Similarly, therapies for neuropathic pain, such as gabapentin or tricyclic antidepressants, are not indicated for ALBP. Nonpharmacologic treatments for ALBP include spinal manipulation, exercise, physical therapy, massage, acupuncture, transcutaneous electrical nerve stimulation, and ultrasound. Spinal manipulation appears to be roughly equivalent to conventional medical treatments and may be a useful alternative for patients who wish to avoid or who cannot tolerate drug therapy. There is little evidence to support the use of physical therapy, massage, acupuncture, laser therapy, therapeutic ultrasound, corsets, or lumbar traction. Although important for

TABLE II-16 Acute Low Back Pain: Risk Factors for an Important Structural Cause

History
Pain worse at rest or at night
Prior history of cancer
History of chronic infection (especially lung, urinary tract, skin)
History of trauma
Incontinence
Age >70 years
Intravenous drug use
Glucocorticoid use
History of a rapidly progressive neurologic deficit
Examination
Unexplained fever
Unexplained weight loss
Percussion tenderness over the spine
Abdominal, rectal, or pelvic mass
Internal/external rotation of the leg at the hip; heel percussion sign
Straight-leg or reverse straight-leg raising signs
Progressive focal neurologic deficit

chronic pain, back exercises for ALBP are generally not supported by clinical evidence. There is no convincing evidence regarding the value of ice or heat applications for ALBP; however, many patients report temporary symptomatic relief from ice or frozen gel packs, and heat may produce a short-term reduction in pain after the first week.

II-18. The answer is D. *(Chap. 23)* Hyperthermia occurs when exogenous heat exposure or an endogenous heat-producing process, such as neuroleptic malignant syndrome or malignant hyperthermia, leads to high internal temperatures despite a normal hypothalamic temperature set point. Fever occurs when a pyrogen such as a microbial toxin, microbe particle, or cytokine resets the hypothalamus to a higher temperature. A particular temperature cutoff point does not define hyperthermia. Rigidity and autonomic dysregulation are characteristic of malignant hyperthermia, a subset of hyperthermia. Fever, not hyperthermia, responds to antipyretics.

II-19. The answer is C. *(Chap. 23)* The normal daily temperature variation is approximately 0.5°C. However, in individuals recovering from a febrile illness, this daily variation can be as high as 1.0°C. Body temperature has a predictable diurnal variation in normal individuals. The lowest levels on average occur at 6 AM, and the highest levels occur at 4–6 PM. During a febrile illness, the diurnal variation is usually maintained but at higher levels. In women who menstruate, the morning temperature is generally lower in the 2 weeks before ovulation; it then rises by ~0.6°C (1°F) with ovulation and remains at that level until menses occur. Oral temperature may not be an accurate measurement of body core temperature, particularly in low-output states and during hyperventilation.

II-20. The answer is A. *(Chap. 23)* For patients on anticytokine therapy (anti-TNF, anti–IL-1, IL-6, and IL-12), even a low-grade fever is concerning. In nearly all reported cases of infection associated with anticytokine therapy, fever is among the presenting signs. However, the extent to which the febrile response is blunted in these patients remains unknown. Measurement of specific cytokines is not diagnostically useful. A similar situation is seen in patients receiving high-dose glucocorticoid therapy or anti-inflammatory agents such as ibuprofen. Therefore, low-grade fever is of considerable concern in patients receiving anticytokine therapies. The physician should conduct an early and rigorous diagnostic evaluation in these patients and not presume a likely benign cause. The opportunistic infections reported in patients treated with agents that neutralize TNF-α are similar to those reported in the HIV-1–infected population (e.g., a new infection with or reactivation of *Mycobacterium tuberculosis*, with dissemination). Even a negative test for latent *M tuberculosis* does not rule out active tuberculosis as a cause of fever in a patient on anticytokine therapy. There are no data that indicate that antipyretics delay the resolution of viral or bacterial infections.

II-21. The answer is E. *(Chap. 23)* As effective antipyretics, glucocorticoids act at two levels. First, glucocorticoids reduce prostaglandin E2 (PGE2) synthesis by inhibiting the activity of phospholipase A2, which is needed to release arachidonic acid from the cell membrane. Second, glucocorticoids block the transcription of the mRNA for the pyrogenic cytokines. Ibuprofen, aspirin, and celecoxib are all direct cyclooxygenase inhibitors, which in turn reduce the production of PGE2 from the hypothalamic endothelium. Acetaminophen is a poor COX inhibitor in peripheral tissue and lacks noteworthy anti-inflammatory activity; in the brain, however, acetaminophen is oxidized by the P450 cytochrome system, and the oxidized form inhibits COX activity. Moreover, in the brain, the inhibition of another enzyme, COX-3, by acetaminophen may account for the antipyretic effect of this agent.

II-22. The answer is A. *(Chap. 23)* In children, aspirin increases the risk of Reye syndrome and should be avoided except in very select circumstances. It is appropriate to aim for aggressive antipyrexia in patients with underlying impairment in cardiac, pulmonary, or central nervous system (CNS) function. Fever increases the demand for oxygen (for every increase of 1°C over 37°C, there is a 13% increase in oxygen consumption), and for patients with borderline ventilatory function, the increased oxygen demand may precipitate decompensation (option E). For pediatric patients with a history of febrile seizures, aggressive therapy with antipyretics is reasonable, although there is no correlation between absolute temperature elevation and the onset of a febrile seizure in susceptible children (option B). For patients with hyperpyrexia (temperature >40.5°C), the use of cooling blankets can facilitate reduction of temperature, but they must always be used with oral antipyretics (option C). Particularly for patients with CNS disease or trauma, reducing core temperature aggressively can mitigate detrimental effects of high temperature on the brain (option D).

II-23. **The answer is A.** *(Chap. 24)* Based on the characteristic rash and Koplik spots, this patient has measles. A rare but feared complication of measles is subacute sclerosing panencephalitis. His examination does not support epiglottitis as he has no drooling or dysphagia. His rash is not characteristic of acute HIV infection, and he lacks the pharyngitis and arthralgias commonly seen with this diagnosis. The rash is not consistent with herpes zoster, and he is quite young to invoke this diagnosis. Splenic rupture occasionally occurs with infectious mononucleosis, but this patient has no pharyngitis, lymphadenopathy, or splenomegaly to suggest this diagnosis. Due to widespread (and in some cases mandatory) vaccination, measles is very uncommon in the United States (as well as Central and South America); almost all cases are imported. However, countries with lower rates of vaccination still have endemic measles. Recent cases in the United States in unvaccinated children make this an important diagnosis for clinicians to consider in appropriate situations.

II-24. **The answer is C.** *(Chap. 24)* This patient likely has toxic shock syndrome, given the clinical appearance of septic shock with no positive blood cultures. The characteristic diffuse rash, as well as the lack of a primary infected site, make *Staphylococcus* the more likely inciting agent. Streptococcal toxic shock usually has a prominent primary site of infection, but the diffuse rash is usually much more subtle than in this case. Staphylococcal toxic shock can be associated with immunosuppression, surgical wounds, or retained tampons. Mere *Staphylococcus aureus* colonization (with an appropriate toxigenic strain) can incite toxic shock; overt infection is not necessary. Centers for Disease Control and Prevention guidelines state that measles, Rocky Mountain spotted fever, and leptospirosis need to be ruled out serologically to confirm the diagnosis. However, this patient is at very low risk for these diagnoses based on vaccination and travel history. Juvenile rheumatoid arthritis would be a consideration only if the fevers were more prolonged and there was documented evidence of organomegaly and enlarged lymph nodes.

II-25. **The answer is B.** *(Chap. 24)* This case is classic for infection mononucleosis due to Ebstein-Barr virus (EBV). Often confused with streptococcal pharyngitis, it is not unusual for patients with EBV to receive empiric antibiotics. Curiously, 90% of patients with mononucleosis due to EBV develop a rash when given ampicillin. This is one of several groups of patients who have an elevated risk of exanthematous drug eruptions. In another example, 50% of patients with HIV will develop a rash in response to sulfa drugs. Fifth disease, or erythema infectiosum, is due to parvovirus B19 and tends to effect children age 3–12. Nicknamed "slapped cheek disease," it appears after a febrile illness as a bright blanchable erythema on the cheeks ("slapped cheeks") with perioral pallor (option C). The rash of rubeola (measles) starts at the hairline 2–3 days into the illness and moves down the body, typically sparing the palms and soles (option E). Rubella (German measles) also spreads from the hairline downward; unlike that of measles, however, the rash of rubella tends to clear from originally affected areas as it migrates, and it may be pruritic (option D). Chikungunya fever is associated with a maculopapular eruption, but prominently features painful polyarticular arthralgias and is primarily present in Africa and the Indian Ocean regions (option A).

II-26. **The answer is B.** *(Chap. 24)* This patient likely has Rocky Mountain spotted fever (RMSF), which is caused by *Rickettsia rickettsii*. Most common in the southwestern and southeastern United States, it is spread by tick vector. The patient likely was exposed by tick bite when clearing the field; many patients neither notice nor report a history of tick bite. The absence of noted tick exposure should not rule out this serious disease. The rash of RMSF classically begins on the wrists and ankles and spreads centripetally, appearing on palms and soles later in disease. Lesions can evolve from blanchable macules to petechiae. RMSF requires prompt treatment because mortality of the untreated disease is approximately 40%. *Borrelia burgdorferi* causes Lyme disease, which is classically associated with the erythema migrans rash, a papule expanding to an erythematous annular lesion with central clearing. *Spirillum minis* is an etiologic agent of rat-bite fever. Its rash is characterized by an eschar at bite site and then a blotchy violaceous or red-brown rash involving the trunk and extremities. *Salmonella typhi* is the etiologic agent in typhoid fever, which is usually contracted via contaminated food or water (though it is rare in the United States). Its rash usually consists of transient, blanchable erythematous macules and papules, 2–4 mm, usually on the trunk. Finally, although *Vibrio vulnificus* is classically associated with exposure to contaminated saltwater (e.g., raw oysters) and carries a high mortality, its rash is characterized by hemorrhagic bullae. It is often most common in patients with underlying liver disease, diabetes, or renal failure.

II-27. **The answer is C.** *(Chap. 25e)* This is a classic picture of erythema migrans due to *B burgdorferi*, or Lyme disease. The rash is an early manifestation of Lyme disease and is characterized by erythematous annular patches, often with a central erythematous focus at the tick bite site. The sequelae of Lyme disease are myriad and include CNS, articular, and cardiac complications. One of the classic cardiac complications is conduction system disease, most concerning the possibility of progression to complete heart block. Option B describes the classic cutaneous manifestations of Kawasaki disease, most commonly seen in children. When seen in conjunction with painful or nonpainful purpuric lesions on the hands or feet, the murmur of mitral regurgitation would suggest infectious endocarditis (option A). Option D describes a toxic shock syndrome, which is unlikely in this patient with erythema migrans. Option E describes Koplik spots, the pathognomic buccal mucosal finding in measles.

II-28. **The answer is A.** *(Chaps. 24 and 25e)* This patient exhibits classic findings of the drug reaction with eosinophilia and systemic symptoms syndrome (DRESS). Some individuals are genetically unable to detoxify arene oxides present in some anticonvulsants (e.g., phenobarbital) and are susceptible to this dire syndrome. The confluence of this desquamative rash, eosinophilia, hepatic involvement, facial edema, and hypotension are all typical of this disease. Sweet syndrome, or acute febrile neutrophilic dermatosis, is characterized by erythematous indurated plaque with a pseudovesicular border. In 20% of cases, it is associated with malignancy (usually hematologic) but can also be associated with infections, inflammatory bowel disease, or pregnancy. Erythema multiforme is characterized by target lesions (central erythema surrounded by area of clearing and another rim of erythema) up to 2 cm, which are symmetric on the knees, elbows, palms, and soles and spread centripetally. It is often confused with Stevens-Johnson syndrome, although erythema multiforme lacks the marked skin sloughing seen in Stevens-Johnson syndrome. *Staphylococcus* toxic shock syndrome is a consideration here, as the hypotension and skin rash are typical. However, the lack of a cutaneous lesion or other risk factors and the concomitant eosinophilia and hepatitis make DRESS the more likely diagnosis.

II-29. **The answer is C.** *(Chaps. 24 and 25e)* This is erythema nodosum, a panniculitis classically found on the lower extremities characterized by exquisitely tender nodules and plaques. It has several associated disease etiologies including infections (streptococcal, fungal, mycobacterial, yersinial), drugs (sulfas, penicillins, oral contraceptives), sarcoidosis, and other autoimmune diseases such as inflammatory bowel disease. Lung cancer is not a classically associated disease for erythema nodosum.

II-30. **The answer is D.** *(Chap. 26)* Many clinicians incorrectly employ the term fever of unknown origin (FUO), using it to mean any fever without an initially obvious etiology. However, the term FUO connotes a very specific set of criteria and should be reserved for prolonged febrile illnesses without an established etiology despite intensive evaluation and diagnostic testing. These criteria are:

1. Fever >38.3°C (101°F) on at least two occasions
2. Illness duration of ≥3 weeks
3. No known immunocompromised state

4. Diagnosis that remains uncertain after a thorough history taking, physical examination, and the following obligatory investigations: determination of erythrocyte sedimentation rate (ESR) and C-reactive protein (CRP) level; platelet count; leukocyte count and differential; measurement of levels of hemoglobin, electrolytes, creatinine, total protein, alkaline phosphatase, alanine aminotransferase, aspartate aminotransferase, lactate dehydrogenase, creatine kinase, ferritin, antinuclear antibodies, and rheumatoid factor; protein electrophoresis; urinalysis; blood cultures (n = 3); urine culture; chest x-ray; abdominal ultrasonography; and tuberculin skin test (TST)

Only the patient described in option D meets these criteria. The patient described in option A meets criteria for a diagnosis of systemic lupus erythematosus, so the etiology is not unknown for her fever. The patient described in option B is no longer having fevers, and his duration of febrile illness was not >3 weeks. The patient in option C has no objective evidence of fever and has not undergone any of the obligatory evaluations for obvious etiologies. The patient in option E is immunocompromised. These patients' workup requires an entirely different diagnostic and therapeutic approach, and they are not included in the diagnosis of FUO.

II-31. **The answer is A.** *(Chap. 26)* Studies of FUO have shown that a diagnosis is more likely in elderly patients than in younger age groups. In many cases, FUO in the elderly results from an atypical manifestation of a common disease, among which giant cell arteritis and polymyalgia rheumatica are most frequently involved. Tuberculosis is the most common infectious disease associated with FUO in elderly patients, occurring much more often than in younger patients. Because many of these diseases are treatable, it is well worth pursuing the cause of fever in elderly patients. In Western countries, infection is the most common single cause of FUO, at 22% of cases, but remains far less common than in non-Western countries (43%) (option C). As diagnostic serologic and imaging techniques improve, many patients who previously would have remained undiagnosed for >3 weeks (and thus qualified for an FUO diagnosis) are now being diagnosed earlier. Thus, the patients who remain febrile beyond 3 weeks have a greater chance of remaining undiagnosed than in previous decades (option E). Fortunately, patients with FUO who remain ultimately undiagnosed have a good prognosis (option D). In one study, none of 37 FUO patients without a diagnosis died during a follow-up period of at least 6 months; 4 of 36 patients with a diagnosis died during follow-up due to infection (n = 1) or malignancy (n = 3). In general, FUO is more often caused by an unusual presentation of a common disease than by a usual presentation of a very rare disease (option B).

II-32. **The answer is C.** *(Chap. 26)* FUO is defined as the presence of fevers >38.3°C (101.0°F) on several occasions occurring for >3 weeks without a defined cause after appropriate investigation into potential causes have failed to yield a diagnosis. Initial laboratory investigation into an FUO should include a complete blood count with differential, peripheral blood smear, ESR, CRP, electrolytes, creatinine, calcium, liver function tests, urinalysis, and muscle enzymes. In addition, specific testing for a variety of infections should be performed, including Venereal Disease Research Laboratory (VDRL) test for syphilis; HIV, cytomegalovirus (CMV), EBV, and positive protein derivative (PPD) testing; and blood, sputum, and urine cultures, if appropriate. Finally, the workup should include evaluation for inflammatory disorders. These tests include antinuclear antibodies, rheumatoid factor, ferritin, iron, and transferrin. This patient has had a significant workup that has demonstrated primarily nonspecific findings, including elevation in the erythrocyte sedimentation rate and ferritin as well as borderline enlargement of multiple lymph nodes. The only finding that may help define further workup is the elevation in calcium levels. When combined with the clinical symptoms and prominent lymph nodes, this could suggest granulomatous diseases, including disseminated tuberculosis, fungal infections, or sarcoidosis. The next step in the workup of this patient would be to obtain a sample from an enlarged lymph node for cultures and pathology to confirm granulomatous inflammation and provide additional samples for microbiology. In recent studies, up to 30% of individuals will not have an identified cause of FUO, and infectious etiologies continue to comprise approximately 25% of all FUO in the United States. The most common infection causing FUO is extrapulmonary tuberculosis, which may be difficult to diagnose because PPD is often negative in these individuals. However, one would not consider empirical therapy if the possibility to obtain definitive diagnosis exists through a procedure such as a needle biopsy because it is prudent to have not only the diagnosis but also the sensitivity profile of the organism to ensure appropriate therapy. Even in the presence of granulomatous infection, sarcoidosis would be considered a diagnosis of exclusion and would require definitive negative mycobacterial cultures prior to considering therapy with corticosteroids. Serum angiotensin-converting enzyme levels are neither appropriately sensitive nor specific for diagnosis of sarcoidosis and should not be used to determine if therapy is needed. PET-CT imaging would be unlikely to be helpful to diagnose malignancy in this situation as the presence of granulomatous inflammation can lead to false-positive results or will confirm the presence of already characterized abnormal lymph nodes.

II-33. The answer is A. *(Chap. 28)* Dizziness is a common but imprecise symptom that may include vertigo, light-headedness, faintness, and imbalance. Patients often have difficulty distinguishing these various symptoms, and the quality of dizziness does not reliably reflect the underlying cause. Distinguishing between dangerous and benign causes as well as between peripheral and central causes of dizziness is critical. Dangerous causes of dizziness include arrhythmia and stroke. The duration of symptoms can be helpful. Causes of brief episodes of dizziness lasting seconds include benign paroxysmal position vertigo and orthostatic hypotension. Longer lasting dizziness can be caused by either peripheral or central disease such as vestibular migraine, Meniere disease, or transient ischemic attack (TIA)/stroke in the posterior circulation. The cause of dizziness can be clarified by the company it keeps. Unilateral hearing loss or other aural symptoms (ear pain, pressure, fullness) suggest a peripheral cause. Neurologic findings such as diplopia, paresthesias or limb ataxia suggest a central cause. The head impulse test assesses the vestibulo-ocular reflex (VOR). The head impulse sign is positive if the VOR is deficient and suggests vestibular hypofunction. In this case, the absence of a head impulse sign in a patient with acute prolonged vertigo suggests a central, not peripheral, cause of her dizziness. Further, this patient has multiple risk factors for stroke including tobacco use, dyslipidemia, hypertension, and diabetes. Therefore, brain MRI is the next most appropriate step. Vestibular suppressant therapy (meclizine) or glucocorticoid therapy would not be appropriate. Although the Dix-Hallpike maneuver worsened her dizziness, no nystagmus was observed. The critical finding in a positive test is transient upbeating torsional nystagmus and not the subjective experience of dizziness. Because her presentation is not consistent with benign paroxysmal positional vertigo (BPPV), the Epley maneuver is not appropriate.

II-34. The answer is E. *(Chap. 28)* Vertigo describes a perceived sense of spinning or other motion. Vestibular causes of vertigo may be caused by peripheral lesions affecting the labyrinths or the vestibular nerves or caused by disease in the central vestibular pathways. Peripheral lesions usually present with unidirectional horizontal nystagmus. Although conjugate horizontal jerk nystagmus may be seen in either peripheral or central causes of vertigo, all of the other forms of nystagmus implicate a central etiology. Downbeat nystagmus is a pure vertical nystagmus associated with cerebellar disease. Gaze-evoked nystagmus describes nystagmus that changes direction with gaze. It is characteristic of cerebellar disease. Rebound nystagmus is a type of primary position nystagmus provoked by eccentric gaze. It is found in cerebellar or brainstem disease. Pure torsional nystagmus is also a central sign.

II-35. The answer is C. *(Chap. 28)* Bilateral defects in the vestibular system can cause both imbalance and oscillopsia. The head impulse test is a bedside assessment of the VOR used to assess vestibular hypofunction. In the test, the patient fixates on a target while the examiner rapidly rotates the head. When the VOR is intact, a patient is able to maintain focused gaze despite head movements to the side. When the VOR is deficient, the eyes deviate with the head movement, and a corrective saccade opposite in direction to the head movement returns the eyes to the focus point. In this case, injury to the peripheral vestibular system is suggested by the bilaterally abnormal head impulse test. Of the listed drugs, gentamicin is most associated with vestibular toxicity.

II-36. The answer is E. *(Chap. 29)* Fatigue describes the near universal human experience of weariness or exhaustion. Fatigue may be a nonspecific manifestation of psychiatric disease, neurologic disease, sleep disorders, endocrine disorders, kidney or liver disease, rheumatologic disorders, infection, malignancy, anemia, obesity, malnutrition, pregnancy, or diseases of unclear cause. A suggested approach to screening includes a complete blood count with differential, electrolytes, glucose, renal function, liver function, and thyroid function tests. Testing for HIV and adrenal function can also be considered. However, extensive laboratory testing infrequently identifies the cause of chronic fatigue and may more often lead to false-positive findings and prolonged workups. Because low-titer positive antinuclear antibodies (ANAs) are not uncommon in otherwise healthy adults, ANA testing is unlikely to be helpful in isolation. Electromyography with nerve conduction studies may have a role if the presence of muscle weakness cannot be determined by physical examination. Testing for viral or bacterial infections is often unhelpful. Although complete resolution of fatigue is uncommon, longitudinal and multidisciplinary follow-up sometimes identifies a previously undiagnosed serious cause of chronic fatigue.

II-37. **The answer is D.** *(Chap. 30)* Complaints of weakness in a patient have a multitude of causes, and it is important to perform a thorough history and physical examination to help localize the site of weakness. Lower motor neuron diseases occur when there is destruction of the cell bodies of the lower motor neurons in the brainstem or the anterior horn of the spinal cord. Lower motor neuron diseases can also occur due to direct axonal dysfunction and demyelination. The primary presenting symptoms are those of distal muscle weakness such as tripping or decreased hand grip strength. When a motor neuron becomes diseased, it may discharge spontaneously, leading to muscle fasciculations that are not seen in disease of the upper motor neurons or myopathies. Additionally, on physical examination, lower motor neuron disease leads to decreases in muscle tone and decreased or absent deep tendon reflexes. Over time, severe muscle atrophy can occur. A Babinski sign should not be present. If there is evidence of a Babinski sign in the presence of lower motor neuron disease, this should raise the suspicion of a disorder affecting both upper and lower motor neurons such as amyotrophic lateral sclerosis.

II-38, II-39, and II-40. **The answers are A, D, and B, respectively.** *(Chap. 30)* Lesions of the upper motor neurons or their descending axons to the spinal cord produce weakness through decreased activation of lower motor neurons. In general, distal muscle groups are affected more severely than proximal ones, and axial movements are spared unless the lesion is severe and bilateral. Spasticity is typical but may not be present acutely. Lower motor neuron weakness results from disorders of lower motor neurons in the brainstem motor nuclei and the anterior horn of the spinal cord or from dysfunction of the axons of these neurons as they pass to skeletal muscle. Weakness is due to a decrease in the number of muscle fibers that can be activated through a loss of the upper motor neurons or their descending axons to the spi An absent stretch reflex suggests involvement of spindle afferent fibers. When a motor unit becomes diseased, especially in anterior horn cell diseases, it may discharge spontaneously, producing fasciculations. Myopathic weakness is produced by a decrease in the number or contractile force of muscle fibers activated within motor units. With muscular dystrophies, inflammatory myopathies, or myopathies with muscle fiber necrosis, the number of muscle fibers is reduced within many motor units. Proximal muscle weakness may be present. A good physical examination focusing on tone, reflexes, assessment of atrophy, fasciculations, and the distribution of weakness may give insight into the diagnosis (Table II-40).

TABLE II-40 Signs That Distinguish the Origin of Weakness

Sign	Upper Motor Neuron	Lower Motor Neuron	Myopathic	Psychogenic
Atrophy	None	Severe	Mild	None
Fasciculations	None	Common	None	None
Tone	Spastic	Decreased	Normal/decreased	Variable/paratonia
Distribution of weakness	Pyramidal/regional	Distal/segmental	Proximal	Variable/inconsistent with daily activities
Muscle stretch reflexes	Hyperactive	Hypoactive/absent	Normal/hypoactive	Normal
Babinski sign	Present	Absent	Absent	Absent

II-41. **The answer is D.** *(Chap. 31)* Cutaneous sensory receptors are classified by the type of stimulus that optimally excites them. They consist of naked nerve endings (nociceptors, which respond to tissue-damaging stimuli, and thermoreceptors, which respond to noninjurious thermal stimuli) and encapsulated terminals (several types of mechanoreceptor, activated by physical deformation of the skin). Each type of receptor has its own set of sensitivities to specific stimuli, size and distinctness of receptive fields, and adaptational qualities. Afferent fibers in peripheral nerve trunks traverse the dorsal roots and enter the dorsal horn of the spinal cord. From there, the polysynaptic projections of the smaller fibers (unmyelinated and small myelinated), which subserve mainly nociception, itch, temperature sensibility, and touch, cross and ascend in the opposite anterior and lateral columns of the spinal cord, through the brainstem, to the ventral posterolateral (VPL) nucleus of the thalamus and ultimately project to the postcentral gyrus of the parietal cortex. This is the spinothalamic pathway or anterolateral system. The larger fibers, which subserve tactile and position sense and kinesthesia, project rostrally in the posterior and posterolateral columns on the same side of the spinal cord and make their first synapse in the gracile or cuneate nucleus of the lower medulla. Axons of second-order neurons decussate and ascend in the medial lemniscus located medially in the medulla and in the tegmentum of the pons and midbrain and synapse in the VPL nucleus; third-order neurons project to parietal cortex as well as to other cortical areas. This large-fiber system is referred to as the posterior column–medial lemniscal pathway (lemniscal, for short). Although the fiber types and functions that make up the spinothalamic and lemniscal systems are relatively well known, many other fibers, particularly those associated with touch, pressure, and position sense, ascend in a diffusely distributed pattern both ipsilaterally and contralaterally in the anterolateral quadrants of the spinal cord. This explains why a complete lesion of the posterior columns of the spinal cord may be associated with little sensory deficit on examination. Nerve conduction studies and nerve biopsy are important means of investigating the peripheral nervous system, but they do not evaluate the function or structure of cutaneous receptors and free nerve endings or of unmyelinated or thinly myelinated nerve fibers in the nerve trunks. Skin biopsy can be used to evaluate these structures in the dermis and epidermis.

II-42 and II-43. The answers are C and D, respectively. *(Chap. 31)* In focal nerve trunk lesions, sensory abnormalities are readily mapped and generally have discrete boundaries. Root ("radicular") lesions frequently are accompanied by deep, aching pain along the course of the related nerve trunk. With compression of a fifth lumbar (L5) or first sacral (S1) root, as from a ruptured intervertebral disk, sciatica (radicular pain relating to the sciatic nerve trunk) is a common manifestation. With a lesion affecting a single root, sensory deficits may be minimal or absent because adjacent root territories overlap extensively; however, close examination may reveal the likely involved nerve root (Figure II-43).

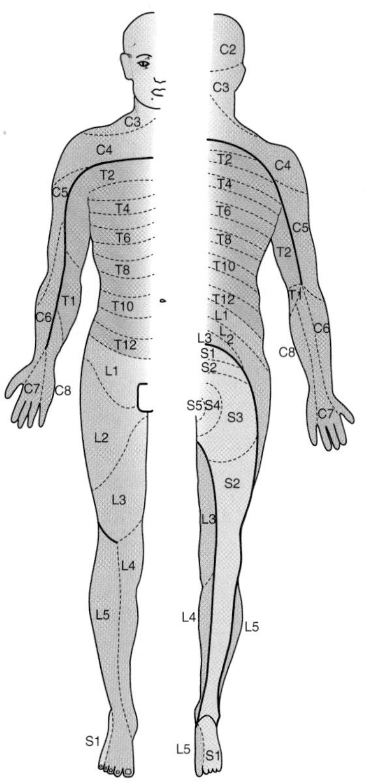

FIGURE II-43 Distribution of the sensory spinal roots on the surface of the body (dermatomes). From D Sinclair: *Mechanisms of Cutaneous Sensation*. Oxford, UK, Oxford University Press, 1981; with permission from Dr. David Sinclair.

II-44. The answer is E. *(Chap. 32)* Approximately 15% of individuals older than 65 years have an identifiable gait disorder. By age 80, 25% of individuals will require a mechanical aid to assist ambulation. Proper maintenance of gait requires a complex interaction between central nervous system centers to integrate postural control and locomotion. The cerebellum, brainstem, and motor cortex are simultaneously processing information regarding the environment and purpose of the motion to allow for proper gait and avoidance of falls. Any disorder affecting either sensory input regarding the environment or central nervous system output has the potential to affect gait. In most case series, the most common cause of gait disorders is a sensory deficit. The causes of sensory deficits can be quite broad, including peripheral sensory neuropathy from a variety of causes including diabetes mellitus, peripheral vascular disease, and vitamin B_{12} deficiency, among many others (Table II-44). Other common causes of gait disorders include myelopathy and multiple cerebrovascular infarcts. While Parkinson disease is almost inevitably marked by gait abnormalities, it occurs less commonly in the general population than the previously discussed disorders. Likewise, cerebellar degeneration is frequently associated with gait disturbance but is a less common disorder in the general population.

TABLE II-44 Etiology Of Gait Disorders

Etiology	No. of Cases	Percent
Sensory deficits	22	18.3
Myelopathy	20	16.7
Multiple infarcts	18	15.0
Parkinsonism	14	11.7
Cerebellar degeneration	8	6.7
Hydrocephalus	8	6.7
Toxic/metabolic causes	3	2.5
Psychogenic causes	4	3.3
Other	6	5.0
Unknown causes	17	14.2
Total	120	100

Source: Reproduced with permission from J Masdeu, L Sudarsky, L Wolfson: *Gait Disorders of Aging*. Lippincott Raven, 1997.

II-45. The answer is B. *(Chap. 32)* Characteristics on neurologic examination can assist with the localization of disease in gait disorders. In this case, the patient presents with signs of a frontal gait disorder or parkinsonism. The specific characteristics that would be seen with a frontal gait disorder are a wide-based stance with a slow and short shuffling steps. The patient may have difficulty rising from a chair and has a slow hesitating start. Likewise, there is great difficulty with turning, with multiple steps required to complete a turn. The patient has very significant postural instability. However, cerebellar signs are typically absent. Romberg sign may or may not be positive, and seated cerebellar testing is normal, including heel-to-shin testing and rapid alternating movements. Additionally, there should otherwise be normal muscle bulk and tone without sensory or strength deficits. The most common cause of frontal gait disorders (sometimes known as gait apraxia) is cerebrovascular disease, especially small-vessel subcortical disease. Communicating hydrocephalus also presents with a gait disorder of this type. In some individuals, the gait disorder precedes other typical symptoms such as incontinence or mental status change. Alcoholic cerebellar degeneration and multiple system atrophy present with signs of cerebellar ataxia. Characteristics of cerebellar ataxia include wide-based gait with variable velocity. Gait initiation is normal, but the patient is hesitant during turns. The stride is lurching and irregular. Falls are a late event. The heel-to-shin test is abnormal and the Romberg is variably positive. Neurosyphilis and lumbar myelopathy are examples of sensory ataxia. Sensory ataxia presents with frequent falls. The gait with sensory ataxia, however, is narrow based. Often the patient is noted to be looking down while walking. The patient tends to walk slowly but have path deviation. Gait is initiated normal, but the patient may have some difficulty with turning. The Romberg is typically unsteady and may result in falls.

II-46. The answer is C. *(Chap. 34)* Delirium is an acute and fluctuating decline in cognition typified by inattention, disorganized thinking, and an altered level of consciousness. Delirium can be subdivided into hyperactive and hypoactive phenotypes. Delirium, especially of the hypoactive subtype, is often unrecognized on the medical wards and in the intensive care unit (ICU). Collateral history obtained from family may be especially important in identifying hypoactive delirium. The confusion assessment method (CAM) is a tool developed for nonpsychiatrists to screen for delirium (Table II-46). According to this method, the diagnosis of delirium requires the presence of both the acute-onset and fluctuating course of mental status changes (feature 1) and inattention (feature 2) together with either disorganized thinking (feature 3) or altered level of consciousness (feature 4).

The patient in this vignette demonstrates an acute change in mental status (feature 1) and altered level of consciousness (feature 4). However, evidence of inattention (feature 2) is required to diagnosis delirium. Inattention would be suggested by observing easy distractibility or difficulty keeping track of what was being said. Poor performance on the digit span test (i.e., digit span ≤4) in the absence of hearing or language barriers also supports inattention. While psychomotor agitation may be seen in the hyperactive subtype of delirium, it is neither necessary nor sufficient for the diagnosis. Similarly, disorientation, alternations in sleep-wake cycles, and perceptional disturbances are common in delirium but are not cardinal manifestations of delirium used in the CAM.

TABLE II-46 The Confusion Assessment Method (CAM) Diagnostic Algorithm[a]

The diagnosis of delirium requires the presence of features 1 and 2 and of *either* feature 3 or 4.
Feature 1. Acute onset and fluctuating course
This feature is satisfied by positive responses to the following questions: Is there evidence of an acute change in mental status from the patient's baseline? Did the (abnormal) behavior fluctuate during the day, i.e., tend to come and go, or did it increase and decrease in severity?
Feature 2. Inattention
This feature is satisfied by a positive response to the following question: Did the patient have difficulty focusing attention, e.g., being easily distractible, or have difficulty keeping track of what was being said?
Feature 3. Disorganized thinking
This feature is satisfied by a positive response to the following question: Was the patient's thinking disorganized or incoherent, such as rambling or irrelevant conversation, unclear or illogical flow of ideas, or unpredictable switching from subject to subject?
Feature 4. Altered level of consciousness
This feature is satisfied by any answer other than "alert" to the following question: Overall, how would you rate the patient's level of consciousness: alert (normal), vigilant (hyperalert), lethargic (drowsy, easily aroused), stupor (difficult to arouse), or coma (unarousable)?

[a]Information is usually obtained from a reliable reporter, such as a family member, caregiver, or nurse.

Source: Modified from SK Inouye et al: Clarifying confusion: The Confusion Assessment Method. A new method for detection of delirium. *Ann Intern Med* 113:941, 1990.

II-47. The answer is A. *(Chap. 34)* Delirium is an acute and fluctuating decline in cognition typified by inattention, disorganized thinking, and an altered level of consciousness. The common etiologies of delirium are manifold, and in many patients, the cause is multifactorial. Nearly one-third of cases of delirium are due to medications. Especially in older adults, drugs with anticholinergic properties may precipitate delirium. Deficiency of acetylcholine may play a key role in the pathogenesis of delirium. Diphenhydramine is a sedating antihistamine with substantial anticholinergic activity. Diphenhydramine does not significantly antagonize the activity of serotonin, dopamine, or norepinephrine.

II-48. The answer is D. *(Chap. 34)* Delirium is an acute and fluctuating decline in cognition typified by inattention, disorganized thinking, and altered level of consciousness. Potential risk factors for delirium include older age, baseline cognitive dysfunction or neurologic illness, sensory deprivation, immobility, malnutrition, polypharmacy, sleep deprivation, and the use of physical restraints. Systemic infections and critical illness are frequently associated with delirium. In addition to the deliriogenic effect of proinflammatory cytokines, routine ICU care with its unfamiliar environment, frequent interventions, interrupted sleep, and use of multiple medications may promote delirium. Benzodiazepines have been most consistently associated with delirium in the ICU. In contrast, dexmedetomidine is a sedative that may be less likely to lead to delirium in critically ill patients.

II-49. The answer is B. (*Chap 34*) The causes of delirium are many. No definitive algorithm applies to all cases. The etiology of delirium is best determined in a stepwise approach that begins with a careful history and physical examination with special attention to medication history including over-the-counter medications, herbals, and drugs of abuse (Table II-49). Collateral informants such as family members, friends, and staff are essential because delirious patients are often unable to provide reliable information. It is reasonable to screen basic laboratories including a complete blood count; electrolyte panel including calcium, magnesium, phosphorus, and glucose; as well as liver and renal function tests in the initial evaluation of delirium. Alterations in serum electrolytes such as sodium, potassium, bicarbonate, calcium, magnesium, and phosphorus may contribute or cause delirium. Especially in the elderly, screening for systemic infection with urinalysis, cultures, and chest imaging is important. In younger patients, toxicology may be appropriate earlier in the workup. Guided by the initial evaluation, further evaluation may include additional testing for systemic infections, other toxic/metabolic etiologies, ischemia, vitamin deficiencies, endocrinopathies, autoimmune disorders, neoplastic disorders, cerebrovascular disorders, or seizure-related disorders. Although screening for vitamin B_{12} deficiency, syphilis, or hyperammonemia may have a role in the subsequent evaluation of delirium, these tests are not routinely recommended in the initial evaluation. Brain imaging in delirium is often unhelpful but may be considered if the initial evaluation is unrevealing.

TABLE II-49 Stepwise Evaluation of a Patient with Delirium

Initial evaluation
History with special attention to medications (including over-the-counter and herbals)
General physical examination and neurologic examination
Complete blood count
Electrolyte panel including calcium, magnesium, phosphorus
Liver function tests, including albumin
Renal function tests
First-tier further evaluation guided by initial evaluation
Systemic infection screen
Urinalysis and culture
Chest radiograph
Blood cultures
Electrocardiogram
Arterial blood gas
Serum and/or urine toxicology screen (perform earlier in young persons)
Brain imaging with MRI with diffusion and gadolinium (preferred) or CT
Suspected CNS infection: lumbar puncture after brain imaging
Suspected seizure-related etiology: electroencephalogram (EEG) (if high suspicion, should be performed immediately)
Second-tier further evaluation
Vitamin levels: B_{12}, folate, thiamine
Endocrinologic laboratories: thyroid-stimulating hormone (TSH) and free T_4; cortisol
Serum ammonia
Sedimentation rate
Autoimmune serologies: antinuclear antibodies (ANA), complement levels; p-ANCA, c-ANCA. consider paraneoplastic serologies
Infectious serologies: rapid plasmin reagin (RPR); fungal and viral serologies if high suspicion; HIV antibody
Lumbar puncture (if not already performed)
Brain MRI with and without gadolinium (if not already performed)

Abbreviations: c-ANCA, cytoplasmic antineutrophil cytoplasmic antibody; CNS, central nervous system; CT, computed tomography; MRI, magnetic resonance imaging; p-ANCA, perinuclear antineutrophil cytoplasmic antibody.

II-50. The answer is B. *(Chap. 35)* Approximately 10% of all persons over the age of 70 have significant memory loss, and in more than half, the cause is Alzheimer disease (AD). AD can occur in any decade of adulthood, but it is the most common cause of dementia in the elderly. AD most often presents with an insidious onset of memory loss followed by a slowly progressive dementia over several years. Pathologically, atrophy is distributed throughout the medial temporal lobes, as well as lateral and medial parietal lobes and lateral frontal cortex. Microscopically, there are neurofibrillary tangles composed of hyperphosphorylated tau filaments, and accumulation of amyloid in blood vessel walls in cortex and leptomeninges. The cognitive changes of AD tend to follow a characteristic pattern, beginning with memory impairment and spreading to language and visuospatial deficits. Yet, approximately 20% of patients with AD present with nonmemory complaints such as word-finding, organizational, or navigational difficulty. In the early stages of the disease, the memory loss may go unrecognized or be ascribed to benign forgetfulness. Slowly the cognitive problems begin to interfere with daily activities, such as keeping track of finances, following instructions on the job, driving, shopping, and housekeeping. Some patients are unaware of these difficulties (*anosognosia*), whereas others remain acutely attuned to their deficits. Social graces, routine behavior, and superficial conversation may be surprisingly intact. Language becomes impaired—first naming, then comprehension, and finally fluency. In some patients, *aphasia* is an early and prominent feature. Word-finding difficulties and circumlocution may be a problem even when formal testing demonstrates intact naming and fluency. Visuospatial deficits begin to interfere with dressing, eating, or even walking, and patients fail to solve simple puzzles or copy geometric figures. Simple calculations and clock reading become difficult in parallel. Loss of judgment and reasoning is inevitable. Delusions are common and usually simple, with common themes of theft, infidelity, or misidentification. In end-stage AD, patients become rigid, mute, incontinent, and bedridden. Hyperactive tendon reflexes and myoclonic jerks may occur spontaneously or in response to physical or auditory stimulation. Generalized seizures may also occur. Often death results from malnutrition, secondary infections, pulmonary emboli, heart disease, or, most commonly, aspiration. The typical duration of AD is 8–10 years, but the course can range from 1 to 25 years. For unknown reasons, some AD patients show a steady decline in function, while others have prolonged plateaus without major deterioration.

II-51. The answer is D. *(Chap. 35)* There is currently no robust or curative medical therapy for AD. The acetylcholinesterase inhibitors donepezil, rivastigmine, and galantamine, as well as the *N*-Methyl-D-aspartate (NMDA) receptor antagonist, memantine, are approved by the U.S. Food and Drug Administration (FDA) for treatment of AD. Double-blind, placebo-controlled, crossover studies with these agents have shown improved caregiver ratings of patients' functioning and an apparent decreased rate of decline in cognitive test scores over periods of up to 3 years. The average patient on an anticholinesterase compound maintains his or her Mini Mental State Examination (MMSE) score for close to a year, whereas a placebo-treated patient declines 2–3 points over the same time period. Memantine, used in conjunction with cholinesterase inhibitors or by itself, slows cognitive deterioration and decreases caregiver burden for patients with moderate to severe AD but is not approved for mild AD. Each of these compounds has only modest efficacy for AD. Some studies have suggested a protective effect of estrogen replacement in women. However, a prospective study of an estrogen-progesterone combination increased the prevalence of AD in previously asymptomatic women. A randomized, double-blind, placebo-controlled trial of an extract of *Ginkgo biloba* found modest improvement in cognitive function in subjects with AD and vascular dementia. Unfortunately, a comprehensive 6-year multicenter prevention study using *Ginkgo biloba* found no slowing of progression to dementia in the treated group. Recent work has focused on developing antibodies against Aβ42 as a treatment for AD. Although the initial randomized controlled trials failed, there was some evidence for efficacy in the mildest patient groups. Therefore, researchers have begun to focus on patients with very mild disease and asymptomatic individuals at risk for AD, such as those who carry autosomal dominantly inherited genetic mutations or healthy elders with cerebrospinal fluid (CSF) or amyloid imaging biomarker evidence supporting presymptomatic AD. Newer generation antipsychotics (risperidone, quetiapine, olanzapine) in low doses may benefit neuropsychiatric symptoms. Medications with strong anticholinergic effects should be vigilantly avoided, including prescription and over-the-counter sleep aids (e.g., diphenhydramine) or incontinence therapies (e.g., oxybutynin).

II-52. **The answer is D.** *(Chap. 35)* All the choices given in the question are causes of or may be associated with dementia. Binswanger disease, the cause of which is unknown, often occurs in patients with longstanding hypertension and/or atherosclerosis; it is associated with diffuse subcortical white matter damage and has a subacute insidious course. Alzheimer disease, the most common cause of dementia, is also slowly progressive and can be confirmed at autopsy by the presence of amyloid plaques and neurofibrillary tangles. Creutzfeldt-Jakob disease, a prion disease, is associated with a rapidly progressive dementia, myoclonus, rigidity, a characteristic electroencephalogram (EEG) pattern, and death within 1–2 years of onset. Vitamin B_{12} deficiency, which often is seen in the setting of chronic alcoholism, most commonly produces a myelopathy that results in loss of vibration and joint position sense and brisk deep tendon reflexes (dorsal column and lateral corticospinal tract dysfunction). This combination of pathologic abnormalities in the setting of vitamin B_{12} deficiency is also called subacute combined degeneration. Vitamin B_{12} deficiency may also lead to a subcortical type of dementia. Recent studies have demonstrated that elevated levels of methylmalonic acid (MMA), which is a more sensitive measure of vitamin B_{12} deficiency, may increase the risk of cognitive decline in elderly patients. The therapeutic implications of this finding are not yet clear, but emphasize the importance of adequate vitamin B_{12} intake. Multi-infarct dementia, as in this case, presents with a history of sudden stepwise declines in function associated with the accumulation of bilateral focal neurologic deficits. Brain imaging demonstrates multiple areas of stroke.

II-53. **The answer is D.** *(Chap. 35)* Based on initial symptoms, mental status, neuropsychiatric evaluation, neurologic examination, and imaging, it is often possible to differentiate the major causes of dementia (Table II-53). In this case, the combination of apathy, poor judgement, disinhibition, and overeating makes frontotemporal dementia the most likely diagnosis.

TABLE II-53 Clinical Differentiation of the Major Dementias

Disease	First Symptom	Mental Status	Neuropsychiatry	Neurology	Imaging
AD	Memory loss	Episodic memory loss	Irritability, anxiety, depression	Initially normal	Entorhinal cortex and hippocampal atrophy
FTD	Apathy; poor judgment/insight, speech/language; hyperorality	Frontal/executive and/or language; spares drawing	Apathy, disinhibition, overeating, compulsivity	May have vertical gaze palsy, axial rigidity, dystonia, alien hand, or MND	Frontal, insular, and/or temporal atrophy; usually spares posterior parietal lobe
DLB	Visual hallucinations, REM sleep behavior disorder, delirium, Capgras syndrome, parkinsonism	Drawing and frontal/executive; spares memory; delirium-prone	Visual hallucinations, depression, sleep disorder, delusions	Parkinsonism	Posterior parietal atrophy; hippocampi larger than in AD
CJD	Dementia, mood, anxiety, movement disorders	Variable, frontal/executive, focal cortical, memory	Depression, anxiety, psychosis in some	Myoclonus, rigidity, parkinsonism	Cortical ribboning and basal ganglia or thalamus hyperintensity on diffusion/FLAIR MRI
Vascular	Often but not always sudden; variable; apathy, falls, focal weakness	Frontal/executive, cognitive slowing; can spare memory	Apathy, delusions, anxiety	Usually motor slowing, spasticity; can be normal	Cortical and/or subcortical infarctions, confluent white matter disease

Abbreviations: AD, Alzheimer disease; CBD, cortical basal degeneration; CJD, Creutzfeldt-Jakob disease; DLB, dementia with Lewy bodies; FLAIR, fluid-attenuated inversion recovery; FTD, frontotemporal dementia; MND, motor neuron disease; MRI, magnetic resonance imaging; PSP, progressive supranuclear palsy; REM, rapid eye movement.

II-54. **The answer is B.** *(Chap. 36)* When evaluating someone who reports difficulty with language, it is important to assess speech in several different domains: spontaneous speech, comprehension, repetition, naming, reading, and writing. Anomia refers to the inability to name common objects and is the most common finding in aphasic patients.

Indeed anomia is present in all types of aphasia except pure word deafness or pure alexia. Anomia can be present in many fashions including complete inability to name, provision of a related word ("pen" for "pencil"), a description of the word ("a thing for writing"), or the wrong word. Fluency is assessed by listening to spontaneous speech. Fluency is decreased in Broca or global aphasia but is relatively preserved in other forms of aphasia. Comprehension is assessed by asking patients to follow conversation and provide simple answers (yes/no, pointing to appropriate objects). The most common aphasia presenting with deficits of comprehension is Wernicke aphasia, in which fluent but nonsensical spontaneous speech (word salad) is present. Repetition asks patients to repeat a string of words, sentences, or a single word and is impaired in many types of aphasia. In addition, repetition of tongue twisters can be useful in the evaluation of dysarthria or palilalia as well. Alexia refers to the inability to read aloud or comprehend written language.

II-55. The answer is C. *(Chap. 36)* The parietofrontal area of the brain is responsible for spatial orientation. The major components of the network include the cingulate cortex, posterior parietal cortex, and the frontal eye fields. In addition, subcortical areas in the striatum and thalamus are also important. Together, these systems integrate information to maintain spatial cognition, and a lesion in any of these areas can lead to hemispatial neglect. In neglect syndromes, three behavioral manifestations are seen: sensory events in the neglected hemisphere have less overall impact; there is a paucity of conscious acts directed toward the neglected hemisphere; and the patient behaves as if the neglected hemisphere is devalued. In the figure, almost all of the A's (the target) represented on the left half of the figure are missed. This is an example of a target detection task. Hemianopia alone is not sufficient to cause this finding because the individual can turn his or her head left and right to identify the targets. Bilateral disorders of the parietofrontal area of the brain can lead to severe spatial disorientation known as Balint syndrome. In Balint syndrome, there is inability to orderly scan the environment (oculomotor apraxia) and inaccurate manual reaching for objects (optic apraxia). A third finding in Balint syndrome is simultanagnosia. Simultanagnosia refers to the inability to integrate information in the center of the gaze with peripheral information. An example would be a target detection test where only the A's present in the outer portion of the figure would be indicated. Individuals with this finding also tend to miss the larger objects in a figure and would not be able to accurately identify the target when it was made much larger than the surrounding letters. Construction apraxia refers to the inability to copy a simple line drawing like a house or star and occurs most commonly in association with parietal lesions. Object agnosia refers to the inability to name a generic object or describe its use, in contrast to anomia, where an individual should be able to describe the use of the object even if it cannot be named. The defect in the object agnosia is usually in the territory of the bilateral posterior cerebral arteries.

II-56. The answer is C. *(Chap. 38)* Shift work sleep disorder is a disorder of the circadian rhythm that is common in any individual who has to commonly work at night. At present, an estimated 7 million individuals in the United States work permanently at night or on rotating shifts. Increasing research devoted to sleep disorders in night shift workers has demonstrated that the circadian rhythm never fully shifts to allow one to perform at full alertness at night. The reason for this is likely multifactorial and includes the fact that most individuals who work at night try to abruptly shift their sleep schedules to a more normal pattern on days when they are not working. Consequently, night shift workers often have chronic sleep deprivation, increased length of time awake prior to starting work, and misalignment of their circadian phase with the intrinsic circadian phase, which result in decreased alertness and increased errors during night shifts. In an estimated 5%–10% of individuals working night shifts, the excessive sleepiness during the night and insomnia during the day are deemed to be clinically significant. Strategies for treating shift work sleep disorder utilize a combination of behavioral and pharmacologic strategies. Caffeine does promote wakefulness, but the effects are not long-lasting and tolerance develops over time. Brief periods of exercise frequently boost alertness and can be used prior to starting a night shift or during the shift at times of increased sleepiness. Many sleep experts support strategic napping during shifts for no more than 20 minutes at times of circadian nadirs. Naps longer than 20 minutes can lead to sleep inertia during which an individual may feel very disoriented, groggy, and experience a decline in motor skills upon abrupt awakening from sleep. Bright lights prior to and during night shift work may improve alertness, but one must be careful to avoid bright lights in the morning following a night shift as light entrainment is a powerful stimulus of the internal circadian clock. If an individual is exposed to bright light in the morning, it will interfere with the ability to fall asleep during the day. Night shift workers should be encouraged to wear dark sunglasses in the morning on the way home. Sleep during the day is frequently disrupted in night shift workers. Creating a quiet, dark, and comfortable environment is important, and sleep should be a priority for the individual during the day. The only pharmacologic therapy approved by the FDA for treatment of shift work sleep disorder is modafinil 200 mg taken 20–30 minutes prior to the start of a night shift. Modafinil has been demonstrated to increase sleep latency and decrease attentional failures during night shifts, but it does not alleviate the feelings of excessive sleepiness. Melatonin is not one of the recommended therapies for shift work sleep disorder. If used, it should be taken 2–3 hours prior to bedtime, rather than right before bedtime, to simulate the normal peaks and troughs of melatonin secretion.

II-57. **The answer is C.** *(Chap. 38)* This patient complains of symptoms that are consistent with restless legs syndrome (RLS). This disorder affects 1%–5% of young to middle-aged individuals and as many as 20% of older individuals. The symptoms of RLS are a nonspecific uncomfortable sensation in the legs that begins during periods of quiescence and is associated with the irresistible urge to move. Patients frequently find it difficult to describe their symptoms but usually describe the sensation as deep within the affected limb. Rarely is the sensation described as distinctly painful unless an underlying neuropathy is also present. The severity of the disorder tends to wax and wane over time and tends to worsen with sleep deprivation, caffeine intake, pregnancy, and alcohol. Renal disease, neuropathy, and iron deficiency are known secondary causes of RLS symptoms. In this patient, correcting the iron deficiency is the best choice for initial therapy because this may entirely relieve the symptoms of RLS. For individuals with primary RLS (not related to another medical condition), the dopaminergic agents are the treatment of choice. Pramipexole and ropinirole are recommended as first-line treatment. While carbidopa/levodopa is highly effective, individuals have a high risk of developing augmented symptoms over time, with increasingly higher doses needed to control the symptoms. Other options for treating RLS include narcotics, benzodiazepines, and gabapentin. Hormone replacement therapy has no role in the treatment of RLS.

II-58. **The answer is A.** *(Chap. 38)* Narcolepsy is a sleep disorder characterized by excessive sleepiness with intrusion of rapid eye movement (REM) sleep into wakefulness. Narcolepsy affects ~1 in 4000 individuals in the United States with a genetic predisposition. Recent research has demonstrated that narcolepsy with cataplexy is associated with low or undetectable levels of the neurotransmitter hypocretin (orexin) in the cerebrospinal fluid. This neurotransmitter is released from a small number of neurons in the hypothalamus. Given the association of narcolepsy with the major histocompatibility complex (MHC) antigen HLA DQB1*0602, it is thought that narcolepsy is an autoimmune process that leads to destruction of the hypocretin-secreting neurons in the hypothalamus. The classic symptom tetrad of narcolepsy is: (1) cataplexy; (2) hypnagogic or hypnopompic hallucinations; (3) sleep paralysis; and (4) excessive daytime somnolence. Of these symptoms, cataplexy is the most specific for the diagnosis of narcolepsy. Cataplexy refers to the sudden loss of muscle tone in response to strong emotions. It most commonly occurs with laughter or surprise but may be associated with anger as well. Cataplexy can have a wide range of symptoms, from mild sagging of the jaw lasting for a few seconds to a complete loss of muscle tone lasting several minutes. During this time, individuals are aware of their surroundings and are not unconscious. This symptom is present in 76% of individuals diagnosed with narcolepsy and is the most specific finding for the diagnosis. Hypnagogic and hypnopompic hallucinations and sleep paralysis can occur from any cause of chronic sleep deprivation, including sleep apnea and chronic insufficient sleep. Excessive daytime somnolence is present in 100% of individuals with narcolepsy but is not specific for the diagnosis because this symptom may be present with any sleep disorder as well as with chronic insufficient sleep. The presence of two or more REM periods occurring during a daytime multiple sleep latency test is suggestive but not diagnostic of narcolepsy. Other disorders that may lead to presence of REM during short daytime nap periods include sleep apnea, sleep phase delay syndrome, and insufficient sleep.

II-59. **The answer is B.** *(Chap. 38; http://www.sleepfoundation.org/site/c.huIXKjM0IxF/b.2417355/k.143E/2002_Sleep_in_America_Poll.htm, accessed May 12, 2011)* Insomnia is the most common sleep disorder in the population. In the 2002 Sleep in America Poll, 58% of respondents reported at least one symptom of insomnia on a weekly basis, and a third of individuals experienced these symptoms on a nightly basis. Insomnia is defined clinically as the inability to fall asleep or stay asleep, which leads to daytime sleepiness or poor daytime function. These symptoms occur despite adequate time and opportunity for sleep. Insomnia can be further characterized as primary or secondary. Primary insomnia occurs in individuals with an identifiable cause of insomnia and is often a longstanding diagnosis for many years. Within the category of primary insomnia is adjustment insomnia, which is typically of short duration with a well-defined stressor. Secondary causes of insomnia include comorbid medical or psychiatric conditions and also can be related to caffeine or illegal and prescribed drugs. Obstructive sleep apnea is thought to affect as much as 10%–15% of the population and is currently underdiagnosed in the United States. In addition, because of the rising incidence of obesity, obstructive sleep apnea is also expected to increase in incidence over the coming years. Obstructive sleep apnea occurs when there is ongoing effort to inspire against an occluded oropharynx during sleep. It is directly related to obesity and also has an increased incidence in men and in older populations. Narcolepsy affects 1 in 4000 people and is due to a deficit of hypocretin (orexin) in the brain. Symptoms of narcolepsy include sudden loss of tone in response to emotional stimuli (cataplexy), hypersomnia, sleep paralysis, and hallucinations with sleep onset and waking. Physiologically, there is intrusion or persistence of REM sleep during wakefulness that accounts for the classic symptoms of narcolepsy. RLS is estimated to affect 1%–5% of young to middle-aged adults and as much as 10–20% of the elderly. RLS is marked by uncomfortable sensations in the legs that are difficult to describe. The symptoms have an onset with quiescence, especially at night, and are relieved with movement. Delayed sleep phase syndrome is a circadian rhythm disorder that commonly presents with a complaint of insomnia and accounts for as much as 10% of individuals referred to the sleep clinic for evaluation of insomnia. In delayed sleep phase syndrome, the intrinsic circadian rhythm is delayed such that sleep onset occurs much later than normal. When allowed to sleep according to the intrinsic circadian rhythm, individuals with delayed sleep phase syndrome sleep normally and do not experience excessive somnolence. This disorder is most common in adolescence and young adulthood.

II-60. **The answer is C.** *(Chap. 38)* Parasomnias are abnormal behaviors or experiences that arise from slow-wave sleep. Also known as confusional arousals, the electroencephalogram during a parasomnia event frequently shows persistence of slow-wave (delta) sleep into arousal. Non-REM (NREM) parasomnias may also include more complex behavior, including eating and sexual activity. Treatment of NREM parasomnias is usually not indicated, and a safe environment should be assured for the patient. In cases where injury is likely to occur, treatment with a drug that decreases slow-wave sleep will treat the parasomnia. Typical treatment is a benzodiazepine. There are no typical parasomnias that arise from stage I or stage II sleep. REM parasomnias include nightmare disorder and REM-behavior disorder. REM-behavior disorder is increasingly recognized as associated with Parkinson disease and other parkinsonian syndromes. This disorder is characterized by the absence of decreased muscle tone in REM sleep, which leads to the acting out of dreams, sometimes resulting in violence and injury.

II-61. **The answer is C.** *(Chap. 38)* Polysomnographic profiles define two basic states of sleep: (1) REM sleep and (2) NREM sleep. NREM sleep is further subdivided into three stages: N1, N2, and N3, characterized by increasing arousal threshold and slowing of the cortical EEG. REM sleep is characterized by a low-amplitude, mixed-frequency EEG similar to that of NREM stage N1 sleep with bursts of rapid eye movements similar to those seen during eyes-open wakefulness. EMG activity is absent in nearly all skeletal muscles, reflecting the brainstem-mediated muscle atonia that is characteristic of REM sleep.

Normal nocturnal sleep in adults displays a consistent organization from night to night. After sleep onset, sleep usually progresses through NREM stages N1–N3 sleep within 45–60 minutes. NREM stage N3 sleep (also known as slow-wave sleep) predominates in the first third of the night and comprises 15%–25% of total nocturnal sleep time in young adults. Sleep deprivation increases the rapidity of sleep onset and both the intensity and amount of slow-wave sleep. The first REM sleep episode usually occurs in the second hour of sleep. NREM and REM sleep alternate through the night with an average period of 90–110 minutes (the "ultradian" sleep cycle). Overall, in a healthy young adult, REM sleep constitutes 20%–25% of total sleep, and NREM stages N1 and N2 constitute 50%–60%. Age has a profound impact on sleep state organization. N3 sleep is most intense and prominent during childhood, decreasing with puberty and across the second and third decades of life. N3 sleep declines during adulthood to the point where it may be completely absent in older adults. The remaining NREM sleep becomes more fragmented, with many more frequent awakenings from NREM sleep. It is the increased frequency of awakenings, rather than a decreased ability to fall back asleep, that accounts for the increased wakefulness during the sleep episode in older people. While REM sleep may account for 50% of total sleep time in infancy, the percentage falls off sharply over the first postnatal year as a mature REM–NREM cycle develops; thereafter, REM sleep occupies about 25% of total sleep time. Sleep deprivation degrades cognitive performance, particularly on tests that require continual vigilance. Paradoxically, older people are less vulnerable to the neurobehavioral performance impairment induced by acute sleep deprivation than young adults, maintaining their reaction time and sustaining vigilance with fewer lapses of attention. However, it is more difficult for older adults to obtain recovery sleep after staying awake all night, as the ability to sleep during the daytime declines with age. After sleep deprivation, NREM sleep is generally recovered first, followed by REM sleep. However, because REM sleep tends to be most prominent in the second half of the night, sleep truncation (e.g., by an alarm clock) results in selective REM sleep deprivation. This may increase REM sleep pressure to the point where the first REM sleep may occur much earlier in the nightly sleep episode.

II-62. **The answer is D.** *(Chap. 39)* Bitemporal hemianopia is caused by a lesion at the optic chiasm because fibers there decussate into the contralateral optic tract. Crossed fibers are more damaged by compression than uncrossed fibers. This finding is usually caused by symmetric compression in the sellar region by a pituitary adenoma, meningioma, craniopharyngioma, glioma, or aneurysm. These lesions are often insidious and may be unnoticed by the patient. They will escape detection by the physician unless each eye is tested separately. Lesions anterior to the chiasm (retinal injury, optic nerve injury) will cause unilateral impairment and an abnormal pupillary response. Postchiasmic lesions (temporal, parietal, occipital cortex) will cause homonymous lesions (similar field abnormalities in both eyes) that vary with location. Occlusion of the posterior cerebral artery supplying the occipital lobe is a common cause of total homonymous hemianopia.

II-63. **The answer is D.** *(Chap. 39)* This girl has classic myopia, or "near-sightedness." In this condition, the globe is too long, causing light rays to be focused in front of the retina. Patients can clearly see objects near to them, but farther object are out of focus. They require a diverging lens in front of the eye to bring objects into focus. As an alternative to eyeglasses or contact lenses, refractive error can be corrected by performing laser in situ keratomileusis (LASIK) or photorefractive keratectomy (PRK) to alter the curvature of the cornea. Emmetropia (option A) is the situation where the globe is the appropriate length and parallel rays are focused perfectly on the retina. These patients do not require corrective lenses. Hyperopia is the opposite of myopia; in this condition, the globe is too short, and light rays have a focal point "behind" the retina. These patients suffer from "far-sightedness," where objects nearby are preferentially out of focus. This condition is corrected with converging lenses in front of the eye. Presbyopia is the condition that often begins in middle age, where the lens loses refractive power, particularly for near objects, and is treated with reading glasses.

II-64. **The answer is D.** *(Chap. 39)* This is a classic representation of a left relative afferent pupillary defect, or the Marcus Gunn pupil. In this case, the left eye does not perceive the light stimulus as strongly. Thus, when the light is shined in the left eye, the bilateral constriction stimulus is less than when the light is shined in the right eye. This finding is sometimes the only clue to the presence of an optic neuritis, which can subsequently uncover neurodemyelinating disease. The patient has equally sized pupils in dim light, ruling out Adie tonic pupil, where anisocoria is present due to parasympathetic denervation of the iris ciliary muscle in the affected eye. Thus, the anisocoria would worsen in bright light (the affected eye would be unable to constrict). Curiously, while the pupillary response to light in this condition is poor, the response to near stimulus is often relatively preserved. This can be due to oculomotor nerve palsy or be idiopathic. A similar light–near dissociation can be seen in the Argyll-Robertson pupil of neurosyphilis with involvement of the midbrain. The opposite dissociation (where a pupil reacts to light but does not accommodate to near stimulus) does not occur. Likewise, Horner syndrome would present with anisocoria with miosis (constriction) of the affected eye due to sympathetic denervation, which is not present in this patient. In this condition, the anisocoria would worsen in dim light, and the unaffected eye is free to dilate, while the affected eye is miotic. Often, concomitant ptosis and anhidrosis are seen in Horner syndrome. A homonymous hemianopsia is a defect in visual fields and cannot be assessed with the swinging flashlight test.

II-65. **The answer is C.** *(Chap. 39)* This patient has a classic bitemporal hemianopsia. In this condition, the nasal ganglion cells decussate to the contralateral optic tract. Decussating fibers are sensitive to pressure and thus more easily damaged. Because the nasal ganglion cells are responsible for vision in the temporal fields, damage produces a bitemporal hemianopsia. Associated conditions include pituitary lesions or other sellar lesions such as craniopharyngiomas or aneurysms. Prompt CNS imaging is warranted. Damage to the right retina would produce loss of vision in only the right eye. Similarly, damage to the left optic nerve would produce loss of vision in only the left eye; both of these lesions are termed "pre-chiasmatic" because they are present anterior to the optic chiasm. Right occipital lobe lesions such as a stroke would produce a homonymous hemianopsia on the left visual fields, often with macular sparing. Damage to the left parietal lobe would produce a right inferior quadrantanopsia as seen in Figure II-65B.

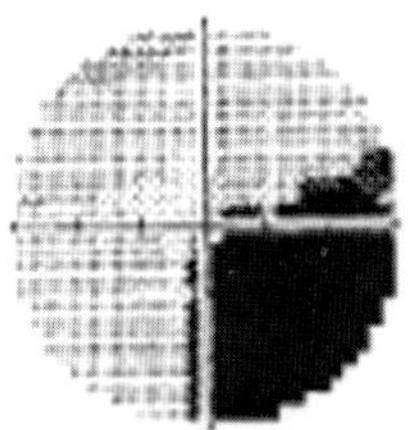
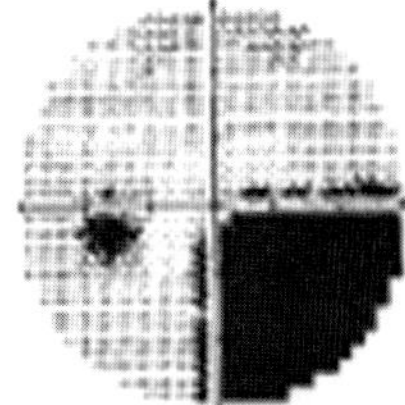

FIGURE II-65B

II-66. **The answer is B.** *(Chap. 39)* This patient has a classic presentation of anterior ischemic optic neuritis (AION) due to giant cell arteritis (GCA). Occurring almost exclusively in patients older than 60, GCA is an important etiology to evaluate for cases of AION. The patient's concomitant symptoms of polymyalgia rheumatica with fatigue and proximal muscle pain/weakness can often coexist with GCA. One would expect an elevation in inflammatory markers (ESR and CRP). Temporal artery biopsy is the diagnostic test of choice, and it is important to take an adequate-sized (>3 cm) sample. However, high-dose steroids should be initiated immediately without waiting for the biopsy to occur or its results, as delay in therapy may lead to permanent vision loss. In Figure II-66, one sees acute disc swelling and splinter hemorrhages classic for AION.

II-67. **The answer is A.** *(Chap. 42)* Olfaction is unique in that its initial afferent projections bypass the thalamus. However, persons with damage to the thalamus can exhibit olfactory deficits, particularly ones of odor identification. Such deficits likely reflect the involvement of thalamic connections between the primary olfactory cortex and the orbitofrontal cortex (OFC), where odor identification occurs. The close anatomic ties between the olfactory system and the amygdala, hippocampus, and hypothalamus help to explain the intimate associations between odor perception and cognitive functions such as memory, motivation, arousal, autonomic activity, digestion, and sex. The sense of taste also employs chemoreceptors.

II-68. The answer is D. *(Chap. 42)* Taste information is sent to the brain via three cranial nerves (CNs): CN VII (the *facial nerve*, which involves the intermediate nerve with its branches, the greater petrosal and chorda tympani nerves), CN IX (the *glossopharyngeal nerve*), and CN X (the *vagus nerve*). CN VII innervates the anterior tongue and all of the soft palate; CN IX innervates the posterior tongue; and CN X innervates the laryngeal surface of the epiglottis, larynx, and proximal portion of the esophagus. The mandibular branch of CN V (V3) conveys somatosensory information (e.g., touch, burning, cooling, irritation) to the brain. Although not technically a gustatory nerve, CN V shares primary nerve routes with many of the gustatory nerve fibers and adds temperature, texture, pungency, and spiciness to the taste experience.

II-69. The answer is C. *(Chap. 42)* Presbyosmia (age-related olfactory deficits) and anosmia (olfactory deficit at any age) are relatively common. The ability to smell is influenced, in everyday life, by such factors as age, gender, general health, nutrition, smoking, and reproductive state. Women typically outperform men on tests of olfactory function and retain normal smell function to a later age than do men. Significant decrements in the ability to smell are present in over 50% of the population between 65 and 80 years of age and in 75% of those 80 years of age and older. Presbyosmia is much more than a nuisance and can confer real health risk. Such presbyosmia helps to explain why many elderly report that food has little flavor, a problem that can result in nutritional disturbances. This also helps to explain why a disproportionate number of elderly die in accidental gas poisonings. While rare, patients with trauma-related anosmia can indeed recover olfactory function. Ten percent of posttraumatic anosmic patients will recover age-related normal function over time. This increases to nearly 25% of those with less than total loss. Olfactory impairment can be an early sign of Parkinson disease, often predating the clinical diagnosis by at least 4 years.

II-70. The answer is C. *(Chaps. 42 and 455)* Mr. McEvoy is suffering from Bell palsy, a dysfunction of CN VII. Since CN VII is involved in gustatory sensation, taste disturbance is occasionally present. The most common etiology of Bell palsy is likely a viral involvement (often varicella-zoster virus or herpes simplex virus) of the cranial nerve, and patients recover spontaneously or with steroid therapy. Clinicians should also consider more dire etiologies, such as Lyme disease or demyelinating diseases, in the differential diagnosis.

II-71. The answer is E. *(Chap. 43)* Hearing loss is a common complaint, particularly in older individuals. In this age group, 33% of people have hearing loss to a degree that requires hearing aids. When evaluating hearing loss, the physician should attempt to determine whether the cause is conductive, sensorineural, or mixed. Sensorineural hearing loss results from injury of the cochlear apparatus or disruption of the neural pathways from the inner ear to the brain. The primary site of damage is the hair cells of the inner ear. Common causes of hair cell injury include prolonged exposure to loud noises, viral infections, ototoxic drugs, cochlear otosclerosis, Meniere disease, and aging. In contrast, conductive hearing loss results from impairment of the external ear and auditory canal to transmit and amplify sound through the middle ear to the cochlea. Causes of conductive hearing loss include cerumen impaction, perforations of the tympanic membrane, otosclerosis, cholesteatomas, large middle ear effusions, and tumors of the external auditory canal or middle ear among others. The initial physical examination can often differentiate between conductive and sensorineural hearing loss. Examination of the external auditory canal can identify cerumen or foreign body impaction. On otoscopic examination, it is more important to assess the topography of the tympanic membrane than look for the presence of a light reflex. Of particular attention is the area in the upper third of the tympanic membrane known as the pars flaccida. This area can develop chronic retraction pockets that are indicative of Eustachian tube dysfunction or a cholesteatoma, a benign tumor comprised of keratinized squamous epithelium. Bedside tests with a tuning fork also are useful for differentiating conductive from sensorineural hearing loss. In the Rinne test, air conduction is compared with bony conduction of sound. A tuning fork is placed over the mastoid process and then in front of the external ear. In conductive hearing loss, the intensity of sound is louder when placed upon the bone, whereas in sensorineural hearing loss, the intensity is maximum at the external ear. In the Weber test, the tuning fork is placed in the midline of the head. In unilateral conductive hearing loss, the intensity of sound is loudest in the affected ear, whereas in unilateral sensorineural hearing loss, the intensity of sound is loudest in the unaffected ear. This patient reports left greater than right hearing loss that is suspected to be sensorineural in nature. Thus, the sound would be expected to be loudest in the right ear on the Weber test.

II-72. **The answer is C.** *(Chap. 43)* Once hearing loss is established, the next diagnostic test is pure tone audiometry that plots hearing threshold versus frequency. Pure tone audiometry establishes the severity, type, and laterality of hearing loss. In this gentleman, high-frequency hearing loss would be expected based on his complaints of inability to hear the alarm tone of his digital watch. Tympanometry measures the impedance of the middle ear to sound and is useful in diagnosis of middle ear effusions. Radiologic studies are indicated for suspected anatomic abnormalities. Axial and coronal CT of the temporal bone is ideal for determining the caliber of the external auditory canal, integrity of the ossicular chain, and presence of middle ear or mastoid disease; it can also detect inner ear malformations. CT is also ideal for the detection of bone erosion with chronic otitis media and cholesteatoma. MRI is superior to CT for imaging of retrocochlear pathology such as vestibular schwannoma, meningioma, other lesions of the cerebellopontine angle, demyelinating lesions of the brainstem, and brain tumors. Both CT and MRI are equally capable of identifying inner ear malformations and assessing cochlear patency for preoperative evaluation of patients for cochlear implantation. Schirmer test is a test for the evaluation of dry eyes to quantify adequate tear production.

II-73. **The answer is A.** *(Chap. 44)* While the patient likely has a middle ear infection, the CT shows an acute fluid collection in the left mastoid air cells consistent with acute mastoiditis. In typical acute mastoiditis, purulent exudate collects in the mastoid air cells, producing pressure that may result in erosion of the surrounding bone and formation of abscess-like cavities that are usually evident on CT. Patients typically present with pain, erythema, and swelling of the mastoid process along with displacement of the pinna, usually in conjunction with the typical signs and symptoms of acute middle ear infection. Rarely, patients can develop severe complications if the infection tracks under the periosteum of the temporal bone to cause a subperiosteal abscess, erodes through the mastoid tip to cause a deep neck abscess, or extends posteriorly to cause septic thrombosis of the lateral sinus. Purulent fluid should be cultured whenever possible to help guide antimicrobial therapy. Initial empirical therapy usually is directed against the typical organisms associated with acute otitis media, such as *Streptococcus pneumoniae*, *Haemophilus influenzae*, and *Moraxella catarrhalis*. Patients with more severe or prolonged courses of illness should be treated for infection with *S aureus* and gram-negative bacilli (including *Pseudomonas*). Most patients can be treated conservatively with IV antibiotics; surgery (cortical mastoidectomy) is reserved for complicated cases and those in which conservative treatment has failed. The CT does not show a mass suggesting meningioma. In the absence of diabetes, poorly controlled hyperglycemia, and a destructive invasive inflammatory process, mucormycosis is not likely.

II-74. **The answer is E.** *(Chap. 44)* Acute sinusitis is a common complication of upper respiratory tract infections and is defined as sinusitis lasting less than 4 weeks. Acute sinusitis typically presents nasal drainage and congestion, facial pain or pressure, and headache that is worse with lying down or bending forward. Presence of purulent drainage does not differentiate bacterial from viral causes of sinusitis. The vast majority of cases of acute sinusitis are due to viral infection. However, when patients with acute sinusitis present to a medical profession, antibiotics are prescribed more than 85% of the time. Indeed, this should not be the preferred treatment as most cases improve without antibiotic therapy. Rather, the initial approach to a patient with acute sinusitis should be symptomatic treatment with nasal decongestants and nasal saline lavage. If a patient has a history of allergic rhinitis or chronic sinusitis, nasal glucocorticoids can be prescribed as well. Antibiotic therapy is recommended in adults for symptom duration greater than 7–10 days and in children with symptom duration greater than 10–14 days. In addition, any patient with concerning features such as unilateral or focal facial pain or swelling should be treated with antibiotics. The initial antibiotic of choice for acute sinusitis is amoxicillin 500 mg orally three times daily or 875 mg twice daily. If a patient has prior exposure to antibiotics within the past 30 days or treatment failure, a respiratory fluoroquinolone can be given. Ten percent of individuals do not respond to initial antibiotic therapy. In this case, one can consider referral to otolaryngology for sinus aspiration and culture. Radiologic imaging of the sinuses is not recommended for evaluation of acute disease unless the sinusitis is nosocomially acquired because the procedures (CT or radiograph) do not differentiate between bacterial or viral causes.

II-75. **The answer is B.** *(Chap. 44)* Approximately 5%–15% of all cases of acute pharyngitis in adults are caused by *Streptococcus pyogenes*. Appropriate identification and treatment of *S pyogenes* with antibiotic therapy is recommended to decrease the small risk of acute rheumatic fever. In addition, treatment with antibiotics within 48 hours of onset of symptoms decreases symptom duration and, importantly, decreases transmission of streptococcal pharyngitis. In adults, the recommended diagnostic procedure by the Centers for Disease Control and Prevention and the Infectious Diseases Society of America is a rapid antigen detection test for group A streptococci only. In children, however, the recommendation is to perform a throat culture for confirmation if the rapid screen is negative to limit spread of disease and minimize potential complications. Throat culture generally is regarded as the most appropriate diagnostic method but cannot discriminate between colonization and infection. In addition, it takes 24–48 hours to get a result. Because most cases of pharyngitis at all ages are viral in origin, empiric antibiotic therapy is not recommended.

II-76 and II-77. **The answers are E and E, respectively.** *(Chaps. 45 and 46e)* The clue to diagnosis in this patient is a painless mouth ulcer. Ulceration is the most common oral mucosal lesion. Most acute ulcers are painful and self-limited. Recurrent aphthous ulcers and herpes simplex account for the majority. Persistent and deep aphthous ulcers can be idiopathic or can accompany HIV/AIDS. Aphthous lesions are often the presenting symptom in Behçet syndrome. Similar-appearing, though less painful, lesions may occur in reactive arthritis, and aphthous ulcers are occasionally present during phases of discoid or systemic lupus erythematosus. Aphthous-like ulcers are seen in Crohn disease, but, unlike the common aphthous variety, they may exhibit granulomatous inflammation on histologic examination. Recurrent aphthae are more prevalent in patients with celiac disease and have been reported to remit with elimination of gluten. Of major concern are chronic, relatively painless ulcers and mixed red/white patches (erythroplakia and leukoplakia) of >2 weeks in duration. Squamous cell carcinoma and premalignant dysplasia should be considered early and a diagnostic biopsy performed. High-risk sites include the lower lip, floor of the mouth, ventral and lateral tongue, and soft palate–tonsillar pillar complex. Significant risk factors for oral cancer in Western countries include sun exposure (lower lip), tobacco and alcohol use, and human papillomavirus infection. Syphilitic chancre may also present with a painless oral ulcer.

II-78. **The answer is A.** *(Chap. 48)* Although common in everyday life, the cough reflex is really quite intricate. First, some sensory input must trigger it. Spontaneous cough is triggered by stimulation of sensory nerve endings that are thought to be primarily rapidly adapting receptors and C fibers. Both chemical (e.g., capsaicin) and mechanical (e.g., particulates in air pollution) stimuli may initiate the cough reflex. Afferent nerve endings richly innervate the pharynx, larynx, and airways to the level of the terminal bronchioles and extend into the lung parenchyma. In some patients, they may also be located in the external auditory meatus (the auricular branch of the vagus nerve, or the Arnold nerve). To initiate the cough, the vocal cords adduct, leading to transient upper-airway occlusion. Expiratory muscles contract, generating positive intrathoracic pressures as high as 300 mmHg. With sudden release of the laryngeal contraction, rapid expiratory flows are generated, exceeding the normal "envelope" of maximal expiratory flow seen on the flow-volume curve (Figure II-78).

Bronchial smooth muscle contraction, together with dynamic compression of airways, narrows airway lumens and maximizes the velocity of exhalation. The kinetic energy available to dislodge mucus from the inside of airway walls is directly proportional to the square of the velocity of expiratory airflow.

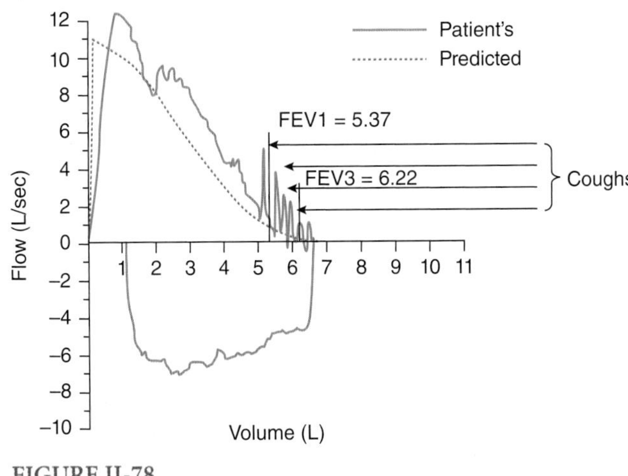

FIGURE II-78

II-79. The answer is B. *(Chap. 48)* Chronic cough is defined as cough existing longer than 8 weeks. In a patient with chronic productive cough, examination of expectorated sputum is warranted. Purulent-appearing sputum should be sent for routine bacterial culture and, in certain circumstances, mycobacterial culture as well. Cytologic examination of mucoid sputum may be useful to assess for malignancy and to distinguish neutrophilic from eosinophilic bronchitis. Chronic eosinophilic bronchitis causes chronic cough with a normal chest radiograph. This condition is characterized by sputum eosinophilia in excess of 3% without airflow obstruction or bronchial hyperresponsiveness and is successfully treated with inhaled glucocorticoids. The mechanism of angiotensin-converting enzyme (ACE) inhibitor–associated cough may involve sensitization of sensory nerve endings due to accumulation of bradykinin (option A). It is commonly held that (alone or in combination) the use of an ACE inhibitor, postnasal drainage, gastroesophageal reflux, and asthma account for more than 90% of cases of chronic cough with a normal or noncontributory chest radiograph. However, clinical experience does not support this contention, and strict adherence to this concept discourages the search for alternative explanations by both clinicians and researchers (option C). Regardless of cause, cough often worsens upon first lying down at night (option D), with talking, or with the hyperpnea of exercise (option E); it frequently improves with sleep.

II-80. The answer is B. *(Chap. 48)* Patients with bronchiectasis (a permanent dilation of the airways with loss of mucosal integrity) are particularly prone to hemoptysis due to chronic inflammation and anatomic abnormalities that bring the bronchial arteries closer to the mucosal surface. One common presentation of patients with advanced cystic fibrosis—the prototypical bronchiectatic lung disease—is hemoptysis, which can be life-threatening. Significant hemoptysis can result from the proximity of the bronchial artery and vein to the airway, with these vessels and the bronchus running together in what is often referred to as the *bronchovascular bundle.* In the smaller airways, these blood vessels are close to the airspace, and lesser degrees of inflammation or injury can therefore result in their rupture into the airways. While alveolar hemorrhage arises from capillaries that are part of the low-pressure pulmonary circulation, bronchial bleeding generally originates from bronchial arteries, which are under systemic pressure and thus are predisposed to larger volume bleeding.

II-81. The answer is C. *(Chap. 48)* Mr. Boyle is suffering from a large-volume life-threatening hemoptysis. As noted in the prior question, in this patient with cystic fibrosis and bronchiectasis, the culprit vessel is likely a bronchial artery. After initial stabilization, which almost always requires establishment of a patent airway with endotracheal intubation and mechanical ventilation and volume resuscitation, the goals are to isolate the bleeding to one lung and not to allow the preserved airspaces in the other lung to be filled with blood so that gas exchange is further impaired. Patients should be placed with the bleeding lung in a dependent position (i.e., bleeding side down), and if possible, dual lumen endotracheal tubes or an airway blocker should be placed in the proximal airway of the bleeding lung.

This patient should be placed in the right lateral decubitus position. Ultimate therapy of a bronchial arterial bleed may require bronchoscopically directed therapies such as cauterization or laser. In very severe cases, angiography and bronchial artery embolization can be employed. This carries a risk of spinal artery embolization requiring specialized interventional radiologic expertise.

II-82. **The answer is C.** *(Chap. 49)* In the evaluation of cyanosis, the first step is to differentiate central from peripheral cyanosis. In central cyanosis, because the etiology is either reduced oxygen saturation or abnormal hemoglobin, the physical findings include bluish discoloration of both mucous membranes and skin. In contrast, peripheral cyanosis is associated with normal oxygen saturation but slowing of blood flow and an increased fraction of oxygen extraction from blood; subsequently, the physical findings are present only in the skin and extremities. Mucous membranes are spared. Peripheral cyanosis is commonly caused by cold exposure with vasoconstriction in the digits. Similar physiology is found in Raynaud phenomenon. Peripheral vascular disease and deep venous thrombosis result in slowed blood flow and increased oxygen extraction with subsequent cyanosis. Methemoglobinemia causes abnormal hemoglobin that circulates systemically. Consequently, the cyanosis associated with this disorder is systemic. Other common causes of central cyanosis include severe lung disease with hypoxemia, right-to-left intracardiac shunting, and pulmonary arteriovenous malformations.

II-83. **The answer is C.** *(Chap. 49)* Chronic hypoxia leads to multiple adaptive changes in human physiology. It is believed that upregulation of hypoxia-inducible factor 1 (HIF-1) leads to increased expression of vascular endothelial growth factor (VEGF), which augments angiogenesis, and erythropoietin, which enhances erythrocyte production. Systemic arterioles dilate in the setting of hypoxia, leading to a reduction in systemic vascular resistance. However, in pulmonary arterioles, inhibition of potassium channels causes depolarization, contraction of smooth muscle cells, and arteriolar constriction. In times of local hypoxia in the lungs (areas with, for example, poor ventilation), this can serve to shunt blood flow toward areas with better ventilation and improve ventilation-perfusion matching. In the setting of systemic hypoxia, pulmonary vasoconstriction will lead to elevated pulmonary vascular resistance.

II-84. **The answer is A.** *(Chap. 49)* Options B–E all are examples of hypoxia due to respiratory failure and characterized by elevated $PaCO_2$. In instances of elevated partial pressure of carbon dioxide, the oxygen–hemoglobin dissociation curve shifts to the right. Thus, for any given arterial partial pressure of oxygen, the arterial hemoglobin will be lower. In normal physiologic circumstances, this is advantageous as hemoglobin is more likely to release oxygen (become less saturated) in areas where CO_2 is most prevalent (the target tissues of perfusion). As opposed to the other choices, the woman in option A will actually be hyperventilating and thus have a lower $PaCO_2$. This will shift the oxygen–hemoglobin dissociation curve to the left from baseline (known as the Bohr effect). Thus, for the given PaO_2 of 60 mmHg, she will have a higher arterial hemoglobin oxygen saturation.

II-85. **The answer is C.** *(Chap. 49)* Cyanosis is most importantly determined by the *absolute*, not relative, quantity of reduced hemoglobin (deoxygenated hemoglobin) or hemoglobin derivative (methemoglobin or sulfhemoglobin) in the capillary blood. In general, cyanosis becomes apparent when the concentration of reduced hemoglobin exceeds 4 g/dL. Thus, if two patients have identical relative concentrations of reduced hemoglobin (e.g., these patients with a hemoglobin saturation of 80% have 20% deoxygenated, or reduced, hemoglobin in their arterial blood), the patient with the highest absolute hemoglobin concentration will appear most cyanotic. As an example, we can consider the arterial blood of the patients in options A and C (although it is capillary blood that determines the appearance of cyanosis). The patient in option A has a hemoglobin concentration of 8 g/dL. If 20% of that is reduced, he will have an absolute amount of reduced hemoglobin of 1.6 g/dL; he may not appear cyanotic at all. However, the patient in option C, with the same relative 20% of his hemoglobin reduced, will have an absolute amount of reduced hemoglobin of 4 g/dL and will readily appear cyanotic. Thus, in a patient with severe anemia, the *relative* quantity of reduced hemoglobin in the venous blood may be very large when considered in relation to the total quantity of hemoglobin in the blood. However, since the concentration of the latter is markedly reduced, the *absolute* quantity of reduced hemoglobin may still be low, and therefore, patients with severe anemia and even *marked* arterial desaturation may not display cyanosis. Conversely, the higher the total hemoglobin content, the greater is the tendency toward cyanosis; thus, patients with marked polycythemia tend to be cyanotic at higher levels of SaO_2 than patients with normal hematocrit values.

II-86. **The answer is B.** *(Chap. 50)* The forces that regulate the disposition of fluid between these two components of the lung extracellular compartment frequently are referred to as the *Starling forces*. Increases in the hydrostatic pressure within the capillaries and the colloid oncotic pressure in the interstitial fluid tend to promote movement of fluid from the vascular to the extravascular space. By contrast, increases in the colloid oncotic pressure contributed by plasma proteins and the hydrostatic pressure within the interstitial fluid promote the movement of fluid into the vascular compartment. As a consequence, there is net movement of water and diffusible solutes from the vascular space at the arteriolar end of the capillaries. Fluid is returned from the interstitial space into the vascular system at the venous end of the capillaries and by way of the lymphatics. These movements are usually balanced so that there is a steady state in the sizes of the intravascular and interstitial compartments, yet a large exchange between them occurs. However, if either the capillary hydrostatic pressure is increased (as in left heart failure) and/or the capillary oncotic pressure is reduced, a further net movement of fluid from the intravascular to the interstitial spaces will take place, resulting in pulmonary edema. Pulmonary edema may also develop due to a decrease in lung permeability or protein reflection coefficient as seen in acute respiratory distress syndrome (ARDS). In isolation, atmospheric pressure changes will not have an effect because the pressure is equally distributed to the intra- and extravascular spaces.

II-87. **The answer is C.** *(Chap. 50)* Mr. Johnson has edema (option E) and signs of heart failure due to his reduced left ventricular function. In heart failure, the impaired systolic emptying of the ventricle(s) and/or the impairment of ventricular relaxation promotes an accumulation of blood in the venous circulation at the expense of the effective arterial volume (option C). In addition, the heightened tone of the sympathetic nervous system causes renal vasoconstriction (option D) and reduction of glomerular filtration. Renin is increased and subsequently increases the production of angiotensin I and II. Circulating angiotensin II stimulates the production of aldosterone from the zona glomerulosa of the adrenal cortex (option A). Circulating arginine vasopressin (AVP) is elevated in patients with heart failure secondary to a nonosmotic stimulus associated with decreased effective arterial volume (option C) and reduced compliance of the left atrium. Brain natriuretic peptide (pre-prohormone BNP) is stored primarily in ventricular myocytes and is released when ventricular diastolic pressure rises (option B). BNP (which is derived from its precursor) binds to the natriuretic receptor A, which causes: (1) excretion of sodium and water by augmenting glomerular filtration rate, inhibiting sodium reabsorption in the proximal tubule, and inhibiting release of renin and aldosterone; and (2) dilation of arterioles and venules by antagonizing the vasoconstrictor actions of angiotensin II, AVP, and sympathetic stimulation. Although circulating levels of atrial natriuretic peptide (ANP) and BNP are elevated in heart failure and in cirrhosis with ascites, the natriuretic peptides are not sufficiently potent to prevent edema formation. Indeed, in edematous states, resistance to the actions of natriuretic peptides may be increased, further reducing their effectiveness.

II-88. **The answer is D.** *(Chap. 51e)* Acute, severe mitral regurgitation (MR) into a normal-sized, relatively noncompliant left atrium results in an early decrescendo systolic murmur best heard at or just medial to the apical impulse. This murmur is often very soft, and indeed, approximately 50% of cases of acute severe mitral regurgitation have no murmur at all. These characteristics reflect the progressive attenuation of the pressure gradient between the left ventricle and the left atrium during systole owing to the rapid rise in left atrial pressure caused by the sudden volume load into an unprepared, noncompliant chamber and contrast sharply with the auscultatory features of chronic MR. Clinical settings in which acute, severe MR occur include (1) papillary muscle rupture complicating acute myocardial infarction, (2) rupture of chordae tendineae in the setting of myxomatous mitral valve disease, (3) infective endocarditis (which is likely the case for Mr. Carpentier), and

(4) blunt chest wall trauma. The murmur is to be distinguished from that associated with post–myocardial infarction ventricular septal rupture, which is accompanied by a systolic thrill at the left sternal border in nearly all patients and is holosystolic in duration. The holosystolic murmur of chronic MR is best heard at the left ventricular apex and radiates to the axilla (Figure II-88); it is usually high-pitched and plateaud in configuration because of the wide difference between left ventricular and left atrial pressure throughout systole. In contrast to acute MR, left atrial compliance is normal or even increased in chronic MR. As a result, there is only a small increase in left atrial pressure for any increase in regurgitant volume.

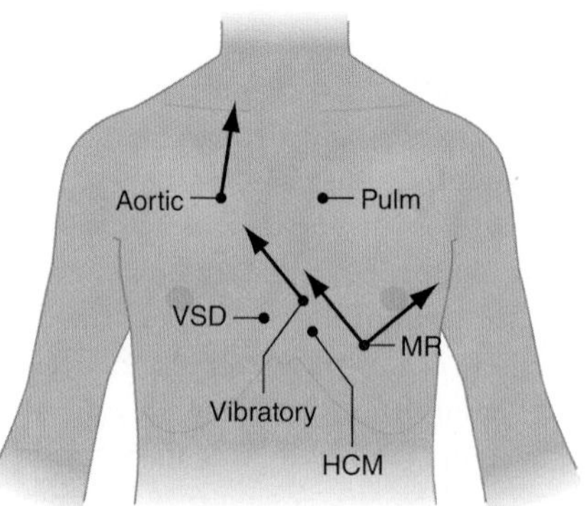

FIGURE II-88 From JB Barlow: *Perspectives on the Mitral Valve*. Philadelphia, FA Davis, 1987, p 140.

II-89. **The answer is D.** *(Chap. 51e)* Auscultatory findings of severe aortic stenosis (AS) include a soft or absent A_2, paradoxical splitting of S_2 (as the aortic valve closes later due to the prolonged ventricular-aortic gradient), an apical S_4, and a late-peaking systolic murmur. In children, adolescents, and young adults with congenital valvular AS, an early ejection sound (click) is usually audible, more often along the left sternal border than at the base. Its presence does not signify severity of the obstruction but signifies a flexible, noncalcified bicuspid valve (or one of its variants) and localizes the left ventricular outflow obstruction to the valvular (rather than sub- or supravalvular) level. Other, nonauscultatory findings can provide clues to the severity of AS. Assessment of the volume and rate of rise of the carotid pulse can provide additional information. A small and delayed upstroke (*parvus et tardus*) is consistent with severe AS. The carotid pulse examination is less discriminatory, however, in older patients with stiffened arteries. The electrocardiogram shows signs of left ventricular hypertrophy as the severity of the stenosis increases. Transthoracic echocardiography is indicated to assess the anatomic features of the aortic valve, the severity of the stenosis, left ventricular size, wall thickness and function, and the size and contour of the aortic root and proximal ascending aorta.

II-90. **The answer is E.** *(Chap. 51e)* The obstructive form of hypertrophic cardiomyopathy (HOCM) is associated with a midsystolic murmur that is usually loudest along the left sternal border or between the left lower sternal border and the apex. The murmur is produced by both dynamic left ventricular outflow tract obstruction and MR, and thus, its configuration is a hybrid between ejection and regurgitant phenomena. The intensity of the murmur may vary from beat to beat and after provocative maneuvers but usually does not exceed grade 3. The murmur classically will increase in intensity with maneuvers that result in increasing degrees of outflow tract obstruction, such as a reduction in preload or afterload (Valsalva, standing, vasodilators) or with an augmentation of contractility (inotropic stimulation such as milrinone). However, augmentation of contractility will also increase the intensity of the murmur of aortic stenosis and thus is not useful for differentiation. Augmentation of afterload (hand grip) is associated with diminished murmur intensity in both aortic stenosis and obstructive hypertrophic cardiomyopathy. Maneuvers that increase preload (squatting, passive leg raising, volume administration) or afterload (squatting, vasopressors) or agents that reduce contractility (β-adrenoceptor blockers) decrease the intensity of the murmur of hypertrophic cardiomyopathy. In contrast to AS, the carotid upstroke is rapid and of normal volume. Rarely, it is bisferiens or bifid in contour due to midsystolic closure of the aortic valve.

II-91. **The answer is A.** *(Chap. 51e)* Chronic, severe atrial regurgitation (AR) may produce a lower-pitched mid to late, grade 1 or 2 diastolic murmur at the apex (Austin Flint murmur), which is thought to reflect turbulence at the mitral inflow area from the admixture of regurgitant (aortic) and forward (mitral) blood. This lower-pitched, apical diastolic murmur can be distinguished from that due to MS by the absence of an opening snap and the response of the murmur to a vasodilator challenge. Lowering afterload with an agent such as amyl nitrite will decrease the duration and magnitude of the aortic–left ventricular diastolic pressure gradient, and thus, the Austin Flint murmur of severe AR will become shorter and softer. Increasing afterload (hand grip or phenylephrine) will have the opposite effect as the regurgitant volume through the incompetent aortic valve increases. The intensity of the diastolic murmur of MS may either remain constant or increase with afterload reduction (amyl nitrate or a calcium channel blocker such as nifedipine) because of the reflex increase in cardiac output and mitral valve flow.

II-92. **The answer is B.** *(Chap. 51e)* Rheumatic fever is the most common cause of MS. In younger patients with pliable valves, S_1 is loud and the murmur begins after an opening snap, which is a high-pitched sound that occurs shortly after S_2. The interval between the pulmonic component of the second heart sound (P_2) and the opening snap is inversely related to the magnitude of the left atrial–left ventricular pressure gradient. The murmur of MS is low-pitched and thus is best heard with the bell of the stethoscope. It is loudest at the left ventricular apex and often is appreciated only when the patient is turned in the left lateral decubitus position. It is usually of grade 1 or 2 intensity but may be absent when the cardiac output is severely reduced despite significant obstruction. The intensity of the murmur increases during maneuvers that increase cardiac output and mitral valve flow, such as exercise. The duration of the murmur reflects the length of time over which left atrial pressure exceeds left ventricular diastolic pressure. An increase in the intensity of the murmur just before S_1, a phenomenon known as *presystolic accentuation*, occurs in patients in sinus rhythm and is due to a late increase in transmitral flow with atrial contraction. Presystolic accentuation does not occur in patients with atrial fibrillation, as is the case with Mrs. Edwards, because of the lack of effective atrial contraction.

II-93. **The answer is A.** *(Chap. 52)* While the first sentence of option B is a correct statement for the general population—most patients with palpitations do *not* have serious arrhythmias or structural heart disease—this patient has some features that are concerning that the palpitations may be due to a life-threatening etiology. The association of palpitations with syncope or presyncope is concerning for a ventricular arrhythmia (either idiopathic or ischemic in origin) or another tachyarrhythmia in a patient with structural heart disease. In this patient with multiple coronary risk factors, the onset of dyspnea and palpitations leading to presyncope/syncope during physical exertion is concerning for myocardial ischemia. Further evaluation with an exercise stress test is appropriate. The suggestion of swimming (option C) would be potentially very dangerous as he runs the risk of passing out while in the water. Counseling tobacco cessation is always correct (option D), although the red-flag symptoms of syncope and dyspnea with his palpitations warrant further workup. Holter monitoring (option E) can be useful for a patient who has frequent arrhythmias, but this patient reliably has his palpitations with exertion, not at rest.

II-94. **The answer is D.** *(Chap. 56)* Involuntary weight loss (IWL) is frequently insidious and can have important implications, often serving as a harbinger of serious underlying disease. It is a common sign observed in outpatient practice, occurring in approximately 8% of all adult outpatients and 27% of the elderly or frail. Clinically important weight loss is defined as the loss of 10 lb (4.5 kg) or >5% of one's body weight over a period of 6–12 months. This patient has lost approximately 20% of her body weight in 9 months and therefore merits further evaluation. Documentation of the weight loss (weight record, clothing size) is important because up to 50% of people who claim to have lost weight have no documented weight loss. Most patients with IWL have a malignant neoplasm, chronic inflammatory or infectious disease, metabolic disorder (e.g., hyperthyroidism and diabetes), or psychiatric disorder. Not infrequently, more than one cause is responsible. There is no identifiable cause of IWL in up to 25% of cases despite investigation. Based on this differential, initial evaluation should include a comprehensive history and physical examination, neurologic/cognitive/mood screening, medication review, appropriate cancer screening, and the laboratory examinations listed in the question. At this time, despite the increase in lung cancers in female nonsmokers, low-dose CT scan is not recommended as part of age-appropriate cancer screening. If lung cancer is suspected after the initial evaluation, a lung CT may be indicated at a later date. In this patient, bone density assessment is indicated given her recent hip fracture. It is likely that the hip fracture was related to the IWL.

II-95. **The answer is E.** *(Chap. 59)* The normal small intestine contains approximately 200 mL of gas comprised of nitrogen, oxygen, carbon dioxide, hydrogen, and methane. Nitrogen and oxygen are consumed (swallowed), whereas carbon dioxide, hydrogen, and methane are produced intraluminally by bacterial fermentation. Increased intestinal gas can occur in a number of conditions. Aerophagia, the swallowing of air, can result in increased amounts of oxygen and nitrogen in the small intestine and lead to abdominal swelling. Aerophagia typically results from gulping food; chewing gum; smoking; or as a response to anxiety, which can lead to repetitive belching. In some cases, increased intestinal gas is the consequence of bacterial metabolism of excess fermentable substances such as lactose and other oligosaccharides, which can lead to production of hydrogen, carbon dioxide, or methane.

II-96. **The answer is E.** *(Chap. 59)* This patient presents with abdominal swelling due to ascites (one of the 6 "F's"—fluid, fetus, fat, feces, flatus, fatal mass) as is evidenced by the fluid wave and dullness to percussion on physical examination. A careful examination can often determine the underlying cause of ascites, particularly if it is due to elevated portal pressures. In this case, the patient has evidence of elevated pressure in the jugular veins (Kussmaul sign, where the jugular venous pulse fails to decrease with inspiration) and right ventricle (right ventricular heave and loud P_2 accompanied by the murmur of tricuspid regurgitation). These elevated right-sided cardiac pressures will back up into the hepatic veins. By necessity, the pressure in the portal vein must also elevate (as measured by the hepatic vein wedge pressure) to keep blood flowing forward.

II-97. **The answer is B.** *(Chap. 59)* This patient has ascites due to cirrhosis. The most telling laboratory value to calculate when assessing the etiology of ascites is the serum-ascites albumin gradient (SAAG). The SAAG is useful for distinguishing ascites caused by portal hypertension from non–portal hypertensive ascites. The SAAG reflects the pressure within the hepatic sinusoids and correlates with the hepatic venous pressure gradient. The SAAG is calculated by subtracting the ascitic albumin concentration from the serum albumin level and does not change with diuresis. A SAAG ≥1.1 g/dL reflects the presence of portal hypertension and indicates that the ascites is due to increased pressure in the hepatic sinusoids, as in cirrhosis. According to Starling's law, a high SAAG reflects the oncotic pressure that counterbalances the portal pressure. Possible causes include cirrhosis, cardiac ascites, hepatic vein thrombosis (chronic Budd-Chiari syndrome), sinusoidal obstruction syndrome (veno-occlusive disease), or massive liver metastases. A SAAG <1.1 g/dL indicates that the ascites is not related to portal hypertension, as in tuberculous peritonitis, peritoneal carcinomatosis, or pancreatic ascites. For high-SAAG (≥1.1) ascites, the ascitic protein level can provide further clues to the etiology. An ascitic protein level of ≥2.5 g/dL indicates that the hepatic sinusoids are normal and are allowing passage of protein into the ascites, as occurs in cardiac ascites, acute Budd-Chiari syndrome, or sinusoidal obstruction syndrome. An ascitic protein level <2.5 g/dL indicates that the hepatic sinusoids have been damaged and scarred and no longer allow passage of protein, as occurs with cirrhosis. In this patient, the SAAG is elevated (3.6 – 1.1 = 2.5) and ascitic protein is very low (0.9).

II-98. **The answer is D.** *(Chap. 59)* Cirrhotic patients with a history of spontaneous bacterial peritonitis (SBP), an ascitic fluid total protein concentration <1 g/dL, or active gastrointestinal bleeding should receive prophylactic antibiotics to prevent SBP. Oral daily norfloxacin is commonly used for this indication. Lactulose is often used to prevent and treat hepatic encephalopathy, which this patient does not have. Propranolol and other β-blockers are effective in preventing variceal bleeds; however, this patient is not known to have varices and has not had a bleeding episode. In cases of refractory ascites (need for repeated paracentesis despite adequate sodium restriction and maximally tolerated doses of diuretics), clonidine or midodrine may be used to attempt to reverse splanchnic vasoconstriction.

II-99. **The answer is D.** *(Chap. 61)* Acute renal failure can result from processes that affect renal blood flow (prerenal azotemia), intrinsic renal diseases (affecting small vessels, glomeruli, or tubules), or postrenal processes (obstruction of urine flow in ureters, bladder, or urethra). Differentiating between the processes narrows the differential diagnosis significantly. In this patient, the lack of hydronephrosis rules out obstructive uropathy, and the bland urinalysis and lack of urinary casts make glomerulonephritis, interstitial nephritis, or tubular necrosis unlikely. Control of vascular tone of the afferent glomerular arterioles is via prostaglandins. Prostaglandin antagonism with NSAIDs (such as naproxen) leads to afferent arteriolar constriction and reduction in glomerular flow/pressure. Angiotensin II causes efferent arteriolar vasoconstriction. Blocking angiotensin II (with ACE inhibitors or angiotensin receptor blockers [ARBs]) can cause efferent arteriolar vasodilation and a decrement in glomerular flow/pressure. For this patient, both mechanisms are likely active. Patients with bilateral renal artery stenosis are particularly prone to reductions in glomerular filtration rate with ACE inhibitor or ARB therapy because they rely heavily on vasoconstriction of the efferent arterioles to maintain glomerular pressure.

II-100. **The answer is C.** *(Chap. 61)* The dipstick protein measurement detects only albumin and gives false-positive results at pH >7.0 or when the urine is very concentrated or contaminated with blood. Proteinuria that is not predominantly due to albumin will be missed by dipstick screening. This information is particularly important for the detection of Bence-Jones proteins in the urine of patients with multiple myeloma. Tests to measure total urine protein concentration accurately rely on precipitation with sulfosalicylic or trichloracetic acid. Plasma cell dyscrasias (multiple myeloma) can be associated with large amounts of excreted light chains in the urine, which may not be detected by dipstick but will be measured by the direct test. The light chains are filtered by the glomerulus and overwhelm the reabsorptive capacity of the proximal tubule. Renal failure from these disorders occurs through a variety of mechanisms, including proximal tubule injury, tubule obstruction (cast nephropathy), and light chain deposition.

II-101. **The answer is D.** *(Chap. 63)* Osmolality and water homeostasis are jealously guarded within the body. Vasopressin secretion, water ingestion, and renal water transport collaborate to maintain human body fluid osmolality between 280 and 295 mOsm/kg. Vasopressin (AVP) is synthesized in magnocellular neurons within the hypothalamus; the distal axons of these neurons project to the posterior pituitary or neurohypophysis, from which AVP is released into the circulation. A network of central "osmoreceptor" neurons, which includes the AVP-expressing magnocellular neurons themselves, sense circulating osmolality via nonselective, stretch-activated cation channels. These osmoreceptor neurons are activated or inhibited by modest increases and decreases in circulating osmolality, respectively; activation leads to AVP release and thirst. AVP secretion is stimulated as systemic osmolality increases above a threshold level of ~285 mOsm/kg, above which there is a linear relationship between osmolality and circulating AVP. Thirst and thus water ingestion are also activated at ~285 mOsm/kg, beyond which there is an equivalent linear increase in the perceived intensity of thirst as a function of circulating osmolality. The excretion or retention of electrolyte-free water by the kidney is modulated by circulating AVP. AVP acts on renal, V2-type receptors in the thick ascending limb of Henle and principal cells of the collecting duct (CD), increasing intracellular levels of cyclic AMP and activating protein kinase A (PKA)–dependent phosphorylation of multiple transport proteins. The AVP- and PKA-dependent activation of Na^+-Cl^- and K^+ transport by the thick ascending limb of the loop of Henle (TALH) is a key participant in the countercurrent mechanism. The countercurrent mechanism ultimately increases the interstitial osmolality in the inner medulla of the kidney, driving water absorption across the renal CD. However, water, salt, and solute transport by both proximal and distal nephron segments participates in the renal concentrating mechanism. AVP-induced, PKA-dependent phosphorylation of the aquaporin-2 water channel in principal cells stimulates the insertion of active water channels into the lumen of the CD, resulting in transepithelial water absorption down the medullary osmotic gradient. Under "antidiuretic" conditions, with increased circulating AVP, the kidney reabsorbs water filtered by the glomerulus, equilibrating the osmolality across the CD epithelium to excrete a hypertonic, "concentrated" urine (osmolality of up to 1200 mOsm/kg). In the absence of circulating AVP, insertion of aquaporin-2 channels and water absorption across the CD are essentially abolished, resulting in secretion of a hypotonic, dilute urine (osmolality as low as 30–50 mOsm/kg). Abnormalities in this "final common pathway" are involved in most disorders of water homeostasis (e.g., a reduced or absent insertion of active aquaporin-2 water channels into the membrane of principal cells in diabetes insipidus).

II-102. The answer is D. *(Chap. 63)* It is indeed true that normal renal glomeruli filter approximately ~1.5 kg of salt daily, which would occupy roughly 10 times the extracellular space; 99.6% of filtered Na^+-Cl^- must be reabsorbed to excrete 100 mM per day. Minute changes in renal Na^+-Cl^- excretion will thus have significant effects on the extracellular fluid volume, leading to edema syndromes or hypovolemia. Approximately two-thirds of filtered Na^+-Cl^- is reabsorbed by the renal proximal tubule, via both paracellular and transcellular mechanisms. The thick ascending limb of Henle subsequently reabsorbs another 25%–30% of filtered Na^+-Cl^- via the apical, furosemide-sensitive Na^+-K^+-$2Cl^-$ co-transporter. The adjacent aldosterone-sensitive distal nephron, comprising the distal convoluted tubule (DCT), connecting tubule (CNT), and collecting duct, accomplishes the "fine-tuning" of renal Na^+-Cl^- excretion. The thiazide-sensitive apical Na^+-Cl^- co-transporter (NCC) reabsorbs 5%–10% of filtered Na^+-Cl^- in the DCT. Principal cells in the CNT and CD reabsorb Na^+ via electrogenic, amiloride-sensitive epithelial Na^+ channels (ENaC); Cl^- ions are primarily reabsorbed by adjacent intercalated cells, via apical Cl^- exchange (Cl^--OH^- and Cl^--HCO_3^- exchange), mediated by the SLC26A4 anion exchanger.

II-103. The answer is E. *(Chap. 63)* This patient is dehydrated (hypovolemic) from vomiting and has a hypochloremic metabolic alkalosis in response. Because gastric secretions have a low pH (high H^+ concentration), whereas biliary, pancreatic, and intestinal secretions are alkaline (high HCO_3^- concentration), vomiting and diarrhea are often accompanied by metabolic alkalosis and acidosis, respectively. The neurohumoral response to hypovolemia stimulates an increase in renal tubular Na^+ and water reabsorption, with a urine osmolality of >450 mOsm/kg. The reduction in both glomerular filtration rate and distal tubular Na^+ delivery may cause a defect in renal potassium excretion, with an increase in plasma K^+ concentration. Of note, patients with hypovolemia and a hypochloremic alkalosis due to vomiting or diuretics will typically have a urine Na^+ concentration >20 mM and urine pH of >7.0, due to the increase in filtered HCO_3^-; the urine Cl^- concentration in this setting is a more accurate indicator of volume status, with a level <25 mM suggestive of hypovolemia. Patients with uncomplicated hypovolemia, such as after insufficient oral intake or diarrhea, will have urine sodium <20mM. The urine Na^+ concentration is also often >20 mM in patients with intrinsic renal injury. Urine specific gravity increases as osmolality increases; in this case, it would be elevated, or >1.020.

II-104. The answer is C. *(Chap. 63)* This patient is hypovolemic. Hypovolemia causes a marked neurohumoral activation, increasing circulating levels of AVP. The increase in circulating AVP helps preserve blood pressure via vascular and baroreceptor V1A receptors and increases water reabsorption via renal V2 receptors; activation of V2 receptors can lead to hyponatremia in the setting of increased free water intake. Nonrenal causes of hypovolemic hyponatremia include GI loss (e.g., vomiting, diarrhea, tube drainage) and insensible loss (sweating, burns) of Na^+-Cl^- and water, in the absence of adequate oral replacement; urine Na^+ concentration is typically <20 mM. Notably, these patients may be clinically classified as euvolemic, with only the reduced urinary Na^+ concentration to indicate the cause of their hyponatremia. Indeed, a urine Na^+ concentration <20 mM, in the absence of a cause of hypervolemic hyponatremia, predicts a rapid increase in plasma

Na^+ concentration in response to intravenous normal saline; saline therapy thus induces a water diuresis in this setting, as circulating AVP levels plummet. A cognitive framework for thinking through etiologies of hyponatremia is shown in Figure II-104.

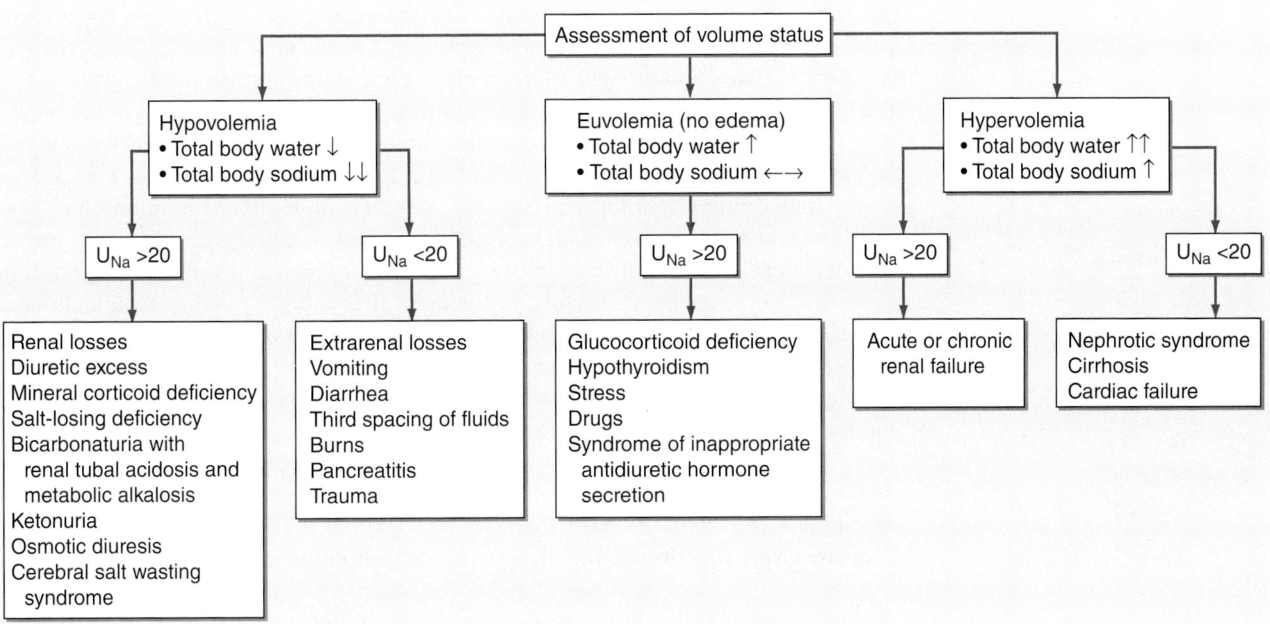

FIGURE II-104

II-105. The answer is E. *(Chap. 63)* Largely, hyponatremia is due to a dyscrasia in water homeostasis. There are some conditions (e.g., beer potomania) where very low intake of dietary solutes leads to hyponatremia, although antidiuretic hormone (ADH) levels are likely initially elevated in this condition (though they have never been measured). In most cases of hyponatremia (dehydration, heart failure, cirrhosis), the effective arterial circulating volume is reduced, leading to excess ADH signaling and water reabsorption. However, in psychogenic polydipsia, the patient drinks massive amounts of solute-free water, overwhelming the body's ability to excrete free water. In this setting, ADH is suppressed. Central diabetes insipidus is a failure of manufacture or release of ADH and thus is associated with a reduction in ADH levels. However, it is associated with hypernatremia.

II-106. The answer is E. *(Chap. 63)* This patient has pseudohyponatremia. Laboratory investigation should include a measurement of serum osmolality to exclude pseudohyponatremia, which is defined as the coexistence of hyponatremia with a normal or increased plasma tonicity. Most clinical laboratories measure plasma Na^+ concentration by testing diluted samples with automated ion-sensitive electrodes, correcting for this dilution by assuming that plasma is 93% water. This correction factor can be inaccurate in patients with pseudohyponatremia due to extreme hyperlipidemia and/or hyperproteinemia, in whom serum lipid or protein makes up a greater percentage of plasma volume. This patient likely has a type of familial hyperlipidemia associated with elevated triglycerides (thus explaining his seemingly idiopathic pancreatitis) and accounting for his pseudohyponatremia.

II-107. The answer is C. *(Chap. 63)* Exercise-associated hyponatremia, an important clinical issue at marathons and other endurance events, has similarly been linked to both a "nonosmotic" increase in circulating AVP and excessive free water intake. The first major consideration guiding the therapy of hyponatremia is the presence and/or severity of symptoms. This determines the urgency and goals of therapy. Patients with acute hyponatremia, such as Mr. Jones, present with symptoms that can range from headache, nausea, and/or vomiting, to seizures, obtundation, and central herniation; patients with chronic hyponatremia, present for >48 hours, are less likely to have severe symptoms. Treatment of acute symptomatic hyponatremia should include hypertonic 3% saline (513 mM) to acutely increase plasma Na^+ concentration by 1–2 mM/hr to a total of 4–6 mM; this modest increase is typically sufficient to alleviate severe acute symptoms, after which corrective guidelines for chronic hyponatremia are appropriate (see below). A number of equations have been developed to estimate the required rate of hypertonic saline, which has an Na^+-Cl^- concentration of 513 mM. The traditional approach is to calculate an Na^+ deficit, where the Na^+ deficit = 0.6 × body weight × (target plasma Na^+ concentration – starting plasma Na^+ concentration), followed by a calculation of the required rate. Regardless of the method used to determine the rate of administration, the increase in plasma Na^+ concentration can be highly unpredictable during treatment with hypertonic saline, due to rapid changes in the underlying physiology; plasma Na^+ concentration should be monitored every 2–4 hours during treatment, with appropriate changes in therapy based on the observed rate of change. The administration of supplemental oxygen and ventilatory support are also critical in acute hyponatremia, in the event that patients develop acute pulmonary edema or hypercapneic respiratory failure. Intravenous loop diuretics will help treat acute pulmonary edema and will also increase free water excretion, by interfering with the renal countercurrent multiplication system. AVP antagonists do not have an approved role in the management of acute hyponatremia. The rate of correction should be comparatively slow in chronic hyponatremia (<8–10 mM in the first 24 hours and <18 mM in the first 48 hours), so as to avoid osmotic demyelination syndrome (ODS); lower target rates are appropriate in patients at particular risk for ODS, such as alcoholics or hypokalemic patients. Overcorrection of the plasma Na^+ concentration can occur when AVP levels rapidly normalize, for example following the treatment of patients with chronic hypovolemic hyponatremia with intravenous saline or following glucocorticoid replacement of patients with hypopituitarism and secondary adrenal failure. Approximately 10% of patients treated with vaptans, such as conivaptan, will overcorrect; the risk is increased if water intake is not liberalized. In the event that the plasma Na^+ concentration overcorrects following therapy, be it with hypertonic saline, isotonic saline, or a vaptan, hyponatremia can be safely reinduced or stabilized by the administration of the AVP agonist desmopressin acetate (DDAVP) and/or the administration of free water, typically intravenous D5W; the goal is to prevent or reverse the development of ODS. Alternatively, the treatment of patients with marked hyponatremia can be initiated with the twice-daily administration of DDAVP to maintain constant AVP bioactivity, combined with the administration of hypertonic saline to slowly correct the serum sodium in a more controlled fashion, thus reducing upfront the risk of overcorrection.

II-108. **The answer is E.** *(Chap. 63)* This patient has severe hypernatremia after being denied free water. In the state of nephrogenic diabetes insipidus, the kidneys fail to respond to ADH and excrete dilute urine regardless of serum osmolality. To correct this hyponatremia, you must first calculate the patient's total free water deficit. This is calculate as: ([Na] – 140/140) × (total body water) where total body water is roughly 50%–60% of body weight (60% in men, or 60 kg for Mr. Matherli). Thus, Mr. Matherli's free water deficit is ~8.5 L (or 8500 mL). To replace this in 24 hours requires approximately 350 mL/hr of free water administration.

II-109. **The answer is D.** *(Chap. 65)* The first step in the diagnostic evaluation of hyper- or hypocalcemia is to ensure that the alteration in serum calcium levels is not due to abnormal albumin concentrations. About 50% of total calcium is ionized, and the rest is bound principally to albumin. Although direct measurements of ionized calcium are possible, they are easily influenced by collection methods and other artifacts; thus, it is generally preferable to measure total calcium and albumin to "correct" the serum calcium. When serum albumin concentrations are reduced, a corrected calcium concentration is calculated by adding 0.2 mM (0.8 mg/dL) to the total calcium level for every decrement in serum albumin of 1.0 g/dL below the reference value of 4.1 g/dL for albumin and, conversely, for elevations in serum albumin. This patient's albumin is 2.5, or ~1.5 below the reference value. Thus, we would add 1.6 (or 0.8 × 1.5) to the measured calcium level, arriving at a corrected value of 9.4 mg/dL—a value requiring no treatment for the hypocalcemia. Additional evaluation may be in order for the symptoms and reduced serum albumin.

II-110. The answer is B. *(Chap. 65)* When serum albumin concentrations are reduced, a corrected calcium concentration is calculated by adding 0.2 mM (0.8 mg/dL) to the total calcium level for every decrement in serum albumin of 1.0 g/dL below the reference value of 4.1 g/dL for albumin and, conversely, for elevations in serum albumin. For this patient, the corrected serum calcium is elevated at 12.7 (11.5 + [4 – 2.5] × 0.8). Significant symptomatic hypercalcemia usually requires therapeutic intervention independent of the etiology of hypercalcemia. Initial therapy of significant hypercalcemia begins with volume expansion because hypercalcemia invariably leads to dehydration; 4–6 L of intravenous saline may be required over the first 24 hours, keeping in mind that underlying comorbidities (e.g., congestive heart failure) may require the use of loop diuretics to enhance sodium and calcium excretion. However, loop diuretics should not be initiated until the volume status has been restored to normal. If there is increased calcium mobilization from bone (as in malignancy or severe hyperparathyroidism), drugs that inhibit bone resorption should be considered. Zoledronic acid (e.g., 4 mg intravenously over ~30 minutes), pamidronate (e.g., 60–90 mg intravenously over 2–4 hours), and ibandronate (2 mg intravenously over 2 hours) are bisphosphonates that are commonly used for the treatment of hypercalcemia of malignancy in adults. In patients with 1,25(OH)2D-mediated hypercalcemia, glucocorticoids are the preferred therapy, as they decrease 1,25(OH)2D production. Intravenous hydrocortisone (100–300 mg daily) or oral prednisone (40–60 mg daily) for 3–7 days is used most often.

II-111. The answer is B *(Chap. 66)* This patient has evidence of an acidosis with serum pH <7.35; thus both choices invoking alkalosis are ruled out. The next step is to evaluate which physiologic determinant of pH accounts for the acidosis. The $PaCO_2$ is low (normal ~40 mmHg); thus it is not compatible with a respiratory acidosis. The HCO_3^- is low, accounting for a metabolic acidosis. Thus, this is a pure metabolic acidosis, likely due to ketoacidosis given the patient's diabetes history and elevated anion gap (sodium – [chloride + HCO_3^-]).

II-112. The answer is E. *(Chap. 66)* While all of the choices listed can cause lactic acidosis, short gut syndrome is the only associated with D-lactic acidosis, instead of L-lactic acidosis. D-Lactic acid acidosis, which may be associated with jejunoileal bypass, short bowel syndrome, or intestinal obstruction, is due to formation of D-lactate by gut bacteria. The other forms of lactic acidosis typically seen in situations of inadequate oxygen delivery to tissues are due to elevations of intrinsically produced L-lactic acid.

II-113. The answer is A. *(Chap. 66)* This patient is suffering from ethylene glycol toxicity. Ingestion of ethylene glycol (commonly used in antifreeze) leads to a metabolic acidosis and severe damage to the CNS, heart, lungs, and kidneys. The increased anion gap and osmolar gap are attributable to ethylene glycol; its metabolites oxalic acid and glycolic acid; and other organic acids. Lactic acid production increases secondary to inhibition of the tricarboxylic acid cycle and altered intracellular redox state. Diagnosis is facilitated by recognizing oxalate crystals in the urine, the presence of an osmolar gap in serum, and a high anion gap metabolic acidosis. Although use of a Wood lamp to visualize the fluorescent additive to commercial antifreeze in the urine of patients with ethylene glycol ingestion is suggested, this is rarely reproducible. The combination of a high anion gap and high osmolar gap in a patient suspected of ethylene glycol ingestion should be taken as evidence of ethylene glycol toxicity. This patient's osmolar gap is 20. Calculated serum osmolality is 2(Na) + BUN/2.8 + glucose/18 = 300 in this case. Therefore the osmolar gap is 20 (320 – 300). Treatment should not be delayed while awaiting measurement of ethylene glycol levels in this setting. Treatment includes the prompt institution of a saline or osmotic diuresis, thiamine and pyridoxine supplements, fomepizole, and occasionally, hemodialysis. The IV administration of the alcohol dehydrogenase inhibitor fomepizole (4-methylpyrazole; 15 mg/kg as a loading dose) is the treatment of choice and offers the advantages of a predictable decline in ethylene glycol levels without excessive obtundation as seen during ethyl alcohol infusion. If used, ethanol IV should be infused to achieve a blood level of 22 mmol/L (100 mg/dL). Both fomepizole and ethanol reduce toxicity because they compete with ethylene glycol for metabolism by alcohol dehydrogenase. Hemodialysis is indicated when the arterial pH is <7.3 or the osmolar gap exceeds 20 mOsm/kg.

II-114. The answer is A. *(Chap. 67)* Normal male sexual function requires (1) an intact libido, (2) the ability to achieve and maintain penile erection, (3) ejaculation, and (4) detumescence. Libido refers to sexual desire and is influenced by a variety of visual, olfactory, tactile, auditory, imaginative, and hormonal stimuli. Sex steroids, particularly testosterone, act to increase libido. Libido can be diminished by hormonal or psychiatric disorders and by medications. Nitric oxide, which induces vascular relaxation, promotes erection. Nitric oxide increases the production of cyclic GMP, which induces relaxation of smooth muscle. Cyclic GMP is gradually broken down by phosphodiesterase type 5 (PDE-5). Inhibitors of PDE-5, such as the oral medications sildenafil, vardenafil, and tadalafil, maintain erections by reducing the breakdown of cyclic GMP. Ejaculation is stimulated by the sympathetic nervous system; this results in contraction of the epididymis, vas deferens, seminal vesicles, and prostate, causing seminal fluid to enter the urethra. Seminal fluid emission is followed by rhythmic contractions of the bulbocavernosus and ischiocavernosus muscles, leading to ejaculation. Detumescence is mediated by norepinephrine from the sympathetic nerves, endothelin from the vascular surface, and smooth muscle contraction induced by postsynaptic α-adrenergic receptors and activation of Rho kinase. These events increase venous outflow and restore the flaccid state.

II-115. The answer is D. *(Chap. 67)* The phosphodiesterase-5 inhibitors, including sildenafil, tadalafil, vardenafil, and avanafil, are the only approved and effective oral agents for the treatment of erectile dysfunction (ED). They are effective for the treatment of a broad range of causes, including psychogenic, diabetic, vasculogenic, post–radical prostatectomy (nerve-sparing procedures), and spinal cord injury. Androgen therapy with testosterone may be effective to improve libido and erectile function in patients with low serum testosterone, but this patient has a normal serum testosterone for age. 5α-Reductase inhibitors, such as finasteride, are used to treat prostatic hypertrophy and act as antiandrogens; thus, they may cause ED. Corticosteroids and selective serotonin reuptake inhibitor (SSRI) medications are associated with causing ED.

II-116. The answer is B. *(Chap. 67)* In postmenopausal women, estrogen replacement therapy may be helpful in treating vaginal atrophy, decreasing coital pain, and improving clitoral sensitivity. Estrogen replacement in the form of local cream is the preferred method, as it avoids systemic side effects. There is no proven efficacy of phosphodiesterase-5 inhibitors, such as sildenafil, in female sexual dysfunction despite similar sexual response physiology in women as men. Selective serotonin reuptake inhibitors used for depression, such as paroxetine, may cause sexual dysfunction in women. Tamoxifen and anastrozole are antiestrogens used to treat breast cancer and may cause vaginal atrophy and female sexual dysfunction.

II-117. The answer is D. *(Chap. 68)* Hirsutism, which is defined as androgen-dependent excessive male pattern hair growth, affects approximately 10% of women. Hirsutism is most often idiopathic or the consequence of androgen excess associated with the polycystic ovarian syndrome (PCOS). Less frequently, it may result from adrenal androgen overproduction as occurs in nonclassic congenital adrenal hyperplasia (CAH). Historic elements relevant to the assessment of hirsutism include the age at onset and rate of progression of hair growth and associated symptoms or signs (e.g., acne). Depending on the cause, excess hair growth typically is first noted during the second and third decades of life. The growth is usually slow but progressive. Sudden development and rapid progression of hirsutism suggest the possibility of an androgen-secreting neoplasm, in which case virilization also may be present. Physical examination should include measurement of height and weight and calculation of body mass index (BMI). A BMI >30 kg/m^2 is often seen in association with hirsutism, probably the result of increased conversion of androgen precursors to testosterone. Notation should be made of blood pressure, because adrenal causes may be associated with hypertension. Cutaneous signs sometimes associated with androgen excess and insulin resistance include acanthosis nigricans and skin tags. An objective clinical assessment of hair distribution and quantity is central to the evaluation in any woman presenting with hirsutism. This assessment permits the distinction between hirsutism and hypertrichosis and provides a baseline reference point to gauge the response to treatment. A simple and commonly used method to grade hair growth is the modified scale of Ferriman and Gallwey (Figure II-117), in which each of nine androgen-sensitive

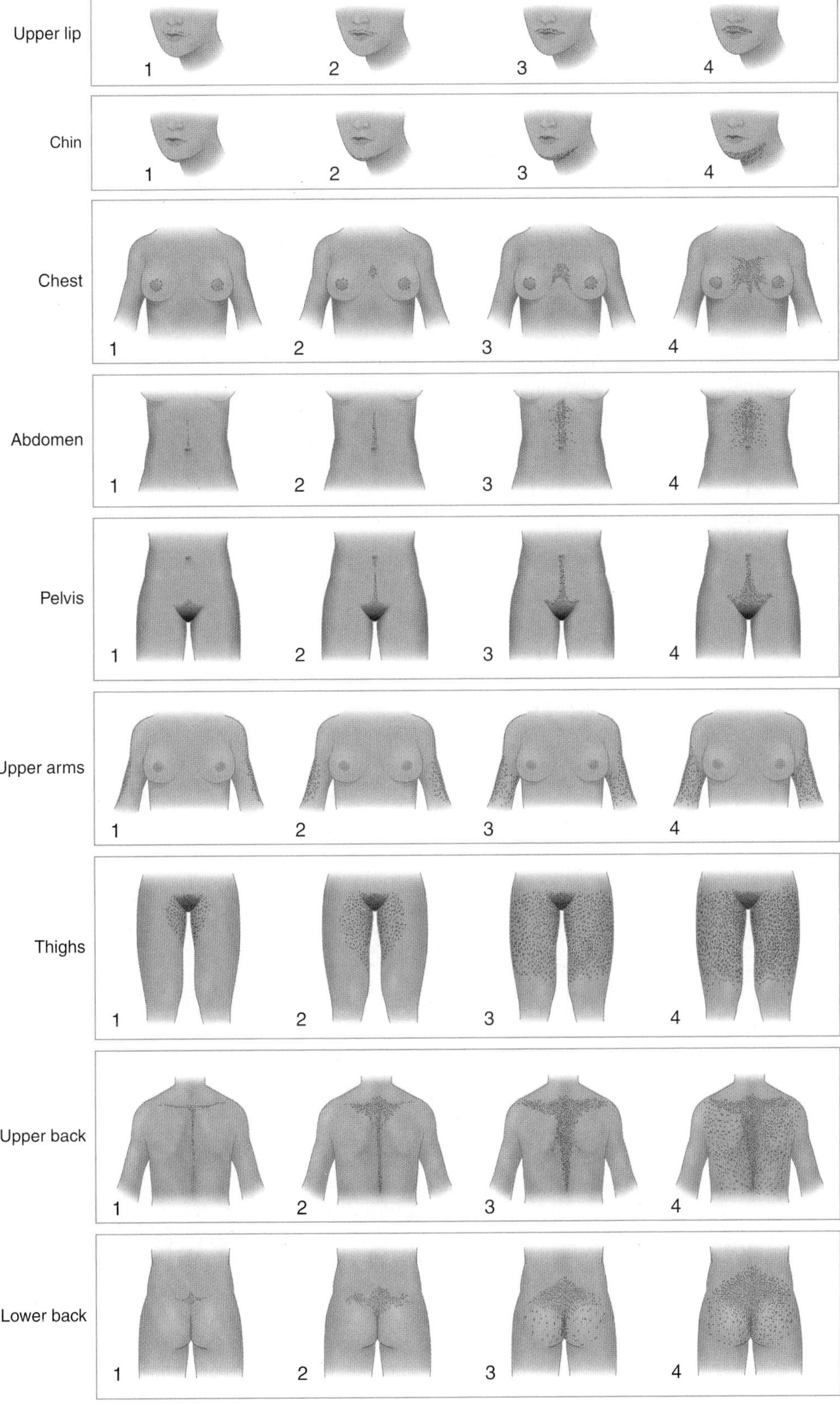

FIGURE II-117 Modified from DA Ehrmann et al: Hyperandrogenism, hirsutism, and polycystic ovary syndrome, in LJ DeGroot and JL Jameson (eds.), *Endocrinology*, 5th ed. Philadelphia, Saunders, 2006; with permission.

sites is graded from 0 to 4. Approximately 95% of white women have a score below 8 on this scale; thus, it is normal for most women to have some hair growth in androgen-sensitive sites. Scores above 8 suggest excess androgen-mediated hair growth, a finding that should be assessed further by means of hormonal evaluation. In racial/ethnic groups that are less likely to manifest hirsutism (e.g., Asian women), additional cutaneous evidence of androgen excess should be sought, including pustular acne and thinning scalp hair.

II-118. The answer is E. *(Chap. 68)* Androgens are secreted by the ovaries and adrenal glands in response to their respective tropic hormones: luteinizing hormone (LH) and adrenocorticotropic hormone (ACTH). The principal circulating steroids involved in the etiology of hirsutism are testosterone, androstenedione, and dehydroepiandrosterone (DHEA) and its sulfated form (DHEAS). The ovaries and adrenal glands normally contribute about equally to testosterone production. The initial evaluation of hirsutism includes measurement of serum testosterone, free testosterone, and DHEAS. High levels of testosterone suggest a virilizing tumor, and high levels of DHEAS suggest an adrenal source or polycystic ovarian syndrome. A suggested diagnostic algorithm is shown in Figure II-118.

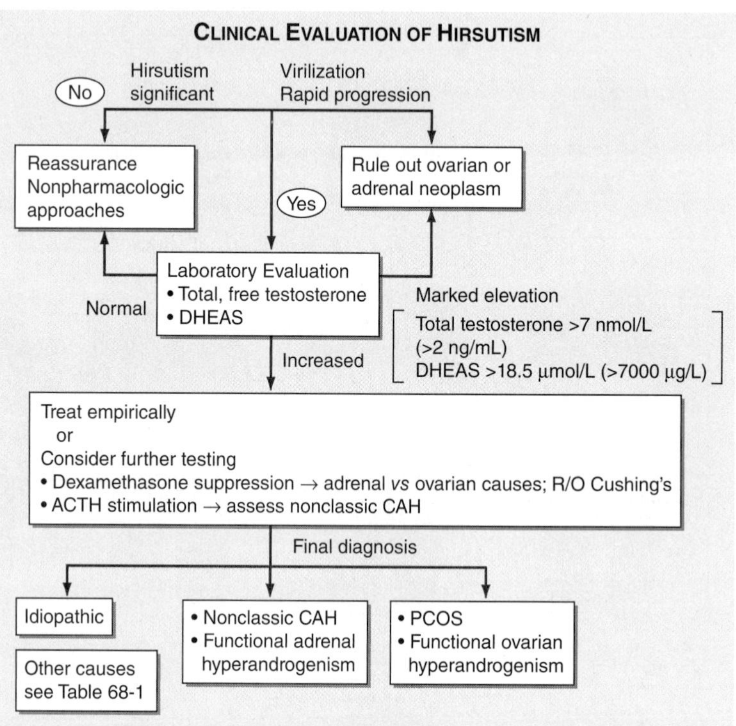

FIGURE II-118 *Abbreviations:* ACTH, adrenocorticotropic hormone; CAH, congenital adrenal hyperplasia; DHEAS, sulfated form of dehydroepiandrosterone; PCOS, polycystic ovarian syndrome.

II-119. The answer is D. *(Chap. 69)* Amenorrhea refers to the absence of menstrual periods. Amenorrhea is classified as primary if menstrual bleeding has never occurred in the absence of hormonal treatment or secondary if menstrual periods cease for 3–6 months. Primary amenorrhea is a rare disorder that occurs in <1% of the female population. However, between 3% and 5% of women experience at least 3 months of secondary amenorrhea in any specific year. There is no evidence that race or ethnicity influences the prevalence of amenorrhea. However, because of the importance of adequate nutrition for normal reproductive function, both the age at menarche and the prevalence of secondary amenorrhea vary significantly in different parts of the world. The absence of menses by age 16 has been used traditionally to define primary amenorrhea. However, other factors, such as growth, secondary sexual characteristics, the presence of cyclic pelvic pain, and the secular trend toward an earlier age of menarche, particularly in African American girls, also influence the age at which primary amenorrhea should be investigated. Thus, an evaluation for amenorrhea should be initiated by age 15 or 16 in the presence of normal growth and secondary sexual characteristics; age 13 in the absence of secondary sexual characteristics or if height is less than the third percentile; age 12 or 13 in the presence of breast development and cyclic pelvic pain; or within 2 years of breast development if menarche, defined by the first menstrual period, has not occurred. Anovulation and irregular cycles are relatively common for up to 2 years after menarche and for 1–2 years before the final menstrual period. In the intervening years, menstrual cycle length is ~28 days, with an intermenstrual interval normally ranging between 25 and 35 days. Cycle-to-cycle variability in an individual woman who is ovulating consistently is generally +/– 2 days. Pregnancy is the most common cause of amenorrhea and should be excluded early in any evaluation of menstrual irregularity. However, many women occasionally miss a single period. Three or more months of secondary amenorrhea should prompt an evaluation, as should a history of intermenstrual intervals >35 or <21 days or bleeding that persists for >7 days.

II-120. The answer is B. *(Chap. 69)* The first step in the evaluation of amenorrhea is assessment of the uterus and outflow tract. If normal, subsequent evaluation should include ruling out pregnancy followed by measurement of androgens (testosterone and DHEAS), follicle-stimulating hormone (FSH), and prolactin. As shown in the Figure II-120 below, this patient has findings consistent with a neuroendocrine tumor and should receive an MRI. Androgen resistance syndrome requires gonadectomy because there is risk of gonadoblastoma in the dysgenetic gonads. Whether this should be performed in early childhood or after completion of breast development is controversial.

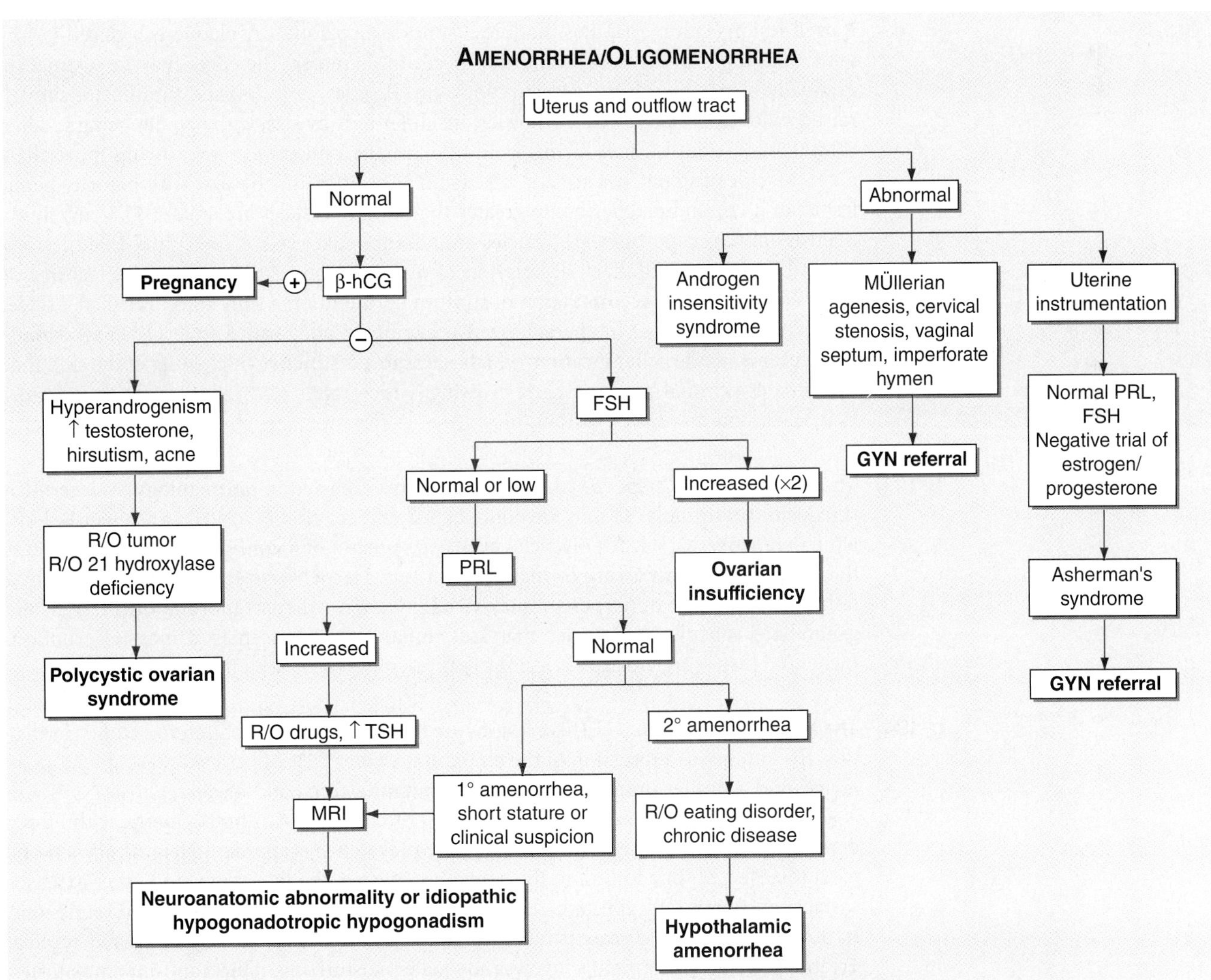

FIGURE II-120 Algorithm for evaluation of amenorrhea. β-hCG, human chorionic gonadotropin; FSH, follicle-stimulating hormone; GYN, gynecologist; MRI, magnetic resonance imaging; PRL, prolactin; R/O, rule out; TSH, thyroid-stimulating hormone.

II-121. The answer is D. *(Chap. 69)* Polycystic ovarian syndrome (PCOS) is diagnosed based on a combination of clinical or biochemical evidence of hyperandrogenism, amenorrhea or oligomenorrhea, and the ultrasound appearance of polycystic ovaries. Approximately half of patients with PCOS are obese, and abnormalities in insulin dynamics are common, as is metabolic syndrome. Symptoms generally begin shortly after menarche and are slowly progressive. Patients may develop dysfunctional uterine bleeding as defined by frequent or heavy uterine bleeding. A major abnormality in patients with PCOS is the failure of regular predictable ovulation. Thus, these patients are at risk for the development of dysfunctional bleeding and endometrial hyperplasia associated with unopposed estrogen exposure. Endometrial protection can be achieved with the use of oral contraceptives or progestins (medroxyprogesterone acetate, 5–10 mg, or Prometrium, 200 mg daily for 10–14 days of each month). Oral contraceptives are also useful for management of hyperandrogenic symptoms, as is spironolactone, which functions as weak androgen receptor blocker. Clomiphene and letrozole are used in PCOS patients who are interested in fertility. Corticosteroids will worsen this patient's obesity and hyperglycemia. Testosterone will worsen the PCOS because the disorder is driven by androgen excess.

II-122. The answer is D. *(Chap. 70)* Rashes and skin lesions are one of the most common reasons for visits to primary care physicians. Accurately characterizing a skin lesion is important for determining the underlying cause of the disease. Four basic features that are important when describing a skin lesion are the distribution, types of primary and secondary lesions, shape, and arrangement of lesions. The primary description of a skin lesion takes into account size, whether the lesion is raised or flat, and whether the lesion is fluid-filled. Raised lesions can be papules, nodules, tumors, or plaques. A plaque is a raised lesion with a flat top that measures more than 1 cm in diameter. The edges may be distinct or gradually blend in with the surrounding skin. Papules, nodules, and tumors are similar raised solid lesions of the skin. These lesions differ only by size, with papules being smaller than 0.5 cm, nodules measuring from 0.5–5.0 cm, and tumors measuring more than 5 cm. Macules and patches are not raised and also differ only by size, with macules being less than 2 cm and patches being greater than 2 cm. Vesicles are small (<0.5 cm) fluid-filled lesions, and pustules are vesicles containing leukocytes. Larger fluid-filled lesions are called bullae. Secondary description of a skin lesion takes into account features of the lesion. An excess accumulation of stratum corneum on a skin lesion is called a scale. Thus, this patient would be characterized as having a plaque with a scale. Other secondary descriptors include lichenification, which refers to a distinctive thickening of the skin that accentuates skinfold markings, and crusting, which refers to dried body fluids. In addition, the lesion may have erosions, ulceration, excoriation, atrophy, or scarring.

II-123. The answer is D. *(Chap. 70)* Characteristic terms are used in dermatology to describe a skin lesion. Nummular lesions are coin-shaped and are closely related to annular lesions, which are ring-shaped. A polycyclic eruption consists of a configuration of skin lesions that coalesce to form a ring or incomplete rings. Herpetiform lesions are grouped in a fashion that is seen in herpes simplex virus infection, whereas morbilliform lesions are generalized macules or papules that are similar to those seen in a measles eruption. Lichenoid rashes are violaceous lesions that resemble those seen in lichen planus.

II-124. The answer is D. *(Chap. 71)* These lesions are typical examples of childhood atopic dermatitis, the cutaneous expression of the atopic state. Over 75% of patients present by 5 years of age, and a similar proportion have concomitant asthma and/or allergic rhinitis. There is a strong genetic predisposition. Over 80% of children with both parents with atopic dermatitis will have similar skin findings; the prevalence is approximately 50% when one parent is affected. In addition to the antecubital fossae, the face, neck, and other extensor surfaces are commonly affected. The typical course involves exacerbations and remissions. In the adult form, the disease is often localized lichen simplex chronicus or hand eczema. Treatment of atopic dermatitis involves adequate moisturizing, topical anti-inflammatories, and avoidance of secondary bacterial infection. Topical tacrolimus and pimecrolimus are approved as therapy. They do not cause some of the complications of topical corticosteroids, but recent reports have raised the concern of a potentially increased risk of lymphoma. Children with atopic dermatitis may have spontaneous resolution, but about 40% of children with symptoms will have dermatitis as adults. Interestingly, for unknown reasons, the worldwide prevalence of atopic dermatitis is increasing.

II-125. The answer is E. *(Chap. 71)* All patients with psoriasis should be advised to avoid excessive drying of the skin and maintain hydration. Secondary bacterial infection should be suspected with local worsening and treated appropriately. Topical glucocorticoids often cause skin atrophy and lose effectiveness over time. Topical vitamin D analogues and retinoids have effectively replaced topical coal tar, salicylic acid, and anthralin as local adjunctive therapies. UVA (with psoralen) and/or UVB light is an effective therapy for widespread psoriasis in many cases. These therapies may be associated with an increased risk of skin cancer, particularly in patients who are immunocompromised. Methotrexate is often effective in patients with psoriatic arthritis (up to 30% of patients with psoriasis). Cyclosporine and other modulators of T-cell–mediated immunity are effective in psoriasis. Alefacept is an intramuscular biologic that is anti-CD2 and is indicated in psoriasis. It may cause lymphopenia, increased risk of infection, or secondary malignancy. Infliximab, etanercept, and adalimumab are anti-TNF biologics indicated for use in psoriasis arthritis (etanercept is indicated for psoriasis). They are associated with an increased risk of serious systemic infection, neurologic events (progressive multifocal leukoencephalopathy), and hypersensitivity reactions. Oral glucocorticoids should not be used for the treatment of psoriasis due to the potential for developing life-threatening pustular psoriasis when the therapy is discontinued.

II-126. The answer is C. *(Chap. 71)* The figure shows findings typical of stasis dermatitis with erythematous, scaly, and oozing patches over the lower leg and noninfected stasis ulcers. Stasis dermatitis develops on the lower extremities secondary to venous incompetence and chronic edema. Patients may give a history of deep venous thrombosis and may have evidence of vein removal or varicose veins. Early findings in stasis dermatitis consist of mild erythema and scaling associated with pruritus. The typical initial site of involvement is the medial aspect of the ankle, often over a distended vein. Stasis dermatitis may become acutely inflamed, with crusting and exudate. In this state, it is easily confused with cellulitis. Chronic stasis dermatitis is often associated with dermal fibrosis that is recognized clinically as brawny edema of the skin. As the disorder progresses, the dermatitis becomes progressively pigmented due to chronic erythrocyte extravasation leading to cutaneous hemosiderin deposition. Stasis dermatitis may be complicated by secondary infection and contact dermatitis. Patients with stasis dermatitis and stasis ulceration benefit greatly from leg elevation and the routine use of compression stockings with a gradient of at least 30–40 mmHg. Stockings providing less compression, such as antiembolism hose, are poor substitutes. Topical steroids may help the itching of dermatitis but should not be applied to the stasis ulcers, as they may slow healing. There is no indication for systemic corticosteroids. In the absence of active infection, there is no indication for antibiotics. The lesions of stasis ulcers should not be confused with zoster; thus, there is no indication for acyclovir. Calciphylaxis or calcific uremic arteriolopathy causes skin necrosis in patients with advanced chronic renal insufficiency.

II-127. The answer is A. *(Chap. 72)* This patient presents with clinical characteristics consistent with telogen effluvium, a common cause of diffuse, nonscarring hair loss. Telogen effluvium occurs when typically asynchronous hair growth cycles become synchronous, and therefore, a large number of hairs simultaneously change from a cycle of growth (anagen) to death (telogen). Common causes of telogen effluvium include stressors such as high fever or infection, medications, and changes in hormone levels. The postpartum period is a common time when telogen effluvium occurs. On physical examination, a practitioner may not notice any visible hair thinning, although examination of pictures of the patient from prior to the onset may allow the changes to become clinically recognizable. More importantly, the clinician should not find evidence of broken or brittle hair or scalp changes, including scaling or scarring. The hair pull test may yield an increased number of intact hairs (>6–10) with light pressure. Telogen effluvium does not require any treatment and is reversible. Any potential offending medication should be stopped, and the patient should be examined for underlying metabolic disorders.

II-128. The answer is E. *(Chap. 72)* Purpura is seen when red blood cells extravasate into the dermis, resulting in the characteristic lack of blanching with pressure. Purpura can be either palpable or nonpalpable, and this distinction helps to identify the underlying etiology. This patient has palpable purpura, which is caused by either a vasculitis or emboli. Leukocytoclastic vasculitis (LCV) is a cutaneous small-vessel vasculitis and one of the most common causes of palpable purpura. There are many etiologies of LCV including drugs, infections, and autoimmune disease. The most likely etiology in this patient would be the recent use of cefuroxime causing immune complex deposition. Henoch-Schönlein purpura also causes LCV with a lower extremity predominance. However, the age of onset is most often in children and adolescents, and there are associated symptoms including fever, arthralgias, abdominal pain, gastrointestinal bleeding, and nephritis. Ecthyma gangrenosum is an embolic phenomenon associated with gram-negative infection. These lesions are edematous and erythematous papules or plaques that can develop central purpura and necrosis. Both capillaritis and drug-induced thrombocytopenia are associated with nonpalpable purpura.

II-129. The answer is A. *(Chap. 73)* A variety of immunologically mediated skin diseases are recognized by their clinical and pathologic features. This patients presents with features consistent with pemphigus vulgaris, which is an autoimmune blistering disease characterized by loss of adhesion between epidermal cells. Clinically, most patients with pemphigus vulgaris present after age 40, and the initial lesions are on mucosal surfaces, predominantly the oral mucosa. These lesions erode quickly to ulcers and are typically quite painful. They may be the only manifestation or precede the development of blistering skin lesions by several months. The typical skin lesions are fragile, flaccid blisters on the scalp, face, neck, axilla, groin, and trunk. Due to the fragile nature of the blisters, they rupture quickly, leaving behind denuded skin with ulcerations that can be extensive and quite painful. Pruritus may or may not be present. Lesions typically heal without scarring unless there is secondary infection or mechanically induced dermal wounds. Manual pressure to the skin of these patients may elicit the separation of the epidermis, a phenomenon known as Nikolsky sign. However, this finding is nonspecific. Characteristic lesions are shown in Figure II-129. Biopsy of the lesion will show acantholytic blister formation in the suprabasal layer of the epidermis with intradermal vesicle formation. Basal keratinocytes remain attached to the epidermal basement membrane. Dermal alterations are minimal. On immunopathology, deposits of IgG are found on the surface of keratinocytes. Deposits of complement may be found in lesional but not uninvolved skin. The autoantibody in pemphigus vulgaris is directed toward desmoglein-3 in those who have only mucosal involvement. If skin involvement is also present, antibodies to desmoglein-1 are demonstrated as well. Pemphigus vulgaris can be life-threatening when there is diffuse skin involvement. Mortality rates prior to use of systemic steroids were as high as 60%–90%, but currently, mortality rates are only ~5%. The most common causes of death in pemphigus vulgaris are secondary infection and complications of treatment with systemic glucocorticoids. Initial treatment is prednisone at a dose of 1 mg/kg daily. Additional immunosuppressive treatment including azathioprine, cyclophosphamide, mycophenolate mofetil, rituximab, or plasmapheresis may be required in severe cases. Other diseases have distinct immunopathologic features as well. Cell surface deposits of IgG and C3 on keratinocytes with variable deposition of immunoreactants on the epidermal basement membrane zone (option B) are characteristic of paraneoplastic pemphigus. These patients develop painful mucosal erosive lesions as well as papulosquamous and/or lichenoid eruptions that may progress to blistering lesions. These individuals have an array of autoantibodies to members of the plakin family. Individuals who are found to have granular deposits of IgA in the dermal papillae (option C) present with dermatitis herpetiformis, a profoundly pruritic papulovesicular rash on extensor surfaces that is associated with gluten-sensitive enteropathy. Mucous membrane pemphigoid is a rare disease characterized by erosive lesions of mucous membranes and skin, including scalp, face, and upper trunk, with demonstration of deposit of IgG, IgA, and/or C3 in the epidermal basement membrane (option D). Finally, a linear band of IgG and/or C3 (option E) in the epidermal basement membrane is seen in epidermolysis bullosa acqusita, another rare chronic blistering disease. Lesions in this disorder generally occur at sites of minor trauma and are associated with widespread inflammatory scarring.

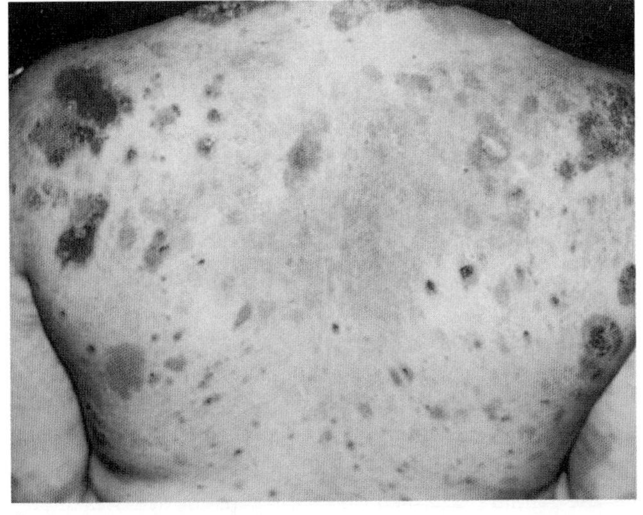

A

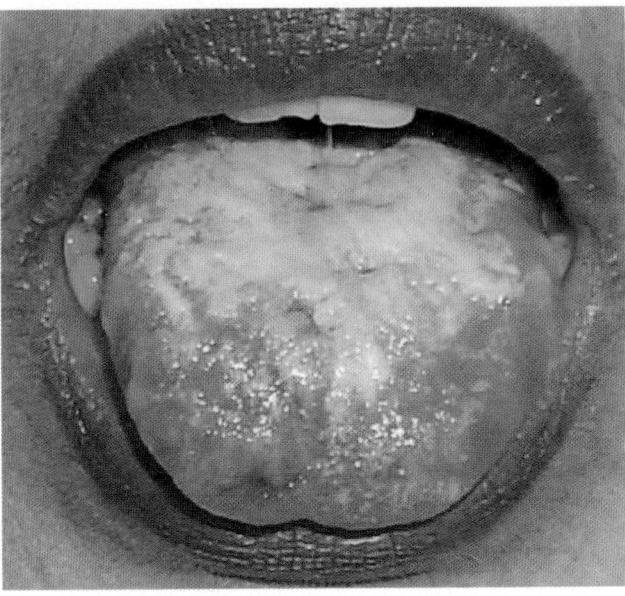

B

FIGURE II-129 **B.** Courtesy of Robert Swerlick, MD; with permission.

II-130. The answer is A. *(Chap. 73)* Bullous pemphigoid is an autoimmune cutaneous disease that primarily presents in elderly individuals. Although the initial lesions may consist of urticarial plaques, most patients eventually develop tense blisters on either a normal or erythematous base. Typical lesions of bullous pemphigoid are demonstrated in the figure. The most common sites of bullous pemphigoid are the lower abdomen, groin, and flexor surfaces of the extremities. Oral mucosal lesions may be seen but are not the common presenting lesion that is typically seen in pemphigus vulgaris. Pruritus may or may not be present. However, if present, it may be severe. Nontraumatized blisters will heal without scarring. It should be noted that there is no epidemiologic link between bullous pemphigoid and undiagnosed malignancy despite some initial case studies suggesting this might be so. Biopsies of the lesions of bullous pemphigoid demonstrate a subepidermal blister with a dense eosinophil-rich infiltrate. Mononuclear cells and neutrophils are also seen. Biopsies of normal-appearing skin will also show minimal perivascular leukocytic infiltrate with some eosinophils. Direct immunofluorescence microscopy of normal-appearing skin, however, will demonstrate linear deposits of IgG and/or C3 in the epidermal basement membrane, and about 70% of individuals with bullous pemphigoid have IgG autoantibodies that bind the epidermal basement membrane of normal human skin in indirect immunofluorescence microscopy. Bullous pemphigoid may persist for many months to years, with relapses and remissions. Most patients are treated with oral glucocorticoids. Additional immunosuppression may be needed in extensive disease.

II-131. The answer is D. *(Chap. 73)* Dermatitis herpetiformis (DH) is an immunologic skin disorder characterized by severe pruritus with skin lesions symmetrically distributed along the extensor surfaces, buttocks, back, scalp, and posterior neck. The lesions of DH may be papular, papulovesicular, or urticarial plaques. Because of the severity of the associated pruritus, many patients do not exhibit the primary skin lesions but have excoriations and crusted papules. Burning and stinging are also frequently reported along with the pruritus, and these symptoms are present prior to the manifestation of skin lesions. Almost all patients have an associated gluten-sensitive enteropathy, although it may be clinically unrecognized on presentation. Pathologically, the lesions demonstrate a neutrophilic inflammatory infiltrate in the dermal papillae. On immunofluorescence, granular deposits of IgA are found in the papillary dermis and along the epidermal basement membrane. The primary treatment of DH is dapsone at doses of 50–200 mg daily, with most patients reporting remarkable improvement within 24–48 hours. At doses greater than 100 mg daily, one must pay close attention to side effects because methemoglobinemia and hemolysis frequently occur. In addition to dapsone, gluten-free diets are recommended. However, many months of the diet are required to achieve a clinical benefit, so diet is not recommended as the sole treatment. Corticosteroids are not used in the treatment of DH.

II-132. The answer is E. *(Chap. 75)* Sunburn is an acute inflammatory reaction of the skin to sunlight, predominantly to the UVB rays of the sun. The body's response to the sun depends primarily on the amount of melanin in the skin, which is produced in melanocytes in the dermis. The melanocortin-1 receptor (MC1R) is central to determining the genetic differences in skin coloration and response to sunlight. Individuals with fair skin and red hair typically have low MC1R levels and thus produce little melanin upon exposure to sunlight. These individuals may always burn in response to sun exposure and never tan. In contrast, high MC1R activity is associated with increased melanocyte activity and resultant melanin production, resulting in tanning of the skin. Sunburn erythema is caused by vasodilation of dermal blood vessels and has a lag time of 4–12 hours after sun exposure to the development of visible redness. Both UVA and UVB radiation can cause sunburn, but UVB is much more efficient at causing burns. However, at midday, UVA rays are much more prevalent and thus contribute more to the response at this time. Tanning beds, used for cosmetic tanning, administer >90% UVA radiation but are still associated with the toxicities of excessive sun exposure such as skin cancer and premature skin aging. Sunscreens are now required to protect against both UVA and UVB radiation and are labelled as broad spectrum to indicate this.

II-133. The answer is E. *(Chap. 75)* Sulfonylurea medications can cause both photoallergy and phototoxicity reactions, but several clinical manifestations should allow one to distinguish between the two disorders. Phototoxicity is a nonimmunologic reaction that can occur without a latency period after taking a drug. The response resembles a sunburn and occurs in sun-exposed areas. Like a sunburn, a phototoxic reaction can blister and desquamate. A photoallergic reaction is much less common and occurs when the UV rays transform the drug into an unstable hapten capable of stimulating an immune response. This delayed hypersensitivity response is intensely pruritic. Sun-exposed skin appears lichenified and leathery. In some individuals, non–sun-exposed skin is also involved. Mucous membranes are not involved. In rare cases (5%–10%), persistent hypersensitivity to light will persist even after the offending drug is discontinued, a condition known as persistent light reaction.

II-134. The answer is D. *(Chap. 77)* Normal erythropoiesis requires proper erythropoietin production, proliferative capacity of the bone marrow, availability of iron and other cofactors, and effective maturation of red blood cell (RBC) precursors. The physiologic regulator of RBC production is erythropoietin (EPO), a glycoprotein produced in the peritubular capillary lining cells of the kidney. EPO production and gene regulation are controlled by hypoxia-inducible factor-1α, which is upregulated in response to hypoxia. EPO then stimulates the early progenitor cells in the bone marrow to increase in number and, in turn, to produce more RBCs. The first morphologically recognizable RBC precursor is the pronormoblast. This cell divides four to five times to generate a total of 16–32 mature RBCs. With EPO stimulation, RBC production increases markedly up to four- to fivefold, reaching maximum capacity within a 1–2 week period. In the absence of EPO, however, erythroid progenitor cells will undergo apoptosis or programmed cell death. Overall, normal RBC production and turnover results in the replacement of 0.8%–1.0% of the RBC population on a daily basis.

II-135. The answer is E. *(Chap. 77)* This patient presents with a microcytic anemia in the setting of heavy menses and a vegetarian diet that may be low in iron. She is most likely to have an iron deficiency anemia, which results in a hypoproliferative bone marrow relative to the degree of anemia. At least 75% off all anemias are hypoproliferative in nature, with iron deficiency being the most common cause. Iron deficiency anemia results in a characteristic microcytic hypochromic anemia. On laboratory examination, this is manifest as a low mean corpuscular volume (MCV), low mean corpuscular hemoglobin (MCH), and low mean corpuscular hemoglobin concentration. The peripheral blood smear in iron deficiency anemia characteristically shows microcytosis (small cells) and hypochromia (pale cells) with small cells with central pallor. However, there is also marked anisocytosis (unequal size cells) and poikilocytosis (abnormal shape cells), with cells of many different sizes and shapes. The degree of anisocytosis typically correlates with the red cell distribution width (RDW) as measured on the complete blood count. Poikilocytosis results in cells of many different shapes and represents a defect of red cell maturation in the bone marrow or fragmentation of circulating red cells. Thus, all of the findings can be seen in severe iron deficiency anemia. The next step in the workup of this patient would be to perform iron studies, including ferritin, iron, transferrin, and total iron-binding capacity.

II-136. The answer is E. *(Chap. 77)* This patient has an asymptomatic microcytosis and hypochromia, as evidenced by a low MCV and low MCH, but is not anemic. This is typical of individuals with α-thalassemia trait. Thalassemias are inherited disorders of hemoglobin production that result in production of an abnormal α- or β-globin. α-Thalassemias are most common in individuals of African, Asian, Middle Eastern, or Mediterranean descent. The production of α-globulin is encoded by four α-globin genes, two each on chromosome 16 (αα/αα). α-Thalassemia trait results when there is a defect in two of the α-globin genes (-α/-α or --/αα). Overall, the production of the α-globin is adequate to yield a normal hemoglobin and not result in excessive hemolysis. However, microcytosis and hypochromia are seen. Hematocrit is normal or only minimally reduced while RBC count may be increased. In addition, to microcytosis and hypochromia, the characteristic finding on peripheral smear is the target cell. These cells have a bulls-eye appearance and can also be seen in liver disease. Burr cells are typically seen in uremia and show multiple spiny projections. Howell-Jolly bodies are nuclear remnants that can be seen in some RBCs in individuals who have undergone splenomegaly as these proteins are not easily cleared in these individuals. Schistocytes are RBC fragments that can be seen in individuals who are experiencing intravascular hemolysis. Spherocytes are small dense RBCs that lack central pallor and biconcavity. They are typically seen in hereditary spherocytosis, but can also be seen in other autoimmune hemolytic anemias.

II-137. The answer is C. *(Chap. 77)* This blood smear shows fragmented RBCs of varying size and shape. In the presence of a foreign body within the circulation (prosthetic heart valve, vascular graft), RBCs can become destroyed. Such intravascular hemolysis will also cause serum lactate dehydrogenase to be elevated and hemoglobinuria. In isolated extravascular hemolysis, there is no hemoglobin or hemosiderin released into the urine. The characteristic peripheral blood smear in splenomegaly is the presence of Howell-Jolly bodies (nuclear remnants within RBCs). Certain diseases are associated with extramedullary hematopoiesis (e.g., chronic hemolytic anemias), which can be detected by an enlarged spleen, thickened calvarium, myelofibrosis, or hepatomegaly. The peripheral blood smear may show teardrop cells or nucleated RBCs. Hypothyroidism is associated with macrocytosis, which is not demonstrated here. Chronic gastrointestinal blood loss will cause microcytosis, not schistocytes.

II-138. The answer is B. *(Chap. 77)* The first step in diagnosing polycythemia vera is to document an elevated RBC mass. A normal RBC mass suggests spurious polycythemia. Next, serum EPO levels should be measured. If EPO levels are low, the diagnosis is polycythemia vera. Confirmatory tests include *JAK-2* mutation analysis, leukocytosis, and thrombocytosis. Elevated EPO levels are seen in the normal physiologic response to hypoxia as well as in autonomous production of EPO. Further steps in the workup include evaluation for hypoxia with an arterial blood gas, consideration of smoker's polycythemia (elevated carboxyhemoglobin levels) and disorders of increased hemoglobin affinity for oxygen. Low serum EPO levels with low oxygen saturation suggest inadequate renal production (renal failure). High RBC mass and high EPO levels with normal oxygen saturation may be seen with autonomous EPO production, such as in renal cell carcinoma.

II-139. The answer is E. *(Chap. 78)* Upon injury, hemostasis is achieved via platelet adhesion and aggregation along with fibrin clot formation. The initial step in the process of hemostasis is platelet adhesion. This is primarily mediated by von Willebrand factor (vWF). vWF is a very large multimeric protein that is found in both the plasma and in the extracellular matrix of the subendothelial vessel wall. It acts almost like a "molecular glue" as it binds the platelets with enough strength to allow them to withstand shear stress and prevent detachment. Platelet adhesion also occurs to a lesser degree with subendothelial collagen through specific platelet membrane collagen receptors.

II-140, II-141, II-142, and II-143. The answers are B, D, C, and A, respectively. *(Chap. 78)* Hemostasis involves a balance of procoagulant and anticoagulant forces. The procoagulant forces include platelet adhesion and aggregation and fibrin clot formation, whereas the anticoagulant system includes the natural inhibitors of coagulation and the process of fibrinolysis. There are many proteins required to balance this system, which is finely tuned to be ready to initiate coagulation upon injury and arrest bleeding quickly. Upon injury, platelets quickly adhere to the site of injury by binding to von Willebrand factor primarily and to exposed subepithelial collagen to a lesser extent. After the initial platelet adhesion, platelets become activated to promote further aggregation to promulgate the clot. This process is mediated in part through the action of the glycoprotein IIb/IIIa receptor on the platelet surface. The protein is the most abundant receptor on the platelet surface. Upon platelet activation, the glycoprotein IIb/IIIa receptor can bind von Willebrand factor and fibrinogen, furthering platelet aggregation. Fibrin clot formation is classically thought of as occurring via the intrinsic and extrinsic pathways. It is now known that coagulation is normally initiated through exposure to tissue factor (the classic extrinsic pathway) with important amplification through the element of the intrinsic pathway. There are many dynamic interactions that occur with tissue factor activation. Tissue factor binds the cofactor VIIa and can act to directly activate factor X, or it can activate factor IX, which in turn acts with factor VIIIa to activate factor X. Activated factor X then converts prothrombin to thrombin, which in turn has a positive feedback on the coagulant system by activating factor XI (the classic intrinsic pathway). (See Figure II-143.) Thrombin is a multifunctional enzyme that also converts fibrinogen to fibrin to promulgate clot formation. The body has several antithrombotic mechanisms to counteract the coagulant system. Antithrombin is the major protease inhibitor of thrombin and the other clotting factors of the coagulation system. Protein C is a plasma glycoprotein that is activated by thrombin and acts to inactivate factors V and VIII. This process is accelerated by the cofactor protein S, which is a glycoprotein that, like protein C, undergoes vitamin K–dependent posttranslational modification. Tissue factor pathway inhibitor (TFPI) is a protease that acts near the binding site for tissue factor (TF) and factor VIIa to downregulate the coagulation pathway. In addition to these anticoagulants, there is an active process of fibrin degradation. Plasmin is the major protease of the fibrinolytic system, breaking fibrin down to fibrin degradation products.

II-144. The answer is E. *(Chap. 78)* This individual has experienced significant bleeding that is primarily mucosal in origin (postpartum hemorrhage, prior oral bleeding). This suggests

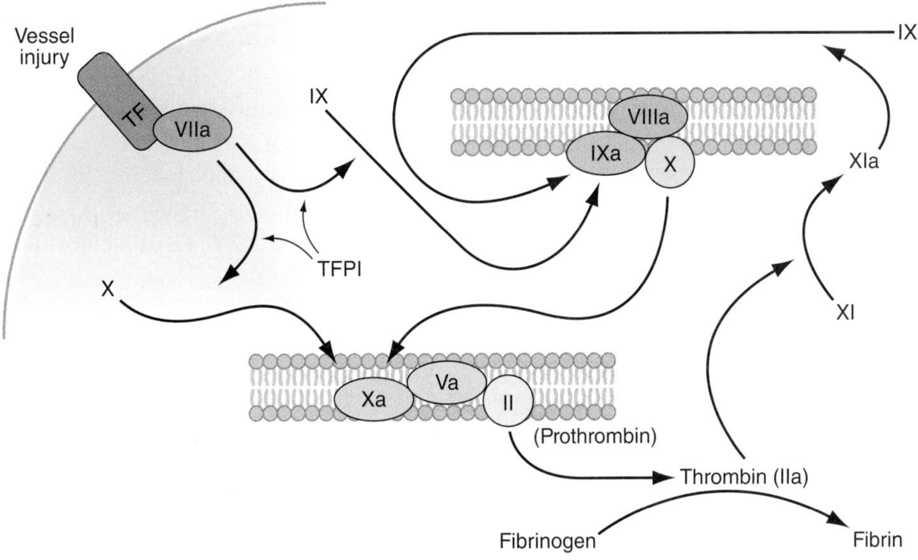

FIGURE II-143

a disorder of primary hemostasis, or platelet plug formation. von Willebrand disease (vWD) is the only disease listed that is a disorder of primary hemostasis. Bleeding symptoms that are common in vWD include prolonged bleeding after surgery, including dental procedures, menorrhagia, postpartum hemorrhage, and large bruises or hematomas, even with minor trauma. Epistaxis is also common but occurs in many other diseases as well. Therefore, a clinician should assess for other symptoms prior to ascribing the symptom to a disorder of platelet function. The postpartum hemorrhage can be delayed beyond the immediate period of delivery. Hemarthroses are rare in vWD unless the disease is very severe. All of the other disorders listed affect anticoagulant levels.

II-145. The answer is C. *(Chap. 78)* The most important part of determining bleeding risk prior to surgery is a careful history and physical examination. Routine testing for preoperative evaluation should include a prothrombin time because this test may detect a previously unknown vitamin K deficiency or unsuspected liver disease. Although it is common to concomitantly assess the activated partial thromboplastin time, the utility of this practice has not been validated in patients undergoing surgery in the absence of a bleeding history. The bleeding time has previously been used to assess bleeding risk but has not been shown to have any predictive value in determining individuals at increased bleeding risk during surgery. Thus, it should not be ordered.

II-146. The answer is A. *(Chap. 78)* Deciding which individuals require workup for hypercoagulability and the timing of the workup is a difficult diagnostic dilemma. This scenario presents an individual with two clotting episodes separated in time by a prolonged period and with clear risk factors. It is not likely that she would have a hypercoagulable state and would not require further workup. However, limited testing could be performed at this point. Laboratory assays for thrombophilia include both molecular diagnostics for inherited risk factors for thrombophilia as well as immunologic and functional assays. Molecular diagnostics are not indicated in the absence of a strong family history of thrombosis. Levels of coagulation factors are affected by acute thrombosis, acute illness, inflammatory conditions, pregnancy, and medications. Antithrombin levels are decreased by heparin and in the setting of acute thrombosis. Protein C and S levels are decreased by warfarin and increased in the setting of acute thrombosis. Antiphospholipid antibody levels may even be transiently positive in acute illness. In most instances of acute thrombosis, anticoagulation with warfarin would be continued for 3–6 months. If a decision is made to perform a workup for a hypercoagulable state, it can be done at least 3 weeks after discontinuation of warfarin.

II-147. The answer is E. *(Chap. 79)* Evaluation of enlarged lymph nodes is a common reason for evaluation in a primary care practice. Most of the time, the cause of an enlarged lymph node is benign. In one study, 84% of patients were found to have benign causes of lymphadenopathy, and only 16% had malignancy. Moreover, in more than half of cases, the lymphadenopathy is deemed to be "reactive," and no specific cause is identified. When evaluating an individual for lymphadenopathy, a careful history and physical examination often provides clues to whether the individual is at risk for a malignant cause of disease. Children and young adults usually have benign causes of lymphadenopathy, including viral or bacterial upper respiratory tract infections, infectious mononucleosis, toxoplasmosis, or tuberculosis. After the age of 50, however, the incidence of malignant disorders increases. Other factors in medical history that favor a benign diagnosis include sore throat, cough, fever, night sweats, and fatigue. Localized or regional lymphadenopathy implies involvement of a single anatomic area, whereas generalized lymphadenopathy involves three or more noncontiguous lymph node areas. Many etiologies of lymphadenopathy can cause either localized/regional or generalized lymphadenopathy. So the distinction is of limited utility in determining benign from malignant disorders. Size, texture, and the presence of pain can be helpful in assessing whether a lymph node may be malignant, and size is often the most useful of these. Lymph nodes that are <1 cm in size are almost always due to benign causes, whereas size greater than 2–2.25 cm carries a much greater likelihood of malignancy or granulomatous disease. If the size is ≤1 cm, then watchful waiting is prudent. When describing the texture of a lymph node, typical descriptions include *soft, firm, rubbery, hard, discrete, matted, tender, movable*, or *fixed*. It can be difficult to use these terms to distinguish benign from malignant disease by description alone, specifically in the case of lymphoma. Lymphomatous lymph nodes are most often firm, rubbery, discrete, and mobile. Depending on the rapidity of enlargement, they may or may not be tender. In comparison, lymph nodes in infection or infectious mononucleosis appear similarly but are frequently tender. However, metastatic lymph nodes often feel distinctly different. They are often hard, fixed, and nontender. In this patient, the diagnosis was most likely a benign case of infectious mononucleosis with the only concerning factor being a single lymph node that is 2 cm in size. A simple blood test will provide a diagnostic answer, but you would want to follow up the lymph node to ensure that the size diminished as the patient healed from her disease.

II-148. The answer is A. *(Chap. 79)* This patient presents with splenomegaly and a constellation of finding suggestive of autoimmune hemolytic anemia (AIHA) including anemia, indirect hyperbilirubinemia, and a peripheral blood smear showing spherocytosis and anisocytosis. The presenting clinical symptoms may be nonspecific and are related to the degree of anemia. These include fatigue, dyspnea on exertion, weakness, tachycardia, and angina. In longstanding cases of AIHA, the patient may be asymptomatic. Physical examination often reveals mild jaundice and scleral icterus. Laboratory studies would confirm the findings as noted earlier. Additional testing would include a positive direct Coombs test, low serum haptoglobin, and elevated lactate dehydrogenase testing. The most likely cause of AIHA in this case would be the use of methyldopa as an antihypertensive agent. This drug is a known cause of AIHA, typically within a few months of starting the medication, although some cases have been described as long as several years later. All of the other choices are associated with splenomegaly that may be massive, but are associated with other abnormalities that are not described in this patient. Chronic myeloid leukemia results in an elevation of the white blood cell count, predominantly neutrophils, typically to the range of 20,000–60,000/μL. A mild increase in basophils and eosinophils may also be seen, whereas the lymphocytes numbers are normal. Lymphoma of all types can be associated with splenomegaly, but the patient would be expected to have other symptoms of lymphoma, including fever, chills, night sweats, and weight loss. Hodgkin lymphoma is also not frequently associated with evidence of hemolysis, which was present in this case. Myelofibrosis with myeloid metaplasia is a clonal disorder that is associated with massive splenomegaly. It may be asymptomatic or associated with symptoms related to the splenomegaly, anemia, or bleeding related to platelet dysfunction. The anemia related to myelofibrosis is due to bone marrow fibrosis and would not be expected to be associated with hemolysis. The peripheral smear in myelofibrosis typically demonstrates teardrop red blood cells, nucleated red blood cells, and immature myeloid cells. Passive congestion of the spleen due to portal hypertension is also a common cause of splenomegaly, but this patient has normal liver function testing. The elevated bilirubin is due to indirect hyperbilirubinemia due to hemolysis rather than elevated direct bilirubin that would be expected with liver disease.

II-149. The answer is A. *(Chap. 79)* The presence of Howell-Jolly bodies (nuclear remnants), Heinz bodies (denatured hemoglobin), basophilic stippling, and nucleated red blood cells in the peripheral blood implies that the spleen is not properly clearing senescent or damaged red blood cells from the circulation. This usually occurs because of surgical splenectomy but is also possible when there is diffuse infiltration of the spleen with malignant cells. Hemolytic anemia can have various peripheral smear findings depending on the etiology of the hemolysis. Spherocytes and bite cells are an example of damaged red cells that might appear due to autoimmune hemolytic anemia and oxidative damage, respectively. Disseminated intravascular coagulation is characterized by schistocytes and thrombocytopenia on smear, with elevated international normalized ratio (INR) and activated partial thromboplastin time as well. However, in these conditions, damaged red cells are still cleared effectively by the spleen. Transformation to acute leukemia does not lead to splenic damage.

II-150. The answer is A. *(Chap. 79)* Splenectomy leads to an increased risk of overwhelming postsplenectomy sepsis, an infection that carries an extremely high mortality rate. The most commonly implicated organisms are encapsulated. *Streptococcus pneumoniae*, *Haemophilus influenzae*, and sometime gram-negative enteric organisms are most frequently isolated. There is no known increased risk for any viral infections. Vaccination for *S pneumoniae*, *H influenzae*, and *Neisseria meningitidis* is indicated for any patient who may undergo splenectomy. The vaccines should be given at least 2 weeks *before* surgery. The highest risk of sepsis occurs in patients under 20 because the spleen is responsible for first-pass immunity and younger patients are more likely to have primary exposure to implicated organisms. The risk is highest during the first 3 years after splenectomy and persists at a lower rate until death.

II-151. The answer is E. *(Chap. 80)* The figure shows the characteristic bilobed nucleus of a neutrophil in the Pelger-Hüet anomaly. This finding has been described as appearing like spectacles or a pince-nez, popular 19th-century reading glasses that did not have earpieces. The Pelger-Hüet anomaly can be inherited or acquired. The inherited form is a benign autosomal dominant trait, whereas the acquired form is called the pseudo Pelger-Hüet anomaly. It occurs following acute infections or in myelodysplastic syndromes. Because this patient did not have a differential or peripheral smear performed prior to his acute infection, it is not possible to determine from the information provided whether he has the inherited or acquired anomaly.

II-152. The answer is B. *(Chap. 80)* Chronic granulomatous disease (CGD) is a rare disorder of granulocyte and monocyte oxidation with an incidence of 1 in 200,000 individuals. In about two-thirds of individuals, it is inherited in an X-linked recessive fashion, and 30% inherit the disorder as an autosomal recessive trait. Leukocytes affected by CGD have impaired function of NADPH oxidase and severely diminished ability to produce hydrogen peroxide. Clinically, individuals with CGD typically present in early childhood with recurrent infections with *S aureus*, *Burkholderia cepacia*, and *Aspergillus* species. The sites of infection in CGD are most commonly skin and lungs. Granulomas are frequent, and gastrointestinal inflammation, including chronic abdominal pain, nausea, and diarrhea, is common. Symptoms of inflammatory bowel disease can occur with obstruction of the bowel. Diagnosis of CGD is made through either the nitroblue tetrazolium dye test (NBT) or the dihydrorhodamine (DHR) oxidation test. The fundamental property underlying these tests is the ability of the neutrophil to respond with an oxidative burst when stimulated, and these oxidative responses can be detected microscopically (NBT) or by flow cytometry (DHR). Treatment of CGD includes use of prophylactic trimethoprim-sulfamethoxazole and itraconazole to decrease the frequency of life-threatening infections. In addition, interferon-γ at a dose of 50 $\mu g/m^2$ subcutaneously three times weekly has been demonstrated to decrease the frequency of infections in CGD by 70% and also decreases the severity of infections. The mechanism of action of interferon-γ is to nonspecifically improve phagocytic cell function, and its effect is additive to the effect of prophylactic antibiotics. Glucocorticoids, initially at doses of 1 mg/kg/d, are used for treating inflammatory bowel disease and bowel obstructions due to CGD. TNF-α–blocking agents such as infliximab are successful in relieving these symptoms as well. However, they markedly increase the risk of life-threatening infections and should not be used as first-line treatment in this disease.

II-153. The answer is E. *(Chap. 80)* Many drugs can lead to neutropenia, most commonly via retarding neutrophil production in the bone marrow. Of the drugs listed in the question, trimethoprim-sulfamethoxazole is the most likely culprit. Other common causes of drug-induced neutropenia include alkylating agents such as cyclophosphamide or busulfan, antimetabolites including methotrexate and 5-flucytosine, penicillin and sulfonamide antibiotics, antithyroid drugs, antipsychotics, and anti-inflammatory agents. Prednisone, when used systemically, often causes an increase in the circulating neutrophil count because it leads to demargination of neutrophils and bone marrow stimulation. Ranitidine, an H_2 blocker, is a well-described cause of thrombocytopenia but has not been implicated in neutropenia. Efavirenz is a nonnucleoside reverse transcriptase inhibitor whose main side effects include a morbilliform rash and central nervous system effects including strange dreams and confusion. The presence of these symptoms does not require drug cessation. Darunavir is a protease inhibitor that is well tolerated. Common side effects include a maculopapular rash and lipodystrophy, a class effect for all protease inhibitors.

II-154, II-155, II-156, II-157, and II-158. The answers are C, E, D, A, and B, respectively. *(Chap. 81e)* Patients with homozygous sickle cell disease have RBCs that are less pliable and more "sticky" than normal RBCs. Vaso-occlusive crisis is often precipitated by infection, fever, excessive exercise, anxiety, abrupt changes in temperature, hypoxia, or hypertonic dyes. Peripheral blood smear will show the typical elongated, crescent-shaped red cells. There is also a nucleated red cell at the bottom of the figure, which may occur due to increased bone marrow production. Howell-Jolly bodies, small nuclear remnants normally removed by the intact spleen, are seen in red cells in patients after splenectomy and with maturation/dysplastic disorders characterized by excess production. Acanthocytes are contracted dense red cells with irregular membrane projections that vary in width and length. They are seen in patients with severe liver disease or abetalipoproteinemia and in rare patients with McLeod blood group. Iron deficiency, often due to chronic stool blood loss in patients with colonic polyps or adenocarcinoma, causes a hypochromic microcytic anemia characterized by small pale red cells (a small lymphocyte is present on the smear to assess red cell size). Red cells are never hyperchromic; if more than the normal amount of hemoglobin is made, the cells get larger not darker. Fragmented red cells, or schistocytes, are helmet-shaped cells that reflect microangiopathic hemolytic anemia (e.g., thrombotic thrombocytopenic purpura, disseminated intravascular coagulation, hemolytic uremic syndrome, scleroderma crisis) or shear damage from a prosthetic heart valve.

SECTION III

Oncology and Hematology

QUESTIONS

DIRECTIONS: Choose the one best response to each question.

III-1. Which of the following statements regarding the epidemiology of cancer is true?

A. Cancer has equal mortality rates across all racial groups.
B. Cancer is responsible for one out of four deaths in the United States.
C. Cancer is the third leading cause of death in the United States.
D. Since 1992, the incidence of cancer has been increasing by about 2% each year.
E. The greatest number of cancers in the world occurs in Europe or North America.

III-2. A 42-year-old woman is treated with carboplatin and paclitaxel for stage III ovarian cancer. Computed tomography (CT) imaging after completing six cycles of therapy shows that the tumor burden has decreased by 25%. What is the best assessment of her response to therapy?

A. Complete response
B. Partial response
C. Progressive disease
D. Stable disease

III-3. A 68-year-old woman is diagnosed with stage II breast cancer. She has a history of severe chronic obstructive pulmonary disease with a forced expiratory volume in 1 second (FEV_1) of 32% predicted, coronary artery disease with prior stenting of the left anterior descending artery, peripheral vascular disease, and obesity. She continues to smoke one to two packs of cigarettes every day. She requires oxygen at 2 L/min continuously and is functionally quite limited. She currently is able to attend to all of her activities of daily living, including showering and dressing. She retired from her work as a waitress 10 years previously due to her lung disease. At home, she does perform some of the household chores but is not able to use a vacuum. She does go out once or twice weekly to run typical errands and does drive. She feels short of breath with most of these activities and often uses a motorized cart when out and about. How would you categorize her performance status and prognosis for treatment taking this into consideration?

A. She has an Eastern Cooperative Oncology Group (ECOG) performance status of 1 and has a good prognosis with appropriate therapy.
B. She has an ECOG performance status of 2 and has a good prognosis with appropriate therapy.
C. She has an ECOG performance status of 3 and has a good prognosis with appropriate therapy.
D. She has an ECOG performance status of 3 and has a poor prognosis despite therapy.
E. She has an ECOG performance status of 4 and has a poor prognosis that precludes therapy.

III-4. Among women younger than 60 who die from cancer, which of the following is the most common organ of origin?

A. Breast
B. Cervix
C. Colon
D. Blood
E. Lung

III-5. A 24-year-old woman is seen in follow-up 12 months after an allogeneic stem cell transplantation for acute myeloid leukemia. She is doing well without evidence of recurrent disease but has had manifestations of chronic graft-versus-host disease. She should be administered all of the following vaccines EXCEPT:

A. Diphtheria-tetanus
B. Influenza
C. Measles, mumps, and rubella
D. Poliomyelitis via injection
E. 23-Valent pneumococcal polysaccharide

III-6. A 63-year-old man is treated with paclitaxel and carboplatin chemotherapy for stage IIIB adenocarcinoma of the lung. He presents for evaluation of a fever to 38.3°C (100.9°F). He is found to have erythema at the exit site of his tunneled catheter, although the tunnel itself is not tender or red. Blood cultures are negative at 48 hours. His neutrophil count is 1550/μL. What is the best approach to the management of this patient?

A. Removal of catheter alone
B. Treatment with ceftazidime and vancomycin
C. Treatment with topical antibiotics at the catheter site
D. Treatment with vancomycin alone
E. Treatment with vancomycin and removal of catheter

III-7. A 44-year-old woman has myelodysplastic syndrome and has undergone myeloablative allogeneic stem cell transplantation. She has been neutropenic for 10 days and has developed a fever to 39.5°C (103.1°F). She has had a Port-a-Cath inserted for her intravenous access for the past 6 months. Her catheter site does not appear inflamed, and she has never tested positive for methicillin-resistant *Staphylococcus aureus*. What is the best initial choice of antibiotics for this patient?

A. Cefepime
B. Meropenem
C. Piperacillin-tazobactam
D. Any of the above would be an acceptable choice
E. Any of the above would be an acceptable choice with the addition of vancomycin

III-8. A 42-year-old man is diagnosed with a stage I malignant melanoma on his left upper arm. Which of the following represents the strongest risk factor(s) for the development of this disease?

A. First-degree relative with melanoma
B. Light skin/hair/eye color
C. Number of total body nevi
D. Poor tanning ability
E. A and C

III-9. A 55-year-old woman presents to her dermatologist with a lesion on her leg that is 8 mm in largest diameter and irregular in shape. She reports this mole has become larger and darker and wants to have it evaluated. Biopsy confirms melanoma that extends 0.5 mm from the surface and into the dermis with <1 mitosis/mm. Which of the following factors has the greatest impact on the patient's prognosis?

A. Anatomic site
B. Breslow thickness
C. Clark level
D. Number of mitoses
E. Sex

III-10. A 46-year-old woman has previously had stage IIB melanoma removed from her upper back. She presents to the emergency department with dyspnea and is found to have multiple lung lesions concerning for metastatic disease. Prior to embarking upon chemotherapy for her disease, the presence of which genetic mutation is an indication for specific therapy?

A. *BRAF*
B. *C-KIT*
C. *ERK*
D. *N-RAS*
E. *MEK*

III-11. You confirm the patient in Question III-10 has the mutation of interest. Which of the following is recommended?

A. Dacarbazine
B. Interleukin-2
C. Ipilimumab
D. Vemurafenib
E. The specific therapy depends on the functional status and desires of the patient

III-12. All of the following statements regarding nonmelanoma skin cancer are true EXCEPT:

A. Actinic keratoses and cheilitis are both premalignant forms of squamous cell carcinoma.
B. All forms of ultraviolet light exposure, including tanning beds, increase the risk of nonmelanoma skin cancers.
C. Basal cell carcinoma is most likely to become a metastatic malignancy.
D. Keratoacanthomas that regress spontaneously should be treated as aggressively as other squamous cell cancers as they progress to metastatic disease.
E. Solid organ transplantation is associated with a marked increased risk of both squamous and basal cell carcinoma that can be aggressive and lead to death.

III-13. A 65-year-old man presents to his primary care physician complaining of a hoarse voice for 6 months. He smokes one pack of cigarettes daily and also drinks at least a six pack of beer daily. His physical examination reveals a thin man with a weak voice in no distress. No stridor is heard. The head and neck examination is normal. No cervical lymphadenopathy is present. He is referred to an otolaryngologist who discovers a laryngeal lesion during flexible laryngoscopy. Biopsy reveals squamous cell carcinoma. On imaging, the mass measures 2.8 cm.

No suspicious lymphadenopathy is present on positron emission tomography (PET) imaging. What is the best choice of therapy in this patient?

A. Concomitant chemotherapy and radiation therapy
B. Chemotherapy alone
C. Radiation therapy alone
D. Radical neck dissection alone
E. Radical neck dissection followed by concomitant chemotherapy and radiation

III-14. All of the following have been identified as risk factors for the development of head and neck cancers EXCEPT:

A. Alcohol consumption
B. Epstein Barr virus infection
C. *Helicobacter pylori* infection
D. Human papillomavirus infection
E. Tobacco consumption

III-15. Which of the following statements regarding a solitary pulmonary nodule is true?

A. A lobulated and irregular contour is more indicative of malignancy than a smooth one.
B. About 80% of incidentally found pulmonary nodules are benign.
C. Absence of growth over a period of 6–12 months is sufficient to determine whether a solitary pulmonary nodule is benign.
D. Ground glass nodules should be regarded as benign.
E. Multiple nodules indicate malignant disease.

III-16. A 64-year-old man seeks evaluation for a solitary pulmonary nodule that was found incidentally. He had presented to the emergency department for shortness of breath and chest pain. A CT pulmonary angiogram did not show any evidence of pulmonary embolism; however, a 9-mm nodule is seen in the periphery of the left lower lobe. No enlarged mediastinal lymph nodes are present. He is a current smoker of two packs of cigarettes daily and has done so since the age of 16. He generally reports no functional limitation related to respiratory symptoms. His FEV_1 is 88% predicted, forced vital capacity is 92% predicted, and diffusion capacity is 80% predicted. He previously had a normal chest x-ray 3 years previously. What is the next best step in the evaluation and treatment of this patient?

A. Perform a bronchoscopy with biopsy for diagnosis
B. Perform a combined PET/CT to assess for uptake in the nodule and assess for lymph node metastases
C. Perform a follow-up CT scan in 3 months to assess for interval growth
D. Refer the patient to radiation oncology for stereotactic radiation of the dominant nodule
E. Refer the patient to thoracic surgery for video-assisted thoracoscopic biopsy and resection of lung nodule if malignancy is diagnosed

III-17. A 62-year-old man presents to the emergency department complaining of a droopy right eye and blurred vision for the past day. The symptoms started abruptly, and he denies any antecedent illness. For the past 4 months, he has been complaining of increasing pain in his right arm and shoulder. His primary care physician has treated him for shoulder bursitis without relief. His past medical history is significant for chronic obstructive pulmonary disease and hypertension. He smokes one pack of cigarettes daily. He has chronic daily sputum production and stable dyspnea on exertion. On physical examination, he has right eye ptosis with unequal pupils. His pupil is 2 mm on the right and not reactive, whereas the pupil is 4 mm and reactive on the left. However, his ocular movements appear intact. His lung fields are clear to auscultation. On extremity examination, there is wasting of the intrinsic muscles of the hand. Which of the following would be most likely to explain the patient's constellation of symptoms?

A. Enlarged mediastinal lymph nodes causing occlusion of the superior vena cava
B. Metastases to the midbrain from small-cell lung cancer
C. Paraneoplastic syndrome caused by antibodies to voltage-gated calcium channels
D. Presence of a cervical rib on chest x-ray
E. Right apical pleural thickening with a mass-like density measuring 1 cm in thickness

III-18. As an oncologist, you are considering treatment options for your patients with lung cancer, including small-molecule therapy targeting the epidermal growth factor receptor (EGFR). Which of the following patients is most likely to have an EGFR mutation?

A. A 23-year-old man with a hamartoma
B. A 33-year-old woman with a carcinoid tumor
C. A 45-year-old woman who has never smoked with an adenocarcinoma
D. A 56-year-old man with a 100-pack-year history of tobacco use with small-cell lung carcinoma
E. A 76-year-old man with squamous cell carcinoma and a history of asbestos exposure

III-19. You are meeting today with Mr. Takei to discuss his recent diagnosis of small-cell lung cancer (SCLC). On reviewing his PET/CT results from earlier today, you note that he has a mass in the hilar region of his left lung and that he has a moderate pleural effusion there. You know that he underwent thoracentesis of that effusion last week, and so you call the pathologist to get a cytopathology report. He reports the presence of hyperchromic, small basophilic atypical cells in the pleural fluid, consistent with SCLC. Which of the following statements is true?

A. Thirty percent of patients with SCLC are diagnosed with the same stage of disease as Mr. Takei.
B. Mr. Takei has extensive-stage disease.
C. Surgical therapy alone has a high curative rate for Mr. Takei's stage of SCLC.
D. The majority of patients with SCLC of this stage respond to chemotherapy alone and go into remission with a high 2-year survival.
E. Radiation plays no role in therapy for this disease.

III-20. Which of the following statements regarding screening for lung cancer in the National Lung Screening Trial using low-dose CT scanning is true?

A. Greater than 80% of positive results were found to be malignant after biopsy.
B. Positive results were found in approximately 5% of patients over the 3-year trial.
C. The trial compared the use of chest radiograph versus low-dose CT scan in patients 30–50 years old.
D. There was a reduction in lung cancer mortality in the low-dose CT group.
E. There was no difference in all-cause mortality between the CT and radiograph groups.

III-21. A 34-year-old woman is seen by her internist for evaluation of right breast mass. This was noted approximately 1 week ago when she was showering. She has not had any nipple discharge or discomfort. She has no other medical problems. On examination, her right breast has a soft 1 cm × 2 cm mass in the right upper quadrant. There is no axillary lymphadenopathy present. The contralateral breast is normal. The breast is reexamined in 3 weeks, and the same findings are present. The cyst is aspirated, and clear fluid is removed. The mass is no longer palpable. Which of the following statements is true?

A. Breast magnetic resonance imaging (MRI) should be obtained to discern for residual fluid collection.
B. Mammography is required to further evaluate the lesion.
C. She should be evaluated in 1 month for recurrence.
D. She should be referred to a breast surgeon for resection.
E. She should not breastfeed any more children.

III-22. Which of the following women has the lowest risk of breast cancer?

A. A woman with menarche at 12 years, first child at 24 years, and menopause at 47 years
B. A woman with menarche at 14 years, first child at 17 years, and menopause at 52 years
C. A woman with menarche at 16 years, first child at 17 years, and menopause at 42 years
D. A woman with menarche at 16 years, first child at 32 years, and menopause at 52 years
E. They are all equal

III-23. Which of the following history or physical examination findings should prompt investigation for hereditary nonpolyposis colon cancer screening in a 32-year-old man?

A. Father, paternal aunt, and paternal cousin with colon cancer with ages of diagnosis of 54, 68, and 37 years, respectively
B. Innumerable polyps visualized on routine colonoscopy
C. Mucocutaneous pigmentation
D. New diagnosis of ulcerative colitis
E. None of the above

III-24. A 64-year-old woman presents with complaints of a change in stool caliber for the past 2 months. The stools now have a diameter of only the size of her fifth digit. Over this same period, she feels she has to exert increasing strain to have a bowel movement and sometimes has associated abdominal cramping. She often has blood on the toilet paper when she wipes. During this time, she has lost about 20 lb with a decreased appetite. On physical examination, the patient appears cachectic with a body mass index of 22.5 kg/m^2. The abdomen is flat and nontender. The liver span is 12 cm to percussion. On digital rectal examination, a mass lesion is palpated approximately 6 cm into the rectum. A colonoscopy is attempted, which demonstrates a 2.5-cm sessile mass that narrows the distal colonic lumen. The biopsy confirms adenocarcinoma. The colonoscope is not able to traverse the mass. A CT scan of the abdomen does not show evidence of metastatic disease. Liver function tests are normal. A carcinoembryonic antigen level is 4.2 ng/mL. The patient is referred for surgery and undergoes rectosigmoidectomy with pelvic lymph node dissection. Final pathology demonstrates extension of the primary tumor into the muscularis propria, but not the serosa. Of 15 lymph nodes removed, 2 are positive for tumor. What do you recommend for this patient following surgery?

A. Chemotherapy with a regimen containing 5-fluorouracil
B. Complete colonoscopy within 3 months
C. Measurement of carcinoembryonic antigen levels at 3-month intervals
D. Radiation therapy to the pelvis
E. All of the above

III-25. A 56-year-old man presents to a physician with weight loss and dysphagia. He feels that food gets stuck in his mid-chest such that he no longer is able to eat meats. He reports his diet consists primarily of soft foods and liquids. The symptoms have progressively worsened over 6 months. During this time, he has lost about 50 lb. He occasionally gets pain in his mid-chest that radiates to his back and also occasionally feels that he regurgitates undigested foods. He does not have a history of gastroesophageal reflux disease. He does not regularly seek medical care. He is known to have hypertension but takes no medications. He drinks 500 mL or more of whiskey daily and also smokes 1.5 packs of cigarettes per day. On physical examination, the patient appears cachectic with temporal wasting. He has a body mass index of 19.4 kg/m^2. His blood pressure is 198/110 mmHg, heart rate is 110 bpm, respiratory rate is 18 breaths/min, temperature is 37.4°C (99.2°F), and oxygen saturation is 93% on room air. His pulmonary examination shows decreased breath sounds at the apices with scattered expiratory wheezes. His cardiovascular examination demonstrates an S_4 gallop with a hyperdynamic precordium. A regular tachycardia is present. Blood pressures are equal in both arms. Liver span is not enlarged. There are no palpable abdominal masses. What is the most likely cause of the patient's presentation?

A. Adenocarcinoma of the esophagus
B. Ascending aortic aneurysm
C. Esophageal stricture
D. Gastric cancer
E. Squamous cell carcinoma of the esophagus

III-26. Which of the following risk factors is associated with both adenocarcinoma and squamous cell carcinoma of the esophagus?

A. Barrett esophagus
B. Chronic gastroesophageal reflux disease
C. Cigarette smoking
D. Lye ingestion
E. Male sex

III-27. All of the following conditions are known to increase the risk of developing hepatocellular carcinoma EXCEPT:

A. Cirrhosis from any cause
B. Hepatitis C infection
C. Malaria
D. Nonalcoholic fatty liver
E. Nonalcoholic steatohepatitis

III-28. A 59-year-old man with known cirrhosis due to prior hepatitis C infection is brought to the clinic by his family due to complaints of 1 month of worsening malaise, abdominal bloating, and nausea with 1 week of right upper quadrant pain. His physical examination is notable for normal vital signs (baseline low blood pressure) and new hepatomegaly. Which of the following statements is true regarding the possibility of hepatocellular carcinoma?

A. Fluorodeoxyglucose (FDG)-PET scan is more sensitive for showing primary tumor than CT or ultrasound.
B. Hepatomegaly is an uncommon finding in hepatocellular carcinoma.
C. Imaging criteria alone (without biopsy) have a <75% specificity for the diagnosis.
D. Serum α-fetoprotein is the most sensitive test but is not specific.
E. Ultrasound is an excellent screening test for this patient.

III-29. The patient described in Question III-28 is found to have a 4-cm single hepatocellular carcinoma lesion. His performance status is excellent despite his recent decline. He still works as a web designer and walks over 10,000 steps daily. Based on this information, he may be eligible for all of the following therapies EXCEPT:

A. Cadaveric liver transplantation
B. Living donor liver transplantation
C. Local ablation with ethanol injection
D. Local radiofrequency ablation
E. Primary resection

III-30. All of the following statements regarding cholangiocarcinoma are true EXCEPT:

A. Asians infected with liver flukes have an increased risk of cholangiocarcinoma.
B. In eligible patients with cholangiocarcinoma, liver transplant plus radiation has a >60% 5-year recurrence-free survival.
C. Most patients present due to an abnormal screening ultrasound, without symptoms.
D. Primary biliary cirrhosis and hepatitis C virus infection are associated with cholangiocarcinoma.
E. The incidence of cholangiocarcinomas has been increasing in recent years.

III-31. All of the following statements regarding pancreatic cancer are true EXCEPT:

A. Alcohol consumption is not a risk factor for pancreatic cancer.
B. Cigarette smoking is a risk factor for pancreatic cancer.
C. Despite accounting for <5% of malignancies diagnosed in the United States, pancreatic cancer is the fourth leading cause of cancer death.
D. If detected early, the 5-year survival is up to 20%
E. The 5-year survival rates for pancreatic cancer have improved substantially in the last decade.

III-32. A 65-year-old man is evaluated in clinic for 1 month of progressive painless jaundice and a 10-lb unintentional weight loss. His physical examination is unremarkable. A dual-phase contrast CT shows a suspicious mass in the head of the pancreas with biliary ductal dilation. Which of the following is the best diagnostic test to evaluate for suspected pancreatic cancer?

A. CT-guided percutaneous needle biopsy
B. Endoscopic ultrasound–guided needle biopsy
C. Endoscopic retrograde cholangiopancreatography with pancreatic juice sampling for cytopathology
D. FDG-PET imaging
E. Serum CA 19-9

III-33. A 63-year-old man presents to his internist with 3 months of worsening painless jaundice and anorexia. Further evaluation reveals a 1.5-cm obstructing lesion in the head of the pancreas that is confirmed as pancreatic adenocarcinoma by endoscopic ultrasound biopsy. The patient undergoes a modified Whipple procedure and is found to have a 1.6-cm primary tumor with no microscopic residual disease and negative lymph nodes. Which of the following statements regarding this patient is true?

A. He has a >75% expected 5-year survival after surgery.
B. He has pathologic stage II disease.
C. He should receive adjuvant chemotherapy.
D. The presence of *SMAD4* gene inactivation in the tumor is a positive prognostic sign.
E. This presentation accounts for approximately 25% of patients with pancreatic cancer.

III-34. A 63-year-old man complains of notable pink-tinged urine for the last month. At first he thought it was due to eating beets, but it has not cleared. His medical history is notable for hypertension and cigarette smoking. He does report some worsening urinary frequency and hesitancy over the last 2 years. Physical examination is unremarkable. Urinalysis is notable for gross hematuria with no white cells or casts. Renal function is normal. Which of the following statements regarding this patient is true?

A. Cigarette smoking is not a risk for bladder cancer.
B. Gross hematuria makes prostate cancer more likely than bladder cancer.
C. If invasive bladder cancer with nodal involvement but no distant metastases is found, 5-year survival is 20%.
D. If superficial bladder cancer is found, intravesicular Bacillus Calmette-Guerin may be used as adjuvant therapy.
E. Radical cystectomy is generally recommended for invasive bladder cancer.

III-35. A 68-year-old man comes to his physician complaining of 2 months of increasing right flank pain with 1 month of worsening hematuria. He was treated for cystitis at a walk-in clinic 3 weeks ago with no improvement. He also reports poor appetite and 5-lb weight loss. His physical examination is notable for a palpable mass in the right flank measuring >5 cm. His renal function is normal. All of the following are true about this patient's likely diagnosis EXCEPT:

A. Anemia is more common than erythrocytosis.
B. Cigarette smoking increased his risk.
C. If his disease has metastasized, with best therapy, 5-year survival is >50%.
D. If his disease is confined to the kidney, 5-year survival is >80%.
E. The most likely pathology is clear cell carcinoma.

III-36. In the patient described in Question III-35, imaging shows a 10-cm solid mass in the right kidney and multiple nodules in the lungs consistent with metastatic disease. Needle biopsy of a lung lesion confirms the diagnosis of renal cell carcinoma. Which of the following is recommended therapy?

A. Gemcitabine
B. Interferon-γ
C. Interleukin-2
D. Radical nephrectomy
E. Sunitinib

III-37. Which of the following has been shown in randomized trials to reduce the future risk of prostate cancer?

A. Finasteride
B. Selenium
C. Testosterone
D. Vitamin C
E. Vitamin E

III-38. A 54-year-old man is evaluated in an executive health program. On physical examination, he is noted to have an enlarged prostate with a right lobe nodule. He does not recall his last digital rectal examination and has never had prostate-specific antigen (PSA) tested. Based on this evaluation, which of the following is recommended next?

A. Bone scan to evaluate for metastasis
B. PSA
C. PSA now and in 3 months to measure PSA velocity
D. Repeat digital rectal examination in 3 months
E. Transrectal ultrasound-guided biopsy

III-39. Which of the following statements regarding use of PSA is true?

A. Asymptomatic men with an elevated PSA should receive a 2-week course of antibiotics before repeating PSA and considering biopsy.
B. Most prostate cancer deaths occur in men with PSA levels below the top quartile.
C. PSA is produced by malignant and nonmalignant prostate cells.
D. The American Urological Association recommends PSA screening in men 40–55 years of age.
E. The US Preventive Services Task Force recommends PSA screening in men between 55 and 69 years of age.

III-40. All of the following medications may be useful in the treatment of benign prostatic hypertrophy EXCEPT:

A. Alfuzosin
B. Bosentan
C. Dutasteride
D. Finasteride
E. Sildenafil

III-41. A 26-year-old man presents with pain and swelling of his right testicle that has persisted after an empiric treatment for epididymitis. Ultrasound confirms a 1.5 × 2 cm solid mass, suspicious for testicular cancer. Radical inguinal orchiectomy confirms the mass as a seminoma with disease limited to the testis (tumor stage pT1). Chest, abdomen, and pelvis CT shows no evidence of metastatic disease or lymphadenopathy. Results of serum tumor markers demonstrate the following (normal values in parentheses): α-fetoprotein (AFP) 5 ng/mL (<10 ng/mL), β-human chorionic gonadotropin (β-hCG) 182 U/L (0.2–0.8 U/L), and lactate dehydrogenase (LDH) 432 U/L (100–190 U/L). Following resection, all tumor markers become undetectable after an appropriate interval. Which is the next best step in this patient's treatment?

A. Immediate retroperitoneal radiation therapy
B. Nerve-sparing retroperitoneal lymph node dissection
C. Single-dose therapy with cisplatin
D. Surveillance alone with treatment only if relapse detected
E. Either A or D, because both are associated with a near 100% cure rate

III-42. Which of the following statements describes the relationship between testicular tumors and serum markers?

A. β-hCG and AFP should be measured when following the progress of a tumor.
B. β-hCG is limited in its usefulness as a marker because it is identical to human luteinizing hormone.
C. Measurement of tumor markers the day after surgery for localized disease is useful in determining completeness of the resection.
D. More than 40% of nonseminomatous germ cell tumors produce no cell markers.
E. Pure seminomas produce AFP or β-hCG in more than 90% of cases.

III-43. All of the following statements regarding the risk of ovarian cancer are true EXCEPT:

A. Ten percent of women with ovarian cancer have a germline mutation in either *BRCA1* or *BRCA2*.
B. Early prophylactic oophorectomy in women with *BRCA1* or *BRCA2* mutations reduces the risk of developing subsequent breast cancer.
C. Individuals with a single copy of a *BRCA1* or *BRCA2* mutant allele have an increased risk of breast and ovarian cancer.
D. Women with a mutation in *BRCA1* have a higher risk of ovarian cancer than woman with a mutation in *BRCA2*.
E. Women with *BRCA1*, *BRCA2*, or other at-risk germline mutations should be screened with serial measurement of the CA-125 tumor marker.

III-44. A 42-year-old woman seeks evaluation for over 6 months of postcoital bleeding without dyspareunia. She also notes some recent spotting between her regular menses. She has no past medical history, is unmarried with multiple sexual partners and practicing unprotected sex, and works as an accountant. She has not sought gynecologic evaluation for over 10 years. Pelvic examination reveals an abnormal appearance of the cervix with an abnormal Pap smear, positive human papillomavirus (HPV) test, and negative human immunodeficiency virus (HIV), chlamydia, gonorrhea, and syphilis studies. A cervical biopsy shows squamous cell carcinoma confined to the cervix. All of the following statements regarding this woman's condition are true EXCEPT:

A. Cervical cancer is an uncommon cancer worldwide.
B. Her cancer is related to HPV infection.
C. HPV vaccination before initiation of sexual activity can decrease the risk of developing an abnormal Pap smear.
D. She has stage I cervical cancer.
E. With surgical therapy, her 5-year survival is >80%.

III-45. Which of the following statements regarding the presentation and evaluation of suspected brain malignancy is true?

A. A low-grade glioma is more likely to present with a new seizure than a high-grade glioma.
B. Approximately half of all malignant brain lesions are metastatic, with the other half being all primary brain tumors combined.
C. CT with intravenous contrast is the preferred radiologic study to evaluate a suspected intracranial tumor.
D. Headache is present at presentation in over 75% of patients with brain tumors.
E. High-grade gliomas are more likely to present with headache and alteration in cognitive function than metastatic lesions.

III-46. A 63-year-old woman presents to the emergency department after developing a new-onset seizure. Family members came to her when they heard a commotion in her bedroom and found her having a tonic-clonic seizure that spontaneously ended after about 1 minute. She has no prior neurologic history, and her medical history is only notable for hypertension controlled with a diuretic and 40 pack-years of cigarette smoking. There is no history of illicit drug use, and she has been in excellent health until this episode. She works as a congressional staffer in a legislative office. Her physical examination is unremarkable, and she is somnolent and disoriented after receiving lorazepam by the emergency medical team. She receives an urgent head MRI with contrast (Figure III-46). The largest lesion visualized is less than 3 cm in diameter. Which of the following statements is true about her likely diagnosis?

A. Metastatic lesions due to ovarian carcinoma are more likely to be present than metastatic lesions due to a lung carcinoma.
B. She is likely a candidate for platinum-based chemotherapy.
C. She likely has a primary brain malignancy.
D. She may be a candidate for stereotactic radiosurgery.
E. Stereotactic radiosurgery and whole-brain radiation have similar mortality outcomes for metastatic disease.

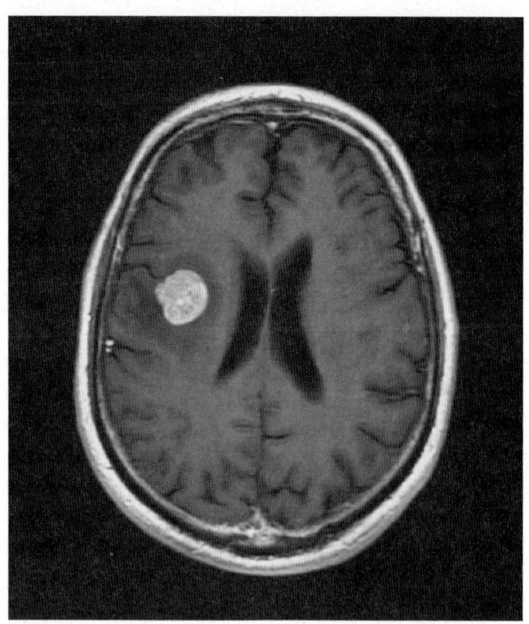
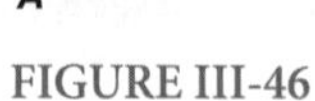
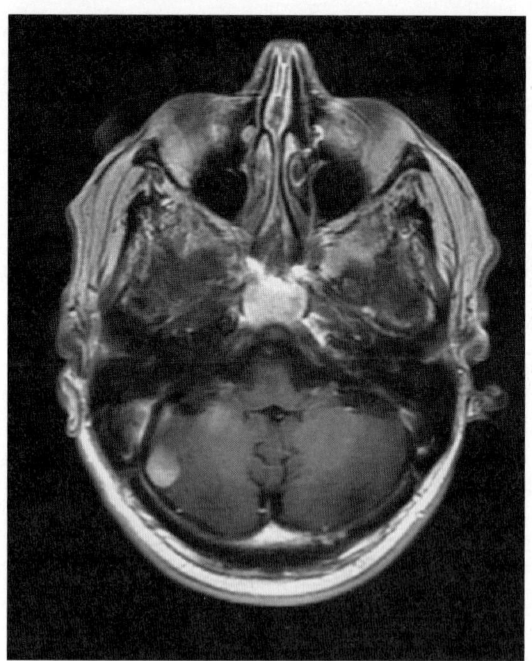

A B

FIGURE III-46

III-47. A 55-year-old woman presents to the emergency department after a minor motorcycle collision complaining of diffuse chest pain. Her chest radiograph shows multiple 2- to 4-cm nodules and masses without cavitation in all lobes. Her physical examination is totally normal other than some diffuse chest. She has no past medical history and takes no medications, other than a multivitamin. She exercises regularly and had a negative colonoscopy and mammogram within the last 2 years. She works as a librarian and rides motorcycles for recreation. There is no history of cigarette or illicit drug use. Abdominal, pelvic, and head imaging shows no likely primary lesions. A bronchoscopic biopsy of a lung lesion is performed and shows histology consistent with moderately well-differentiated adenocarcinoma. There were no airway abnormalities. Her FDG-PET scan shows no lesions other than those in the lung, and repeat colonoscopy and mammography are normal. All of the following statements regarding her carcinoma are true EXCEPT:

A. Gene expression profiles may help determine the original primary carcinoma and aid in determining the most appropriate therapy.
B. Immunohistochemical staining of cytokeratin 7 (CK 7) and cytokeratin 20 (CK 20) may help determine the most appropriate therapy.
C. Median survival of patients with carcinoma of uncertain primary is approximately 18 months.
D. Moderately differentiated adenocarcinoma is the most common histology of carcinoma of unknown primary.
E. Prognostic factors including performance status and LDH level may identify patients most amenable to therapy.

III-48. A 63-year-old woman is brought to the emergency department by her nephew because of severe confusion and obtundation. Her vital signs are normal, and there are no focal physical findings. She is found to have hypercalcemia with a serum level of 14.8 mg/dL, along with minimal elevation of blood urea nitrogen (BUN) and creatinine. Initial evaluation reveals a chest radiograph with multiple nodules suggestive of metastatic disease. Unfortunately the nephew does not know anything about his aunt's medical history. He reports that she was in town attending a healing yoga conference. Subsequent laboratory testing reveals a normal parathyroid hormone level and an elevated parathyroid hormone–related protein level. All of the following are a likely primary malignancy in this woman EXCEPT:

A. Adenocarcinoma of the breast
B. Mantle cell lymphoma
C. Squamous cell of the lung
D. Squamous cell of the piriform sinus
E. Transitional cell of the bladder

III-49. The patient described in Question III-49 should receive treatment with all of the following for her hypercalcemia EXCEPT:

A. Calcitonin
B. Furosemide
C. Normal saline
D. Pamidronate
E. Prednisone

III-50. A 61-year-old woman is diagnosed with stage II breast carcinoma. She receives a mastectomy, where she is found to have one positive lymph node. The tumor is positive for estrogen receptor, progestin receptor, and overexpression of HER2/Neu. She receives adjuvant chemotherapy with doxorubicin, cisplatin, and trastuzumab. Match the concerning toxicity with the appropriate agent.

1. Cisplatin
2. Doxorubicin
3. Trastuzumab

A. Reversible cardiomyopathy
B. Irreversible cardiomyopathy
C. Sensorimotor neuropathy

III-51. Which of the following proteins is most responsible for iron transport in the plasma?

A. Albumin
B. Ferritin
C. Haptoglobin
D. Hemoglobin
E. Transferrin

III-52. A 38-year-old woman with a history of inflammatory bowel disease complains of worsening fatigue over the last 1–2 months. Her gastrointestinal disease has been stable for the past year on infliximab. Physical examination is unremarkable, including heme-negative stool. Her hemoglobin has fallen from 11 g/dL to 8 g/dL since last checked 6 months ago. Additionally, her serum iron and ferritin, which were both normal 6 months ago, are now low. Her blood smear is shown in Figure III-52. Which of the following is the most likely etiology of her new anemia?

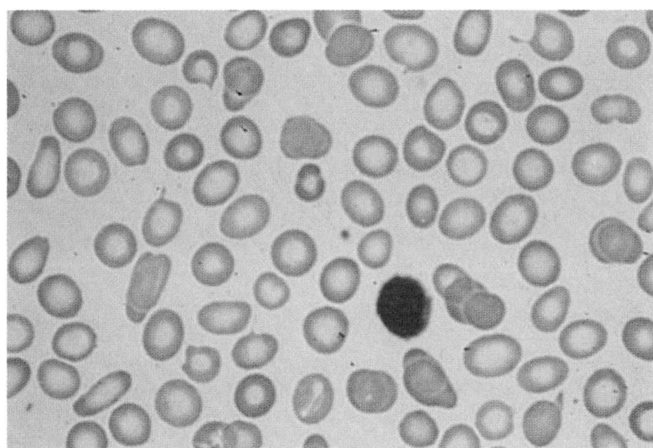

FIGURE III-52 From Lichtman M, Beutler E, Kaushansky K, Kipps T (eds): *Williams Hematology*, 7th ed, New York, NY: McGraw-Hill, 2005.

A. Folate deficiency
B. Inflammation
C. Iron deficiency
D. Sideroblastic anemia
E. Vitamin B_{12} deficiency

III-53. All of the following statements regarding hemoglobinopathies are true EXCEPT:

A. Approximately 15% of African Americans are silent carriers of α-thalassemia.
B. Approximately 15% of African Americans are heterozygous for sickle cell disease.
C. Hemoglobinopathies are especially common in areas where malaria is endemic.
D. Sickle cell disease is the most common structural hemoglobinopathy.
E. Thalassemias are the most common genetic disorders in the world.

III-54. A 22-year-old man with known sickle cell anemia is admitted to the intensive care unit with diffuse body pain, shortness of breath, fever, and cough. He started having a bone pain crisis 1 day ago and tried to treat it at home with oral hydration. On examination, his blood pressure and heart rate are elevated, and he is in obvious pain and respiratory discomfort. His room air arterial oxygen saturation (SaO_2) is 83% and increases to 91% on a nonrebreather oxygen face mask. His chest radiograph shows bilateral diffuse alveolar infiltrates. This is his third similar episode in the last 12 months. All of the statements regarding his condition are true EXCEPT:

A. Chronic therapy with oral hydroxyurea should be considered.
B. He is having a sickle cell acute chest syndrome.
C. He should receive daily sildenafil.
D. Hematocrit should be maintained at >30%.
E. Hydration should be continued.

III-55. A 28-year-old woman is referred to your clinic for evaluation of anemia that was found on a life insurance screening examination. She reports being healthy, takes no medications other than a multivitamin with iron, and only admits some recent fatigue on exertion in the past 6–9 months. She menstruates regularly with 3- to 4-day menses that have not changed in years. She eats a normal omnivorous diet, smokes one pack per day of cigarettes, and does not use illicit drugs. The results of her complete blood count (CBC) reveal a white blood cell (WBC) count of 4.0/μL, platelet count of 235,000/μL, and hemoglobin of 8 g/dL with a mean corpuscular volume (MCV) of 105. Her blood smear is shown in Figure III-55. She has normal renal and liver function. Which of the following is the most likely diagnosis?

A. Acute myeloblastic anemia
B. Hereditary spherocytosis
C. Iron deficiency anemia
D. Nutritional megaloblastic anemia
E. Pernicious anemia

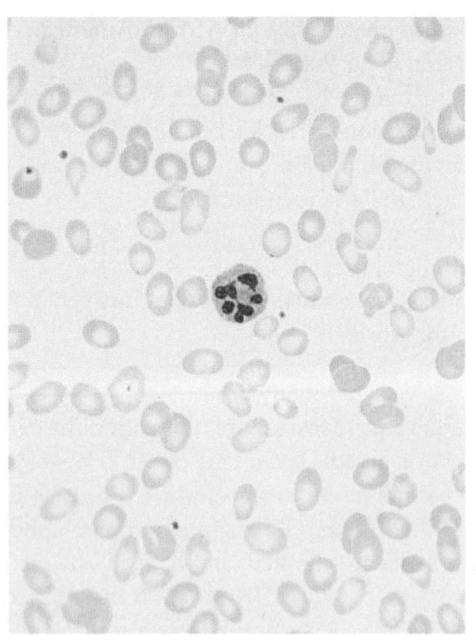

FIGURE III-55 Reprinted from Hoffbrand AV, Catovsky D, Tuddenham EGD (eds): *Postgraduate Haematology*, 5th ed. Oxford, UK: Blackwell Publishing, 2005; with permission.

III-56. In the patient from Question III-55, which of the following is the next best study to confirm the diagnosis?

A. Bone marrow biopsy
B. Hemoglobin electrophoresis
C. Serum homocysteine level
D. Serum iron and transferrin levels
E. Serum vitamin B_{12} level

III-57. All of the following are typically increased in a patient with hemolytic anemia EXCEPT:

A. Aspartate aminotransferase (AST)
B. Haptoglobin
C. LDH
D. MCV
E. Reticulocytes

III-58. A 24-year-old man returns to the acute care clinic complaining of 1 day of worsening malaise, weakness, abdominal pain, and discolored dark urine. He was at the clinic yesterday where he was diagnosed with a possible staphylococcal skin carbuncle and treated with empiric trimethoprim/sulfamethoxazole. His physical examination is notable for mild jaundice, normal vital signs, and no focal findings other than the carbuncle in his left axilla. His CBC shows that his hemoglobin has fallen from 13 g/dL to 8 g/dL and his bilirubin has gone from normal to 3.0 mg/dL. His urine dipstick is positive for bilirubin. A peripheral blood smear is shown in Figure III-58. Which of the following is the most likely cause of his new anemia?

A. Glucose 6-phosphate dehydrogenase (G6PD) deficiency
B. Hemolytic-uremic syndrome
C. Hereditary spherocytosis
D. Iron deficiency anemia
E. Thrombotic thrombocytopenic purpura (TTP)

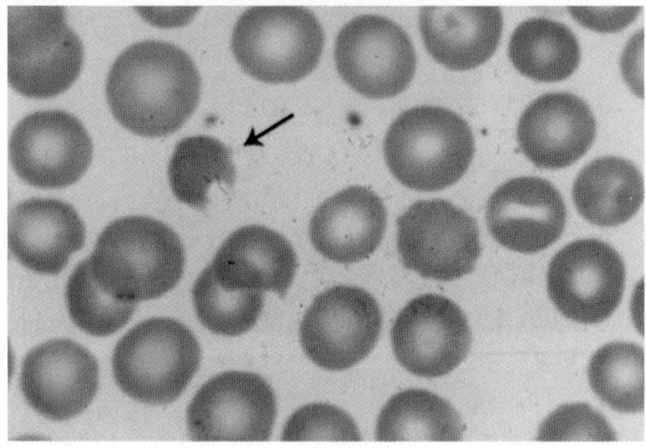

FIGURE III-58 From MA Lichtman et al: *Lichtman's Atlas of Hematology*. http://www.accessmedicine.com. Copyright © The McGraw-Hill Companies, Inc. All rights reserved.

III-59. You are seeing Ms. Stoked, a 19-year-old collegiate rower who has been in excellent health and takes no chronic medications, for new-onset severe fatigue and left upper abdominal pain. She was treated 2 days ago in the health center for presumed gonorrhea with ceftriaxone and azithromycin. Her past medical history is only notable for one prior episode of presumed gonorrhea when she was 17 years old. Her physical examination is notable for a heart rate of 100 bpm and a palpable spleen. Stool is negative for heme. Laboratory examination is notable for a hemoglobin of 5 g/dL with normal WBC and platelets. Peripheral blood smear shows an excess of spherocytes. Which of the following tests will most likely confirm the diagnosis?

A. ADAMTS-13 activity assay
B. Direct antiglobulin (Coombs) test
C. Flow cytometry
D. G6PD deficiency assay
E. Hemoglobin electrophoresis

III-60. A 73-year-old man comes to primary care clinic complaining of 4–6 weeks of increasing malaise, fatigue, dyspnea on exertion, and occasional night sweats. His past medical history is notable for hypertension and hyperlipidemia. Medications include lisinopril and atorvastatin. He had a screening colonoscopy 6 months ago, at which time his laboratory studies were normal. His physical examination today is only notable for a heart rate of 105 bpm and pale mucous membranes. Lungs are clear, and there are no new cardiac findings. Electrocardiogram (ECG) shows sinus tachycardia but no acute changes. Laboratory studies show normal electrolytes, but his WBC is 1300/μL, platelet count is 35,000/μL, and hemoglobin is 7.5 g/dL. Examination of his peripheral smear confirms the pancytopenia and notes the red blood cells are macrocytic, and there are 3% blasts present. All of the following statements regarding his condition are true EXCEPT:

A. Azacitidine may improve his blood counts and prolong survival.
B. Children with Down syndrome are also at risk.
C. He is at high risk of developing acute myeloid leukemia.
D. Hematopoietic stem cell transplantation is contraindicated.
E. Increasing percentages of bone marrow blasts correlate with worsening prognosis.

III-61. All of the following disorders are considered by World Health Organization classification as chronic myeloproliferative neoplasms EXCEPT:

A. Chronic myeloid leukemia (Bcr-Abl positive)
B. Essential thrombocytosis
C. Polycythemia vera
D. Primary myelofibrosis
E. All are chronic myeloproliferative neoplasms

III-62. A 53-year-old man is sent to you for evaluation of an elevated hematocrit found incidentally on lab testing. He was removing dry wall in a house and cut his upper arm. A CBC before his arm was stitched revealed a hematocrit of 59% with hemoglobin of 20 g/dL, WBC count of 15.4/μL with a normal differential, and platelet count of 445,000/μL. His physical examination is notable for a room air oxygen saturation of 95%, blood pressure of 145/85 mmHg, and a palpable spleen. He has no past medical history, is a nonsmoker, drinks rarely on social occasions, and is taking no medications. The patient reports his last contact with a physician was 2–3 years ago, and he recalls no abnormalities reported on blood testing. Which of the following is the next diagnostic step?

A. Arterial blood gas
B. Erythropoietin (EPO) level
C. Red blood cell (RBC) mass
D. Pulmonary function tests
E. Renal ultrasound

III-63. In the patient described in Question III-62, if secondary causes of elevated hemoglobin are ruled out, which of the following is the recommended therapy?

A. Aspirin
B. Hydroxyurea
C. Imatinib
D. Phlebotomy to maintain hemoglobin <14 g/dL
E. Warfarin

III-64. Exposure to all of the following has been associated with the development of acute myelogenous leukemia EXCEPT:

A. Benzene
B. Cyclophosphamide
C. Doxorubicin
D. Herpes virus infection
E. High-dose radiation

III-65. A 64-year-old man presents with 3 weeks of increasing fatigue and bleeding while brushing his teeth. Physical examination is notable for low-grade fever and normal heart rate, blood pressure, and respiratory rate. He has splenomegaly. A CBC shows marked pancytopenia with blasts present on peripheral smear. A bone marrow aspirate and biopsy result in the diagnosis of acute promyelocytic leukemia with the t(15;17)(q22;q12) cytogenetic rearrangement. Which of the following medications that is specific to acute promyelocytic leukemia will be included in his induction chemotherapy?

A. Acyclovir
B. Daunorubicin
C. Rituximab
D. Sildenafil
E. Tretinoin

III-66. All of the following statements are true regarding chronic myelogenous leukemia (CML) EXCEPT:

A. Allogeneic stem cell transplantation is first-line therapy.
B. Current therapy includes use of a tyrosine kinase inhibitor.
C. Half of afflicted individuals are children.
D. The disease is driven by a mutation in the *HFE* gene.
E. With treatment, the 5-year median survival is 50%.

III-67. Which of the following is the most common lymphoid malignancy?

A. Acute lymphoid leukemia
B. Chronic lymphoid leukemia
C. Hodgkin lymphoma
D. Multiple myeloma
E. Non-Hodgkin lymphoma

III-68. All of the following infectious agents are associated with the development of a lymphoid malignancy EXCEPT:

A. Epstein-Barr virus
B. *H pylori*
C. HIV
D. Human herpesvirus 8
E. JC virus

III-69. Which of the following is the most likely finding in a patient with a "dry" bone marrow aspiration?

A. Chronic myeloid leukemia
B. Hairy cell leukemia
C. Metastatic carcinoma infiltration
D. Myelofibrosis
E. Normal marrow

III-70. All of the following statements are true regarding the criteria to diagnose hypereosinophilic syndrome EXCEPT:

A. Increased bone marrow eosinophils must be demonstrated.
B. It is not necessary to have increased circulating eosinophils.
C. Primary myeloid leukemia must be excluded.
D. Reactive eosinophilia (e.g., parasitic infection, allergy, collagen vascular disease) must be excluded.
E. There must be <20% myeloblasts in blood or bone marrow.

III-71. All of the following statements regarding mastocytosis are true EXCEPT:

A. Elevated serum tryptase suggests aggressive disease.
B. Eosinophilia is common.
C. It is often associated with myeloid neoplasm.
D. Over 90% of cases are confined to the skin.
E. Urticaria pigmentosa is the most common clinical manifestation.

III-72. A 58-year-old man is evaluated for sudden-onset cough with yellow sputum production and dyspnea in the emergency department. Aside from systemic hypertension, he is otherwise healthy. His only medication is amlodipine. Chest radiograph shows a right upper lobe alveolar infiltrate, and labs are notable for a BUN of 53 mg/dL, creatinine of 2.8 mg/dL, calcium of 12.3 mg/dL, total protein of 9 g/dL and albumin of 3.1 g/dL. Sputum culture grows *Streptococcus pneumoniae*. Which of the following tests will confirm the underlying condition predisposing him to pneumococcal pneumonia?

A. Bone marrow biopsy
B. CT of chest, abdomen, and pelvis with contrast
C. HIV antibody
D. Sweat chloride testing
E. Videoscopic swallow study

III-73. In patients with multiple myeloma, which of the following results is the most powerful predictor of survival?

A. Bone involvement on radiograph
B. Renal function
C. Serum albumin
D. Serum β_2-microglobulin
E. Serum calcium

III-74. You are evaluating a 72-year-old man who has been diagnosed with monoclonal gammopathy of undetermined significance (MGUS) after finding an elevated gamma gap on routine blood testing. His bone marrow biopsy demonstrated 5% clonal plasma cells, and he has no evidence of end-organ or bone damage. He reports his appetite is excellent, and he has had no weight gain or loss in the past 1 year. His past medical history is notable for mild hypertension treated only with a diuretic and hyperlipidemia treated with atorvastatin. He has no history of latent or active tuberculosis. He still works as an international travel consultant and walks at least 2 miles three times per week. Calcium and renal function are normal on laboratory testing. His physical examination is unremarkable. Which of the following treatments is indicated at this time?

A. Low-dose prednisone
B. Rituximab
C. Thalidomide
D. Twice-yearly plasmapheresis
E. Yearly serum protein electrophoresis, blood count, creatine, and calcium

III-75. A 64-year-old African American male is evaluated in the hospital for congestive heart failure, renal failure, and polyneuropathy. Physical examination on admission was notable for these findings and raised waxy papules in the axilla and inguinal region. Admission laboratories showed a BUN of 90 mg/dL and a creatinine of 6.3 mg/dL. Total protein was 9.0 g/dL, with an albumin of 3.2 g/dL. Hematocrit was 24%, and WBC and platelet counts were normal. Urinalysis was remarkable for 3+ proteinuria but no cellular casts. Further evaluation included an echocardiogram with a thickened left ventricle and preserved systolic function. Which of the following tests is most likely to diagnose the underlying condition?

A. Bone marrow biopsy
B. Electromyogram (EMG) with nerve conduction studies
C. Fat pad biopsy
D. Right heart catheterization
E. Renal ultrasound

III-76. You are caring for a 65-year-old African American man who was recently told by a cardiologist that he likely has heart failure due to familial amyloidosis based on echocardiography. He has a strong family history of nonsystolic heart failure including his father and a brother who both died in their 60s. Which of the following statements regarding this patient's condition is true?

A. Bone marrow transplantation is curative.
B. Heart failure with diminished systolic function is more typical than heart failure with preserved systolic function.
C. The most common form involves a mutation in the transthyretin gene.
D. This disorder is more common in Hispanic Americans than African Americans.
E. Without intervention, the median survival is <2 years.

III-77. A 28-year-old man comes to your clinic with an abnormal laboratory report. He was seen in an urgent care center after a motor vehicle accident where he sustained a minor chest trauma. All studies were unremarkable, and he was discharged without any specific therapy. However, he was told that he had a low platelet count. He is asymptomatic, has no excessive bleeding, has no past medical history, takes no medications, and does not use alcohol or illicit drugs. His physical examination is totally normal. A CBC reveals normal hemoglobin and WBC with a platelet count of 80,000/μL. His peripheral blood smear is shown

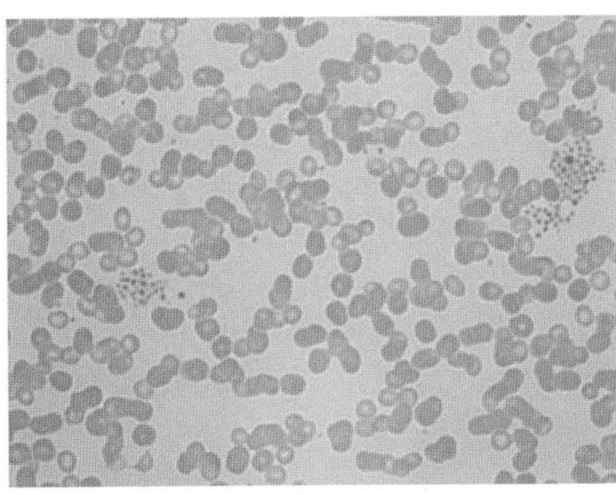

A

FIGURE III-77A

in Figure III-77A. Which of the following is the most likely diagnosis?

A. Congenital thrombocytopenia
B. Disseminated intravascular coagulopathy
C. Drug-induced thrombocytopenia
D. Idiopathic immune thrombocytopenia
E. Pseudothrombocytopenia

III-78. A 75-year-old man is hospitalized for treatment of a deep venous thrombosis. He had recently been discharged from the hospital about 2 months ago. At that time, he had been treated for community-acquired pneumonia complicated by acute respiratory failure requiring mechanical ventilation. He was hospitalized for 21 days at that time and was discharged from a rehabilitation facility 2 weeks ago. On the day prior to admission, he developed painful swelling of his left lower extremity. A lower extremity Doppler ultrasound confirmed an occlusive thrombus of his deep femoral vein. After an initial bolus, he is started on a continuous infusion of unfractionated heparin at 1600 U/hr as he has end-stage renal disease on hemodialysis. His activated partial thromboplastin time (aPTT) is maintained in the therapeutic range. On day 5, it is noted that his platelets have fallen from 150,000/μL to 88,000/μL. What is the most appropriate action at this time?

A. Continue heparin infusion at the current dose and assess for anti-heparin/platelet factor 4 antibodies.
B. Stop all anticoagulation while awaiting results of anti-heparin/platelet factor 4 antibodies.
C. Stop heparin infusion and initiate argatroban.
D. Stop heparin infusion and initiate enoxaparin.
E. Stop heparin infusion and initiate lepirudin.

III-79. A 48-year-old woman is evaluated by her primary care physician for a complaint of gingival bleeding and easy bruising. She has noted the problem for about 2 months. Initially, she attributed it to aspirin that she was taking intermittently for headaches, but she stopped all aspirin and nonsteroidal anti-inflammatory drug use 6 weeks ago. Her only medical history is an automobile accident 12 years previously that caused a liver laceration. It required surgical repair, and she received several transfusions of red blood cells and platelets at that time. She currently takes no prescribed medications and otherwise feels well. On physical examination, she appears well and healthy. She has no jaundice or scleral icterus. Her cardiac and pulmonary examinations are normal. The abdominal examination shows a liver span of 12 cm to percussion, and the edge is palpable 1.5 cm below the right costal margin. The spleen tip is not palpable. There are petechiae present on her extremities and hard palate with a few small ecchymoses on her extremities. A CBC shows a hemoglobin of 12.5 g/dL, hematocrit of 37.6%, WBC count of 8400/μL with a normal differential, and platelet count of 7500/μL. What tests are indicated for the workup of this patient's thrombocytopenia?

A. Antiplatelet antibodies
B. Bone marrow biopsy
C. Hepatitis C antibody
D. HIV antibody
E. C and D
F. All of the above

III-80. A 54-year-old woman presents acutely with alterations in mental status and fever. She was well until 4 days previously when she began to develop complaints of myalgia and fever. Her symptoms progressed rapidly, and today her husband noted her to be lethargic and unresponsive when he awakened. She has recently felt well otherwise. Her only current medication is atenolol 25 mg daily for hypertension. On physical examination, she is responsive only to sternal rub and does not vocalize. Her vital signs are as follows: blood pressure 165/92 mmHg, heart rate 114 bpm, temperature 38.7°C (101.7°F), respiratory rate 26 breaths/min, and oxygen saturation 92% on room air. Her cardiac examination shows a regular tachycardia. Her lungs have bibasilar crackles. The abdominal examination is unremarkable. No hepatosplenomegaly is present. There are petechiae on the lower extremities. Her CBC shows a hemoglobin of 8.8 g/dL, hematocrit of 26.4%, WBC count of 10.2/μL (89% polymorphonuclear cells, 10% lymphocytes, 1% monocytes), and a platelet count of 54,000/μL. A peripheral blood smear is shown in Figure III-80. Her basic metabolic panel shows a sodium of 137 mEq/L, potassium of 5.4 mEq/L, chloride of 98 mEq/L, bicarbonate of 18 mEq/L, BUN of 89 mg/dL, and creatinine of 2.9 mg/dL. Which of the following most correctly describes the pathogenesis of the patient's condition?

A. Development of autoantibodies to a metalloproteinase that cleaves von Willebrand factor
B. Development of autoantibodies to the heparin/platelet factor 4 complex
C. Direct endothelial toxicity initiated by an infectious agent
D. Inherited disorder of platelet granule formation
E. Inherited disorder of von Willebrand factor that precludes binding with factor VIII

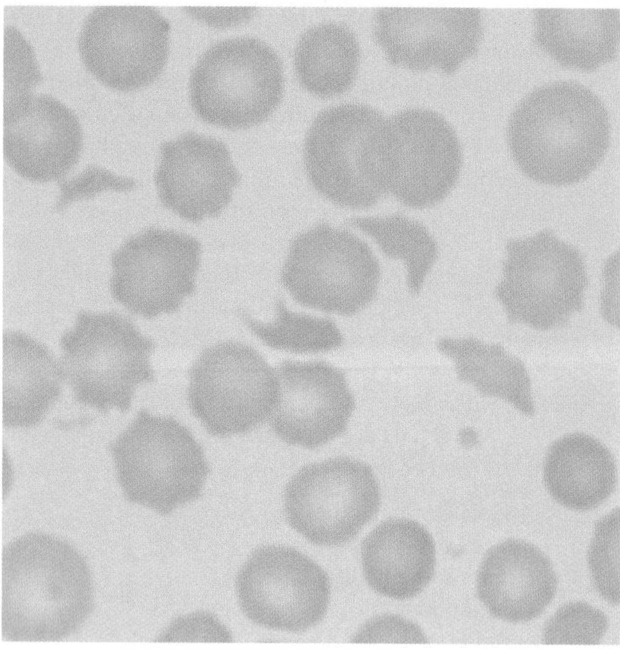

FIGURE III-80

III-81. What is the best initial treatment for the patient in Question III-80?

A. Acyclovir 10 mg/kg intravenously every 8 hours
B. Ceftriaxone 2 g intravenously daily plus vancomycin 1 g intravenously twice daily
C. Hemodialysis
D. Methylprednisolone 1 g intravenously
E. Plasma exchange

III-82. All of the following genetic mutations are associated with an increased risk of deep venous thrombosis EXCEPT:

A. Factor V Leiden mutation
B. Glycoprotein 1b platelet receptor
C. Heterozygous protein C deficiency
D. Prothrombin 20210G
E. Tissue plasminogen activator

III-83. A 76-year-old man presents to an urgent care clinic with pain in his left leg for 4 days. He also describes swelling in his left ankle, which has made it difficult for him to ambulate. He is an active smoker and has a medical history remarkable for gastroesophageal reflux disease, prior deep venous thrombosis (DVT) 9 months ago that resolved, and well-controlled hypertension. Physical examination is revealing for 2+ edema in his left ankle. A D-dimer is ordered and is elevated. Which of the following makes D-dimer less predictive of DVT in this patient?

A. Age >70
B. History of active tobacco use
C. Lack of suggestive clinical symptoms
D. Negative Homan sign on examination
E. Previous DVT in the past year

III-84. A 22-year-old woman comes to the emergency department complaining of 12 hours of shortness of breath. The symptoms began toward the end of a long car ride home from college. She has no past medical history, and her only medication is an oral contraceptive. She smokes occasionally, but the frequency has increased recently because of midterm examinations. On physical examination, she is afebrile with a respiratory rate of 22 breaths/min, blood pressure of 120/80 mmHg, heart rate of 110 bpm, and oxygen saturation of 92% (room air). The rest of her physical examination is normal. A chest radiograph and CBC are normal. Her serum pregnancy test is negative. Which of the following is the indicated management strategy?

A. Check D-dimer and, if normal, discharge with nonsteroidal anti-inflammatory therapy.
B. Check D-dimer and, if normal, obtain lower extremity ultrasound.
C. Check D-dimer and, if abnormal, treat for DVT/pulmonary embolism (PE).
D. Check D-dimer and, if abnormal, obtain contrast multislice CT of chest.
E. Obtain contrast multislice CT of chest.

ANSWERS

III-1. **The answer is B.** *(Chap. 99)* Worldwide, there are more than 12.7 million new cases of cancer and 7.6 million cancer deaths each year, according to estimates provided by the International Agency for Research on Cancer. Most new cases of cancer occur in Asia (45%), with 26% occurring in Europe and 14.5% in North America. Worldwide, lung cancer is both the most common cause of cancer and the most common cause of cancer deaths. In the United States, lung cancer is the most common cause of cancer death but is not the most commonly diagnosed cancer. For men, the most commonly diagnosed cancer is prostate cancer, and for women, it is breast cancer. However, overall, in the United States, the incidence of cancer has been declining by about 2% each year since 1992. Despite the declining incidence, cancer is the second leading cause of death in the United States behind heart disease and is responsible for one out every four deaths. In individuals younger than 85 years, cancer is the leading cause of death. However, 5-year survival rates for cancer are generally improving over time. In 1960–1963, the 5-year survival for all cancers in white patients was 39%. By 2003–2009, this had increased to 69%. African American individuals with cancer fare more poorly with cancer. Over the same interval from 2003–2009, the 5- year survival was only 61% for black individuals. However, racial differences in survival are narrowing over time.

III-2. **The answer is D.** *(Chap. 99)* Assessing response to treatment is an essential component of cancer treatment and compares repeat imaging to the imaging that was used to initially stage the disease. A complete response (option A) is defined as the disappearance of all evidence of disease. To qualify as a partial response (option B), an individual must experience at least a 50% reduction in tumor burden. This reduction is measured as the sum of the products of the perpendicular diameters of all measurable lesions. Another way that partial response can be measured is based upon a 30% decrease in the sum of the longest diameters of the lesions. Progressive disease (option C) is identified when there are any new lesions or if there has been a >25% increase in the sum of the products of the perpendicular diameters of all measurable lesions. The scenario proposed in the clinical history meets none of these criteria and, therefore, would be classified as stable disease (option D), which refers to tumor growth or shrinkage that fails to meet any of the definitions for response or progression.

III-3. **The answer is B.** *(Chap. 99)* While tumor burden is certainly a major factor in determining cancer outcomes, it is also important to consider the functional status of the patient when generating a therapeutic plan. The physiologic stresses of undergoing surgical interventions, radiation therapy, and chemotherapy can exhaust the limited reserves of a patient with multiple medical problems. It is clearly difficult to adequately measure the physiologic reserves of a patient, and most oncologists use performance status measures as a surrogate. Two of the most commonly used measures of performance status are the Eastern Cooperative Oncology Group (ECOG) and Karnofsky performance status. The ECOG scale provides a grade between 0 (fully active) and 5 (dead). Most patients are considered to have adequate reserve for undergoing treatment if the performance status is 0–2, with a status of 2 indicating someone who is ambulatory and capable of all self-care but unable carry out work activities. These individuals are up and about more than 50% of waking hours. A grade 3 performance score would indicate someone who is capable of only limited self-care and is confined to bed or chair more than 50% of waking hours. The Karnofsky score ranges from 0 (dead) to 100 (normal) and is graded at 10-point intervals. A Karnofsky score of <70 also indicates someone with poor performance status and would confer a worse prognosis.

III-4. **The answer is A.** *(Chap. 99)* The cause of cancer death differs across the lifespan and between sexes. In both men and women who are under 20, the primary cause of cancer death is leukemia. In women between the ages of 20 and 59, breast cancer (option A) becomes the leading cause of cancer death. In men, leukemia remains the leading cause of cancer death until the age of 40. After age 40, lung cancer becomes the leading cause of cancer death in men, and in women, it becomes the leading cause of cancer death after age 60.

III-5. **The answer is C.** *(Chap. 104)* Patients who have undergone allogeneic stem cell transplantation remain at risk for infectious complications for an extended period despite engraftment and apparent return of normal hematopoietic capacity. Individuals with graft-versus-host disease (GVHD) often require immunosuppressive treatment that further increases infectious risk. Prevention of infection is the goal in these individuals, and the clinician should ensure appropriate vaccinations for all patients who have undergone intensive chemotherapy, have been treated for Hodgkin disease, or have undergone hematopoietic stem cell transplantation. In hematopoietic stem cell transplantations, the timeline for vaccination varies after transplantation. Pneumococcal vaccination (PCV13) can be given as early as 3–6 months after transplantation, but most vaccines are delayed until 6–12 months after transplantation. In general, the only vaccines that are given contain inactivated organisms. Therefore, oral vaccines for poliomyelitis and the varicella-zoster vaccine are contraindicated. The measles, mumps, and rubella vaccine is also a live virus vaccine, but can be safely given after 24 months if the patient does not have GVHD. Other recommended vaccines include diphtheria-tetanus, inactivated poliomyelitis (by injection), *Haemophilus influenzae* type B, hepatitis B, and 23-valent pneumococcal polysaccharide vaccine. Meningococcal vaccination is recommended in splenectomized patients and in those living in endemic areas, including college dormitories.

III-6. **The answer is D.** *(Chap. 104)* Clinicians are often faced with treatment decisions regarding catheter-related infections in patients who are immunocompromised from cancer and chemotherapy. Because many patients require several weeks of chemotherapy, tunneled catheters are often placed, and determining the need for catheter removal is an important consideration. When blood cultures are positive or there is evidence of infection along the track of the tunnel, catheter removal is recommended. When the erythema is limited to the exit site only, then it is not necessary to remove the catheter unless the erythema fails to respond to treatment. The recommended treatment for an exit site infection should be directed against coagulase-negative staphylococci. In the options presented, vancomycin alone is the best option for treatment. There is no need to add therapy for gram-negative organisms because the patient does not have neutropenia and has negative cultures.

III-7. **The answer is D.** *(Chap. 104)* General guidelines for the treatment of febrile neutropenia depend on the expected duration of neutropenia, previous infections, and recent antibiotic exposures. Each febrile neutropenic patient should be approached as a unique problem. However, several general guidelines can help in treating these patients. The initial regimen should include antibiotics with activity against both gram-negative and gram-positive bacteria. If the expected duration of neutropenia is expected to be greater than 7 days, as in this scenario, then the initial antibiotic choice could be (1) ceftazidime or cefepime, (2) piperacillin/tazobactam, or (3) imipenem/cilastatin or meropenem; all of these regimens have shown equal efficacy in large clinical trials. These antibiotics exhibit broad-spectrum efficacy against gram-positive and gram-negative organisms, including *Pseudomonas aeruginosa*. Double coverage of *P aeruginosa* is not necessary, and use of aminoglycosides alone is contraindicated because these do not provide coverage of gram-positive organisms. Other antibiotics not providing adequate gram-positive coverage include aztreonam and fluoroquinolones. In addition, routine addition of vancomycin is also not indicated because studies have not shown improved outcomes with increased toxic effects. Vancomycin should only be added when there is high suspicion of coagulase-negative staphylococcal infection or specific concerns regarding methicillin-resistant *Staphylococcus aureus* infection. However, the treating physician needs to be knowledgeable about his or her local epidemiology and resistance patterns and prescribe in accordance with this knowledge. Antifungal therapy is often added when there is persistent fevers at 4–7 days without a known source of infection. The choice of specific antifungal agent (echinocandin, azole, lipid formulation of amphotericin B) would depend on whether the patient was receiving antifungal prophylaxis and whether there were reasons to suspect a specific source of infection, such as a pulmonary source.

III-8. The answer is E. *(Chap. 105)* Melanoma is an aggressive malignancy of the melanocytes that is seen predominantly in white-skinned individuals (~98% of cases) and has had a more than 17-fold increase in men and 9-fold increase in women in recent years. The strongest risk factors for the development of melanoma are the presence of multiple benign or atypical nevi and a family or personal history of the disease. Atypical nevi are often referred to as precursor lesions to melanoma, although the specific risk for any individual nevus is quite low. Only about 25% of melanomas arise from nevi; most arise de novo. Other risk factor for melanoma include presence of dysplastic nevi, ultraviolet exposure (including tanning beds), fair complexion, poor tanning ability, freckling, and specific genetic mutations, including *CDKN2A*, *CDK4*, and *MITF*.

III-9. The answer is B. *(Chap. 105)* The best predictor of metastatic risk in melanoma is Breslow thickness, which defines the absolute extent of tumor extension into the tissue. The Clark level defines the extent of invasion of the melanoma based on the layer of the skin involved but does not add significant prognostic information beyond the Breslow thickness. The number of mitoses is used in staging of tumors <1 mm in thickness to provide additional prognostic information about the likelihood of metastatic disease because patients with fewer mitoses have better long-term outcomes. Favorable anatomic sites for prognosis are the forearm and leg, with less favorable sites being the scalp, hands, feet, and mucous membranes. Women generally have better outcomes than men and are frequently diagnosed at earlier stages than men. The effect of age is not straightforward. Older patients are usually diagnosed with thicker primary tumors and have a later diagnosis, but younger patients have a greater risk of lymph node metastases.

III-10 and III-11. The answers are A and E, respectively. *(Chap. 105)* Treatment of metastatic melanoma has largely shown little improvement in mortality in this disease, with median survival following diagnosis of metastatic disease of 6–15 months depending on organs involved. The prognosis is better for those with skin or subcutaneous metastases (M1a) than for those with lung metastases (M1b) and worst for those with liver, bone, or brain disease (M1c). Historically, no traditional chemotherapy regimen has had any effect on the outcome of metastatic melanoma, and these drugs are typically used only for symptom palliation. The agent with the most use in metastatic melanoma is interleukin-2 (IL-2). This cytokine requires individuals to be in good performance status, and the drug is often administered in an intensive care–like setting due to the high incidence of serious, but expected, side effects. IL-2 is not chemotherapy in the traditional sense, and the mechanism by which it kills tumor cells is not fully explained. It is thought to induce the activity of melanoma-specific T cells and leads to long-term disease-free survival in about 5% of treated patients. Other agents that alter the immune response to the tumor cells are the agents that cause immune checkpoint blockade. The only US Food and Drug Administration (FDA)–approved agent in this class is ipilimumab. This treatment is a monoclonal antibody that blocks CTLA-4 and results in improved T-cell function with eradication of tumor cells. This medication was the first treatment of any kind to show a survival benefit in metastatic melanoma. However, the response rate is only ~10%, and there is a significant side effect profile including induced autoimmunity that has limited the enthusiasm for the clinical use of the drug. In the past few years, two new classes of targeted therapies for melanoma have been introduced that have had fewer side effects, although the durability of response is unknown. It is now recommended that all newly diagnosed metastatic lesions undergo molecular testing for *BRAF* mutation. *BRAF* mutations are found in 40%–60% of melanomas and result in constitutive activation of the MAP kinase pathway. There are two currently approved *BRAF* inhibitors, vemurafenib and dabrafenib. These oral medications have shown tumor regression in approximately 50% of treated patients, although they are associated with a class-specific complication of the development of numerous skin lesions, which can include squamous cell cancer. An MEK inhibitor acts one step farther down the MAP kinase pathway and has also been approved by the FDA. Trametinib is less effective than the *BRAF* inhibitors as single-agent therapy but may improve survival when added to the *BRAF* inhibitors. Thus, the current recommended approach to the patient with metastatic melanoma is to test every patient for the presence of a "drugable" (*BRAF*) mutation. If the mutation is not present, the immunotherapy would be offered if the patient had an acceptable functional status. If the mutation is present, then the patient and physician would have to consider the pros and cons of the targeted therapy versus immunotherapy, as either could be acceptable. Targeted therapy has fewer side effects, but long-term durability of response is unknown. In contrast, immunotherapy has many more side effects and a lower initial response rate, but among responders, long-term durable responses can be achieved.

III-12. **The answer is C.** *(Chap. 105)* Nonmelanoma skin cancer (NMSC) is the most common cancer in the United States, with an estimated annual incidence of 1.5–2 million cases yearly. However, most of these cases represent very limited disease with a low metastatic potential and account for only 2400 deaths yearly. The vast majority of NMSCs are basal cell carcinomas (BCC, 70%–80%) or squamous cell carcinomas (SCC, ~20%). The primary risk factor for all NMSCs is ultraviolet (UV) light exposure. UV exposure can occur either through direct exposure to sunlight (UVA and UVB exposure) or via tanning beds (97% UVA exposure). Other risk factors for NMSC include inherited disorders of nucleotide excision repair such as xeroderma pigmentosum, fair complexion, light hair/eyes, cigarette smoking, human immunodeficiency virus (HIV) infection, exposure to ionizing radiation, thermal burn scars, albinism, and chronic ulcerations. In addition, recipients of solid organ transplantations on chronic immunosuppression have a 65-fold increase in SCC and 10-fold increase in BCC. Moreover, NMSC in those with solid organ transplantation is more likely to be aggressive with higher rates of local recurrence, metastasis, and mortality. When comparing BCC to SCC, BCC is the less aggressive of the NMSCs and is typically a slowly enlarging, locally invasive neoplasm. The metastatic potential of BCC is <0.1%. SCC has a more variable natural history, depending on the lesion and host factors. Keratoacanthomas are rapidly growing, low-grade SCCs that can regress spontaneously without therapy. However, progression to metastatic disease has been reported after regression, so treatment for keratoacanthoma should be similar to that for other SCCs. Actinic keratoses and cheilitis are premalignant forms of SCC with transformation to malignancy occurring in 0.25%–20%. In general, the metastatic potential of SCC ranges from 0.3%–5.2%, with the greatest risk of metastases in tumors arising from non–sun-exposed tissues. The approach to treating NMSC depends on the size, depth, location, and host factors, with the primary goal being eradication of tumor with wide local margins.

III-13. **The answer is C.** *(Chap. 106)* Cancers of the larynx often present with the subacute onset of hoarseness that does not resolve over time, but symptoms of head and neck cancer can be rather nonspecific. In more advanced cases, pain, stridor, dysphagia, odynophagia, and cranial neuropathies can occur. Diagnosis of head and neck cancer should include a computed tomography (CT) scan of the head and neck and endoscopic examination under anesthesia to perform biopsies. Positron emission tomography (PET) scans may be used as adjunctive therapy. The staging of head and neck cancers follows a tumor-node-metastasis (TNM) staging guideline (see Figure III-13). This patient would be staged as T2N0M0 based on tumor size without evidence of lymph node involvement or distant metastatic disease. With this designation, the patient's overall stage would be stage II, and the disease would be classified as localized disease. The intent of therapy at this stage of disease is cure of cancer, and overall 5-year survival is 60%–90%. The choice of therapy for laryngeal cancer is radiation therapy to preserve voice. Surgical therapy could be chosen by the patient as well, but is less desirable. In locally or regionally advanced disease, patients can still be approached with curative intent, but this requires multimodality therapy with surgery followed by concomitant chemotherapy and radiation treatment.

III-14. **The answer is C.** *(Chap. 106)* The number of new cases of head and neck cancers (oral cavity, pharynx, and larynx) in the United States was 53,640 in 2013, accounting for about 3% of adult malignancies; 11,520 people died from the disease. The worldwide incidence exceeds half a million cases annually. In North America and Europe, the tumors usually arise from the oral cavity, oropharynx, or larynx. The incidence of oropharyngeal cancers has been increasing in recent years. Nasopharyngeal cancer is more commonly seen in the Mediterranean countries and in the Far East, where it is endemic in some areas. Alcohol and tobacco use are the most significant risk factors for head and neck cancer, and when used together, they act synergistically. Smokeless tobacco is an etiologic agent for oral cancers. Other potential carcinogens include marijuana and occupational exposures

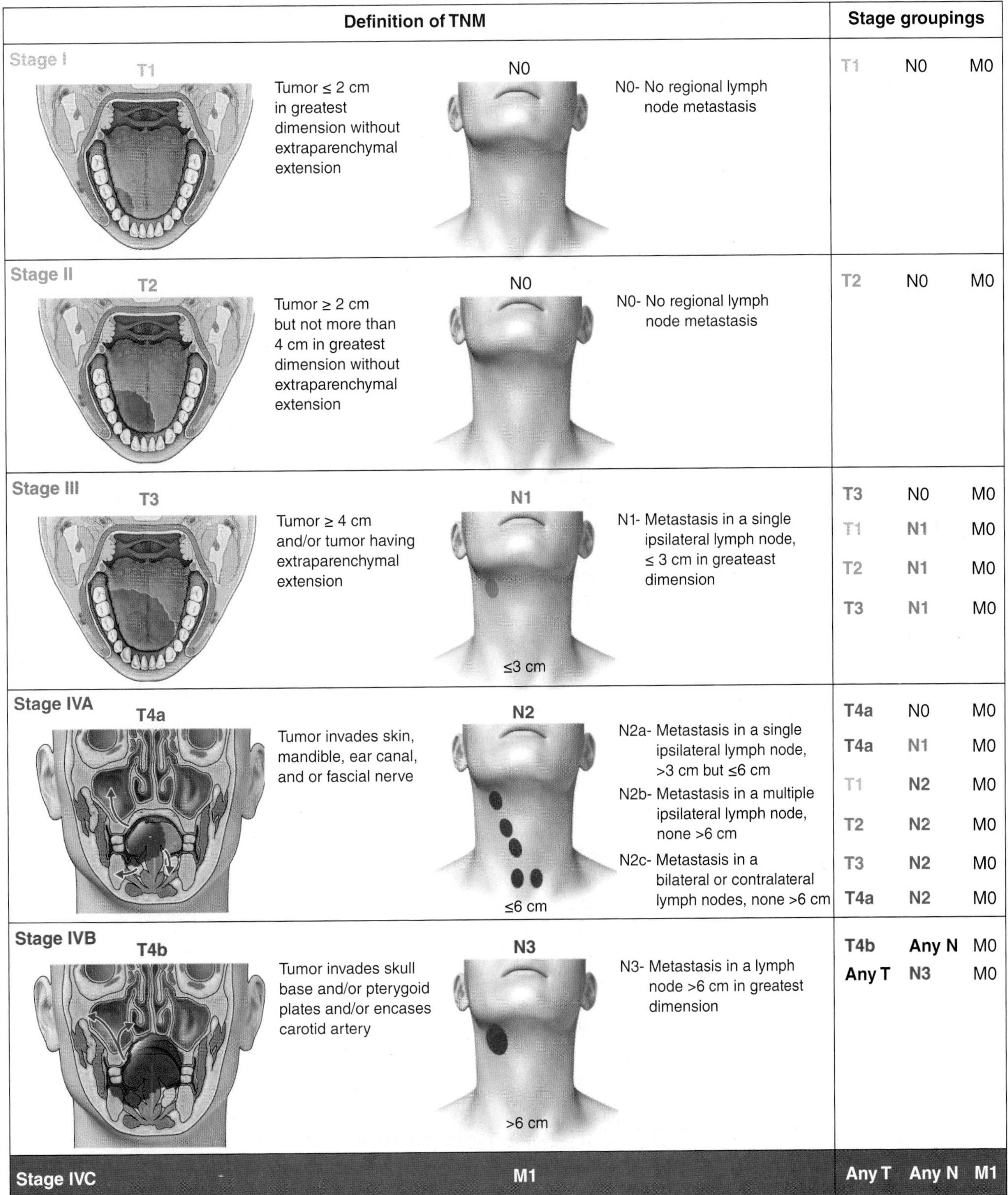

Stage	T	Definition of TNM	N		Stage groupings
Stage I	T1	Tumor ≤ 2 cm in greatest dimension without extraparenchymal extension	N0	N0- No regional lymph node metastasis	T1 N0 M0
Stage II	T2	Tumor ≥ 2 cm but not more than 4 cm in greatest dimension without extraparenchymal extension	N0	N0- No regional lymph node metastasis	T2 N0 M0
Stage III	T3	Tumor ≥ 4 cm and/or tumor having extraparenchymal extension	N1 (≤3 cm)	N1- Metastasis in a single ipsilateral lymph node, ≤ 3 cm in greateast dimension	T3 N0 M0 T1 N1 M0 T2 N1 M0 T3 N1 M0
Stage IVA	T4a	Tumor invades skin, mandible, ear canal, and or fascial nerve	N2 (≤6 cm)	N2a- Metastasis in a single ipsilateral lymph node, >3 cm but ≤6 cm N2b- Metastasis in a multiple ipsilateral lymph node, none >6 cm N2c- Metastasis in a bilateral or contralateral lymph nodes, none >6 cm	T4a N0 M0 T4a N1 M0 T1 N2 M0 T2 N2 M0 T3 N2 M0 T4a N2 M0
Stage IVB	T4b	Tumor invades skull base and/or pterygoid plates and/or encases carotid artery	N3 (>6 cm)	N3- Metastasis in a lymph node >6 cm in greatest dimension	T4b Any N M0 Any T N3 M0
Stage IVC			M1		Any T Any N M1

FIGURE III-13 Tumor-node-metastasis (TNM) staging system.

such as nickel refining, exposure to textile fibers, and woodworking. Some head and neck cancers have a viral etiology. Epstein-Barr virus (EBV) infection is frequently associated with nasopharyngeal cancer, especially in endemic areas of the Mediterranean and Far East. In Western countries, the human papillomavirus (HPV) is associated with a rising incidence of tumors arising from the oropharynx (i.e., the tonsillar bed and base of tongue). Over 50% of oropharyngeal tumors are caused by HPV in the United States. HPV-16 is the dominant viral subtype, although HPV-18 and other oncogenic subtypes are seen as well. Alcohol- and tobacco-related cancers, on the other hand, have decreased in incidence.

HPV-related oropharyngeal cancer occurs in a younger patient population and is associated with increased numbers of sexual partners and oral sexual practices. It is associated with a better prognosis, especially for nonsmokers.

III-15. **The answer is A.** *(Chap. 107)* A solitary pulmonary nodule is a frequent reason for referral to a pulmonologist, but most solitary pulmonary nodules are benign. In fact, over 90% of incidentally identified nodules are of benign origin. Features that are more likely to be present in a malignant lesion are size >3 cm, eccentric calcification, rapid doubling time, and lobulated and irregular contour. Ground glass appearance on CT imaging can be either malignant or benign. Among malignant lesions, ground glass infiltrate is seen more commonly in bronchoalveolar cell carcinoma. When multiple pulmonary nodules are identified, this most commonly represents prior granulomatous disease from healed infections. If multiple nodules are malignant in origin, this usually indicates disease metastatic to the lung, but can be simultaneous lung primary lesions or lesions metastatic from a primary lung cancer. Many incidentally identified nodules are too small to be diagnosed by biopsy and are nonspecific in nature. In this situation, it is prudent to follow the lesions for a period of 2 years, especially in a patient who is high risk for lung cancer, to allow for a proper doubling time to occur. If the lesion remains stable for 2 years, it is most likely benign, although some slow-growing tumors such bronchoalveolar cell carcinoma can have a slower growth rate.

III-16. **The answer is E.** *(Chap. 107)* The evaluation and treatment of solitary pulmonary nodules are important to understand. This patient has a long smoking history with a new nodule that was not apparent by chest x-ray 3 years previously. This should be assumed to be a malignant nodule, and definitive diagnosis and treatment should be attempted. The option for diagnostic and staging procedures include PET/CT, bronchoscopic biopsy, percutaneous needle biopsy, or surgical biopsy with concomitant resection if positive. PET/CT would be low yield in this patient given the small size of the primary lesion (<1 cm) and the lack of enlarged mediastinal lymph nodes. Likewise, bronchoscopy would not provide a good yield because the lesion is very peripheral in origin, and a negative biopsy for malignancy would not be definitive. Appropriate approaches would be to either perform a percutaneous needle biopsy with CT guidance or perform a surgical biopsy with definitive resection if positive. Because this patient has preserved lung function, surgical biopsy and resection are good treatment options for this patient. A repeat CT scan assessing for interval growth would only be appropriate if the patient declined further workup at this time. Referral for treatment with radiation therapy is not appropriate in the absence of tissue diagnosis of malignancy, and surgical resection is the preferred primary treatment because the patient has no contraindications to surgical intervention.

III-17. **The answer is E.** *(Chap. 107)* Pancoast syndrome results from apical extension of a lung mass into the brachial plexus with frequent involvement of the eighth cervical and first and second thoracic nerves. As the tumor continues to grow, it will also involve the sympathetic ganglia of the thoracic chain. The clinical manifestations of a Pancoast tumor include shoulder and arm pain and Horner syndrome (ipsilateral ptosis, miosis, and anhidrosis). Often, the shoulder and arm pain present several months prior to diagnosis. The most common cause of Pancoast syndrome is an apical lung tumor, usually non–small-cell lung cancer. Other causes include mesothelioma and infection, among others. Although midbrain lesions can cause Horner syndrome, other cranial nerve abnormalities would be expected.

Enlarged mediastinal lymph nodes and masses in the middle mediastinum can occlude the superior vena cava, leading to superior vena cava syndrome. Individuals with superior vena cava syndrome typically present with dyspnea and have evidence of facial and upper extremity swelling. Eaton-Lambert myasthenic syndrome is caused by antibodies to voltage-gated calcium channels and is characterized by generalized weakness of muscles that increases with repetitive nerve stimulation. Cervical ribs can cause thoracic outlet syndrome by compression of nerves or vasculature as they exit the chest. This typically presents with ischemic symptoms to the affected limb, but intrinsic wasting of the muscles of the hand can be seen due to neurologic compromise.

III-18. The answer is C. *(Chap. 107)* Mutations of the epidermal growth factor receptor (EGFR) have recently been recognized as important mutations that affect the response of non–small-cell lung cancers to treatment with EGFR tyrosine kinase inhibitors. Initial studies of erlotinib in all patients with advanced non–small-cell lung cancer failed to show a treatment benefit; however, when only those patients with EGFR mutations were considered, treatment with anti-EGFR therapy improved progression-free and overall survival. Patients who are more likely to have EGFR mutations are women, nonsmokers, Asians, and patients with adenocarcinoma histopathology.

III-19. The answer is B. *(Chap. 107)* The Veterans Administration staging system for small-cell lung cancer (SCLC) is a distinct two-stage system dividing patients into those with limited- or extensive-stage disease. Patients with limited-stage disease (LD) have cancer that is confined to the ipsilateral hemithorax and can be encompassed within a tolerable radiation port. Thus, contralateral supraclavicular nodes, recurrent laryngeal nerve involvement, and superior vena caval obstruction can all be part of LD. Patients with extensive-stage disease (ED) have overt metastatic disease by imaging or physical examination. Cardiac tamponade, malignant pleural effusion, and bilateral pulmonary parenchymal involvement generally qualify disease as ED, because the involved organs cannot be encompassed safely or effectively within a single radiation therapy port. Sixty to 70% of patients are diagnosed with ED at presentation. In general, surgical resection is not routinely recommended for patients because even patients with LD-SCLC still have occult micrometastases. Chemotherapy significantly prolongs survival in patients with SCLC. Despite response rates to first-line therapy as high as 80%, the median survival ranges from 12 to 20 months for patients with LD and from 7 to 11 months for patients with ED. Regardless of disease extent, the majority of patients relapse and develop chemotherapy-resistant disease. Only 6%–12% of patients with LD-SCLC and 2% of patients with ED-SCLC live beyond 5 years. The role of radiotherapy in ED-SCLC is largely restricted to palliation of tumor-related symptoms such as bone pain and bronchial obstruction.

III-20. The answer is D. *(Chap. 107 and N Engl J Med 2011;365:395–409)* The National Lung Screening Trial (NLST), a randomized study designed to determine whether low-dose CT scan (LDCT) screening could reduce mortality from lung cancer in high-risk populations as compared with standard posterior-anterior chest x-ray (CXR), was published in 2011. High-risk patients were defined as individuals between 55 and 74 years of age with a ≥30 pack-year history of cigarette smoking; former smokers must have quit within the previous 15 years. Excluded from the trial were individuals with a previous lung cancer diagnosis, a history of hemoptysis, an unexplained weight loss of >15 lb in the preceding year, or a chest CT within 18 months of enrollment. A total of 53,454 persons were enrolled and randomized to annual screening yearly for 3 years (LDCT screening, n = 26,722; CXR screening, n = 26,732). Any noncalcified nodule measuring ≥4 mm in any diameter found on LDCT and CXR images with any noncalcified nodule or mass was classified as "positive." Overall, 39.1% of participants in the LDCT group and 16% in the CXR group had at least one positive screening result. Of those who screened positive, the

TABLE III-20 Results of National Lung Screening Trial

	Event Number		Rates of Events per 100,000 Person-Years			
	LDCT (n = 26,772)	CXR (n = 26,732)	LDCT	CXR	Relative Risk (95% CI)	*p*
Lung cancer mortality	356	443	247	309	0.80 (0.73–0.93)	.004
All-cause mortality	1877	2000	1303	1395	0.93 (0.86–0.99)	.02
Mortality not due to lung cancer	1521	1557	1056	1086	0.99 (0.95–1.02)	.51

Abbreviations: CI, confidence interval; CXR, chest x-ray; LDCT, low-dose computed tomography; RR, rate ratio.
Source: Modified from PB Bach et al: *JAMA* 307:2418, 2012.

false-positive rate was 96.4% in the LDCT group and 94.5% in the CXR group. A greater number of cancers were found in the LDCT group. Nearly twice as many early stage IA cancers were detected in the LDCT group compared with the CXR group (40% vs. 21%). The overall rates of lung cancer death were 247 and 309 deaths per 100,000 participants in the LDCT and CXR groups, respectively, representing a 20% reduction in lung cancer mortality in the LDCT-screened population (95% confidence interval [CI], 6.8%–26.7%; $p = .004$). Compared with the CXR group, the rate of death in the LDCT group from any cause was reduced by 6.7% (95% CI, 1.2–13.6; $p = .02$). Despite the aforementioned caveats, screening of individuals who meet the NLST criteria for lung cancer risk seems warranted, provided comprehensive multidisciplinary coordinated care and follow-up similar to those provided to NLST participants are available.

III-21. **The answer is C.** *(Chap. 108)* The patient has a breast cyst. This has a benign feel on examination, and aspiration of the mass showed nonbloody fluid with resolution of the mass. If there were residual mass or bloody fluid, mammogram and biopsy would be the next step. In patients such as this with nonbloody fluid in whom aspiration clears the mass, reexamination in 1 month is indicated. If the mass recurs, then aspiration should be repeated. If fluid recurs, mammography and biopsy would be indicated at that point. There is no indication at this point to refer for advanced imaging or surgical evaluation. Breastfeeding is not affected by breast cyst presence.

III-22. **The answer is C.** *(Chap. 108)* Breast cancer risk is related to many factors, but age of menarche, age of first full-term pregnancy, and age and menopause together account for 70%–80% of all breast cancer risk. The lowest risk patients have the shortest duration of total menses (i.e., later menarche and earlier menopause), as well as early first full-term pregnancy. Specifically, the lowest risks are menarche at age 16 years old or older, first pregnancy by the age of 18 years, and menopause that begins 10 years before the median age of menopause of 52 years. Thus, patient C meets these criteria.

III-23. **The answer is A.** *(Chap. 109)* A strong family history of colon cancer should prompt consideration for hereditary nonpolyposis colon cancer (HNPCC), or Lynch syndrome, particularly if diffuse polyposis is *not* noted on colonoscopy. HNPCC is characterized by (1) three or more relatives with histologically proven colorectal cancer, one of whom is a first-degree relative and of the other two, at least one had the diagnosis before age 50; and (2) colorectal cancer in at least two generations. The disease is an autosomal dominant trait and is associated with other tumors, including in the endometrium and ovary. The proximal colon is most frequently involved, and cancer occurs with a median age of 50 years, 15 years earlier than in sporadic colon cancer. Patients with HNPCC are recommended to receive biennial colonoscopy and pelvic ultrasound beginning at age 25. Innumerable polyps suggest the presence of one of the autosomal dominant polyposis syndromes, many of which carry a high malignant potential. These include familial adenomatous polyposis, Gardner syndrome (associated with osteomas, fibromas, epidermoid cysts), or Turcot syndrome (associated with brain cancer). Peutz-Jeghers syndrome is associated with mucocutaneous pigmentation and hamartomas. Tumors may develop in the ovary, breast, pancreas, and endometrium; however, malignant colon cancers are not common. Ulcerative colitis is strongly associated with development of colon cancer, but it is unusual for colon cancer to be the presenting finding in ulcerative colitis. Patients are generally symptomatic from their inflammatory bowel disease long before cancer risk develops.

III-24. **The answer is E.** *(Chap. 109)* Colorectal cancer is the second most common cause of cancer death in the United States, and the mortality related to the disease has been decreasing in recent years. When colorectal cancer is identified, patients should be referred for surgical intervention because proper staging and prognosis cannot be determined without pathologic specimens if there is no gross evidence of metastatic disease. The preoperative workup to assess for metastatic or synchronous disease includes a complete colonoscopy if possible, chest radiograph, liver function testing, carcinoembryonic antigen (CEA) testing, and CT imaging of the abdomen. Staging of colorectal cancer follows a TNM staging system. However, the tumor staging is not based on absolute size of the tumor; rather, it is based on the extension of the tumor through the colonic wall. T1 tumors can extend into the submucosa but not beyond, T2 tumors extend into the muscularis propria, and

T3 tumors involve the serosa and beyond. Nodal metastases are graded as N1 (one to three positive lymph nodes) and N2 (four or more positive lymph nodes). This patient's stage of cancer would be T2N1M0 and would stage this as a stage III cancer. Despite the relatively advanced stage, the overall 5-year survival would be 50%–70% due to improvements in overall care of the patient with colorectal cancer. Since the patient has an occluding lesion that prevents preoperative colonoscopy, the patient needs to have a complete colonoscopy performed within the first several months following surgery and every 3 years thereafter. Serial measurements of CEA every 3 months have also been advocated by some specialists. Annual CT scanning may be performed for the first 3 years following resection, although the utility of the practice is debated. Radiation therapy to the pelvis is recommended for all patients with rectal cancer because it reduces local recurrence rate, especially in stage II and III tumors. When postoperative radiation therapy is combined with chemotherapeutic regimens containing 5-fluorouracil, the local recurrence rate is further reduced and overall survival is increased as well.

III-25. **The answer is E.** *(Chap. 109)* Esophageal cancer has a high mortality rate as most patients do not present until advanced disease is present. The typical presenting symptoms of esophageal cancer are dysphagia and significant weight loss. Dysphagia is typically fairly rapidly progressive over a period of weeks to months. Dysphagia initially is only to solid foods but progresses to include semisolids and liquids. For dysphagia to occur, an estimated 60% of the esophageal lumen must be occluded. Weight loss occurs due to decreased oral intake in addition to the cachexia that is common with cancer. Associated symptoms may include pain with swallowing that can radiate to the back, regurgitation or vomiting of undigested food, and aspiration pneumonia. The two major cell types of esophageal cancer in the United States are adenocarcinoma and squamous cell carcinoma, which have different risk factors. Individuals with squamous cell carcinomas typically have a history of both tobacco and alcohol abuse, whereas those with adenocarcinoma more often have a history of long-standing gastroesophageal reflux disease and Barrett esophagitis. Among those with a history of alcohol and tobacco abuse, there is an increased risk with increased intake, and interestingly, risk is more associated with whiskey drinking when compared to wine or beer. Other risk factors for squamous cell carcinoma of the esophagus include ingestion of nitrites, smoked opiates, fungal toxins in pickled vegetables, and physical insults that include long-standing ingestion of very hot tea or lye.

III-26. **The answer is C.** *(Chap. 109)* A variety of causative factors have been implicated in the development of squamous cell cancers of the esophagus. In the United States, the etiology of such cancers is primarily related to excess alcohol consumption and/or cigarette smoking. The relative risk increases with the amount of tobacco smoked or alcohol consumed, with these factors acting synergistically. Squamous cell esophageal carcinoma has also been associated with the ingestion of nitrates, smoked opiates, and fungal toxins in pickled vegetables, as well as mucosal damage caused by such physical insults as long-term exposure to extremely hot tea, the ingestion of lye, radiation-induced strictures, and chronic achalasia. The presence of an esophageal web in association with glossitis and iron deficiency (i.e., Plummer-Vinson or Paterson-Kelly syndrome) and congenital hyperkeratosis and pitting of the palms and soles (i.e., tylosis palmaris et plantaris) have each been linked with squamous cell esophageal cancer, as have dietary deficiencies of molybdenum, zinc, selenium, and vitamin A. Several strong etiologic associations have been observed to account for the development of adenocarcinoma of the esophagus. Such tumors arise in the distal esophagus in association with chronic gastric reflux, often in the presence of Barrett esophagus (replacement of the normal squamous epithelium of the distal esophagus by columnar mucosa), which occurs more commonly in obese individuals. Adenocarcinomas arise within dysplastic columnar epithelium in the distal esophagus. Cigarette smoking is associated with the development of adenocarcinoma of the esophagus as well.

III-27. **The answer is C.** *(Chap. 111)* Hepatitis B virus (HBV) and hepatitis C virus (HCV) infection both have a clear relationship with the subsequent development of hepatocellular carcinoma (HCC). Both case-control and cohort studies have shown a strong association between chronic hepatitis B carrier rates and increased incidence of HCC. In Taiwanese male postal carriers who were hepatitis B surface antigen (HBsAg) positive, a 98-fold greater risk for HCC was found compared to HBsAg-negative individuals. HBV-based

HCC may involve rounds of hepatic destruction with subsequent proliferation and not necessarily frank cirrhosis. The latency of HCV infection and development of HCC is approximately 30 years. Patients with HCV-associated HCC tend to have more frequent and advanced cirrhosis, but in HBV-associated HCC, only half the patients have cirrhosis, with the remainder having chronic active hepatitis. Approximately 75%–80% of patients with HCC have cirrhosis, and other liver conditions without cirrhosis, such as nonalcoholic fatty liver and nonalcoholic steatohepatitis, are associated with the development of HCC. Natural chemical carcinogens, such as aflatoxin B_1, are strongly associated with HCC. It can be found in a variety of stored grains in hot, humid places, where peanuts and rice are stored in unrefrigerated conditions. Aflatoxin contamination of foodstuffs correlates well with incidence rates in Africa and to some extent in China. In endemic areas of China, even farm animals such as ducks have HCC. Malaria is not associated with HCC.

TABLE III-27 **Factors Associated with an Increased Risk of Developing Hepatocellular Carcinoma**

Common	Unusual
Cirrhosis from any cause	Primary biliary cirrhosis
Hepatitis B or C chronic infection	Hemochromatosis
Ethanol chronic consumption	α_1-Antitrypsin deficiency
NASH/NAFL	Glycogen storage diseases
Aflatoxin B_1 or other mycotoxins	Citrullinemia
	Porphyria cutanea tarda
	Hereditary tyrosinemia
	Wilson disease

Abbreviations: NAFL, nonalcoholic fatty liver; NASH, nonalcoholic steatohepatitis.

III-28. The answer is E. *(Chap. 111)* Hepatomegaly is the most common physical sign in patients with HCC, occurring in 50%–90% of the patients. Abdominal bruits are noted in 6%–25%, and ascites occurs in 30%–60% of patients. α-Fetoprotein (AFP) is a serum tumor marker for HCC; however, it is only increased in approximately one-half of U.S. patients. Rising AFP in a patient at risk of HCC may be a marker of development of disease, and in some cases, serial measurement of AFP may be used as a marker of response to therapy. An ultrasound examination of the liver is an excellent screening tool. The two characteristic vascular abnormalities are hypervascularity of the tumor mass (neovascularization or abnormal tumor-feeding arterial vessels) and thrombosis by tumor invasion of otherwise normal portal veins. To determine tumor size and extent and the presence of portal vein invasion accurately, a helical/triphasic CT scan of the abdomen and pelvis, with fast-contrast bolus technique, should be performed to detect the vascular lesions typical of HCC. Portal vein invasion is normally detected as an obstruction and expansion of the vessel. Magnetic resonance imaging (MRI) can also provide detailed information, especially with the newer contrast agents. A prospective comparison of triphasic CT, gadolinium-enhanced MRI, ultrasound, and fluorodeoxyglucose (FDG)-PET showed similar results for CT, MRI, and ultrasound; PET imaging appears to be positive in only a subset of HCC patients. MRI is better able to distinguish dysplastic or regenerative nodules from HCC. Imaging criteria have been developed for HCC that do not require biopsy proof, as they have >90% specificity. The criteria include nodules >1 cm with arterial enhancement and portal venous washout and, for small tumors, specified growth rates on two scans performed less than 6 months apart (Organ Procurement and Transplant Network). Nevertheless, explant pathology after liver transplant for HCC has shown that approximately 20% of patients diagnosed without biopsy did not actually have a tumor.

III-29. The answer is E. *(Chap. 111)* Because this patient has a tumor >3 cm, he is not a candidate for primary radical resection. However, with his otherwise good prognosis and excellent performance status, he may be a candidate for liver transplantation that would cure his cirrhosis and his carcinoma. There are also evolving local ablative modalities that he would be eligible to receive (Figure III-29).

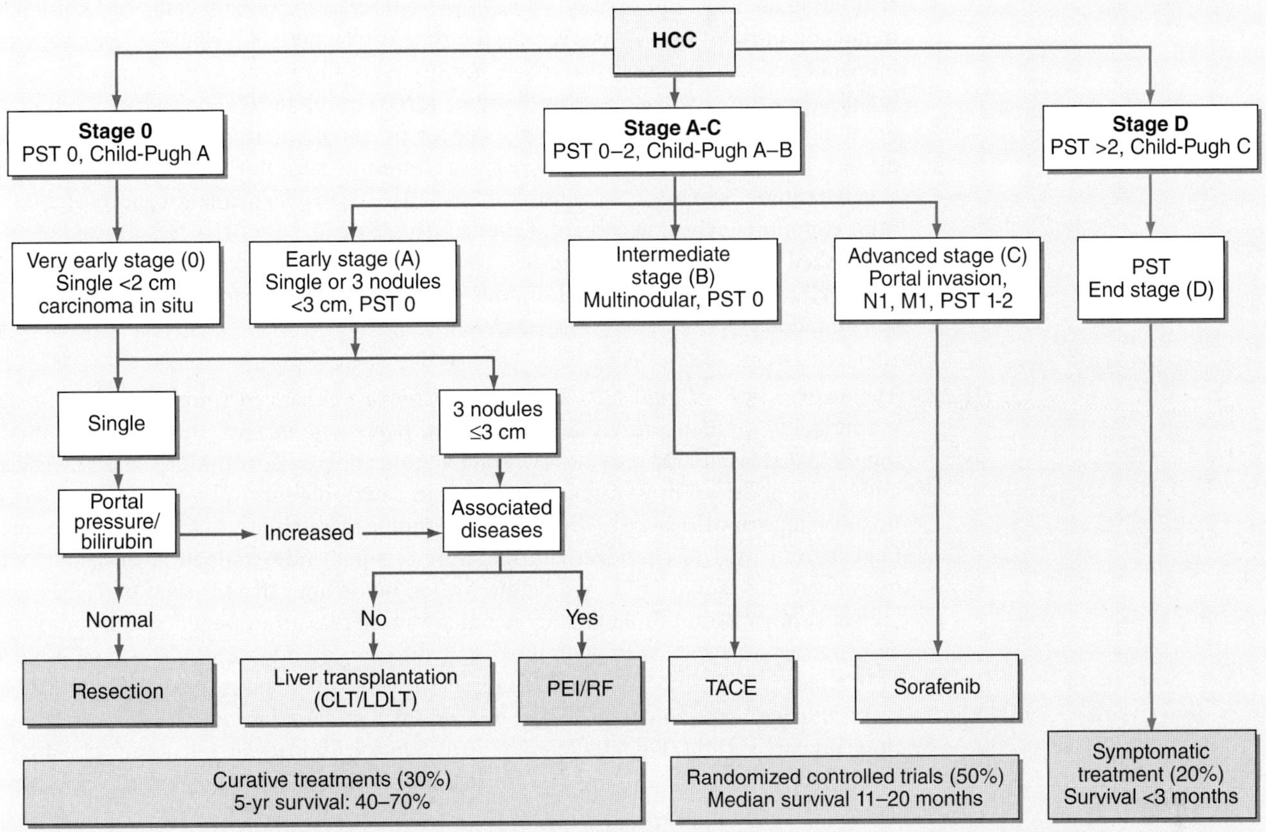

FIGURE III-29 Barcelona Clinic Liver Cancer (BCLC) staging classification and treatment schedule. Patients with very early hepatocellular carcinoma (HCC) (stage 0) are optimal candidates for resection. Patients with early HCC (stage A) are candidates for radical therapy (resection, liver transplantation [LT], or local ablation via percutaneous ethanol injection [PEI] or radiofrequency [RF] ablation). Patients with intermediate HCC (stage B) benefit from transcatheter arterial chemoembolization (TACE). Patients with advanced HCC, defined as presence of macroscopic vascular invasion, extrahepatic spread, or cancer-related symptoms (Eastern Cooperative Oncology Group performance status 1 or 2) (stage C), benefit from sorafenib. Patients with end-stage disease (stage D) will receive symptomatic treatment. Treatment strategy will transition from one stage to another on treatment failure or contraindications for the procedures. CLT, cadaveric liver transplantation; LDLT, living donor liver transplantation; PST, Performance Status Test. (*Modified from JM Llovet et al: JNCI* 100:698, 2008.)

III-30. The answer is C. *(Chap. 111)* Cholangiocarcinoma (CCC) typically refers to mucin-producing adenocarcinomas (different from HCC) that arise from the biliary tract and have features of cholangiocyte differentiation. They are grouped by their anatomic site of origin, as intrahepatic (IHC), perihilar (central, ~65% of CCCs), and peripheral (or distal, ~30% of CCCs). IHC is the second most common primary liver tumor. They arise as a result of cirrhosis less frequently than HCC, but may complicate primary biliary cirrhosis. However, cirrhosis and both primary biliary cirrhosis and HCV predispose to IHC. Nodular tumors arising at the bifurcation of the common bile duct are called *Klatskin* tumors and are often associated with a collapsed gallbladder, a finding that mandates visualization of the entire biliary tree. Incidence is increasing. Although most CCCs have no obvious cause, a number of predisposing factors have been identified, including primary sclerosing cholangitis (10%–20% of primary sclerosing cholangitis patients), an autoimmune disease, and liver fluke in Asians, especially *Opisthorchis viverrini* and *Clonorchis sinensis*. CCC also seems to be associated with any cause of chronic biliary inflammation and injury, including alcoholic liver disease, choledocholithiasis, choledochal cysts (10%), and Caroli disease (a rare inherited form of bile duct ectasia). CCC most typically presents as painless jaundice, often with pruritus or weight loss. Incidence has been increasing in recent decades; few patients survive 5 years. The usual treatment is surgical, but combination systemic chemotherapy may be effective. After complete surgical resection for IHC, 5-year survival is 25%–30%. Combination radiation therapy with liver transplantation has produced a 5-year recurrence-free survival rate of 65%.

III-31. The answer is E. *(Chap. 112)* Pancreatic cancer is the fourth leading cause of cancer death in the United States, despite representing only 3% of all newly diagnosed malignancies.

Infiltrating ductal adenocarcinomas account for the vast majority of cases and arise most frequently in the head of pancreas. At the time of diagnosis 85%–90% of patients have inoperable or metastatic disease, which is reflected in the 5-year survival rate of only 5% for all stages combined. An improved 5-year survival of up to 20% may be achieved when the tumor is detected at an early stage and when complete surgical resection is accomplished. Over the past 30 years, 5-year survival rates have not improved substantially. Cigarette smoking may be the cause of up to 20%–25% of all pancreatic cancers and is the most common environmental risk factor for this disease. Other risk factors are not well established due to inconsistent results from epidemiologic studies, but include chronic pancreatitis and diabetes. Alcohol does not appear to be a risk factor unless excess consumption gives rise to chronic pancreatitis.

III-32. **The answer is B.** *(Chap. 112)* Dual-phase, contrast-enhanced spiral CT is the imaging modality of choice to visualize suspected pancreatic masses. In addition to imaging the pancreas, it also provides accurate visualization of surrounding viscera, vessels, and lymph nodes. In most cases, this study can determine surgical resectability. There is no advantage of MRI over CT in predicting tumor resectability, but selected cases may benefit from MRI to characterize the nature of small indeterminate liver lesions and to evaluate the cause of biliary dilatation when no obvious mass is seen on CT. Preoperative confirmation of malignancy is not always necessary in patients with radiologic appearances consistent with operable pancreatic cancer. Endoscopic ultrasound–guided needle biopsy is the most effective technique to evaluate the mass for malignancy. It has an accuracy of approximately 90% and has a smaller risk of intraperitoneal dissemination compared with CT-guided percutaneous biopsy. Endoscopic retrograde cholangiopancreatography is a useful method for obtaining ductal brushings, but the diagnostic value of pancreatic juice sampling is only 25%–30%. CA 19-9 is elevated in approximately 70%–80% of patients with pancreatic carcinoma but is not recommended as a routine diagnostic or screening test because its sensitivity and specificity are inadequate for accurate diagnosis. Preoperative CA 19-9 levels correlate with tumor stage and prognosis. They are also an indicator of asymptomatic recurrence in patients with completely resected tumors. FDG-PET should be considered before surgery for detecting distant metastases.

III-33. **The answer is C.** *(Chap. 112)* This patient has a <2-cm tumor with no microscopic residual disease and, therefore, has stage I disease, with a 20% 5-year survival after surgery and a gemcitabine-containing adjuvant chemotherapy regimen (Figure III-33). This presentation accounts for <10% of patients with newly diagnosed pancreatic cancer. Most patients present with advanced disease (stage IV), with a <5% 5-year survival. The four genes most commonly mutated or inactivated in pancreatic cancer are *KRAS* and the tumor-suppressor genes *p16* (deleted in 95% of tumors), *p53* (inactivated or mutated in 50%–70% of tumors), and *SMAD4* (deleted in 55% of tumors). Typically, the cancer precursor lesions acquire these genetic abnormalities in a progressive manner that is associated with increasing dysplasia. *SMAD4* gene inactivation is associated with a pattern of widespread metastatic disease in advanced-stage patients and poorer survival in patients with surgically resected pancreatic adenocarcinoma.

III-34. **The answer is D.** *(Chap. 114)* Bladder cancer is the 4th most common cancer in men and the 13th most common cancer in women. Cigarette smoking has a strong association with bladder cancer, particularly in men. The increased risk persists for at least 10 years after quitting. Bladder cancer is a small cause of cancer deaths because most detected cases are superficial with an excellent prognosis. Most cases of bladder cancer come to medical attention by the presence of gross hematuria emanating from exophytic lesions. Microscopic hematuria is more likely due to prostate cancer than bladder cancer. Cystoscopy under anesthesia is indicated to evaluate for bladder cancer. In cases of superficial disease, bacillus Calmette-Guerin is an effective adjuvant to decrease recurrence or treat unresectable superficial disease. In the United States, cystectomy is generally recommended for invasive disease. Even invasive cancer with nodal involvement has a >40% 10-year survival after surgery and adjuvant therapy.

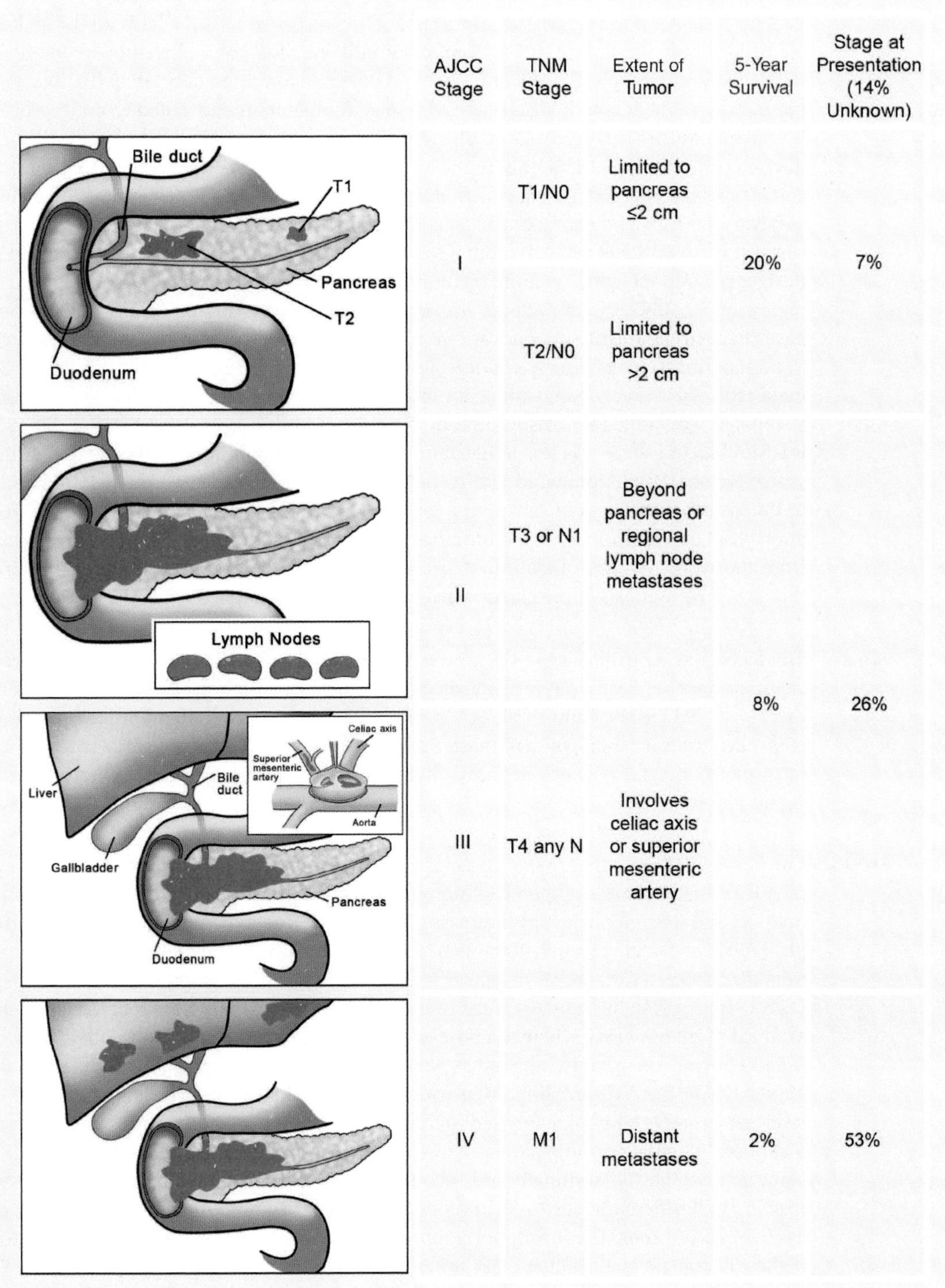

AJCC Stage	TNM Stage	Extent of Tumor	5-Year Survival	Stage at Presentation (14% Unknown)
I	T1/N0	Limited to pancreas ≤2 cm	20%	7%
	T2/N0	Limited to pancreas >2 cm		
II	T3 or N1	Beyond pancreas or regional lymph node metastases	8%	26%
III	T4 any N	Involves celiac axis or superior mesenteric artery		
IV	M1	Distant metastases	2%	53%

FIGURE III-33 AJCC, American Joint Committee on Cancer: TNM, tumor-node-metastasis. Illustration by Stephen Millward.

III-35 and III-36. The answers are C and E, respectively. *(Chap. 114)* The incidence of renal cell carcinoma continues to rise and is now nearly 58,000 cases annually in the United States, resulting in 13,000 deaths. The male-to-female ratio is 2:1. Incidence peaks between the ages of 50 and 70 years, although this malignancy may be diagnosed at any age. Many environmental factors have been investigated as possible contributing causes; the strongest association is with cigarette smoking. Risk is also increased for patients who have acquired cystic disease of the kidney associated with end-stage renal disease and for those with tuberous sclerosis. Most renal cell carcinomas are clear cell tumors (60%), with papillary and chromophobic tumors being less common. Clear cell tumors account for >80% of patients that develop metastases. The classic triad of hematuria, flank pain, and palpable mass is only present in 10%–20% of cases initially. Most cases currently are found as incidental findings on CT scans or ultrasound obtained for different reasons. The increasing number of incidentally discovered low-stage tumors has contributed to an improved 5-year survival. The paraneoplastic phenomenon of erythrocytosis due to increased production of erythropoietin is only found in 3% of cases; anemia due to advanced disease is far more common. Stage I and II tumors are confined to the kidney and have a >80% survival after radical nephrectomy. Stage IV tumors with distant metastases have a 5-year survival of 10%. Renal cell carcinoma is notably resistant to traditional chemotherapeutic agents. Until recently, cytokine therapy with IL-2 or interferon-γ was used to produce regression in 10%–20% of patients with metastatic disease. Antiangiogenic medications have changed the treatment of advance renal cell carcinoma. Sunitinib was demonstrated to be superior to interferon-γ, and it is now first-line therapy for patients with advanced metastatic disease. Pazopanib and axitinib are newer agents of the same class as sunitinib. Pazopanib was compared to sunitinib in a randomized first-line phase III trial. Efficacy was similar, and there was less fatigue and skin toxicity, resulting in better quality of life scores for pazopanib compared with sunitinib. Temsirolimus and everolimus, inhibitors of the mammalian target of rapamycin (mTOR), show activity in patients with untreated poor-prognosis tumors and in sunitinib/sorafenib-refractory tumors. Patients may benefit from the sequential use of axitinib and everolimus following progression after first-line therapy. The prognosis of metastatic renal cell carcinoma is variable.

III-37. **The answer is A.** *(Chap. 115)* The results from several large, double-blind, randomized chemoprevention trials have established 5α-reductase inhibitors as the predominant therapy to reduce the future risk of a prostate cancer diagnosis. Randomized placebo-controlled trials have shown that finasteride and dutasteride reduce the period prevalence of prostate cancer. Trials of selenium, vitamin C, and vitamin E have shown no benefit versus placebo.

III-38. **The answer is E.** *(Chap. 115)* Transrectal ultrasound-guided biopsy is recommended for men with an abnormal digital rectal examination. Carcinomas are characteristically hard, nodular, and irregular, whereas induration may also be due to benign prostatic hypertrophy (BPH) or calculi. Overall, 20%–25% of men with an abnormal digital rectal examination have cancer. A diagnosis of cancer is established by an image-guided needle biopsy. Direct visualization by transrectal ultrasound or MRI assures that all areas of the gland are sampled. Contemporary schemas advise an extended pattern 12-core biopsy that includes sampling from the peripheral zone as well as a lesion-directed palpable nodule or suspicious image-guided sampling. Men with an abnormal prostate-specific antigen (PSA) level and negative biopsy are advised to undergo a repeat biopsy. When prostate cancer is diagnosed, a measure of histologic aggressiveness is assigned using the Gleason grading system, in which the dominant and secondary glandular histologic patterns are scored from 1 (well differentiated) to 5 (undifferentiated) and summed to give a total score of 2–10 for each tumor. The most poorly differentiated area of tumor (i.e., the area with the highest histologic grade) often determines biologic behavior. The presence or absence of perineural invasion and extracapsular spread is also recorded.

III-39. **The answer is C.** *(Chap. 115)* PSA is a serine protease that causes liquefaction of seminal coagulum. It is produced by both nonmalignant and malignant epithelial cells and, as such, is prostate specific, not prostate cancer specific. Serum levels may also increase from prostatitis and benign prostatic hypertrophy. Serum levels are not significantly affected by digital rectal examination, but the performance of a prostate biopsy can increase PSA levels up to 10-fold for 8–10 weeks. PSA testing was approved by the U.S. FDA in 1994 for early detection of prostate cancer, and the widespread use of the test has played a significant role in the proportion of men diagnosed with early-stage cancers: more than 70%–80% of newly diagnosed cancers are clinically organ confined. The level of PSA in blood is strongly associated with the risk and outcome of prostate cancer. Most prostate cancer deaths (90%) occur among men with PSA levels in the top quartile (>2 ng/mL), although only a minority of men with PSA >2 ng/mL will develop lethal prostate cancer.

Despite this and mortality rate reductions reported from large randomized prostate cancer screening trials, routine use of the test remains controversial. The U.S. Preventive Services Task Force (USPSTF) recently made a clear recommendation against screening. By giving a grade of D in the recommendation statement that was based on this review, the USPSTF concluded that "there is moderate or high certainty that this service has no net benefit or that the harms outweigh the benefits." Whether the harms of screening, overdiagnosis, and overtreatment are justified by the benefits in terms of reduced prostate cancer mortality is open to reasonable doubt. In response to the USPSTF, the American Urological Association (AUA) updated their consensus statement regarding prostate cancer screening. They concluded that the quality of evidence for the benefits of screening was moderate, and evidence for harm was high for men age 55–69 years. For men outside this age range, evidence was lacking for benefit, but the harms of screening, including overdiagnosis and overtreatment, remained. The AUA recommends shared decision making considering PSA-based screening for men age 55–69, a target age group for whom benefits may outweigh harms. Outside this age range, PSA-based screening as a routine test was not recommended based on the available evidence. The PSA criteria used to recommend a diagnostic prostate biopsy have evolved over time. However, based on the commonly used cut point for prostate biopsy (a total PSA ≥4 ng/mL), most men with a PSA elevation do not have histologic evidence of prostate cancer at biopsy. In addition, many men with PSA levels below this cut point harbor cancer cells in their prostate. There is no PSA below which the risk of prostate cancer is zero. The routine use of antibiotics in an asymptomatic man with an elevated PSA level is strongly discouraged and should not affect the decision to pursue further evaluation.

III-40. **The answer is B.** *(Chap. 115)* Benign prostatic hypertrophy (BPH) is a pathologic process that contributes to the development of lower urinary tract symptoms in men. Such symptoms, arising from lower urinary tract dysfunction, are further subdivided into obstructive symptoms (urinary hesitancy, straining, weak stream, terminal dribbling, prolonged voiding, incomplete emptying) and irritative symptoms (urinary frequency, urgency, nocturia, urge incontinence, small voided volumes). Lower urinary tract symptoms and other sequelae of BPH are not just due to a mass effect, but are also likely due to a combination of the prostatic enlargement and age-related detrusor dysfunction. Asymptomatic patients do not require treatment regardless of the size of the prostate gland. Symptomatic relief is the most common reason men seek treatment for BPH, and therefore, the goal of therapy for BPH is usually relief of these symptoms. Selective α-adrenergic receptor antagonists, such as alfuzosin, are thought to treat the dynamic aspect of BPH by reducing sympathetic tone of the bladder outlet, thereby decreasing resistance and improving urinary flow. 5α-Reductase inhibitors, such as dutasteride and finasteride, are thought to treat the static aspect of BPH by reducing prostate volume and having a similar, albeit delayed effect. They have also proven to be beneficial in the prevention of BPH progression, as measured by prostate volume, the risk of developing acute urinary retention, and the risk of having BPH-related surgery. The use of an α-adrenergic receptor antagonist and a 5α-reductase inhibitor as combination therapy seeks to provide symptomatic relief while preventing progression of BPH.

Another class of medications that has shown improvement in lower urinary tract symptoms secondary to BPH is phosphodiesterase-5 (PDE5) inhibitors, used currently in the treatment of erectile dysfunction. All three of the PDE5 inhibitors available in the United States, sildenafil, vardenafil, and tadalafil, appear to be effective in the treatment of symptoms secondary to BPH. The use of PDE5 inhibitors is not without controversy, however, given the fact that short-acting PDE5 inhibitors such as sildenafil need to be dosed separately from α-blockers because of potential hypotensive effects. Bosentan is a nonselective endothelin receptor antagonist used in the treatment of pulmonary arterial hypertension.

III-41. **The answer is E.** *(Chap. 116)* Pure seminomas have the best survival of all forms of testicular cancer and represent approximately 50% of all germ cell tumors. The median age of presentation is the fourth decade of life, and approximately 80% of individuals present with stage I disease, indicating any disease limited to the testis no matter the size at initial presentation. All men presenting with a testicular mass should be referred for radical inguinal orchiectomy as this approach mirrors the embryonic development of the testis and does not breach anatomic barriers to allow for other pathways of spread. In the staging workup of testicular cancers, men should undergo CT imaging of the chest, abdomen, and pelvis as well as measurement of the serum tumor markers AFP and β-human chorionic gonadotropin (β-hCG), in addition to lactate dehydrogenase (LDH) levels. These tumor markers assist with both diagnosis and prognosis in testicular cancer and help with determining the appropriate postorchiectomy treatment. In pure seminomas, AFP levels should not be elevated. If the AFP level is elevated, this indicates an occult nonseminomatous component, which may require more aggressive initial treatment with either retroperitoneal lymph node dissection or adjuvant chemotherapy depending on local surgical expertise and preference of the patient and treating physician. β-hCG levels may be elevated in pure seminomas, although this too is infrequent in men without advanced disease. LDH levels are less specific, but are increased in up to 80% of patients with advanced seminoma. After resection, the tumor markers should return to normal values within their expected half-lives following first-order kinetics. The half-life of β-hCG is 24–36 hours, and that of AFP is 5–7 days. In stage I seminoma, survival is near 100% with either immediate postorchiectomy radiation or with surveillance alone (option E). Given the concern about secondary malignancy due to radiation exposure, many providers chose watchful waiting with surveillance alone in men who are compliant with follow-up. However, approximately 15% of patients will experience relapse, and 5% of relapses occur after 5 years. Thus, extended follow-up is required. A single dose of carboplatin has been investigated as an alternative to radiation therapy, but long-term outcomes are as yet unknown.

III-42. **The answer is A.** *(Chap. 116)* Ninety percent of persons with nonseminomatous germ cell tumors produce either AFP or β-hCG; in contrast, persons with pure seminomas usually produce neither. These tumor markers are present for some time after surgery; if the presurgical levels are high, 30 days or more may be required before meaningful postsurgical levels can be obtained. The half-lives of AFP and β-hCG are 6 days and 1 day, respectively. After treatment, unequal reduction of β-hCG and AFP may occur, suggesting that the two markers are synthesized by heterogeneous clones of cells within the tumor; thus, both markers should be followed. β-hCG is similar to luteinizing hormone except for its distinctive β subunit.

III-43. **The answer is E.** *(Chap. 117)* A variety of genetic syndromes substantially increase a woman's risk of developing ovarian cancer. Approximately 10% of women with ovarian cancer have a germline mutation in one of two DNA repair genes: *BRCA1* (chromosome 17q12-21) or *BRCA2* (chromosome 13q12-13). Individuals inheriting a single copy of a mutant allele have a very high incidence of breast and ovarian cancer. Most of these women have a family history that is notable for multiple cases of breast and/or ovarian cancer, although inheritance through male members of the family can camouflage this genotype through several generations. The most common malignancy in these women is breast carcinoma, although women harboring germline *BRCA1* mutations have a marked increased risk of developing ovarian malignancies in their 40s and 50s with a 30%–50% lifetime risk of developing ovarian cancer. Women harboring a mutation in *BRCA2* have a lower penetrance of ovarian cancer with perhaps a 20%–40% chance of developing this malignancy, with onset typically in their 50s or 60s. Women with a *BRCA2* mutation also are at slightly increased risk of pancreatic cancer. Likewise, women with mutations in the DNA mismatch repair genes associated with Lynch syndrome type 2 (*MSH2*, *MLH1*, *MLH6*, *PMS1*, *PMS2*) may have a risk of ovarian cancer as high as 1% per year in their 40s and 50s. Finally, a small group of women with familial ovarian cancer may have mutations in other *BRCA*-associated genes such as *RAD51*, *CHK2*, and others. Screening studies in this select population suggest that current screening techniques, including serial evaluation of the CA-125 tumor marker and ultrasound, are insufficient at detecting early-stage and curable disease, so women with these germline mutations are advised to undergo prophylactic removal of ovaries and fallopian tubes typically after completing childbearing and ideally before age 35–40 years. Early prophylactic oophorectomy also protects these women from subsequent breast cancer, with a reduction of breast cancer risk of approximately 50%.

III-44. **The answer is A.** *(Chap. 117)* Cervical cancer is the second most common and most lethal malignancy in women worldwide likely due to the widespread infection with high-risk strains of HPV and limited utilization of or access to Pap smear screening in many nations throughout the world. Nearly 500,000 cases of cervical cancer are expected worldwide, with approximately 240,000 deaths annually. Cancer incidence is particularly high in women residing in Central and South America, the Caribbean, and southern and eastern Africa. Mortality rate is disproportionately high in Africa. In the United States, 12,360 women were diagnosed with cervical cancer, and 4020 women died of the disease in 2014. HPV is the primary neoplastic-initiating event in the vast majority of women with invasive cervical cancer. This double-strand DNA virus infects epithelium near the transformation zone of the cervix. More than 60 types of HPV are known, with approximately 20 types having the ability to generate high-grade dysplasia and malignancy. HPV-16 and -18 are the types most frequently associated with high-grade dysplasia and targeted by both U.S. FDA–approved vaccines. The large majority of sexually active adults are exposed to HPV, and most women clear the infection without specific intervention. Risk factors for HPV infection and, in particular, dysplasia include a high number of sexual partners, early age of first intercourse, and history of venereal disease. Smoking is a cofactor; heavy smokers have a higher risk of dysplasia with HPV infection. HIV infection, especially when associated with low CD4+ T-cell counts, is associated with a higher rate of high-grade dysplasia and likely a shorter latency period between infection and invasive disease. The administration of highly active antiretroviral therapy reduces the risk of high-grade dysplasia associated with HPV infection. Currently approved vaccines include the recombinant proteins to the late proteins, L1 and L2, of HPV-16 and -18. Vaccination of women before the initiation of sexual activity dramatically reduces the rate of HPV-16 and -18 infection and subsequent dysplasia. Stage I disease, which accounts for almost half of staging at presentation, is defined by carcinoma confined to the cervix and has a >80% 5-year survival (Figure III-44).

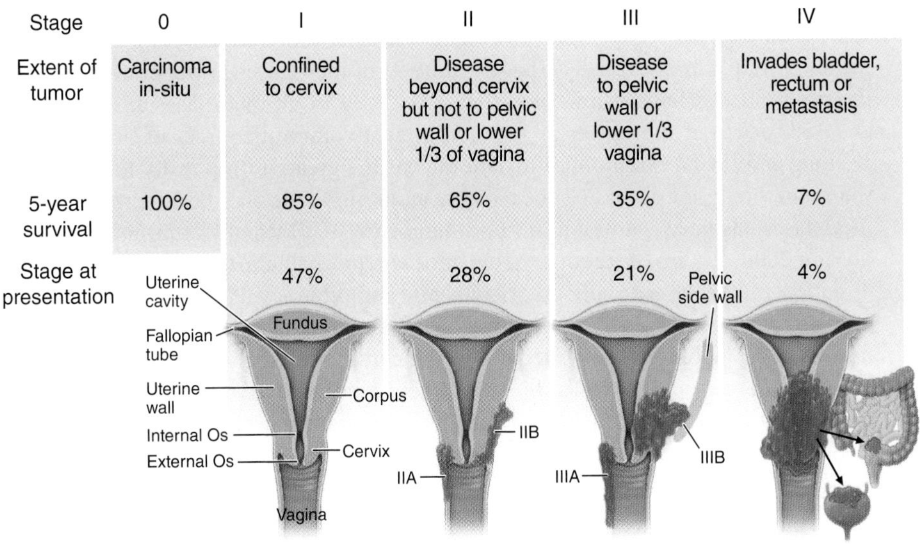

FIGURE III-44

III-45. **The answer is A.** *(Chap. 118)* Primary brain tumors are diagnosed in approximately 52,000 people each year in the United States. At least one-half of these tumors are malignant and associated with a high mortality. Glial tumors account for about 30% of all primary brain tumors, and 80% of those are malignant. Meningiomas account for 35%, vestibular schwannomas 10%, and central nervous system (CNS) lymphomas about 2%. Brain metastases are three times more common than all primary brain tumors combined and are diagnosed in approximately 150,000 people each year. Brain tumors of any type can present with a variety of symptoms and signs that fall into two categories: general and focal; patients often have a combination of the two (Table III-45).

TABLE III-45 Symptoms and Signs at Presentation of Brain Tumors

	High-Grade Glioma (%)	Low-Grade Glioma (%)	Meningioma (%)	Metastases (%)
Generalized				
Impaired cognitive function	50	10	30	60
Hemiparesis	40	10	36	60
Headache	50	40	37	50
Lateralizing				
Seizures	20	70+	17	18
Aphasia	20	<5	—	18
Visual field deficit	—	—	—	7

Seizures are a common presentation of brain tumors, occurring in about 25% of patients with brain metastases or malignant gliomas, but can be the presenting symptom in up to 90% of patients with a low-grade glioma. All seizures that arise from a brain tumor will have a focal onset whether or not it is apparent clinically. Cranial MRI is the preferred diagnostic test for any patient suspected of having a brain tumor and should be performed with gadolinium contrast administration. CT scan should be reserved for patients unable to undergo MRI (e.g., pacemaker). Malignant brain tumors—whether primary or metastatic—typically enhance with gadolinium and may have central areas of necrosis; they are characteristically surrounded by edema of the neighboring white matter. Low-grade gliomas usually do not enhance with gadolinium and are best appreciated on fluid-attenuated inversion recovery (FLAIR) MRIs. Meningiomas have a characteristic appearance on MRI because they are dural based with a dural tail and compress, but do not invade, the brain.

III-46. The answer is D. *(Chap. 118)* This patient presents with at least two presumed metastatic lesions in the right frontal and right cerebellar lobes. The multiple lesions make a primary brain tumor unlikely. The distribution of metastases in the brain approximates the proportion of blood flow such that about 85% of all metastases are supratentorial and 15% occur in the posterior fossa. The most common sources of brain metastases are lung and breast carcinomas; melanoma has the greatest propensity to metastasize to the brain, being found in 80% of patients at autopsy. The standard treatment for brain metastases has been whole-brain radiotherapy (WBRT) usually administered to a total dose of 3000 cGy in 10 fractions. This affords rapid palliation, and approximately 80% of patients improve with glucocorticoids and radiotherapy. However, it is not curative. Median survival is only 4–6 months. More recently, stereotactic radiosurgery (SRS) delivered through a variety of techniques, including the gamma knife, linear accelerator, proton beam, and CyberKnife, can deliver highly focused doses of radiation therapy, usually in a single fraction. SRS can effectively sterilize the visible lesions and afford local

TABLE III-46 Frequency of Nervous System Metastases by Common Primary Tumors

	Brain (%)	LM (%)	ESCC (%)
Lung	41	17	15
Breast	19	57	22
Melanoma	10	12	4
Prostate	1	1	10
GIT	7	—	5
Renal	3	2	7
Lymphoma	<1	10	10
Sarcoma	7	1	9
Other	11	—	18

Abbreviations: ESCC, epidural spinal cord compression; GIT, gastrointestinal tract; LM, leptomeningeal metastases.

disease control in 80%–90% of patients. In addition, there are some patients who have clearly been cured of their brain metastases using SRS, whereas this is distinctly rare with WBRT. However, SRS can be used only for lesions 3 cm or less in diameter and should be confined to patients with only one to three metastases. The addition of WBRT to SRS improves disease control in the nervous system but does not prolong survival. Randomized controlled trials have demonstrated that surgical extirpation of a single brain metastasis followed by WBRT is superior to WBRT alone. Removal of two lesions or a single symptomatic mass, particularly if compressing the ventricular system, can also be useful. Chemotherapy is rarely useful for brain metastases.

III-47. **The answer is C.** *(Chap. 120e)* Carcinoma of unknown primary (CUP) is a biopsy-proven malignancy for which the anatomic site of origin remains unidentified after an intensive search. CUP is one of the 10 most frequently diagnosed cancers worldwide, accounting for 3%–5% of all cancers. CUP is limited to epithelial cancers and does not include lymphomas, metastatic melanomas, and metastatic sarcomas because these cancers have specific histology- and stage-based treatments that guide management. The emergence of sophisticated imaging, robust immunohistochemistry (IHC), and genomic and proteomic tools has challenged the "unknown" designation. Additionally, effective targeted therapies in several cancers have moved the paradigm from empiricism to considering an individualized approach to CUP management. The reasons cancers present as CUP remain unclear. One hypothesis is that the primary tumor either regresses after seeding the metastasis or remains so small that it is not detected. It is possible that CUP falls on the continuum of cancer presentation where the primary has been contained or eliminated by the natural immune defenses. Alternatively, CUP may represent a specific malignant event that results in an increase in metastatic spread or survival relative to the primary tumor. Most tumor markers, including CEA, CA-125, CA 19-9, and CA 15-3, when elevated, are nonspecific and not helpful in determining the primary tumor site. Men who present with adenocarcinoma and osteoblastic metastasis should undergo a PSA test. In patients with undifferentiated or poorly differentiated carcinoma (especially with a midline tumor), elevated β-hCG and AFP levels suggest the possibility of an extragonadal germ cell (testicular) tumor. Monoclonal antibodies to specific cytokeratin (CK) subtypes have been used to help classify tumors according to their site of origin; commonly used CK stains in adenocarcinoma CUP are CK7 and CK20. CK7 is found in tumors of the lung, ovary, endometrium, breast, and upper gastrointestinal tract including pancreaticobiliary cancers, whereas CK20 is normally expressed in the gastrointestinal epithelium, urothelium, and Merkel cells. Gene expression profiling offers the promise of substantially increasing the yield of CUP.

The median survival duration of most patients with disseminated CUP is approximately 6–10 months. Systemic chemotherapy is the primary treatment modality in most patients with disseminated disease, but the careful integration of surgery, radiation therapy, and even periods of observation is important in the overall management of this condition (Figure III-47). Prognostic factors include performance status, site and number of metastases, response to chemotherapy, and serum LDH levels.

III-48. **The answer is B.** *(Chap. 121)* Humoral hypercalcemia of malignancy (HHM) occurs in up to 20% of patients with cancer. HHM is most common in cancers of the lung, head and neck, skin, esophagus, breast, and genitourinary tract and in multiple myeloma and lymphomas. There are several distinct humoral causes of HHM, but it is caused most commonly by overproduction of parathyroid hormone–related protein (PTHrP). In addition to acting as a circulating humoral factor, bone metastases (e.g., breast, multiple myeloma) may produce PTHrP, leading to local osteolysis and hypercalcemia. PTHrP is structurally related to parathyroid hormone (PTH) and binds to the PTH receptor, explaining the similar biochemical features of HHM and hyperparathyroidism. Metastatic lesions to bone are more likely to produce PTHrP than are metastases in other tissues. Another relatively common cause of HHM is excess production of 1,25-dihydroxyvitamin D. Like granulomatous disorders associated with hypercalcemia, lymphomas can produce an enzyme that converts 25-hydroxyvitamin D to the more active 1,25-dihydroxyvitamin D, leading to enhanced gastrointestinal calcium absorption. Other causes of HHM include tumor-mediated production of osteolytic cytokines and inflammatory mediators. In this

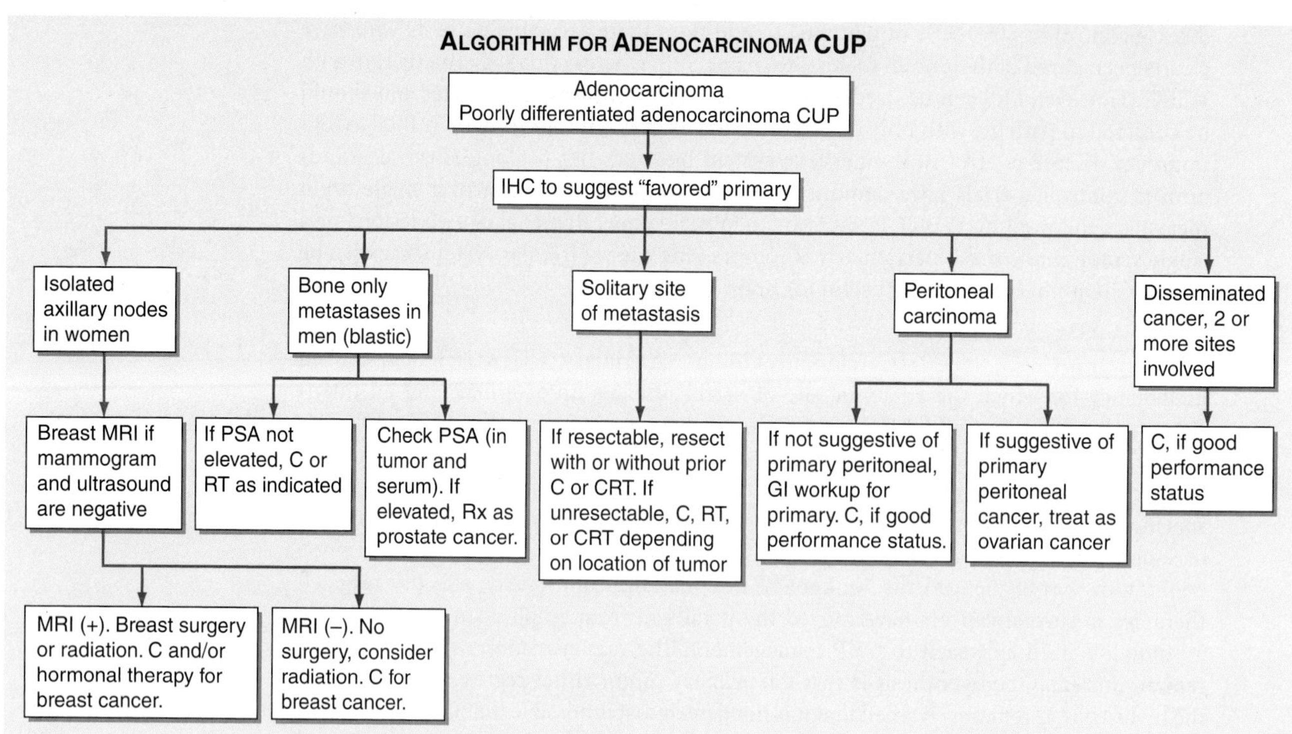

FIGURE III-47 C, chemotherapy; CRT, chemoradiation; CUP, cancer of unknown primary; GI, gastrointestinal; IHC, immunohistochemistry; MRI, magnetic resonance imaging; PSA, prostate-specific antigen; RT, radiation.

case, the multiple metastatic nodules and elevated PTHrP make lymphoma the least likely malignancy.

III-49. The answer is E. *(Chap. 121)* The management of severe HHM begins with saline rehydration (typically 200–500 mL/hr) to dilute serum calcium and promote calciuresis. Forced diuresis with furosemide or other loop diuretics can enhance calcium excretion but provides relatively little value except in life-threatening hypercalcemia. When used, loop diuretics should be administered only after complete rehydration and with careful monitoring of fluid balance. Oral phosphorus should be given until serum phosphorus is >1 mmol/L (>3 mg/dL). Bisphosphonates such as pamidronate, zoledronate, and etidronate can reduce serum calcium within 1–2 days and suppress calcium release for several weeks. Bisphosphonate infusions can be repeated, or oral bisphosphonates can be used for chronic treatment. Dialysis should be considered in severe hypercalcemia when saline hydration and bisphosphonate treatments are not possible or are too slow in onset. Previously used agents such as calcitonin and mithramycin have little utility now that bisphosphonates are available. Calcitonin should be considered when rapid correction of severe hypercalcemia is needed. Hypercalcemia associated with lymphomas, multiple myeloma, or leukemia may respond to glucocorticoid treatment. This patient most likely does not have lymphoma, so initial treatment should not include corticosteroids.

III-50. The answers are: 1-C; 2-B; 3-A. *(Chap. 125)* Dose-dependent myocardial toxicity of anthracyclines with characteristic myofibrillar dropout is pathologically pathognomonic on endomyocardial biopsy. Anthracycline cardiotoxicity occurs through a root mechanism of chemical free radical damage. $Fe3^{+}$-doxorubicin complexes damage DNA, nuclear and cytoplasmic membranes, and mitochondria. About 5% of patients receiving >450–550 mg/m^2 of doxorubicin will develop congestive heart failure (CHF). Cardiotoxicity in relation to the dose of anthracycline is clearly not a step function, but rather a continuous function, and occasional patients are seen with CHF at substantially lower doses. Advanced age, other concomitant cardiac disease, hypertension, diabetes, and thoracic radiation therapy are all important cofactors in promoting anthracycline-associated CHF. The risk of cardiac failure appears to be substantially lower when doxorubicin is administered by continuous infusion. Anthracycline-related CHF is difficult to reverse and has a mortality rate as high as

50%, making prevention crucial. Monitoring patients for cardiac toxicity typically involves periodic gated nuclear cardiac blood pool ejection fraction testing (multigated acquisition scan [MUGA]) or cardiac ultrasonography. More recently, cardiac MRI has been used, but MRI is not standard or widespread. After anthracyclines, trastuzumab is the next most frequent cardiotoxic drug currently in use. Trastuzumab is frequently used as adjuvant breast cancer therapy, sometimes in conjunction with anthracyclines, which is believed to result in additive or possibly synergistic toxicity. In contrast to anthracyclines, cardiotoxicity is not dose related, is usually reversible, is not associated with pathologic changes of anthracyclines on cardiac myofibrils, and has a different biochemical mechanism inhibiting intrinsic cardiac repair mechanisms. Toxicity is typically routinely monitored every three to four doses using functional cardiac testing as mentioned earlier for anthracyclines. Cisplatin is associated with sensorimotor neuropathy and hearing loss, especially at doses >400 mg/m^2, requiring audiometry in patients with preexisting hearing compromise. Carboplatin is often substituted in such cases given its lesser effect on hearing.

III-51. The answer is E. *(Chap. 126)* Iron absorbed from the diet or released from stores circulates in the plasma bound to transferrin, the iron transport protein. Transferrin that carries iron exists in two forms—monoferric (one iron atom) or diferric (two iron atoms). The turnover (half-clearance time) of transferrin-bound iron is very rapid—typically 60–90 minutes. Because almost all of the iron transported by transferrin is delivered to the erythroid marrow, the clearance time of transferrin-bound iron from the circulation is affected most by the plasma iron level and the erythroid marrow activity. Ferritin is an iron storage protein, and levels represent an indirect measure of total-body iron stores. Free iron, which is toxic to cells, may also be stored intracellularly bound to hemosiderin. Haptoglobin binds free hemoglobin in the plasma, and low levels are consistent intravascular hemolysis. Albumin, which binds many serum proteins, does not bind significant amounts of free iron in plasma.

III-52. The answer is C. *(Chap. 126)* The peripheral blood smear is consistent with a hypochromic microcytic anemia. There are only three conditions that need to be considered in the differential diagnosis of hypochromic microcytic anemia: thalassemia, inflammation, and sideroblastic anemia related to a myelodysplastic syndrome. Thalassemia is an inherited defect of globin chain synthesis and will have normal or increased serum iron levels. The anemia of inflammation (AI; also referred to as the anemia of chronic disease) is characterized by inadequate iron supply to the erythroid marrow. The distinction between true iron deficiency anemia and AI is a common diagnostic problem. Usually, AI is normocytic and normochromic. The iron values usually make the differential diagnosis clear, as the ferritin level is normal or increased and the percent transferrin saturation and total iron-binding capacity are typically below normal. Sideroblastic anemia is the least common microcytic hypochromic anemia condition. Occasionally, patients with myelodysplasia have impaired hemoglobin synthesis with mitochondrial dysfunction, resulting in impaired iron incorporation into heme. The iron values again reveal normal stores and more than an adequate supply to the marrow, despite the microcytosis and hypochromia. Vitamin B_{12} deficiency and folate deficiency cause macrocytic anemia. This patient has low iron and low ferritin, consistent with iron deficiency.

TABLE III-52 Diagnosis of Microcytic Anemia

Tests	Iron Deficiency	Inflammation	Thalassemia	Sideroblastic Anemia
Smear	Micro/hypo	Normal micro/hypo	Micro/hypo with targeting	Variable
Serum iron (μg/dL)	<30	<50	Normal to high	Normal to high
TIBC (μg/dL)	>360	<300	Normal	Normal
Percent saturation	<10	10–20	30–80	30–80
Ferritin (μg/L)	<15	30–200	50–300	50–300
Hemoglobin pattern on electrophoresis	Normal	Normal	Abnormal with β-thalassemia; can be normal with α-thalassemia	Normal

Abbreviation: TIBC, total iron-binding capacity.

III-53. The answer is B. *(Chap. 127)* Hemoglobinopathies are especially common in areas in which malaria is endemic. This clustering of hemoglobinopathies is assumed to reflect a selective survival advantage for the abnormal red blood cell (RBC), which presumably provides a less hospitable environment during the obligate RBC stages of the parasitic life cycle. Very young children with α-thalassemia are *more* susceptible to infection with the nonlethal *Plasmodium vivax*. Thalassemia might then favor a natural protection against infection with the more lethal *Plasmodium falciparum*.

Thalassemias are the most common genetic disorders in the world, affecting nearly 200 million people worldwide. About 15% of African Americans are silent carriers for α-thalassemia; α-thalassemia trait (minor) occurs in 3% of African American and in 1%–15% of persons of Mediterranean origin. β-Thalassemia has a 10%–15% incidence in individuals from the Mediterranean and Southeast Asia and 0.8% in African Americans. The number of severe cases of thalassemia in the United States is about 1000. Sickle cell disease is the most common structural hemoglobinopathy, occurring in heterozygous form in approximately 8% of African Americans and in homozygous form in 1 in 400. Between 2% and 3% of African Americans carry a hemoglobin C allele.

III-54. The answer is C. *(Chap. 127)* Acute chest syndrome is a distinctive manifestation characterized by chest pain, tachypnea, fever, cough, and arterial oxygen desaturation. It can mimic pneumonia, pulmonary emboli, bone marrow infarction and embolism, myocardial ischemia, or in situ lung infarction. Acute chest syndrome is thought to reflect in situ sickling within the lung, producing pain and temporary pulmonary dysfunction. Often it is difficult or impossible to distinguish among other possibilities. Pulmonary infarction and pneumonia are the most frequent underlying or concomitant conditions in patients with this syndrome. Repeated episodes of acute chest pain correlate with reduced survival. Chronic acute or subacute pulmonary crises lead to pulmonary hypertension and cor pulmonale, an increasingly common cause of death as patients survive longer. Considerable controversy exists about the possible role played by free plasma hemoglobin S in scavenging nitrogen dioxide (NO_2), thus raising pulmonary vascular tone. Trials of sildenafil to restore NO_2 levels were terminated because of adverse effects. Acute chest syndrome is a medical emergency that may require management in an intensive care unit. Hydration should be monitored carefully to avoid the development of pulmonary edema, and oxygen therapy should be administered to avoid hypoxemia. Critical interventions are transfusion to maintain a hematocrit >30% and emergency exchange transfusion if arterial saturation drops to <90%. The most significant advance in the therapy of sickle cell anemia has been the introduction of hydroxyurea as a mainstay of therapy for patients with severe symptoms. Hydroxyurea (10–30 mg/kg/d) increases fetal hemoglobin and may also exert beneficial effects on RBC hydration, vascular wall adherence, and suppression of the granulocyte and reticulocyte counts; dosage is titrated to maintain a white cell count between 5000 and 8000/μL. White cells and reticulocytes may play a major role in the pathogenesis of sickle cell crisis, and their suppression may be an important side benefit of hydroxyurea therapy.

Hydroxyurea should be considered in patients experiencing repeated episodes of acute chest syndrome or with more than three crises per year requiring hospitalization. Hydroxyurea offers broad benefits to most patients whose disease is severe enough to impair their functional status, and it may improve survival. Fetal hemoglobin levels increase in most patients within a few months.

III-55 and III-56. The answers are E and E, respectively. *(Chap. 128)* The peripheral blood smear shows macrocytosis, anisocytosis, and poikilocytosis with a hypersegmented (greater than five lobes) polymorphonuclear cell. These findings are diagnostic of megaloblastic anemia. In cases of severe anemia, there may also be reduction in white blood cell (WBC) and platelet count. The most common causes of megaloblastic anemia are folate and cobalamin deficiency (Tables III-55 and III-56). This patient most likely has pernicious anemia given her normal diet and absence of other symptoms. The next best test will be a serum vitamin B_{12} level. In patients with cobalamin deficiency sufficient to cause anemia or neuropathy, the serum methylmalonic acid (MMA) level is raised. Sensitive methods for measuring MMA and homocysteine in serum have been introduced and recommended for the early diagnosis of cobalamin deficiency, even in the absence of hematologic abnormalities or subnormal levels of serum cobalamin. Serum MMA levels fluctuate, however, in patients with renal failure. Serum homocysteine is raised in both early cobalamin and folate deficiency but may be raised in other conditions (e.g., chronic renal disease, alcoholism, smoking, pyridoxine deficiency, hypothyroidism, and therapy with steroids, cyclosporine, and other drugs).

TABLE III-55 Causes of Cobalamin Deficiency Sufficiently Severe to Cause Megaloblastic Anemia

Nutritional	Vegans
Malabsorption	Pernicious anemia
Gastric causes	Congenital absence of intrinsic factor or functional abnormality
	Total or partial gastrectomy
Intestinal causes	Intestinal stagnant loop syndrome: jejunal diverticulosis, ileocolic fistula, anatomic blind loop, intestinal stricture, etc.
	Ileal resection and Crohn disease
	Selective malabsorption with proteinuria
	Tropical sprue
	Transcobalamin II deficiency
	Fish tapeworm

TABLE III-56 Causes of Folate Deficiency

Dietary[a]

Particularly in: old age, infancy, poverty, alcoholism, chronic invalids, and the psychiatrically disturbed; may be associated with scurvy or kwashiorkor

Malabsorption

Major causes of deficiency

Tropical sprue, gluten-induced enteropathy in children and adults, and in association with dermatitis herpetiformis, specific malabsorption of folate, intestinal megaloblastosis caused by severe cobalamin or folate deficiency

Minor causes of deficiency

Extensive jejunal resection, Crohn disease, partial gastrectomy, congestive heart failure, Whipple disease, scleroderma, amyloid, diabetic enteropathy, systemic bacterial infection, lymphoma, sulfasalazine (Salazopyrin)

Excess utilization or loss

Physiologic

Pregnancy and lactation, prematurity

Pathologic

Hematologic diseases: chronic hemolytic anemias, sickle cell anemia, thalassemia major, myelofibrosis

Malignant diseases: carcinoma, lymphoma, leukemia, myeloma

Inflammatory diseases: tuberculosis, Crohn disease, psoriasis, exfoliative dermatitis, malaria

Metabolic disease: homocystinuria

Excess urinary loss: congestive heart failure, active liver disease

Hemodialysis, peritoneal dialysis

Antifolate drugs[b]

Anticonvulsant drugs (phenytoin, primidone, barbiturates), sulfasalazine

Nitrofurantoin, tetracycline, antituberculosis (less well documented)

Mixed causes

Liver diseases, alcoholism, intensive care units

[a]In severely folate-deficient patients with causes other than those listed under Dietary, poor dietary intake is often present.

[b]Drugs inhibiting dihydrofolate reductase are discussed in the text of Chapter 128 in *Harrison's Principles of Internal Medicine*, 19th edition.

III-57. The answer is B. *(Chap. 129)* What differentiates hemolytic anemias (HAs) from other anemias is that the patient has signs and symptoms arising directly from hemolysis. At the clinical level, the main sign is jaundice; in addition, the patient may report discoloration of the urine. In many cases of HA, the spleen is enlarged, because it is a preferential site of hemolysis; and in some cases, the liver may be enlarged as well. The laboratory features of HA are related to hemolysis per se and the erythropoietic response of the bone marrow. Hemolysis regularly produces an increase in unconjugated bilirubin and aspartate aminotransferase (AST) in the serum; urobilinogen will be increased in both urine and stool. If hemolysis is mainly intravascular, the telltale sign is hemoglobinuria (often associated with hemosiderinuria); in the serum, there is hemoglobin, LDH is increased, and haptoglobin is reduced. In contrast, the bilirubin level may be normal or only mildly elevated. The main sign of the erythropoietic response by the bone marrow is an increase in reticulocytes (a test all too often neglected in the initial workup of a patient with anemia). Usually the increase will be reflected in both the percentage of reticulocytes (the more commonly quoted figure) and the absolute reticulocyte count (the more definitive parameter). The increased number of reticulocytes is associated with an increased mean corpuscular volume (MCV) in the blood count. On the blood smear, this is reflected in the presence of macrocytes; there is also polychromasia, and sometimes, one sees nucleated red cells.

III-58. The answer is A. *(Chap. 129)* The peripheral blood smear shows bite cells (arrow in Figure III-58), anisocytosis, and spherocytes. The combination of the smear, jaundice, and hyperbilirubinemia 1 day after receiving sulfamethoxazole makes glucose 6-phosphate dehydrogenase (G6PD) deficiency most likely. G6PD deficiency is widely distributed in tropical and subtropical parts of the world (Africa, southern Europe, the Middle East, Southeast Asia, and Oceania) and wherever people from those areas have migrated. A conservative estimate is that at least 400 million people have a *G6PD* deficiency gene. In several of these areas, the frequency of a *G6PD* deficiency gene may be as high as 20% or more. The *G6PD* gene is X-linked; thus, males have only one *G6PD* gene (i.e., they are hemizygous for this gene); therefore, they must be either normal or G6PD deficient. Hemolytic anemia in patients with G6PD deficiency can develop as a result of fava beans, infections, and drugs. Common drugs include primaquine, dapsone, sulfamethoxazole, and nitrofurantoin. Typically, a hemolytic attack starts with malaise, weakness, and abdominal or lumbar pain. After an interval of several hours to 2–3 days, the patient develops jaundice and often dark urine. The onset can be extremely abrupt, especially with favism in children. There may be hemoglobinemia, hemoglobinuria, high LDH, and low or absent plasma haptoglobin. G6PD deficiency may be diagnosed by semiquantitative or quantitative RBC tests or by DNA testing. Hemolytic-uremic syndrome and thrombotic thrombocytopenic purpura cause microangiopathic hemolytic anemia with prominent schistocytes. Iron deficiency causes a microcytic and hypochromic anemia.

III-59. The answer is B. *(Chap. 129)* This patient has autoimmune hemolytic anemia (AIHA) with development of warm immunoglobulin G (IgG) antibodies due to ceftriaxone exposure (Table III-59).

AIHA is a serious condition; without appropriate treatment, it may have a mortality of approximately 10%. The onset is often abrupt and can be dramatic. The hemoglobin level can drop within days to as low as 4 g/dL; the massive red cell removal will produce jaundice; and sometimes the spleen is enlarged. When this triad is present, the suspicion of AIHA must be high. The diagnostic test for AIHA is the direct antiglobulin (Coombs) test, which detects the presence of antibody on the red cells. When the test is positive, it clinches the diagnosis; when it is negative, the diagnosis is unlikely. The immediate treatment almost invariably includes transfusion of red cells. This may pose a special problem because, if the antibody involved is nonspecific, all of the blood units cross-matched will be incompatible. Whenever the anemia is not immediately life threatening, blood transfusion should be withheld (because compatibility problems may increase with each unit of blood transfused), and medical treatment started immediately with prednisone (1 mg/kg/d), which will produce a remission promptly in at least one-half of patients. Rituximab (anti-CD20) was regarded as second-line treatment, but it is increasingly likely that a relatively low dose (100 mg/wk × 4) of rituximab together with prednisone will become a first-line standard. It is especially encouraging that this approach seems to reduce the rate of relapse, a common occurrence in AIHA. G6PD deficiency is unlikely in this previously healthy female only exposed to ceftriaxone. ADAMTS-13 activity assay is used to diagnose thrombotic thrombocytopenic purpura. Flow cytometry may be used to diagnose paroxysmal nocturnal hemoglobinuria. Hemoglobin electrophoresis is used to diagnose congenital hemoglobinopathies.

TABLE III-59 Classification of Acquired Immune Hemolytic Anemias

	Type of Antibody	
Clinical Setting	Cold, Mostly IgM, Optimal Temperature 4–30°C	Warm, Mostly IgG, Optimal Temperature 37°C; or Mixed
Primary	CAD	AIHA (idiopathic)
Secondary to viral infection	EBV CMV Other	HIV Viral vaccines
Secondary to other infection	*Mycoplasma* infection: paroxysmal cold hemoglobinuria	
Secondary to/associated with other disease	CAD in: Waldenström disease Lymphoma	AIHA in: SLE CLL Other malignancy Chronic inflammatory disorders (e.g., IBD) After allogeneic HSCT
Secondary to drugs: drug-induced immune hemolytic anemia	Small minority (e.g., with lenalidomide)	Majority: currently most common culprit drugs are cefotetan, ceftriaxone, piperacillin
	Drug-dependent: antibody destroys red cells only when drug present (e.g., rarely penicillin)	
	Drug-independent: antibody can destroy red cells even when drug no longer present (e.g., methyldopa)	

Abbreviations: AIHA, autoimmune hemolytic anemia; CAD, cold agglutinin disease; CLL, chronic lymphocytic leukemia; CMV, cytomegalovirus; EBV, Epstein-Barr virus; HIV, human immunodeficiency virus; HSCT, hematopoietic stem cell transplantation; IBD, inflammatory bowel disease; SLE, systemic lupus erythematosus.

III-60. The answer is D. *(Chap. 130)* This patient likely has idiopathic myelodysplastic syndrome. The myelodysplastic syndromes (MDS) are a heterogeneous group of hematologic disorders broadly characterized by both (1) cytopenias due to bone marrow failure and (2) a high risk of development of acute myeloid leukemia (AML; Table III-60). Anemia, often with thrombocytopenia and neutropenia, occurs with dysmorphic (abnormal-appearing) and usually cellular bone marrow, which is evidence of ineffective blood cell production. In patients with "low-risk" MDS, marrow failure dominates the clinical course. In other patients, myeloblasts are present at diagnosis, chromosomes are abnormal, and the "high risk" is due to leukemic progression. MDS may be fatal due to the complications of pancytopenia or the incurability of leukemia, but a large proportion of patients will die of concurrent disease, the comorbidities typical in an elderly population. Idiopathic MDS is a disease of the elderly; the mean age at onset is older than 70 years. There is a slight male predominance. MDS is a relatively common form of bone marrow failure, with reported incidence rates of 35 to >100 per million persons in the general population and 120 to >500 per million persons in older adults. MDS is rare in children but is increased in children with Down syndrome. MDS is associated with environmental exposures such as radiation and benzene. Secondary MDS occurs as a late toxicity of cancer treatment, usually a combination of radiation and the radiomimetic alkylating agents such as busulfan, nitrosourea, or procarbazine (with a latent period of 5–7 years) or the DNA topoisomerase inhibitors (2-year latency). Anemia dominates the early course of MDS. Most symptomatic patients complain of the gradual onset of fatigue and weakness, dyspnea, and pallor, but at least one-half of patients are asymptomatic, and their MDS is discovered only incidentally on routine blood counts. The physical examination is typical for signs of anemia, with approximately 20% of patients having splenomegaly.

Some unusual skin lesions, including Sweet syndrome (febrile neutrophilic dermatosis), occur with MDS. Median survival times of patients with MDS vary widely, but prognosis worsens with increasing percent blasts in bone marrow, cytogenetic abnormalities, and lineages affected by cytopenia. Only hematopoietic stem cell transplantation offers cure of MDS. The current survival rate in selected patient cohorts is approximately 50% at 3 years and is improving. New epigenetic modulator drugs are believed to act through a demethylating mechanism to alter gene regulation and allow differentiation to mature blood cells from the abnormal MDS stem cell. Azacitidine and decitabine are two epigenetic modifiers frequently used in bone marrow failure clinics. Azacitidine improves blood counts and survival in MDS, compared to best supportive care.

TABLE III-60 World Health Organization (WHO) Classification of Myelodysplastic Syndromes (MDS)/Neoplasms

Name	WHO Estimated Proportion of Patients with MDS	Peripheral Blood: Key Features	Bone Marrow: Key Features
Refractory cytopenias with unilineage dysplasia (RCUD):			
Refractory anemia (RA)	10%–20%	Anemia <1% of blasts	Unilineage erythroid dysplasia (in ≥10% of cells) <5% blasts
Refractory neutropenia (RN)	<1%	Neutropenia <1% blasts	Unilineage granulocytic dysplasia <5% blasts
Refractory thrombocytopenia (RT)	<1%	Thrombocytopenia <1% blasts	Unilineage megakaryocytic dysplasia <5% blasts
Refractory anemia with ringed sideroblasts (RARS)	3%–11%	Anemia No blasts	Unilineage erythroid dysplasia ≥15% of erythroid precursors are ringed sideroblasts <5% blasts
Refractory cytopenias with multilineage dysplasia (RCMD)	30%	Cytopenia(s) <1% blasts No Auer rods	Multilineage dysplasia ± ringed sideroblasts <5% blasts No Auer rods
Refractory anemia with excess blasts, type 1 (RAEB-1)	40%	Cytopenia(s) <5% blasts No Auer rods	Unilineage or multilineage dysplasia
Refractory anemia with excess blasts, type 2 (RAEB-2)		Cytopenia(s) 5%–19% blasts ± Auer rods	Unilineage or multilineage dysplasia 10%–19% blasts ± Auer rods
MDS associated with isolated del(5q) [del(5q)]	Uncommon	Anemia Normal or high platelet count <1% blasts	Isolated 5q31 chromosome deletion Anemia; hypolobated megakaryocytes <5% blasts
Childhood MDS, including refractory cytopenia of childhood (*provisional*) (RCC)	<1%	Pancytopenia	<5% marrow blasts for RCC Marrow usually hypocellular
MDS, unclassifiable (MDS-U)	?	Cytopenia ≤1% blasts	Does not fit other categories Dysplasia <5% blasts If no dysplasia, MDS-associated karyotype

Note: If peripheral blood blasts are 2%–4%, the diagnosis is RAEB-1 even if marrow blasts are <5%. If Auer rods are present, the WHO considers the diagnosis RAEB-2 if the blast proportion is <20% (even if <10%), or acute myeloid leukemia (AML) if at least 20% blasts. For all subtypes, peripheral blood monocytes are $<1 \times 10^9$/L. Bicytopenia may be observed in RCUD subtypes, but pancytopenia with unilineage marrow dysplasia should be classified as MDS-U. Therapy-related MDS (t-MDS), whether due to alkylating agents or topoisomerase II inhibitors (t-MDS/t-AML), is now included in the WHO classification of myeloid neoplasms. The listing in this table excludes MDS/myeloproliferative neoplasm overlap categories, such as chronic myelomonocytic leukemia, juvenile myelomonocytic leukemia, and the provisional entity RARS with thrombocytosis.

III-61. The answer is E. *(Chap. 131)* The World Health Organization (WHO) classification of the chronic myeloproliferative neoplasms (MPNs) includes eight disorders, some of which are rare or poorly characterized but all of which share an origin in a multipotent hematopoietic progenitor cell; overproduction of one or more of the formed elements of the blood without significant dysplasia; and a predilection to extramedullary hematopoiesis, myelofibrosis, and transformation at varying rates to acute leukemia (Table III-61).

Within this broad classification, however, significant phenotypic heterogeneity exists. Some diseases such as chronic myelogenous leukemia (CML), chronic neutrophilic leukemia (CNL), and chronic eosinophilic leukemia (CEL) express primarily a myeloid phenotype, whereas in other diseases, such as polycythemia vera (PV), primary myelofibrosis (PMF), and essential thrombocytosis (ET), erythroid or megakaryocytic hyperplasia predominates. The latter three disorders, in contrast to the former three, also appear capable of transforming into each other. Such phenotypic heterogeneity has a genetic basis; CML is the consequence of the balanced translocation between chromosomes 9 and 22 [t(9;22)(q34;11)]; CNL has been associated with a t(15;19) translocation; and CEL occurs with a deletion or balanced translocations involving the *PDGFRα* gene. By contrast, to a greater or lesser extent, PV, PMF, and ET are characterized by a mutation, V617F, that causes constitutive activation of JAK2, a tyrosine kinase essential for the function of the erythropoietin and thrombopoietin receptors but not the granulocyte colony-stimulating factor receptor. This important distinction is also reflected in the natural histories of CML, CNL, and CEL, which are usually measured in years, and their high rate of leukemic transformation. By contrast, the natural history of PV, PMF, and ET is usually measured in decades, and transformation to acute leukemia is uncommon in PV and ET in the absence of exposure to mutagenic drugs.

TABLE III-61 World Health Organization Classification of Chronic Myeloproliferative Neoplasms

Chronic myeloid leukemia, Bcr-Abl positive
Chronic neutrophilic leukemia
Chronic eosinophilic leukemia, not otherwise specified
Polycythemia vera
Primary myelofibrosis
Essential thrombocytosis
Mastocytosis
Myeloproliferative neoplasms, unclassifiable

III-62. The answer is C. *(Chaps. 77 and 131)* This patient has polycythemia, likely due to PV, with the elevation of hemoglobin, WBC count, and platelets. The next step in his evaluation is measurement of RBC mass. After finding an elevated RBC mass, measurement of erythropoietin levels will distinguish between PV and other causes of polycythemia such as renal cell carcinoma, lung disease, hypoxemic states, or chronic carbon monoxide poisoning (Figure III-62).

PV is a clonal disorder involving a multipotent hematopoietic progenitor cell in which phenotypically normal red cells, granulocytes, and platelets accumulate in the absence of a recognizable physiologic stimulus. The etiology of PV is unknown. A mutation in the autoinhibitory pseudokinase domain of the tyrosine kinase JAK2, that replaces valine with phenylalanine (V617F) causing constitutive kinase activation, appears to have a central role in the pathogenesis of PV.

III-63. The answer is D. *(Chap. 131)* The patient described in Question III-62 had a red cell mass that was markedly elevated, with a low erythropoietin level confirming the diagnosis of PV. PV is generally an indolent disorder, the clinical course of which is measured in decades, and its management should reflect its tempo. Thrombosis due to erythrocytosis is the most significant complication and often the presenting manifestation, and maintenance of the hemoglobin level at ≤140 g/L (14 g/dL; hematocrit <45%) in men and ≤120 g/L (12 g/dL; hematocrit <42%) in women is mandatory to avoid thrombotic complications. Phlebotomy serves initially to reduce hyperviscosity by bringing the red

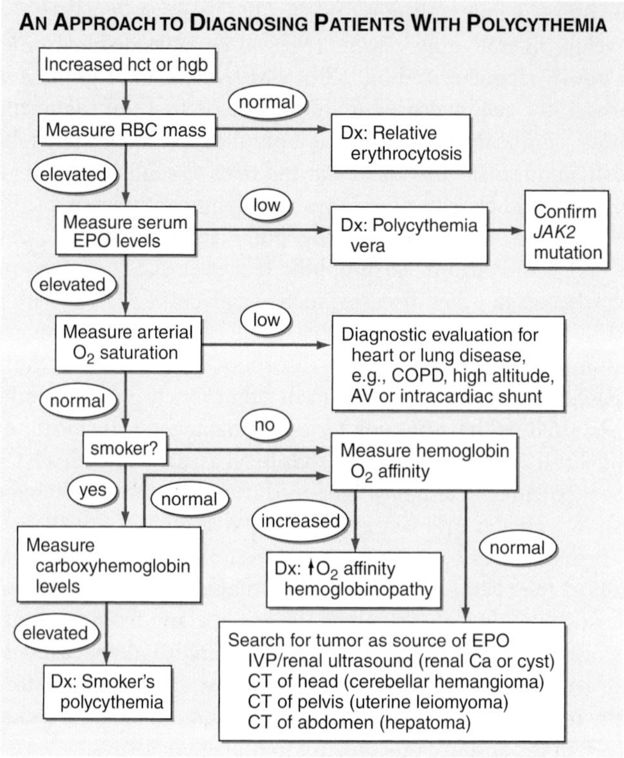

AN APPROACH TO DIAGNOSING PATIENTS WITH POLYCYTHEMIA

Increased hct or hgb
Measure RBC mass
normal → Dx: Relative erythrocytosis
elevated
Measure serum EPO levels
low → Dx: Polycythemia vera → Confirm *JAK2* mutation
elevated
Measure arterial O_2 saturation
low → Diagnostic evaluation for heart or lung disease, e.g., COPD, high altitude, AV or intracardiac shunt
normal
smoker?
no → Measure hemoglobin O_2 affinity
yes
Measure carboxyhemoglobin levels
normal → Measure hemoglobin O_2 affinity
elevated → Dx: Smoker's polycythemia
increased → Dx: ↑O_2 affinity hemoglobinopathy
normal → Search for tumor as source of EPO
IVP/renal ultrasound (renal Ca or cyst)
CT of head (cerebellar hemangioma)
CT of pelvis (uterine leiomyoma)
CT of abdomen (hepatoma)

FIGURE III-62 AV, atrioventricular; COPD, chronic obstructive pulmonary disease; CT, computed tomography; EPO, erythropoietin; hct, hematocrit; hgb, hemoglobin; IVP, intravenous pyelogram; RBC, red blood cell.

cell mass into the normal range while further expanding the plasma volume. Periodic phlebotomies thereafter serve to maintain the red cell mass within the normal range and to induce a state of iron deficiency that prevents an accelerated reexpansion of the red cell mass. Neither phlebotomy nor iron deficiency increases the platelet count relative to the effect of the disease itself, and thrombocytosis is not correlated with thrombosis in PV, in contrast to the strong correlation between erythrocytosis and thrombosis in this disease. The use of salicylates as a tonic against thrombosis in PV patients is not only potentially harmful if the red cell mass is not controlled by phlebotomy, but is also an unproven remedy. Anticoagulants are only indicated when a thrombosis has occurred and can be difficult to monitor if the red cell mass is substantially elevated owing to the artifactual imbalance between the test tube anticoagulant and plasma that occurs when blood from these patients is assayed for prothrombin or partial thromboplastin activity. Imatinib is a Bcr-Abl tyrosine kinase inhibitor typically used in cases of CML and is not efficacious in PV.

III-64. **The answer is D.** *(Chap. 132)* Anticancer drugs are the leading cause of therapy-associated acute myelogenous leukemia (AML). Alkylating agent–associated leukemias, such as cyclophosphamide, occur on average 4–6 years after exposure, and affected individuals have aberrations in chromosomes 5 and 7. Topoisomerase II inhibitor–associated leukemias, such as doxorubicin, occur 1–3 years after exposure, and affected individuals often have aberrations involving chromosome 11q23. High-dose radiation, like that experienced by survivors of the atomic bombs in Japan or nuclear reactor accidents, increases the risk of myeloid leukemias that peaks 5–7 years after exposure. Therapeutic radiation alone seems to add little risk of AML but can increase the risk in people also exposed to alkylating agents. Exposure to benzene, a solvent used in the chemical, plastic, rubber, and pharmaceutical industries, is associated with an increased incidence of AML. Smoking and exposure to petroleum products, paint, embalming fluids, ethylene oxide, herbicides, and pesticides have also been associated with an increased risk of AML. In contrast to B-cell lymphomas, there is no direct evidence linking viral infection to AML.

III-65. The answer is E. *(Chap. 132)* Acute promyelocytic leukemia (APL) is a highly curable subtype of acute myelogenous leukemia, and approximately 85% of these patients achieve long-term survival with current approaches. APL has long been shown to be responsive to cytarabine and daunorubicin, but previously, patients treated with these drugs alone frequently died from disseminated intravascular coagulation (DIC) induced by the release of granule components by the chemotherapy-treated leukemia cells. However, the prognosis of APL patients has changed dramatically from adverse to favorable with the introduction of tretinoin, an oral drug that induces the differentiation of leukemic cells bearing the characteristic translocation [t(15;17)], where disruption of the *RARA* gene encoding a retinoid acid receptor occurs. Tretinoin decreases the frequency of DIC but produces another complication called the APL differentiation syndrome. Occurring within the first 3 weeks of treatment, it is characterized by fever, fluid retention, dyspnea, chest pain, pulmonary infiltrates, pleural and pericardial effusions, and hypoxemia. The syndrome is related to adhesion of differentiated neoplastic cells to the pulmonary vasculature endothelium. Glucocorticoids, chemotherapy, and/or supportive measures can be effective for management of the APL differentiation syndrome. Temporary discontinuation of tretinoin is necessary in cases of severe APL differentiation syndrome (i.e., patients developing renal failure or requiring admission to the intensive care unit due to respiratory distress). The mortality rate of this syndrome is about 10%. Acyclovir is used to treat herpes virus infection. Daunorubicin is an anthracycline chemotherapy agent commonly used in the therapy of AML and ALL; it is not specific to APL. Rituximab is a monoclonal antibody against CD20 used in a wide assortment of autoimmune and malignant diseases. Sildenafil is a PDE5 inhibitor used for treatment of erectile dysfunction and pulmonary arterial hypertension.

III-66. The answer is B. *(Chap. 133)* Chronic myeloid leukemia (CML) is a clonal hematopoietic stem cell disorder. The disease is driven by the *BCR-ABL1* chimeric gene product, a constitutively active tyrosine kinase, resulting from a reciprocal balanced translocation between the long arms of chromosomes 9 and 22, t(9;22) (q34;q11.2), cytogenetically detected as the Philadelphia chromosome. Untreated, the course of CML may be biphasic or triphasic, with an early indolent or chronic phase, followed often by an accelerated phase and a terminal blastic phase. Before the era of selective BCR-ABL1 tyrosine kinase inhibitors (TKIs), the median survival in CML was 3–7 years, and the 10-year survival rate was 30% or less. Introduced into CML therapy in 2000, TKIs, such as imatinib, nilotinib, and dasatinib, have revolutionized the treatment, natural history, and prognosis of CML. Today, the estimated 10-year survival rate with imatinib mesylate, the first BCR-ABL1 TKI approved, is 85%. Allogeneic stem cell transplantation, a curative but risky treatment approach, is now offered as second- or third-line therapy after failure of TKIs. The median age at diagnosis is 55–65 years. CML is uncommon in children; only 3% of patients with CML are younger than 20 years. Mutations of the *HFE* gene are associated with primary hemochromatosis.

III-67. The answer is E. *(Chap. 134)* Non-Hodgkin lymphoma is the most common lymphoid malignancy (Figure III-67).

Chronic lymphoid leukemia (CLL) is the most prevalent form of leukemia in Western countries. It occurs most frequently in older adults and is exceedingly rare in children. In contrast to CLL, acute lymphoid leukemias (ALLs) are predominantly cancers of children and young adults. The Burkitt leukemia occurring in children in developing countries seems to be associated with infection by the Epstein-Barr virus (EBV) in infancy. The etiology of ALL in adults is also uncertain. ALL is unusual in middle-aged adults but increases in incidence in the elderly. However, acute myelogenous leukemia (AML) is still much more common in older patients. The preponderance of evidence suggests that Hodgkin lymphoma is of B-cell origin. The incidence of Hodgkin lymphoma appears fairly stable, with 9190 new cases diagnosed in 2014 in the United States. Hodgkin lymphoma is more common in whites than in blacks and more common in males than in females. A bimodal distribution of age at diagnosis has been observed, with one peak incidence occurring in patients in their 20s and the other in those in their 80s. Patients in the younger age groups diagnosed in the United States largely have the nodular sclerosing subtype of Hodgkin lymphoma. Elderly patients, patients infected with HIV, and patients

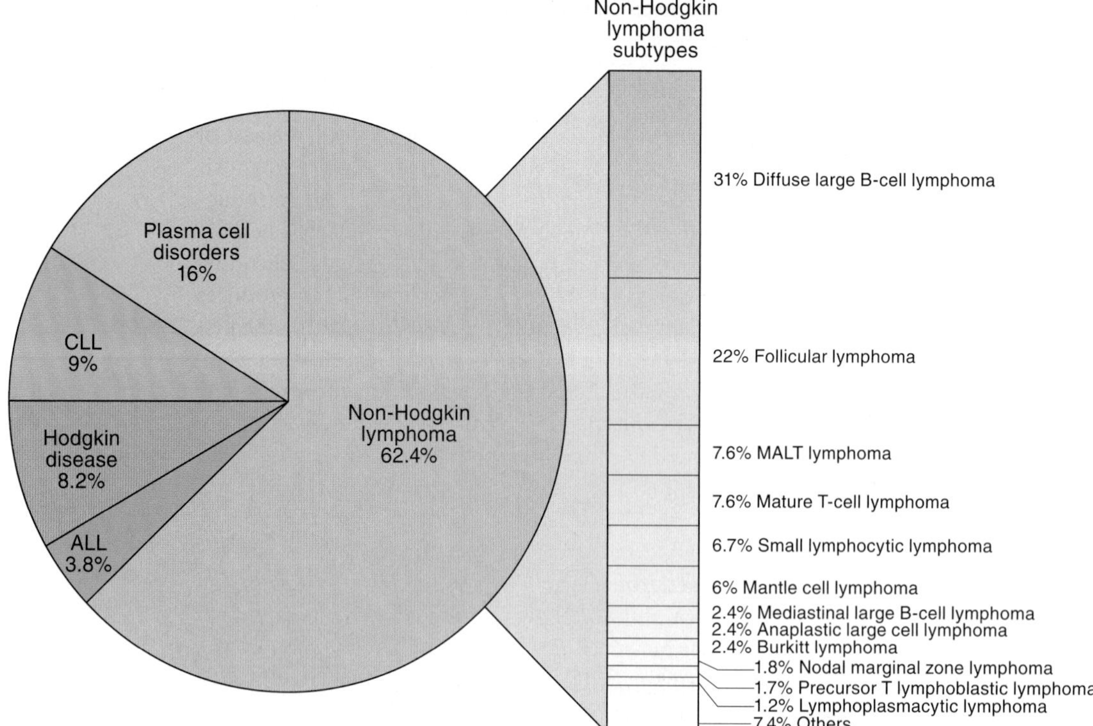

FIGURE III-67 ALL, acute lymphoid leukemia; CLL, chronic lymphoid leukemia; MALT, mucosa-associated lymphoid tissue.

in third-world countries more commonly have mixed-cellularity Hodgkin lymphoma or lymphocyte-depleted Hodgkin lymphoma. Non-Hodgkin lymphomas are more frequent in the elderly and more frequent in men. Patients with both primary and secondary immunodeficiency states are predisposed to developing non-Hodgkin lymphomas. These include patients with HIV infection; patients who have undergone organ transplantation; and patients with inherited immune deficiencies, the sicca syndrome, and rheumatoid arthritis. The incidence of non-Hodgkin lymphomas and the patterns of expression of the various subtypes differ geographically. T-cell lymphomas are more common in Asia than in Western countries, whereas certain subtypes of B-cell lymphomas, such as follicular lymphoma, are more common in Western countries. A specific subtype of non-Hodgkin lymphoma, known as the angiocentric nasal T/natural killer (NK) cell lymphoma, has a striking geographic occurrence, being most frequent in southern Asia and parts of Latin America. A number of environmental factors have been implicated in the occurrence of non-Hodgkin lymphoma, including infectious agents, chemical exposures, and medical treatments. Several studies have demonstrated an association between exposure to agricultural chemicals and an increased incidence of non-Hodgkin lymphoma. Patients treated for Hodgkin lymphoma can develop non-Hodgkin lymphoma; it is unclear whether this is a consequence of the Hodgkin lymphoma or its treatment.

III-68. **The answer is E.** *(Chap. 134)* A number of infectious agents are associated with the development of lymphoid malignancies. JC virus is associated with progressive multifocal leukoencephalopathy (PML) in immunodeficient individuals (Table III-68).

III-69. **The answer is E.** *(Chap. 135e)* A "dry tap" is defined as the inability to aspirate bone marrow and is reported in approximately 4% of attempts (Table III-69). It is rare in the case of normal bone marrow. The differential diagnosis includes metastatic carcinoma infiltration (17%), chronic myeloid leukemia (15%), myelofibrosis (14%), hairy cell leukemia (10%), acute leukemia (10%), and lymphomas including Hodgkin disease (9%).

III-70. **The answer is B.** *(Chap. 135e)* The diagnostic criteria for chronic eosinophilic leukemia and the hypereosinophilic syndrome first require the presence of persistent eosinophilia ≥1500/μL in blood, increased marrow eosinophils, and <20% myeloblasts in blood or marrow. Additional disorders that must be excluded include all causes of reactive eosinophilia,

TABLE III-68 Infectious Agents Associated with the Development of Lymphoid Malignancies

Infectious Agent	Lymphoid Malignancy
Epstein-Barr virus	Burkitt lymphoma
	Post–organ transplant lymphoma
	Primary CNS diffuse large B-cell lymphoma
	Hodgkin lymphoma
	Extranodal NK/T-cell lymphoma, nasal type
HTLV-1	Adult T-cell leukemia/ lymphoma
HIV	Diffuse large B-cell lymphoma
	Burkitt lymphoma
Hepatitis C virus	Lymphoplasmacytic lymphoma
Helicobacter pylori	Gastric MALT lymphoma
Human herpesvirus 8	Primary effusion lymphoma
	Multicentric Castleman disease

Abbreviations: CNS, central nervous system; HIV, human immunodeficiency virus; HTLV, human T-cell lymphotropic virus; MALT, mucosa-associated lymphoid tissue; NK, natural killer.

TABLE III-69 Differential Diagnosis of "Dry Tap"—Inability to Aspirate Bone Marrow

Dry taps occur in about 4% of attempts and are associated with:	
Metastatic carcinoma infiltration	17%
Chronic myeloid leukemia	15%
Myelofibrosis	14%
Hairy cell leukemia	10%
Acute leukemia	10%
Lymphomas, Hodgkin disease	9%
Normal marrow	Rare

primary neoplasms associated with eosinophilia (e.g., T-cell lymphoma, Hodgkin disease, ALL, mastocytosis, CML, AML, myelodysplasia, myeloproliferative syndromes), and T-cell reaction with increased IL-5 or cytokine production. If these entities have been excluded and the myeloid cells show a clonal chromosome abnormality and blast cells (>2%) are present in peripheral blood or are increased in marrow (but <20%), then the diagnosis is chronic eosinophilic leukemia. Patients with hypereosinophilic syndrome and chronic eosinophilic leukemia may be asymptomatic (discovered on routine testing) or present with systemic findings such as fever, shortness of breath, new neurologic findings, or rheumatologic findings. The heart, lungs, and CNS are most often affected by eosinophil-mediated tissue damage.

III-71. **The answer is D.** *(Chap. 135e)* Mastocytosis is a proliferation and accumulation of mast cells in one or more organ systems. Only the skin is involved in approximately 80% of cases, with the other 20% being defined as systemic mastocytosis due to the involvement of another organ system. The most common manifestation of mastocytosis is cutaneous urticaria pigmentosa, a maculopapular pigmented rash involving the papillary dermis. Other cutaneous forms include diffuse cutaneous mastocytosis (almost entirely in children) and mastocytoma. Clinical manifestations of systemic mastocytosis are related to either cellular infiltration of organs and/or release of histamine, proteases, eicosanoids, or heparin from mast cells. Therefore, signs and symptoms may include constitutional symptoms, skin manifestations (pruritus, dermatographia, rash), mediator-related symptoms (abdominal pain, flushing, syncope, hypertension, diarrhea), or bone-related symptoms (fracture, pain, arthralgia). In a recent series, 40% of patients with systemic mastocytosis had an associated myeloid neoplasm, most commonly myeloproliferative syndrome, CML, and MDS. Eosinophilia was present in approximately one-third of patients. Elevated serum tryptase, bone marrow involvement, splenomegaly, skeletal involvement, cytopenia, and malabsorption predict more aggressive disease and worse prognosis. Many patients with systemic mastocytosis have an activating mutation of c-KIT, a kinase inhibited by imatinib; however, the mutation appears relatively resistant to this agent.

III-72. The answer is A. *(Chap. 136)* The patient presents with pneumococcal pneumonia and evidence of hypercalcemia, renal failure, and a wide protein gap suggestive of an M protein. These findings are classic for multiple myeloma (Table III-72). Although patients appear

TABLE III-72 Diagnostic Criteria for Multiple Myeloma, Myeloma Variants, and Monoclonal Gammopathy of Undetermined Significance

Monoclonal Gammopathy of Undetermined Significance (MGUS)
M protein in serum <30 g/L
Bone marrow clonal plasma cells <10%
No evidence of other B-cell proliferative disorders
No myeloma-related organ or tissue impairment (no end-organ damage, including bone lesions)[a]
Smoldering Multiple Myeloma (Asymptomatic Myeloma)
M protein in serum ≥30 g/L *and/or*
Bone marrow clonal plasma cells ≥10%
No myeloma-related organ or tissue impairment (no end-organ damage, including bone lesions)[a] or symptoms
Symptomatic Multiple Myeloma
M protein in serum and/or urine
Bone marrow (clonal) plasma cells[b] or plasmacytoma
Myeloma-related organ or tissue impairment (end-organ damage, including bone lesions)
Nonsecretory Myeloma
No M protein in serum and/or urine with immunofixation
Bone marrow clonal plasmacytosis ≥10% or plasmacytoma
Myeloma-related organ or tissue impairment (end-organ damage, including bone lesions)[a]
Solitary Plasmacytoma of Bone
No M protein in serum and/or urine[c]
Single area of bone destruction due to clonal plasma cells
Bone marrow not consistent with multiple myeloma
Normal skeletal survey (and magnetic resonance imaging of spine and pelvis if done)
No related organ or tissue impairment (no end-organ damage other than solitary bone lesion)[a]
POEMS Syndrome
All of the following four criteria must be met: 1. Polyneuropathy 2. Monoclonal plasma cell proliferative disorder 3. Any one of the following: (a) sclerotic bone lesions; (b) Castleman disease; (c) elevated levels of vascular endothelial growth factor (VEGF) 4. Any one of the following: (a) organomegaly (splenomegaly, hepatomegaly, or lymphadenopathy); (b) extravascular volume overload (edema, pleural effusion, or ascites); (c) endocrinopathy (adrenal, thyroid, pituitary, gonadal, parathyroid, and pancreatic); (d) skin changes (hyperpigmentation, hypertrichosis, glomeruloid hemangiomata, plethora, acrocyanosis, flushing, and white nails); (e) papilledema; (f) thrombocytosis/polycythemia[d]

[a]Myeloma-related organ or tissue impairment (end-organ damage): calcium levels increased: serum calcium >0.25 mmol/L above the upper limit of normal or >2.75 mmol/L; renal insufficiency: creatinine >173 mmol/L; anemia: hemoglobin 2 g/dL below the lower limit of normal or hemoglobin <10 g/dL; bone lesions: lytic lesions or osteoporosis with compression fractures (magnetic resonance imaging or computed tomography may clarify); other: symptomatic hyperviscosity, amyloidosis, recurrent bacterial infections (>2 episodes in 12 months).
[b]If flow cytometry is performed, most plasma cells (>90%) will show a "neoplastic" phenotype.
[c]A small M component may sometimes be present.
[d]These features should have no attributable other causes and have temporal relation with each other.
Abbreviation: POEMS, polyneuropathy, organomegaly, endocrinopathy, M protein, and skin changes.

to be making large quantities of immunoglobulins, they are in fact generally monoclonal, and patients actually have functional hypogammaglobulinemia related to both decreased production and increased destruction of normal antibodies. This hypogammaglobulinemia predisposes patients to infections, most commonly pneumonia with pneumococcus or *S aureus* or gram-negative pyelonephritis. Bone marrow biopsy would confirm the presence of clonal plasma cells and define the quantity, which will help define treatment options. A serum protein electrophoresis would also be indicated to prove the presence of the M protein suspected by the wide protein gap. While HIV may be associated with kidney injury, both acute and chronic, hypercalcemia would be an unusual feature. There is no clinical history of aspiration, and the location of infiltrate (upper lobe) is unusual for aspiration. Sweat chloride testing is not indicated because there is no suspicion for cystic fibrosis. Because solid organ malignancy is not suspected, CT of the body is unlikely to be helpful.

III-73. **The answer is D.** *(Chap. 136)* Serum β_2-microglobulin is the single most powerful predictor of survival and can substitute for staging. Patients with β_2-microglobulin levels <0.004 g/L have a median survival of 43 months, and those with levels >0.004 g/L have a survival of only 12 months. Combination of serum β_2-microglobulin and albumin levels forms the basis for a three-stage International Staging System (ISS) that predicts survival. Other factors that may influence prognosis are the presence of cytogenetic abnormalities and hypodiploidy by karyotype, fluorescent in situ hybridization (FISH)–identified chromosome 17p deletion, and translocations t(4;14), (14;16), and t(14;20) (Table III-73). Chromosome 13q deletion, previously thought to predict poor outcome, is not a predictor following the use of newer agents. Microarray profiling and comparative genomic hybridization have formed the basis for RNA- and DNA-based prognostic staging systems, respectively. The ISS system, along with cytogenetic changes, is the most widely used method for assessing prognosis.

TABLE III-73 Risk Stratification in Myeloma

	Chromosomal Abnormalities	
Method	Standard Risk (80%) (expected survival 6–7+ years)	High Risk (20%) (expected survival 2–3 years)
Karyotype	No chromosomal aberration	Any abnormality on conventional karyotype
FISH	t(11;14)	Del(17p)
	t(6:14)	t(4:14)
	del(13)	t(14:16)
		t(14;20)
	International Staging System	
	Stage	Median Survival, Months
β_2M <3.5, alb ≥3.5	I (28%)[a]	62
β_2M <3.5, alb <3.5 *or* β_2M = 3.5–5.5	II (39%)	44
β_2M >5.5	III (33%)	29
Other features suggesting high-risk disease:		
De novo plasma cell leukemia		
Extramedullary disease		
Elevated lactate dehydrogenate (LDH)		
High-risk gene expression profile		

[a]Percentage of patients presenting at each stage.
Abbreviations: β_2M, serum β_2-microglobulin in mg/L; alb, serum albumin in g/dL; FISH, fluorescent in situ hybridization.

III-74. **The answer is E.** *(Chap. 136)* Monoclonal gammopathy of undetermined significance (MGUS) is diagnosed in patients with abnormal serum protein electrophoresis, elevated serum M protein, <10% clonal plasma cells in bone marrow, no evidence of other B-cell proliferative disease, and no myeloma-related bone lesions or organ damage. No specific intervention is indicated for patients with MGUS. Follow-up once a year or less frequently is adequate except in higher risk MGUS, where serum protein electrophoresis, complete blood count, creatinine, and calcium should be repeated every 6 months. A patient with MGUS and severe polyneuropathy is considered for therapeutic intervention if a causal relationship can be assumed, especially in absence of any other potential causes for neuropathy. Therapy can include plasmapheresis and occasionally rituximab in patients with IgM MGUS or myeloma-like therapy in those with IgG or IgA disease.

III-75. **The answer is A.** *(Chap. 137)* This patient presents with a multisystem illness involving the heart, kidneys, and peripheral nervous system. The physical examination is suggestive of amyloidosis with classic waxy papules in the folds of his body. The laboratories are remarkable for renal failure of unclear etiology with significant proteinuria but no cellular casts. A possible etiology of the renal failure is suggested by the elevated gamma globulin fraction and low hematocrit, bringing to mind a monoclonal gammopathy perhaps leading to renal failure through amyloid AL deposition. This could also account for the enlarged heart seen on the echocardiogram and the peripheral neuropathy. The fat pad biopsy is generally reported to be 60%–80% sensitive for amyloid; however, it would not allow a diagnosis of this patient's likely myeloma. A right heart catheterization probably would prove that the patient has restrictive cardiomyopathy secondary to amyloid deposition; however, it too would not diagnose the underlying plasma cell dyscrasia. Renal ultrasound, although warranted to rule out obstructive uropathy, would not be diagnostic. Similarly, the electromyogram and nerve conduction studies would not be diagnostic. The bone marrow biopsy is about 50%–60% sensitive for amyloid, but it would allow evaluation of the percentage of plasma cells in the bone marrow and allow the diagnosis of multiple myeloma to be made. Multiple myeloma is associated with amyloid AL in approximately 20% of cases. Light chains most commonly deposit systemically in the heart, kidneys, liver, and nervous system, causing organ dysfunction. In these organs, biopsy would show the classic eosinophilic material that, when exposed to Congo red stain, has a characteristic apple-green birefringence. Extensive multisystemic involvement typifies AL amyloidosis, and the median survival period without treatment is usually only approximately 1–2 years from the time of diagnosis.

III-76. **The answer is C.** *(Chap. 137)* The most common form of familial amyloidosis is ATTRm in the updated nomenclature, caused by mutation of the abundant plasma protein transthyretin (TTR, also known as *prealbumin*). More than 100 TTR mutations are known, and most are associated with ATTR amyloidosis. One variant, V122I, has a carrier frequency that may be as high as 4% in the African American population and is associated with late-onset cardiac amyloidosis. The actual incidence and penetrance of disease in the African American population are the subject of ongoing research, but ATTR amyloidosis warrants consideration in the differential diagnosis of African American patients who present with concentric cardiac hypertrophy and evidence of diastolic dysfunction, particularly in the absence of a history of hypertension. DNA sequencing is the standard for diagnosis of ATTR. Without intervention, the survival period after onset of ATTR disease is 5–15 years. Standard treatment for nonsystolic heart failure is indicated. Orthotopic liver transplantation replaces the major source of variant TTR production with a source of normal TTR. Although liver transplantation can slow disease progression and improve chances of survival, it does not reverse sensorimotor neuropathy. Liver transplantations are most successful in young patients with early peripheral neuropathy; older patients with familial amyloidotic cardiomyopathy or advanced polyneuropathy often experience end-organ disease progression despite successful liver transplantation.

III-77. **The answer is E.** *(Chap. 140)* The peripheral blood smear is not consistent with true thrombocytopenia because of the clumped enlarged platelets. A repeat platelet count after the patient's blood was collected in sodium citrate revealed a normal platelet count. Pseudothrombocytopenia is an in vitro artifact resulting from platelet agglutination via antibodies (usually IgG, but also IgM and IgA) when the calcium content is decreased by blood collection in ethylenediaminetetraacetic acid (EDTA) (the anticoagulant present in tubes [purple top] used to collect blood for complete blood counts). If a low platelet count is obtained in EDTA-anticoagulated blood, a blood smear should be evaluated and a platelet count determined in blood collected into sodium citrate (blue top tube) or heparin (green top tube), or a smear of freshly obtained unanticoagulated blood, such as from a finger stick, can be examined (Figure III-77B). The other options cause true thrombocytopenia.

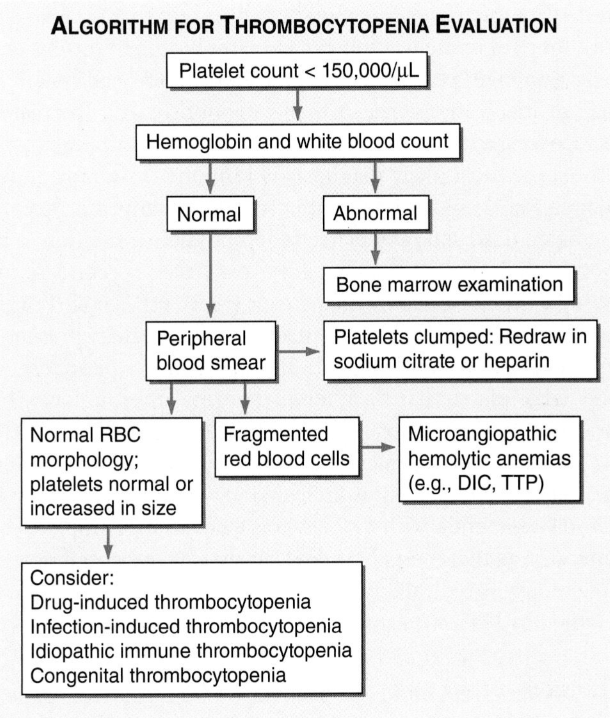

FIGURE III-77B DIC, disseminated intravascular coagulation; RBC, red blood cell; TTP, thrombotic thrombocytopenic purpura.

III-78. The answer is C. *(Chap. 140)* Heparin-induced thrombocytopenia (HIT) is a clinical diagnosis that must not be missed because life-threatening thrombosis can occur if not treated appropriately. The cause of HIT is the formation of antibodies to the complex of heparin and platelet factor 4 (PF4). This complex is able to activate platelets, monocytes, and endothelial cells. Many patients exposed to heparin will develop antibodies to the heparin/PF4 complex, but only a few of these will progress to develop thrombocytopenia or thrombocytopenia with thrombosis (HITT). The typical patient will develop evidence of HIT 5–14 days after exposure to heparin, although it can occur within 5 days in individuals exposed to heparin within the previous approximately 100 days, as would be expected in this patient given his recent hospitalization. The nadir platelet count is typically greater than 20,000/μL. When HIT is suspected, one should not delay treatment for laboratory testing as no currently available test has adequate sensitivity or specificity for the diagnosis. The anti-heparin/PF4 antibody test is positive in many individuals who have been exposed to heparin regardless of whether HIT is present. The platelet activation assay is more specific but less sensitive for HIT. As soon as HIT is suspected, heparin should be discontinued and replaced with an alternative form of anticoagulation to protect against development of new thromboses. Low-molecular-weight heparins (LMWH) such as enoxaparin are not appropriate treatment options in individuals with HIT. Although heparin is 10 times more likely to cause HIT, LMWHs also cause the illness and should not be used. The primary agents used for HIT in the United States are the direct thrombin inhibitors argatroban and lepirudin. Argatroban is the preferred agent for this patient because of his renal failure. The drug is not excreted by the kidneys, and no dosage adjustment is required. In contrast, lepirudin is markedly increased in renal failure, and significant dosage adjustment is required. Danaparoid has previously been used frequently for HIT/HITT, but this medication is no longer available in the United States. Other anticoagulants that are used for treatment of HITT include bivalirudin and fondaparinux, but these are not currently approved by the U.S. FDA for this indication.

III-79. The answer is E. *(Chap. 140)* This patient presents with symptoms of thrombocytopenia including bleeding gums and easy bruising. The only finding on physical examination may be petechiae at points of increased venous pressure, especially in the feet and ankles. The laboratory findings confirm thrombocytopenia but show no abnormalities in other cell lines. When evaluating isolated thrombocytopenia, one must initially consider whether there is an underlying infection or medication that is causing the platelet count to fall. There is a long list of medications that are implicated in thrombocytopenia, including aspirin, acetaminophen, penicillins, H_2-blockers, heparin, and many others. This patient discontinued all medications over 6 weeks previously, and the platelet count would be expected to recover if a medication reaction were the cause. She gives no signs of any acute infection. Thus, the most likely diagnosis is immune thrombocytopenia purpura (ITP). This disorder is also known as idiopathic thrombocytopenia purpura and refers to an immune-mediated destruction of platelets and possible inhibition of platelet release from megakaryocytes. ITP can truly be idiopathic, or it can be secondary to an underlying disorder including systemic lupus erythematosus (SLE), HIV, or chronic HCV infection. The platelet count can be quite low (<5000/μL) in ITP and usually presents with mucocutaneous bleeding. Laboratory testing for ITP should include a peripheral smear that typically demonstrates large platelets with otherwise normal morphology. Initial testing should evaluate for secondary causes of ITP, including HIV antibodies, HCV antibodies, serologic testing for SLE, serum protein electrophoresis, and immunoglobulins. If anemia is also present, a direct Coombs test is indicated to assess whether there is a combined autoimmune hemolytic anemia with ITP (Evans syndrome). Antiplatelet antibody testing is not recommended as these tests have low sensitivity and specificity for ITP. In addition, bone marrow biopsy is typically not performed unless there are other abnormalities that are not explained by ITP or the patient has failed to respond to usual therapy.

III-80 and III-81. The answers are A and E, respectively. *(Chap. 140)* This patient presents with the classic pentad of thrombotic thrombocytopenic purpura (TTP): fever, neurologic symptoms, acute renal failure, thrombocytopenia, and microscopic angiopathic hemolytic anemia (MAHA). The peripheral blood smear shows schistocytes and decreased platelets consistent with MAHA. Although this is the classic presentation of TTP, it is not necessary to have all five characteristics for an individual to be diagnosed with TTP. In recent years, the pathogenesis of inherited and idiopathic TTP has been discovered to be due to a deficiency of antibodies directed against the ADAMTS13 protein. The ADAMTS13 protein is a metalloproteinase that cleaves von Willebrand factor (vWF). In the absence of ADAMTS13, ultra-large vWF multimers circulate in the blood and can cause pathogenic platelet adhesion and activation, resulting in microvascular ischemia and microangiopathic hemolytic anemia. However, it appears as if there is a necessary inciting event because not all individuals with an inherited deficiency of ADAMTS13 develop TTP. Some drugs have been implicated as causative agents in TTP. Ticlopidine and possibly clopidogrel cause TTP by inducing antibody formation. Other drugs including mitomycin C, cyclosporine, and quinine can cause TTP by causing direct endothelial toxicity.

In patients presenting with new thrombocytopenia, with or without evidence of renal insufficiency and other elements of classic TTP, laboratory data should be obtained to rule out DIC and to evaluate for evidence of MAHA. Findings to support the TTP diagnosis include an increased lactate dehydrogenase and indirect bilirubin, decreased haptoglobin, and increased reticulocyte count, with a negative direct antiglobulin test. The peripheral smear should be examined for evidence of schistocytes. Polychromasia is usually also present due to the increased number of young RBCs, and nucleated RBCs are often present, which is thought to be due to infarction in the microcirculatory system of the bone marrow. A diagnosis of TTP can be made based on clinical factors. It should be differentiated from DIC, which causes MAHA but has a predominant coagulopathy. Hemolytic-uremic syndrome also causes MAHA and appears very similar to TTP in clinical presentation, although neurologic symptoms are less prominent. Often a preceding diarrheal illness alerts one to hemolytic-uremic syndrome as the cause of MAHA. It is important to make a prompt and correct diagnosis as the mortality of TTP without treatment is 85%–100%, decreasing to 10%–30% with treatment. The primary treatment for TTP remains plasma exchange. Plasma exchange should be continued until the platelet count returns to the normal range and there is no further evidence of hemolysis for at least

2 days. Glucocorticoids can be used as adjunctive treatment in TTP but are not effective as the sole therapy. Additionally, other immunomodulatory therapies have been reported to be successful in refractory or relapsing TTP, including rituximab, vincristine, cyclophosphamide, and splenectomy. A significant relapse rate is noted; 25%–45% of patients relapse within 30 days of initial "remission," and 12%–40% of patients have late relapses. Relapses are more frequent in patients with severe ADAMTS13 deficiency at presentation.

III-82. The answer is B. *(Chap. 142)* Venous thrombosis occurs through activation of the coagulation cascade primarily through the exposure to tissue factor, and the genetic factors that contribute to a predisposition to venous thrombosis typically are those polymorphisms affecting procoagulant or fibrinolytic pathways. In contrast, arterial thrombosis occurs in the setting of a platelet activation, and the genetic predisposition for arterial thrombosis includes mutations that affect platelet receptors or redox enzymes. The most common inherited risk factors for venous thrombosis are the factor V Leiden mutation and the prothrombin 20210 mutation. Other mutations predisposing an individual to venous thrombosis include inherited deficiency of protein C or S and mutations of fibrinogen, tissue plasminogen activator, thrombomodulin, or plasminogen activator inhibitor. The glycoprotein Ib platelet receptor mutation would increase the risk of arterial, but not venous, thrombosis.

III-83. The answer is A. *(Chap. 142)* D-dimer is a degradation product of cross-linked fibrin and is elevated in conditions of ongoing thrombosis. Low concentrations of D-dimer are considered to indicate the absence of thrombosis. Patients over the age of 70 will frequently have elevated D-dimers in the absence of thrombosis, making this test less predictive of acute disease. Clinical symptoms are often not present in patients with deep venous thrombosis (DVT) and do not affect interpretation of a D-dimer. Tobacco use, while frequently considered a risk factor for DVT, and previous DVT should not affect the predictive value of D-dimer. Homan sign, calf pain elicited by dorsiflexion of the foot, is not predictive of DVT and is unrelated to D-dimer.

III-84. The answer is E. *(Chaps. 142 and 300)* The clinical probability of pulmonary embolism (PE) can be delineated into likely versus unlikely using the clinical decision rule shown in Table III-84. In those with a score ≤4, PE is unlikely and a D-dimer test

TABLE III-84 Clinical Decision Rules

Low clinical likelihood of DVT if point score is 0 or less; moderate likelihood if score is 1 to 2; high likelihood if score is 3 or greater	
Clinical Variable	DVT Score
Active cancer	1
Paralysis, paresis, or recent cast	1
Bedridden for >3 days; major surgery <12 weeks	1
Tenderness along distribution of deep veins	1
Entire leg swelling	1
Unilateral calf swelling >3 cm	1
Pitting edema	1
Collateral superficial nonvaricose veins	1
Alternative diagnosis at least as likely as DVT	−2
High clinical likelihood of PE if point score exceeds 4	
Clinical Variable	PE Score
Signs and symptoms of DVT	3.0
Alternative diagnosis less likely than PE	3.0
Heart rate >100/min	1.5
Immobilization >3 days; surgery within 4 weeks	1.5
Prior PE or DVT	1.5
Hemoptysis	1.0
Cancer	1.0

should be performed. A normal D-dimer combined with an unlikely clinical probability of PE identifies patients who do not need further testing or anticoagulation therapy. Those with either a likely clinical probability (score >4) or an abnormal D-dimer (with unlikely clinical probability) require an imaging test to rule out PE. Currently the most attractive imaging method to detect PE is the multislice CT scan. It is accurate and, if normal, safely rules out PE. This patient has a clinical probability score of 4.5 because of her resting tachycardia and the lack of an alternative diagnosis at least as likely as PE. Therefore, there is no indication for measuring D-dimer, and she should proceed directly to multislice CT of the chest. If this cannot be performed expeditiously, she should receive one dose of LMWH while awaiting the test.

SECTION IV

Infectious Diseases

QUESTIONS

DIRECTIONS: Choose the one best response to each question.

IV-1. Deficits in the complement membrane attack complex (C5–8) are associated with infections of what variety?

A. Catalase-positive bacteria
B. *Neisseria meningitidis*
C. *Pseudomonas aeruginosa*
D. *Salmonella* spp
E. *Streptococcus pneumoniae*

IV-2. All of the following statements regarding global infectious diseases are true EXCEPT:

A. Drug-resistant tuberculosis is common in the former Soviet bloc countries.
B. Infectious diseases are the leading cause of death worldwide.
C. Over 60% of deaths in sub-Saharan Africa were related to infectious diseases (2010).
D. The absolute number of infectious disease–related deaths has remained relatively constant in the past 20 years.
E. The rate of infectious disease–related death has dropped notably in the past 20 years.

IV-3. Which of the following infectious organisms is most likely to cause relative bradycardia during a febrile event?

A. *P aeruginosa*
B. *Salmonella typhi*
C. *Staphylococcus aureus*
D. *S pneumoniae*
E. *Streptococcus pyogenes*

IV-4. A 42-year-old man has a history of splenectomy following trauma at the age of 20. He received appropriate vaccinations immediately after his trauma but has not had any medical care for more than 10 years. He is homeless. He presents to the emergency department with a fever of 102.3°F (39.1°C), blood pressure (BP) of 70/40 mmHg, heart rate (HR) of 130 bpm, respiratory rate (RR) of 30 breaths/min, and oxygen saturation (SaO_2) of 95% on room air. What is the best initial antibiotic therapy for this patient?

A. Ceftriaxone and vancomycin
B. Ceftriaxone, ampicillin, and vancomycin
C. Ceftriaxone, vancomycin, and amphotericin B
D. Clindamycin, gentamicin, and vancomycin
E. Clindamycin and quinine

IV-5. The patient described in Question IV-4 subsequently develops multisystem organ failure due to overwhelming sepsis and dies despite appropriate medical management. Which of the following organisms would be MOST likely to cause the patient's presentation?

A. *Escherichia coli*
B. *Haemophilus influenzae*
C. *N meningitidis*
D. *P aeruginosa*
E. *S pneumoniae*

IV-6. A 44-year-old woman with relapsed acute myelogenous leukemia has undergone a myeloablative allogeneic stem cell transplantation. She has been profoundly neutropenic for 21 days and has had a persistent fever for the past 7 days. Today, she has appeared septic with hypotension, tachycardia, and a new oxygen requirement. A nurse calls you to evaluate a new rash. On examination, the patient looks ill. She is tachypneic and is rigoring. Skin examination reveals a few scattered areas of hemorrhagic vesicles, the largest measuring 3 cm in diameter, on the hands and legs (Figure IV-6). What is the most likely causative organism?

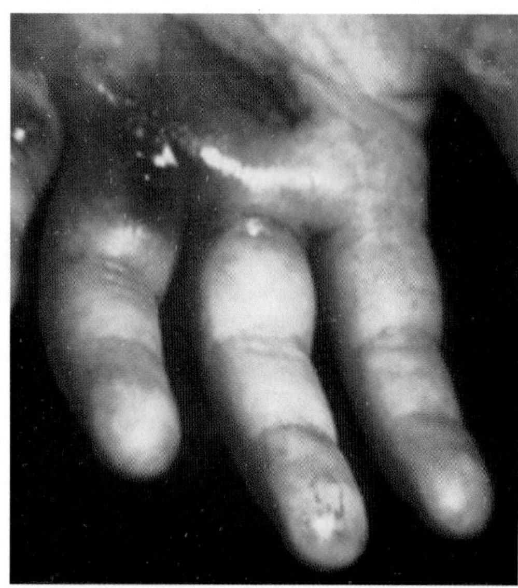

FIGURE IV-6

A. *N meningitidis*
B. *P aeruginosa*
C. *Rickettsia rickettsii*
D. *S aureus*
E. *Vibrio vulnificus*

IV-7. A 32-year-old woman is admitted to the hospital complaining of right thigh pain. She is treated empirically with oxacillin intravenously for a cellulitis. The admitting physician notes that the degree of pain appears to be disproportionate to the amount of overlying cellulitis. Over the course of the next 24 hours, the patient develops profound septic shock complicated by hypotension, acute renal failure, and evidence of disseminated intravascular coagulation. A computed tomography (CT) scan of her right leg demonstrates a collection of fluid with gas in the deep fascia of her right leg. Emergent surgical evacuation is planned. What changes to the patient's antibiotic therapy should be recommended?

A. Continue oxacillin and add clindamycin
B. Continue oxacillin and add clindamycin and gentamicin
C. Discontinue oxacillin and add clindamycin, vancomycin, and gentamicin
D. Discontinue oxacillin and add piperacillin/tazobactam and vancomycin
E. Discontinue oxacillin and add vancomycin and gentamicin

IV-8. In 2012, there were 55 reported cases of measles in the United States. In 2014, there were 644 cases reported to the Centers for Disease Control and Prevention's (CDC) National Center for Immunization and Respiratory Diseases. This was the highest reported number since the disease was considered to be eliminated in 2000 (http://www.cdc.gov/measles/cases-outbreaks.html). In late 2014 and early 2015, there was another large outbreak of measles with more than 100 cases reported in the first 2 months of 2015 alone. In the case of the recent outbreaks of measles in the United States, which of the following was the source of the infection?

A. Indigenous transmission from unvaccinated individuals
B. Importation of the disease from an endemic area
C. Spontaneous mutation of measles vaccine virus to a virulent form
D. Spontaneous outbreak from an environmental source

IV-9. Once the measles infection was established in the United States, what was the source of sustained transmission?

A. Transmission of disease among individuals too young to undergo vaccination
B. Transmission of disease among individuals who had chosen to forego vaccination for personal or religious reasons
C. Transmission of disease among individuals with medical contraindications
D. Transmission of disease among unvaccinated foreign travelers or immigrants
E. Viral breakthrough in vaccinated individuals

IV-10. A 63-year-old man has chronic obstructive pulmonary disease and presents to your office for routine follow-up. He has no complaints currently and feels well. His most recent forced expiratory volume in 1 second (FEV_1) was 55% predicted, and he is not on oxygen. He received one dose of pneumococcal vaccine 7 years previously. He is asking whether he should receive another dose of pneumococcal vaccine. According to the guidelines of the CDC, what is your recommendation?

A. He does not require further vaccination unless his FEV_1 drops below 50% predicted.
B. He does not require further vaccination until he reaches age 65.
C. He should be revaccinated today.
D. He should be revaccinated 10 years after his initial vaccine.
E. No further vaccination is recommended as a single dose is all that is required.

IV-11. In which of the following patients is it appropriate to administer the vaccination against herpes zoster?

A. A 35-year-old woman who has never had varicella-zoster infection who is 12 weeks pregnant with her first child
B. A 54-year-old man who has never had varicella-zoster infection and is otherwise healthy
C. A 62-year-old man who had a car accident resulting in splenectomy
D. A 64-year-old woman with dermatomyositis-associated interstitial lung disease treated with prednisone 20 mg daily and azathioprine 150 mg daily
E. A 66-year-old woman who was recently diagnosed with non-Hogkin lymphoma

IV-12. Which of the following immunizations is required for entry into many countries in sub-Saharan Africa?

A. Cholera
B. Hepatitis A
C. Meningococcus
D. Typhoid fever
E. Yellow fever

IV-13. A 48-year-old woman is traveling to Haiti with a humanitarian aid group. What is the recommended prophylaxis against malaria for this patient?

A. Atovaquone-proguanil
B. Chloroquine
C. Doxycycline
D. Mefloquine
E. Any of the above can be used

IV-14. A 46-year-old man wishes to travel to Kenya for a 2-week vacation. He is human immunodeficiency virus (HIV) positive and is taking antiretroviral therapy. His last CD4+ count was 625/μL and viral load was undetectable. His nadir CD4+ count was 250/μL. He has never had an acquired immunodeficiency syndrome (AIDS)-defining illness. In addition to HIV, he has a history of hypertension and is known to have proteinuria due to HIV-associated nephropathy. What is your recommendation to this patient regarding his travel plans?

A. He should not receive the live measles vaccine prior to travel.
B. He should receive the yellow fever vaccine prior to travel.
C. He will be required to show proof of HIV testing upon entry into the country.
D. His likelihood of response to the influenza vaccine would be less than 50%.
E. With a CD4+ count greater than 500/μL, he is at no greater risk during travel than persons without HIV.

IV-15. All of the following are reasons that troops deployed on foreign soil are at risk of acquiring infectious diseases endemic to those foreign areas EXCEPT:

A. Crowded social conditions engendered by mass troop deployments
B. Immunologic naiveté with regard to local endemic or enzootic pathogens
C. Lapses in hygiene and sanitation that accompany armed conflicts
D. Medical facilities that are decreased in quantity and often inadequate
E. Population displacements

IV-16. Which of the following diseases had the highest incidence in the specified population?

A. Cutaneous leishmaniasis cases in U.S. troops deployed to Afghanistan and Iraq over the past decade
B. Malaria cases among U.S. troops returning from Vietnam
C. Rabies infections among U.S. troops deployed to Afghanistan and Iraq between 2001 and 2010
D. Viral hepatitis cases among Soviet troops serving in Afghanistan in the 1980s
E. Visceral leishmaniasis (kala-azar) cases in U.S. troops deployed to Afghanistan and Iraq over the past decade

IV-17. Chronic dialysis is associated with an increased risk of healthcare-associated pneumonia caused by which of the following?

A. *Acinetobacter* species
B. *Candida* species
C. Methicillin-resistant *S aureus* (MRSA)
D. Multidrug-resistant Enterobacteriaceae
E. *P aeruginosa*

IV-18. Which of the following bacteria are a common cause of community-acquired pneumonia in hospitalized patients but not in patients treated as outpatients?

A. *Chlamydia pneumoniae*
B. *H influenzae*
C. *Legionella* species
D. *Mycoplasma pneumoniae*
E. *S pneumoniae*

IV-19. Which of the following statements regarding the diagnosis of community-acquired pneumonia is true?

A. Directed therapy specific to the causative organism is more effective than empiric therapy in hospitalized patients who are not in intensive care.
B. Five to 15% of patients hospitalized with community-acquired pneumonia will have positive blood cultures.
C. In patients who have bacteremia caused by *S pneumoniae*, sputum cultures are positive in more than 80% of cases.
D. Polymerase chain reaction tests for identification of *Legionella pneumophila* and *M pneumoniae* are widely available and should be used for diagnosis in patients hospitalized with community-acquired pneumonia.
E. The etiology of community-acquired pneumonia is typically identified in about 70% of cases.

IV-20. A 55-year-old man presents to his primary care physician with a 2-day history of cough and fever. His cough is productive of thick dark green sputum. His past medical history is significant for hypercholesterolemia treated with rosuvastatin. He does not smoke cigarettes and is generally quite healthy, exercising several times weekly. He has no ill contacts and cannot recall the last time he was treated with any antibiotics. On presentation, his vital signs are: temperature 102.1°F (38.9°C); BP 132/78 mmHg; HR 87 bpm; RR 20 breaths/min; and SaO_2 95% on room air. Crackles are present in the right lung base, as is egophony. A chest radiograph demonstrates segmental consolidation of the right lower lobe with air bronchograms. What is the most appropriate approach to the ongoing care of this patient?

A. Obtain a sputum culture and await results prior to initiating treatment.
B. Perform a chest CT to rule out postobstructive pneumonia.
C. Refer to the emergency department for admission and treatment with intravenous antibiotics.
D. Treat with azithromycin.
E. Treat with moxifloxacin.

IV-21. A 65-year-old woman was admitted to the intensive care unit for management of septic shock associated with an infected hemodialysis catheter. She was initially intubated on hospital day 1 with the acute respiratory distress syndrome. She had slowly been improving such that her fraction of inspired oxygen (FiO2) had been weaned to 0.40, and she was no longer febrile or requiring vasopressors. On hospital day 7, however, she develops a new fever to 39.4°C (102.9°F) with increased thick yellow-green sputum in her endotracheal tube. You suspect the patient has ventilator-associated pneumonia (VAP). Which of the following makes the most definitive diagnosis of VAP in this patient?

A. An endotracheal aspirate yielding a new organism typical of VAP
B. The presence of a new infiltrate on chest radiograph
C. Quantitative cultures from an endotracheal aspirate yielding more than 10^6 organisms typical of VAP
D. Quantitative culture from a protected brush specimen yielding more than 10^3 organisms typical of VAP
E. There is no single set of criteria that is reliably diagnostic of pneumonia in a ventilated patient.

IV-22. You admit a patient with severe community-acquired pneumonia who requires intubation and mechanical ventilation. She has decreased breath sounds and dullness to percussion halfway up her right lung. Chest x-ray and ultrasound confirm the presence of a large pleural effusion. You perform a diagnostic thoracentesis, but fluid remains. All of the following are indications for complete drainage of the pleural fluid EXCEPT:

A. Pleural fluid pH <7
B. Pleural fluid glucose <2.2 mmol/L
C. Pleural fluid protein >5 g/dL
D. Pleural fluid lactate dehydrogenase concentration >1000 units/L
E. Bacteria seen or cultured from pleural fluid

IV-23. Which of the following represents the recommended duration for treatment of uncomplicated community-acquired pneumonia and improving VAP?

A. 7 days; 7–14 days
B. 5 days; 8 days
C. 7 days; 10 days
D. 5 days; 10–14 days
E. 10–14 days for both

IV-24. All of the following statements regarding lung abscesses are true EXCEPT:

A. Lemierre syndrome is a lung abscess due to septic thrombophlebitis originating in the pharynx.
B. Lung abscesses are typically characterized by a >2-cm single dominant cavity.
C. Primary lung abscesses are often principally caused by anaerobic bacteria.
D. Primary lung abscesses typically are related to oropharyngeal aspiration.
E. Radiographically, primary lung abscesses most commonly involve the middle lobe and the lingula.

IV-25. A 50-year-old man is admitted to the hospital with 3 weeks of progressive malaise, weight loss, and purulent cough. He has a history of alcoholism and frequent emergency department visits due to intoxication. He is a former subprime mortgage broker who is now unemployed and lives with his elderly parents. On examination, he appears disheveled and chronically ill. His temperature is 38.5°C, HR is 110 bpm, BP is 110/65 mmHg, and RR is 18 breaths/min, with room air SaO_2 of 93%. He has extremely poor dentition, is coughing up foul-smelling phlegm, and has rhonchi over his right lung base. There is no diffuse adenopathy and the only other remarkable finding is an enlarged liver. His chest radiograph is shown in Figure IV-25. Which of the following is the most appropriate therapy?

A. Aztreonam
B. Clindamycin
C. Metronidazole
D. Micafungin
E. Penicillin

IV-26. Which of the following is the most common cause of native valve infective endocarditis in the community?

A. Coagulase-negative staphylococci
B. Coagulase-positive staphylococci
C. Enterococci
D. Fastidious gram-negative coccobacilli
E. Nonenterococcal streptococci

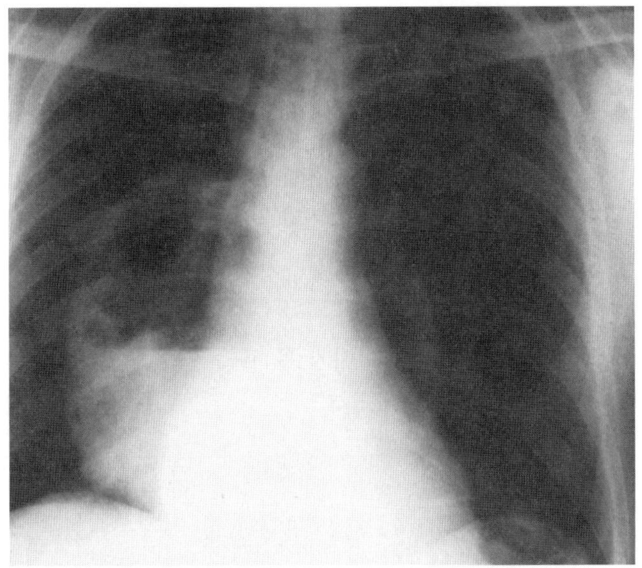

FIGURE IV-25 From Mandell GL (ed): *Atlas of Infectious Diseases*, Vol VI. Philadelphia, PA: Current Medicine Inc, Churchill Livingstone, 1996; with permission.

IV-27. All of the following are minor criteria in the Modified Duke Criteria for the clinical diagnosis of infective endocarditis EXCEPT:

A. Immunologic phenomena (glomerulonephritis, Osler nodes, Roth spots)
B. New valvular regurgitation on transthoracic echocardiogram
C. Predisposing condition (heart condition, intravenous drug use)
D. Temperature >38°C
E. Vascular phenomena (e.g., arterial emboli, septic pulmonary emboli, Janeway lesions)

IV-28. Which of the following patients should receive antibiotic prophylaxis prior to prevent infective endocarditis?

A. A 23-year-old woman with known mitral valve prolapse having a tooth cavity filled
B. A 24-year-old woman who had an atrial septal defect completely corrected 22 years ago who is undergoing elective cystoscopy for painless hematuria
C. A 30-year-old man with a history of intravenous drug use and prior endocarditis undergoing gingival surgery
D. A 45-year-old man who received a prosthetic mitral valve 5 years ago undergoing routine dental cleaning
E. A 63-year-old woman who received a prosthetic aortic valve 2 years ago undergoing screening colonoscopy

IV-29. A 38-year-old homeless man presents to the emergency department with a transient ischemic attack characterized by a facial droop and left arm weakness lasting 20 minutes and left upper quadrant pain. He reports intermittent subjective fevers, diaphoresis, and chills for the past 2 weeks. He has had no recent travel or contact with animals. He has no recent history of taking antibiotics. Physical examination reveals a slightly distressed man with disheveled appearance. His temperature is 38.2°C; HR is 90 bpm; and BP is 127/74 mmHg. He has poor dentition. Cardiac examination reveals an early diastolic murmur over the left third intercostal space. His spleen is tender and 2 cm descended below the costal margin. He has tender painful red nodules on the tips of the third finger of his right hand and on the fourth finger of his left hand that are new. He has nits evident on his clothes, consistent with body louse infection. White blood cell count is 14,500, with 5% band forms and 93% polymorphonuclear cells. Blood cultures are drawn followed by empirical vancomycin therapy. These cultures remain negative for growth 5 days later. He remains febrile but hemodynamically stable but does develop a new lesion on his toe similar to those on his fingers on hospital day 3. A transthoracic echocardiogram reveals a 1-cm mobile vegetation on the cusp of his aortic valve and moderate aortic regurgitation. A CT scan of the abdomen shows an enlarged spleen with wedge-shaped splenic and renal infarctions. What test should be sent to confirm the most likely diagnosis?

A. *Bartonella* serology
B. Epstein-Barr virus (EBV) heterophile antibody
C. HIV polymerase chain reaction (PCR)
D. Peripheral blood smear
E. Q fever serology

IV-30. In a patient with bacterial endocarditis, which of the following echocardiographic lesions is most likely to lead to embolization?

A. 5-mm mitral valve vegetation
B. 5-mm tricuspid valve vegetation
C. 11-mm aortic valve vegetation
D. 11-mm mitral valve vegetation
E. 11-mm tricuspid valve vegetation

IV-31. A 58-year-old man is admitted to the hospital with fevers, malaise, and diffuse joint pains. He had a mechanical mitral valve placed 3 years ago due to chronic mitral regurgitation. His initial blood cultures reveal methicillin-sensitive *S aureus* (MSSA) in all culture bottles. The isolates are also sensitive to gentamicin. He has no arthritis on examination, and his renal function is normal. Echocardiogram shows a 5-mm vegetation on the prosthetic valve. Which of the following antibiotic regimens is recommended?

A. Ampicillin plus gentamicin
B. Cefazolin
C. Nafcillin plus gentamicin
D. Nafcillin plus gentamicin plus rifampin
E. Vancomycin plus gentamicin

IV-32. All of the following infectious clinical syndromes typically cause vesicular lesions EXCEPT:

A. Cold sores
B. Hand-foot-and-mouth disease
C. Rickettsialpox
D. Scalded skin syndrome
E. Shingles

IV-33. A 49-year-old man with a history of alcoholism is admitted to the hospital with sepsis syndrome. He is somnolent, febrile to 40°C, hypotensive, and tachycardic. His room air oxygen saturation is 95% on nasal oxygen. He is disheveled with multiple skin excoriations on his arms, legs, and trunk. There is tenderness and swelling over his left chest but no other focal findings. Laboratory studies and blood cultures are pending. After receiving fluids, vasopressors, and empiric antibiotics, a chest CT is performed and shown in Figure IV-33. Which of the following is the most likely causative organism?

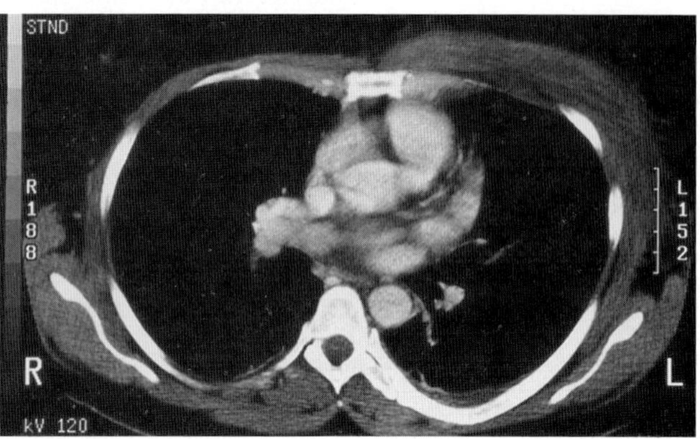

FIGURE IV-33

A. *Actinomyces israelii*
B. *Klebsiella pneumoniae*
C. Oral anaerobic bacteria
D. *S pneumoniae*
E. *S pyogenes*

IV-34. A 45-year-old man with a history of alcoholism and presumed cirrhosis is brought to the emergency department by his friend complaining of 2–3 days of increasing lethargy and confusion. He has not consumed alcohol in the past 2 years. He currently takes no medications and works at home as a video game designer. He has no risk factors for HIV. He was referred by his primary care physician for a liver transplant evaluation and is scheduled to begin his evaluation next month. His vital signs are as follows: BP 90/60 mmHg, HR 105 bpm, temperature 38.5°C, RR 10 breaths/min, and SaO_2 97% on room air. He is somnolent but is able to answer questions accurately. His skin is notable for many spider telangiectasias and palmar erythema. He has a distended diffusely tender abdomen with a positive fluid wave. Paracentesis reveals slightly cloudy fluid with white blood cell (WBC) count of 1000/μL and 40% neutrophils. His BP increases to 100/65 mmHg, and his HR decreases to 95 bpm after 1 of L intravenous fluids. Which of the following statements regarding his condition and treatment is true?

A. Fever is present in >50% of cases.
B. Initial empiric therapy should include metronidazole or clindamycin for anaerobes.
C. The diagnosis of primary (spontaneous) bacterial peritonitis is not confirmed because the percentage of neutrophils in the peritoneal fluid is <50%.
D. The mostly causative organism for his condition is *Enterococcus*.
E. The yield of peritoneal fluid cultures for diagnosis is >90%.

IV-35. A 48-year-old woman with a history of end-stage renal disease due to diabetic renal disease is admitted to the hospital with 1 day of abdominal pain and fever. She has been on continuous ambulatory peritoneal dialysis for the last 6 months. She reports that for the last day she has had poor return of dialysate and is feeling bloated. She has had complications from her diabetes including retinopathy and peripheral neuropathy. She is uncomfortable but not toxic. Her vital signs include the following: temperature 38.8°C, BP 130/65 mmHg, HR 105 bpm, RR 15 breaths/min, and room air SaO_2 98%. Her abdomen is slightly distended and diffusely tender with rebound tenderness. A sample of dialysate reveals WBC of 400/μL with 80% neutrophils. Empiric intraperitoneal antibiotic therapy should include which of the following?

A. Cefoxitin
B. Fluconazole
C. Metronidazole
D. Vancomycin
E. Voriconazole

IV-36. A 77-year-old man presents to the hospital with a week of fever, chills, nausea, and right upper quadrant pain. His temperature is 39°C, and he appears toxic. His BP is 110/70 mmHg, HR is 110 bpm, and RR is 22 breaths/min with room air SaO_2 of 92%. He has diminished breath sounds at the right base and diffuse tenderness in the right upper quadrant. He has a history of cholelithiasis but has declined elective cholecystectomy. His CT scan of the abdomen is shown in Figure IV-36A. Which of the following statements regarding his condition or therapy is true?

A. Concomitant bacteremia is rare (<10%).
B. He should receive empiric antibiotics targeting *Candida* species.
C. He should receive empiric antibiotics targeting anaerobic organisms.
D. He should undergo percutaneous drainage.
E. His serum alkaline phosphatase is most likely normal.

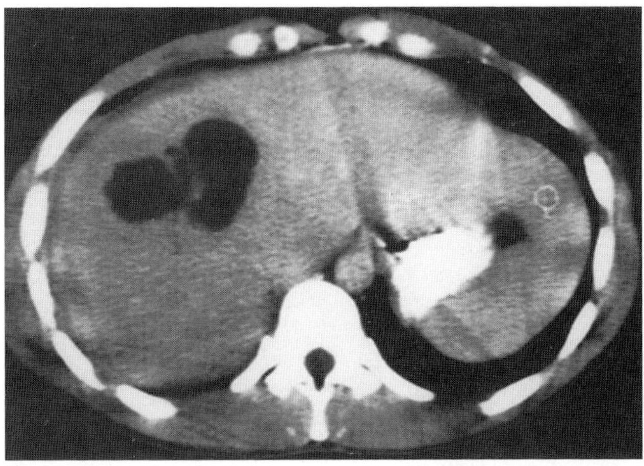

A

FIGURE IV-36A Reprinted with permission from Lorber B (ed): *Atlas of Infectious Diseases, Volume VII: Intra-Abdominal Infections, Hepatitis, and Gastroenteritis.* Philadelphia, PA: Current Medicine, 1996, Fig. 1.22.

IV-37. A 78-year-old woman presents to the hospital from her nursing home with complaints of diarrhea. She has been in the nursing home for the past 5 years following a stroke with residual right-sided hemiplegia. She was recently treated with ceftriaxone for pyelonephritis due to *E coli*. Yesterday, she developed a temperature of 100.6°F with a complaint of diffuse abdominal pain. Over the past 24 hours, she has had worsening abdominal pain and abdominal distention. In addition, she has had eight bowel movements. The bowel movements are loose and have become bloody. Six months ago, she was treated with oral metronidazole for a documented *Clostridium difficile* infection. Additionally, her past medical history is significant for cerebrovascular disease, atrial fibrillation, coronary artery disease requiring angioplasty, hypertension, and hyperlipidemia. On presentation to the hospital, she appears uncomfortable and has a temperature of 101.2°F. Her BP is 98/60 mmHg, and HR is 115 bpm. Her abdomen appears distended and tympanitic with diffuse tenderness to palpation. An abdominal x-ray shows distention of the colon with ileus. Initial laboratory examination shows a WBC count of 27,200/μL with 92% neutrophils and 3% band forms. Her hemoglobin is 9.2 g/dL, and hematocrit is 28.1%. One month ago, her hemoglobin was 10.1 g/dL. Given her recent antibiotic use, you consider the possibility of *C difficile* infection. Which of the following findings is unlikely to be found in *C difficile* infection?

A. Bloody diarrhea
B. Fever
C. Ileus
D. Leukocytosis
E. Recurrence after therapy

IV-38. All of the following patients should be treated for *C difficile* infection EXCEPT:

A. A 57-year-old nursing home resident with diarrhea for 2 weeks and pseudomembranes found on colonoscopy with no evidence of toxin A or B in the stool
B. A 63-year-old woman with fever, leukocytosis, adynamic ileus, and a positive PCR for *C difficile* in the stool
C. A 68-year-old woman with recent course of antibiotics admitted to the medical intensive care unit after presentation to the emergency department with abdominal pain and diarrhea; she was found to have severe abdominal tenderness with absent bowel sounds, systemic hypotension, and colonic wall thickening on CT of the abdomen
D. A 75-year-old woman who completed therapy with amoxicillin for an upper respiratory tract infection yesterday and now has had two loose bowel movements per day for the last 3 days; she is afebrile and has a WBC count of 8600/μL

IV-39. An 82-year-old woman with dementia has been living in a nursing home for 5 years. She was been seen by her primary care provider for evaluation of diarrhea 4 weeks ago. At that time, a stool sample was positive by PCR for *C difficile*, and she was treated with oral metronidazole with some improvement in her symptoms. However, she has had five loose bowel movements per day starting 4 days ago and now has abdominal tenderness. Stool PCR remains positive. Which of the following is the most appropriate therapy?

A. Fecal microbiota transplantation
B. Intravenous (IV) immunoglobulin
C. Oral metronidazole
D. Oral nitazoxanide
E. Oral vancomycin

IV-40. Which of the following antibiotics has the weakest association with the development of *C difficile*–associated disease?

A. Ceftriaxone
B. Ciprofloxacin
C. Clindamycin
D. Moxifloxacin
E. Piperacillin-tazobactam

IV-41. Which of the following statements regarding the epidemiology of and risk factors for urinary tract infections (UTIs) is true?

A. About one-third of all women will experience at least one UTI in their lifetime.
B. Across all ages, UTI is 2–3 times more common among females.
C. Asymptomatic bacteriuria is a common and incidental finding in pregnancy that does not require treatment.
D. Contrary to popular wisdom, sexual intercourse is not a risk factor for UTI.
E. In infancy, UTI is more common among males than females.

IV-42. A 28-year-old woman is admitted to the intensive care unit with temperature to 103.2°F, back pain, and hypotension. She began to feel ill approximately 36 hours previously when she developed pain in her right upper back. She noticed increased urinary frequency and urgency as well. She denies suprapubic discomfort. Over the next 24 hours, she began to feel more ill with ongoing fevers, nausea, and vomiting. She has a past medical history of type 1 diabetes mellitus since the age of 10 years. She takes insulin glargine 24 units daily and insulin aspartate based on carbohydrate counting. When she last checked a fingerstick blood glucose, her meter read "high." She ultimately presented to the emergency department 2 hours previously. On presentation, her initial BP was 75/44 mmHg, and HR was 138 bpm. After 3 L of normal saline, her BP is 88/44 mmHg, and HR is 126 bpm. She remains febrile. She appears uncomfortable. Her mucous membranes are dry. Chest and cardiovascular examinations are normal. Her abdomen is soft and without tenderness or guarding. There is focal severe pain at the right costovertebral angle. Her basic metabolic panel shows evidence of an anion gap metabolic acidosis. Urinalysis has too numerous to count bacteria; shows 30–50 WBCs per high-power field; and is positive for ketones, leukocyte esterase, and nitrites. What is the best initial therapy for this patient?

A. Ceftriaxone 1 g IV daily
B. Ciprofloxacin 400 mg IV twice daily
C. Ciprofloxacin 500 mg orally twice daily
D. Piperacillin-tazobactam 3.375 g IV every 6 hours
E. Trimethoprim-sulfamethoxazole double strength, 1 tablet orally twice daily

IV-43. A 23-year-old woman is seen for routine follow-up of an uncomplicated pregnancy. She had one prior visit at 10 weeks when pregnancy was confirmed. She is currently at week 16. What is the recommendation for screening and treatment of asymptomatic bacteriuria in this patient?

A. She should be screened and treated in the third trimester only.
B. She should be screened at this time with a urine culture but not treated unless symptomatic.
C. She should be screened at this time and treated if the culture is positive.
D. She should be screened now and again in the third trimester. Treatment is recommended only if both cultures are positive.
E. She should not be screened unless she has comorbid medical conditions that increase the risk of UTI.

IV-44. A 64-year-old man presents with urinary frequency, dysuria, and perineal pain. He has also been having fevers to as high as 101.5°F at home. Prior to the current symptoms, he has noted some intermittent symptoms of hesitancy and decreased urine stream that has developed over the past 1–2 years. He has had one prior episode of febrile UTI about 6 weeks ago. At that time, he was treated with ciprofloxacin 500 mg twice daily for 7 days. It was recommended he see a urologist and begin taking tamsulosin 0.4 mg daily following this, but he has not followed through on these recommendations. A rectal examination demonstrates a warm, edematous prostate that is tender to palpation. A urinalysis and urine culture demonstrate ongoing pyuria and presence of $>10^5$ *E coli*. The patient is initiated on treatment with ciprofloxacin 500 mg twice daily. What is the appropriate duration of therapy for this patient?

A. 1 week
B. 2 weeks
C. 4 weeks
D. 12 weeks

IV-45. All of the following are common causes of urethritis in men EXCEPT:

A. *Gardnerella vaginalis*
B. *Mycoplasma genitalium*
C. *Neisseria gonorrhoeae*
D. *Trichomonas vaginalis*
E. *Ureaplasma urealyticum*

IV-46. A 25-year-old woman presents with 2 days of urinary frequency, urgency, and pelvic discomfort. She has no pain in her vulva on urination. She has no other medical problems and does not have fevers. She is sexually active. A microscopic examination of her urine shows pyuria but no pathogens. After 24 hours, her urine culture does not grow any pathogens. Which of the following tests will likely confirm her diagnosis?

A. Cervical culture
B. Clue cells on microscopy of vaginal secretions
C. Nucleic acid amplification test of urine for *Chlamydia trachomatis*
D. Physical examination of the vulva and vagina
E. Vaginal pH ≥5.0

IV-47. Which of the following diagnostic features characterizes bacterial vaginosis?

A. Scant vaginal secretions, erythema of vaginal epithelium, and clue cells
B. Vaginal fluid pH >4.5, clue cells, and profuse mixed microbiota on microscopic exam
C. Vaginal fluid pH ≥5.0, motile trichomonads on microscopic exam, and fishy odor with 10% KOH
D. Vaginal fluid pH <4.5, lactobacilli predominate on microscopic exam, and scant clear secretions
E. Vaginal fluid pH <4.5, clue cells, and profuse mixed microbiota on microscopic exam

IV-48. Which of the following is most likely to be identified in a woman seen at a sexually transmitted disease clinic with leukocytosis and cervicitis?

A. *C trachomatis*
B. *Herpes simplex virus*
C. *N gonorrhoeae*
D. *T vaginalis*
E. No organism identified

IV-49. A 19-year-old woman is seen in the emergency department for pelvic pain. She reports 1 week of pain but has developed more severe pain on the right side of her lower abdomen over the past day with accompanying fever. Additionally, she reports pain in her right upper abdomen for the past day that is worsened by deep breathing. She is sexually active with multiple partners and only reports a past medical history of asthma. Examination is notable for fever, normal breath sounds, mild tachycardia, and a tender right upper quadrant without rebound, guarding, or masses. Pelvic exam shows a normal cervical appearance, but cervical motion tenderness and adnexal tenderness are present. No masses are palpated. A urine pregnancy test is negative and leukocytosis is present, but otherwise, renal and liver function labs are normal. Which of the following is true regarding her right upper quadrant tenderness?

A. Acute cholecystitis is likely present, and a tech HIDA scan should be ordered to confirm the diagnosis.
B. If a liver biopsy were preformed, herpes simplex virus could be cultured from the liver tissue.
C. Laparoscopic examination would show inflammation of her liver capsule.
D. Plasma PCR is indicated for diagnosis of acute hepatitis C virus (HCV) infection as the etiology of her hepatitis.
E. CT scan of the chest would confirm the presence of septic pulmonary emboli.

IV-50. A 23-year-old college student is seen in the student health clinic for evaluation of multiple genital ulcers that he noted developing over the past week. They started as pustules and, after suppuration, are now ulcers. The ulcers are extremely tender and occasionally bleed. Examination shows multiple bilateral deep ulcers with purulent bases that bleed easily. They are exquisitely tender but are soft to palpation. Which of the following organisms is likely to be found on culture of the lesions?

A. *Haemophilus ducreyi*
B. Herpes simplex virus
C. HIV
D. *N gonorrhoeae*
E. *Treponema pallidum*

IV-51. A 21-year-old college student with no significant past medical history comes to the student health clinic reporting 1–2 days of malaise and 12 hours of worsening headache, fever, and mild neck stiffness. He is a varsity swimmer and takes no medications. He is heterosexually active and has had unprotected intercourse with four different partners in the last 6 months. His examination is notable for BP 110/60 mmHg, HR of 105 bpm, RR of 20 breaths/min, and temperature of 103.8°F. His mental status examination is entirely normal. There is pain on neck movement, but his neurologic and funduscopic examinations are unremarkable with no focal findings. Based on these findings, which of following is the most likely diagnosis?

A. Acute disseminated encephalomyelitis
B. Encephalopathy
C. Mass lesion
D. Meningoencephalitis
E. Viral meningitis

IV-52. All of the following are predisposing conditions that increase the risk for development of acute bacterial meningitis due to *S pneumoniae* EXCEPT:

A. Alcoholism
B. Pneumococcal pneumonia
C. Pneumococcal sinusitis
D. Pregnancy
E. Splenectomy

IV-53. A 28-year-old army recruit is brought to the local hospital with 12 hours of worsening headache and mild confusion. She has no significant past medical history, takes no medications, does not use cigarettes, alcohol, or illicit drugs, and is not recently sexually active. Over the past 1–2 days, she has had low-grade fever, malaise, dyspnea on exertion, and a productive cough. Her vital signs are as follows: BP 90/50 mmHg, HR 110 bpm, RR 24 breaths/min, oxygen saturation 88% on room air, and temperature 104°F. She is oriented to person and place, but thinks the year is 1999. Kernig and Brudzinski signs are positive, but the remainder of the neurologic examination shows no focal findings. There is no papilledema. Chest examination reveals bronchial breath sounds at the right base. Her abdomen and skin examinations are normal. Portable chest radiograph demonstrates a small right lower lobe infiltrate. All of the following medications should be administered immediately EXCEPT:

A. Acyclovir
B. Ampicillin
C. Ceftriaxone
D. Dexamethasone
E. Vancomycin

IV-54. A 45-year-old woman presents with an 8-week history of new-onset headache that is persistent and daily. She describes the pain as a diffuse ache and rates it 6–7 out of 10. It has been worsening over time. She had seen her primary doctor who reassured her that her physical examination was normal, and he prescribed ibuprofen 600 mg as needed for pain. This treatment did not alleviate her symptoms. Yesterday, she awoke with double vision and a facial droop. The patient lives in Pennsylvania and hikes frequently along the Appalachian Trial. She does not recall any tick bites. She has intermittently had joint pain over this past month. She denies rash. She presents to the emergency department for further evaluation. On physical examination, the patient has a temperature of 99.4°F. Vital signs are normal. Neurologic examination demonstrates a complete right facial droop. The left eye fails to abduct when looking laterally, although the right eye has full range of motion. Which of the following findings is most likely to be present in the cerebrospinal fluid?

A. Elevated angiotensin-converting enzyme level
B. Elevated neutrophil count
C. Elevated protein level
D. Low glucose
E. Positive VDRL (Venereal Disease Research Laboratory) test

IV-55. The use of an alcohol-based hand rub would be inadequate after leaving the room of which of the following patients?

A. A 20-year-old renal transplant recipient with varicella pneumonia
B. A 40-year-old man with MRSA furunculitis
C. A 35-year-old woman with advanced HIV and cavitary pulmonary tuberculosis
D. A 54-year-old quadriplegic man admitted with a UTI due to extended-spectrum β-lactamase–producing bacteria
E. A 78-year-old nursing home resident with recent antibiotic use and *C difficile* infection

IV-56. During the first 2 weeks following solid organ transplantation, which family of infection is most common?

A. Cytomegalovirus (CMV) and EBV reactivation
B. Humoral immunodeficiency–associated infections (e.g., meningococcemia, invasive *S pneumoniae* infection)
C. Neutropenia-associated infection (e.g., aspergillosis, candidemia)
D. T-cell deficiency–associated infections (e.g., *Pneumocystis jiroveci*, nocardiosis, cryptococcosis)
E. Typical hospital-acquired infections (e.g., central line infection, hospital-acquired pneumonia, UTI)

IV-57. A 22-year-old woman underwent cadaveric renal transplantation 3 months ago for congenital obstructive uropathy. After a demanding college exam schedule in which she forgot to take some of her medications for at least a week, she is admitted to the hospital with a temperature of 102°F, arthralgias, lymphopenia, and a rise in creatinine from her baseline of 1.2 mg/dL to 2.4 mg/dL. Which of the following medications did she most likely forget?

A. Acyclovir
B. Isoniazid
C. Itraconazole
D. Trimethoprim-sulfamethoxazole
E. Valganciclovir

IV-58. Which of the following pathogens are cardiac transplant patients at unique risk for acquiring from the donor heart early after transplant when compared to other solid organ transplant patients?

A. *Cryptococcus neoformans*
B. Cytomegalovirus
C. *P jiroveci*
D. *S aureus*
E. *Toxoplasma gondii*

IV-59. A 43-year-old woman undergoes allogeneic stem cell transplantation for acute myelogenous leukemia. Two weeks after the date of her transplantation, she is admitted to the hospital with a temperature of 101.1°F, pulse of 115 bpm, BP of 110/83 mmHg, and oxygen saturation of 89% on room air. Her WBC count is 0.5 thousand/μL, and 20% are polymorphonuclear cells. Because of hypoxia and infiltrates on plain chest radiograph, a CT scan is ordered. She is found to have diffuse nodules and masses, some with a halo sign. Which of the following tests is most likely to be diagnostic of her disease?

A. Microscopic exam of buffy coat
B. Plasma CMV viral load
C. Serum galactomannan antigen test
D. Sputum culture
E. Urine *Legionella* assay

IV-60–64. Match each class of antibiotic with its mechanism of action.

IV-60. Ampicillin

IV-61. Azithromycin

IV-62. Ciprofloxacin

IV-63. Tobramycin

IV-64. Trimethoprim-sulfamethoxazole

A. Binds to 30S ribosomal subunit of bacteria to inhibit protein synthesis
B. Binds to 50S ribosomal subunit of bacteria to inhibit protein synthesis
C. Inhibits cell wall synthesis by binding to transpeptidase enzymes involved in peptide cross-linking
D. Inhibits DNA gyrase and topoisomerase to inhibit DNA synthesis
E. Inhibits folate synthesis to disrupt bacterial

IV-65. A 48-year-old woman has been hospitalized for 30 days following a stabbing with penetrating chest and abdominal trauma. She had a right-sided hemopneumothorax as well as large bowel injury requiring hemicolectomy and hepatic contusion. She presented in hemodynamic shock and subsequently developed multiorgan failure due to septic shock. She remains critically ill on mechanical ventilation via a tracheostomy tube and on hemodialysis. She had been off vasopressors for 1 week but acutely became febrile over night with a drop in her BP to 72/38 mmHg and HR of 148 bpm. The patient has new infiltrates on chest radiograph and increased thick yellow secretions from her tracheostomy tube. Recently, the surgical intensive care unit has had multiple cases of *K pneumoniae* that produce an extended-spectrum β-lactamase (ESBL). Which of the following statements regarding the ESBL bacteria is true?

A. An ESBL-producing organism is unlikely to be the cause of the patient's recurrent sepsis because bacteria that produce ESBL rarely cause ventilator-associated pneumonia.
B. An ESBL-producing organism is unlikely to cause the patient's recurrent sepsis because the resistance mechanism does not promote easy transmission of organisms among patients within the intensive care unit.
C. The resistance mechanism in ESBL-producing bacteria is related to a genetic mutation that passes down generations.
D. The resistance mechanism in ESBL-producing organisms is plasmid-mediated and is easily passed among bacteria.

IV-66. In the patient described in Question IV-65, which of the following empiric antibiotics would have the most likely efficacy against a presumed ESBL infection?

A. Aztreonam
B. Cefazolin
C. Cefepime
D. Meropenem
E. Nafcillin

IV-67. A 22-year-old man with cystic fibrosis was admitted to the hospital for an exacerbation of his underlying disease. He is known to be colonized with *P aeruginosa*. His empiric antibiotic regimen is ceftazidime 2 g IV every 8 hours and tobramycin 10 mg/kg once daily. Which statement best describes the pharmacokinetics and pharmacodynamics of this combination of agents in the treatment of a patient with cystic fibrosis?

A. Aminoglycoside antibiotics such as tobramycin kill bacteria in a time-dependent fashion and thus need higher concentrations of antibiotics.
B. Assessing trough levels of aminoglycosides will help determine if the appropriate drug level to achieve optimal killing of organisms has occurred.
C. For β-lactam antibiotics, the duration of time with a concentration of drug above the minimal inhibitory concentration determines the killing effect.
D. Lower doses of antibiotics are typically required because cystic fibrosis patients have a higher volume of distribution of antibiotics.
E. Steady-state concentration of the drugs will be reached in three to four half-lives of the drug.

IV-68. A woman is 24 weeks pregnant with her first child. She develops a cellulitis in the right leg and requires antibiotic treatment. Which of the following antibiotics should not be used during the second and third trimesters of pregnancy?

A. Amoxicillin
B. Cephalexin
C. Clindamycin
D. Doxycycline
E. Penicillin

IV-69. A 73-year-old woman has recurrent UTIs. She is placed on suppressive antibiotic therapy by her primary physician. One year later, she is complaining of progressive dyspnea, and a chest radiograph shows development of pulmonary fibrosis. Which antibiotic could explain development of this complication?

A. Cefaclor
B. Cephalexin
C. Ciprofloxacin
D. Nitrofurantoin
E. Trimethoprim-sulfamethoxazole

IV-70. All of the following statements regarding pneumococcus (*S pneumoniae*) are true EXCEPT:

A. Asymptomatic colonization does not occur.
B. Infants (<2 years old) and the elderly are at greatest risk of invasive disease.
C. Pneumococcal vaccination has impacted the epidemiology of disease.
D. The likelihood of death within 24 hours of hospitalization for patients with invasive pneumococcal pneumonia has not changed since the introduction of antibiotics.
E. There is a clear association between prior viral upper respiratory infection and secondary pneumococcal pneumonia.

IV-71. You are examining a blood culture from a recently admitted 75-year-old man with fever. You note that the bacteria growing on the blood agar plate have produced a greenish color and seem to be inhibited by an optochin disc (pictured in Figure IV-71). They appear shiny. On microscopic examination, you note chains of spherical gram-positive organisms. On direct testing, you note a positive Quellung reaction. What bacteria are causing the patient's fever?

A. *P aeruginosa*
B. *S aureus*
C. *Staphylococcus epidermidis*
D. *S pneumoniae*
E. *S pyogenes*

IV-72. Which of the following statements regarding pneumococcal (*S pneumoniae*) pneumonia is true?

A. An infiltrate on chest radiograph is invariably present and required for diagnosis.
B. Blood cultures are positive in a minority of cases.
C. Pneumococcal pneumonia is unilobar in over 90% of cases.
D. The gold standard for etiologic diagnosis for pneumococcal pneumonia is sputum culture and Gram staining.
E. The high colonization rates of pneumococcus in adults prohibit the use of urinary pneumococcal antigen assays diagnostically.

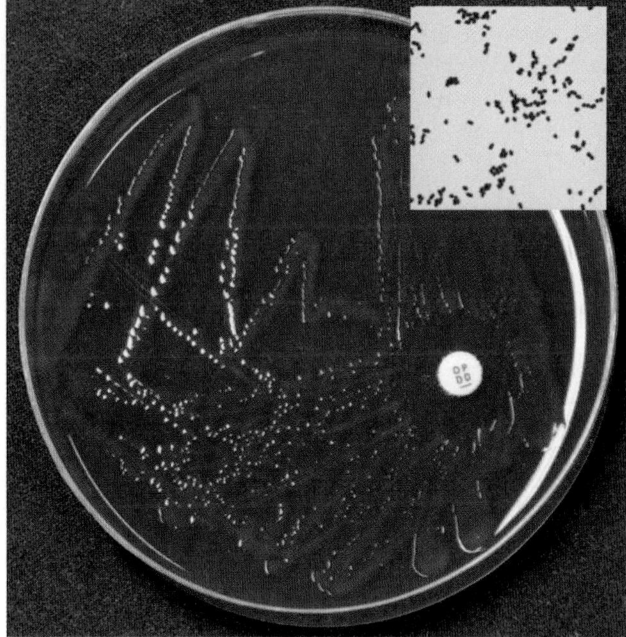

FIGURE IV-71 Photographs courtesy of Paul Turner, University of Oxford, United Kingdom.

IV-73. Which of the following statements regarding infections due to pneumococcus (*S pneumoniae*) is true?

A. An appropriate therapy for an adult believed to have pneumococcal meningitis is vancomycin in combination with ceftriaxone.
B. Azithromycin provides as much treatment efficacy for pneumococcal infections as amoxicillin.
C. Fluoroquinolone resistance has yet to be observed for pneumococcus.
D. For outpatient management of noninvasive pneumococcal infections, fluoroquinolones provide an efficacy advantage over amoxicillin.
E. Penicillin resistance has yet to be observed for pneumococcus.

IV-74. You are taking care of a 92-year-old man with a history of hypertension and prior transient ischemic attacks. He presented to the emergency department with 2 days of rigors and fever, along with shortness of breath and purulent sputum production. You collect an expectorated sputum sample and perform a Gram stain, visualizing the bacteria shown in Figure IV-74 under the microscope. The organisms are reported as catalase positive and produce coagulase and protein A. Which of the following organisms is likely responsible for this patient's infection?

A. *H influenzae*
B. *P aeruginosa*
C. *S aureus*
D. *S epidermidis*
E. *S pneumoniae*

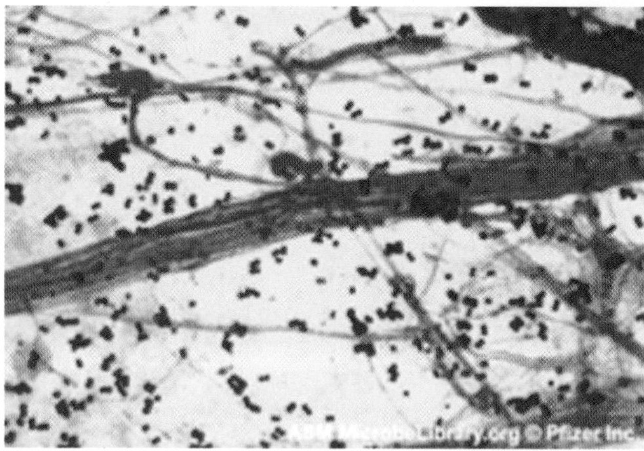

FIGURE IV-74 From ASM MicrobeLibrary.org.© Pfizer, Inc.

IV-75. Which of the following statements regarding *S aureus* is true?

A. Infections due to *S aureus* among colonized individuals are almost always due to a strain distinct from their colonizing strain.
B. *S aureus* is always a pathogen when detected in any human culture.
C. The anterior nares and oropharynx are the most common sites of colonization with *S aureus*.
D. The colonization rate in the population is independent of patient factors.
E. The majority of people in the United States are colonized with *S aureus*.

IV-76. Ms. Jung is an 18-year-old previously healthy woman who presents with fever and hypotension. On the morning of admission, she felt quite ill with fevers, rigors, nausea, vomiting, and diarrhea. As the day progressed, she developed redness of her skin all over and became lethargic and ultimately quite difficult to arouse. She has no notable past medical history and takes no medications. She does not use alcohol or illicit drugs and is not sexually active. Her parents brought her to the emergency department in the late afternoon where her BP was noted to be 70/50 mmHg, with a HR of 140 bpm, temperature of 39.5°C, and RR of 24 breaths/min. Oxygen saturation is 94% on room air. She is minimally responsive. Skin examination reveals generalized erythroderma but no signs of skin tears or infection. Genitourinary examination reveals a retained tampon that is immediately removed. Blood Gram stain and culture are negative at 12 hours. You suspect staphylococcal toxic shock syndrome (TSS). Which of the following statements regarding staphylococcal TSS is true?

A. A skin site infection is clinically apparent in most cases.
B. Blood cultures will likely return positive by 24–36 hours given her grave clinical presentation.
C. Desquamation of the skin will occur within 1–2 days.
D. High-dose IV penicillin should be started immediately.
E. It is caused by a toxin that binds to the invariant region of the major histocompatibility complex and directly stimulates T-cell replication.

IV-77. A 30-year-old healthy woman presents to the hospital with severe dyspnea, confusion, productive cough, and fevers. She had been ill 1 week prior with a flulike illness characterized by fever, myalgias, headache, and malaise. Her illness almost entirely improved without medical intervention until 36 hours ago, when she developed new rigors followed by progression of the respiratory symptoms. On initial examination, her temperature is 39.6°C, pulse is 130 bpm, BP is 95/60 mmHg, RR is 40 breaths/min, and oxygen saturation is 88% on 100% face mask. On examination, she is clammy, confused, and very dyspneic. Lung examination reveals amphoric breath sounds over her left lower lung fields. She is intubated and resuscitated with fluid and antibiotics. Chest CT scan reveals necrosis of her left lower lobe. Blood and sputum cultures grow *S aureus*. This isolate is likely to be resistant to which of the following antibiotics?

A. Doxycycline
B. Linezolid
C. Methicillin
D. Trimethoprim-sulfamethoxazole
E. Vancomycin

IV-78. Which of the following organisms is most likely to cause infection of a shunt implanted for the treatment of hydrocephalus?

A. *Bacteroides fragilis*
B. *Corynebacterium diphtheriae*
C. *E coli*
D. *S aureus*
E. *S epidermidis*

IV-79. A 42-year-old man with poorly controlled diabetes (hemoglobin A1C = 13.3%) presents with thigh pain and fever over several weeks. Physical examination reveals erythema and warmth over the thigh with notable woody nonpitting edema. There are no cutaneous ulcers. CT of the thigh reveals several abscesses located between the muscle fibers of the thigh. Orthopedics is consulted to drain and culture the abscesses. Which of the following is the most likely pathogen?

A. *Clostridium perfringens*
B. Group A *Streptococcus*
C. Polymicrobial flora
D. *S aureus*
E. *Streptococcus milleri*

IV-80. A 19-year-old woman from Guatemala presents to your office for a routine screening physical examination. At age 4 years, she was diagnosed with acute rheumatic fever. She does not recall the specifics of her illness and remembers only that she was required to be on bed rest for 6 months. She has remained on penicillin V orally at a dose of 250 mg twice a day since that time. She asks if she can safely discontinue this medication. She has had only one other flare of her disease, at age 8, when she stopped taking penicillin at the time of her emigration to the United States. She is currently working as a day care provider. Her physical examination is notable for normal point of maximal impulse (PMI) with a grade III/VI holosystolic murmur that is heard best at the apex of the heart and radiates to the axilla. What do you advise the patient to do?

A. An echocardiogram should be performed to determine the extent of valvular damage before deciding if penicillin can be discontinued.
B. Penicillin prophylaxis can be discontinued because she has had no flares in 5 years.
C. She should change her dosing regimen to intramuscular benzathine penicillin every 8 weeks.
D. She should continue on penicillin indefinitely as she had a previous recurrence, has presumed rheumatic heart disease, and is working in a field with high occupational exposure to group A *Streptococcus*.
E. She should replace penicillin prophylaxis with polyvalent pneumococcal vaccine every 5 years.

IV-81. A 36-year-old man is brought to the hospital by his wife because of a rapidly worsening skin infection. The patient has a history of type 1 diabetes, and his last documented hemoglobin A1C was 5.5%. His wife reports that he had a small insect bite on his calf a few days ago with some redness. Over the course of today, he has developed severe thigh pain initially with no redness, but over the last 1 hour, there has been worsening pain and swelling with some mottling of the skin. He also reports that he feels like his thigh and calf are numb. He is febrile and tachycardic. Physical examination reveals marked tenderness and tenseness of the right leg from the thigh down. There is some redness and mottling. A femoral and posterior tibial pulse are present. CT scan of the leg shows extensive inflammation of the fascial planes but no evidence of muscle inflammation. Which of the following organisms is most likely responsible for his infection?

A. *C difficile*
B. *S aureus*
C. *S epidermidis*
D. *S pneumoniae*
E. *S pyogenes*

IV-82. You are seeing a 17-year-old adolescent with no notable past medical history or medication allergies. He states that for the past 3 days, he has noticed an increasingly sore throat, cough, runny nose, and painful "knots" on his neck. On examination, he is afebrile, has pharyngeal erythema without exudate, and bilateral tender cervical adenopathy (nodes <1.5 cm). A rapid latex agglutination test for group A streptococci is negative. Which of the following statements is true?

A. Azithromycin orally should be initiated given the clinical suspicion for streptococcal pharyngitis.
B. If antibiotic therapy is initiated, a 5-day duration is generally sufficient.
C. Pharyngeal swab for culture should be performed.
D. The clinical scenario is classic for streptococcal pharyngitis.
E. The negative rapid test effectively rules out streptococcal pharyngitis.

IV-83. A 32-year-old woman with no medication allergies presents in active labor at 36 weeks of gestation. While her labor is progressing normally, you review her chart and note that a genitourinary culture for group B streptococci was not performed during this pregnancy, despite the fact that the patient had a previous child with infectious complications due to group B *Streptococcus*. What is the most appropriate course of action for this delivery?

A. Immediately perform a swab and rapid nucleic acid amplification test for group B *Streptococcus* to determine the need for treatment.
B. Initiate therapy with penicillin G.
C. Perform a perineal swab and gram stain. The presence of any gram-positive cocci should prompt antibiotic prophylaxis.
D. Provided that the patient does not have prolonged rupture of membranes or fever, no testing or treatment is required.

IV-84. Which of the following statements regarding the epidemiology of enterococcal infections is true?

A. Enterococcal infections are rare as a cause of nosocomial infections.
B. Human colonization with enterococci is rare.
C. Resistance to vancomycin among *Enterococcus faecium* isolates remains rare.
D. The majority of *Enterococcus faecalis* isolates are sensitive to β-lactams, particularly ampicillin.
E. The risk of mortality is equivalent among patients infected with vancomycin-resistant and vancomycin-susceptible strains of *Enterococcus*.

IV-85. Which of the following statements regarding enterococcal infections is true?

A. *E faecalis* is the most frequently isolated enteroccal species in surgical site infections.
B. Enterococci are the most common causative organisms in community-acquired endocarditis.
C. Most enterococcal UTIs occur de novo with no prior known underlying risk factor.
D. Poor dentition and gingival disease are the usual proximal sources for enterococcal bacteremia.
E. Presence of enterococci in a sterilely obtained urine culture invariably indicates infection and warrants treatment.

IV-86. A 74-year-old man with a recent history of diverticulitis is admitted to the hospital with 1 week of fever, malaise, and generalized weakness. His physical examination is notable for a temperature of 38.5°C, a new mitral heart murmur, and splinter hemorrhages. Three blood cultures grow *E faecalis*, and an echocardiogram shows a small vegetation on the mitral valve. The organism is reported as being sensitive to ampicillin with no high-level resistance to aminoglycosides. Based on this information, which of the following is recommended therapy?

A. Ampicillin
B. Ampicillin plus gentamicin
C. Daptomycin
D. Linezolid
E. Tigecycline

IV-87. Which of the following statements regarding *C diphtheriae* infections is true?

A. Alcoholism is a risk factor for adult diphtheria infections.
B. Birds and horses provide animal reservoirs for *C diphtheriae.*
C. Childhood vaccination imparts lifelong protective immunity to patients who receive the proper vaccination course.
D. Cutaneous diphtheria is almost always caused by a toxigenic strain.
E. Development of an effective vaccination has eliminated adult diphtheria infections in the United States.

IV-88. You are evaluating a 7-year-old boy in the emergency department who was brought from school for fever and sore throat. On examination, he has extensive submandibular and cervical swelling, foul breath, and a tenacious well-demarcated white/gray exudative substance adherent to his oropharynx (seen in Figure IV-88). Attempts to remove this pseudomembranous substance result in bleeding. A rapid strep test is negative. On asking for the patient's vaccination records, the school notes that he has not undergone routine vaccinations by parental choice. The patient is at risk for which of the following complications of this disease?

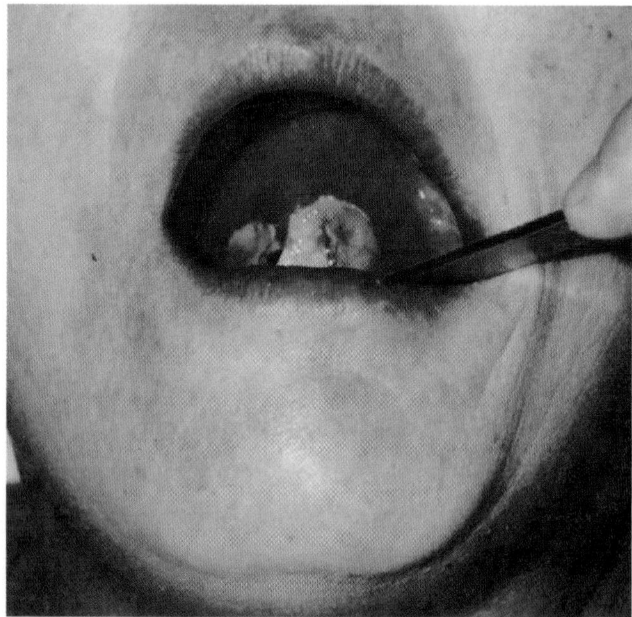

FIGURE IV-88 Photograph by P. Strebel, MD, used by permission. From R. Kadirova et al: *J Infect Dis* 181:S110, 2000. With permission of Oxford University Press.

A. Epidural abscess
B. Hepatitis
C. Meningitis
D. Myocarditis
E. Rheumatic fever

IV-89. You are caring for a 34-year-old pregnant woman with fever, backache, myalgias, headache, and bacteremia. Blood cultures show *Listeria monocytogenes,* and she is promptly initiated on appropriate antibiotic therapy. What mode of transmission is most likely the source of her listeriosis?

A. Aerosol person-to-person transmission
B. Fecal-oral route
C. Ingestion of contaminated food
D. Sexually transmitted
E. Waterborne

IV-90. An 84-year-old woman with diabetes mellitus and chronic kidney disease is admitted to the hospital for 2–4 days of altered mental status and headaches. She denies photophobia but does have mild neck stiffness. CT scan of the head reveals a 1-cm focal abscess in the right temporal lobe, and cerebrospinal fluid (CSF) analysis shows WBC count of 800/μL (75% polymorphonuclear leukocytes) with a low-normal glucose level. Gram stain of the CSF reveals gram-positive rods. Which of the following antibiotics is the most appropriate choice for this patient?

A. Ampicillin
B. Azithromycin
C. Cefazolin
D. Ciprofloxacin
E. Moxifloxacin

IV-91. A 26-year-old woman presents late in the third trimester of her pregnancy with high fevers, myalgias, backache, and malaise. She is admitted and started on empirical broad-spectrum antibiotics. Blood cultures return positive for *L monocytogenes*. She delivers a 5-lb infant 24 hours after admission. Which of the following statements regarding antibiotic treatment for this infection is true?

A. Clindamycin should be used in patients with penicillin allergy.
B. Neonates should receive weight-based ampicillin and gentamicin.
C. Penicillin plus gentamicin is first-line therapy for the mother.
D. Quinolones should be used for *Listeria* bacteremia in late-stage pregnancy.
E. Trimethoprim-sulfamethoxazole has no efficacy against *Listeria*.

IV-92. A 4-day-old female infant is brought emergently to the hospital after her parents noticed behavioral changes and shallow breathing. The infant was born by normal vaginal delivery after an uncomplicated full-term delivery and received normal antenatal care for 48 hours in the hospital, and hospital notes indicate that she had a normal suck and cry during her time inpatient. On examination, you note a generalized hypertonia and rigidity throughout the infant's body and occasional spasms. You note a foul-smelling brown material on and around the umbilical stump. Which of the following is true regarding the etiologic agent responsible for this infant's severe illness?

A. At the time of initial clinical presentation, death is most commonly due to cardiovascular complications with this disease.
B. Blood cultures will yield gram-positive rods.
C. Diagnosis of this illness requires laboratory confirmation of the causative organism.
D. The toxin responsible for this illness is active at the peripheral neuromuscular junctions.
E. The toxin responsible for this illness works by inhibiting inhibitory presynaptic neurons, leading to upregulated activity in the motor nervous system.

IV-93. A 64-year-old man with a long history of heroin abuse is brought to the hospital because of fever and worsening muscle spasms and pain over the last day. Because of longstanding venous sclerosis, he no longer injects intravenously but "skin-pops," often with dirty needles. On examination, he is extremely sweaty and febrile to 101.4°F. There are widespread muscle spasms including of the face. He is unable to open his jaw due to muscle spasm and has severe back pain due to diffuse spasm. On his leg, there is a skin wound that is tender and erythematous. All of the following statements regarding this patient are true EXCEPT:

A. Culture of the wound may reveal *Clostridium tetani.*
B. Intrathecal antitoxin administration is recommended therapy.
C. Metronidazole is recommended therapy.
D. Permanent muscle dysfunction is likely after recovery.
E. Strychnine poisoning and antidopaminergic drug toxicity should be ruled out.

IV-94. A 6-month-old male infant is brought emergently to the hospital for evaluation of altered behavior and cyanosis. On examination, he is taking only shallow respirations, and you note a flaccid muscle tone throughout. The parents note no preceding fever, cough, coryza, rash, or new medications. He had an uncomplicated pre- and antenatal course and was growing and progressing normally through his cognitive and motor milestones prior to this. He recently started eating soft and pureed foods including yogurt, pureed broccoli, spinach, carrots, and bananas with small amounts of added honey. He has had no scheduled vaccinations within the past month. Deep tendon reflexes are absent. Which of the following is the most likely cause of his presentation?

A. Botulinum toxicity
B. Guillain-Barré syndrome
C. Hypokalemic periodic paralysis
D. Tetanus toxicity
E. Tick paralysis

IV-95. A 34-year-old injection drug user presents with a 2-day history of slurred speech, blurry vision that is worse with bilateral gaze deviation, dry mouth, and difficulty swallowing both liquids and solids. He states that his arms feel weak as well but denies any sensory deficits. He has had no recent illness but does describe a chronic ulcer on his left lower leg that has felt slightly warm and tender of late. He frequently injects heroin into the edges of the ulcer. On review of systems, he reports mild shortness of breath but denies any gastrointestinal symptoms, urinary retention, or loss of bowel or bladder continence. Physical examination reveals a frustrated, non–toxic-appearing man who is alert and oriented but noticeably dysarthric. He is afebrile with stable vital signs. Cranial nerve examination reveals bilateral cranial nerve VI deficits and an inability to maintain medial gaze in both eyes. He has mild bilateral ptosis, and both pupils are reactive but sluggish. His strength is 5/5 in all extremities except for his shoulder shrug, which is 4/5. Sensory examination and deep tendon reflexes are within normal limits in all four extremities. His oropharynx is dry. Cardiopulmonary and abdominal examinations are normal. He has a 4 cm × 5 cm well-granulated lower extremity ulcer with redness, warmth, and erythema noted on the upper margin of the ulcer. What is the treatment of choice?

A. Glucocorticoids
B. Equine antitoxin to *Clostridium botulinum* neurotoxin
C. IV heparin
D. Naltrexone
E. Plasmapheresis

IV-96. You are a medical resident completing a clinical rotation in Papua New Guinea. Today, two adults present only hours apart to the emergency department with remarkably similar cases. Both had attended a pig feast yesterday and awoke today with excruciating abdominal pain. Both CT scans show extensive necrosis of the intestinal wall, most severely in the jejunum. The causative organism of these infections is also most commonly causative in cases of which of the following?

A. Cellulitis
B. Gas gangrene myonecrosis
C. Meningitis
D. Pharyngitis
E. Pneumonia

IV-97. A 19-year-old man presents to the emergency department with 4 days of watery diarrhea, nausea, vomiting, and low-grade fever. He recalls no unusual meals, sick contacts, or travel. He is hydrated with IV fluid, given antiemetics, and discharged home after feeling much better. Three days later, two out of three blood cultures are positive for *C perfringens*. He is called at home and says that he feels fine and is back to work. What should your next instruction to the patient be?

A. Reassurance
B. Return for IV penicillin therapy
C. Return for IV penicillin therapy plus echocardiogram
D. Return for IV penicillin therapy plus colonoscopy
E. Return for surveillance blood culture

IV-98. During your freshman year of college, you perform an experiment for your microbiology class. You obtain nasopharyngeal swab cultures on your roommates to analyze the colonizing bacteria there. You find that one of your roommates has evidence of *N meningitidis* from his culture. When he returns from class, he says he has been feeling fine. He does not think he has been vaccinated against meningococcus. What treatment, if any, should this student receive?

A. Ceftriaxone 1 g intramuscularly
B. Mupirocin cream to the bilateral nares twice daily
C. Quadrivalent meningococcal vaccine
D. Admit to the hospital for IV ceftriaxone 2 g daily for 14 days
E. No action

IV-99. A 21-year-old college student is admitted to the hospital with meningitis. CSF cultures reveal *N meningitides* type B. The patient lives in a dormitory suite with five other students. Which of the following is recommended for the close household contacts?

A. Culture all close contacts and offer prophylaxis to those with positive cultures
B. Immediate administration of ceftriaxone to all close contacts
C. Immediate administration of rifampin to all close contacts
D. Immediate vaccination with conjugate vaccine
E. No therapy necessary

IV-100. Which of the following is the most common clinical manifestation of *N meningitidis* infection?

A. Asymptomatic nasopharyngeal colonization
B. Chronic meningitis
C. Meningitis
D. Petechial or purpuric rash
E. Septicemia

IV-101. Ms. Jones is a 27-year-old telephone repair technician who is 4 months pregnant. She is sexually active with her boyfriend. For the past 2 days, she has been experiencing dysuria and vaginal discharge. Gram stain of her vaginal discharge is shown in Figure IV-101. She has no known medication allergies. Which of the following is the most reasonable medical regimen for the treatment of her infection?

A. Ceftriaxone 250 mg intramuscularly (IM) once
B. Ceftriaxone 250 mg IM and azithromycin 1 g orally once
C. Ceftriaxone 250 mg IM and doxycycline 100 mg orally once
D. Ciprofloxacin 500 mg twice daily for 10 days
E. Vancomycin 1 g daily for 7 days

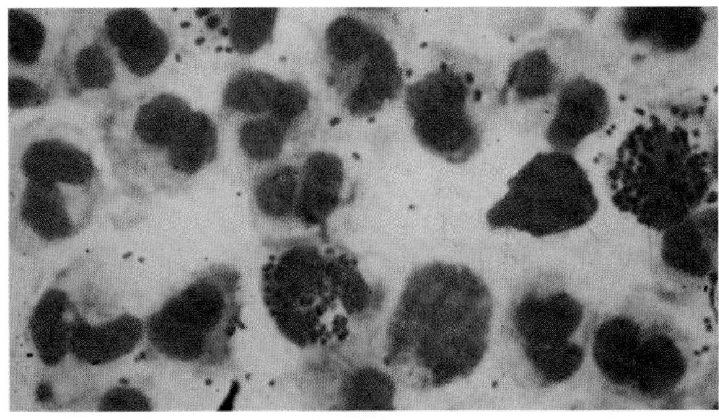

FIGURE IV-101 From the Public Health Agency of Canada. © All rights reserved. Reproduced with permission from the Minister of Health, 2016.

IV-102. A 27-year-old man presents to the hospital with fever, chills, and migratory polyarthralgias. You note skin lesions including papules and pustules with a hemorrhagic component on the extremities (pictured in Figure IV-102). Aspiration of a painful knee reveals gram-negative diplococci, and you make the diagnosis of disseminated gonococcal infection/arthritis (DGI). Oddly, this is his second bout of DGI in the past 2 years. What immunodeficiency should be particularly screened for in this patient?

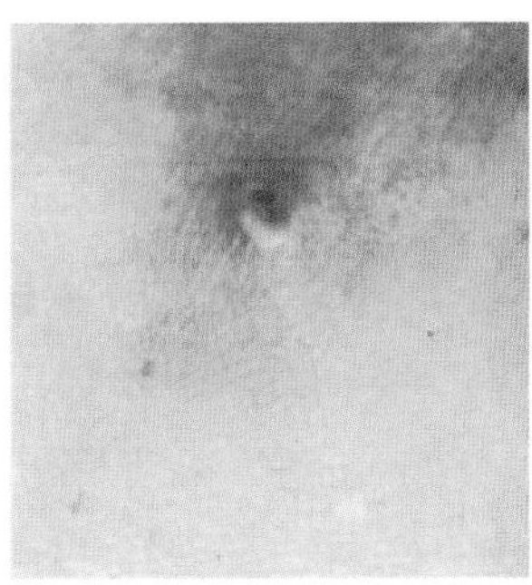

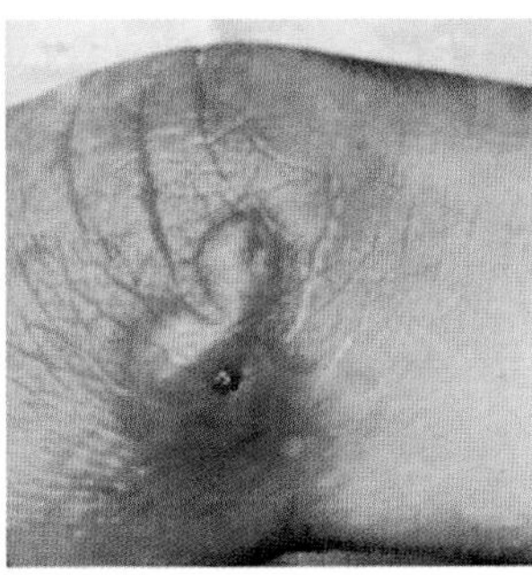

FIGURE IV-102 Reprinted with permission from KK Holmes et al: Disseminated gonococcal infection. *Ann Intern Med* 74:979, 1971.

A. Chédiak-Higashi syndrome
B. Common variable immunodeficiency
C. Leukemia
D. Neutropenia
E. Total hemolytic complement activity

IV-103. Which of the following is the most common bacterial cause of chronic obstructive pulmonary disease exacerbations?

A. *S pneumoniae*
B. *Moraxella catarrhalis*
C. *P aeruginosa*
D. Nontypable *H influenzae*
E. *Acinetobacter* species

IV-104. A 44-year-old man presents to the emergency department for evaluation of a severe sore throat. His symptoms began this morning with mild irritation on swallowing and have gotten progressively severe over the course of 12 hours. He has been experiencing a fever to as high as 39°C at home and also reports progressive shortness of breath. He denies antecedent rhinorrhea or tooth or jaw pain. He has had no ill contacts. On physical examination, the patient appears flushed and in respiratory distress with use of accessory muscles of respiration. Inspiratory stridor is present. He is sitting leaning forward and is drooling with his neck extended. His vital signs are as follows: temperature 39.5°C, BP 116/60 mmHg, HR 118 bpm, RR 24 breaths/min, and SaO_2 95% on room air. Examination of his oropharynx shows erythema of the posterior oropharynx without exudates or tonsillar enlargement. The uvula is midline. There is no sinus tenderness and no cervical lymphadenopathy. His lung fields are clear to auscultation, and cardiovascular examination reveals a regular tachycardia with a II/VI systolic ejection murmur heard at the upper right sternal border. Abdominal, extremity, and neurologic examinations are normal. Laboratory studies reveal a WBC count of 17,000/μL with a differential of 87% neutrophil, 8% band forms, 4% lymphocytes, and 1% monocytes. Hemoglobin is 13.4 g/dL, with a hematocrit of 44.2%. An arterial blood gas on room air has a pH of 7.32, a partial pressure of carbon dioxide (PCO_2) of 48 mmHg, and a partial pressure of oxygen (PO_2) of 92 mmHg. A lateral neck film shows an edematous epiglottis. What is the next most appropriate step in evaluation and treatment of this individual?

A. Ampicillin 500 mg IV every 6 hours
B. Ceftriaxone 1 g IV every 24 hours
C. Endotracheal intubation and ampicillin 500 mg IV every 6 hours
D. Endotracheal intubation, ceftriaxone 1 g IV every 24 hours, and clindamycin 600 mg IV every 6 hours
E. Laryngoscopy and close observation

IV-105. All of the following statements regarding the HACEK organisms are true EXCEPT:

A. HACEK-associated endocarditis tends to occur in younger patients than non-HACEK endocarditis.
B. HACEK organisms require an oxygen-enriched environment for growth.
C. Most cultures that ultimately yield a HACEK organism become positive within the first week.
D. The most common clinical manifestation of the HACEK organisms is endocarditis.
E. They are fastidious slow-growing organisms.

IV-106. A 38-year-old woman with frequent hospital admissions related to alcoholism comes to the emergency department after being bitten by a dog. There are open wounds on her arms and right hand that are purulent and have necrotic borders. She is hypotensive and is admitted to the intensive care unit. She is found to have disseminated intravascular coagulation and soon develops multiorgan failure. Which of the following is the most likely organism to have caused her rapid decline?

A. *Aeromonas* spp
B. *Capnocytophaga* spp
C. *Eikenella* spp
D. *Haemophilus* spp
E. *Staphylococcus* spp

IV-1-7. *Legionella* outbreaks are usually tied to which of the following?

A. A significant population of unvaccinated individuals
B. Bioterrorism attacks
C. Contaminated aquatic reservoir
D. Equine animal reservoir and zoonotic transmission
E. Surgical wound infections

IV-108. Which of the following statements regarding is *Legionella* pneumonia (Legionnaires' disease) is true?

A. Gastrointestinal complaints are more common in Legionnaires' disease than other types of bacterial pneumonia.
B. Hypernatremia is common in patients with Legionnaires' disease.
C. Most patients with Legionnaires' disease do not have fever.
D. Myocarditis is the most severe extrapulmonary sequela of Legionnaires' disease.
E. The prognosis of Legionnaires' disease is similar to that of other "atypical" pneumonias.

IV-109. A 56-year-old man with a history of hypertension and cigarette smoking is admitted to the intensive care unit after 1 week of fever and nonproductive cough. Imaging shows a new pulmonary infiltrate, and urine antigen test for *Legionella* is positive. Each of the following is likely to be an effective antibiotic EXCEPT:

A. Azithromycin
B. Aztreonam
C. Levofloxacin
D. Tigecycline
E. Trimethoprim-sulfamethoxazole

IV-110. A 72-year-old woman is admitted to the intensive care unit with respiratory failure. She has fever, obtundation, and bilateral parenchymal consolidation on chest imaging. Her family notes 3–4 days of abdominal pain, nausea, and vomiting prompting strong consideration of *Legionella* pneumonia. Which of the following is true regarding the diagnosis of *Legionella* pneumonia?

A. Acute and convalescent antibodies are not helpful due to the presence of multiple serotypes.
B. *Legionella* can never be seen on a Gram stain.
C. *Legionella* cultures grow rapidly on the proper media.
D. *Legionella* urinary antigen maintains utility after antibiotic use.
E. PCR for *Legionella* DNA is the "gold standard" diagnostic test.

IV-111. Which of the following statements regarding the epidemiology of pertussis infection is true?

A. Completing the pertussis vaccination series confers lifelong immunity for immune-competent patients.
B. In North America, pertussis infection rates are highest in summer and autumn.
C. Pertussis infection rates have remained relatively stable year to year after the widespread adoption of vaccination.
D. Pertussis is uniquely a disease of childhood; adults and adolescents suffer no symptoms from pertussis infection.
E. Worldwide vaccination has made infant mortality from pertussis exceedingly rare globally.

IV-112. An 18-year-old man seeks attention for a severe cough. He reports no past medical history and excellent health. Approximately 7 days ago, he developed an upper respiratory syndrome with low-grade fever, coryza, some cough, and malaise. The fever and coryza have improved but over the last 2 days, but he has an episodic cough that is often severe enough to result in vomiting. He reports receiving all infant vaccinations, but only tetanus in the last 12 years. He is afebrile, and while not coughing, his chest examination is normal. During a coughing episode, there is an occasional inspiratory whoop. Chest radiograph is unremarkable. Which of the following is true regarding his likely illness?

A. A fluoroquinolone is recommended therapy.
B. Cold agglutinins may be positive.
C. Nasopharyngeal aspirate for DNA testing is likely to be diagnostic.
D. Pneumonia is a common complication.
E. Urinary antigen testing remains positive for up to 3 months.

IV-113. In healthy individuals, which of the following bacteria species is the predominant gram-negative bacillus in the colonic flora?

A. *Klebsiella*
B. *Proteus*
C. *E coli*
D. *Staphylococcus*
E. *Clostridium*

IV-114. A 54-year-old man with a history of alcohol abuse and hepatic cirrhosis presents to the emergency department after being found unconscious in his apartment by his next-door neighbors. On presentation, his temperature is 34.7°C, HR is 120 bpm, and BP is 77/45 mmHg. He is jaundiced, and abdominal exam reveals a small liver span and moderate ascites. Early laboratory results include an elevated serum and ascitic fluid WBC count, both with a neutrophilic predominance. Gram stain on the ascitic fluid rapidly returns positive for gram-negative bacilli. You suspect that the patient is suffering from gram-negative sepsis with bacterial peritonitis as an initial source. Of the following choices, which antibiotic choice is most appropriate for initial therapy?

A. Imipenem
B. Penicillin G
C. Tigecycline
D. Trimethoprim-sulfamethoxazole
E. Vancomycin

IV-115. Ms. Posada is a 32-year-old sexually active woman with no past medical history. She presents to your acute care clinic with a complaint of burning urination for the past 4 days. Yesterday, she noticed that her left flank and her back were also painful, and she began having fevers up to 102°F. She has three sexual partners and frequently has unprotected vaginal intercourse with them, although she does not consider any of them high risk for sexually transmitted infections. Her examination is notable for temperature of 39°C, HR of 105 bpm, and BP of 105/65 mmHg, left costophrenic angle tenderness, and an otherwise benign abdominal/pelvic examination. Clean catch urinalysis shows positive leukocyte esterase, a high WBC count, and no epithelial cells. You suspect pyelonephritis. Which of the following organisms is the most common cause of this infection?

A. *E coli*
B. *Klebsiella oxytoca*
C. *Proteus mirabilis*
D. *S aureus*
E. *Staphylococcus saprophyticus*

IV-116. All of the following statements regarding intestinal disease caused by strains of Shiga toxin–producing and enterohemorrhagic *E coli* are true EXCEPT:

A. Antibiotic therapy lessens the risk of developing hemolytic-uremic syndrome.
B. Ground beef is the most common source of contamination.
C. Gross bloody diarrhea without fever is the most common clinical manifestation.
D. Infection is more common in industrialized than developing countries.
E. O157:H7 is the most common serotype.

IV-117. You are a medical resident partaking in a visiting clinical rotation in Vietnam. Today, a 54-year-old man presented to the local hospital with agonizing abdominal pain, fever, chills, jaundice, and hypotension. He is resuscitated in the intensive care unit, and CT of the abdomen reveals the striking abnormalities denoted by the red and black arrows in Figure IV-117. Your very experienced intensivist attending tells you that the epidemiology of this infection has changed recently in this part of the world. Which of the following organisms is now the most likely etiologic agent in this infection?

A. *C difficile*
B. ESBL-producing *Salmonella*
C. *E coli*
D. Hypervirulent *K pneumoniae*
E. *S aureus*

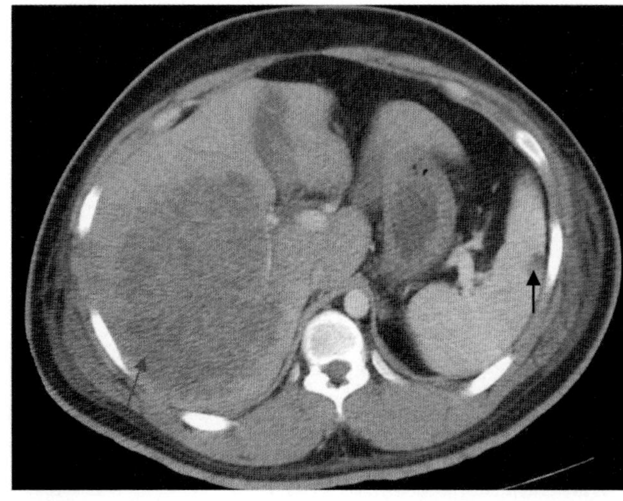

FIGURE IV-117 Courtesy of Drs. Chiu-Bin Hsaio and Diana Pomakova.

IV-118. A 63-year-old man has been in the intensive care unit for 3 weeks with slowly resolving acute respiratory distress syndrome after an episode of acute pancreatitis. He remains on mechanical ventilation through a tracheostomy. Over the last week, he has had gradual lessening of his mechanical ventilator needs and slight improvement of his radiograph. He has been afebrile with a normal WBC for the last 10 days. Over the last 24 hours, his FiO_2 has been increased from 0.60 to 0.80 to maintain adequate oxygenation. In addition, he has developed newly purulent sputum with a right lower lobe infiltrate, fever to 101.5°C, and a rising WBC. Sputum Gram stain shows gram-negative plump coccobacilli that are identified as *Acinetobacter baumannii*. All of the following statements regarding infections due to this organism are true EXCEPT:

A. It is a growing cause of hospital-acquired pneumonia and bloodstream infections in the United States.
B. It is not yet a significant problem in Asia/Australia.
C. Mortality from bloodstream infection approaches 40%.
D. Multidrug resistance is characteristic.
E. Tigecycline is the treatment of choice for bloodstream infection.

IV-119. You are taking care of Mrs. Brosius, a 74-year-old woman who was admitted to the intensive care unit 12 days prior with a chronic obstructive pulmonary disease exacerbation. Unfortunately, she has remained dependent on mechanical ventilation and is still sedated and intubated. Today, her nurse noted that her tracheal suction secretions have increased in volume and tenacity, and a chest x-ray confirms a new infiltrate. Laboratory values reveal a rising serum WBC count, and her oxygen requirement has increased slightly. Sputum culture confirms *A baumannii*. You know that this is a particularly difficult organism to treat due to which of the following properties?

A. Chronic carrier status in the biliary system of many critically ill patients
B. The ability to acquire or upregulate a wide range of antibiotic resistance determinants
C. The ability to form antibiotic-resistants spores
D. The ability to form biofilms that are nearly impenetrable to most antibiotics
E. Very slow growth requiring long courses (>4 weeks) of antibiotics

IV-120. You are conducting a research study to determine if socioeconomic status is correlated with *Helicobacter pylori* colonization. Today, your subject is a 35-year-old high school teacher. The subject drinks a solution of urea labeled with nonradioactive ^{13}C isotope. He then blows into a tube. Your instruments detect carbon dioxide containing ^{13}C. Which of the following is true regarding this patient?

A. Histologic examination of gastric tissue is unlikely to reveal gastritis in this patient.
B. The results of this test indicate that this patient has a higher risk of gastric adenocarcinoma.
C. The same test performed a year later in the absence of treatment will likely not detect carbon dioxide containing ^{13}C in the patient's exhalation.
D. This patient has a higher risk of colon cancer.
E. This patient is not colonized with *H pylori*.

IV-121. One month after receiving a 14-day course of omeprazole, clarithromycin, and amoxicillin for *H pylori*–associated gastric ulcer disease, a 44-year-old woman still has mild dyspepsia and pain after meals. What is the appropriate next step in management?

A. Empirical long-term proton pump inhibitor therapy
B. Endoscopy with biopsy to rule out gastric adenocarcinoma
C. *H pylori* serology testing
D. Second-line therapy for *H pylori* with omeprazole, bismuth subsalicylate, tetracycline, and metronidazole
E. Urea breath test

IV-122. A 42-year-old man with heme occult-positive stools and a history of epigastric pain is found to have a duodenal ulcer that is biopsy-proven positive for *H pylori*. All of the following are effective eradication regimens EXCEPT:

A. Amoxicillin and levofloxacin for 10 days
B. Omeprazole, clarithromycin, and metronidazole for 14 days
C. Omeprazole, clarithromycin, and amoxicillin for 14 days
D. Omeprazole, bismuth, tetracycline, and metronidazole for 14 days
E. Omeprazole, amoxicillin for 5 days followed by omeprazole, clarithromycin, and tinidazole for 5 days

IV-123. Ms. Murdock is a 67-year-old smoker who is being treated in the intensive care unit for a severe community-acquired pneumonia. She continues to require intubation and mechanical ventilation despite 8 days of therapy with meropenem and azithromycin. Her temperature today on rounds is reported as 38.5°C, which is notable as she has been afebrile for the past 6 days. Also, her sputum production has increased. Sputum cultures obtained through the endotracheal tube reveal *Stenotrophomonas maltophilia*. Which of the following is true regarding this patient and *S maltophilia*?

A. It is almost certain that this organism is a colonizer and not a pathogen; therapy specific for *S maltophilia* is not warranted.
B. *S maltophilia* is almost universally susceptible to most antibiotic classes; meropenem continuation should effectively eradicate this organism.
C. *S maltophilia* is an important cause of community-acquired pneumonia.
D. *S maltophilia* is found in aquatic reservoirs in nature.
E. Treatment is warranted and should be initiated with a combination of trimethoprim-sulfamethoxazole and ticarcillin-clavulanate.

IV-124. You are taking care of Mr. Tanaka, an 18-year-old baseball player undergoing a myeloablative bone marrow transplant for acute myelogenous leukemia. He is day 2 after transplantation and remains deeply neutropenic. While you are on call, you receive a page that he has spiked a fever to 38.7°C. You immediately order blood, urine, and sputum cultures and initiate appropriate antibiotic coverage. In cases of febrile neutropenia worldwide, which single organism causes a larger proportion of infections in febrile neutropenic patients than any other single organism and necessitates consideration when choosing empiric antibiotic coverage?

A. *Candida albicans*
B. *E coli*
C. *P aeruginosa*
D. *S aureus*
E. *S pneumoniae*

IV-125. A sputum culture from a patient with cystic fibrosis showing which of the following organisms has been associated with a rapid decline in pulmonary function and a poor clinical prognosis?

A. *Burkholderia cepacia*
B. *P aeruginosa*
C. *S aureus*
D. *S epidermidis*
E. *S maltophilia*

IV-126. You are taking care of a 65-year-old zoo employee who presents with fever and diarrhea. Ultimately, you diagnose her with nontyphoidal salmonellosis. You know that she must have contracted the infection via what route?

A. Contact with contaminated fomites
B. Oral ingestion of organisms
C. Respiratory secretions
D. Sexually transmitted
E. Any of the above routes

IV-127. You are caring for Mr. Munoz, a previously healthy 65-year-old man who was admitted to the hospital yesterday after having fevers for a week at home. He states that he just got off vacation where he traveled through South Asia, visiting India, Malaysia, and Thailand. He denied any risky sexual or gastronomic behaviors during his travels. On admission, his temperature was 39.7°C, HR was 68 bpm, and BP was 110/60 mmHg. Examination of his skin reveals a faint, salmon-colored, blanching, maculopapular rash located primarily on the trunk and chest, pictured in Figure IV-127. He complains of moderate abdominal pain and nausea. While blood culture reveals no organisms, bone marrow culture grows gram-negative rods. The bacteria produce acid on glucose fermentation, reduce nitrates, and do not produce cytochrome oxidase or ferment lactose. Closer inspection shows that they are motile by means of flagella. Which of the following organisms is Mr. Munoz most likely infected with?

A. *C difficile*
B. *Entamoeba histolytica*
C. *E coli*
D. *K pneumoniae*
E. *S typhi*

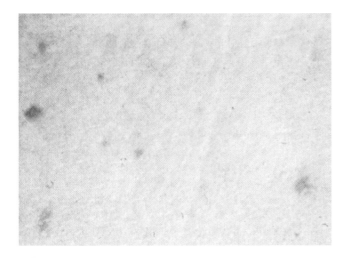

FIGURE IV-127

IV-128. 128. Five healthy college roommates develop rapid (<8 hours) onset of abdominal pain, cramping, fever to 38.5°C, vomiting, and copious nonbloody diarrhea while camping. They immediately return for hydration and diagnosis. A stool culture grows *Salmonella enteritidis.* All of the following statements regarding their clinical syndrome are true EXCEPT:

A. Antibiotic therapy is not indicated.
B. Bacteremia occurs in less than 10% of cases.
C. The most likely source was undercooked eggs.
D. There is no vaccine available for this illness.
E. They have enteric (typhoid) fever.

IV-129. Two days after returning from a trip to Thailand, a 36-year-old woman develops severe crampy abdominal pain, fever to 40°C, nausea, and malaise. The next day, she begins having bloody mucopurulent diarrhea with worsening abdominal pain and continued fever. She reports she was in Bangkok during monsoonal flooding and ate fresh food from stalls. A stool examination shows many neutrophils, and culture grows *Shigella flexneri.* Which of the following statements regarding her clinical syndrome is true?

A. An effective vaccine for travelers is available.
B. Antibiotic therapy prolongs the carrier state and should not be administered unless she develops bacteremia.
C. Antimotility agents are effective in reducing the risk of dehydration.
D. Ciprofloxacin is recommended therapy.
E. Her disease can be distinguished from illness due to *Campylobacter jejuni* on clinical grounds by the presence of fever.

IV-130. A 45-year-old healthy businessman just returned from a trip to Vietnam where he was traveling on vacation. Five days after his return, he developed fever and a headache followed 12 hours later by diarrhea and abdominal pain. The next day, he had >10 bowel movements in 12 hours, the final two with gross blood in the stool, prompting his presentation to the emergency department. His vital signs are as follows: temperature 37.8°C, HR 90 bpm, RR 14 breaths/min, and oxygen saturation 98% on room air. Gram stain of a stool specimen identifies a small curved helical-shaped gram-negative rod. You suspect a *Campylobacter* spp. Which of the following statements regarding his most likely infection is true?

A. A single dose of azithromycin is effective therapy.
B. Antibiotics are not helpful. He should receive supportive fluid and electrolyte repletion.
C. Ciprofloxacin for 7 days is the therapy of choice.
D. If the *Campylobacter* subtype is *jejuni*, the patient should be monitored closely for systemic infection and distal organ involvement (seeding).
E. The *Campylobacter* subtype *fetus* carries a more favorable prognosis than other subtypes.

IV-131. You are leading a medical aid team in a country in central Africa when a cholera epidemic strikes a nearby village. As you ride to the village to assist in caring for the ill, one of the medical students on your team asks what causes the severe diarrhea. Which of the following statements regarding diarrhea in cholera is true?

A. Cholera toxin causes a disruption in the adenylate cyclase pathway in the intestinal epithelial cells.
B. Diarrhea in cholera is due to massive neutrophilic colonic inflammation.
C. Diarrhea due to cholera occurs due to an inability of the intestine to absorb glucose.
D. Fever often precedes the onset of diarrhea in cholera.
E. The stool in cholera diarrhea is often dark brown or black.

IV-132. While you are caring for villagers stricken with cholera in Central Africa, you encounter Mr. Zi, a 22-year-old truck driver with cholera. He has the typical rice-water stools and has had seven bowel movements today before noon. He is thirsty but is able to hold a coherent conversation with you and can stand up without feeling lightheaded. His HR is 87 bpm, and BP is 105/70 mmHg. What is the most appropriate treatment for Mr. Zi?

A. Erythromycin 250 mg orally four times daily for 3 days
B. IV fluid replacement with normal saline 100 mL/kg over 3 hours
C. IV fluid replacement with lactated Ringer's solution 100 mg/kg over 3 hours
D. Mix 0.5 teaspoon of table salt and 6 teaspoons of table sugar with 1 L of sterile water and have the patient drink up to 2 L of this solution daily
E. No treatment is necessary

IV-133. Mr. Hou is a 56-year-old former pig farmer from China who has been in the United States for the past year visiting his sister. Shortly after arriving, he began experiencing fevers. Curiously, he has noted that while the fever has persisted for a year, it has followed the unusual undulating pattern. The fever would usually last for 2 weeks and then relent for about 2 weeks at a time before returning. He also experienced joint pains and myalgias during his times of fever. More recently, he has experienced lower back pain with movement and at rest. He denies any weakness or numbness. A serologic investigation returns positive for immunoglobulin (Ig) G antibodies for *Brucella*. Which of the following statements regarding his condition is true?

A. A safe and effective human vaccine is available for brucellosis.
B. In this patient, *Brucella melitensis* is more likely than *Brucella suis*.
C. Prior to starting treatment, coinfection with tuberculosis should be excluded.
D. The presence of IgG antibodies is nonspecific. Given the atypical presentation, this likely is not a true *Brucella* infection
E. With appropriate treatment, the patient's relapse rate from his disease is 1%–2%.

IV-134. A 45-year-old man from western Kentucky presents to the emergency department in September complaining of fevers, headaches, and muscle pains. He recently had been on a camping trip with several friends during which they hunted for their food, including fish, squirrels, and rabbits. He did not recall any tick bites during the trip, but does recall having several mosquito bites. For the past week, he has had an ulceration on his right hand with redness and pain surrounding it. He also has noticed some pain and swelling near his right elbow. None of the friends he camped with have been similarly ill. His vital signs are as follows: BP 106/65 mmHg, HR 116 bpm, RR 24 breaths/min, and temperature 38.7°C. His oxygen saturation is 93% on room air. He appears mildly tachypneic and flushed. His conjunctiva are not injected, and his mucous membranes are dry. The chest examination reveals crackles in the right mid-lung field and left base. His heart rate is tachycardic but regular. There is a II/VI systolic ejection murmur heard best at the lower left sternal border. His abdominal examination is unremarkable. On the right hand, there is an erythematous ulcer with a punched-out center covered by a black eschar. He has no cervical lymphadenopathy, but there are markedly enlarged and tender lymph nodes in the right axillae and epitrochlear regions. The epitrochlear node has some fluctuance with palpation. A chest x-ray shows fluffy bilateral alveolar infiltrates. Over the first 12 hours of his hospitalization, the patient becomes progressively hypotensive and hypoxic, requiring intubation and mechanical ventilation. What is the most appropriate therapy for this patient?

A. Ampicillin 2 g IV every 6 hours
B. Ceftriaxone 1 g IV daily
C. Ciprofloxacin 400 mg IV twice daily
D. Doxycycline 100 mg IV twice daily
E. Gentamicin 5 mg/kg twice daily

IV-135. You are working as a physician in northern New Mexico when a case of human infection with *Yersinia pestis* is reported in a nearby hospital. You know that this patient most likely contracted the disease through what method?

A. Consumption of undercooked beef, pork, or mutton
B. Direct handling of an infected small mammal
C. Direct bite from an infected wild carnivore
D. Fleabite
E. Person-to-person contact

IV-136. You are seeing a 19-year-old undergraduate student in your office in northern New Mexico for left axillary pain. During the current summer break, he is assisting one of his University professors in research that involves trapping, tagging, and releasing prairie dogs. Today, he presents with fever (38.7°C), malaise, myalgias, and exquisite left axillary pain. On examination, he is uncomfortable, and his left axilla has a tender swelling with a boggy consistency and a hard core. There is an eschar in the patient's left upper abdominal quadrant (Figure IV-136A). Gram stain of an aspirate of this swelling is shown in Figure IV-136B. What organism is responsible for this patient's infection?

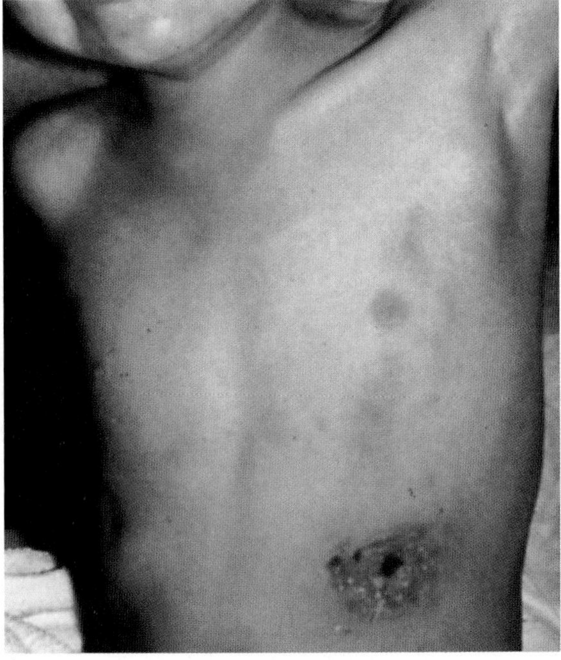

A

FIGURE IV-136A Reprinted with permission from *Harrison's Principles of Internal Medicine*, 17th ed, AS Fauci et al (eds). New York, NY: McGraw-Hill, Chap. 152, 2008.

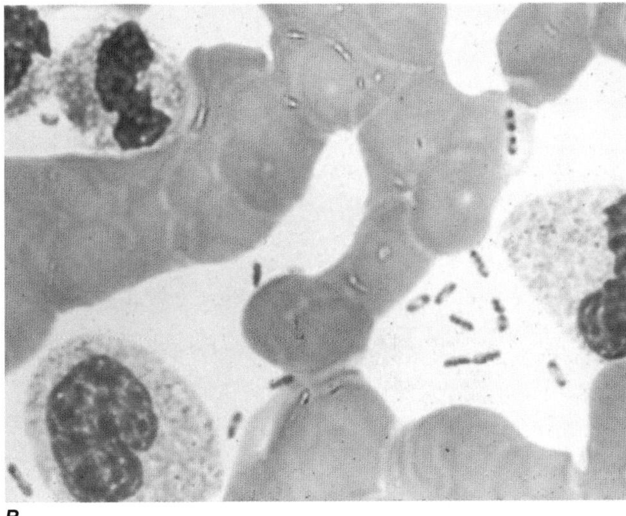

B

FIGURE IV-136B Reprinted with permission from *Harrison's Principles of Internal Medicine*, 17th ed, AS Fauci et al (eds). New York, NY: McGraw-Hill, Chap. 152, 2008.

A. *Clostridium gangrenosum*
B. *P aeruginosa*
C. *Rhizopus arrhizus*
D. *S aureus*
E. *Y pestis*

IV-137. You are caring for a 15-year-old student who presented to the emergency department with left lower quadrant pain yesterday. Given his presentation, he was taken emergently to the operating room for appendectomy. However, on exploratory laparotomy, his appendix appeared quite normal, and the surgeon visualized striking mesenteric adenitis and terminal ileitis. The operation was aborted without further intervention, and he was admitted to the medical intensive care unit. On further questioning, the patient endorsed eating barely cooked chitterlings at a party a week prior. You suspect his infection is due to which of the following?

A. *C difficile*
B. *E coli*
C. *S aureus*
D. *Trichinella spiralis*
E. *Yersinia enterocolitica*

IV-138. The *Bartonella* species have adapted to survive in animals by existing in what immunologically protected site within the body?

A. Bone marrow
B. Central nervous system
C. Erythrocytes
D. Eyes
E. Gonads

IV-139. Mr. Sisson is a 40-year-old automobile mechanic. Two weeks ago, he went to a local "minute-clinic" after a cat bite on his right ring finger. The wound was irrigated, and he was sent home with instructions for local wound care. Today, he presents to your clinic with 2 days of right axillary swelling (shown in Figure IV-139). His temperature is 38.4°C, and he has complained of general malaise over the past few days. You palpate no other lymphadenopathy on examination, and his finger has healed nicely without signs of overlying infection. He has no visual or neurologic complaints or abnormalities on examination. What is the most appropriate course of action?

A. Admit for blood cultures and empirically initiate vancomycin IV
B. Check *Bartonella* serologies, electrolytes, and liver and renal function tests; do not initiate antibiotics
C. Initiate azithromycin for a 5-day course
D. Obtain peripheral blood thick and thin blood smears
E. Refer for bone marrow aspirate and flow cytometry

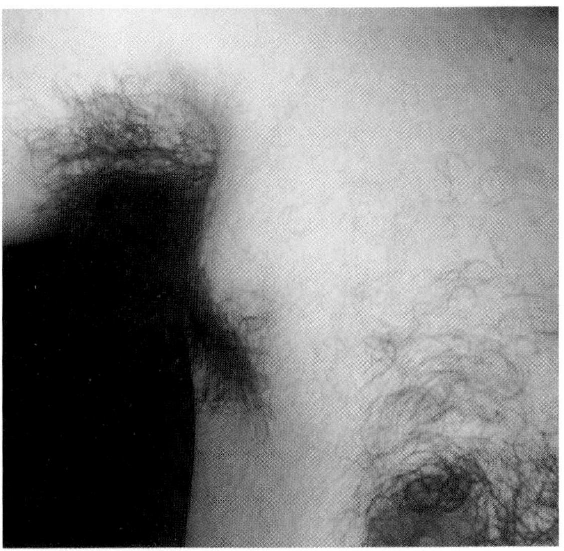

FIGURE IV-139

IV-140. Mr. Pelosa is a 42-year-old man with HIV who is not on antiretroviral therapy and has a recent CD4 cell count of 43/μL. He presents with several nontender red, ulcerated plaques (one is shown in Figure IV-140). He endorses a couple weeks of fever and malaise. Pathologic examination of a biopsy of one of the lesions reveals lobular proliferations of small blood vessels lined by enlarged endothelial cells interspersed with mixed infiltrates of neutrophils and lymphocytes, and blood cultures are positive for *Bartonella henselae*. What condition is causing the patient's skin lesions?

A. Bacillary angiomatosis
B. Bubonic plague
C. Kaposi sarcoma
D. Pyoderma gangrenosum
E. Verruga peruana

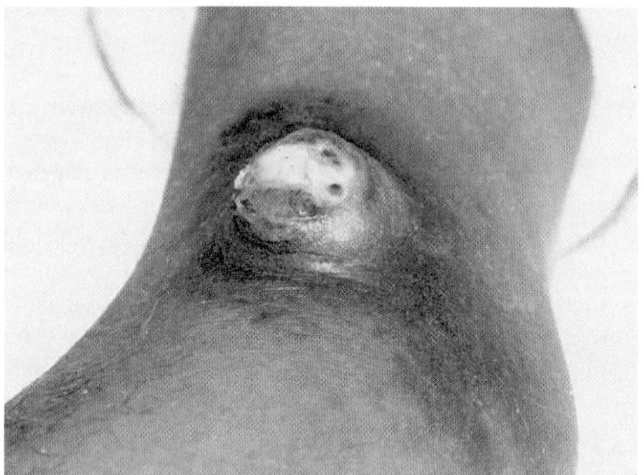

FIGURE IV-140 Reprinted with permission from *Harrison's Principles of Internal Medicine*, 17th ed, AF Fauci et al (eds). New York, NY: McGraw-Hill, 2008, p 989.

IV-141. Mr. Awayab is a 54-year-old truck driver in the Dominican Republic. He presents to the local health department with a penile lesion (shown in Figure IV-141A). He denies fever or chills but has had several unprotected sexual encounters in the past 6 months. You swab the lesion and stain the collected material with a rapid Giemsa stain, visualizing the cell in Figure IV-141B. You know that Mr. Awayab's infection is caused by which organism?

A. *C trachomatis*
B. *Haemophilus ducreyi*
C. *Klebsiella granulomatis*
D. *Mycobacterium leprae*
E. *N gonorrhea*

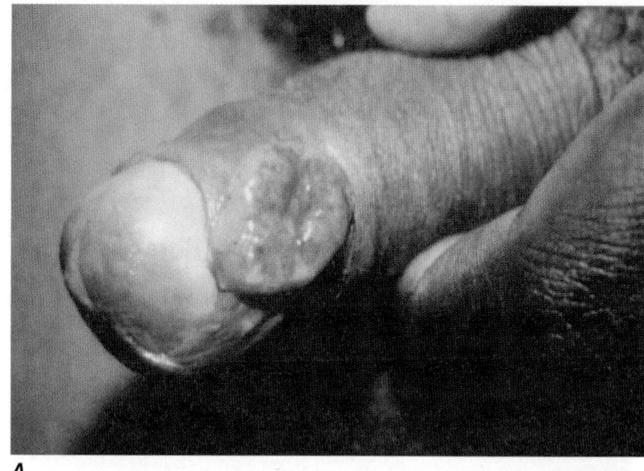

A

FIGURE IV-141A

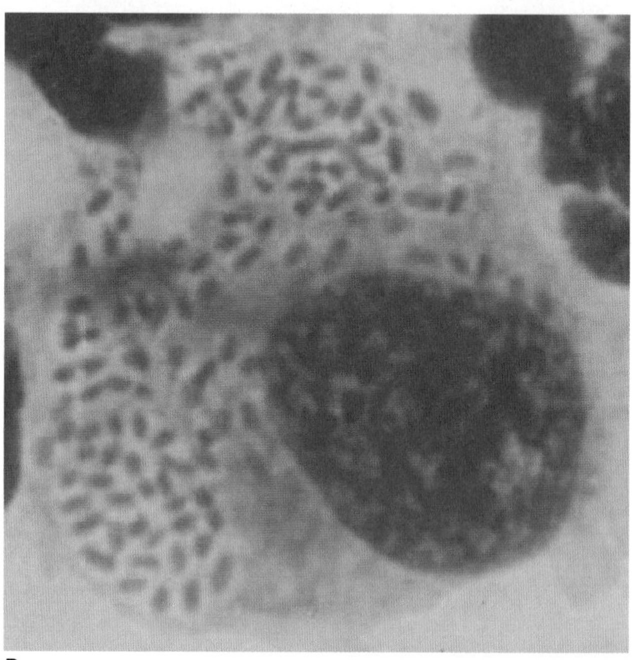

B

FIGURE IV-141B

IV-142. A 35-year-old man is seen 6 months after a cadaveric renal allograft. The patient has been on tacrolimus and prednisone since that procedure. He has felt poorly for the past 2 weeks with fever to 38.6°C (101.5°F), anorexia, and a cough productive of thick sputum. Chest x-ray reveals a left lower lobe (50-cm) mass with central cavitation. Examination of the sputum reveals long, crooked, branching, beaded gram-positive filaments (Figure IV-142A). The sputum is also weakly acid-fast on a smear. The most appropriate initial therapy would include the administration of which of the following antibiotics?

A. Ceftazidime
B. Erythromycin
C. Penicillin
D. Tobramycin
E. Trimethoprim-sulfamethoxazole

IV-143. A 67-year-old woman presents to her local emergency department with 2 weeks of right jaw pain that now has developed an area of purulent drainage into her mouth. She reports accompanying fever. She has poor dentition and has not seen a dentist in more than a decade. Her only medications are alendronate and lisinopril. Physical

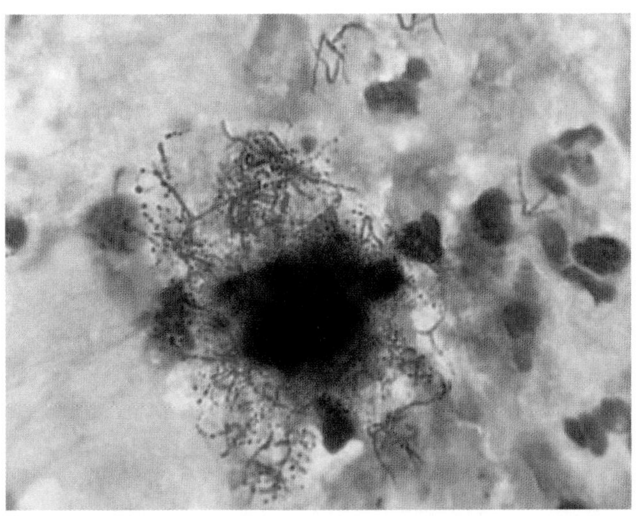

FIGURE IV-142A Image provided by Charles Cartwright and Susan Nelson, Hennepin County Medical Center, Minneapolis, MN.

examination is notable for a temperature of 101.1°F, right-sided facial swelling, diffuse mandibular tenderness, and an area of yellow purulent drainage through the buccal mucosa on the right side. Microscopic examination of the purulent secretions is likely to show which of the following?

A. Auer rods
B. Sialolith
C. Squamous cell carcinoma
D. Sulfur granules
E. Weakly acid-fast branching, beaded filaments

IV-144. In the patient described in Question IV-143, what is the most appropriate therapy?

A. Amphotericin B
B. Itraconazole
C. Penicillin
D. Surgical debridement
E. Tobramycin

IV-145. A 68-year-old homeless man with a long history of alcohol abuse presents to his primary care physician with several weeks of fever, night sweats, and sputum production. He denies nausea, vomiting, or other gastrointestinal symptoms. Examination is notable for low-grade temperature, weight loss of 15 lb since the last visit, and foul breath, but is otherwise normal. Blood work, including complete blood count and serum chemistries, is unremarkable. An interferon-γ release assay is negative. His chest radiograph is shown in Figure IV-145. Which of the following is appropriate as initial therapy?

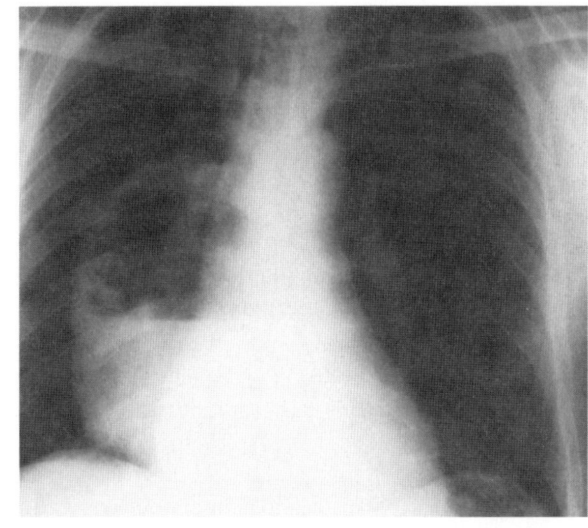

FIGURE IV-145 From GL Mandell (ed): *Atlas of Infectious Diseases*, Vol VI. Philadelphia, PA: Current Medicine Inc, Churchill Livingstone, 1996; with permission.

A. Bronchoscopy with biopsy of the cavity to diagnose squamous cell lung cancer
B. Esophagogastroduodenoscopy to diagnose hiatal hernia with aspiration
C. Immediate hospitalization and isolation to prevent spread of *Mycobacterium tuberculosis*
D. IV meropenem for lung abscess
E. IV penicillin for lung abscess

IV-146. Which of the following is a major reservoir for anaerobic organisms in the human body?

A. Duodenum
B. Female genital tract
C. Gallbladder
D. Lung
E. Prostate

IV-147. All of the following factors influence the likelihood of transmitting active tuberculosis EXCEPT:

A. Duration of contact with an infected person
B. Environment in which contact occurs
C. Presence of extrapulmonary tuberculosis
D. Presence of laryngeal tuberculosis
E. Probability of contact with an infectious person

IV-148. Which of the following individuals with a known history of prior latent tuberculosis infection (without therapy) has the lowest likelihood of developing reactivation tuberculosis?

A. A 28-year-old woman with anorexia nervosa, a body mass index of 16 kg/m^2, and a serum albumin of 2.3 g/dL
B. A 36-year-old IV drug user who does not have HIV but is homeless
C. A 42-year-old man who is HIV-positive with a CD4 count of 350/μL on highly active antiretroviral therapy
D. A 52-year-old man who works as a coal miner
E. An 83-year-old man who was infected while stationed in Korea in 1958

IV-149. A 42-year-old Nigerian man comes to the emergency department because of fevers, fatigue, weight loss, and cough for 3 weeks. He complains of fevers and a 4.5-kg weight loss. He describes his sputum as yellow in color. It has rarely been blood streaked. He emigrated to the United States 1 year ago and is an undocumented alien. He has never been treated for tuberculosis, has never had a purified protein derivative (PPD) skin test placed, and does not recall receiving bacillus Calmette–Guérin (BCG) vaccination. He denies HIV risk factors. He is married and reports no ill contacts. He smokes a pack of cigarettes daily and drinks a pint of vodka on a daily basis. On physical examination, he appears chronically ill with temporal wasting. His body mass index is 21 kg/m^2. Vital signs are as follows: BP 122/68 mmHg, HR 89 bpm, RR 22 breaths/min, SaO_2 95% on room air, and temperature 37.9°C. There are amphoric breath sounds posteriorly in the right upper lung field with a few scattered crackles in this area. No clubbing is present. The examination is otherwise unremarkable. His chest radiograph is shown in Figure IV-149. A stain for acid-fast bacilli is negative. What is the most appropriate approach to the ongoing care of this patient?

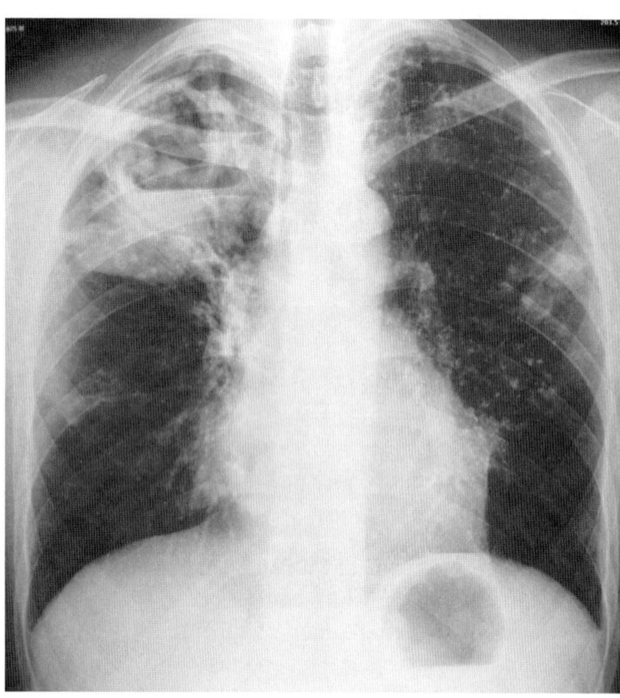

FIGURE IV-149 Courtesy of Dr. Andrea Gori, Department of Infectious Diseases, S. Paolo University Hospital, Milan, Italy; with permission.

A. Admit the patient on airborne isolation until three expectorated sputums show no evidence of acid-fast bacilli.
B. Admit the patient without isolation as he is unlikely to be infectious with a negative acid-fast smear.
C. Perform a biopsy of the lesion and consult oncology.
D. Place a PPD test on his forearm and have him return for evaluation in 3 days.
E. Start a 6-week course of antibiotic treatment for anaerobic bacterial abscess.

IV-150. An 18-year-old man is brought to a clinic in South Africa complaining of 2 weeks of progressive malaise with low-grade fevers. He was unable to get out of bed this morning to go to work. He has known HIV infection and is not on therapy. He denies cough or sputum. His chest radiograph is shown in Figure IV-150. Given his HIV infection and the high prevalence of tuberculosis in the man's neighborhood, you are concerned he has tuberculosis. Which of the following forms of tuberculosis is most likely in this case?

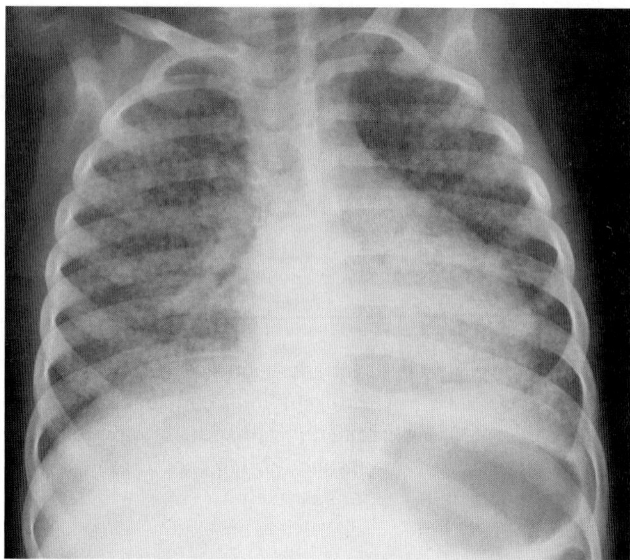

FIGURE IV-150 Courtesy of Prof. Robert Gie, Department of Paediatrics and Child Health, Stellenbosch University, South Africa; with permission.

A. Disseminated
B. Extrapulmonary
C. Lymphadenitis
D. Pleural
E. Postprimary cavitary

IV-151. A 50-year-old man is admitted to the hospital for active pulmonary tuberculosis with a positive sputum acid-fast bacilli smear. He is HIV positive with a CD4 count of 85/μL and is not on highly active antiretroviral therapy. In addition to pulmonary disease, he is found to have disease in the L4 vertebral body. What is the most appropriate initial therapy?

A. Isoniazid, rifampin, ethambutol, and pyrazinamide
B. Isoniazid, rifampin, ethambutol, and pyrazinamide; initiate antiretroviral therapy
C. Isoniazid, rifampin, ethambutol, pyrazinamide, and streptomycin
D. Isoniazid, rifampin, and ethambutol
E. Withhold therapy until sensitivities are available.

IV-152. All of the following individuals receiving tuberculin skin PPD reactions should be treated for latent tuberculosis EXCEPT:

A. A 23-year-old injection drug user who is HIV negative and has a 12-mm PPD reaction
B. A 38-year-old fourth grade teacher who has a 7-mm PPD reaction and no known exposures to active tuberculosis; she has never been tested with a PPD previously
C. A 43-year-old individual in the Peace Corps working in sub-Saharan Africa who has a 10-mm PPD reaction; 18 months ago, the PPD reaction was 3 mm
D. A 55-year-old man who is HIV positive and has a negative PPD; his partner was recently diagnosed with cavitary tuberculosis
E. A 72-year-old man who is receiving chemotherapy for non-Hodgkin lymphoma and has a 16-mm PPD reaction

IV-153. All of the following statements regarding interferon-γ release assays for the diagnosis of latent tuberculosis are true EXCEPT:

A. There is no booster (repeated testing) phenomenon.
B. They are more specific than tuberculin skin testing.
C. They have a higher sensitivity than tuberculin skin testing in high HIV-burden areas.
D. They have less cross-reactivity with BCG and nontuberculous mycobacteria than tuberculin skin testing.
E. They may be used to screen for latent tuberculosis in adults working in low-prevalence U.S. settings.

IV-154. All of the following statements regarding BCG vaccination are true EXCEPT:

A. BCG dissemination may occur in severely immunosuppressed patients.
B. BCG vaccination is recommended at birth in countries with high TB prevalence.
C. BCG vaccination may cause a false-positive tuberculin skin test.
D. BCG vaccine provides protection for infants and children from TB meningitis and military disease.
E. BCG vaccine provides protection from TB in HIV-infected patients.

IV-155. A 76-year-old woman is brought in to clinic by her son. She complains of a chronic nonproductive cough and fatigue. Her son adds that she has had low-grade fevers, progressive weight loss over months, and "just doesn't seem like herself." A representative slice from her chest CT is shown in Figure IV-155. She was treated for tuberculosis when she was in her 20s. A sputum sample is obtained, as are blood cultures. Two weeks later, both culture sets grow acid-fast bacilli consistent with *Mycobacterium avium* complex. Which of the following is the best treatment option?

A. Bronchodilators and pulmonary toilet
B. Clarithromycin, ethambutol, and rifampin
C. Clarithromycin and rifampin
D. Moxifloxacin and rifampin
E. Pyrazinamide, isoniazid, rifampin, and ethambutol

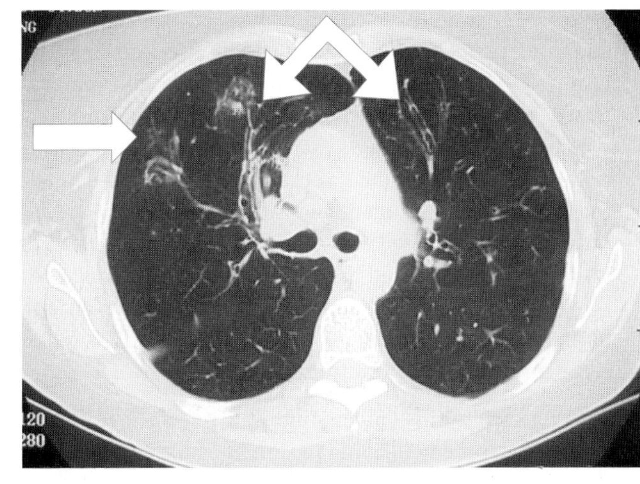

FIGURE IV-155

IV-156. A 45-year-old patient with HIV/AIDS presents to the emergency department. He complains of a rash that has been slowly spreading up his right arm and is now evident on his chest and back. The rash consists of small nodules that have a reddish-blue appearance. Some of them are ulcerated, but there is minimal fluctuance or drainage. He is unsure when these began. He notes no foreign travel or unusual exposures. He is homeless and unemployed but occasionally gets work as a day laborer doing landscaping and digging. A culture of a skin lesion grows *Mycobacterium* in 5 days. Which of the following is the most likely organism?

A. *M abscessus*
B. *M avium*
C. *M kansasii*
D. *M marinum*
E. *M ulcerans*

IV-157. All of the following statements regarding antituberculosis therapeutic agents are true EXCEPT:

A. In the United States, *M tuberculosis* resistance to isoniazid remains <10%.
B. Optic neuritis is the most severe adverse effect of ethambutol.
C. Pyrazinamide has utility in the therapy of *M avium* complex and *M kansasii* infections.
D. Rifabutin should be used instead of rifampin in patients receiving concurrent treatment with protease inhibitors or nevirapine.
E. Rifampin can decrease the half-life of warfarin, cyclosporine, prednisone, oral contraceptives, clarithromycin, and other important drugs.

IV-158. A 22-year-old college student presents for the evaluation of a painless nonpruritic rash of 1 week in duration (Figure IV-158). Three months ago, he engaged in unprotected sexual intercourse. Two months ago, he noted a penile papule that evolved to a painless, clean-based, and indurated ulcer. He did not seek medical attention because the ulcer healed spontaneously. Subsequently, he developed the rash pictured in Figure IV-158. He complains of no other symptoms and has no stigmata of ocular or neurologic involvement. He reports no new medications and has no known drug allergies. He does not have HIV. What is the most appropriate antibiotic regimen?

A. Azithromycin 1000 mg orally for one dose
B. Benzathine penicillin G 2.4 mU IM for one dose
C. Doxycycline 100 mg orally twice a day for 14 days
D. Doxycycline 200 mg orally for one dose
E. Penicillin G 18–24 mU/d IV for 14 days

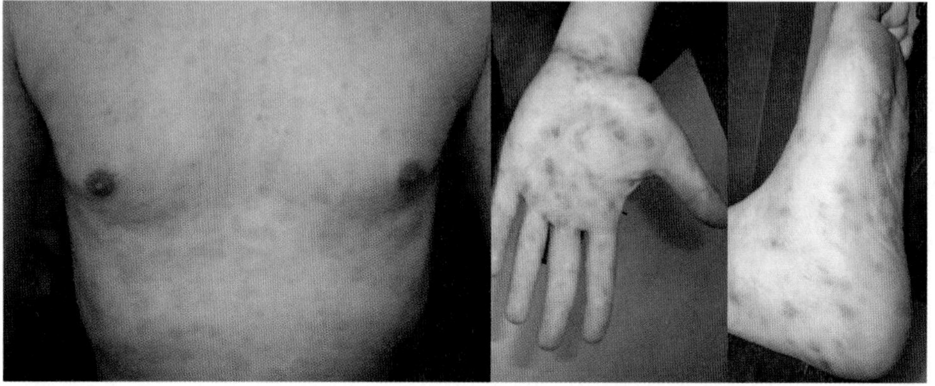

FIGURE IV-158 Courtesy of Jill McKenzie and Christina Marra.

IV-159. A 68-year-old man is referred for evaluation of gait instability. He complains of lightning-like pains lancinating to his thighs that last minutes. Exam is notable for impaired proprioceptive and vibratory sense in his feet. He has a wide-based, ataxic gait and a positive Romberg sign. His family reports that his wife had treated syphilis 35 years ago, but that he was never tested or treated for syphilis. Which ocular finding would be most consistent with neurosyphilis?

A. Pupils that react to accommodation but not light
B. Pupils that react to light but not accommodation
C. Pupils that react to both light and accommodation
D. Pupils that do not react to light or accommodation

IV-160. A 74-year-old woman with mild cognitive impairment is screened for syphilis. She has no history of recent sexual activity or of prior exposure to syphilis. The prevalence of syphilis in her local population is low. Her rapid plasma reagin (RPR) is reactive with a titer of ≤1:2. Her fluorescent treponemal antibody absorption test (FTA-ABS) is nonreactive. The reactive RPR is most likely:

A. False negative because the nontreponemal test is negative
B. False negative because the treponemal test is positive
C. False positive because the nontreponemal test is negative
D. False positive because the treponemal test is negative
E. True positive because the nontreponemal test is positive

IV-161. A 47-year-old man undergoes lumbar puncture to evaluate asymptomatic neurosyphilis. He tested positive for syphilis with serum RPR titer of 1:256. He has no history of HIV. He has no ocular disease. His CSF studies resulted with WBC of 10/μL, red blood cells (RBCs) of 1/μL, CSF-glucose of 55 mg/dL, and CSF-protein of 50 mg/dL. CSF-VDRL is negative. He has no history of penicillin allergy. Which of the following is the most appropriate next therapeutic regimen?

A. Aqueous crystalline penicillin G 18–24 MU/d IV for 14 days
B. Aqueous procaine penicillin G 2.4 MU/d IM daily for 14 days
C. Benzathine penicillin G 2.4 MU IM for one dose
D. Benzathine penicillin G 2.4 MU IM every 7 days for 3 weeks
E. No therapy is indicated

IV-162. All of the following are indications for CSF examination in adults infected with syphilis EXCEPT:

A. HIV infection with CD4+ count ≤ 350/μL
B. Maculopapular rash involving the palms and soles
C. RPR titer ≥1:32
D. Sensorineural hearing loss
E. Suspected treatment failure

IV-163. What proportion of sexual contacts of persons with infectious syphilis become infected?

A. 5%–10%
B. 10%–33%
C. 33%–50%
D. 50%–67%
E. 67%–90%

IV-164. A 52-year-old man presents for evaluation of fever and jaundice. Flu-like symptoms including fever, chills, headache, and myalgias started suddenly 2 days ago. Yesterday, he noted scleral icterus and darkened urine. Today, he developed new cough, chest discomfort, dyspnea, and hemoptysis. He resides in Baltimore City and works as an exterminator. Two weeks ago, he suffered a minor leg injury while abating a rat infestation in a dilapidated home also plagued with standing water. He has no other travel or exposure history. Which pattern of electrolytes is typical of acute kidney injury in the severe form of this spirochetal zoonosis?

A. Hyperkalemia and hyponatremia
B. Hyperkalemia and hypernatremia
C. Hypokalemia and hyponatremia
D. Hypokalemia and hypernatremia

IV-165. A 26-year-old man presents to your office complaining of recurrent episodes of fever and malaise. He returned from a camping trip in the northwestern part of Montana about 3 weeks ago. While he was hiking, he denies eating or drinking any unpasteurized milk products. He sterilized all of his water prior to drinking. He had multiple insect bites, but did not identify any ticks. He primarily slept in cabins or tents and did not notice any rodent droppings in the areas where he camped. Two friends that accompanied him on the trip have not been ill. He initially experienced fevers as high as 104.7°F (40.4°C), with myalgias, headache, nausea, vomiting, and diarrhea beginning 5 days after his return home. These symptoms lasted for about 3 days and resolved spontaneously. He attributed his symptoms to the "flu" and returned to his normal functioning. Seven days later, the fevers returned with temperatures to 105.1°F (40.6°C). With these episodes, his family noted him to have intermittent confusion. Today is day 4 of his current illness, and the patient feels that his fevers have again subsided. What is the most likely cause of the patient's recurrent fevers?

A. Brucellosis
B. Colorado tick fever
C. Leptospirosis
D. Lymphocytic choriomeningitis
E. Tick-borne relapsing fever

IV-166. Infection by what organism causes the rash shown in Figure IV-166?

A. *Anaplasma phagocytophilum*
B. *B henselae*
C. *Borrelia burgdorferi*
D. *Ehrlichia chaffeensis*
E. *R rickettsii*

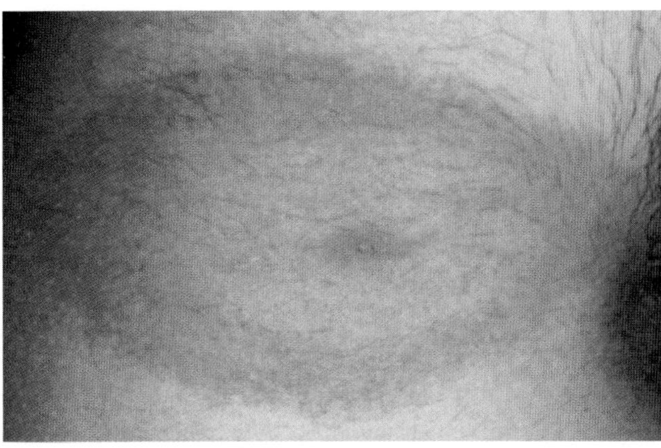

FIGURE IV-166 Courtesy of Vijay K. Sikand, MD; with permission.

IV-167. A 36-year-old man presents to the emergency department in Pennsylvania complaining of lightheadedness and dizziness. On physical examination, the patient is found to have an HR of 38 bpm, and the electrocardiogram (ECG) demonstrates acute heart block. On further questioning, he reports that he lives in a wooded area. He has two dogs that often roam in the woods and have been found with ticks on many occasions. He takes no medications and is otherwise healthy. He is an avid hiker and is also training for a triathlon. He denies any significant childhood illness. His family history is positive for an acute myocardial infarction in his father at age 42. His physical examination is normal with the exception of the slow but regular heartbeat. His chemistry panel shows no abnormalities. His chest radiograph is normal. What is the most likely cause of complete heart block in this individual?

A. Acute myocardial infarction
B. Chagas disease
C. Lyme disease
D. Sarcoidosis
E. Subacute bacterial endocarditis

IV-168. *B burgdorferi* serology testing is indicated for which of the following patients, all of whom reside in Lyme-endemic regions?

A. A 19-year-old female camp counselor who presents with her second episode of an inflamed, red, and tender left knee and right ankle
B. A 23-year-old male house painter who presents with a primary erythema migrans lesion at the site of a witnessed tick bite
C. A 36-year-old female state park ranger who presents with a malar rash; diffuse arthralgias/arthritis of her shoulders, knees, and metacarpophalangeal and proximal interphalangeal joints; pericarditis; and acute glomerulonephritis
D. A 42-year-old woman with chronic fatigue, myalgias, and arthralgias
E. A 46-year-old male gardener who presents with fevers, malaise, migratory arthralgias/myalgias, and three erythema migrans lesions

IV-169. A previously healthy 17-year-old girl presents in early October with profound fatigue and malaise, as well as fevers, headache, nuchal rigidity, diffuse arthralgias, and a rash. She lives in a small town in Massachusetts and spent her summer as a camp counselor at a local day camp. She participated in daily hikes in the woods but did not travel outside of the area during the course of the summer. Physical examination reveals a well-developed young woman who appears extremely fatigued but not in extremis. Her temperature is 37.4°C; pulse is 86 bpm; BP is 96/54 mmHg; and RR is 12 breaths/min. Physical examination documents clear breath sounds, no cardiac rub or murmur, normal bowel sounds, a nontender abdomen, no organomegaly, and no evidence of synovitis. Several erythema migrans lesions are noted on her lower extremities, bilateral axillae, right thigh, and left groin. All of the following are possible complications of her current disease state EXCEPT:

A. Bell palsy
B. Large-joint oligoarticular arthritis
C. Meningitis
D. Progressive dementia
E. Third-degree heart block

IV-170. In the patient described in Question 169, which of the following is appropriate therapy?

A. Azithromycin 500 mg orally (PO) daily
B. Ceftriaxone 2 g IV daily
C. Cephalexin 500 mg PO twice a day (bid)
D. Doxycycline 100 mg PO bid
E. Vancomycin 1 g IV bid

IV-171. A 48-year-old man is admitted to the intensive care unit in July with hypotension and fever. He lives in a suburban area of Arkansas. He became ill yesterday with a fever as high as 104.0°F (40.0°C). Today, his wife noted increasing confusion and lethargy. Over this same time, he has complained of headaches and myalgias. He has had nausea with two episodes of vomiting. Prior to the acute onset of illness, he had no medical complaints. He has no other medical history and takes no medications. He works as a landscape architect. The history is obtained from the patient's wife, and she does not know if he has suffered any recent insect or tick bites. No one else in the family is ill, nor are the patient's coworkers. On presentation, the vital signs are as follows: BP 88/52 mmHg, HR 135 bpm, RR 22 breaths/min, temperature 101.9°F (38.8°C), and oxygen saturation 94% on room air. His physical examination reveals an ill-appearing man, moaning quietly. He is oriented to person only. No meningismus is present. His cardiac examination reveals a regular tachycardia. His chest and abdominal examinations are normal. He has no rash. His laboratory values are listed in Table IV-171.

He is fluid resuscitated and treated with IV ceftriaxone and vancomycin. A lumbar puncture shows no pleocytosis and normal protein and glucose. Despite this treatment, the patient develops worsening thrombocytopenia, neutropenia, and lymphopenia over the next 2 days. A bone marrow biopsy shows a hypercellular marrow with noncaseating granulomas. Which test is most likely to suggest the cause of the patient's illness?

TABLE IV-171 Laboratory Values

WBC count	4200/μL	Sodium	132 mEq/L
PMNs	88%	Potassium	4.6 mEq/L
Lymphocytes	10%	Chloride	98 mEq/L
Monocytes	2%	Bicarbonate	22 mEq/L
Eosinophils	0%	Blood urea nitrogen	38 g/dL
Hemoglobin	12.3 g/dL	Creatinine	1.6 mg/dL
Hematocrit	37%	Glucose	102 mg/dL
Platelets	82,000/μL		
AST	215 U/L		
ALT	199 U/L		
Bilirubin	1.2 mg/dL		
Alkaline phosphatase	98 U/L		

A. Antibodies to double-stranded DNA and Smith antigens
B. Chest radiography
C. Levels of IgM and IgG on CSF
D. Peripheral blood smear
E. PCR on peripheral blood

IV-172. A 27-year-old man who lives in North Carolina presents to his primary care physician complaining of fever, headache, myalgias, nausea, and anorexia 7 days after returning from hiking on the Appalachian Trail. Physical examination is remarkable for a temperature of 101.5°F (38.6°C). He appears generally fatigued but not toxic and does not have a rash. He is reassured by his primary care physician that this likely represents a viral illness, but returns to clinic 3 days later with a progressive rash and ongoing fevers. He states that small red spots began to appear on the wrists and ankles within 24 hours of the prior visit and have now progressed up his extremities and onto the trunk. (See Figure IV-172.) He also notes an increasing headache, and his wife thinks he has had some confusion. On physical examination, the patient is noted to be lethargic and answers questions slowly. What would be a reasonable course of action?

A. Admit the patient to the hospital for treatment with IV ceftriaxone 1 g twice daily and vancomycin 1 g twice daily
B. Admit the patient to the hospital for treatment with doxycycline 100 mg twice daily
C. Initiate treatment with doxycycline 100 mg orally twice daily as an outpatient
D. Initiate treatment with trimethoprim-sulfamethoxazole double strength twice daily
E. Order rickettsial serologies and withhold treatment until a firm diagnosis is made

IV-173. A previously healthy 20-year-old college student presents with several days of headache, extensive cough with scant sputum, and fever of 101.5°F (38.6°C) in September.

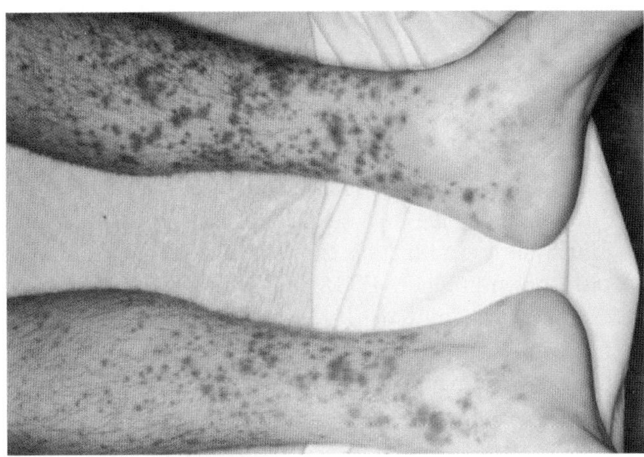

A

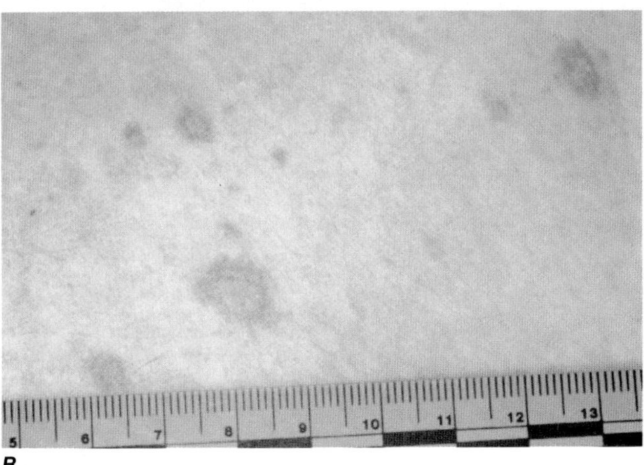

B

FIGURE IV-172 Photos courtesy of Dr. Lindsey Baden; with permission.

Several individuals in his dormitory have also been ill with a similar illness. On examination, pharyngeal erythema is noted, and lung examination reveals bilateral expiratory wheezing and scattered crackles in the lower lung zones. He coughs frequently during the examination. Chest radiograph reveals bilateral peribronchial pneumonia with increased interstitial markings. No lobar consolidation is seen. Which organism is most likely to cause the patient's presentation?

A. Adenovirus
B. *C pneumoniae*
C. *L pneumophila*
D. *M pneumoniae*
E. *S pneumoniae*

IV-174. A previously healthy 19-year-old man presents with several days of headache, cough with scant sputum, dyspnea, and fever of 38.6°C. On examination, pharyngeal erythema is noted, and lung fields showed scattered wheezes and some crackles. Chest radiograph shows bilateral peribronchial interstitial infiltrates. His hematocrit is 24.7%, down from a baseline measure of 46%. The only other laboratory abnormality is an indirect bilirubin of 3.4. A peripheral smear reveals no abnormalities. A cold agglutinin titer is measured at 1:64. What is the most likely infectious agent?

A. *Coxiella burnetii*
B. *L pneumophila*
C. Methicillin-resistant *S aureus*
D. *M pneumoniae*
E. *S pneumoniae*

IV-175. A 42-year-old woman is admitted to the intensive care unit with hypoxemic respiratory failure and pneumonia in August. She was well until 2 days prior to admission when she developed fevers, myalgias, and headache. She works in a poultry processing plant and is originally from El Salvador. She has been in the United States for 15 years. She has no major health problems. Her PPD was negative upon arrival to the United States. Several other workers have been ill with a similar illness, although no one else has developed respiratory failure. She is currently intubated and sedated. Her oxygen saturation is 93% on an FiO_2 of 0.80 and positive end-expiratory pressure of 12 cm H_2O. On physical examination, crackles are present in both lung fields. There is no cardiac murmur. Hepatosplenomegaly is present. Laboratory studies reveal a mild transaminitis. Influenza nasal swab is negative for the presence of influenza A. Which of the following tests is most likely to be positive in this patient?

A. Acid-fast bacilli stain and mycobacterial culture for *Mycobacterium tuberculosis*
B. Blood cultures growing *S aureus*
C. Microimmunofluorescence testing for *Chlamydia psittaci*
D. Urine *Legionella* antigen
E. Viral cultures of bronchoscopic samples for influenza A

IV-176. A 20-year-old woman is 36 weeks pregnant and presents for her first evaluation. She is diagnosed with *C trachomatis* infection of the cervix. Upon delivery, what complication is her infant most at risk for?

A. Jaundice
B. Hydrocephalus
C. Hutchinson triad
D. Conjunctivitis
E. Sensorineural deafness

IV-177. A 19-year-old man presents to an urgent care clinic with urethral discharge. He reports three new female sexual partners over the past 2 months. What should his management be?

A. Nucleic acid amplification test for *N gonorrhoeae* and *C trachomatis* and return to clinic in 2 days
B. Ceftriaxone 250 mg IM × 1 and azithromycin, 1 g PO × 1 for the patient and his recent partners
C. Nucleic acid amplification test for *N gonorrhoeae* and *C trachomatis* plus ceftriaxone 250 mg IM × 1 and azithromycin 1 g PO × 1 for the patient
D. Nucleic acid amplification test for *N gonorrhoeae* and *C trachomatis* plus ceftriaxone 250 mg IM × 1 and azithromycin 1 g PO × 1 for the patient and his recent partners
E. Nucleic acid amplification test for *N gonorrhoeae* and *C trachomatis* plus ceftriaxone 250 mg IM × 1, azithromycin 1 g PO × 1, and metronidazole 2 g PO × 1 for the patient and his partners

IV-178. All of the following regarding herpes simplex virus (HSV)-2 infection are true EXCEPT:

A. Approximately one in five Americans harbors HSV-2 antibodies.
B. Asymptomatic shedding of HSV-2 in the genital tract occurs nearly as frequently in those with no symptoms as in those with ulcerative disease.
C. Asymptomatic shedding of HSV-2 is associated with transmission of virus.
D. HSV-2 seropositivity is an independent risk factor for HIV transmission.
E. Seroprevalence rates of HSV-2 are lower in Africa than in the United States.

IV-179. A 23-year-old woman is newly diagnosed with genital HSV-2 infection. What is her chance of reactivation of disease during the first year after infection?

A. 5%
B. 25%
C. 50%
D. 75%
E. 90%

IV-180. A 65-year-old man is brought to the hospital by his wife because of new-onset fever and confusion. He was well until 3 days ago, when he developed high fever, somnolence, and progressive confusion. His current medical history is unremarkable except for elevated cholesterol, and his only medication is atorvastatin. He is a civil engineer at an international construction company. His wife reports he obtains regular health screening and has always been PPD negative. On admission, his temperature is 40°C, and his vital signs are otherwise normal. He is confused and hallucinating. Soon after admission, he develops a tonic-clonic seizure that requires lorazepam to terminate. His head CT shows no acute bleeding or elevated intracranial pressure. An electroencephalogram shows an epileptiform focus in the left temporal lobe and diffusion-weighted magnetic resonance imaging (MRI) shows bilateral temporal lobe inflammation. Which of the following is most likely to be diagnostic?

A. CSF acid-fast staining
B. CSF India ink stain
C. CSF PCR for herpes virus
D. CSF oligoclonal band testing
E. Serum cryptococcal antigen testing

IV-181. Which of the following statements regarding administration of varicella-zoster vaccine to patients >60 years old is true?

A. It is a killed virus vaccine, so it is safe in immunocompromised patients.
B. It is not recommended for patients in this age group.
C. It will decrease the risk of developing post-herpetic neuralgia.
D. It will not decrease the risk of developing shingles.
E. It will not decrease the burden of disease.

IV-182. Mr. Brian is a 29-year-old man who comes to the emergency department complaining of a painful red rash on his left back and buttocks that has worsened over the past 3 days. He reports it started as a few small red bumps but has grown and become more painful. His history is notable for HIV infection and medical noncompliance. He does not take any medications. He is afebrile, and his physical examination is unremarkable other than the rash shown in Figure IV-182. Of note, the rest of his skin examination is unremarkable, and the painful rash does not cross the midline. Which of the following is the most effective treatment?

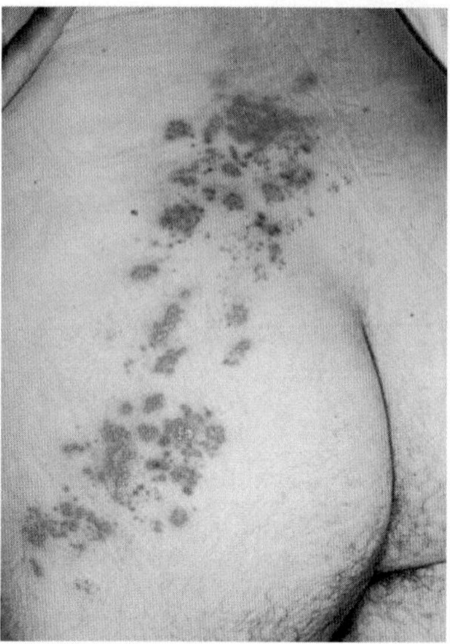

FIGURE IV-182

A. Doxycycline
B. Ganciclovir
C. Penicillin
D. Piperacillin-tazobactam
E. Valacyclovir

IV-183. A 19-year-old college student comes to clinic reporting that she has been ill for 2 weeks. About 2 weeks ago, she developed notable fatigue and malaise that prevented her from her usual exercise regimen and caused her to miss some classes. Last week, she developed low-grade fevers, sore throat, and swollen lymph nodes in her neck. She has a history of strep pharyngitis, so 3 days ago, she took some ampicillin that she had in her possession. Over the last 2 days, she has developed a worsening slightly itchy rash, as shown in Figure IV-183. Her physical examination is notable for a temperature of 38.1°C, pharyngeal erythema, bilateral tonsillar enlargement without exudates, bilateral tender cervical adenopathy, and a palpable spleen. All of the following statements regarding her illness are true EXCEPT:

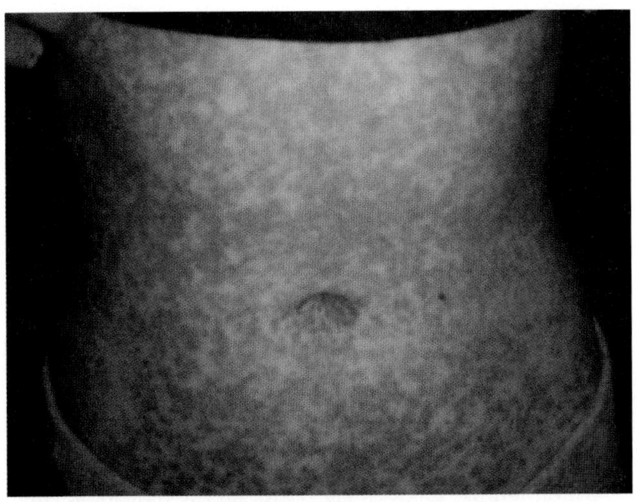

FIGURE IV-183 Reprinted from RP Usatine et al: *Color Atlas of Family Medicine*, 2nd ed. New York, McGraw-Hill, 2013. Courtesy of Richard P. Usatine, MD.

A. Greater than 10% atypical lymphocytosis is likely.
B. Heterophile antibody testing will likely be diagnostic.
C. If heterophile antibody testing is negative, testing for IgG antibodies against viral capsid antigen will likely be diagnostic.
D. It is spread via contaminated saliva.
E. The patient can receive ampicillin in the future if indicated.

IV-184. For the patient described in Question IV-183, which of the following is the indicated treatment?

A. Acyclovir
B. Acyclovir plus prednisone
C. Ganciclovir
D. Prednisone
E. Rest, supportive measures, and reassurance

IV-185. Which of the following manifestations of CMV infection is least likely to occur following lung transplantation?

A. Bronchiolitis obliterans
B. CMV esophagitis
C. CMV pneumonia
D. CMV retinitis
E. CMV syndrome (fever, malaise, cytopenias, transaminitis, and CMV viremia)

IV-186. Which of the following serology patterns places a transplant recipient at the lowest risk of developing CMV infection after renal transplantation?

A. Donor CMV IgG negative, recipient CMV IgG negative
B. Donor CMV IgG negative, recipient CMV IgG positive
C. Donor CMV IgG positive, recipient CMV IgG negative
D. Donor CMV IgG positive, recipient CMV IgG positive
E. The risk is equal regardless of serology results.

IV-187. All of the following statements regarding human herpesvirus (HHV)-8 are true EXCEPT:

A. It has been implicated causally in invasive cervical carcinoma.
B. It has been implicated causally in Kaposi sarcoma.
C. It has been implicated causally in multicentric Castleman disease.
D. It has been implicated causally in primary pleural lymphoma.
E. Primary infection may manifest with fever and maculopapular rash.

IV-190. A 42-year-old man with AIDS and a CD4+ lymphocyte count of 23 presents with shortness of breath and fatigue in the absence of fevers. On examination, he appears chronically ill with pale conjunctiva. Hematocrit is 16%. Mean corpuscular volume is 84. Red cell distribution width is normal. Bilirubin, lactose dehydrogenase, and haptoglobin are all within normal limits. Reticulocyte count is zero. WBC count is 4300, with an absolute neutrophil count of 2500. Platelet count is 105,000. Which of the following tests is most likely to produce a diagnosis?

A. Bone marrow aspirate and biopsy
B. Parvovirus B19 IgG
C. Parvovirus B19 PCR
D. Parvovirus B19 IgM
E. Peripheral blood smear

IV-189. A 22-year-old woman presents with diffuse arthralgias and morning stiffness in her hands, knees, and wrists. Two weeks earlier, she had a self-limited febrile illness notable for a red facial rash and lacy reticular rash on her extremities. On examination, her bilateral wrists, metacarpophalangeal joints, and proximal interphalangeal joints are warm and slightly boggy. Which of the following tests is most likely to reveal her diagnosis?

A. Antinuclear antibody
B. *C trachomatis* ligase chain reaction of the urine
C. Joint aspiration for crystals and culture
D. Parvovirus B19 IgM
E. Rheumatoid factor

IV-190. Which of the following statements regarding the currently licensed human papillomavirus (HPV) vaccines is true?

A. Both protect against genital warts.
B. Once sexually active, women will derive little protective benefit from vaccination.
C. They are inactivated live virus vaccines.
D. They are targeted toward all oncogenic strains of HPV but are only 70% effective at decreasing infection in an individual.
E. Those who have been vaccinated should continue to receive standard Pap smear testing.

IV-191. A 32-year-old woman experiences an upper respiratory illness that began with rhinorrhea and nasal congestion. She also complains of a sore throat but has no fever. Her illness lasts for about 5 days and resolves. Just prior to her illness, her 4-year-old child who attends daycare also experienced a similar illness. All of the following statements regarding the most common etiologic agent causing this illness are true EXCEPT:

A. Following the primary illness in a household, a secondary case of illness will occur is 25%–70% of cases.
B. The seasonal peak of the infection is in early fall and spring in temperate climates.
C. The virus can be isolated from plastic surfaces up to 3 hours following exposure.
D. The virus grows best at a temperature of 37°C, the temperature within the nasal passages
E. The virus is a single-stranded RNA virus of the Picornaviridae family.

IV-192. All of the following respiratory viruses may cause a common cold syndrome in children or adults EXCEPT:

A. Adenoviruses
B. Coronaviruses
C. Enteroviruses
D. Human respiratory syncytial viruses
E. Rhinoviruses

IV-193. All of the following viruses are correctly matched with their primary clinical manifestation EXCEPT:

A. Adenovirus—Gingivostomatitis
B. Coronavirus—Severe acute respiratory syndrome
C. Human respiratory syncytial virus—Bronchiolitis in infants and young children
D. Parainfluenza—Croup
E. Rhinovirus—Common cold

IV-194. A 9-month-old infant is admitted to the hospital with a febrile respiratory illness with wheezing and cough. Upon admission to the hospital, the baby is tachypneic and tachycardic with an oxygen saturation of 75% on room air. Rapid viral diagnostic testing confirms the presence of human respiratory syncytial virus. All of the following treatments should be used as part of the treatment plan for this child EXCEPT:

A. Aerosolized ribavirin
B. Hydration
C. Immunoglobulin with high titers of antibody directed against human respiratory syncytial virus
D. Nebulized albuterol
E. Oxygen therapy to maintain oxygen saturation greater than 90%

IV-195. In March 2009, the H1N1 strain of the influenza A virus emerged in Mexico and quickly spread worldwide over the next several months. Ultimately, over 18,000 people died due to the pandemic. This virus had genetic components of swine influenza viruses, an avian virus, and a human influenza virus. The genetic process by which this pandemic strain of influenza A emerged is an example of which of the following?

A. Antigenic drift
B. Antigenic shift
C. Genetic reassortment
D. Point mutation
E. Both B and C

IV-196. A 65-year-old woman is admitted to the hospital in January with a 2-day history of fevers, myalgias, headache, and cough. She has a history of end-stage kidney disease, diabetes mellitus, and hypertension. Her medications include darbepoetin, selamaver, calcitriol, lisinopril, aspirin, amlodipine, and insulin. She receives hemodialysis three times weekly. Upon admission, her BP is 138/65 mmHg, HR is 122 bpm, temperature is 39.4°C, RR is 24 breaths/min, and oxygen saturation is 85% on room air. On physical examination, diffuse crackles are heard, and a chest radiograph confirms the presence of bilateral lung infiltrates concerning for pneumonia. It is known that the most common cause of seasonal influenza in this area is an H3N2 strain of influenza A. All of the following should be included in the initial management of this patient EXCEPT:

A. Amantadine
B. Assessment of the need for close household contacts to receive chemoprophylaxis if influenza swab is positive
C. Droplet precautions
D. Nasal swab for influenza
E. Oxygen therapy

IV-197. A 17-year-old patient with a medical history of mild intermittent asthma presents to your clinic in February with several days of cough, fever, malaise, and myalgias. She notes that her symptoms started 3 days earlier with a headache and fatigue and that several students and teachers at her high school have been diagnosed recently with "the flu." She did not receive a flu shot this year. Which of the following medication treatment plans is the best option for this patient?

A. Aspirin and a cough suppressant with codeine
B. Oseltamivir 75 mg PO bid for 5 days
C. Rimantadine 100 mg PO bid for 1 week
D. Symptom-based therapy with over-the-counter agents
E. Zanamivir 10 mg inhaled bid for 5 days

IV-198. All of the following statements regarding influenza vaccination are true EXCEPT:

A. An egg-free influenza vaccine is available for individuals with true egg hypersensitivity.
B. In 2016, the U.S. CDC recommended not using the live attenuated influenza vaccine administered by nasal spray for the 2016–2017 season.
C. Inactivated influenza virus vaccine is less immunogenic in the elderly.
D. Influenza vaccination is recommended for all U.S. residents over 6 months of age.
E. There are rare reports of a possible association between the inactivated influenza vaccine and the development of the Guillain-Barré syndrome as recently as 2009.

IV-199. All of the following statements regarding HIV transmission are true EXCEPT:

A. Genital ulcerations increase the risk of HIV transmission.
B. HIV may be transmitted to infants in maternal breast milk.
C. HIV may be transmitted via a mosquito or tick bite.
D. The probability of acquiring HIV is greater during receptive anal intercourse than insertive anal intercourse.
E. The quantity of HIV in plasma is a primary determinant of the risk of HIV transmission.

IV-200. A 36-year-old man with HIV/AIDS (CD4+ lymphocyte count = 112/μL) develops a scaly, waxy, yellowish, patchy, crusty, pruritic rash on and around his nose. The rest of his skin examination is normal. Which of the following is the most likely diagnosis?

A. Molluscum contagiosum
B. Kaposi sarcoma
C. Psoriasis
D. Reactivation herpes zoster
E. Seborrheic dermatitis

IV-201. Which of the following scenarios is most likely associated with the lowest risk of HIV transmission to a healthcare provider after an accidental needle stick from a patient with HIV?

A. The needle is visibly contaminated with the patient's blood.
B. The needle stick injury is a deep tissue injury to the healthcare provider.
C. The patient whose blood is on the contaminated needle has been on antiretroviral therapy for many years with a history of resistance to many available agents but most recently has had successful viral suppression on current therapy.
D. The patient whose blood is on the contaminated needle was diagnosed with acute HIV infection 2 weeks ago.

IV-202. Abacavir is a nucleoside transcription inhibitor that carries which side effect unique for HIV antiretroviral agents?

A. Fanconi anemia
B. Granulocytopenia
C. Lactic acidosis
D. Lipoatrophy
E. Severe hypersensitivity reaction

IV-203. A 38-year-old man with HIV/AIDS presents with 4 weeks of diarrhea, fever, and weight loss. Which of the following tests makes the diagnosis of CMV colitis?

A. CMV IgG
B. Colonoscopy with biopsy
C. Serum CMV PCR
D. Stool CMV antigen
E. Stool CMV culture

IV-204. A 40-year-old man is admitted to the hospital with 2–3 weeks of fever, tender lymph nodes, and right upper quadrant abdominal pain. He reports progressive weight loss and malaise for over a year. On examination, he is found to be febrile and frail with temporal wasting and oral thrush. Matted, tender anterior cervical lymphadenopathy <1 cm and tender hepatomegaly are noted. He is diagnosed with AIDS (CD4+ lymphocyte count = 12/μL and HIV RNA 650,000 copies/mL). Blood cultures grow *M avium*. He is started on rifabutin and clarithromycin, as well as dapsone for *Pneumocystis* prophylaxis, and discharged home 2 weeks later after his fevers subside. He follows up with an HIV provider 4 weeks later and is started on tenofovir, emtricitabine, and efavirenz. Two weeks later, he returns to clinic with fevers, neck pain, and abdominal pain. His temperature is 39.2°C, HR is 110 bpm, BP is 110/64 mmHg, and oxygen saturations are normal. His cervical nodes are now 2 cm in size and extremely tender, and one has fistulized to his skin and is draining yellow pus that is acid-fast bacillus stain positive. His hepatomegaly is pronounced and tender. What is the most likely explanation for his presentation?

A. Cryptococcal meningitis
B. HIV treatment failure
C. Immune reconstitution syndrome to *M avium*
D. Kaposi sarcoma
E. *M avium* treatment failure due to drug resistance

IV-205. Current CDC recommendations are that screening for HIV be performed in which of the following?

A. All high-risk groups (injection drug users, men who have sex with men, and high-risk heterosexual women)
B. All U.S. adults
C. Injection drug users
D. Men who have sex with men
E. Women who have sex with more than two men per year

IV-206. A 38-year-old woman is seen in clinic for a decrease in cognitive and executive function. Her husband is concerned because she is no longer able to pay bills, keep appointments, or remember important dates. She also seems to derive considerably less pleasure from caring for her children and participating in her hobbies. She is unable to concentrate for long enough to enjoy movies. This is a clear change from her functional status 6 months prior. A workup reveals a positive HIV antibody by enzyme immunoassay and Western blot. Her CD4+ lymphocyte count is 378/μL with a viral load of 78,000/mL. She is afebrile with normal vital signs. Her affect is blunted, and she seems disinterested in the medical interview. Neurologic examination for strength, sensation, cerebellar function, and cranial nerve function is nonfocal. Funduscopic examination is normal. Mini-Mental Status Examination score is 22/30. A serum RPR test is negative. MRI of the brain shows only cerebral atrophy disproportionate to her age but no focal lesions. What is the next step in her management?

A. Antiretroviral therapy
B. CSF JV virus PCR
C. CSF mycobacterial PCR
D. CSF VDRL test
E. Serum cryptococcal antigen
F. *Toxoplasma* IgG

IV-207. Indinavir is a protease inhibitor that carries which side effect unique for HIV antiretroviral agents?

A. Abnormal dreams
B. Benign hyperbilirubinemia
C. Hepatic necrosis in pregnant women
D. Nephrolithiasis
E. Pancreatitis

IV-208. In an HIV-infected patient, *Isospora belli* infection is different from *Cryptosporidium* infection in which of the following ways?

A. *Isospora* causes a more fulminant diarrheal syndrome, leading to rapid dehydration and even death in the absence of rapid rehydration.
B. *Isospora* infection may cause biliary tract disease, whereas cryptosporidiosis is strictly limited to the lumen of the small and large bowel.
C. *Isospora* is more likely to infect immunocompetent hosts than *Cryptosporidium*.
D. *Isospora* is less challenging to treat and generally responds well to trimethoprim-sulfamethoxazole treatment.
E. *Isospora* occasionally causes large outbreaks among the general population.

IV-209. A 27-year-old man presents to your clinic with 2 weeks of sore throat, malaise, myalgias, night sweats, fevers, and chills. He visited an urgent care center and was told that he likely had the flu. He was told that he had a "negative test for mono." The patient is homosexual, states that he is in a monogamous relationship, and has unprotected receptive and insertive anal and oral intercourse with one partner. He had several partners prior to his current partner 4 years ago but none recently. He reports a negative HIV-1 test 2 years ago and recalls being diagnosed with *Chlamydia* infection 4 years ago. He is otherwise healthy with no medical problems. You wish to rule out the diagnosis of acute HIV. Which blood test should you order?

A. CD4+ lymphocyte count
B. HIV enzyme immunoassay (EIA)/Western blot combination testing
C. HIV resistance panel
D. HIV RNA by PCR
E. HIV RNA by ultrasensitive PCR

IV-210. A 47-year-old woman with known HIV/AIDS (CD4+ lymphocyte = 106/μL and viral load = 35,000/mL) presents with painful growths on the side of her tongue as shown in Figure IV-210. What is the most likely diagnosis?

A. Aphthous ulcers
B. Hairy leukoplakia
C. Herpes stomatitis
D. Oral candidiasis
E. Oral Kaposi sarcoma

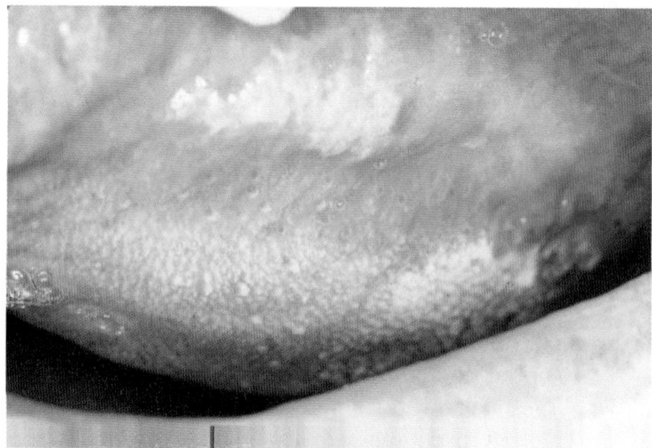

FIGURE IV-210

IV-211. Which of the following patients should receive HIV antiretroviral therapy?

A. A 24-year-old man with newly diagnosed acute HIV infection by viral PCR
B. A 44-year-old man who reports having unprotected anal intercourse with another man who has active HIV infection
C. A 26-year-old pregnant women found at screening to have HIV infection of unknown duration and a CD4 lymphocyte count of 700/μL
D. A 51-year-old man found at screening to have HIV infection of unknown duration and a CD4 lymphocyte count of 150/μL
E. All of the patients should receive antiretroviral therapy.

IV-212. All of the following statements regarding antiretroviral therapy for HIV are true EXCEPT:

A. CD4+ lymphocyte count should rise by >100 within 2 months of initiation of therapy.
B. Intermittent administration regimens have equivalent efficacy to constant administration regimens.
C. Plasma HIV RNA should fall by 1 log order within 2 months of initiation of therapy
D. Recommended initial regimens include three drugs.
E. Viral genotype should be checked prior to initiation of therapy.

IV-213. You are working as a physician on a cruise ship that has traveled to the eastern coast of Mexico. The cruise stopped in the Yucatan Peninsula yesterday. Since that stop, you have evaluated 54 people with nausea, vomiting, and watery diarrhea. Many patients have also complained of abdominal cramping and mild fever. All of the affected individuals disembarked yesterday but were not traveling together. They also have all eaten at the evening buffet on the ship. Physical examination of affected individuals generally shows no abdominal tenderness. A few patients have required IV rehydration. What organism do you suspect as the cause of the outbreak?

A. *Bacillus cereus*
B. Enterotoxigenic *E coli*
C. Group A rotavirus
D. Norovirus
E. *S aureus*

IV-214. A 28-year-old woman is evaluated for fever, anorexia, and malaise. She has a 4-year-old son who recently has had a similar illness and now has the findings shown in Figure IV-214. What is the most likely etiologic agent for this patient's presentation?

A. Contact dermatitis
B. Coxsackievirus
C. Enterovirus D68
D. Herpes simplex virus 1
E. Varicella

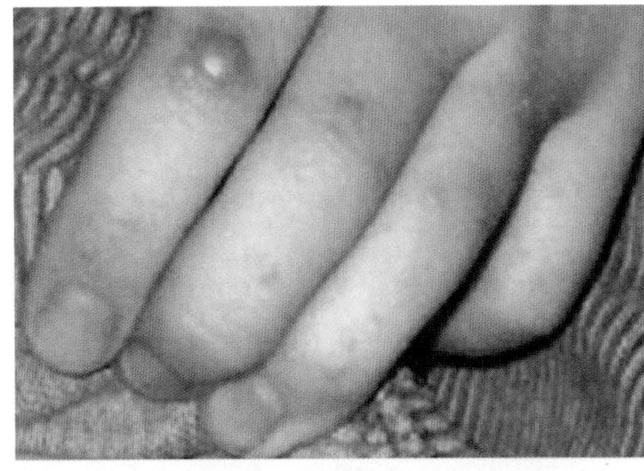

A

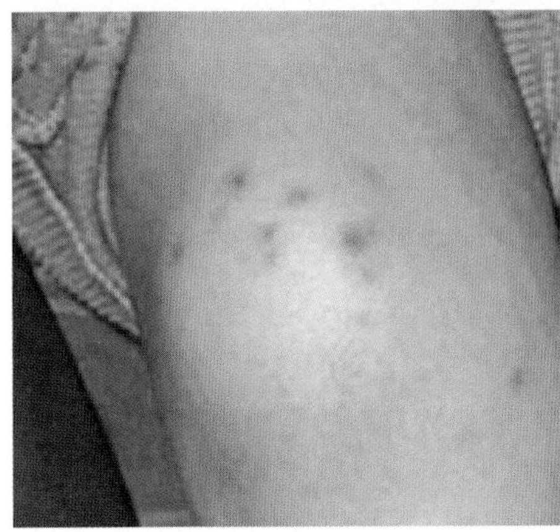

B

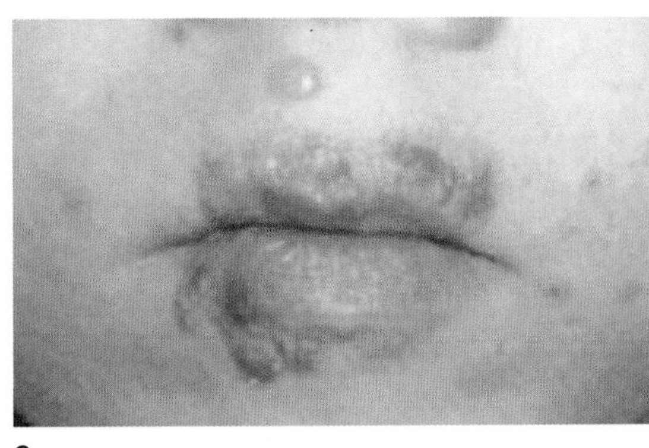

C

FIGURE IV-214 Images reprinted courtesy of Centers for Disease Control and Prevention/Emerging Infectious Diseases.

IV-215. You are working as a public health practitioner in a county of 100,000 individuals. You are asked to investigate an outbreak of a febrile illness accompanied by rash at a small, private preschool. The initial case of illness occurred in a 28-year-old teacher who had recently returned from visiting her family in India. She was born in India and moved to the United States at the age of 4 years. She received her usual childhood immunizations at that time. Her illness began with fever and fatigue about 14 days ago. She stayed home from work until the fever subsided 6 days ago. She had onset of rash that is erythematous and macular. It began on the face, neck, and near the hairline but has become generalized and confluent on the trunk. When examining her oral mucosa, the lesion shown in Figure IV-215 is seen. There are now four children in the preschool exhibiting a high fever, and two have developed a similar rash. Review of medical records at this school shows nonvaccination rates of 25%. Which of the following vaccine-preventable illnesses is most likely?

A. Measles
B. Mumps
C. Poliovirus
D. Rubella
E. Varicella

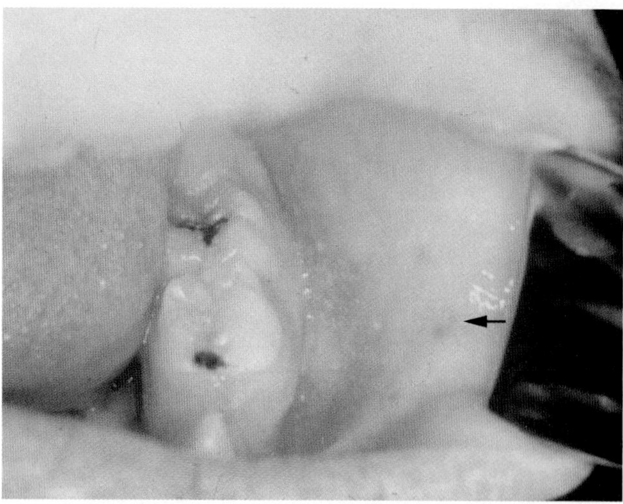

FIGURE IV-215 Courtesy of the Centers for Disease Control and Prevention.

IV-216. You are treating a 5-year-old child who was not vaccinated for measles. The child was exposed at a playground where an individual who had the disease was present. The child is having fevers to 102.1°F, has a diffuse erythematous macular rash, and has Koplik spots. What treatment do you recommend at this time?

A. IV immunoglobulin
B. Ribavirin
C. Prophylactic antibacterial therapy with a penicillin or cephalosporin to prevent pneumonia
D. Supportive care only
E. Vitamin A

IV-217. A 23-year-old previously healthy female letter carrier works in a suburb in which the presence of rabid foxes and skunks has been documented. She is bitten by a bat, which then flies away. Initial examination reveals a clean break in the skin in the right upper forearm. She has no history of receiving treatment for rabies and is unsure about vaccination against tetanus. What should the physician do next?

A. Clean the wound with a 20% soap solution
B. Clean the wound with a 20% soap solution and administer tetanus toxoid
C. Clean the wound with a 20% soap solution, administer tetanus toxoid, and administer human rabies immune globulin intramuscularly
D. Clean the wound with a 20% soap solution, administer tetanus toxoid, administer human rabies immune globulin IM, and administer human diploid cell vaccine
E. Clean the wound with a 20% soap solution and administer human diploid cell vaccine

IV-218. While working at a new medical school in Kuala Lumpur, Malaysia, a 40-year-old previously healthy male from Baltimore develops sudden-onset malaise, fever, headache, retro-orbital pain, backache, and myalgias. On examination, his temperature is 39.6°C with normal BP and slight tachycardia. He has some vesicular lesions on his palate and scleral injection. Laboratory studies are notable for a platelet count of 80,000/μL. All of the following are true regarding his illness EXCEPT:

A. A second infection could result in hemorrhagic fever.
B. After resolution, he has lifelong immunity.
C. IgM enzyme-linked immunosorbent assay (ELISA) may be diagnostic.
D. In equatorial areas, year-round transmission occurs.
E. The disease is transmitted by mosquito.

IV-219. All of the following statements regarding chikungunya virus disease are true EXCEPT:

A. *Aedes aegypti* mosquitoes are the usual vectors for the disease in urban areas.
B. Fever and arthralgia are common symptoms.
C. HLA-B27–positive individuals are at greater risk of prolonged joint symptoms.
D. Oseltamivir shortens the duration of illness.
E. Small joint migratory arthralgia is common.

IV-220. All of the following statements regarding Ebola virus disease (EVD) are true EXCEPT:

A. Abdominal pain and diarrhea are common manifestations of EVD.
B. EVD is frequently spread human-to-human via respiratory aerosols.
C. Patients who survive EVD often have severe sequelae such as arthralgias and asthenia.
D. Treatment of EVD is entirely supportive.
E. Viruses of the Filoviridae family cause EVD.

IV-221. A 24-year-old female student at the Ohio State University is seen in the emergency department for shortness of breath and chest pain. She has no significant past medical history and grew up Cincinnati. Her only medication is an oral contraceptive. As a component of her evaluation, she receives a contrast-enhanced CT scan of the chest. Fortunately, there is no pulmonary embolism (she is diagnosed with viral pleuritis), but there are numerous lung, mediastinal, and splenic calcifications. Based on these findings, which of the following remote infections was most likely?

A. Blastomycosis
B. Coccidioidomycosis
C. Cryptococcosis
D. Histoplasmosis
E. Tuberculosis

IV-222. A 43-year-old woman with a history of rheumatoid arthritis is admitted to the hospital with respiratory failure. She was started on infliximab 2 months ago due to refractory disease. Prior to initiation of the medication, her physician found no evidence of latent tuberculosis infection. She reports 2 days of fever and worsening shortness of breath. On admission, she is hypotensive and hypoxemic with a chest radiograph showing bilateral interstitial and reticulonodular infiltrates. After administration of fluids and broad-spectrum antibiotics, intubation, and initiation of mechanical ventilation, a bronchoalveolar lavage (BAL) is performed. A silver stain of the BAL fluid shows the organisms shown in Figure IV-222. Which of the following is the most likely causative organism?

A. *Aspergillus fumigatus*
B. CMV
C. *Histoplasma capsulatum*
D. *M avium* complex
E. Mycobacterial tuberculosis

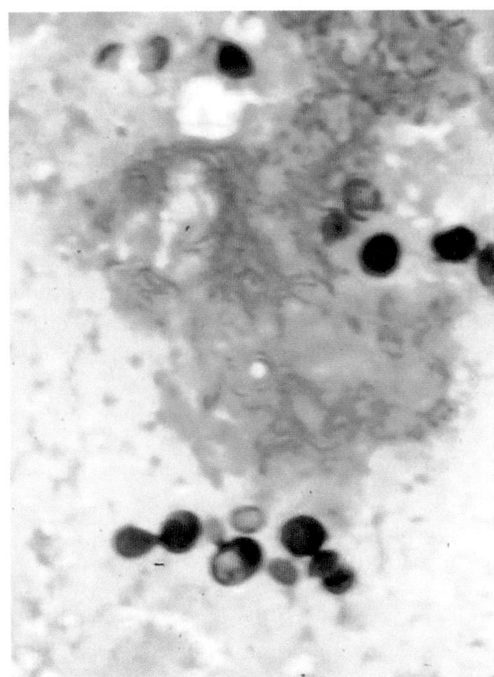

FIGURE IV-222

IV-223. In the patient described in Question IV-222, which of the following therapies should be continued?

A. Caspofungin
B. Clarithromycin/rifampin/ethambutol
C. Ganciclovir
D. Isoniazid (INH)/rifampin/pyrazinamide (PZA)/ ethambutol
E. Liposomal amphotericin B

IV-224. A 24-year-old man is brought to the emergency department by his friends because of worsening mental status, confusion, and lethargy. He has been complaining of a severe headache for over a week. The patient works as a migrant farm worker, most recently in the Fresno, California, area. He is originally from the Philippines and has been in the United States for 4 years with no medical therapy. Vital signs include the following: BP 95/45 mmHg, HR 110 bpm, RR 22 breaths/min, oxygen saturation 98%, and temperature 101.1°F. He appears cachectic and is confused. There is minimal nuchal rigidity but notable photophobia. His complete blood count (CBC) is notable for a WBC of 2000 (95% neutrophils) and a hemoglobin of 9 g/dL. A lumbar puncture reveals 300 WBC (90% lymphocytes), glucose 10 mg/dL, and protein 130 mg/dL. Silver stain of the CSF reveals large (30–100 μm) round structures measuring with thick walls, containing small round spores and internal septations. Which of the following is the most appropriate therapy?

A. Caspofungin
B. Ceftriaxone plus vancomycin
C. Fluconazole
D. INH/rifampin/ethambutol/PZA
E. Penicillin G

IV-225. You are a physician for an undergraduate university health clinic in Arizona. You have evaluated three students with similar complaints of fever, malaise, diffuse arthralgias, cough without hemoptysis, and chest discomfort, and one of the patients has a skin rash on her upper neck consistent with erythema multiforme. Chest radiography is similar in all three, with hilar adenopathy and small pleural effusions. Her CBC is notable for eosinophilia. Upon further questioning, you learn that all three students are in the same archaeology class and participated in an excavation 1 week ago. What is your leading diagnosis?

A. Mononucleosis
B. Primary pulmonary aspergillosis
C. Primary pulmonary coccidioidomycosis
D. Primary pulmonary histoplasmosis
E. Streptococcal pneumonia

IV-226. A 62-year-old man returns from a vacation to Arizona with fever, pleurisy, and a nonproductive cough. All of the following factors on history and laboratory examination favor a diagnosis of pulmonary coccidioidomycosis rather than community-acquired pneumonia EXCEPT:

A. Eosinophilia
B. Erythema nodosum
C. Mediastinal lymphadenopathy on chest roentgenogram
D. Positive *Coccidioides* complement fixation titer
E. Travel limited to northern Arizona (Grand Canyon area)

IV-227. In a patient with lung and skin lesions, a travel history to which of the following regions would be most compatible with the potential diagnosis of blastomycosis?

A. Brazil (Amazon river basin)
B. Malaysia
C. Northern Wisconsin
D. Southern Arizona
E. Western Washington state

IV-228. A 43-year-old man comes to the physician complaining of 1 month of low-grade fever, malaise, shortness of breath, and a growing skin lesion. He resides in the upper peninsula of Michigan and works as a landscaper. He avoids medical care as much as possible. He is on no medications and smokes 2 packs per day of cigarettes. Over the last month, he notices that his daily productive cough has worsened, and the phlegm is dark yellow. He also reports that he has developed a number of skin lesions that start as painful nodules then, over a week, ulcerate and discharge pus (Figure IV-228). His physical examination is notable for egophony and bronchial breath sounds in the right lower lobe, and approximately 5–10 ulcerating 4- to 8-cm skin lesions on the lower extremities consistent with the one shown in Figure IV-228. His chest radiograph shows right lower lobe consolidation with no pleural effusion and no evidence of hilar or mediastinal adenopathy. After obtaining sputum for cytology and culture and a biopsy of the skin lesion, which is the next most likely diagnostic or therapeutic intervention?

A. Colonoscopy to evaluate for inflammatory bowel disease
B. INH/rifampin/PZA/ethambutol
C. Itraconazole
D. Positron emission tomography (PET) scan to evaluate for metastatic malignant disease
E. Vancomycin

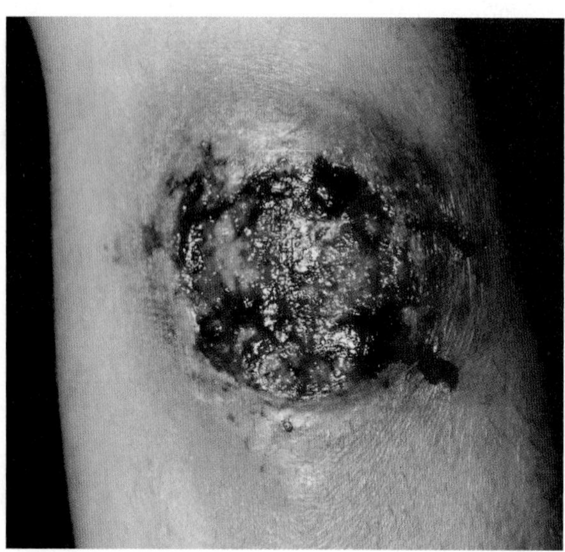

FIGURE IV-228 From Wolff K, Johnson RA, Saavedra AP: *Fitzpatrick's Color Atlas & Synopsis of Clinical Dermatology*, 7th ed. New York, NY: McGraw-Hill, 2013, Fig. C-8. Courtesy of Elizabeth M. Spiers, MD.

IV-229. A 34-year-old female aviary worker who has no significant past medical history, is taking no medications, has no allergies, and is HIV-negative presents to the emergency department with fever, headache, and fatigue. She reports that her headache has been present for at least 2 weeks, is bilateral, and is worsened by bright lights and loud noises. She is typically an active person who has recently been fatigued and has lost 8 lb due to anorexia. Her work involves caring for birds and maintaining their habitat. Her vital signs are notable for a temperature of 101.8°F. Neurologic examination is normal except for notable photophobia. Head CT examination is normal. Lumbar puncture is significant for an opening pressure of 20 cmH_2O, WBC count of 15 cells/μL (90% monocytes), protein of 0.5 g/L (50 mg/mL), glucose of 2.8 mmol/L (50 mg/dL), and positive India ink stain. What is the appropriate therapy for this patient?

A. Amphotericin B for 2 weeks followed by lifelong fluconazole
B. Amphotericin B plus flucytosine for 2 weeks followed by oral fluconazole for 10 weeks
C. Caspofungin for 3 months
D. Ceftriaxone and vancomycin for 2 weeks
E. Voriconazole for 3 months

IV-230. An HIV-positive patient with a CD4 count of 110/μL who is not taking any medications presents to an urgent care center with complaints of a headache for the past week. He also notes nausea and intermittently blurred vision. Examination is notable for normal vital signs without fever but mild papilledema. Head CT does not show dilated ventricles. What is the definitive diagnostic test for this patient?

A. CSF culture
B. MRI with gadolinium imaging
C. Ophthalmologic examination including visual field testing
D. Serum cryptococcal antigen testing
E. Urine culture

IV-231. All of the following have been identified as predisposing factors or conditions associated with the development of hematogenously disseminated candidiasis EXCEPT:

A. Abdominal surgery
B. Indwelling vascular catheters
C. Hyperalimentation
D. Pulmonary alveolar proteinosis
E. Severe burns

IV-232. A 19-year-old young man is undergoing intensive chemotherapy for acute myelogenous leukemia. He has been neutropenic for >5 days and is on prophylactic meropenem and vancomycin for 3 days in addition to parenteral alimentation. His absolute neutrophil count yesterday was 50, and today, it is 200. He had a fever spike to 101°F yesterday. A chest/abdomen CT at that time was unremarkable. You are asked to see him because over the last 3 hours he has developed fever >102°F, severe myalgias and joint pains, and new skin lesions (Figure IV-232). New skin lesions are appearing in all body areas. Initially they are red areas that become macronodular and are mildly painful. Vital signs are otherwise notable for a blood pressure of 100/60 mmHg and heart rate of 105 bpm. An urgent biopsy of the skin lesion is most likely to show which of the following?

A. Branching (45°) septated hyphae on methenamine silver stain
B. Budding yeast on methenamine silver stain
C. Encapsulated yeast on India ink stain
D. Pseudohyphae and hyphae on tissue Gram stain
E. Rounded internally septated spherules on methenamine silver stain

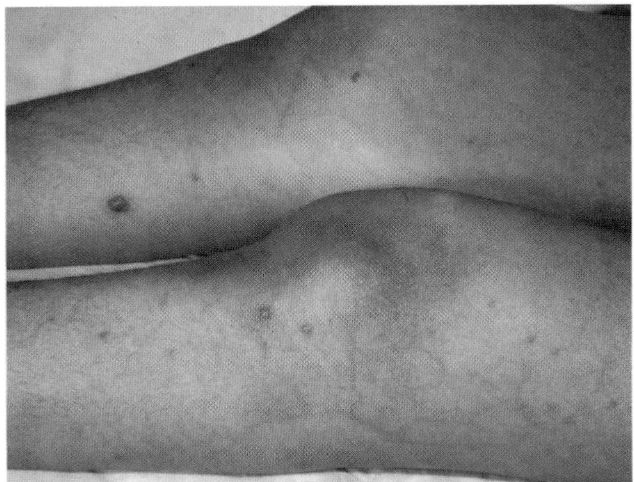

FIGURE IV-232 Image courtesy of Dr. Noah Craft and the Victor Newcomer Collection at UCLA; with permission.

IV-233. In the patient described in Question IV-232, all of the following medications are appropriate additions to the current antibiotic regimen EXCEPT:

A. Amphotericin
B. Caspofungin
C. Fluconazole
D. Flucytosine
E. Voriconazole

IV-234. Which of the following statements regarding the use of antifungal agents to prevent *Candida* infections is true?

A. HIV-infected patients should receive prophylaxis for oropharyngeal candidiasis when CD4 count is <200.
B. Most centers administer fluconazole to recipients of allogeneic stem cell transplants.
C. Most centers administer fluconazole to recipients of living related renal transplants.
D. Voriconazole has been shown to be superior to other agents as prophylaxis in liver transplant recipients.
E. Widespread *Candida* prophylaxis in postoperative patients in the surgical intensive care unit has been shown to be cost effective.

IV-235. A 72-year-old man is admitted to the hospital with bacteremia and pyelonephritis. He is HIV negative and has no other significant past medical history. Two weeks into his treatment with antibiotics, a fever evaluation reveals a blood culture positive for *C albicans*. Examination is unremarkable. WBC count is normal. The central venous catheter is removed, and systemic antifungal agents are initiated. What further evaluation is recommended?

A. Abdominal CT scan to evaluate for abscess
B. Chest x-ray
C. Funduscopic examination
D. Repeat blood cultures
E. Transthoracic echocardiogram

IV-236. A local oncology center is concerned about the occurrence of an outbreak of cases of invasive *Aspergillus* in patients receiving bone marrow transplants. Which of the following is the most likely source of *Aspergillus* infection?

A. Contaminated air source
B. Contaminated water source
C. Patient-to-patient spread in outpatient clinic waiting rooms
D. Provider-to-patient spread due to poor hand washing technique
E. Provider-to-patient spread due to poor utilization of alcohol disinfectant

IV-237. A 23-year-old man receiving chemotherapy for relapsed acute myelogenous leukemia has had persistent neutropenia for the past 4 weeks. Over the past 5 days, his absolute neutrophil count has risen from zero to 200, and he has had persistent fevers despite receiving cefepime/vancomycin empiric therapy. Other than fever, tachycardia, and malaise, he has no focal findings and his vital signs are otherwise unremarkable, including a normal oxygen saturation on room air. A chest/abdomen CT performed due to the fever shows a few scattered 1- to 2-cm nodules with surrounding ground-glass infiltrates in the lower lobes. Which of the following tests will most likely be positive in this patient?

A. Serum cryptococcal antigen
B. Serum galactomannan assay
C. Sputum fungal culture
D. Urine *Histoplasma* antigen
E. Urine *Legionella* antigen

IV-238. In the patient described in Question IV-237, which of the following medications should be initiated immediately?

A. Amphotericin B
B. Caspofungin
C. Fluconazole
D. Trimethoprim-sulfamethoxazole
E. Voriconazole

IV-239. A 40-year-old male smoker with a history of asthma is admitted to the inpatient medical service with fever, cough, brownish-green sputum, and malaise. Physical examination shows an RR of 15 breaths/min, no use of accessory muscles of breathing, and bilateral polyphonic wheezes throughout the lung fields. There is no clubbing or skin lesions. You consider a diagnosis of allergic bronchopulmonary aspergillosis. All of the following clinical features are consistent with allergic bronchopulmonary aspergillosis EXCEPT:

A. Bilateral, peripheral cavitary lung infiltrates
B. Elevated serum IgE
C. Peripheral eosinophilia
D. Positive serum antibodies to *Aspergillus* species
E. Positive skin testing for *Aspergillus* species

IV-240. A 26-year-old asthmatic continues to have coughing fits and dyspnea despite numerous steroid tapers and frequent use of albuterol over the past few months. Persistent infiltrates are seen on chest roentgenogram. A pulmonary consultation suggests an evaluation for allergic bronchopulmonary aspergillosis. Which of the following is the best diagnostic test for this diagnosis?

A. Bronchoalveolar lavage (BAL) with fungal culture
B. Galactomannan enzyme immunoassay (EIA)
C. High-resolution CT
D. Pulmonary function tests
E. Serum IgE level

IV-241. Patients with all of the following conditions have increased risk of developing mucormycosis EXCEPT:

A. Deferoxamine therapy
B. Factitious hypoglycemia
C. Glucocorticoid therapy
D. Metabolic acidosis
E. Neutropenia

IV-242. A 38-year-old woman with a history of diabetes mellitus, hypertension, and chronic renal insufficiency reports comes to the emergency department complaining of double vision for 1 day. She has required chronic hemodialysis for 8 years and often misses appointments, including four of her last eight sessions. She also notes 12 hours of facial swelling and difficulty speaking. She appears to be in moderate distress. Her vital signs are notable for a temperature of 39.0°C, BP of 155/95 mmHg, HR of 110 bpm, and RR of 25 breaths/min. Her head examination demonstrates right-sided proptosis, facial edema, and a facial palsy. (See Figure IV-242.) Laboratory examination reveals a WBC count of 15,000/μL, serum glucose of 225 mg/dL, serum creatinine of 6.3 mg/dL, and hemoglobin A1C of 9.7%. Arterial blood gas on room air is as follows: pH 7.24, PCO_2 20 mmHg, and PO_2 100 mmHg. She is immediately brought to the intensive care unit, and a needle aspirate of a retro-orbital mass is performed. On-site cytopathology reveals wide, thick-walled, ribbon-shaped, nonseptate hyphal organisms that branch at 90 degrees. All of the following are components of the initial therapy for her likely infection EXCEPT:

A. Hemodialysis
B. Insulin
C. Liposomal amphotericin B
D. Surgical debridement
E. Voriconazole

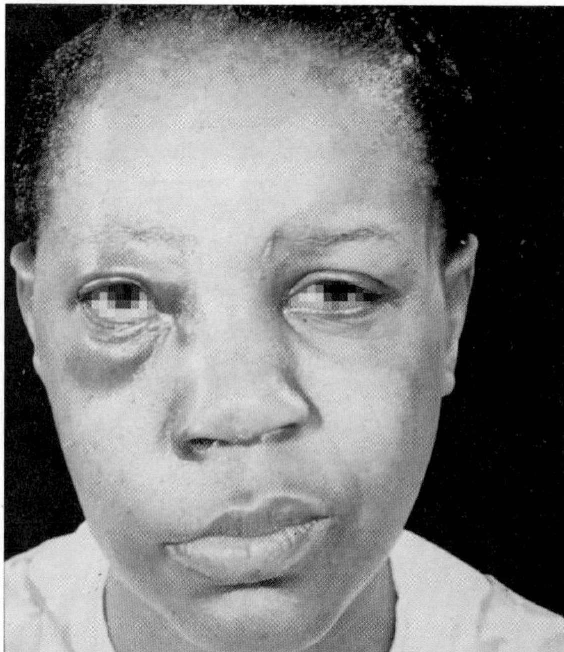

A

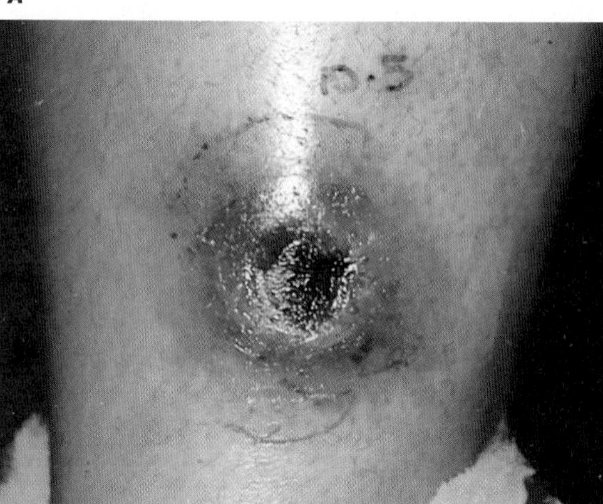

B

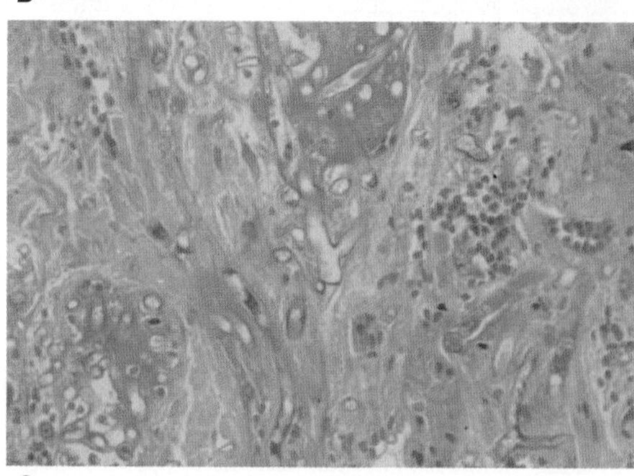

C

FIGURE IV-242 From Goldsmith LA, Katz SI, Gilchrest BA, et al (eds): *Fitzpatrick's Dermatology in General Medicine*, 8th ed. New York, NY: McGraw-Hill, 2012, Fig. 190-19A.

IV-243. Which of the following is the most common form of infection in patients with mucormycosis?

A. Cutaneous
B. Gastrointestinal
C. Hematogenous dissemination
D. Pulmonary
E. Rhinocerebral

IV-244. A 21-year-old college student seeks your opinion because of a lesion on his head. He has no significant medical history and reports a solitary lesion on the crown of his head for over 1 month that has been growing slowly. He has had no fever and reports that while the area is itchy he feels well. On examination, you note a 3-cm round area of alopecia without redness, pain, or inflammation. It is well demarcated with central clearing, scaling, and broken hair shafts at the edges. There is no redness or pain. Which of the following should you recommend?

A. Caspofungin
B. Clindamycin
C. Doxycycline
D. Minoxidil
E. Terbinafine

IV-245. A 34-year-old man seeks the advice of his primary care physician because of an asymptomatic rash on his chest. There are coalescing light brown to salmon-colored macules present on the chest. A scraping of the lesions is viewed after a wet preparation with 10% potassium hydroxide solution. There are both hyphal and spore forms present, giving the slide an appearance of "spaghetti and meatballs." In addition, the lesions fluoresce to a yellow-green appearance under a Wood's lamp. Tinea versicolor is diagnosed. Which of the following microorganisms is responsible for this skin infection?

A. *Fusarium solani*
B. *Malassezia furfur*
C. *Penicillium marneffei*
D. *Sporothrix schenckii*
E. *Trichophyton rubrum*

IV-246. A 16-year-old young man seeks evaluation for an ulcerative lesion on his right hand. He reports that he was playing in the woods and pricked his index finger on a thorn. Three days later, he developed a knot there that ulcerated, and now he has new bumps going up his hand. (See Figure IV-246.) On examination, the only notable findings in addition to his hand are a temperature of 38.5°C and an enlarged and tender epitrochlear lymph node on the right arm. A biopsy of the edge of the finger lesion shows ovoid and cigar-shaped yeasts. Sporotrichosis is diagnosed. What is the most appropriate therapy for this patient?

A. Amphotericin B IV
B. Caspofungin IV
C. Clotrimazole topically
D. Itraconazole PO
E. Selenium sulfide topically

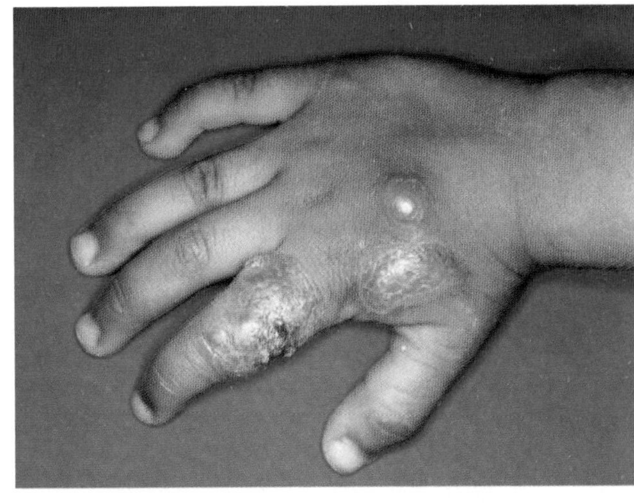

FIGURE IV-246 Courtesy of Dr. Angela Restrepo.

IV-247. A 35-year-old woman with long-standing rheumatoid arthritis has been treated with infliximab for the last 6 months with improvement of her joint disease. She has a history of positive PPD and takes INH prophylaxis. For the past week, she reports worsening dyspnea on exertion with low-grade fevers and a nonproductive cough. On examination, her vital signs are notable for normal BP, temperature of 38.0°C, HR of 105 bpm, RR of 22 breaths/min, and SaO_2 of 91% on room air. Her lungs are clear. Within one flight of steps, she becomes dyspneic and her SaO_2 falls to 80%. A representative image from her chest CT scan is shown in Figure IV-247. Which of the following is the most likely diagnosis?

A. *Aspergillus fumigatus* pneumonia
B. *Nocardia asteroides* pneumonia
C. *Pneumocystis jiroveci* pneumonia
D. Rheumatoid nodules
E. Staphylococcal bacteremia and septic pulmonary emboli

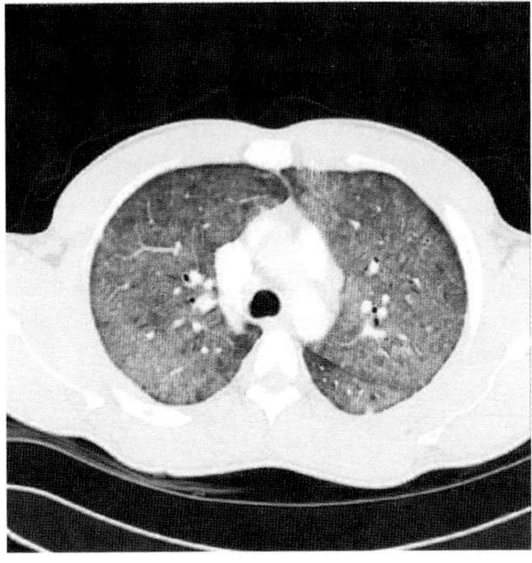

FIGURE IV-247

IV-248. Which of the following patients should receive prophylaxis against *Pneumocystis jiroveci* pneumonia?

A. A 24-year-old man with HIV initiated on HAART therapy 9 months ago when his CD4 count was 200/μL and now has a CD4 count of 700/μLfor the last 4 months
B. A 26-year-old man with asthma receiving 40 mg of prednisone for an acute exacerbation
C. A 36-year-old man with newly diagnosed HIV and a CD4 count of 400/μL
D. A 42-year-old woman who presented with acute respiratory failure and was found to have polymyositis with interstitial lung disease and is being initiated on high-dose corticosteroid therapy for at least 2 months
E. A 69-year-old woman with polymyalgia rheumatica maintained on prednisone 7.5 mg/d

IV-249. A 45-year-old woman with known HIV infection and medical nonadherence to therapy is admitted to the hospital with 2–3 weeks of increasing dyspnea on exertion and malaise. Chest radiograph shows bilateral alveolar infiltrates, and induced sputum is positive for *P jiroveci*. Which of the following clinical conditions is an indication for administration of adjunct glucocorticoids?

A. Acute respiratory distress syndrome
B. CD4+ lymphocyte count <100/μL
C. No clinical improvement 5 days into therapy
D. Pneumothorax
E. Room air PaO_2 <70 mmHg

IV-250. A 28-year-old man is diagnosed with HIV infection during a clinic visit. He has no symptoms of opportunistic infection. His CD4+ lymphocyte count is 150/μL. All of the following are approved regimens for primary prophylaxis against *P jiroveci* infection EXCEPT:

A. Aerosolized pentamidine 300 mg monthly
B. Atovaquone 1500 mg PO daily
C. Clindamycin 900 mg PO every 8 hours plus primaquine 30 mg PO daily
D. Dapsone 100 mg PO daily
E. Trimethoprim-sulfamethoxazole 1 single-strength tablet PO daily

IV-251. A 35-year-old migrant fruit picker originally from El Salvador is evaluated for right upper quadrant pain, fever, and hepatic tenderness. He reports no diarrhea or bloody stool. A representative image from his abdominal CT scan is shown in Figure IV-251. Of note, he has been in the United States for approximately 10 years and was well until approximately 10 days ago. Which of the following tests can be used to confirm the diagnosis?

A. Examination of stool for trophozoites
B. Liver biopsy
C. PCR of stool for *Campylobacter*
D. Response to empiric trial of iodoquinol
E. Serologic test for antibody to *E histolytica*

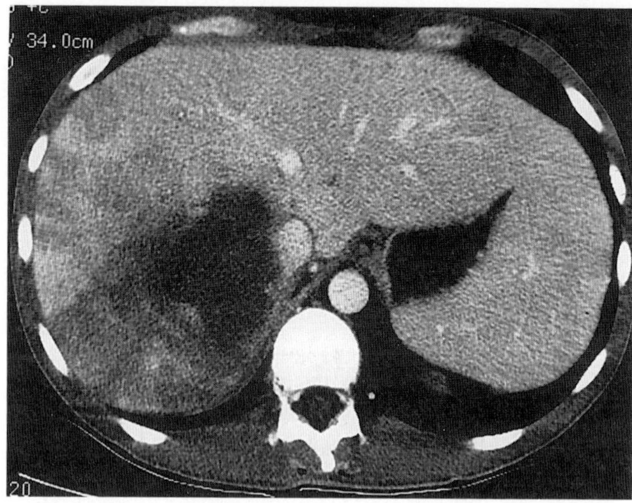

FIGURE IV-251 Courtesy of the Department of Radiology, UCSD Medical Center, San Diego; with permission.

IV-252. A 19-year-old woman is seen in the emergency department for fever and altered mental status. She is from Algeria and arrived in the United States earlier that day. She reported 3 days of episodic fever before leaving home. Over the course of the day, her family describes deteriorating mental status. Now she is confused and lethargic. Her physical examination is notable for a temperature of 40°C, HR of 145 bpm, and systemic BP of 105/62 mmHg. She has a clearly gravid uterus, approximately 24 weeks of gestational age, and neurologic examination shows confusion but no focal findings. Thick and thin smears for malaria are performed. (See Figure IV-252.) Treatment with IV quinidine is started immediately while you are contacting the CDC for artesunate. Which of the following is a potential complication of quinidine therapy?

A. Arrhythmias
B. Hyperthyroidism
C. Nightmares
D. Retinopathy
E. Seizures

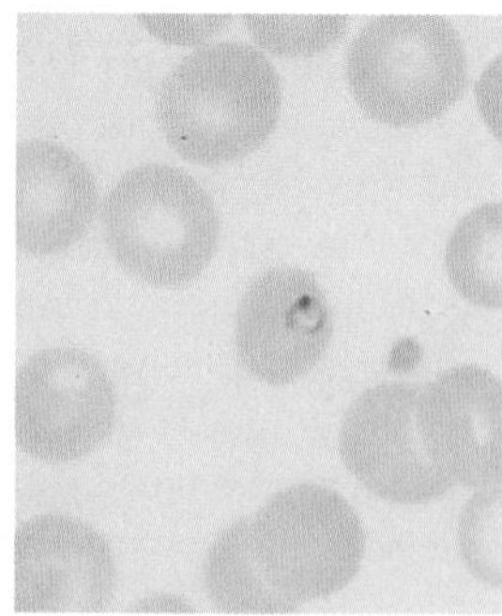

FIGURE IV-252 Reproduced from *Bench Aids for the Diagnosis of Malaria Infections*, 2nd ed, with the permission of the World Health Organization.

IV-253. A 28-year-old woman presents with fevers, headache, diaphoresis, and abdominal pain 2 days after returning from an aid mission to the coast of Papua New Guinea. Several of her fellow aid workers developed malaria while abroad, and she stopped her doxycycline prophylaxis due to a photosensitivity reaction 5 days prior. You send blood cultures, routine labs, and a thick and thin smear to evaluate the source of her fevers. Which of the following statements is accurate in reference to diagnosis of malaria?

A. A thick smear is performed to increase sensitivity in comparison to a thin smear but can only be performed in centers with experienced laboratory personnel and has a longer processing time.
B. Careful analysis of the thin blood film allows for prognostication based on estimation of parasitemia and morphology of the erythrocytes.
C. In the absence of rapid diagnostic information, empirical treatment for malaria should be strongly considered.
D. Morphology on blood smear is the current criterion used to differentiate the four species of *Plasmodium* that infect humans.
E. All of the above are true.

IV-254. Mr. Zachs is planning a college semester abroad in Mongolia, and his mother is worried that he needs malaria prophylaxis. Which of the following statements is true?

A. Chloroquine-resistant malaria is endemic in Mongolia.
B. Chloroquine-sensitive malaria is endemic in Mongolia.
C. Malaria is not endemic in Mongolia.
D. Mefloquine-resistant malaria is endemic in Mongolia.
E. Mr. Zachs should begin prophylactic treatment with atovaquone-proguanil (Malarone) 1 week before starting his semester abroad.

IV-255. A 19-year-old college student is employed during the summer months on Nantucket Island in Massachusetts. She is evaluated in the local emergency department with 5 days of fever, malaise, and generalized weakness. While she does recall a tick bite approximately 6 weeks ago, she denies rash around that time or presently. Physical examination is unremarkable with the exception of a temperature of 39.3°C. Which of the following statements is true regarding her most likely illness?

A. *Babesia duncani* is the most likely organism to be found in her peripheral blood smear.
B. First-line therapy for severe disease in this patient is immediate complete RBC exchange transfusion in addition to clindamycin and quinine.
C. If babesiosis is not demonstrated on thick or thin preparations of peripheral blood, PCR amplification of babesial 18S rRNA is recommended.
D. The ring form of *Babesia microti* seen in RBCs on microscopy is indistinguishable from *Plasmodium falciparum*.
E. Without a current or historical rash, she is unlikely to have babesiosis.

IV-256. A 35-year-old man from India is seen for evaluation of several weeks of fever that has decreased in intensity, but he now has developed abdominal swelling. He has no significant past medical history. Physical examination shows palpable splenomegaly and hepatomegaly and diffuse lymphadenopathy. Diffuse hyperpigmentation is present in his skin. Visceral leishmaniasis is suspected. Which of the following diagnostic techniques is most commonly employed?

A. Culture of peripheral blood for *Leishmania*
B. PCR for *Leishmania infantum* nucleic acid in peripheral blood
C. Rapid immunochromatographic test for recombinant antigen rK39 from *L infantum*
D. Smear of stool for amastigotes
E. Splenic aspiration to demonstrate amastigotes

IV-257. All of the following statements regarding infection with *Trypanosoma cruzi* are true EXCEPT:

A. It is found only in the Americas.
B. It is the causative agent of Chagas disease.
C. It is transmitted to humans by the bite of deer flies.
D. It may be transmitted to humans by blood transfusion.
E. It may cause acute and chronic disease.

IV-258. A 36-year-old man is admitted to the hospital with 3 months of worsening dyspnea on exertion and orthopnea. Over the last 2 weeks, he has been sleeping upright. He denies any chest pain with exertion or syncope. There is no history of hypertension, hyperlipidemia, or diabetes. He is a lifelong nonsmoker and, since arriving to the United States from rural Mexico 16 years ago, works as an electrician. His physical examination is notable for being afebrile with an HR of 105 bpm, BP of 100/80 mmHg, RR of 22 breaths/min, and oxygen saturation of 88% on room air. He has notable jugular venous distension upright with no Kussmaul sign, 3+ pitting edema to the knees, and bilateral crackles two-thirds up the lung fields. Cardiac examination shows a laterally displaced PMI, a 2/6 systolic murmur at the apex and axilla, an S_3, and no friction rub or pericardial knock. Which of the following is likely to reveal the most likely diagnosis?

A. Coronary angiography
B. Right heart catheterization
C. Serum PCR for *T cruzi* DNA
D. Serum *T cruzi* IgG antibodies
E. Serum troponin

IV-259. A 36-year-old medical missionary recently returned from a 2-week trip to rural Honduras. During the trip, she lived in the jungle where she received multiple bug bites and developed open sores. One week after her return, she comes to clinic reporting 2 days of malaise, fever to 38.5°C, and anorexia. There is an indurated swollen area of erythema on her calf and femoral adenopathy. Because of her exposure history, you obtain a thin and thick blood smear that demonstrates organisms consistent with *T cruzi*. Which of the following is the best next intervention?

A. Immediate therapy with benznidazole
B. Immediate therapy with primaquine
C. Immediate therapy with voriconazole
D. Observation only
E. Serologic confirmation with specific *T cruzi* IgG testing

IV-260. A 44-year-old man who recently returned from a safari trip to Uganda seeks attention for a painful lesion on the leg and new fevers. He was on a safari tour where he stayed in the animal park that was populated extensively with antelope, lions, giraffes, and hippos. They often toured savannah and jungle settings. He returned within the last week and noticed a painful lesion on his neck at the site of some bug bites. He reports fever over 38°C, and you find palpable cervical lymphadenopathy. Review of systems is notable for malaise and anorexia for 2 days. A thick and thin smear of the blood reveals protozoa consistent with trypanosomes. All of the following are true about his disease EXCEPT:

A. Humans are the primary reservoir.
B. If untreated, death is likely.
C. It was transmitted by the bite of a tsetse fly.
D. Lumbar puncture should be performed.
E. Suramin is effective treatment.

IV-261. A 36-year-old man with HIV/AIDS is brought to the hospital after a grand mal seizure at home. He has a history of ongoing IV drug use and is not taking highly active antiretroviral therapy (HAART). His last CD4 T-cell count was <50/μL over a month ago. Further medical history is unavailable. Vital signs are normal. On examination, he is barely arousable and disoriented. He is cachectic. There is no nuchal rigidity or focal motor deficits. Serum creatinine is normal. An urgent head MRI with gadolinium is performed, and the results of the T1-gated images are shown in Figure IV-261. Which of the following will be the most effective therapy?

A. Caspofungin
B. INH/rifampin/PZA/ethambutol
C. Pyrimethamine plus sulfadiazine
D. Streptokinase
E. Voriconazole

IV-262. Which of the following intestinal protozoal infections can be diagnosed with stool ova and parasite examination?

A. *Cryptosporidium*
B. *Cyclospora*
C. *Giardia*
D. *Isospora*
E. Microsporidia

IV-263. A 17-year-old woman presents to the clinic complaining of vaginal itchiness and malodorous discharge. She is sexually active with multiple partners, and she is interested in getting tested for sexually transmitted diseases. A wet-mount microscopic examination is performed, and trichomonal parasites are identified. Which of the following statements regarding trichomoniasis is true?

A. A majority of women are asymptomatic.
B. No treatment is necessary as disease is self-limited.
C. The patient's sexual partner need not be treated.
D. Trichomoniasis can only be spread sexually.
E. Trichomoniasis is 100% sensitive to metronidazole

IV-264. A 19-year-old college student presents to the emergency department with crampy abdominal pain and watery diarrhea that has worsened over 3 days. He recently returned from a volunteer trip to Mexico. He has no past medical history and felt well throughout the trip. Stool examination shows small cysts containing four nuclei, and stool antigen immunoassay is positive for *Giardia*. Which of the following is a recommended treatment regimen for this patient?

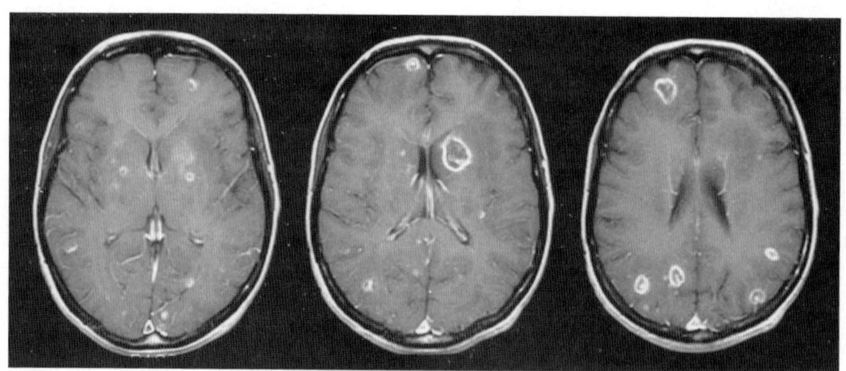

FIGURE IV-261 Courtesy of Clifford Eskey, Dartmouth Hitchcock Medical Center, Hanover, NH; with permission.

A. Albendazole
B. Clindamycin
C. Giardiasis is self-limited and requires no antibiotic therapy
D. Paromomycin
E. Tinidazole

IV-265. A 28-year-old woman is brought to the hospital because of abdominal pain, weight loss, and dehydration. She was diagnosed with HIV/AIDS 2 years ago and has a history of oral candidiasis and pneumocystis pneumonia. She reports voluminous watery diarrhea over the last 2 weeks. Because of medical nonadherence, she has not taken any antiretroviral therapy. Routine stool ova and parasite examination is normal, but stool antigen testing reveals *Cryptosporidium*. Which of the following is the recommended therapy?

A. Metronidazole
B. Nitazoxanide
C. No therapy is recommended because the diarrhea is self-limited
D. There is no effective specific therapy available
E. Tinidazole

IV-266. Which of the following has resulted in a significant decrease in the incidence of trichinellosis in the United States?

A. Adequate therapy that allows for eradication of infection in index cases before person-to-person spread can occur
B. Earlier diagnosis due to a new culture assay
C. Federal laws limiting the import of foreign cattle
D. Laws prohibiting the feeding of uncooked garbage to pigs
E. Requirements for hand washing by commercial kitchen staff who handle raw meat

IV-267. A patient comes to clinic and describes progressive muscle weakness over several weeks. He has also experienced nausea, vomiting, and diarrhea. One month ago, he had been completely healthy and describes a bear hunting trip in Alaska, where they ate some of the game they killed. Soon after he returned, his gastrointestinal (GI) symptoms began, followed by muscle weakness in his jaw and neck that has now spread to his arms and lower back. Examination confirms decreased muscle strength in the upper extremities and neck. He also has slowed extraocular movements. Laboratory examination shows panic values for elevated eosinophils and serum creatine phosphokinase. Which of the following organisms is most likely the cause of his symptoms?

A. *Campylobacter*
B. CMV
C. *Giardia*
D. *Taenia solium*
E. *Trichinella*

IV-268. A 3-year-old boy is brought by his parents to clinic. They state that he has experienced fevers, anorexia, and weight loss, and, most recently, has started wheezing at night. He had been completely healthy until these symptoms started 2 months ago. The family had travelled through Europe several months prior and reported no unusual exposures or exotic foods. They have a puppy at home. On examination, the child is ill-appearing and is noted to have hepatosplenomegaly. Laboratory results show a panic value of 82% eosinophils. Total WBCs are elevated. A CBC is repeated to rule out a laboratory error, and eosinophils are 78%. Which of the following is the most likely organism or process?

A. *Cysticercosis*
B. Giardiasis
C. *Staphylococcus lugdunensis*
D. Toxocariasis
E. Trichinellosis

IV-269. The patient described in Question IV-268 continues to decline over the next 2–3 days, developing worsening respiratory status, orthopnea, and cough. On physical examination, his HR is 120 bpm, BP is 95/80 mmHg, RR is 24 breaths/min, and oxygen saturation is 88% on room air. His neck veins are elevated, there is an apical S_3, and his lungs have bilateral crackles half way up the lung fields. An echocardiogram shows an ejection fraction of 25%. Which of the following therapies should be initiated?

A. Albendazole
B. Methylprednisolone
C. Metronidazole
D. Nafcillin
E. Vancomycin

IV-270. A 28-year-old man is brought to the emergency department by his wife for altered mental status, fevers, vomiting, and headache. He developed a bilateral headache that began about a day ago that has progressively worsened. He hand his wife returned from a trip to Thailand and Vietnam where they spent a lot of time in rural settings eating local mollusks, seafood, and vegetables. His physical examination is notable for fever, nuchal rigidity, confusion, and lethargy. Lumbar puncture reveals elevated opening pressure, elevated protein, normal glucose, and WBC count of 200/μL with 50% eosinophils, 25% neutrophils, and 25% lymphocytes. Which of the following is the most likely etiology of his meningitis?

A. *Angiostrongylus cantonensis*
B. *Gnathostoma spinigerum*
C. *Trichinella murrelli*
D. *Trichinella nativa*
E. *Toxocara canis*

IV-271. While attending the University of Georgia, a group of friends go on a 5-day canoeing and camping trip in rural southern Georgia. A few weeks later, one of the campers develops a serpiginous, raised, pruritic, erythematous eruption on the buttocks. *Strongyloides* larvae are found in his stool. Three of his companions, who are asymptomatic, are also found to have *Strongyloides* larvae in their stool. Which of the following is indicated in the asymptomatic carriers?

A. Fluconazole
B. Ivermectin
C. Mebendazole
D. Mefloquine
E. Treatment only for symptomatic illness

IV-272. All of the following are clinical manifestations of *Ascaris lumbricoides* infection EXCEPT:

A. Asymptomatic carriage
B. Fever, headache, photophobia, nuchal rigidity, and eosinophilia
C. Nonproductive cough and pleurisy with eosinophilia
D. Right upper quadrant pain and fever
E. Small bowel obstruction

IV-273. A 21-year-old college student in Mississippi comes to student health to ask advice about treatment for *Ascaris* infection. He is an education major and works 1 day a week in an elementary school where a number of the students were recently diagnosed with ascariasis over the last 3 months. He feels well and reports being asymptomatic. A stool ova and parasite exam reveals characteristic *Ascaris* eggs. Which of the following should you recommend?

A. Albendazole
B. Diethylcarbamazine (DEC)
C. Fluconazole
D. Metronidazole
E. Vancomycin

IV-274. While on a business trip to Santiago, Chile, a 42-year-old woman presents to the emergency department with severe abdominal pain. She has no past medical or surgical history. She recalls no recent history of abdominal discomfort, diarrhea, melena, bright red blood per rectum, nausea, or vomiting prior to this acute episode. She ate ceviche (lime-marinated raw fish) at a local restaurant 3 hours prior to presentation. On examination, she is in terrible distress and has dry heaves. Temperature is 37.6°C; HR is 128 bpm; BP is 174/92 mmHg. Examination is notable for an extremely tender abdomen with guarding and rebound tenderness. Bowel sounds are present and hyperactive. Rectal examination is normal, and guaiac test is negative. Pelvic examination is unremarkable. WBC count is 6738/μL; hematocrit is 42%. A complete metabolic panel and lipase and amylase levels are all within normal limits. CT of the abdomen shows no abnormality. What is the next step in her management?

A. CT angiogram of the abdomen
B. Pelvic ultrasonography
C. Proton pump inhibitor therapy and observation
D. Right upper quadrant ultrasonography
E. Upper endoscopy

IV-275. While participating in a medical missionary visit to Indonesia, you are asked to see a 22-year-old man with new-onset high fever, groin pain, and a swollen scrotum. His symptoms have been present for about a week and are worsening steadily. His temperature is 38.8°C, and his examination is notable for tender inguinal lymphadenopathy, scrotal swelling with a hydrocele, and lymphatic streaking. All of the following may be useful in diagnosing his condition EXCEPT:

A. Examination of blood
B. Examination of hydrocele fluid
C. Scrotal ultrasound
D. Serum ELISA
E. Stool ova and parasite

IV-276. The patient described in Question IV-275 should be treated with which of the following medications?

A. Albendazole
B. Diethylcarbamazine (DEC)
C. Doxycycline
D. Ivermectin
E. Praziquantel

IV-277. A 45-year-old woman is brought to the emergency department by her daughter because she saw something moving in her mother's eye. The patient is visiting from Zaire where she lives in the rainforest. The patient reports some occasional eye swelling and redness. On examination, you find a worm in the subconjunctiva (see Figure IV-277). Which of the following medications is indicated for therapy?

A. Albendazole
B. Diethylcarbamazine (DEC)
C. Ivermectin
D. Terbinafine
E. Voriconazole

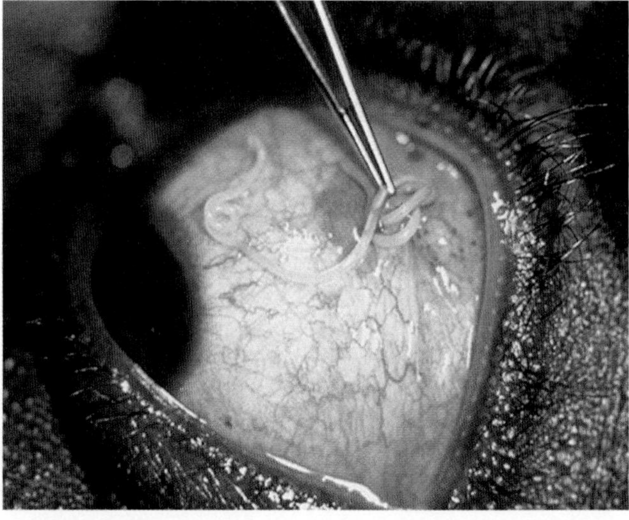

FIGURE IV-277

IV-278. All of the following statements regarding the epidemiology of schistosomal infection are true EXCEPT:

A. *Schistosoma haematobium* infection is seen mostly in South America.
B. *Schistosoma japonicum* infection is seen mostly in China, Philippines, and Indonesia.
C. *Schistosoma mansoni* infection is seen in Africa, South America, and the Middle East.
D. Schistosomal infection causes acute and chronic manifestations.
E. Transmission of all human schistosomal infections is from snails.

IV-279. A 48-year-old woman presents to her physician with a 2-day history of fever, arthralgias, diarrhea, and headache. She recently returned from an ecotour in tropical sub-Saharan Africa, where she went swimming in inland rivers. Notable findings on physical examination include a temperature of 38.7°C (101.7°F); 2-cm tender mobile lymph nodes in the axilla, cervical, and femoral regions; and a palpable spleen. Her WBC count is 15,000/μL with 50% eosinophils. She should receive treatment with which of the following medications?

A. Chloroquine
B. Mebendazole
C. Metronidazole
D. Praziquantel
E. Thiabendazole

IV-280. A person with liver disease caused by *S mansoni* would be most likely to have which of the following?

A. Ascites
B. Esophageal varices
C. Gynecomastia
D. Jaundice
E. Spider nevi

IV-281. A 26-year-old man is brought to the emergency department after the onset of a grand mal seizure. On arrival to the hospital, the seizure had terminated and he was somnolent without focal findings. Vital signs were normal except for tachycardia. The patient has no known medical history and no history of illicit drug or alcohol use. He takes no medications. At a routine clinic visit 3 months prior, he was documented to be HIV antibody and PPD negative. He is originally from rural Guatemala and has been in the United States working as a laborer for the last 3 years. A contrast head CT shows multiple parenchymal lesions in both hemispheres that are identical to the one shown in the posterior right brain (see Figure IV-281). After acute stabilization including anticonvulsant therapy, which of the following is the most appropriate next step in this patient's management?

A. Echocardiogram with Doppler examination of aortic and mitral valves
B. Initiation of praziquantel therapy
C. Initiation of pyrimethamine and sulfadiazine therapy
D. Measurement of HIV viral load
E. Neurosurgical consultation for brain biopsy

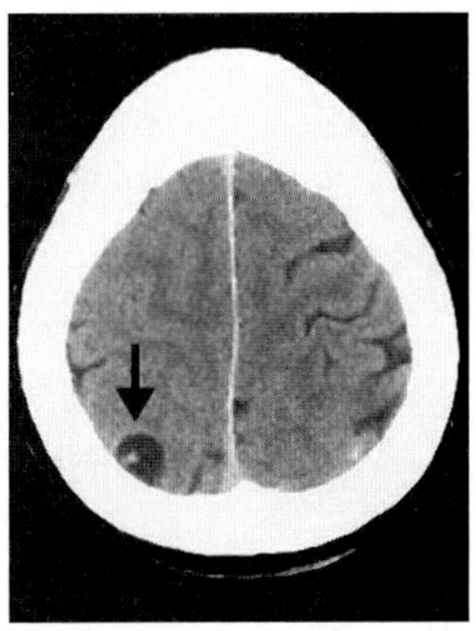

FIGURE IV-281 Modified with permission from JC Bandres et al: *Clin Infect Dis* 15:799, 1992. © The University of Chicago Press.

IV-282. A 44-year-old woman presents to the emergency department with recurrent episodes of right upper quadrant pain, typically soon after meals. These episodes have been present for at least a month and seem to be worsening. The patient emigrated from Lebanon over 20 years ago and works as an attorney. She takes no medications and is physically active. On examination, she is jaundiced and in obvious discomfort due to right upper quadrant pain. She is afebrile and tachycardic. Her physical examination is notable for an enlarged liver. Ultrasound examination confirms the large liver and demonstrates a complex 14-cm cyst with daughter cysts extending to the liver edge with associated biliary tract dilation. Which of the following is the most appropriate management approach to this patient?

A. Albendazole medical therapy
B. Albendazole followed by surgical resection
C. Needle biopsy of the cystic lesion
D. PAIR (percutaneous aspiration, infusion of scolicidal agent, and reaspiration)
E. Serologic testing for *Echinococcus granulosus*

ANSWERS

IV-1. **The answer is B.** *(Chap. 144)* Deficiencies in the complement system predispose patients to a variety of infections. Most of these deficits are congenital. Patients with sickle cell disease have acquired functional defects in the alternative complement pathway. They are at risk of infection from *Streptococcus pneumoniae* and *Salmonella* spp. Patients with liver disease, nephrotic syndrome, and systemic lupus erythematosus may have defects in C3. They are at particular risk for infections with *Staphylococcus aureus, S pneumoniae, Pseudomonas* spp, and *Proteus* spp. Patients with congenital or acquired (usually systemic lupus erythematosus) deficiencies in the terminal complement cascade (C5–8) are at particular risk of infection from *Neisseria* spp, such as *Neisseria meningitidis* or *Neisseria gonorrhoeae.*

IV-2. **The answer is B.** *(Chap. 144)* Infectious diseases remain the second leading cause of death worldwide, with cardiovascular disease the leading cause. Although the rate of infectious disease–related deaths has decreased dramatically over the past 20 years with a growing worldwide population, the absolute numbers of such deaths have remained relatively constant, totaling just over 12 million in 2010. As shown in Figure IV-2, these deaths disproportionately affect low- and middle-income countries; in 2010, 23% of all deaths worldwide were related to infectious diseases, with rates >60% in most sub-Saharan African countries. Given that infectious diseases are still a major cause of global mortality, understanding the local epidemiology of disease is critically important in evaluating patients. Diseases such as human immunodeficiency virus (HIV)/acquired immunodeficiency syndrome (AIDS) have decimated sub-Saharan Africa, with HIV-infected adults representing 15%–26% of the total population in countries like Zimbabwe, Botswana, and Swaziland. Moreover, drug-resistant tuberculosis is rampant throughout the former Soviet bloc countries, India, China, and South Africa. The ready availability of this type of information allows physicians to develop appropriate differential diagnoses and treatment plans for individual patients. Programs such as the Global Burden of Disease seek to quantify human losses (e.g., deaths, disability-adjusted life-years) due to diseases by age, sex, and country over time; these data not only help inform local, national, and international health policy but can also help guide local medical decision making. Even though some diseases (e.g., pandemic influenza, severe acute respiratory syndrome) are seemingly geographically restricted, the increasing ease of rapid worldwide travel has raised concern about their swift spread around the globe. The world's increasing interconnectedness has profound implications not only for the global economy but also for medicine and the spread of infectious diseases.

IV-3. **The answer is B.** *(Chap. 144)* Given that elevations in temperature are often a hallmark of infection, paying close attention to the temperature may be of value in diagnosing an infectious disease. The idea that 37°C (98.6°F) is the normal human body temperature dates back to the 19th century and was initially based on axillary measurements. Rectal temperatures more accurately reflect the core body temperature and are 0.4°C (0.7°F) and 0.8°C (1.4°F) higher than oral and axillary temperatures, respectively. Although the definition of fever varies greatly throughout the medical literature, the most common definition, which is based on studies defining fever of unknown origin, uses a temperature ≥38.3°C (101°F). For every 1°C (1.8°F) increase in core temperature, the heart rate typically rises by 15–20 bpm. Intracellular Gram-negative bacteria, tick-borne organisms, and some viruses cause infections that may be associated with relative bradycardia (*Faget sign*), where patients have a lower heart rate than might be expected for a given body temperature. Although this pulse–temperature dissociation is not highly sensitive or specific for establishing a diagnosis, it is often discussed on rounds and is potentially useful in low-resource settings given its ready availability and simplicity. (See Table IV-3.)

IV-4 and IV-5. **The answers are A and E, respectively.** *(Chap. 147)* Individuals who have had a splenectomy are at increased risk for death due to sepsis, with a death rate 58 times

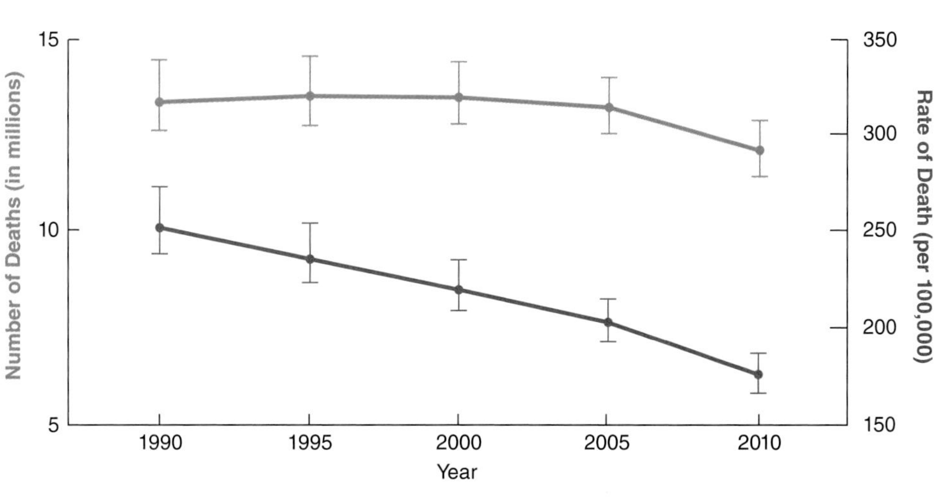

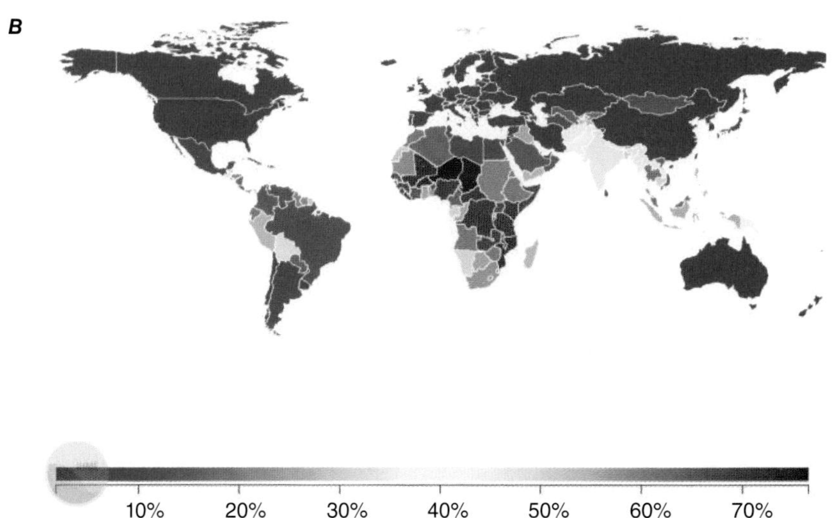

FIGURE IV-2 Magnitude of infectious disease–related deaths globally. **A.** The absolute number (*blue line; left axis*) and rate (*red line; right axis*) of infectious disease–related deaths throughout the world since 1990. **B.** A map depicting country-specific data for the percentages of total deaths that were attributable to communicable, maternal, neonatal, and nutritional disorders in 2010.
Source: Global Burden of Disease Study, Institute for Health Metrics and Evaluation.

higher than that of the general population. Most infections occur within the first 2 years after splenectomy, but the risk remains higher than the general population throughout life despite vaccination. Mortality from sepsis in an individual who has undergone splenectomy is about 50%. The most common organism causing sepsis in individuals who have had splenectomy is *S pneumoniae* (option E), which is responsible for 50%–70% of cases of sepsis in asplenic patients. Other organisms with a high incidence of sepsis in asplenic patients include *Haemophilus influenzae* (option B) and *N meningitidis* (option C), although these are less common than *S pneumoniae*. The recommended antibiotics for individuals with postsplenectomy sepsis are ceftriaxone 2 g intravenously (IV) every 12 hours and vancomycin 15 mg/kg every 12 hours.

IV-6. **The answer is B.** *(Chap. 147)* Ecthyma gangrenosum is a typical rash marked by hemorrhagic vesicles surrounded by a rim of erythema with central necrosis and ulceration. This finding is seen in sepsis caused by *Pseudomonas aeruginosa* most commonly and can also be seen with *Aeromonas hydrophila*. Sepsis due to these organisms most frequently occurs in individuals with prolonged neutropenia, extensive burns, or hypogammaglobulinemia.

TABLE IV-3 **Causes of Relative Bradycardia**

Infectious Causes	
Intracellular organisms	
Gram-negative bacteria	*Salmonella typhi* *Francisella tularensis* *Brucella* spp *Coxiella burnetii* (Q fever) *Leptospira interrogans* *Legionella pneumophila* *Mycoplasma pneumoniae*
Tick-borne organisms	*Rickettsia* spp *Orientia tsutsugamushi* (scrub typhus) *Babesia* spp
Other	*Corynebacterium diphtheriae* *Plasmodium* spp (malaria)
Viruses/viral infections	Yellow fever virus Dengue virus Viral hemorrhagic fevers[a] Viral myocarditis
Noninfectious Causes	
	Drug fever β-Blocker use Central nervous system lesions Malignant lymphoma Factitious fever

[a]Primarily early in the course of infection with Marburg or Ebola virus.

IV-7. **The answer is C.** *(Chap. 147)* Necrotizing fasciitis is a life-threatening infection that leads to extensive necrosis of the subcutaneous tissue and fascia. It is most commonly caused by group A streptococci and mixed facultative and anaerobic flora. Recently, there have been an increasing number of cases of necrotizing fasciitis due to community-acquired methicillin-resistant *S aureus*. Risk factors include diabetes mellitus, IV drug use, and peripheral vascular disease. The infection often arises at a site of minimal trauma, and the physical findings initially are minimal in comparison to the severity of pain and fever. The mortality rate for necrotizing fasciitis is between 15% and 34% but rises to as high as 70% if toxic shock syndrome is present. Wide surgical debridement of the affected tissue is necessary, and without surgery, the mortality is near 100%. A high index of clinical suspicion is important for selecting the appropriate antibiotic therapy and early consultation of surgery. The initial antibiotics should cover the typical organisms and include vancomycin 15 mg/kg IV every 12 hours, clindamycin 600 mg IV every 8 hours, and gentamicin 5 mg/kg IV every 8 hours.

IV-8 and IV-9. **The answers are B and B, respectively.** *(Chap. 148, http://www.cdc.gov/mmwr/preview/mmwrhtml/mm6322a4.htm?s_cid=mm6322a4_w)* Measles and pertussis are two vaccine-preventable illnesses that are making a remarkable reemergence in the United States. Prior to the availability of the combined measles, mumps, and rubella (MMR) vaccine, there were more than 500,000 cases of measles yearly. By 2012, the disease had nearly been eliminated in the United States, with only 55 reported cases; however, in 2014, the number of cases increased to more than 640. The disease is still considered to be eliminated in the United States with no indigenous transmission of the disease because all new cases of the disease arise from importation of the disease from countries outside of the United States. However, with rates of MMR vaccination at historic lows, there has been an unprecedented rise in cases of measles over the past 2 years with distinct outbreaks of measles in unvaccinated communities. The largest outbreak that occurred in 2014 was in an Amish community in Ohio that had low vaccination rates. When one considers all individuals affected in a measles outbreak, the primary individuals who are affected (>75%) are those who are unvaccinated for philosophical or religious beliefs. All components of the MMR vaccine are live attenuated virus, but there are no reports of spontaneous mutation to a virulent form. After two doses of vaccine, >95% of individuals above 1 year of age are immune from measles.

IV-10. **The answer is B.** *(Chap. 148)* Pneumococcal vaccination has been recommended for all individuals at any age with a variety of chronic medical conditions, including chronic respiratory disease, chronic heart disease, chronic liver failure, diabetes mellitus, asplenia, and chronic kidney disease. Determining when to revaccinate individuals has been somewhat controversial. The current recommendations are to revaccinate individuals ages 19 to 64 years old 5 years after the initial vaccine if they have chronic renal failure or nephrotic syndrome, asplenia, or other immunocompromising conditions. All other individuals should receive a one-time revaccination at age 65 and older if they were vaccinated 5 or more years previously and were age less than 65 at the time of original vaccination.

IV-11. **The answer is C.** *(Chap. 148)* The varicella-zoster vaccine is a live virus vaccine that was recently introduced for prevention of shingles in older adults. The current recommendation is that all adults older than 60 years be offered the zoster vaccine regardless of whether they report a childhood history of chickenpox. Because this is a live virus vaccine, it cannot be administered to anyone who has severe immunodeficiency. Specific recommendations for patients for whom the zoster vaccine is either not indicated or contraindicated include the following:

1. Pregnancy
2. Individuals younger than 60 years
3. Patients with leukemia, lymphoma, or other malignant neoplasms affecting the bone marrow. If a patient is in remission and has not received chemotherapy or radiation therapy within 3 months, the vaccine can be given
4. Individuals with AIDS or HIV with a CD4+ count <200/μL or ≤15% peripheral lymphocytes
5. Individuals taking immunosuppressive therapy equivalent to prednisone ≥20 mg daily, methotrexate 0.4 mg/kg/week, or azathioprine <3 mg/kg/d
6. Anyone with suspected cellular immunodeficiency (i.e., hypogammaglobulinemia)
7. Individuals receiving a hematopoietic stem cell transplant
8. Individuals receiving recombinant human immune mediators or modulators, especially anti–tumor necrosis factor agents

IV-12. **The answer is E.** *(Chap. 149)* When traveling abroad, it is important to plan ahead and consider the potential infectious agents to which one might be exposed. The Centers for Disease Control and Prevention (CDC) and the World Health Organization publish guidelines for recommended vaccinations prior to travel to countries around the world. Prior to travel, it is certainly recommended that an individual be up to date on all routine vaccinations, including measles, diphtheria, and polio. Influenza is perhaps the most common preventable illness in travelers, and the influenza vaccine should be administered per routine guidelines. However, there are few required vaccinations in most countries. Yellow fever is one exception, and proof of vaccination is required by many countries in sub-Saharan Africa and equatorial South America. This is especially important for individuals traveling from areas where yellow fever is endemic or epidemic. The only other required vaccinations are meningococcal meningitis and influenza vaccination to travel in Saudi Arabia during the Hajj.

IV-13. **The answer is E.** *(Chap. 149, http://wwwnc.cdc.gov/travel/destinations/haiti.htm)* Malaria remains endemic in many parts of the world, and an estimated 30,000 travelers from the United States and Europe are infected with malaria during travel yearly. The areas of highest risk are in sub-Saharan Africa and Oceania, with the lowest risk in South and Central America, including Haiti and the Dominican Republic. Chloroquine resistance is growing throughout the world and is especially notable in parts of South America, Africa, and Southeast Asia. However, in Haiti, the incidence of chloroquine-resistant malaria is low. For a traveler to Haiti, the CDC states that the traveler has a choice of chloroquine, doxycycline, atovaquone-proguanil, or mefloquine. In addition, the traveler should be cautioned to use appropriate techniques for malarial prevention, including protective clothing, DEET-containing insect repellants, permethrin-impregnated bednets, and screened sleeping accommodations, if possible.

IV-14. **The answer is E.** *(Chap. 149)* Individuals with HIV are generally considered at high risk of infectious complications when traveling abroad. However, individuals who have no symptoms and a CD4+ count >500/μL appear to be at no greater risk than individuals without HIV infection. Prior to travel, it is important to research the travel requirements for the specific country of travel. Many countries routinely deny entry for HIV-positive individuals for prolonged stays, and proof of HIV testing is required in many countries for stays longer than 3 months. Consular offices should be contacted prior to travel to determine if any special documentation is required. The HIV-infected traveler should have all routine immunizations prior to travel, including influenza and pneumococcal vaccinations. The response rate to influenza in an asymptomatic HIV-positive person is >80%. Generally, live attenuated viruses are not given to HIV-infected individuals. However, because measles can be lethal in HIV, this vaccine is recommended unless the CD4+ count is <200/μL, and the expected response rate would be between 50% and 100%. In contrast, the live yellow fever vaccine is not given to HIV-infected travelers, and individuals with a CD4+ count <200/μL should be discouraged from traveling to countries with endemic yellow fever. Some countries in sub-Saharan Africa require yellow fever vaccination. However, as this patient is traveling from a low-risk area, a medical waiver would likely be issued.

IV-15. **The answer is D.** *(Chap. 152e)* Multiple factors contribute to infectious risks for soldiers serving overseas. The clinical spectrum of infectious illness acquired overseas includes acute infections in the combat theater, acute infections with delayed symptoms, and chronic or relapsing infections. Infectious illnesses were once a major cause of noncombat mortality, but the increase in use of preventative vaccines and early antimicrobial therapy has significantly decreased this mortality. Nevertheless, they remain an important source of morbidity. Typically military medical facilities are of high quality and distributed adequately to support the health care needs of troops.

IV-16. **The answer is D.** *(Chap. 152e)* There were 13,000 cases of malaria (mainly *Plasmodium vivax*) imported into the United States after the Vietnam War. More than 115,000 cases of viral hepatitis, mainly due to hepatitis A, were reported among Soviet troops serving in Afghanistan in the 1980s. There were only rare reports of hepatitis A and B infection among U.S. troops serving in the Persian Gulf in the early 1990s. Cutaneous leishmaniasis is caused by *Leishmania major* or *Leishmania tropica*, and there have been approximately 1300 cases diagnosed, but the incidence is likely underreported as lesions may spontaneously resolve. In contrast, visceral leishmaniasis is caused by *Leishmania Donovan*, and there have only been five confirmed reports of this. Between 2001 and 2010, there were 643 animal (mainly dog) bites in troops serving in the combat theaters of Southwest and Central Asia; 18% of bitten personnel received postexposure rabies prophylaxis. One soldier died of rabies in the United States in 2012, 8 months after being bitten by a dog in Afghanistan; this was the first case of a rabies-related death in a member of the U.S. military who caught the infection overseas in nearly 40 years.

IV-17. **The answer is C.** *(Chap. 153)* There are multiple clinical conditions associated with health-care-associated pneumonia (HCAP). Residence in a nursing home or extended-care facility, hospitalizations for 2 or more days in the prior 3 months, and current hospitalizations that have been 48 hours or longer are associated with HCAP due to methicillin-resistant *S aureus* (MRSA), *P aeruginosa*, *Acinetobacter* species, and multidrug-resistant Enterobacteriaceae. HCAP due to *P aeruginosa* is also associated with antibiotic therapy in the preceding 3 months. Chronic dialysis, home infusion therapy, and home wound care place patients at risk for HCAP due to MRSA. Having a family member with a multidrug-resistant infection is associated with HCAP due to both MRSA and multidrug-resistant Enterobacteriaceae.

IV-18. **The answer is C.** *(Chap. 153)* There is an extensive list of potential etiologic agents in community-acquired pneumonia (CAP) including bacteria, fungi, viruses, and protozoa.

However, most cases of CAP are caused by relatively few pathogens. *S pneumoniae* is the most common overall cause of CAP, and 10%-15% of cases are polymicrobial. The most common causes of CAP in outpatients is *S pneumoniae*, *Mycoplasma pneumoniae*, *H influenzae*, *Chlamydia pneumoniae*, and respiratory viruses. In hospitalized patients that are not in the intensive care unit (ICU), this list also includes *Legionella* species. The most common microbial causes of CAP in patients treated in the ICU are *S pneumoniae*, *S aureus*, *Legionella* species, gram-negative bacilli, and *H influenzae*.

IV-19. **The answer is B.** *(Chap. 153)* Diagnosis and treatment of CAP often incorporates a combination of clinical, radiographic, and laboratory features to determine the most likely etiology and treatment. In most instances of CAP, outpatient treatment is sufficient, and definitive etiologic diagnosis of the causative organism is not required and is not cost-effective. However, the outpatient diagnosis of CAP often does require confirmation by chest radiograph as the sensitivity and specificity of physical examination findings are about 58% and 67%, respectively. In addition, chest radiograph may identify risk factors suggestive of a more severe clinical course such as multifocal infiltrates. Moreover, outside of the 2% of individuals admitted to intensive care for treatment of CAP, there are no data that treatment directed against a specific causative organism is superior to empiric therapy. In some instances, one may decide to attempt to determine a causative organism for CAP, particularly in individuals who have risk factors for resistant organisms or in patients who fail to respond appropriate to initial antibiotic therapy. The most common way in which the etiologic organism causing CAP is diagnosed is via sputum culture with Gram stain. The primary purpose of the Gram stain is to ensure that the sputum is an adequate lower respiratory sample for culture with fewer than 10 squamous epithelial cells and more than 25 neutrophils per high-power field. However, at times, Gram stain can suggest a specific diagnosis. Generally, the yield from sputum culture is ≤50%, even in cases of bacteremic pneumococcal pneumonia. The yield from blood cultures is also low, 5%–14%, even when collected prior to initiation of antibiotics. More recently, antigen tests and polymerase chain reaction (PCR) testing directed against specific organisms have gained favor. The most common antigen test that is performed is for *Legionella pneumophila* as this organism does not grow in culture unless performed on specific media. Antigen and PCR tests are also available for *S pneumoniae* and *M pneumoniae*, respectively, but given the costs, they are not frequently performed

IV-20. **The answer is D.** *(Chap. 153)* Determining the appropriate initial treatment for CAP initially requires determining whether the severity of illness warrants admission to the hospital. Clinical rules for determining potential severity of pneumonia have been developed including the Pneumonia Severity Index (PSI) and the CURB-65 criteria. While the PSI has the largest body of research to support its use, the model includes 20 variables that may be impractical to implement in a busy clinical practice. The CURB-65 criteria include only five variables: (1) **c**onfusion; (2) **u**rea > 7 mmol/L; (3) **r**espiratory rate ≥30 breaths/min; (4) **b**lood pressure ≤90/60 mmHg; and (5) age ≥**65**. This patient meets none of these criteria and is not hypoxemic or in a high-risk group for complications from CAP. Therefore, he can safely be treated as an outpatient without further diagnostic workup as his history, physical examination, and chest radiograph are all consistent with the diagnosis of CAP. The empiric antibiotic regimen recommended by the Infectious Diseases Society of America and the American Thoracic Society for individuals who are previously healthy and have not received prior antibiotics in the prior 3 months is either doxycycline or a macrolide such as azithromycin or clarithromycin. In outpatients with significant medical comorbidities or prior antibiotic use within 3 months, the suggested antibiotics are either a respiratory fluoroquinolone (such as moxifloxacin) or a β-lactam plus a macrolide.

IV-21. **The answer is E.** *(Chap. 153)* Ventilator-associated pneumonia (VAP) is a common complication of endotracheal intubation and mechanical ventilation. Prevalence estimates indicate that 70% of patients requiring mechanical ventilation for 30 days or longer will have at least one instance of VAP. However, the epidemiology of VAP has been difficult to accurately study as no single set of criteria is reliably diagnostic of VAP. Generally, it is thought that VAP has a tendency to be overdiagnosed for a variety of reasons, including high rates of tracheal colonization with pathogenic organisms and multiple alternative causes of fevers and/or pulmonary infiltrates in the critically ill patient. Quantitative cultures have gained favor as the quantitative nature is thought to discriminate better between colonization and active infection. A variety of approaches have been advocated including endotracheal aspirates yielding more than 10^6 organisms or protected brush specimens from distal airways yielding more than 10^3 organisms. However, the quantitative yield of these tests can be highly influenced by even a single dose of antibiotics, and antibiotic changes are common in critically ill patients, particularly when a new fever has emerged. Thus, the lack of growth on quantitative culture may be difficult to interpret in this setting. More recently, there has been growing use of the Clinical Pulmonary Infection Score (CPIS) that incorporates a variety of clinical, radiographic, and laboratory factors to determine the likelihood of VAP, although its true utility in clinical practice remains to be fully determined.

IV-22. **The answer is C.** *(Chap. 153)* Pleural effusion is a known complication of severe CAP. A significant pleural effusion should be tapped for both diagnostic and therapeutic purposes. If the pleural fluid grows bacteria or has a pH <7, glucose <2.2 mmol/L, or lactate dehydrogenase concentration >1000 units/L, then the effusion should be completely drained, which sometimes requires chest tube insertion. While pleural fluid protein is a component of the Light criteria and can help determine if an effusion is a transudate or exudate, there is no recommendation for complete drainage based solely on pleural fluid protein result.

IV-23. **The answer is B.** *(Chap. 153)* Patients were previously treated for CAP for 10–14 days, but studies with fluoroquinolones and macrolides have suggested that a 5-day course is sufficient for otherwise uncomplicated CAP. Even a single dose of ceftriaxone has been associated with a significant cure rate. Longer cases may be required for patients with bacteremia or virulent pathogens such as *P aeruginosa*. In cases of ventilator-associated pneumonia, 8-day courses of therapy have been shown to be just as effective as 2-week courses of antibiotics if the CPIS decreased over the first 3 days and are associated with less frequent emergence of antibiotic-resistant strains.

IV-24. **The answer is E.** *(Chap. 154)* Lung abscess represents necrosis and cavitation of the lung following microbial infection. Lung abscesses can be single or multiple but usually are marked by a single dominant cavity >2 cm in diameter. Although the incidence of lung abscesses has decreased in the postantibiotic era, they are still a source of significant morbidity and mortality. Lung abscesses are usually characterized as either primary (~80% of cases) or secondary. Primary lung abscesses usually arise from aspiration, are often caused principally by anaerobic bacteria, and occur in the absence of an underlying pulmonary or systemic condition. Patients at particular risk for aspiration, such as those with altered mental status, alcoholism, drug overdose, seizures, bulbar dysfunction, prior cerebrovascular or cardiovascular events, or neuromuscular disease, are most commonly affected. In addition, patients with esophageal dysmotility or esophageal lesions (strictures or tumors) and those with gastric distention and/or gastroesophageal reflux, especially those who spend substantial time in the recumbent position, are at risk for aspiration. It is widely thought that colonization of the gingival crevices by anaerobic bacteria or microaerophilic streptococci (especially in patients with gingivitis and periodontal disease), combined with a risk of aspiration, is important in the development of lung abscesses. Secondary lung abscesses arise in the setting of an underlying condition, such as a postobstructive process (e.g., a bronchial foreign body or tumor) or a systemic process (e.g., HIV infection or another immunocompromising condition). In Lemierre syndrome, an infection begins in the pharynx (classically involving *Fusobacterium necrophorum*) and then spreads to the neck and the carotid sheath (which contains the jugular vein) to cause septic thrombophlebitis. Because most cases of lung abscess occur in the context of reclining aspiration, the dependent lobes of the lung are most vulnerable. The dependent lobes include the superior segment of the lower lobes and the posterior segment of the upper lobes, with the right lung more commonly involved than the left lung. The middle lobe and the lingula are the most ventral lobes and are therefore nondependent in the supine position.

IV-25. The answer is B. *(Chap. 154)* This patient has a typical right lower lobe lung abscess likely related to alcoholism and aspiration. The history of a few weeks of illness with constitutional findings is typical. The radiograph shows an abscess with air-fluid level in the right lower lobe. Therapy should be directed to the upper airway anaerobic bacteria. For many decades, penicillin was the antibiotic of choice for primary lung abscesses in light of its anaerobic coverage; however, because oral anaerobes can produce β-lactamases, clindamycin has proved superior to penicillin in clinical trials. For primary lung abscesses, the recommended regimens are (1) clindamycin (600 mg IV three times daily; then, with the disappearance of fever and clinical improvement, 300 mg orally [PO] four times daily) or (2) an IV-administered β-lactam/β-lactamase combination, followed—once the patient's condition is stable—by orally administered amoxicillin-clavulanate. This therapy should be continued until imaging demonstrates that the lung abscess has cleared or regressed to a small scar. Treatment duration may range from 3–4 weeks to as long as 14 weeks. One small study suggested that moxifloxacin (400 mg/d PO) is as effective and well tolerated as ampicillin-sulbactam. Notably, metronidazole is not effective as a single agent; it covers anaerobic organisms but not the microaerophilic streptococci that are often components of the mixed flora of primary lung abscesses. Aztreonam has predominant activity against gram-negative bacteria, and micafungin is an antifungal agent; neither has activity against oral anaerobes.

IV-26. The answer is E. *(Chap. 155)* The etiologic agents of infective endocarditis vary by host (Table IV-26). Community-acquired native valve endocarditis remains an important clinical problem, particularly in the elderly. In those patients, streptococci (viridans spp., *Streptococcus gallolyticus*, other non–group A and other group streptococci, and *Abiotrophia* spp.) account for approximately 40% of cases. *S aureus* (28%) is next most common. Enterococci, HACEK group, coagulase-negative, and culture-negative cases each account for <10% of community-acquired native valve cases. In healthcare-associated, injection drug use–associated, and >12-month-old prosthetic valve endocarditis, *S aureus* is most common. Coagulase-negative *Staphylococcus* is the most common organism in prosthetic valve endocarditis <12 months. Enterococci cause endocarditis in approximately 10%–15% of cases in healthcare-associated, 2- to 12-month prosthetic valve, and injection drug use cases. Culture-negative endocarditis accounts for 5%–10% of cases in the aforementioned clinical scenarios.

IV-27. The answer is B. *(Chap. 155)* The Modified Duke criteria for the clinical diagnosis of infective endocarditis are a set of major and minor clinical, laboratory, and echocardiographic criteria that are highly sensitive and specific. The presence of two major criteria, one major criterion and three minor criteria, or five minor criteria allows a clinical diagnosis of definite endocarditis (Table IV-27). Evidence of echocardiographic involvement as evidenced by an oscillating mass (vegetation) on a valve, supporting structure, or implanted material; an intracardiac abscess, partial dehiscence of a prosthetic valve; or new valvular regurgitation is a major criterion in the Duke classification. An increase or change in preexisting murmur by clinical examination is not sufficient. Transthoracic echocardiography is specific for infective endocarditis but only finds vegetations in about 65% of patients with definite endocarditis. It is not adequate for evaluation of prosthetic valves or for intracardiac complications. Transesophageal echocardiography is more sensitive, detecting abnormalities in >90% of cases of definite endocarditis.

IV-28. The answer is C. *(Chap. 155)* To prevent endocarditis, past expert committees have supported systemic antibiotic administration prior to many bacteremia-inducing procedures. A reappraisal of the evidence for antibiotic prophylaxis for endocarditis by the American Heart Association and the European Society of Cardiology culminated in guidelines advising its more restrictive use. At best, the benefit of antibiotic prophylaxis is minimal. Most endocarditis cases do not follow a procedure. Although dental treatments have been widely considered to predispose to endocarditis, such infection occurs no more frequently in patients who are undergoing dental treatment than in matched controls who are not. The relation of gastrointestinal and genitourinary procedures to subsequent endocarditis is even more tenuous than that of dental procedures. In addition, cost-effectiveness and cost-benefit estimates suggest that antibiotic prophylaxis represents a poor use of

TABLE IV-26 Organisms Causing Major Clinical Forms of Endocarditis

	Percentage of Cases							
	Native Valve Endocarditis		Prosthetic Valve Endocarditis at Indicated Time of Onset (Months) after Valve Surgery			Endocarditis in Injection Drug Users		
Organism	**Community Acquired (n = 1718)**	**Healthcare Associated (n = 1110)**	**<2 (n = 144)**	**2–12 (n = 31)**	**>12 (n = 194)**	**Right Sided (n = 346)**	**Left Sided (n = 204)**	**Total (n = 675)[a]**
Streptococci[b]	40	13	1	9	31	5	15	12
Pneumococci	2	—	—	—	—	—	—	—
Enterococci[c]	9	16	8	12	11	2	24	9
Staphylococcus aureus	28	52[d]	22	12	18	77	23	57
Coagulase-negative staphylococci	5	11	33	32	11	—	—	—
Fastidious gram-negative coccobacilli (HACEK group)[e]	3	—	—	—	6	—	—	—
Gram-negative bacilli	1	1	13	3	6	5	13	7
Candida spp	<1	1	8	12	1	—	12	4
Polymicrobial/ miscellaneous	3	3	3	6	5	8	10	7
Diphtheroids	—	<1	6	—	3	—	—	0.1
Culture-negative	9	3	5	6	8	3	3	3

[a]The total number of cases is larger than the sum of right- and left-sided cases because the location of infection was not specified in some cases.
[b]Includes viridans streptococci; *Streptococcus gallolyticus*; other non–group A, groupable streptococci; and *Abiotrophia* and *Granulicatella* spp (nutritionally variant, pyridoxal-requiring streptococci).
[c]Primarily *E faecalis* or nonspeciated isolates; occasionally *E faecium* or other, less likely species.
[d]Methicillin resistance is common among these *S aureus* strains.
[e]Includes *Haemophilus* spp, *Aggregatibacter aphrophilus*, *Aggregatibacter actinomycetemcomitans*, *Cardiobacterium hominis*, *Eikenella* spp, and *Kingella* spp.
Note: Data are compiled from multiple studies.

TABLE IV-27 **The Modified Duke Criteria for the Clinical Diagnosis of Infective Endocarditis**[a]

Major Criteria

1. Positive blood culture

   Typical microorganism for infective endocarditis from two separate blood cultures

   Viridans streptococci, *Streptococcus gallolyticus*, HACEK group organisms, *Staphylococcus aureus, or*

   Community-acquired enterococci in the absence of a primary focus,

   or

   Persistently positive blood culture, defined as recovery of a microorganism consistent with infective endocarditis from:

   Blood cultures drawn >12 h apart; *or*

   All of 3 or a majority of ≥4 separate blood cultures, with first and last drawn at least 1 h apart

   or

   Single positive blood culture for *Coxiella burnetii* or phase I IgG antibody titer of >1:800

2. Evidence of endocardial involvement

   Positive echocardiogram[b]

   Oscillating intracardiac mass on valve or supporting structures or in the path of regurgitant jets or in implanted material, in the absence of an alternative anatomic explanation, *or*

   Abscess, *or*

   New partial dehiscence of prosthetic valve,

   or

   New valvular regurgitation (increase or change in preexisting murmur not sufficient)

Minor Criteria

1. Predisposition: predisposing heart conditions[c] or injection drug use
2. Fever ≥38.0°C (≥100.4°F)
3. Vascular phenomena: major arterial emboli, septic pulmonary infarcts, mycotic aneurysm, intracranial hemorrhage, conjunctival hemorrhages, Janeway lesions
4. Immunologic phenomena: glomerulonephritis, Osler nodes, Roth spots, rheumatoid factor
5. Microbiologic evidence: positive blood culture but not meeting major criterion, as noted previously,[d] *or* serologic evidence of active infection with an organism consistent with infective endocarditis

[a]Definite endocarditis is defined by documentation of two major criteria, of one major criterion and three minor criteria, or of five minor criteria. See text for further details.

[b]Transesophageal echocardiography is required for optimal assessment of possible prosthetic valve endocarditis or complicated endocarditis.

[c]Valvular disease with stenosis or regurgitation, presence of a prosthetic valve, congenital heart disease including corrected or partially corrected conditions (except isolated atrial septal defect, repaired ventricular septal defect, or closed patent ductus arteriosus), prior endocarditis, or hypertrophic cardiomyopathy.

[d]Excluding single positive cultures for coagulase-negative staphylococci and diphtheroids, which are common culture contaminants, or for organisms that do not cause endocarditis frequently, such as gram-negative bacilli.

Source: Adapted from JS Li et al: *Clin Infect Dis* 30:633, 2000. With permission from Oxford University Press.

resources. Nevertheless, studies in animal models suggest that antibiotic prophylaxis may be effective in some circumstances. Weighing the potential benefits, potential adverse events, and costs associated with antibiotic prophylaxis, the American Heart Association and the European Society of Cardiology now recommend prophylactic antibiotics only for patients at highest risk for severe morbidity or death from endocarditis. Maintaining good dental hygiene is essential. Prophylaxis is recommended only when there is manipulation of gingival tissue or the periapical region of the teeth or perforation of the oral mucosa (including surgery on the respiratory tract). Prophylaxis is not advised for patients undergoing routine gastrointestinal or genitourinary tract procedures. High-risk patients should be treated before or when they undergo procedures on an infected genitourinary tract or on infected skin and soft tissue. (See Table IV-28.)

IV-29. **The answer is A.** *(Chap. 155)* This patient has culture-negative endocarditis, a rare entity defined as clinical evidence of infectious endocarditis in the absence of positive blood cultures. Culture-negative endocarditis accounts for <10% of cases in all populations. In this case, evidence for subacute bacterial endocarditis includes valvular regurgitation, an aortic valve vegetation, and embolic phenomena on the extremities, spleen, and kidneys.

TABLE IV-28 **High-Risk Cardiac Lesions for Which Endocarditis Prophylaxis Is Advised Before Dental Procedures**

Prosthetic heart valves
Prior endocarditis
Unrepaired cyanotic congenital heart disease, including palliative shunts or conduits
Completely repaired congenital heart defects during the 6 months after repair
Incompletely repaired congenital heart disease with residual defects adjacent to prosthetic material
Valvulopathy developing after cardiac transplantation[a]

[a]Not a target population for prophylaxis according to recommendations of the European Society for Cardiology.
Source: Table created using the guidelines published by the American Heart Association and the European Society of Cardiology (W Wilson et al: *Circulation* 116:1736, 2007; and G Habib et al: *Eur Heart J* 30:2369, 2009).

A common reason for negative blood cultures is prior antibiotics. In the absence of this, the two most common pathogens (both of which are technically difficult to isolate in blood culture bottles) are Q fever, or *Coxiella burnetii* (typically associated with close contact with livestock), and *Bartonella*. In this case, the patient's homelessness and body louse infestation are clues for *Bartonella quintana* infection. Diagnosis is made by blood culture about 25% of the time. Otherwise, direct PCR of valvular tissue, if available, or acute and convalescent serologies are diagnostic options. Empirical therapy for culture-negative endocarditis usually includes ceftriaxone and gentamicin, with or without doxycycline. For confirmed *Bartonella* endocarditis, optimal therapy is gentamicin plus doxycycline. Ebstein-Barr virus (EBV) and HIV do not cause endocarditis. A peripheral blood smear would not be diagnostic.

IV-30. **The answer is D.** *(Chap. 155)* While any valvular vegetation can embolize, vegetations located on the mitral valve and vegetations >10 mm are at greatest risk of embolizing. Of the choices, options C, D, and E are large enough to increase the risk of embolization. However, only option D demonstrates the risks of both size and location. Hematogenously seeded infection from an embolized vegetation may involve any organ, but particularly affects those organs with the highest blood flow. They are seen in up to 50% of patients with endocarditis. Tricuspid lesions will lead to pulmonary septic emboli, common in injection drug users. Mitral and aortic lesions can lead to embolic infections in the skin, spleen, kidneys, meninges, and skeletal system. A dreaded neurologic complication is mycotic aneurysm, focal dilations of arteries at points in the arterial wall that have been weakened by infection in the vasa vasorum or septic emboli, leading to hemorrhage.

IV-31. **The answer is D.** *(Chap. 155)* The regimens used to treat staphylococcal endocarditis are based not on coagulase production but rather on the presence or absence of a prosthetic valve or foreign device, the native valve(s) involved, and the susceptibility of the isolate to penicillin, methicillin, and vancomycin. All staphylococci are considered penicillin-resistant until shown not to produce penicillinase. Similarly, methicillin resistance has become so prevalent among staphylococci that empirical therapy should be initiated with a regimen that covers methicillin-resistant organisms and should later be revised if the isolate proves to be susceptible to methicillin. The addition of 3–5 days of gentamicin to a β-lactam antibiotic or vancomycin to enhance therapy for native mitral or aortic valve endocarditis has not improved survival rates and may be associated with nephrotoxicity. Neither this addition nor the addition of fusidic acid or rifampin is recommended for native valve endocarditis. Staphylococcal prosthetic valve endocarditis is treated for 6–8 weeks with a multidrug regimen. Rifampin is an essential component because it kills staphylococci that are adherent to foreign material in a biofilm. Two other agents (selected on the basis of susceptibility testing) are combined with rifampin to prevent in vivo emergence of resistance. Because many staphylococci (particularly MRSA and *Staphylococcus epidermidis*) are resistant to gentamicin, the isolate's susceptibility to gentamicin or an alternative agent should be established before rifampin treatment is begun. If the isolate is resistant to gentamicin, then another aminoglycoside, a fluoroquinolone (chosen on the basis of susceptibility), or another active agent should be substituted for gentamicin. (See Table IV-31.)

TABLE IV-31 **Antibiotic Treatment for Infective Endocarditis Caused by Common Organisms**[a]

Organism	Drug (Dose, Duration)	Comments
Streptococci		
Penicillin-susceptible[b] streptococci, *S gallolyticus*	• Penicillin G (2–3 mU IV q4h for 4 weeks)	—
	• Ceftriaxone (2 g/d IV as a single dose for 4 weeks)	Can use ceftriaxone in patients with nonimmediate penicillin allergy.
	• Vancomycin[c] (15 mg/kg IV q12h for 4 weeks)	Use vancomycin in patients with severe or immediate β-lactam allergy.
	• Penicillin G (2–3 mU IV q4h) *or* ceftriaxone (2 g IV qd) for 2 weeks *plus* Gentamicin[d] (3 mg/kg qd IV or IM, as a single dose[e] or divided into equal doses q8h for 2 weeks)	Avoid 2-week regimen when risk of aminoglycoside toxicity is increased and in prosthetic valve or complicated endocarditis.
Relatively penicillin-resistant[f]	• Penicillin G (4 mU IV q4h) *or* ceftriaxone (2 g IV qd) for 4 weeks *plus* Gentamicin[d] (3 mg/kg qd IV or IM, as a single dose[e] or divided into equal doses q8h for 2 weeks)	Penicillin alone at this dose for 6 weeks or with gentamicin during the initial 2 weeks is preferred for prosthetic valve endocarditis caused by streptococci with penicillin MICs of ≤0.1 µg/mL.
	• Vancomycin[c] as noted above for 4 weeks	—
Moderately penicillin-resistant[g] streptococci, nutritionally variant organisms, or *Gemella* species	• Penicillin G (4–5 mU IV q4h) *or* ceftriaxone (2 g IV qd) for 6 weeks *plus* Gentamicin[d] (3 mg/kg qd IV or IM as a single dose[e] *or* divided into equal doses q8h for 6 weeks)	Preferred for prosthetic valve endocarditis caused by streptococci with penicillin MICs of >0.1 µg/mL.
	• Vancomycin[c] as noted above for 4 weeks	Regimen is preferred by some.
Enterococci[h]		
	• Penicillin G (4–5 mU IV q4h) *plus* gentamicin[d] (1 mg/kg IV q8h), both for 4–6 weeks	Can use streptomycin (7.5 mg/kg q12h) in lieu of gentamicin if there is not high-level resistance to streptomycin.
	• Ampicillin (2 g IV q4h) *plus* gentamicin[d] (1 mg/kg IV q8h), both for 4–6 weeks	—
	• Vancomycin[c] (15 mg/kg IV q12h) *plus* gentamicin[d] (1 mg/kg IV q8h), both for 4–6 weeks	Use vancomycin plus gentamicin for penicillin-allergic patients (or desensitize to penicillin) and for isolates resistant to penicillin/ampicillin.
	• Ampicillin (2 g IV q4h) *plus* ceftriaxone (2 g IV q12h), both for 6 weeks	Use for *E faecalis* isolates with high-level resistance to gentamicin and streptomycin or for patients at high risk for aminoglycoside nephrotoxicity (see text).
Staphylococci		
MSSA infecting native valves (no foreign devices)	• Nafcillin, oxacillin, *or* flucloxacillin (2 g IV q4h for 4–6 weeks)	Can use penicillin (4 mU q4h) if isolate is penicillin-susceptible (does not produce β-lactamase).
	• Cefazolin (2 g IV q8h for 4–6 weeks)	Can use cefazolin regimen for patients with nonimmediate penicillin allergy.
	• Vancomycin[c] (15 mg/kg IV q12h for 4–6 weeks)	Use vancomycin for patients with immediate (urticarial) or severe penicillin allergy; see text regarding addition of gentamicin, fusidic acid, or rifampin.
MRSA infecting native valves (no foreign devices)	• Vancomycin[c] (15 mg/kg IV q8–12h for 4–6 weeks)	No role for routine use of rifampin (see text). Consider alternative treatment (see text) for MRSA with vancomycin MIC >1.0 or persistent bacteremia during vancomycin therapy.
MSSA infecting prosthetic valves	• Nafcillin, oxacillin, *or* flucloxacillin (2 g IV q4h for 6–8 weeks) *plus* Gentamicin[d] (1 mg/kg IM or IV q8h for 2 weeks) *plus* • Rifampin[i] (300 mg PO q8h for 6–8 weeks)	Use gentamicin during initial 2 weeks; determine susceptibility to gentamicin before initiating rifampin (see text); if patient is highly allergic to penicillin, use regimen for MRSA; if β-lactam allergy is of the minor nonimmediate type, cefazolin can be substituted for oxacillin/nafcillin.

(*Continued*)

TABLE IV-31 **Antibiotic Treatment for Infective Endocarditis Caused by Common Organisms[a] (*Continued*)**

Organism	Drug (Dose, Duration)	Comments
MRSA infecting prosthetic valves	• Vancomycin[c] (15 mg/kg IV q12h for 6–8 weeks) *plus* Gentamicin[d] (1 mg/kg IM or IV q8h for 2 weeks) *plus* Rifampin[i] (300 mg PO q8h for 6–8 weeks)	Use gentamicin during initial 2 weeks; determine gentamicin susceptibility before initiating rifampin (see text).
HACEK Organisms		
	• Ceftriaxone (2 g/d IV as a single dose for 4 weeks)	Can use another third-generation cephalosporin at comparable dosage.
	• Ampicillin/sulbactam (3 g IV q6h for 4 weeks)	—
Coxiella burnetii		
	• Doxycycline (100 mg PO q12h) *plus* hydroxychloroquine (200 mg PO q8h), both for 18 (native valve) or 24 (prosthetic valve) months	Follow serology to monitor response during treatment (antiphase I IgG and IgA decreased 4-fold and IgM antiphase II negative) and thereafter for relapse.
***Bartonella* spp**		
	• Ceftriaxone (2 g IV q24h) *or* ampicillin (2 g IV q4h) *or* doxycycline (100 mg q12h PO) for 6 weeks *plus* Gentamicin (1 mg/kg IV q8h for 3 weeks)	If patient is highly allergic to β-lactams, use doxycycline.

[a]Doses are for adults with normal renal function. Doses of gentamicin, streptomycin, and vancomycin must be adjusted for reduced renal function. Ideal body weight is used to calculate doses of gentamicin and streptomycin per kilogram (men = 50 kg + 2.3 kg per inch over 5 feet; women = 45.5 kg + 2.3 kg per inch over 5 feet).
[b]MIC ≤0.1 μg/mL.
[c]Vancomycin dose is based on actual body weight. Adjust for trough level of 10–15 μg/mL for streptococcal and enterococcal infections and 15–20 μg/mL for staphylococcal infections.
[d]Aminoglycosides should not be administered as single daily doses for enterococcal endocarditis and should be introduced as part of the initial treatment. Target peak and trough serum concentrations of divided-dose gentamicin 1 h after a 20- to 30-min infusion or IM injection are ~3.5 μg/mL and ≤1 μg/mL, respectively; target peak and trough serum concentrations of streptomycin (timing as with gentamicin) are 20–35 μg/mL and <10 μg/mL, respectively.
[e]Netilmicin (4 mg/kg qd, as a single dose) can be used in lieu of gentamicin.
[f]MIC >0.1 μg/mL and <0.5 μg/mL.
[g]MIC ≥0.5 μg/mL and <8 μg/mL.
[h]Antimicrobial susceptibility must be evaluated; see text.
[i]Rifampin increases warfarin and dicumarol requirements for anticoagulation.
Abbreviations: MIC, minimal inhibitory concentration; MRSA, methicillin-resistant *Staphylococcus aureus*; MSSA, methicillin-sensitive *Staphylococcus aureus.*

IV-32. **The answer is D.** *(Chap. 156)* Vesicle formation due to infection may be caused by viral proliferation within the epidermis. In varicella and variola, viremia precedes the onset of a diffuse centripetal rash that progresses from macules to vesicles, then to pustules, and finally to scabs over the course of 1–2 weeks. Vesicles of varicella have a "dewdrop" appearance and develop in crops randomly about the trunk, extremities, and face over 3–4 days. Herpes zoster occurs in a single dermatome; the appearance of vesicles is preceded by pain for several days. Zoster (shingles) may occur in persons of any age but is most common among immunosuppressed individuals and elderly patients, whereas most cases of varicella occur in young children. Cold sores are typically caused by primary infection or reactivation of herpes simplex virus (HSV). Vesicles due to HSV are found on or around the lips (HSV-1) or genitals (HSV-2) but also may appear on the head and neck of young wrestlers (herpes gladiatorum) or on the digits of healthcare workers (herpetic whitlow). Recurrent herpes labialis (HSV-1) and herpes genitalis commonly follow primary infection. Hand-foot-and-mouth disease is caused by coxsackievirus A16 and characteristically causes vesicles on the hands, feet, and mouth of children. Rickettsialpox begins after mite-bite inoculation of *Rickettsia akari* into the skin. A papule with a central vesicle evolves to form a 1- to 2.5-cm painless crusted black eschar with an erythematous halo and proximal adenopathy. While more common in the northeastern United States and the Ukraine in 1940–1950, rickettsialpox has recently been described in Ohio, Arizona, and Utah. Scalded skin syndrome, typically caused by an *S aureus* toxin, presents with bullae, not vesicles. (See Figure IV-32.)

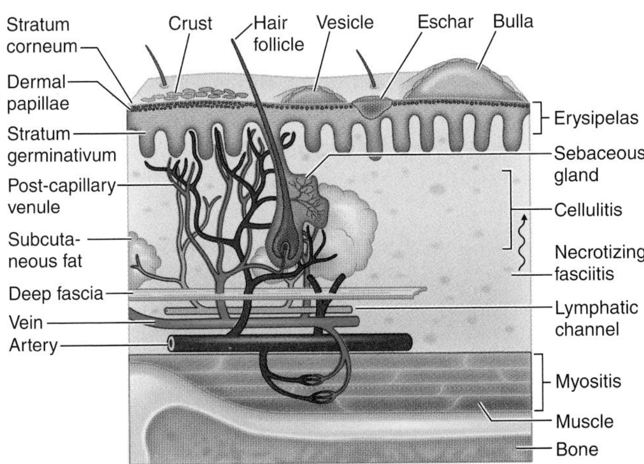

FIGURE IV-32

IV-33. **The answer is E.** *(Chap. 156)* The computed tomography (CT) scan shows edema and inflammation of the left chest wall in a patient with necrotizing fasciitis and myonecrosis consistent with infection by group A *Streptococcus*. The multiple skin excoriations were the most likely portal of entry for the bacteria. There is no evidence on the CT of lung parenchymal infection. *Actinomyces israelii*, *Klebsiella pneumoniae*, and oral anaerobic bacteria may cause necrotizing lung infections, particularly in patients with a history of alcoholism and poor dentition. *S pneumoniae* is the most common cause of bacterial pneumonia and typically shows lobar consolidation on CT scan.

IV-34. **The answer is A.** *(Chap. 159)* Primary (spontaneous) bacterial peritonitis (PBP) occurs when the peritoneal cavity becomes infected without an apparent source of contamination. PBP occurs most often in patients with cirrhosis, usually with preexisting ascites. The bacteria likely invade the peritoneal fluid because of poor hepatic filtration in cirrhosis. While fever is present in up to 80% of cases, abdominal pain, acute onset, and peritoneal signs are often absent. Patients may present with nonspecific findings such as malaise or worsening encephalopathy. A neutrophil count in peritoneal fluid of >250/μL is diagnostic; there is no percent neutrophil differential threshold. Diagnosis is often difficult because peritoneal cultures are often negative. Blood cultures may reveal the causative organism. The most common organisms are enteric gram-negative bacilli, but gram-positive cocci are often found. Anaerobes are not common (in contrast to secondary bacterial peritonitis), and empiric antibiotics targeting them are not necessary if PBP is suspected. Third-generation cephalosporins and piperacillin-tazobactam are reasonable initial empiric therapy. Diagnosis requires exclusion of a primary intra-abdominal source of peritonitis.

IV-35. **The answer is D.** *(Chap. 159)* This patient has chronic ambulatory peritoneal dialysis (CAPD)-associated peritonitis. Unlike primary or secondary bacterial peritonitis, this infection is usually caused by skin organisms, most commonly *Staphylococcus* species. The organisms migrate into the peritoneal fluid via the device. There may not be a tunnel or exit-site infection. Peritonitis is the most common reason for discontinuing CAPD. Y-connectors and diligent technique decrease the risk of CAPD. In contrast to PBP and similar to spontaneous bacterial peritonitis (SPB), the onset of symptoms is usually acute with diffuse pain and peritoneal signs. The dialysate will be cloudy with >100 white blood cells (WBC)/μL and >50% neutrophils. Dialysates should be placed in blood culture media and often are often positive with one organism. Finding more than one organism in culture should prompt an evaluation for SPB. Empirical intraperitoneal coverage for CAPD peritonitis should be directed against staphylococcal species based on local epidemiology. If the patient is severely ill, IV antibiotics should be added. If the patient does not respond within 4 days, catheter removal should be considered.

IV-36. **The answer is D.** *(Chap. 159)* The CT shows a large, complex, multiloculated liver abscess in the right lobe. Liver abscesses may arise from hematogenous spread, biliary disease (most common currently), pylephlebitis, or contiguous infection in the peritoneal cavity. Fever is the only common physical finding in liver abscess. Up to 50% of patients may not have symptoms or signs to direct attention to the liver. Nonspecific symptoms are common, and liver abscess is an important cause of fever of unknown origin (FUO) in the elderly. The only reliably abnormal serum studies are elevated alkaline phosphatase and/or WBC in 70% of patients. Liver abscess may be suggested by an elevated hemidiaphragm on chest radiograph. The most common causative organisms in presumed biliary disease are gram-negative bacilli. Anaerobes are not common unless pelvic or other enteric sources are suspected. Fungal liver abscesses occur following fungemia in immunocompromised patients receiving chemotherapy, often presenting symptomatically with neutrophil reconstitution. Drainage, usually percutaneous, is the mainstay of therapy and is useful initially diagnostically. (See Figure IV-36B.)

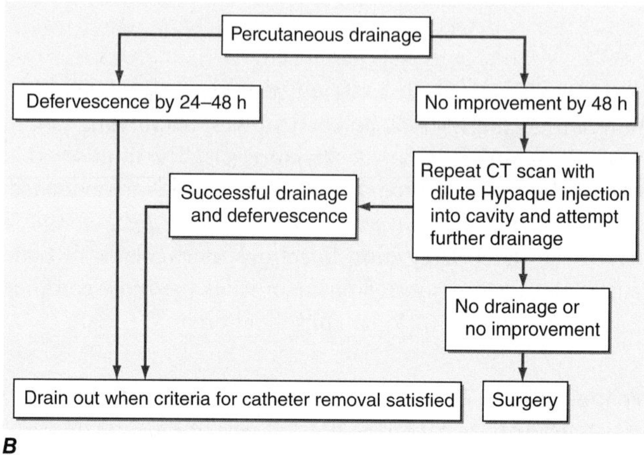

FIGURE IV-36B Algorithm for the management of patients with intraabdominal abscesses using percutaneous drainage. Antimicrobial therapy should be administered concomitantly. CT, computed tomography.
Reprinted with permission from B Lorber (ed): *Atlas of Infectious Diseases,* vol VII: *Intra-abdominal Infections, Hepatitis, and Gastroenteritis.* Philadelphia, Current Medicine, 1996, p 1.30, as adapted from OD Rotstein, RL Simmons, in SL Gorbach et al (eds): *Infectious Diseases.* Philadelphia, Saunders, 1992, p 668.

IV-37. **The answer is A.** *(Chap. 161) Clostridium difficile* infection is a common gastrointestinal illness that is most commonly associated with antimicrobial use and subsequent disruption of normal colonic flora. Cases of *C difficile* infection have been rising since the early 2000s, tripling between the years of 2000 and 2005. Epidemiologically, fecal colonization with *C difficile* is ≥20% after 1 week of hospitalization, but remains lows at 1%–3% among community-dwelling adults. The most common presentation of *C difficile* infection is increased stooling, with stools that may range from soft and unformed to profuse watery diarrhea. Stools are almost never grossly bloody. An individual infected with *C difficile* may have as many as 20 bowel movements per daily. Clinically, fever is present in up to 28% of cases, abdominal pain in 22%, and leukocytosis in 50%. An ileus is often seen on abdominal radiograph. The ileus may be adynamic in origin in 20% of cases. An adynamic ileus occurs when there is an ileus on radiograph with cessation of stooling. *C difficile* infection recurs after treatment in 15%–30% of patients. In this patient, the bloody stools, fever, and abdominal pain suggest ischemic colitis, and the patient has several risk factors for this including atrial fibrillation and cardiovascular disease.

IV-38. **The answer is D.** *(Chap. 161) C difficile* infection (CDI) is diagnosed based on a combination of clinical and microbiologic criteria. Clinically, a patient with CDI is expected to have diarrhea with three or more stools per day for ≥2 days with no other recognized cause. There are a number of different tests for identifying *C difficile* in the stool. However, no single traditional test has a high sensitivity, high specificity, and rapid turnaround. The commonly used tests for diagnosing CDI are demonstration of toxin A or B in the stool, PCR or culture demonstrating presence of toxin-producing *C difficile* in the stool, or identifying pseudomembranes in the colon on endoscopy. Most laboratory tests for toxins have inadequate sensitivity. While finding pseudomembranes on colonoscopy is highly specific, these are not frequently present even in known disease. Nucleic acid amplification tests, including PCR, have been recently approved and have the advantage of being more sensitive than toxin assays and at least as specific. In addition, these tests are rapidly available. Thus, PCR assays are becoming the testing method of choice

IV-39. **The answer is C.** *(Chap. 161)* The patient has evidence of recurrent CDI, which occurs in up to 30% of treated patients. These infections can occur as relapse of the primary infection or as reinfections if the organism remains in the environment. Rates of recurrence of CDI are comparable regardless of whether metronidazole or vancomycin is used as initial treatment. Recurrence rates are higher in individuals ≥65 years old, those who continue to take antibiotics while being treated for CDI, and those who remain hospitalized after the initial infection. Patients who have a first recurrence of CDI should receive the same treatment as in the initial infection (Table IV-39). Fidaxomicin is a new oral macrocyclic antibiotic that is associated with less recurrent disease compared to oral vancomycin. It would also be a consideration in this patient. If there are multiple recurrences, multiple treatment options can be considered including oral vancomycin, oral nitazoxanide, IV immunoglobulin, and fecal microbiota transplantation. Fecal microbiota transplantation is given via nasoduodenal tube, colonoscope, or enema and seeks to restore normal colonic microbial flora. This procedure has been demonstrated in trials to be associated with a lower risk of *C difficile* recurrence but is not currently approved by the U.S. Food and Drug Administration (FDA).

IV-40. **The answer is E.** *(Chap. 161)* Clindamycin, ampicillin, and cephalosporins (including ceftriaxone) were the first antibiotics associated with *C difficile*–associated disease and still are. More recently, broad-spectrum fluoroquinolones, including moxifloxacin and ciprofloxacin, have been associated with outbreaks of *C difficile*, including outbreaks in some locations of a more virulent strain that has caused severe disease among elderly outpatients. For unclear reasons, β-lactams other than the later generation cephalosporins appear to carry a lesser risk of disease. Penicillin/β-lactamase combination antibiotics appear to have lower risk of *C difficile*–associated disease than the other agents mentioned. Cases have even been reported associated with metronidazole and vancomycin administration. Nevertheless, all patients initiating antibiotics should be warned to seek care if they develop diarrhea that is severe or persists for more than a day, as all antibiotics carry some risk for C *difficile*–associated disease.

IV-41. **The answer is E.** *(Chap. 162)* Urinary tract infection (UTI) is one of the most common infections seen in primary care. The term UTI encompasses a number of clinical entities including asymptomatic bacteriuria, cystitis, pyelonephritis, and prostatitis. Acute cystitis is the most common form of UTI that is diagnosed. Except in infancy and in the elderly, UTI is far more common in women. Due to the greater incidence of congenital urinary tract anomalies in males, the incidence of UTI is greater in males in infancy. Between the ages of 1 and 50 years, women far outnumber men with UTI. After the age of 50 years, men have increasing incidence of UTI, and overall, the incidence in men nears that of women. Over a lifetime, 50%–80% of women will experience at least one UTI. Risk factors for UTI in women include prior history of UTI, diabetes mellitus, incontinence, sexual activity, and use of a diaphragm with spermicide. About 20%–30% of women who experience a UTI will have recurrent episodes of UTI. Recent sexual activity is also temporally related to UTI. One episode of intercourse in the preceding week is associated with a relative risk of UTI of 1.4. With five episodes of intercourse in a week, the relative risk increases to 4.8. Men who experience UTI typically have a structural abnormality that contributes to the development of infection. The most common abnormality in men is prostatic hypertrophy that causes urinary obstruction. Lack of circumcision also increases risk of UTI in men as the *Escherichia coli* may colonize the glans and prepuce of an uncircumcised male.

TABLE IV-39 **Recommendations for the Treatment of *Clostridium difficile* Infection (CDI)**[a]

Clinical Setting	Treatment(s)	Comments
Initial episode, mild to moderate	Metronidazole (500 mg tid × 10–14 d)	Vancomycin (125 mg qid × 10–14 d) may be more effective than metronidazole. Fidaxomicin (200 mg bid × 10 d) is another alternative.
Initial episode, severe	Vancomycin (125 mg qid × 10–14 d)	Indicators of severe disease may include leukocytosis (≥15,000 white blood cells/μL) and a creatinine level ≥1.5 times the premorbid value. Fidaxomicin is an alternative.
Initial episode, severe complicated or fulminant	Vancomycin (500 mg PO or via nasogastric tube) *plus* metronidazole (500 mg IV q8h) *plus consider* Rectal instillation of vancomycin (500 mg in 100 mL of normal saline as a retention enema q6–8h)	Severe complicated or fulminant CDI is defined as severe CDI with the addition of hypotension, shock, ileus, or toxic megacolon. The duration of treatment may need to be >2 weeks and is dictated by response. Consider using tigecycline (50 mg IV q12h after a 100-mg loading dose) in place of metronidazole.
First recurrence	Same as for initial episode	Adjust treatment if severity of CDI has changed with recurrence. Consider fidaxomicin, which significantly decreases the likelihood of additional recurrences.
Second recurrence	Vancomycin in taper/pulse regimen	Typical taper/pulse regimen: 125 mg qid × 10–14 d, then bid × 1 week, then daily × 1 week, then q2–3d for 2–8 weeks.
Multiple recurrences	Consider the following options: • Repeat vancomycin taper/pulse • Vancomycin (500 mg qid × 10 d) plus *Saccharomyces boulardii* (500 mg bid × 28 d) • Vancomycin (125 mg qid × 10–14 d); then stop vancomycin and start rifaximin (400 mg bid × 2 weeks) • Nitazoxanide (500 mg bid × 10 d) • Fecal microbiota transplantation • IV immunoglobulin (400 mg/kg)	The only controlled studies that included patients with one or more recurrent CDI episodes were with vancomycin and *S boulardii*, which showed borderline significance compared with vancomycin plus placebo, and fecal microbiota transplantation, which was highly significant compared with a high-dose course of vancomycin. (The vancomycin taper was not compared.)

[a]All agents are given orally unless otherwise specified.

In pregnancy, women should be screened and treated for asymptomatic bacteriuria. The presence of asymptomatic bacteria in a pregnant woman is associated with development of pyelonephritis, preterm birth, and perinatal fetal death.

IV-42. **The answer is D.** *(Chap. 162)* Pyelonephritis is a symptomatic infection of the kidney. Mild cases of pyelonephritis typically present with low-grade fevers with or without lower back or costovertebral angle pain. Symptoms of severe pyelonephritis include high fevers, rigors, nausea, vomiting, and flank and/or loin pain. Up to 20%–30% of cases of pyelonephritis have associated bacteremia. Symptoms can presently acutely without prior symptoms of cystitis. Patients with diabetes mellitus, analgesic nephropathy, or sickle cell disease can present with obstructive uropathy due to acute papillary necrosis with sloughing of renal papillae into the renal pelvis and ureter. Treatment of pyelonephritis depends on the severity of the presentation. Trimethoprim-sulfamethoxazole is not recommended due to high rates of resistant *E coli* in patients with pyelonephritis. Less severe cases are typically treated with fluoroquinolones. Either the oral or parenteral route can be utilized with fluoroquinolones if the patient is tolerating oral therapy, and 7 days of therapy are highly effective for uncomplicated pyelonephritis. Oral β-lactams are less effective than fluoroquinolones and should be used with caution. Options for parenteral therapy for uncomplicated pyelonephritis include fluoroquinolones, extended-spectrum cephalosporins with or without an aminoglycoside, or a carbapenem. However, this patient has diabetes and is presenting with evidence of sepsis and diabetic ketoacidosis.

Therefore, she would have a complicated pyelonephritis. In this case, use of a β-lactam with a β-lactamase inhibitor (ampicillin-sulbactam, piperacillin-tazobactam, ticarcillin-clavulanate) or imipenem-cilastatin would be the initial recommended treatment. Once the patient is stabilized and sensitivities of the causative organism are known, the patient should be switched to oral therapy.

IV-43. **The answer is C.** *(Chap. 162)* Asymptomatic bacteriuria (ASB) occurs when a patient without local or systemic symptoms of infection presents with evidence of bacteria in the urine. The diagnostic cutoff for determining ASB is $>10^5$ colony-forming units (CFU)/mL in spontaneously voiding patients, and $>10^2$ CFU/mL in individuals who have a catheter. Treatment of ASB does not decrease the frequency of symptomatic infections or complications except in pregnant women, individuals undergoing urologic surgery, and perhaps neutropenic patients or those with renal transplants. In pregnant women, screening and treatment of ASB are recommended because pregnant women with untreated ASB have increased risk of preterm birth, perinatal death of the fetus, and pyelonephritis in the mother. A meta-analysis found that treating ASB in pregnant women decreased the risk of pyelonephritis by 75%.

IV-44. **The answer is C.** *(Chap. 162)* Acute bacterial prostatitis presents with dysuria, frequency, and pain in the prostatic or perineal region. Fever and chills are common. Chronic bacterial prostatitis is more indolent and presents as recurrent episodes of cystitis with occasional associated pelvic or perineal pain. Given that this patient had a recent prior episode of cystitis that was treated for 7 days with a fluoroquinolone, chronic prostatitis is suspected and is demonstrated on physical examination by a prostate that is warm and tender on palpation. In one study of men with febrile UTI, early recurrence of UTI, symptoms of urinary retention, hematuria at follow-up, or voiding difficulties predicted individuals with surgically correctable disorders. Acute bacterial prostatitis can be treated with 2–4 weeks of therapy, whereas chronic prostatitis would require a longer course of therapy to between 4 and 6 weeks. If the infection recurs after treatment, then a 12-week course of therapy would be recommended. In addition, treatment of underlying prostatic disorders should help to decrease recurrence.

IV-45. **The answer is A.** *(Chap. 163)* Common causes of urethral discomfort and discharge in men include *Chlamydia trachomatis, N gonorrhoeae, Mycoplasma genitalium, Ureaplasma urealyticum, Trichomonas vaginalis*, and HSV. *Gardnerella* is the usual cause of bacterial vaginosis in women and is not a pathogen in men.

IV-46. **The answer is C.** *(Chap. 163)* The patient has symptoms consistent with the urethral syndrome, characterized by "internal" dysuria with urgency and frequency and pyuria but no uropathogens at counts of $\geq 10^2$/mL in urine. This is most commonly due to *C trachomatis* or *N gonorrhoeae* and can be readily confirmed by nucleic acid amplification testing for these pathogens in the urine. "External" dysuria includes pain in the vulva during urination, often without frequency or urgency. This is found in vulvovaginal candidiasis and HSV infection, which can be visualized on physical examination. Cervical culture would not be useful with her urinary symptoms. Elevated vaginal pH >5.0 is commonly present in trichomonal vaginitis. Clue cells on vaginal secretion microscopy suggest bacterial vaginosis.

IV-47. **The answer is B.** *(Chap. 163)* Bacterial vaginosis is associated with *Gardnerella vaginalis* and various anaerobic and/or noncultured bacteria. It generally has malodorous discharge that is white or gray. There is no external irritation, pH of vaginal fluid is usually >4.5, a fishy odor is present with 10% KOH preparation, and microscopy shows clue cells, few leukocytes, and many mixed microbiota. Normal vaginal findings are described in patient D, with pH <4.5 and lactobacilli seen on microscopic exam. High pH (>5) with external irritation is often found in vulvovaginal candidiasis, whereas the presence of motile trichomonads is diagnostic for trichomonal vaginitis.

IV-48. **The answer is E.** *(Chap. 163)* In a study of leukocytosis cervicitis patients seen at a sexually transmitted disease clinic in the 1980s, more than one-third of cervical samples failed to reveal any etiology. In a recent similar study in Baltimore using nucleic acid amplification testing, more than one half of the cases were not microbiologically identified. *C trachomatis* is the most frequently diagnosed organism, followed by *N gonorrhoeae*. Because of the difficulty in making a microbiologic diagnosis, empiric therapy for *C trachomatis* and, in areas were *N gonorrhoeae* is highly endemic, gonococcus is indicated.

IV-49. **The answer is C.** *(Chap. 163)* The presence of right upper quadrant tenderness in conjunction with classic findings of pelvic inflammatory disease is highly suggestive of Fitz-Hugh-Curtis syndrome, or perihepatitis due to inflammation of the liver capsule due to either *N gonorrhoeae* or *C trachomatis* infection. Although this condition may be easily visualized by laparoscopic examination, the resolution of right upper quadrant symptoms with therapy of pelvic inflammatory disease is the more common proof of the diagnosis. The presence of normal liver function testing is reassuring that hepatitis is not present, making hepatitis C virus (HCV) infection unlikely.

IV-50. **The answer is A.** *(Chap. 163)* The most common causes of genital ulceration are herpes simplex virus, syphilis, and chancroid. Gonorrhea typically manifests as a urethritis, not genital ulcers. Syphilitic ulcers (primary chancre) are firm, shallow single ulcers that are not pustular and are generally not painful. Despite these usual findings, rapid plasma reagin (RPR) testing is indicated in all cases of genital ulceration given the disparate presentations of *Treponema pallidum*. HSV ulcers are quite painful but are vesicular rather than pustular. In primary infection, they may be bilateral, although with reactivation, they are generally unilateral. *Haemophilus ducreyi*, the agent responsible for chancroid, causes multiple ulcers, often starting as pustules, that are soft, friable, and exquisitely tender, as was present in this case. Primary infection with HIV usually will cause an acute febrile illness, not focal ulcers. The presence of genital ulcers increases the likelihood of acquisition and transmission of HIV.

IV-51. **The answer is E.** *(Chap. 164)* In a patient with suspected central nervous system (CNS) infection, the first task is to identify whether an infection predominantly involves the subarachnoid space (*meningitis*) or whether there is evidence of either generalized or focal involvement of brain tissue in the cerebral hemispheres, cerebellum, or brainstem. When brain tissue is directly injured by a bacterial or viral infection, the disease is referred to as *encephalitis*, whereas focal infections involving brain tissue are classified as either *cerebritis* or *abscess*, depending on the presence or absence of a capsule. Nuchal rigidity ("stiff neck") is the pathognomonic sign of meningeal irritation and is present when the neck resists passive flexion. The Kernig and Brudzinski signs are also classic signs of meningeal irritation. *Kernig sign* is elicited with the patient in the supine position. The thigh is flexed on the abdomen, with the knee flexed; attempts to passively extend the knee elicit pain when meningeal irritation is present. *Brudzinski sign* is elicited with the patient in the supine position and is positive when passive flexion of the neck results in spontaneous flexion of the hips and knees. Although commonly tested on physical examinations, the sensitivity and specificity of Kernig and Brudzinski signs are uncertain. Both may be absent or reduced in very young or elderly patients, immunocompromised individuals, or patients with a severely depressed mental status. The high prevalence of cervical spine disease in older individuals may result in false-positive tests for nuchal rigidity.

A significantly depressed level of consciousness (e.g., somnolence, coma), seizures, or focal neurologic deficits does not typically occur in viral meningitis, but may occur in the other options listed. (See Figure IV-51.)

IV-52. **The answer is D.** *(Chaps. 164 and 173) S pneumoniae* is the most common cause of meningitis in adults >20 years of age, accounting for nearly half the reported cases (1.1 per 100,000 persons per year). There are a number of predisposing conditions that increase the risk of pneumococcal meningitis, the most important of which is pneumococcal pneumonia. Additional risk factors include coexisting acute or chronic pneumococcal sinusitis or otitis media, alcoholism, diabetes, splenectomy, hypogammaglobulinemia, complement deficiency, and head trauma with basilar skull fracture and cerebrospinal fluid (CSF) rhinorrhea. The mortality rate remains ~20% despite antibiotic therapy.

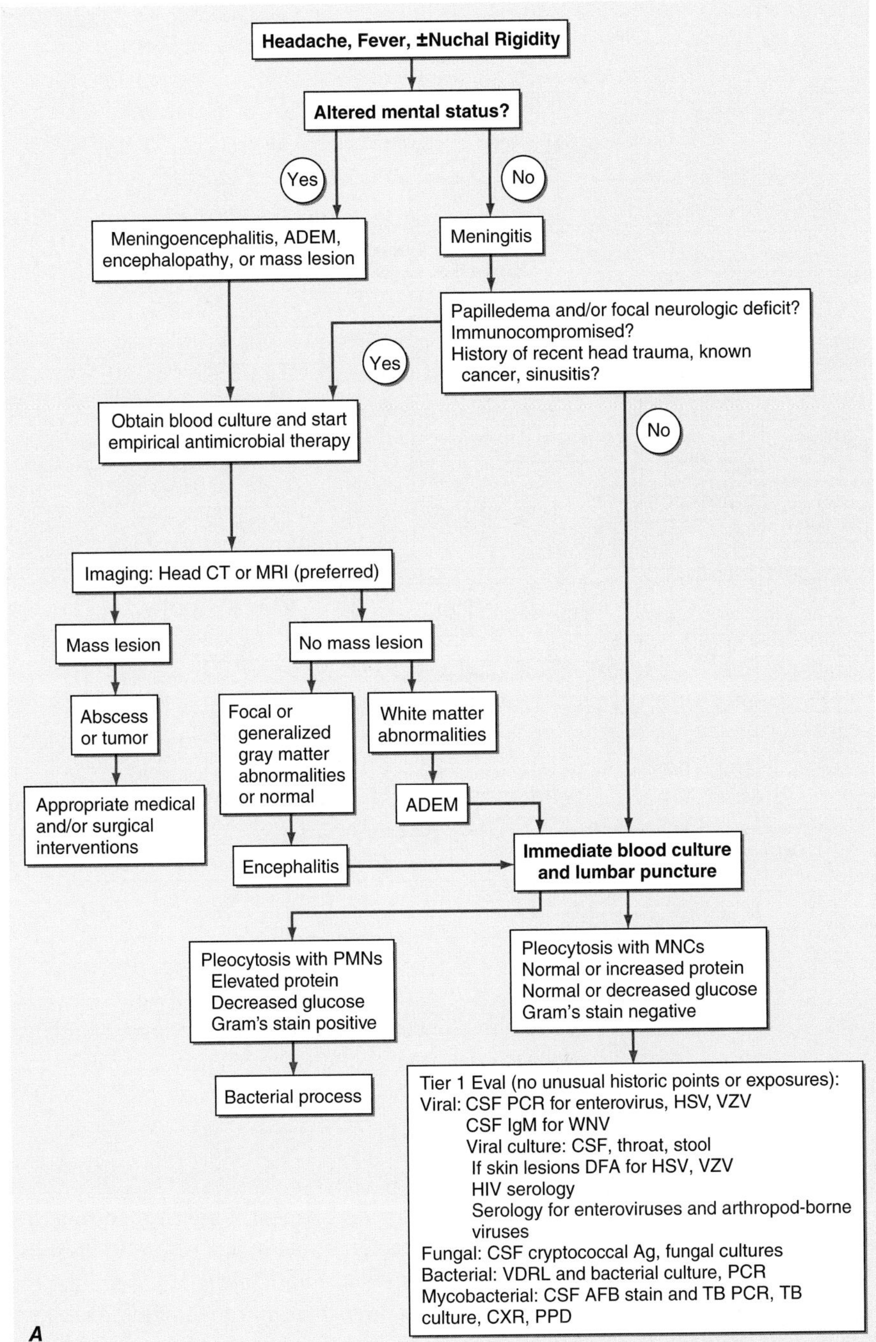

FIGURE IV-51 The management of patients with suspected central nervous system (CNS) infection. ADEM, acute disseminated encephalomyelitis; AFB, acid-fast bacillus; Ag, antigen; CSF, cerebrospinal fluid; CT, computed tomography; CTFV, Colorado tick fever virus; CXR, chest x-ray; DFA, direct fluorescent antibody; EBV, Epstein-Barr virus; HHV, human herpesvirus; HSV, herpes simplex virus; LCMV, lymphocytic choriomeningitis virus; MNCs, mononuclear cells; MRI, magnetic resonance imaging; PCR, polymerase chain reaction; PMNs, polymorphonuclear leukocytes; PPD, purified protein derivative; TB, tuberculosis; VDRL, Venereal Disease Research Laboratory; VZV, varicella-zoster virus; WNV, West Nile virus.

Pregnancy, age >60 years, and immunocompromised status are important risk factors for meningitis due to *Listeria monocytogenes.*

IV-53. **The answer is B.** *(Chap. 164)* This patient presents with a high suspicion of acute bacterial meningitis, likely due to *S pneumoniae* with the presence of concurrent pneumonia. Bacterial meningitis is a medical emergency. The goal is to begin antibiotic therapy within

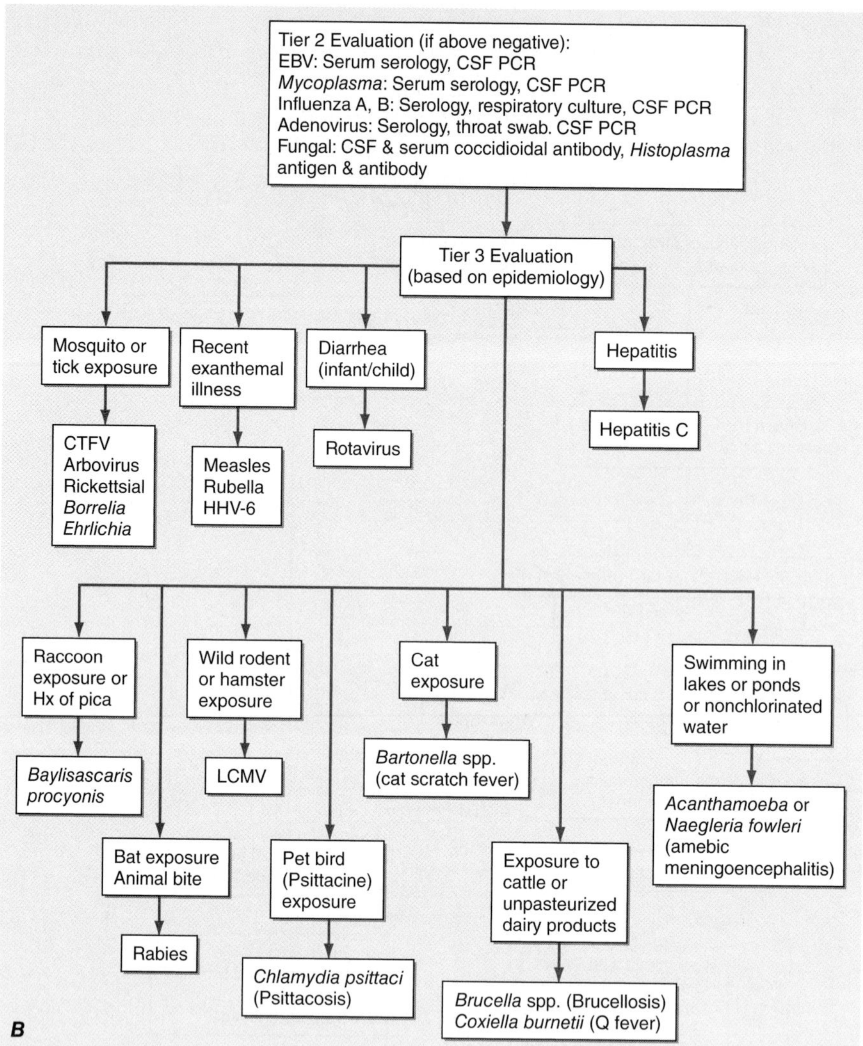

FIGURE IV-51 (*Continued*)

60 minutes of a patient's arrival in the emergency department. Empirical antimicrobial therapy is initiated in patients with suspected bacterial meningitis before the results of CSF Gram stain and culture are known. *S pneumoniae* and *N meningitidis* are the most common etiologic organisms of community-acquired bacterial meningitis. Due to the emergence of penicillin- and cephalosporin-resistant *S pneumoniae*, empirical therapy of community-acquired suspected bacterial meningitis in children and adults should include a combination of dexamethasone, a third- or fourth-generation cephalosporin (e.g., ceftriaxone, cefotaxime, or cefepime), and vancomycin, plus acyclovir (because HSV encephalitis is the leading disease in the differential diagnosis) and doxycycline during tick season to treat tick-borne bacterial infections. Ceftriaxone or cefotaxime provides good coverage for susceptible *S pneumoniae*, group B streptococci, and *H influenzae* and adequate coverage for *N meningitidis*. Cefepime is a broad-spectrum fourth-generation cephalosporin with in vitro activity similar to that of cefotaxime or ceftriaxone against *S pneumoniae* and *N meningitidis* and greater activity against *Enterobacter* species and *P aeruginosa*. In clinical trials, cefepime has been demonstrated to be equivalent to cefotaxime in the treatment of penicillin-sensitive pneumococcal and meningococcal meningitis, and it has been used successfully in some patients with meningitis due to *Enterobacter* species and *P aeruginosa*. Ampicillin should be added to the empirical regimen for coverage of *L monocytogenes* in individuals <3 months of age, those >55, or those with suspected impaired cell-mediated immunity because of chronic illness, organ transplantation, pregnancy, malignancy, or immunosuppressive therapy. Metronidazole is added to the empirical regimen to cover gram-negative anaerobes in patients with otitis, sinusitis,

or mastoiditis. In hospital-acquired meningitis, and particularly meningitis following neurosurgical procedures, staphylococci and gram-negative organisms including *P aeruginosa* are the most common etiologic organisms. In these patients, empirical therapy should include a combination of vancomycin and ceftazidime, cefepime, or meropenem. Ceftazidime, cefepime, or meropenem should be substituted for ceftriaxone or cefotaxime in neurosurgical patients and in neutropenic patients, because ceftriaxone and cefotaxime do not provide adequate activity against CNS infection with *P aeruginosa*. Meropenem is a carbapenem antibiotic that is highly active in vitro against *L monocytogenes*, has been demonstrated to be effective in cases of meningitis caused by *P aeruginosa*, and shows good activity against penicillin-resistant pneumococci. The release of bacterial cell-wall components by bactericidal antibiotics leads to the production of the inflammatory cytokines interleukin (IL)-1β and tumor necrosis factor (TNF)-α in the subarachnoid space. Dexamethasone exerts a beneficial effect by inhibiting the synthesis of IL-1β and TNF-α at the level of mRNA, decreasing CSF outflow resistance, and stabilizing the blood–brain barrier. The rationale for giving dexamethasone 20 minutes before antibiotic therapy is that dexamethasone inhibits the production of TNF-α by macrophages and microglia only if it is administered before these cells are activated by endotoxin. Dexamethasone does not alter TNF-α production once it has been induced. The results of clinical trials of dexamethasone therapy in meningitis due to *H influenzae, S pneumoniae,* and *N meningitidis* have demonstrated its efficacy in decreasing meningeal inflammation and neurologic sequelae such as the incidence of sensorineural hearing loss. A prospective European trial of adjunctive therapy for acute bacterial meningitis in 301 adults found that dexamethasone reduced the number of unfavorable outcomes (15% vs. 25%, $p = .03$) including death (7% vs. 15%, $p = .04$). The benefits were most striking in patients with pneumococcal meningitis. Dexamethasone (10 mg IV) was administered 15–20 minutes before the first dose of an antimicrobial agent, and the same dose was repeated every 6 hours for 4 days. These results were confirmed in a second trial of dexamethasone in adults with pneumococcal meningitis. Therapy with dexamethasone should ideally be started 20 minutes before, or not later than concurrent with, the first dose of antibiotics. It is unlikely to be of significant benefit if started >6 hours after antimicrobial therapy has been initiated. Dexamethasone may decrease the penetration of vancomycin into CSF, and it delays the sterilization of CSF in experimental models of *S pneumoniae* meningitis. As a result, to assure reliable penetration of vancomycin into the CSF, children and adults are treated with vancomycin in a dose of 45–60 mg/kg/d.

IV-54. **The answer is C.** *(Chap. 165)* Chronic meningitis has many causes, including a variety of bacteria, mycobacteria, fungi, viruses, and parasites. In addition, many noninfectious etiologies can cause chronic meningitis as well, and these include systemic lupus erythematosus, sarcoidosis, Behçet syndrome, Mollaret meningitis, drug hypersensitivity, and malignancy, among others. Chronic meningitis is diagnosed when there is a characteristic syndrome of meningitis that has produced symptoms for ≥4 weeks and is associated with inflammation in the CSF. Clinically, a patient with chronic meningitis typically presents with headache, neck pain, or back pain. In this patient also presenting with cranial nerve VI and VII palsy, the lesion can be localized to a basal meningitis affecting cranial nerve roots. Given the patient's geographic location and avidity for hiking, she is at risk for infection with Lyme disease caused by the organism *Borrelia burgdorferi*. Lyme disease causing meningitis typically occurs weeks or months after the tick bite, and many patients cannot recall having a tick bite. Likewise, patients may not recall having the typical target-shaped erythema migrans rash, which occurs early in the disease process. Other features of early disseminated Lyme disease include arthralgias/arthritis, carditis, conjunctivitis or iritis, radiculopathy, and lymphadenopathy. Diagnosis of Lyme disease as a cause of chronic meningitis relies primarily on demonstrating a positive serum Lyme titer and Western blot. The CSF findings are nonspecific, including increased mononuclear cells and elevated protein typically to not greater than 200–300 mg/dL. CSF glucose would be normal. Demonstration of a positive antibody to *B burgdorferi* in the CSF is highly specific for the disease but may be negative. Other diseases that can present with a basal meningitis picture include neurologic sarcoidosis, malignancy, and granulomatosis with polyangiitis. An elevated CSF angiotensin-converting enzyme level may be seen in sarcoidosis but is neither sensitive nor specific for diagnosing disease. *T pallidum* is a spirochete like

B burgdorferi and is the causative organism for syphilis. Untreated syphilis can result in chronic meningitis as well as symptoms of dementia, rather than cranial nerve palsies. Because the causative organisms for both Lyme disease and syphilis are spirochetes, there is a degree of cross-reactivity on serum Lyme titers, but a positive CSF Venereal Disease Research Laboratory (VDRL) test is only positive in syphilis.

IV-55. **The answer is E.** *(Chap. 168)* Nosocomial infections have reservoirs and sources just as do community-acquired pathogens. In hospitalized patients, cross-contamination (i.e., indirect spread of organisms from one patient to the next) accounts for many nosocomial infections. While hand hygiene is uniformly recommended for healthcare practitioners, adherence to hand washing is low, often due to time pressure, inconvenience, and skin damage. Because of improved adherence, alcohol-based hand rubs are now recommended for all heathcare workers except when hands are visibly soiled or after care of a patient with *C difficile* infection, whose spores may not be killed by alcohol and thus require thorough hand washing with soap and water.

IV-56. **The answer is E.** *(Chap. 169)* Ultimately, solid organ transplant patients are at highest risk for infection due to T-cell immunodeficiency from antirejection medicines. As a result, they are also at risk for reactivation of many of the viruses from the herpes virus family, most notably cytomegalovirus (CMV), varicella-zoster virus, and EBV. However, immediately after transplant, these deficits have not yet developed in full. Neutropenia is not common after solid organ transplantation, as it is in bone marrow transplantation. In fact, patients are most at risk of infections typical for all hospitalized patients, including wound infections, UTI, pneumonia, *C difficile* infection, and line-associated infection. Therefore, a standard evaluation of a febrile patient in the first weeks after a solid organ transplant should include a detailed physical examination, blood and urine cultures, urinalysis, chest radiography, *C difficile* stool antigen/toxin studies if warranted, and a transplant-specific evaluation.

IV-57. **The answer is E.** *(Chap. 169)* The patient presents with symptoms suggestive of infection in the middle period after transplantation (1–4 months). In patients with prior CMV exposure or receipt of CMV-positive organ transplant, this is a period of time when CMV infection is most common. The patient presented here has classic signs of CMV disease with generalized symptoms in addition to dysfunction of her transplanted organ (kidney). Often, bone marrow suppression is present, demonstrated here by lymphopenia. Because CMV infection is linked with graft dysfunction and rejection, prophylaxis is frequently used including valganciclovir. Trimethoprim-sulfamethoxazole is used for *Pneumocystis jiroveci* prophylaxis, acyclovir is generally used for varicella-zoster virus prophylaxis, itraconazole may be considered in patients considered at risk for histoplasmosis reactivation, and isoniazid is used for individuals with recent purified protein derivative (PPD) conversion or positive chest imaging and no prior treatment.

IV-58. **The answer is E.** *(Chap. 169) Toxoplasma gondii* commonly achieves latency in cysts during acute infection. Reactivation in the CNS in AIDS patients is well known. However, *Toxoplasma* cysts also reside in the heart. Thus, transplanting a *Toxoplasma*-positive heart into a negative recipient may cause reactivation in the months after transplant. Serologic screening of cardiac donors and recipients for *T gondii* is important. To account for this possibility, prophylactic doses of trimethoprim-sulfamethoxazole, which is also effective prophylaxis against *Pneumocystis* and *Nocardia*, is standard after cardiac transplantation. Cardiac transplant recipients, similar to all other solid organ transplant recipients, are at risk of developing infections related to impaired cellular immunity, particularly >1 month to 1 year posttransplantation. Wound infections or mediastinitis from skin organisms may complicate the early transplant (<1 month) period.

IV-59. **The answer is C.** *(Chaps. 169 and 235)* During the first week after hematopoietic stem cell transplantation, the highest risk of infection comes from aerobic nosocomially acquired bacteria. However, after about 7 days, the risk of fungal infection rises, particularly with prolonged neutropenia. The patient presented here presents with symptoms and signs of a respiratory illness after prolonged neutropenia; fungal infection is high on the differential diagnosis. The CT scan with nodules and associated halo sign is suggestive of *Aspergillus* infection. The halo sign often occurs in *Aspergillus* infection in the context of an increasing neutrophil count after a prolonged nadir. The serum galactomannan antigen test will detect galactomannan, a major component of the *Aspergillus* cell wall that is released during growth of hyphae. The presence of this compound suggests invasion and growth of the mold. This noninvasive test is receiving wider acceptance in the diagnosis of invasive *Aspergillus* in immunocompromised hosts. Additionally, galactomannan assays in bronchoalveolar lavage fluid may aid diagnosis of invasive *Aspergillus* in immunocompromised hosts. In the absence of purulent sputum, sputum cultures are unlikely to be helpful. *Aspergillus* is seldom cultured from the sputum in cases of invasive aspergillosis. Examination of buffy coat is useful for the diagnosis of histoplasmosis, but the focal nodules with halo sign and absence of other systemic symptoms make histoplasmosis less likely. *Legionella* and CMV pneumonia are generally not associated with nodules and have either lobar infiltrates or diffuse infiltrates.

IV-60, IV-61, IV-62, IV-63, and IV-64. **The answers are C, B, D, A, and E, respectively.** Antibacterial agents have a variety of mechanisms of action that target essential components of the bacterial cell structures and metabolism. The targets are typically chosen because they either do not exist in mammalian cells or are sufficiently different to allow for bacterial targeting. One primary target of antibacterial agents is inhibition of cell wall synthesis as mammalian cells have no counterpart to this structure. The cell wall is a cross-linked peptidoglycan that is composed of alternating units of *N*-acetylglucosamine (NAG) and *N*-acetylmuramic acid (NAM). Inhibition of this peptidoglycan synthesis is a target of many antibacterial agents and leads to cell lysis, making these antibiotics bactericidal in nature. Antibacterial drugs that inhibit cell wall synthesis include β-lactams, glycopeptides, bacitracin, and fosfomycin. β-Lactams are a large category of drugs that include penicillins, carbapenems, cephalosporins, and monobactams. All of these agents contain a β-lactam ring that targets transpeptidase enzymes (also called penicillin-binding proteins) to inhibit peptide cross-linking in the formation of peptidoglycan. Glycopeptides bind to the glycosyltransferase enzyme that polymerizes NAG-NAM units. Antibiotics in this class include vancomycin, telavancin, dalbavancin, and oritavancin. Bacitracin and fosfomycin act early in peptidoglycan synthesis to decrease production of the peptidoglycan precursors. Inhibition of bacterial protein synthesis is also a common target of antibacterial drugs. These drugs bind within the bacterial ribosome and are most commonly bacteriostatic, although aminoglycoside antibiotics are bactericidal. Examples of antibacterial drugs that inhibit protein synthesis are aminoglycosides, tetracyclines, macrolides, lincosamides, streptogranins (quinupristin-dalfopristin), chloramphenicol, oxazolidinones (linezolid and tedizolid), and mupirocin. Aminoglycosides bind irreversibly to the 16S ribosomal RNA of the 30S ribosomal subunit to prevent protein synthesis. This class of medication can also cause misreading of messenger RNA codon. Tobramycin, gentamicin, and amikacin are commonly used aminoglycosides. Tetracyclines also bind to the 16S ribosomal RNA of the 30S ribosomal subunit, but in contrast to aminoglycosides, the binding is reversible. Most of the other inhibitors of protein synthesis bind at the 23S ribosomal RNA of the 50S subunit, but all have slightly different mechanisms of inhibition at the site. Mupirocin is only available topically and directly inhibits production of tRNA synthetase. Folate is a required cofactor in the synthesis of some nucleic acids and amino acids. Sulfonamides prevent folate synthesis by inhibiting enzymes within cells that use exogenous precursors to generate folate. Trimethoprim is also a folate synthesis inhibitor that acts farther down the pathway of folate synthesis. When trimethoprim is used in combination with sulfamethoxazole, two subsequent steps in folate synthesis are inhibited. There are also multiple classes of antibiotics that inhibit DNA or RNA synthesis. The most commonly used class of these drugs is the fluoroquinolones, which inhibit DNA gyrase and topoisomerase IV. Rifamycins bind to bacterial RNA polymerase and prevent elongation of mRNA. Nitrofurantoin metabolism within the cell leads to reactive derivatives that cause DNA strand breakage. Metronidazole also creates reactive species that damage DNA and lead to cell death. Finally, two classes of agents act directly to disrupt the integrity of the bacterial cytoplasmic membrane. Polymyxins, including colistin, and daptomycin are the available agents in the class.

IV-65 and IV-66. The answers are D and D, respectively. *(Chap. 170)* Bacteria have a variety of methods to develop resistance to antibacterial therapy. These broadly fall into three categories: (1) altered targets that have reduced binding of the drug; (2) altered access of the drug to its target through decreased uptake or increased active efflux, and (3) a modification of the drug that reduces its activity. For β-lactam antibiotics, the most common mechanism of resistance is for the drugs to be degraded by β-lactamases, enzymes that break down the β-lactam ring and thus destroy drug activity. β-Lactamases may be encoded on the bacterial chromosome, which would affect the susceptibility profile of an entire species of bacteria. Others are acquired through plasmids, and thus, some strains may show susceptibility to a β-lactam, whereas others may not. Most strains of *S aureus* produce a plasmid-encoded β-lactamase that degrades penicillin, but not semisynthetic penicillins such as oxacillin and nafcillin. β-Lactamases acquired by gram-negative bacteria are encoded on plasmids and cause these bacteria to be resistant to penicillins and all early-generation cephalosporins. Most recently, an extended-spectrum β-lactamase (ESBL) has been identified, initially in *Klebsiella* species, but has not been seen in other gram-negative organisms. Presence of an ESBL identifies bacteria that will have resistance to all early (cefazolin) and later-generation cephalosporins (e.g., cefepime, ceftriaxone, ceftazidime), as well as aztreonam. Carbapenems such as meropenem are the drugs of choice to treat an ESBL-producing bacteria.

IV-67. The answer is C. *(Chap. 170)* Pharmacokinetics and pharmacodynamics both play important roles in understanding the appropriate use of antibiotics. Pharmacokinetics refers to the disposition of a drug in the body and includes the absorption, distribution, metabolism, and excretion of the drug. Intravenous use of a drug leads to 100% of absorption of a drug. Other routes of drug administration yield varying degrees of bioavailability and are subject to first-pass effects. Once a drug is in the body, distribution refers to how the drug is passed between the circulation and tissues, and it is important to consider the volume of distribution of a drug. This refers to the amount of drug in the body at a given time relative to the measured serum concentration. Patients with cystic fibrosis are known to have a higher volume of distribution of medications with more rapid drug clearance. Thus, higher doses of antibiotics are often required. Some medications require monitoring to determine if appropriate drugs levels are attained to achieve effective killing while minimizing side effects. It is important to consider drug metabolism and excretion when determining the appropriate time to assess drug levels. Generally, five to seven half-lives of the drug are required for levels to achieve steady state when multiple doses of a medication are given in a time frame shorter than the half-life itself. Trough levels prior to drug administration are performed to ensure that the drug is not accumulating and to prevent side effects. Pharmacodynamics describes the relationship between the serum concentration that achieves the desired drug effect and the serum concentration that can produce toxic effects of the drug. When considering the pharmacodynamics of an antibiotic, it is important to consider whether the drug achieves efficacy through time- or concentration-dependent killing. β-Lactams are an example of a drug that kills in a time-dependent fashion. Thus, these agents do not require high peak levels for efficacy; rather, the important factor in achieving effect is to determine the length of time the drug will be maintained at concentrations greater than the minimal inhibitory concentration (MIC). The longer the concentration of a β-lactam remains above the MIC during the dosing interval, the greater is the killing effect, and using prolonged infusions of β-lactams has been used as a way to improve time-dependent killing. In contrast, concentration-dependent killing requires higher peak concentration of drug to achieve the desired effect. Aminoglycosides are antibiotics that use concentration-dependent pharmacodynamics.

IV-68. The answer is D. *(Chap. 170)* The FDA has a classification system that designates the safety of drugs in pregnancy. The safest class of drugs is class A, which indicates that studies have demonstrated safety of the drug without effects on the fetus. No antibiotic is designated as a class A drug in pregnancy. Class B drugs show no effects in animal reproduction, or if the animal data show effects, there are adequate data in pregnant women to show these drugs can be safely used. Many antibiotics fall into class B drugs in pregnancy, including azithromycin, cephalosporins, clindamycin, meropenem, penicillins, and vancomycin. Class C drugs have more potential risks, but one has to determine if the potential benefits to the health of the mother warrant use despite the potential risk. Antibiotics in this category include fluoroquinolones and linezolid. Class D drugs demonstrate some degree of fetal risk and should be avoided if other safer alternatives exist. Sulfonamides and tetracyclines are class D drugs. The specific concern for use of doxycycline in the second and third trimester is discoloration of the teeth in the fetus.

IV-69. **The answer is D.** *(Chap. 170)* All antibiotics have adverse effects that need to be considered when prescribing a drug. The most common serious side effect of all antibiotic medications is the development of drug allergy, with rash, hives, anaphylaxis or Stevens-Johnson syndrome. Some antibiotics have very specific associated syndromes. Prolonged use of nitrofurantoin is associated with development of pulmonary fibrosis and/or pneumonitis. No other antibiotic has this associated side effect. Cephalosporins and other β-lactams frequently cause hypersensitivity reactions, including anaphylaxis. Fluoroquinolones characteristically are associated with tendinitis. They may also cause dysglycemia, a side effect that caused the withdrawal of one fluoroquinolone (gatifloxacin) from the market. Trimethoprim-sulfamethoxazole is commonly associated with a rash. Prolonged use can lead to nephrotoxicity, and patients commonly develop evidence of a type IV renal tubular acidosis. Other antibiotics with distinct clinical side effect profiles include red-man syndrome with vancomycin infusions, myopathy with daptomycin, myelosuppression with linezolid, and orange discoloration of body fluids with rifampin.

IV-70. **The answer is A.** *(Chap. 171)* Pneumococcal infections, particularly pneumonia, remain a worldwide public health problem. Intermittent colonization of the nasopharynx by pneumococcus transmitted by respiratory droplet is common and is the likely reservoir for invasive disease. Infants and elderly are at greatest risk of developing invasive pneumococcal disease (IPD) and death. In the developed world, children are the most common source of pneumococcal transmission. By 1 year old, 50% of children have had at least one episode of colonization. Prevalence studies show carriage rates of 20%–50% in children up to 5 years old and up to 15% for adults. These numbers approach 90% for children and 40% for adults in the developing world. Pneumococcal vaccination has dramatically impacted the epidemiology, with reduced IPD in the United States attributable to reductions in serotypes included in the vaccine. Similar reductions have been observed in other countries implementing routine childhood vaccinations; however, in certain populations (Alaska native populations and United Kingdom), the reduction in vaccine-covered serotype cases has been offset by increases in nonvaccine serotypes. Case fatality rates due to pneumococcal pneumonia vary by host factors, age, and access to care. Interestingly, there appears to be no reduction in case fatality during the first 24 hours of hospitalization since the introduction of antibiotics. This is likely due to the development of severe multiorgan failure as a result of severe infection. Appropriate care in an intensive care setting can reduce case fatality rate for severe infection. Outbreaks of disease are well recognized in crowded settings with susceptible individuals, such as infant day-care facilities, military barracks, and nursing homes. Furthermore, there is a clear association between preceding viral respiratory disease (especially but not exclusively influenza) and risk of secondary pneumococcal infections. The significant role of pneumococcal pneumonia in the morbidity and mortality associated with seasonal and pandemic influenza is increasingly recognized.

IV-71. **The answer is D.** *(Chap. 171)* The characteristics described are unique to the pneumococcus, or *S pneumoniae*. Pneumococci are spherical gram-positive bacteria of the genus *Streptococcus*. Within this genus, cell division occurs along a single axis, and bacteria grow in chains or pairs—hence the name *Streptococcus*, from the Greek *streptos*, meaning "twisted," and *kokkos*, meaning "berry." At least 22 streptococcal species are recognized and are divided further into groups based on their hemolytic properties. *S pneumoniae* belongs to the α-hemolytic group that characteristically produces a greenish color on blood agar because of the reduction of iron in hemoglobin. The bacteria are fastidious and grow best in 5% CO_2 but require a source of catalase (e.g., blood) for growth on agar plates, where they develop mucoid (smooth/shiny) colonies. Pneumococci without a capsule produce colonies with a rough surface. Unlike that of other α-hemolytic streptococci, their growth is inhibited in the presence of optochin (ethylhydrocupreine hydrochloride), and they are bile soluble.

In common with other gram-positive bacteria, pneumococci have a cell membrane beneath a cell wall, which in turn is covered by a polysaccharide capsule. Pneumococci are divided into serogroups or serotypes based on capsular polysaccharide structure, as distinguished with rabbit polyclonal antisera; capsules swell in the presence of specific antiserum (the Quellung reaction). The staphylococcal organisms grow not in chains, but in clusters. *Streptococcus pyogenes* exhibits a β-hemolytic pattern (complete hemolysis). *Pseudomonas* is gram negative.

IV-72. **The answer is B.** *(Chap. 171)* The gold standard for the etiologic diagnosis of pneumococcal pneumonia is pathologic examination of lung tissue. In lieu of that procedure, evidence of an infiltrate on chest radiography warrants a diagnosis of pneumonia. However, cases of pneumonia without radiographic evidence do occur. An infiltrate can be absent either early in the course of the illness or with dehydration; upon rehydration, an infiltrate usually appears. The radiographic appearance of pneumococcal pneumonia is varied; it classically consists of lobar or segmental consolidation but, in some cases, is patchy. More than one lobe is involved in approximately 30% of cases. Consolidation may be associated with a small pleural effusion or empyema in complicated cases. Blood drawn from patients with suspected pneumococcal pneumonia can be used for supportive or definitive diagnostic tests. Blood cultures are positive for pneumococci in <30% of cases of pneumococcal pneumonia. Urinary pneumococcal antigen assays have facilitated etiologic diagnosis. In adults, among whom the prevalence of pneumococcal nasopharyngeal colonization is relatively low, a positive pneumococcal urinary antigen test has a high predictive value. The same is not true for children, in whom a positive urinary antigen test can reflect the mere presence of *S pneumoniae* in the nasopharynx.

IV-73. **The answer is A.** *(Chap. 171)* Penicillin-resistant pneumococci were first described in the mid-1960s, at which point tetracycline- and macrolide-resistant strains had already been reported. Multidrug-resistant strains were first described in the 1970s, but it was during the 1990s that pneumococcal drug resistance reached pandemic proportions. The use of antibiotics selects for resistant pneumococci, and strains resistant to β-lactam agents and to multiple drugs are now found all over the world. The emergence of high rates of macrolide and fluoroquinolone resistance also has been described in recent years. As a result of the increased prevalence of resistant pneumococci, first-line therapy for persons ≥1 month of age is a combination of vancomycin (adults, 30–60 mg/kg/d; infants and children, 60 mg/kg/d) and cefotaxime (adults, 8–12 g/d in 4–6 divided doses; children, 225–300 mg/kg/d in 1 dose or 2 divided doses) or ceftriaxone (adults, 4 g/d in 1 dose or 2 divided doses; children, 10 mg/kg/d in 1 dose or 2 divided doses). If children are hypersensitive to β-lactam agents (penicillins and cephalosporins), rifampin (adults, 600 mg/d; children, 20 mg/d in 1 dose or 2 divided doses) can be substituted for cefotaxime or ceftriaxone. For outpatient management, amoxicillin (1 g every 8 hours) provides effective treatment for virtually all cases of pneumococcal pneumonia. Neither cephalosporins nor quinolones, which are far more expensive, offer any advantage over amoxicillin. Levofloxacin (500–750 mg/d as a single dose) and moxifloxacin (400 mg/d as a single dose) also are highly likely to be effective in the United States, except in patients who come from closed populations where these drugs are used widely or who have themselves been treated recently with a quinolone. Clindamycin (600–1200 mg/d every 6 hours) is effective in 90% of cases, and azithromycin (500 mg on day 1 followed by 250–500 mg/d) or clarithromycin (500–750 mg/d as a single dose) is ineffective in 80% of cases. Treatment failure resulting in bacteremic disease due to macrolide-resistant isolates has been amply documented in patients given azithromycin empirically.

IV-74. **The answer is C.** *(Chap. 172)* Figure IV-74 shows gram-positive round (cocci) bacteria growing in clumps. *H influenzae* is a gram-negative coccus, and *Pseudomonas* is a gram-negative bacillus (rod). Streptococcal species grow in chains or pairs and do not produce catalase. *S aureus* distinguishes itself from other staphylococcal species, including *S epidermidis*, by the production of coagulase, which contains protein A.

IV-75. **The answer is C.** *(Chap. 172)* *S aureus* is both a commensal and an opportunistic pathogen. Approximately 30% of healthy persons are episodically colonized with *S aureus*, with a smaller percentage (~10%) persistently colonized. The rate of colonization is elevated among insulin-dependent diabetics, HIV-infected patients, patients undergoing hemodialysis, injection drug users, and individuals with skin damage. The anterior nares and oropharynx are frequent sites of human colonization, although the skin (especially when damaged), vagina, axilla, and perineum may also be colonized. These colonization sites serve as a reservoir for future infections. Transmission of *S aureus* most frequently results from direct personal contact. Colonization of different body sites allows transfer from one person to another during contact. Spread of staphylococci in aerosols of respiratory or nasal secretions from heavily colonized individuals has also been reported. Most individuals who develop *S aureus* infections become infected with a strain that is already a part of their own commensal flora. Breaches of the skin or mucosal membrane allow *S aureus* to initiate infection. Some diseases increase the risk of *S aureus* infection; diabetes, for example, combines an increased rate of colonization and the use of injectable insulin with the possibility of impaired leukocyte function. Individuals with congenital or acquired qualitative or quantitative defects of polymorphonuclear leukocytes (PMNs) are at increased risk of *S aureus* infections; this group includes neutropenic patients (e.g., those receiving chemotherapeutic agents), those with chronic granulomatous disease, and those with Job or Chédiak-Higashi syndrome. Other groups at risk include individuals with end-stage renal disease, HIV infection, skin abnormalities, or prosthetic devices.

IV-76. **The answer is E.** *(Chap. 172)* *S aureus* produces three types of toxin: cytotoxins, pyrogenic toxin superantigens, and exfoliative toxins. Toxic shock syndrome (TSS) results from the ability of enterotoxins and TSS toxin-1 to function as T-cell mitogens. In the normal process of antigen presentation, the antigen is first processed within the cell, and peptides are then presented in the major histocompatibility complex (MHC) class II groove, initiating a measured T-cell response. In contrast, enterotoxins bind directly to the invariant region of MHC—outside the MHC class II groove. The enterotoxins can then bind T-cell receptors via the vβ chain; this binding results in a dramatic overexpansion of T-cell clones (up to 20% of the total T-cell population). The consequence of this T-cell expansion is a "cytokine storm," with the release of inflammatory mediators that include interferon-γ, IL-1, IL-6, TNF-α, and TNF-β. The resulting multisystem disease produces a constellation of findings that mimic those in endotoxin shock; however, the pathogenic mechanisms differ. For TSS, investigators recommend a combination of clindamycin and a semisynthetic penicillin or vancomycin (if the isolate is resistant to methicillin). Clindamycin is advocated because, as a protein synthesis inhibitor, it reduces toxin synthesis in vitro. Linezolid also appears to be effective. In most cases of staphylococcal TSS (including nonmenstrual cases), a skin site of infection is not clinically apparent. Because this disease is mediated by toxin formation, blood cultures are almost always negative. Desquamation of the skin often occurs 1–2 weeks after the onset of the illness. Staphylococcal scalded skin syndrome, which affects primarily newborns and children, exhibits skin desquamation very early in the disease.

IV-77. **The answer is C.** *(Chap. 172)* In the past 10 years, numerous outbreaks of community-based infection caused by MRSA in individuals with no prior medical exposure have been reported. These outbreaks have taken place in both rural and urban settings in widely separated regions throughout the world. The reports document a dramatic change in the epidemiology of MRSA infections. The outbreaks have occurred among such diverse groups as children, prisoners, athletes, Native Americans, and drug users. Risk factors common to these outbreaks include poor hygienic conditions, close contact, contaminated material, and damaged skin. The community-associated infections have been caused by a limited number of MRSA strains. In the United States, strain USA300 (defined by pulsed-field gel electrophoresis) has been the predominant clone. While the majority of infections caused by this community-based clone of MRSA have involved the skin and soft tissue, 5%–10% have been invasive, including severe necrotizing lung infections, necrotizing fasciitis, infectious pyomyositis, endocarditis, and osteomylitis. The most feared complication is a necrotizing pneumonia that often follows influenza upper respiratory infection and can affect previously healthy people. This pathogen produces the Panton-Valentine leukocidin protein that forms holes in the membranes of neutrophils as they arrive at the site of infection and serves as a marker for this pathogen. An easy way to identify this strain of MRSA is its sensitivity profile. Unlike MRSA isolates of the past, which were sensitive only to vancomycin, daptomycin, quinupristin/dalfopristin, and linezolid, community-acquired MRSA is almost uniformly susceptible to trimethoprim-sulfamethoxazole and doxycycline. The organism is also usually sensitive to clindamycin. The term *community-acquired* has probably outlived its usefulness because this isolate has become the most common *S aureus* isolate causing infection in many hospitals around the world.

IV-78. **The answer is E.** *(Chap. 172)* Probably because of its ubiquity and ability to stick to foreign surfaces, *S epidermidis* is the most common cause of infections of CNS shunts as well as an important cause of infections on artificial heart valves and orthopedic prostheses. *Corynebacterium* spp (diphtheroids), just like *S epidermidis*, colonize the skin. When these organisms are isolated from cultures of shunts, it is often difficult to be sure if they are the cause of disease or simply contaminants. Leukocytosis in CSF, consistent isolation of the same organism, and the character of a patient's symptoms are all helpful in deciding whether treatment for infection is indicated.

IV-79. **The answer is D.** *(Chap. 172)* This patient has infectious pyomyositis, a disease of the tropics and of immunocompromised hosts such as patients with poorly controlled diabetes mellitus or AIDS. The pathogen is usually *S aureus*. Management includes aggressive debridement, antibiotics, and attempts to reverse the patient's immunocompromised status. *Clostridium perfringens* may cause gas gangrene, particularly in devitalized tissues. Streptococcal infections may cause cellulitis or an aggressive fasciitis, but the presence of abscesses in a patient with poorly controlled diabetes makes staphylococcal infection more likely. Polymicrobial infections are common in diabetic ulcers, but in this case, the imaging and physical examination show intramuscular abscesses.

IV-80. **The answer is D.** *(Chap. 173)* Recurrent episodes of rheumatic fever are most common in the first 5 years after the initial diagnosis. Penicillin prophylaxis is recommended for at least this period. After the first 5 years, secondary prophylaxis is determined on an individual basis. Ongoing prophylaxis is currently recommended for patients who have had recurrent disease, have rheumatic heart disease, or work in occupations that have a high risk for reexposure to group A streptococcal infection. Prophylactic regimens are penicillin V, PO 250 mg twice a day (bid); benzathine penicillin, 1.2 million units intramuscularly (IM) every 4 weeks; and sulfadiazine, 1 g PO daily. Polyvalent pneumococcal vaccine has no cross-reactivity with group A *Streptococcus*.

IV-81. **The answer is E.** *(Chap. 173)* Necrotizing fasciitis involves the superficial and/or deep fascia investing the muscles of an extremity or the trunk. The source of the infection is either the skin, with organisms introduced into tissue through trauma (sometimes trivial), or the bowel flora, with organisms released during abdominal surgery or from an occult enteric source, such as a diverticular or appendiceal abscess. The inoculation site may be unapparent and is often some distance from the site of clinical involvement; for example, the introduction of organisms via minor trauma to the hand may be associated with clinical infection of the tissues overlying the shoulder or chest. Cases originating from the skin are most commonly due to *S pyogenes* (group A *Streptococcus*), sometimes with *S aureus* coinfection. In this case, the presence of fasciitis without myositis (which is more commonly due to *Staphylococcus*) makes *S pyogenes* the most likely organism. The onset of disease is often acute, and the course is fulminant. While pain and tenderness may be severe, physical findings may be subtle initially. Local anesthesia (due to cutaneous nerve infarction) and skin mottling are late findings. Cases associated with the bowel flora are usually polymicrobial, involving a mixture of anaerobic bacteria (such as *Bacteroides fragilis* or anaerobic streptococci) and facultative organisms (usually gram-negative bacilli). Necrotizing fasciitis is a surgical emergency with extensive debridement potentially lifesaving. At surgery, the extent of disease is typically more extensive than clinically or radiologically indicated. Antibiotic therapy is adjunctive. Patients with necrotizing fasciitis may develop streptococcal toxic shock syndrome. *S pneumoniae* and *S epidermidis* are not causes of necrotizing fasciitis. *C difficile* causes antibiotic-associated colitis.

IV-82. The answer is C. *(Chap. 173)* Symptoms of streptococcal pharyngitis include sore throat, fever and chills, malaise, and sometimes abdominal complaints and vomiting, particularly in children. Both symptoms and signs are quite variable, ranging from mild throat discomfort with minimal physical findings to high fever and severe sore throat associated with intense erythema and swelling of the pharyngeal mucosa and the presence of purulent exudate over the posterior pharyngeal wall and tonsillar pillars. Enlarged, tender anterior cervical lymph nodes commonly accompany exudative pharyngitis. Given the presence of cough and coryza, this is not a classic presentation of streptococcal pharyngitis. Streptococcal infection is an unlikely cause when symptoms and signs suggestive of viral infection are prominent (conjunctivitis, coryza, cough, hoarseness, or discrete ulcerative lesions of the buccal or pharyngeal mucosa). The throat culture remains the diagnostic gold standard. Culture of a throat specimen that is properly collected (i.e., by vigorous rubbing of a sterile swab over both tonsillar pillars) and properly processed is the most sensitive and specific means of definitive diagnosis. A rapid diagnostic kit for latex agglutination or enzyme immunoassay of swab specimens is a useful adjunct to throat culture. While precise figures on sensitivity and specificity vary, rapid diagnostic kits generally are >95% specific. Thus, a positive result can be relied upon for definitive diagnosis and eliminates the need for throat culture. However, because rapid diagnostic tests are less sensitive than throat culture (relative sensitivity in comparative studies, 55%–90%), a negative result should be confirmed by throat culture. Azithromycin may be employed therapeutically for streptococcal pharyngitis, but only in patients with serious penicillin allergies (which this patient does not have). Treatment of streptococcal pharyngitis is given mainly to prevent suppurative complications and rheumatic fever. While symptoms often remit in 3–5 days, prevention of rheumatic fever requires complete eradication of the organisms, requiring 10 days of therapy,

IV-83. The answer is B. *(Chap. 173)* Because the usual source of the organisms infecting a neonate is the mother's birth canal, efforts have been made to prevent group B streptococcal infections by the identification of high-risk carrier mothers and treatment with various forms of antibiotic prophylaxis or immunoprophylaxis. Prophylactic administration of ampicillin or penicillin to such patients during delivery reduces the risk of infection in the newborn. This approach has been hampered by logistical difficulties in identifying colonized women before delivery; the results of vaginal cultures early in pregnancy are poor predictors of carrier status at delivery. The CDC recommends screening for anogenital colonization at 35–37 weeks of pregnancy by a swab culture of the lower vagina and anorectum; intrapartum chemoprophylaxis is recommended for culture-positive women. Intrapartum chemoprophylaxis regardless of culture status is also recommended for women who have previously given birth to an infant with group B streptococcal infection (such as this patient) or have a history of group B streptococcal bacteriuria during pregnancy.

IV-84. The answer is D. *(Chap. 174)* Enterococci are normal inhabitants of the large bowel of human adults, although they usually make up <1% of the culturable intestinal microflora. In the healthy human gastrointestinal tract, enterococci are typical symbionts that coexist with other gastrointestinal bacteria. According to the National Healthcare Safety Network of the CDC, enterococci are the second most common organisms (after staphylococci) isolated from hospital-associated infections in the United States. Although *Enterococcus faecalis* remains the predominant species recovered from nosocomial infections, the isolation of *Enterococcus faecium* has increased substantially in the past 20 years. In fact, *E faecium* is now almost as common as *E faecalis* as an etiologic agent of hospital-associated infections. This point is important, because *E faecium* is by far the most resistant and challenging enterococcal species to treat; indeed, more than 80% of *E faecium* isolates recovered in U.S. hospitals are resistant to vancomycin, and more than 90% are resistant to ampicillin (historically the most effective β-lactam agent against enterococci). Resistance to vancomycin and ampicillin in *E faecalis* isolates is much less common (~7% and ~4%, respectively). Two meta-analyses have found that, independent of the patient's clinical status, vancomycin-resistant enterococci infection increases the risk of death over that among individuals infected with a glycopeptide-susceptible enterococcal strain.

IV-85. **The answer is A.** *(Chap. 174)* Enterococci are well-known causes of nosocomial UTI—the most common infection caused by these organisms. Enterococcal UTIs are usually associated with indwelling catheters, instrumentation, or anatomic abnormalities of the genitourinary tract, and it is often challenging to differentiate between true infection and colonization (particularly in patients with chronic indwelling catheters). The presence of leukocytes in the urine in conjunction with systemic manifestations (e.g., fever) or local signs and symptoms of infection with no other explanation suggests the diagnosis. Enterococci are important causes of community- and healthcare-associated endocarditis, ranking second after staphylococci as an etiologic agent. *E faecalis* is the most common species of enterococci in surgical site infections. Enterococcal species colonize the gut (not often the mouth), and thus, most invasive infections are traced back to gut contamination, surgery, or invasive procedures.

IV-86. **The answer is B.** *(Chap. 174)* This patient has enterococcal endocarditis, which often occurs in patients with underlying gastrointestinal or genitourinary pathology. *E faecalis* is a more common causative organism than *E faecium* in community-acquired endocarditis. Patients tend to more commonly be male with underlying chronic disease. The typical presentation is one of subacute bacterial endocarditis with involvement of the mitral and/or aortic valves. Prolonged therapy beyond 4–6 weeks is often necessary for organisms with drug resistance. Complications requiring valve replacement are not uncommon. Enterococci are intrinsically resistant and/or tolerant to several antimicrobial agents (with *tolerance* defined as lack of killing by drug concentrations 16 times higher than the MIC). Monotherapy for endocarditis with a β-lactam antibiotic (to which many enterococci are tolerant) has produced disappointing results, with low cure rates at the end of therapy. However, the addition of an aminoglycoside to a cell wall–active agent (a β-lactam or a glycopeptide) increases cure rates and eradicates the organisms; moreover, this combination is synergistic and bactericidal in vitro. Therefore, combination therapy with a cell wall–active agent and an aminoglycoside is the standard of care for endovascular infections caused by enterococci. This synergistic effect can be explained, at least in part, by the increased penetration of the aminoglycoside into the bacterial cell, presumably as a result of cell wall alterations attributable to the β-lactam or glycopeptide.

IV-87. **The answer is A.** *(Chap. 175)* Immunity to diphtheria induced by childhood vaccination gradually decreases in adulthood. An estimated 30% of men age 60–69 years old have antitoxin titers below the protective level. In addition to older age and lack of vaccination, risk factors for diphtheria outbreaks include alcoholism, low socioeconomic status, crowded living conditions, and Native American ethnic background. An outbreak of diphtheria in Seattle, Washington, between 1972 and 1982 comprised 1100 cases, most of which were cutaneous. *Corynebacterium diphtheriae* is transmitted via the aerosol route, usually during close contact with an infected person. There are no significant reservoirs other than humans. Cutaneous diphtheria is usually a secondary infection that follows a primary skin lesion due to trauma, allergy, or autoimmunity. Most often, these isolates lack the *tox* gene and thus do not express diphtheria toxin.

IV-88. **The answer is D.** *(Chap. 175)* This is a classic clinical description and oral examination of diphtheria. While the development of an effective vaccine has nearly eradicated the disease in developed countries, failure to undergo routine vaccination leaves some patients at risk. The clinical diagnosis of diphtheria is based on the constellation of sore throat; adherent tonsillar, pharyngeal, or nasal pseudomembranous lesions; and low-grade fever. The systemic manifestations of diphtheria stem from the effects of diphtheria toxin and include weakness as a result of neurotoxicity and cardiac arrhythmias or congestive heart failure due to myocarditis. Most commonly, the pseudomembranous lesion is located in the tonsillopharyngeal region as shown in Figure IV-88. Less commonly, the lesions are located in the larynx, nares, and trachea or bronchial passages. Large pseudomembranes are associated with severe disease and a poor prognosis. A few patients develop massive swelling of the tonsils and present with "bull-neck" diphtheria, which results from massive edema of the submandibular and paratracheal region and is further characterized by foul breath, thick speech, and stridorous breathing. The diphtheritic pseudomembrane is gray or whitish and sharply demarcated. Unlike the exudative lesion associated with streptococcal pharyngitis, the pseudomembrane in diphtheria is tightly adherent to the underlying tissues. Polyneuropathy and myocarditis are late toxic manifestations of diphtheria. During a diphtheria outbreak in the Kyrgyz Republic in 1999, myocarditis was found in 22% and neuropathy in 5% of 656 hospitalized patients. The mortality rate was 7% among patients with myocarditis as opposed to 2% among those without myocardial manifestations. The median time to death in hospitalized patients was 4.5 days. Myocarditis is typically associated with dysrhythmia of the conduction tract and dilated cardiomyopathy. Rheumatic fever is a postinfectious complication of group A streptococcal infection, not diphtheria.

IV-89. **The answer is C.** *(Chap. 176) L monocytogenes* usually enters the body via the gastrointestinal tract in foods. Listeriosis is most often sporadic, although outbreaks do occur. No epidemiologic or clinical evidence supports person-to-person transmission (other than vertical transmission from mother to fetus) or waterborne infection. In line with its survival and multiplication at refrigeration temperatures, *L monocytogenes* is commonly found in processed and unprocessed foods of animal and plant origin, especially soft cheeses, delicatessen meats, hot dogs, milk, and cold salads; fresh fruits and vegetables can also transmit the organism. Because food supplies are increasingly centralized and normal hosts tolerate the organism well, outbreaks may not be immediately apparent. The FDA has a zero-tolerance policy for *L monocytogenes* in ready-to-eat foods.

IV-90. **The answer is A.** *(Chap. 176)* This patient has listerial meningitis, a potentially devastating CNS infection particularly prominent in older, chronically ill adults. *L monocytogenes* causes ~5%–10% of all cases of community-acquired bacterial meningitis in adults in the United States. Case fatality rates are reported to be 15%–26% and do not appear to have changed over time. This diagnosis should be considered in all older or chronically ill adults with "aseptic" meningitis. The presentation is more frequently subacute (with illness developing over several days) than in meningitis of other bacterial etiologies, and nuchal rigidity and overt meningeal signs are less common. Photophobia is infrequent. Focal findings and seizures are common in some but not all series. The CSF profile in listerial meningitis most often shows WBC counts in the range of 100–5000/μL (rarely higher); 75% of patients have counts below 1000/μL, usually with a neutrophil predominance more modest than that in other bacterial meningitides. Low glucose levels and positive results on Gram staining are found approximately 30%–40% of the time. No clinical trials have compared antimicrobial agents for the treatment of *L monocytogenes* infections. Data from in vitro and animal studies as well as observational clinical data indicate that ampicillin is the drug of choice, although penicillin also is highly active. Adults should receive IV ampicillin at high doses (2 g every 6 hours).

IV-91. **The answer is B.** *(Chap. 176) Listeria* bacteremia in pregnancy is a relatively rare but serious infection both for mother and fetus. Vertical transmission may occur, with 70%–90% of fetuses developing infection from the mother. Preterm labor is common. Prepartum treatment of the mother increases the chances of a healthy delivery. Mortality among fetuses approaches 50% and is much lower in neonates receiving appropriate antibiotics. First-line therapy is with ampicillin, with gentamicin often added for synergy. This recommendation is the same for mother and child. In patients with true penicillin allergy, the therapy of choice is trimethoprim-sulfamethoxazole. There are case reports of successful therapy with vancomycin, imipenem, linezolid, and macrolides, but there is not enough clinical evidence and some reports of failure that maintain ampicillin as recommended first-line therapy.

IV-92. **The answer is E.** *(Chap. 177)* This clinical scenario describes an unfortunate case of neonatal tetanus. In neonates, infection of the umbilical stump can result from inadequate umbilical cord care; in some cultures, for example, the cord is cut with grass or animal dung is applied to the stump. Circumcision or ear-piercing also can result in neonatal tetanus. It is caused by a powerful neurotoxin produced by the bacterium *Clostridium tetani* and does not result from bacteremia. Tetanus is diagnosed on clinical grounds, and case definitions are often used to facilitate clinical and epidemiologic assessments. The

CDC defines tetanus as "the acute onset of hypertonia or ... painful muscular contractions (usually of the muscles of the jaw and neck) and generalized muscle spasms without other apparent medical cause." Neonatal tetanus is defined by the World Health Organization (WHO) as "an illness occurring in a child who has the normal ability to suck and cry in the first 2 days of life but who loses this ability between days 3 and 28 of life and becomes rigid and has spasms." Tetanus toxin prevents transmitter release and effectively blocks inhibitory interneuron discharge. The result is unregulated activity in the motor nervous system. During the initial symptoms, respiratory failure due to laryngeal and respiratory muscle spasms is the most common cause of death. Later (during the second week), autonomic dysfunction and cardiovascular complications are the most common cause of death.

IV-93. **The answer is D.** *(Chap. 177)* Tetanus is an acute disease manifested by skeletal muscle spasm and autonomic nervous system disturbance. It is caused by a powerful neurotoxin produced by the bacterium *C tetani* and now a rare disease due to widespread vaccination. There were less than 50 cases reported recently in the United States, but a rising frequency in drug users has been seen. Older patients may be at higher risk due to waning immunity. The differential diagnosis of a patient presenting with tetanus includes strychnine poisoning and drug-related dystonic reactions. The diagnosis is clinical. Cardiovascular instability is common due to autonomic dysfunction and is manifest by rapid fluctuation in heart rate and blood pressure. Wound cultures will be positive in approximately 20% of cases. Metronidazole or penicillin should be administered to clear infection. Tetanus immune globulin is recommended over equine antiserum because of a lower risk of anaphylactic reactions. Recent evidence suggests that intrathecal administration is efficacious in inhibiting disease progression and improving outcomes. Muscle spasms may be treated with sedative drugs. With effective supportive care and often respiratory support, muscle function recovers after clearing toxin with no residual damage.

IV-94. **The answer is A.** *(Chap. 178)* The clinical presentation is characteristic of botulinum toxicity. Botulinum toxicity results in a flaccid paralysis by inhibitor presynaptic acetylcholine release. Further, this infant has the history of honey ingestion, which is a risk factor in infants. In adults, the ingestion of *Clostridium botulinum* spores does not lead to clinical botulism, as the pathogenic organisms do not readily grow and produce toxin in that environment. However, the risk is much higher for infants whose gut flora has not yet matured. For this reason, honey should not be given to infants <12 months of age. Tetanus toxicity causes a spastic, not flaccid, paralysis. Guillain-Barré syndrome has been reported in children but is almost always associated with vaccinations or a preceding illness. The absence of mention of a tick found embedded in the skin makes tick paralysis unlikely. In hypokalemic periodic paralysis (a very rare inheritable cause of muscle weakness and paralysis due to a channelopathy), deep tendon reflexes are normal despite the weakness or paralysis.

IV-95. **The answer is B.** *(Chap. 178)* This patient most likely has wound botulism. The use of "black-tar" heroin has been identified as a risk factor for this form of botulism. Typically, the wound appears benign, and unlike in other forms of botulism, gastrointestinal symptoms are absent. Symmetric *descending* paralysis suggests botulism, as does cranial nerve involvement. This patient's ptosis, diplopia, dysarthria, dysphagia, lack of fevers, normal reflexes, and lack of sensory deficits are all suggestive. Botulism can be easily confused with Guillain-Barré syndrome (GBS), which is often characterized by an antecedent infection and rapid, symmetric *ascending* paralysis and treated with plasmapheresis. The Miller Fischer variant of GBS is known for cranial nerve involvement, with ophthalmoplegia, ataxia, and areflexia being the most prominent features. Elevated protein in the CSF also favors GBS over botulism. Both botulism and GBS can progress to respiratory failure, so making a diagnosis by physical examination is critical. Other diagnostic modalities that may be helpful are wound culture, serum assay for toxin, and examination for decreased compound muscle action potentials on routine nerve stimulation studies. Patients with botulism are at risk of respiratory failure due to respiratory muscle weakness or aspiration. They should be followed closely with oxygen saturation monitoring and serial measurement of forced vital capacity.

IV-96. **The answer is B.** *(Chap. 179)* Both of these patients have enteritis necroticans caused by *C perfringens*. In Papua New Guinea during the 1960s, enteritis necroticans (known in that locale as pigbel) was found to be the most common cause of death in childhood; it was associated with pig feasts and occurred both sporadically and in outbreaks. Intramuscular immunization against the β-toxin resulted in a decreased incidence of the disease in Papua New Guinea, although the condition remains common. *C perfringens* is also the cause of gas gangrene myonecrosis, a highly morbid and mortal condition. The most common cause of bacterial pneumonia is the pneumococcus. *N meningitidis* and *S pneumoniae* are the most common causes of meningitis in adults. Group A *Streptococcus* is the most common cause of bacterial pharyngitis, and staphylococcal and streptococcal species are the most common causes of cellulitis.

IV-97. **The answer is A.** *(Chap. 179)* Clostridia are gram-positive spore-forming obligate anaerobes that reside normally in the gastrointestinal (GI) tract. Several clostridial species can cause severe disease. *C perfringens,* which is the second most common clostridial species to normally colonize the GI tract, is associated with food poisoning, gas gangrene, and myonecrosis. *Clostridium septicum* is seen often in conjunction with GI tumors. *Clostridium sordellii* is associated with septic abortions. All can cause a fulminant overwhelming bacteremia, but this condition is rare. The fact that this patient is well several days after his acute complaints rules out this fulminant course. A more common scenario is transient, self-limited bacteremia due to transient gut translocation during an episode of gastroenteritis. There is no need to treat when this occurs, and no further workup is necessary. *Clostridium* spp sepsis rarely causes endocarditis because overwhelming disseminated intravascular coagulation and death occur so rapidly. Screening for GI tumor is warranted when *C septicum* is cultured from the blood or a deep wound infection.

IV-98. **The answer is C.** *(Chap. 180)* A high proportion of young adults and adolescents (up to 25% in some studies) are colonized with *N meningitidis*, likely due to lifestyle and high-risk activities (kissing, crowded living conditions). Changes in living conditions (e.g., freshman year of college) are associated with a higher risk of invasive infections. It is unlikely that treating noninvasive meningococcal colonization would be effective in reducing the risk of invasive disease given the likelihood of recolonization. However, the quadrivalent meningococcal vaccine is effective in preventing invasive meningococcal disease and is recommended for all children older than age 11 years.

IV-99. **The answer is B.** *(Chap. 180)* Close contacts of individuals with known or presumed meningococcal disease are at increased risk of developing secondary disease with reports of secondary cases in up to 3% of primary cases. The rate of secondary cases is highest during the week after presentation of the index case, with most cases presenting within 6 weeks. Increased risk remains for up to 1 year. Prophylaxis is recommended for persons who are intimate with and/or household contacts of the index case and healthcare workers who have been directly exposed to respiratory secretions. Mass prophylaxis is not usually offered. The aim of prophylaxis is to eradicate colonization of close contacts with the strain that has caused invasive disease. Prophylaxis should be given as soon as possible to all contacts at the same time to avoid recolonization. Waiting for culture is not recommended. Ceftriaxone as a single dose is currently the most effective option in reducing carriage. Rifampin is no longer the optimal agent because it requires multiple doses and fails to eliminate carriage in up to 20% of cases. In some countries, ciprofloxacin or ofloxacin is used, but resistance has been reported in some areas. Current conjugated vaccines do not include *N meningitides* serotype B. Most sporadic cases in the United States are now due to this serotype. Vaccination should be offered in cases of meningococcal disease due to documented infection by a serotype included in the current vaccine.

IV-100. **The answer is A.** *(Chap. 180)* *N meningitidis* is an effective colonizer of the human nasopharynx, with asymptomatic infection rates of >25% described in some series of adolescents and young adults and among residents of crowded communities. Despite the high rates of carriage among adolescents and young adults, only 10% of adults carry meningococci, and colonization is very rare in early childhood. Colonization should be considered the normal state of meningococcal infection. Meningeal pharyngitis rarely occurs.

Meningococcal disease occurs when a virulent form of the organism invades a susceptible host. The most important bacterial virulence factor relates to the presence of the capsule. Unencapsulated forms of *N meningitides* rarely cause disease. A nonblanching petechial or purpuric rash occurs in >80% of cases of meningococcal disease. Of patients with meningococcal disease, 30%–50% present with meningitis, approximately 40% with meningitis plus septicemia, and 20% with septicemia alone. Patients with complement deficiency, who are at highest risk of developing meningococcal disease, may develop chronic meningitis.

IV-101. **The answer is B.** *(Chap. 181)* The Gram stain shows gram-negative intracellular mono- and diplococci that, together with the clinical presentation, are diagnostic of the gonococcus. Highly effective single-dose regimens have been developed for uncomplicated gonococcal infections. Quinolone-containing regimens are no longer recommended in the United States as first-line treatment because of widespread resistance. Initial treatment regimens must also incorporate an agent (e.g., azithromycin or doxycycline) that is effective against chlamydial infection because of the high frequency of co-infection. Gonorrhea in pregnancy can have serious consequences for both the mother and the infant. Pregnant women with gonorrhea, who should not take doxycycline, should receive concurrent treatment with a macrolide antibiotic for possible chlamydial infection.

IV-102. **The answer is E.** *(Chap. 181)* The importance of humoral immunity in host defenses against *Neisseria* infections is best illustrated by the predisposition of persons deficient in terminal complement components (C5 through C9) to recurrent bacteremic gonococcal infections and to recurrent meningococcal meningitis or meningococcemia. Gonococcal porin induces T-cell–proliferative responses in persons with urogenital gonococcal disease. A significant increase in porin-specific IL-4–producing CD4+ as well as CD8+ T lymphocytes is seen in individuals with mucosal gonococcal disease. Complement deficiencies, especially of the components involved in the assembly of the membrane attack complex (C5 through C9), predispose to *Neisseria* bacteremia, and persons with more than one episode of disseminated gonococcal infection should be screened with an assay for total hemolytic complement activity. Neutrophil quantitative or qualitative deficiencies (options A and D), immunoglobulin deficiencies (option B), and clonal defective lymphocyte populations (option C) have not been identified as specific risk factors for recurrent gonococcal infections.

IV-103. **The answer is D.** *(Chap. 182)* While most chronic obstructive pulmonary disease (COPD) exacerbations are thought to be due to upper respiratory viral infection, some proportion are associated with culturable pathogenic bacteria. Nontypable *H influenzae* is the most common bacterial cause of exacerbations of COPD; these exacerbations are characterized by increased cough, sputum production, and shortness of breath. Fever is low grade, and no infiltrates are evident on chest x-ray. *Moraxella catarrhalis, S pneumoniae*, and *P aeruginosa* most commonly cause clinical pneumonias instead of COPD exacerbations. *Acinetobacter* can also cause pneumonia, although often in patients with intrinsic airway disease or alterations (e.g., bronchiectasis). Approximately 20%–35% of nontypeable strains produce β-lactamase (with the exact proportion depending on geographic location), and these strains are resistant to ampicillin. Several agents have excellent activity against nontypeable *H influenzae*, including amoxicillin/clavulanic acid, various extended-spectrum cephalosporins, macrolides (azithromycin, clarithromycin), and fluoroquinolones.

IV-104. **The answer is D.** *(Chap. 182)* Generally thought of as a disease of children, epiglottitis is also a disease of adults since the wide use of *H influenzae* type B vaccination. Epiglottitis can cause life-threatening airway obstruction due to cellulitis of the epiglottis and supraglottic tissues, classically due to *H influenzae* type B infection. However, other organisms are also common causes including nontypeable *H influenzae, S pneumoniae, H parainfluenzae, S aureus*, and viral infection. The initial evaluation and treatment for epiglottitis in adults include airway management and intravenous antibiotics. The patient presented here is demonstrating signs of impending airway obstruction with stridor, inability to swallow secretions, and use of accessory muscles of inspiration. A lateral neck x-ray shows the typical thumb sign indicative of a swollen epiglottis. In addition, the patient has evidence of hypoventilation with carbon dioxide retention. Thus, in addition to antibiotics, this patient should also be intubated and mechanically ventilated electively under a controlled setting as he is at high risk for mechanical airway obstruction. Antibiotic therapy should cover the typical organisms outlined above and include coverage for oral anaerobes. In adults presenting without overt impending airway obstruction, laryngoscopy would be indicated to assess airway patency. Endotracheal intubation would be recommended for those with >50% airway obstruction. In children, endotracheal intubation is often recommended as laryngoscopy in children has provoked airway obstruction to a much greater degree than adults, and increased risk of mortality has been demonstrated in some series in children when the airway is managed expectantly.

IV-105. **The answer is B.** *(Chap. 183e)* HACEK organisms are a group of fastidious, slow-growing, gram-negative bacteria whose growth requires an atmosphere of carbon dioxide. Species belonging to this group include several **H***aemophilus* species, **A***ggregatibacter* (formerly *Actinobacillus*) species, **C***ardiobacterium hominis*, **E***ikenella corrodens*, and **K***ingella kingae*. HACEK bacteria normally reside in the oral cavity and have been associated with local infections in the mouth. They are also known to cause severe systemic infections—most often bacterial endocarditis, which can develop on either native or prosthetic valves. Compared with non-HACEK endocarditis, HACEK endocarditis occurs in younger patients and is more frequently associated with embolic, vascular, and immunologic manifestations but less commonly associated with congestive heart failure. The clinical course of HACEK endocarditis tends to be subacute, particularly with *Aggregatibacter* or *Cardiobacterium*. However, *K kingae* endocarditis may have a more aggressive presentation. Systemic embolization is common. The microbiology laboratory should be alerted when a HACEK organism is being considered; however, most cultures that ultimately yield a HACEK organism become positive within the first week, especially with improved culture systems.

IV-106. **The answer is B.** *(Chap. 183e) Capnocytophaga canimorsus* is the most likely organism to have caused fulminant disease in this alcoholic patient following a dog bite. Patients with a history of alcoholism, asplenia, and glucocorticoid therapy are at risk of developing disseminated infection, sepsis, and disseminated intravascular coagulation. Because of increasing β-lactamase expression, recommended treatment is with ampicillin/sulbactam or clindamycin. One of these therapies should be administered to asplenic patients with a dog bite. Other species of *Capnocytophaga* cause oropharyngeal disease and can cause sepsis in neutropenic patients, particularly in the presence of oral ulcers. *Eikenella* and *Haemophilus* are common mouth flora in humans but not in dogs. *Staphylococcus* can cause sepsis but is less likely in this scenario.

IV-107. **The answer is C.** *(Chap. 184)* The natural habitats for *L pneumophila* are aquatic bodies, including lakes and streams. Natural bodies of water contain only small numbers of legionellae. However, once the organisms enter human-constructed aquatic reservoirs (such as drinking-water systems), they can grow and proliferate. Factors known to enhance colonization by and amplification of legionellae include warm temperatures (25–42°C) and the presence of scale and sediment. *L pneumophila* can form microcolonies within biofilms; its eradication from drinking-water systems requires disinfectants that can penetrate the biofilm. Heavy rainfall and flooding can result in the entry of high numbers of legionellae into water-distribution systems, leading to an upsurge of cases. Large buildings over three stories high are commonly colonized with *Legionella*. Sporadic community-acquired Legionnaires' disease has been linked to colonization of hotels, office buildings, factories, and even private homes. Drinking-water systems in hospitals and extended-care facilities have been the source for healthcare-associated Legionnaires' disease. Transmission is via inhalation of bacteria-containing aerosol. The disease is not spread via zoonotic or insect vectors nor via person-to-person transmission. There is no effective vaccination for *L pneumophila*.

IV-108. **The answer is A.** *(Chap. 184)* Legionnaires' disease is often included in the differential diagnosis of "atypical pneumonia," along with pneumonia due to *C pneumoniae*,

Chlamydia psittaci, M pneumoniae, C burnetii, and some viruses. The course and prognosis of *Legionella* pneumonia more closely resembles those of bacteremic pneumococcal pneumonia than those of pneumonia due to other "atypical" pathogens. Patients with community-acquired Legionnaires' disease are significantly more likely than patients with pneumonia of other etiologies to be admitted to an ICU on presentation. Gastrointestinal difficulties are often pronounced; abdominal pain, nausea, and vomiting affect 10%–20% of patients. Diarrhea (watery rather than bloody) is reported in 25%–50% of cases. The most common neurologic abnormalities are confusion or changes in mental status; however, the multitudinous neurologic symptoms reported range from headache and lethargy to encephalopathy. Hyponatremia, elevated values in liver function tests, and hematuria also occur more frequently in Legionnaires' disease than other causes of atypical pneumonia. The most severe extrapulmonary sequela, neurologic dysfunction, is rare but can be debilitating. The most common neurologic deficits in the long term—ataxia and speech difficulties—result from cerebellar dysfunction.

IV-109. **The answer is B.** *(Chap. 184)* Despite antibiotic treatment, pneumonia from all causes remains a major source of mortality in the United States. Mortality from *Legionella* pneumonia varies from 0%–11% in treated immunocompetent patients to approximately 30% if not treated effectively. Because *Legionella* is an intracellular pathogen, antibiotics that reach intracellular MICs are most likely to be effective. Newer macrolides and quinolones are antibiotics of choice and are effective as monotherapy. Doxycycline and tigecycline are active in vitro. Anecdotal reports have described successes and failures with trimethoprim-sulfamethoxazole and clindamycin. Aztreonam, most β-lactams, and cephalosporins cannot be considered effective therapy for *Legionella* pneumonia. For severe cases, rifampin may be initially added to azithromycin or a fluoroquinolone.

IV-110. **The answer is D.** *(Chap. 184) Legionella* urine antigen is detectable within 3 days of symptoms and will remain positive for 2 months. It is not affected by antibiotic use. The urinary antigen test is formulated to detect only *L pneumophilia* (which causes 80% of *Legionella* infections), but cross-reactivity with other *Legionella* species has been reported. The urinary test is sensitive and highly specific. Typically, Gram staining of specimens from sterile sites such as pleural fluid show numerous WBCs but no organisms. However, *Legionella* may appear as faint, pleomorphic gram-negative bacilli. *Legionella* may be cultured from sputum even when epithelial cells are present. Cultures, grown on selective media, take 3–5 days to show visible growth. Antibody detection using acute and convalescent serum is an accurate means of diagnosis. A fourfold rise is diagnostic, but this takes up to 12 weeks and thus is most useful for epidemiologic investigation. *Legionella* PCR has not been shown to be adequately sensitive and specific for clinical use. It is used for environmental sampling.

IV-111. **The answer is B.** *(Chap. 185)* Pertussis is a highly communicable disease, with attack rates of 80%–100% among unimmunized household contacts and 20% within households in well-immunized populations. The infection has a worldwide distribution, with cyclical outbreaks every 3–5 years (a pattern that has persisted despite widespread immunization). Pertussis occurs in all months; however, in North America, its activity peaks in summer and autumn. In developing countries, pertussis remains an important cause of infant morbidity and death. The reported incidence of pertussis worldwide has decreased as a result of improved vaccine coverage. However, coverage rates are still <50% in many developing nations; the WHO estimates that 90% of the burden of pertussis is in developing regions. Although thought of as a disease of childhood, pertussis can affect people of all ages and is increasingly being identified as a cause of prolonged coughing illness in adolescents and adults. The duration of immunity after whole-cell pertussis vaccination is short-lived, with little protection remaining after 10–12 years. Recent studies have demonstrated early waning of immunity—i.e., within 2–4 years after the fifth dose of vaccine in children who received the acellular pertussis vaccine for their primary series in infancy. These data suggest that boosters may be needed more frequently than every 10 years, as previously thought

IV-112. **The answer is C.** *(Chap. 185)* Pertussis, due to the gram-negative bacteria *Bordetella pertussis*, is an upper respiratory infection characterized by a violent cough. Its prevalence has been dramatically reduced, but not eliminated, by widespread infant vaccination. It causes an extremely morbid and often mortal disease in infants <6 months old, particularly in the developing world. The prevalence appears to be increasing in young adults and adolescents due to waning immunity. Some are recommending booster vaccination after 10 years. *B pertussis* is also a growing pathogen in patients with COPD. The clinical manifestations typically include a persistent, episodic cough developing a few days after a cold-like upper respiratory infection. The cough may become persistent. It often wakes the patient from sleep and results in post-tussive vomiting. An audible whoop is only present in less than half the cases. Diagnosis is with nasopharyngeal culture or DNA probe testing. There is no urinary antigen testing available. The goal of antibiotic therapy is to eradicate the organism from the nasopharynx. It does not alter the clinical course. Macrolide antibiotics are the treatment of choice. Pneumonia is uncommon with *B pertussis*. Cold agglutinins may be positive in infection with *M pneumoniae*, which is on the differential diagnosis of *B pertussis*.

IV-113. **The answer is C.** *(Chap. 186)* In healthy humans, *E coli* is the predominant species of gram-negative bacilli (GNB) in the colonic flora; *Klebsiella* and *Proteus* species are less prevalent. Both *Staphylococcus* and *Clostridium* species are gram-positive organisms.

IV-114. **The answer is A.** *(Chap. 186)* Evidence indicates that initiation of appropriate empirical antimicrobial therapy early in the course of GNB infections, particularly serious infections, leads to improved outcomes. The ever-increasing prevalence of multidrug-resistant (MDR) and extensively drug-resistant (XDR) GNB; the lag between published (historical) and current resistance rates; and variations by species, geographic location, regional antimicrobial use, and hospital site (e.g., ICUs vs. wards) necessitate familiarity with evolving patterns of antimicrobial resistance for the selection of appropriate empirical therapy. For a critically ill patient with suspected gram-negative sepsis, it is prudent to choose a broad-spectrum agent initially to ensure adequate antimicrobial coverage. At present, the most reliably active agents against enteric GNB are the carbapenems (e.g., imipenem), the aminoglycoside amikacin, the fourth-generation cephalosporin cefepime, the β-lactam/β-lactamase inhibitor combination piperacillin-tazobactam, and the polymyxins (e.g., colistin or polymyxin B). β-Lactamases, which inactivate β-lactam agents, are the most important mediators of resistance to these drugs in GNB. Decreased permeability and/or active efflux of β-lactam agents, although less common, may occur alone or in combination with β-lactamase–mediated resistance. Broad-spectrum β-lactamases (e.g., TEM, SHV), which mediate resistance to many penicillins and first-generation cephalosporins, are frequently expressed in enteric GNB. Trimethoprim-sulfamethoxazole (TMP-SMX) and tetracycline (and therefore tigecycline) resistance in GNBs has increased drastically in the past several decades. Vancomycin does not provide gram-negative coverage and would be an inappropriate single agent in this case.

IV-115. **The answer is A.** *(Chap. 186)* Uncomplicated cystitis, the most common acute UTI syndrome, is characterized by dysuria, urinary frequency, and suprapubic pain. Fever and/or back pain suggest progression to pyelonephritis. *E coli* is the single most common pathogen for all UTI syndrome/host group combinations. Each year in the United States, *E coli* causes 80%–90% of an estimated 6–8 million episodes of uncomplicated cystitis in premenopausal women. Furthermore, 20% of women with an initial cystitis episode develop frequent recurrences. All of the other organisms can cause UTIs, although de novo infection with *S aureus* is rare and should prompt investigation into prior genitourinary instrumentation procedures or a hematogenous source.

IV-116. **The answer is A.** *(Chap. 186)* Shiga toxic and enterohemorrhagic strains of *E coli* (STEC/EHEC) cause hemorrhagic colitis and the hemolytic-uremic syndrome (HUS). Several large outbreaks resulting from the consumption of fresh produce (e.g., lettuce, spinach, sprouts) and of undercooked ground beef have received significant attention in the media. O157:H7 is the most prominent serotype, but others have been reported to cause similar disease. The ability of STEC/EHEC to produce Shiga toxin (Stx2 and/or Stx1) or related toxins is a critical factor in the expression of clinical disease. Manure from domesticated ruminant animals in industrialized countries serves as the major reservoir for STEC/EHEC. Ground beef—the most common food source of STEC/EHEC strains—is often contaminated during processing. Low bacterial numbers can transmit disease in humans, accounting for widespread infection from environmental sources and person-to-person spread. O157:H7 strains are the fourth most commonly reported cause of bacterial diarrhea in the United States (after *Campylobacter*, *Salmonella*, and *Shigella*). STEC/EHEC characteristically causes grossly bloody diarrhea in >90% of cases. Significant abdominal pain and fecal leukocytes are common (70% of cases), whereas fever is not; absence of fever can incorrectly lead to consideration of noninfectious conditions (e.g., intussusception and inflammatory or ischemic bowel disease). STEC/EHEC disease is usually self-limited, lasting 5–10 days. HUS may develop in the very young or elderly patients within 2 weeks of diarrhea. It is estimated that it occurs in 2%–8% of cases of STEC/EHEC and that >50% of all cases of HUS in the United States and 90% of cases in children are caused by STEC/EHEC. Antibiotic therapy of STEC/EHEC cases of diarrhea should be avoided because antibiotics may increase the likelihood of developing HUS.

IV-117. **The answer is D.** *(Chap. 186)* The abdominal CT (Figure IV-117) shows a primary liver abscess (*red arrow*) with metastatic spread to the spleen (*black arrow*). "Classic" *K pneumoniae* (cKP) causes a spectrum of abdominal infections similar to that caused by *E coli* but is less frequently isolated from these infections. Hypervirulent *K pneumoniae* (hvKP) is a common cause of monomicrobial community-acquired pyogenic liver abscess and, in the Asian Pacific Rim, has been recovered with steadily increasing frequency over the past two decades, replacing *E coli* as the most common pathogen causing this syndrome. hvKP is increasingly described as a cause of spontaneous bacterial peritonitis and splenic abscess. hvKP infection initially was characterized and distinguished from traditional infections due to cKP by (1) presentation as community-acquired pyogenic liver abscess, (2) occurrence in patients lacking a history of hepatobiliary disease, and (3) a propensity for metastatic spread to distant sites (e.g., eyes, CNS, lungs), which occurred in 11%–80% of cases. More recently, this variant has been recognized as the cause of a variety of serious community-acquired extrahepatic abscesses/infections in the absence of liver involvement, including pneumonia, meningitis, endophthalmitis, splenic abscess, and necrotizing fasciitis. The affected individuals often have diabetes mellitus and are of Asian ethnicity; however, nondiabetics and all ethnic groups can be affected. Survivors often suffer catastrophic morbidity, such as loss of vision and neurologic sequelae.

IV-118. **The answer is E.** *(Chap. 187)* Infections with *Acinetobacter* species are a growing cause of hospital-acquired infection worldwide. Surveillance data from Australia and Asia suggest that infections are common, and there are reports of community-acquired *Acinetobacter* infection. *Acinetobacter* typically infects patients receiving long-term care in ICUs by causing ventilator-associated pneumonia, bloodstream infections, or UTIs. They are of particular concern because of their propensity to develop multidrug (or pan-drug) resistance and their ability to colonize units due to healthcare worker transmission. *Acinetobacter baumannii* is the most common isolate and develops drug resistance avidly. Many strains are currently resistant to carbapenems (imipenem, meropenem). Last-line agents such as colistin, polymyxin A, and tigecycline are often the only available therapeutic options. Tigecycline has been used for pneumonia due to carbapenem-resistant strains but is not thought to be efficacious in bloodstream infection because usual dosing does not achieve therapeutic levels against *Acinetobacter*.

IV-119. **The answer is B.** *(Chap. 187)* Treatment of *Acinetobacter* infections is hampered by the remarkable ability of *A baumannii* to upregulate or acquire antibiotic resistance determinants. The most prominent example is that of β-lactamases, including those capable of inactivating carbapenems, cephalosporins, and penicillins. These enzymes, which include the OXA-type β-lactamases (e.g., OXA-23), the metallo-β-lactamases (e.g., NDM), and rarely KPC-type carbapenemases, are typically resistant to currently available β-lactamase inhibitors such as clavulanate or tazobactam. Plasmids that harbor genes encoding these β-lactamases may also harbor genes encoding resistance to aminoglycosides and sulfur antibiotics. The end result is that carbapenem-resistant *A baumannii* may become truly multidrug resistant. Selection of empirical antibiotic therapy when *A baumannii* is suspected is challenging and must rely on knowledge of local epidemiology. Receipt of prompt, effective antibiotic therapy is the goal. Given the diversity of resistance mechanisms in *A baumannii*, definitive therapy should be based on the results of antimicrobial susceptibility testing. Carbapenems (imipenem, meropenem, and doripenem but not ertapenem) have long been thought of as the agents of choice for serious *A baumannii* infections. However, the clinical utility of carbapenems is now widely jeopardized by the production of carbapenemases, as described earlier. Sulbactam may be an alternative to carbapenems. Unlike other β-lactamase inhibitors (e.g., clavulanic acid and tazobactam), sulbactam has intrinsic activity against *Acinetobacter* species; this activity is mediated by the drug's binding to penicillin-binding protein 2 rather than by its ability to inhibit β-lactamases. Sulbactam is commercially available in a combined formulation with either ampicillin or cefoperazone and may also be available as a single agent in some countries. Despite the absence of randomized clinical trials, sulbactam seems to be equivalent to carbapenems in clinical effectiveness against susceptible strains. Therapy for carbapenem-resistant *A baumannii* is particularly problematic. The only currently available choices are polymyxins (colistin and polymyxin B) and tigecycline. Neither option is perfect. Polymyxins may be nephrotoxic and neurotoxic. Definition of the optimal dose and schedule for administration of polymyxins to patients in vulnerable groups (e.g., those requiring renal replacement therapy) remains challenging, and emergence of resistance in association with monotherapy is a concern. Conventional doses of tigecycline may not result in serum concentrations adequate to treat bloodstream infections. Resistance of *A baumannii* to tigecycline may develop during treatment with this drug. *Acinetobacter* species, unlike *C difficile*, do not form spores.

IV-120. **The answer is B.** *(Chap. 188)* This patient has essentially performed a urease breath test. In this simple test, the patient drinks a solution of urea labeled with the nonradioactive isotope ^{13}C and then blows into a collection tube. If *Helicobacter pylori* urease is present, the urea is hydrolyzed, and labeled carbon dioxide is detected in breath samples. This patient's test is "positive"; therefore, he is infected with *H pylori*. Essentially, all *H pylori*–colonized persons have histologic gastritis, but only approximately 10%–15% develop associated illnesses, including gastritis, gastric ulcers, duodenal ulcers, gastric lymphoma, and gastric adenocarcinoma. *H pylori* infection is not correlated with a higher risk of colon cancer. *H pylori* infection is essential for life unless eradicated by antibiotic treatment; thus, the subject's urease breath test will almost certainly remain positive without treatment.

IV-121. **The answer is E.** *(Chap. 188)* It is impossible to know whether the patient's continued dyspepsia is due to persistent *H pylori* as a result of treatment failure or to some other cause. A quick noninvasive test to look for the presence of *H pylori* is a urea breath test. This test can be done as an outpatient and gives a rapid, accurate response. Patients should not have received any proton pump inhibitors or antimicrobials in the meantime. Stool antigen test is another good option if urea breath testing is not available. If the urea breath test is positive >1 month after completion of first-line therapy, second-line therapy with a proton pump inhibitor, bismuth subsalicylate, tetracycline, and metronidazole may be indicated. If the urea breath test is negative, the remaining symptoms are unlikely due to persistent *H pylori* infection. Serology is useful only for diagnosing infection initially, but it can remain positive and therefore be misleading in those who have cleared *H pylori*. Endoscopy is a consideration to rule out ulcer or upper gastrointestinal malignancy but is generally preferred after two failed attempts to eradicate *H pylori*. Figure IV-121 outlines the algorithm for management of *H pylori* infection.

IV-122. **The answer is A.** *(Chap. 188)* In vitro, *H pylori* is susceptible to a wide variety of antibiotics. However, monotherapy is no longer recommended because of inadequate antibiotic delivery to the colonization niche and the development of resistance. All current regimens include either a proton pump inhibitor (omeprazole or equivalent), H2 blocker (ranitidine or equivalent), and/or bismuth. Regimens including quinolones may not be advisable because of common resistance and the risk of developing *C difficile* colitis. Current regimens have an eradication rate of 75%–80%.

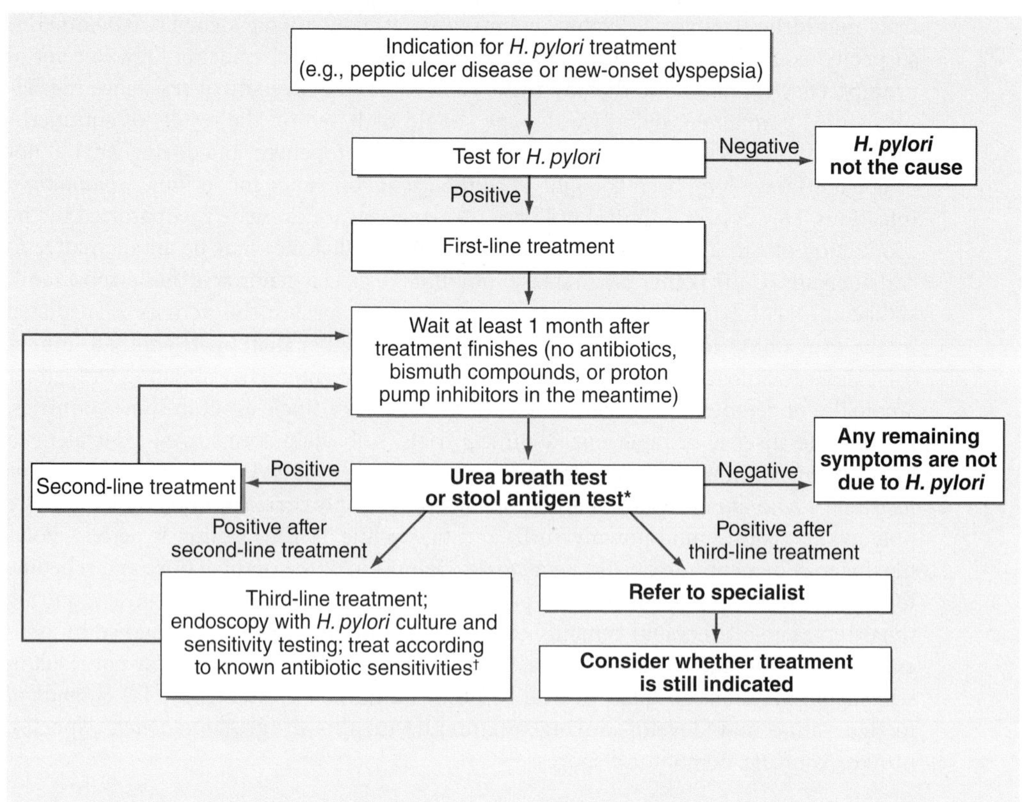

FIGURE IV-121 *Note that either the urea breath test or the stool antigen test can be used in this algorithm. Occasionally, endoscopy and a biopsy-based test are used instead of either of these tests in follow-up after treatment. The main indication for these invasive tests is gastric ulceration; in this condition, as opposed to duodenal ulceration, it is important to check healing and to exclude underlying gastric adenocarcinoma. However, even in this situation, patients undergoing endoscopy may still be receiving proton pump inhibitor therapy, which precludes *H pylori* testing. Thus, a urea breath test or a stool antigen test is still required at a suitable interval after the end of therapy to determine whether treatment has been successful (see text). †Some authorities use empirical third-line regimens, of which several have been described.

IV-123. **The answer is E.** *(Chap. 189) Stenotrophomonas maltophilia* is the only potential human pathogen among a genus of ubiquitous organisms found in the rhizosphere (i.e., the soil that surrounds the roots of plants). An immunocompromised state alone is not sufficient to permit human colonization or infection; rather, major perturbations of the human flora are usually necessary for the establishment of *S maltophilia*. Accordingly, most cases of human infection occur in the setting of very broad-spectrum antibiotic therapy with agents such as advanced cephalosporins and carbapenems, which eradicate the normal flora and other pathogens. The remarkable ability of *S. maltophilia* to resist virtually all classes of antibiotics is attributable to the possession of antibiotic efflux pumps and of two β-lactamases that mediate β-lactam resistance, including that to carbapenems. It is fortunate that the virulence of *S maltophilia* appears to be limited. *S maltophilia* is most commonly found in the respiratory tract of ventilated patients, where the distinction between its roles as a colonizer and as a pathogen is often difficult to make. However, *S maltophilia* does cause pneumonia and bacteremia in such patients, and these infections have led to septic shock. The intrinsic resistance of *S maltophilia* to most antibiotics renders infection difficult to treat. The antibiotics to which it is most often (although not uniformly) susceptible are trimethoprim-sulfamethoxazole (TMP-SMX), ticarcillin-clavulanate, levofloxacin, and tigecycline (Table IV-123). Consequently, a combination of TMP-SMX and ticarcillin-clavulanate is recommended for initial therapy.

IV-124. **The answer is C.** *(Chap. 189)* In febrile neutropenia, *P aeruginosa* has historically been the organism against which empirical coverage is always essential. Although in Western countries these infections are now less common, their importance has not diminished because

TABLE IV-123 **Antibiotic Treatment of Infections due to *Pseudomonas aeruginosa* and Related Species**

Infection	Antibiotics and Dosages	Other Considerations
Bacteremia		
Nonneutropenic host	Monotherapy: Ceftazidime (2 g q8h IV) *or* cefepime (2 g q12h IV) Combination therapy: Piperacillin/tazobactam (3.375 g q4h IV) *or* imipenem (500 mg q6h IV) *or* meropenem (1 g q8h IV) *or* doripenem (500 mg q8h IV) *plus* Amikacin (7.5 mg/kg q12h or 15 mg/kg q24h IV)	Add an aminoglycoside for patients in shock and in regions or hospitals where rates of resistance to the primary β-lactam agents are high. Tobramycin may be used instead of amikacin (susceptibility permitting). The duration of therapy is 7 days for nonneutropenic patients. Neutropenic patients should be treated until no longer neutropenic.
Neutropenic host	Cefepime (2 g q8h IV) *or* all other agents (except doripenem) in above dosages	
Endocarditis	Antibiotic regimens as for bacteremia for 6–8 weeks	Resistance during therapy is common. Surgery is required for relapse.
Pneumonia	Drugs and dosages as for bacteremia, except that the available carbapenems should not be the sole primary drugs because of high rates of resistance during therapy	IDSA guidelines recommend the addition of an aminoglycoside or ciprofloxacin. The duration of therapy is 10–14 days.
Bone infection, malignant otitis externa	Cefepime or ceftazidime at the same dosages as for bacteremia; aminoglycosides not a necessary component of therapy; ciprofloxacin (500–750 mg q12h PO) may be used	Duration of therapy varies with the drug used (e.g., 6 weeks for a β-lactam agent; at least 3 months for oral therapy except in puncture-wound osteomyelitis, for which the duration should be 2–4 weeks).
Central nervous system infection	Ceftazidime or cefepime (2 g q8h IV) or meropenem (1 g q8h IV)	Abscesses or other closed-space infections may require drainage. The duration of therapy is ≥2 weeks.
Eye infection Keratitis/ulcer	Topical therapy with tobramycin/ciprofloxacin/levofloxacin eye drops	Use maximal strengths available or compounded by pharmacy. Therapy should be administered for 2 weeks or until the resolution of eye lesions, whichever is shorter.
Endophthalmitis	Ceftazidime or cefepime as for central nervous system infection *plus* Topical therapy	
Urinary tract infection	Ciprofloxacin (500 mg q12h PO) *or* levofloxacin (750 mg q24h) *or* any aminoglycoside (total daily dose given once daily)	Relapse may occur if an obstruction or a foreign body is present. The duration of therapy for complicated UTI is 7–10 days (up to 2 weeks for pyelonephritis).
Multidrug-resistant *P aeruginosa* infection	Colistin (100 mg q12h IV) for the shortest possible period to obtain a clinical response	Doses used have varied. Dosage adjustment is required in renal failure. Inhaled colistin may be added for pneumonia (100 mg q12h).
Stenotrophomonas maltophilia infection	TMP-SMX (1600/320 mg q12h IV) *plus* ticarcillin/clavulanate (3.1 g q4h IV) for 14 days	Resistance to all agents is increasing. Levofloxacin or tigecycline may be alternatives, but there is little published clinical experience with these agents.
Burkholderia cepacia infection	Meropenem (1 g q8h IV) *or* TMP-SMX (1600/320 mg q12h IV) for 14 days	Resistance to both agents is increasing. Do not use them in combination because of possible antagonism.
Melioidosis, glanders	Ceftazidime (2 g q6h) *or* meropenem (1 g q8h) *or* imipenem (500 mg q6h) for 2 weeks *followed by* TMP-SMX (1600/320 mg q12h PO) for 3 months	

Abbreviations: IDSA, Infectious Diseases Society of America; TMP-SMX, trimethoprim-sulfamethoxazole.

of persistently high mortality rates. In other parts of the world as well, *P aeruginosa* continues to be a significant problem in febrile neutropenia, causing a larger proportion of infections in febrile neutropenic patients than any other single organism. For example, *P aeruginosa* was responsible for 28% of documented infections in 499 febrile neutropenic patients in one study from the Indian subcontinent and for 31% of such infections in another. In a large study of infections in leukemia patients from Japan, *P aeruginosa* was the most frequently documented cause of bacterial infection. The most common clinical syndromes encountered were bacteremia, pneumonia, and soft tissue infections manifesting mainly as ecthyma gangrenosum.

IV-125. **The answer is A.** *(Chap. 189) Burkholderia cepacia* is an opportunistic pathogen that has been responsible for nosocomial outbreaks. It also colonizes and infects the lower respiratory tract of patients with cystic fibrosis, chronic granulomatous disease, and sickle cell disease. In patients with cystic fibrosis, it portends a rapid decline in pulmonary function and a poor clinical prognosis. It also may cause a resistant necrotizing pneumonia. *B cepacia* is often intrinsically resistant to a variety of antimicrobials, including many β-lactams and aminoglycosides. TMP-SMX is usually the first-line treatment. *P aeruginosa* and *S aureus* are common colonizers and pathogens in patients with cystic fibrosis. Repeated infections due to these agents will result in lung function deterioration. However, airway colonization of *B cepacia* has the strongest risk of declining lung function and worsening function. *Stenotrophomonas maltophilia* is an opportunistic pathogen, particularly in patients with cancer, transplants, and critical illness. *S maltophilia* is a cause of pneumonia, UTI, wound infection, and bacteremia. TMP-SMX is usually the treatment of choice for *Stenotrophomonas* infections.

IV-126. **The answer is B.** *(Chap. 190)* All *Salmonella* infections begin with ingestion of organisms, most commonly in contaminated food or water. The infectious dose ranges from 200 CFU to 106 CFU, and the ingested dose is an important determinant of incubation period and disease severity. Conditions that decrease either stomach acidity (an age of <1 year, antacid ingestion, or achlorhydric disease) or intestinal integrity (inflammatory bowel disease, prior gastrointestinal surgery, or alteration of the intestinal flora by antibiotic administration) increase susceptibility to *Salmonella* infection.

IV-127. **The answer is E.** *(Chap. 190)* Mr. Munoz is infected with a *Salmonella* species, most likely *typhi* or *paratyphus*. This infection should be suspected in any individual returning from travel to a developing country, particularly from southern Asia, where the disease remains endemic, despite reporting no known potentially infected ingestion. *Salmonella* species do not ferment lactose. Further, this patient has striking relative bradycardia, a dissociation between the heart rate, and presence of fever. Most patients with such a degree of fever will be tachycardic; however, approximately 50% of patients with *Salmonella* infections will manifest this relative bradycardia. The rash, termed *rose spots*, is also typical for *Salmonella* typhoid or enteric fever. The patient is unlikely to have developed *C difficile* in the absence of antibiotic therapy. Travelers to South Asia are at risk of developing *E coli* infection from ingested food. However, the microbial characteristics rule out the other choices. *E coli* and *K pneumoniae* are both lactose fermenters. *Clostridium* is a gram-positive rod, and *Entamoeba histolytica* is a protozoan, not a bacteria.

IV-128. **The answer is E.** *(Chap. 190) Salmonella enteritidis* is one of the causes of nontyphoidal salmonellosis (NTS) along with *Salmonella typhimurium* and other strains. Enteric (typhoid) fever is caused by *S typhi* or *S paratyphi*. Recent cases of gastroenteritis due to NTS have been associated with undercooked or raw eggs. In contrast to *S typhi* and *S paratyphi*, which only have human reservoirs, the NTS can colonize livestock, accounting for outbreaks related to contaminated water (fresh produce, undercooked ground meat, dairy products). The gastroenteritis caused by NTS is indistinguishable clinically for other enteric pathogens. The diarrhea is nonbloody and may be copious. The disease is typically self-limited in healthy hosts, and antibiotic therapy is not recommended because it does not change the course of disease and promotes resistance. Therapy may be necessary for neonates or debilitated elderly patients who are more likely to develop bacteremia. Bacteremia occurs in less than 10% of cases. Metastatic infections of bone, joint, and endovascular devices may occur. There is no vaccine for NTS. There are oral and parenteral vaccines for *S typhi*.

IV-129. **The answer is D.** *(Chap. 191)* Shigellosis remains a cause of dysentery in the developing world, and sporadic cases due to fecal-oral contamination occur in the developing and developed world. The human intestinal tract is the most prevalent reservoir for the bacteria. Clinical illness due to *Shigella* can be caused by a very small inoculum. Shigellosis typically evolves through four phases: incubation, watery diarrhea, dysentery, and the postinfectious phase. The incubation period is usually 1–4 days, and the dysentery follows within hours to days. The dysentery syndrome is indistinguishable from other invasive enteropathogens (including *Campylobacter*), and inflammatory bowel disease is also in the differential. Because the organism is enteroinvasive, antibiotic therapy is indicated. Ciprofloxacin is generally recommended unless there is proven resistance. Ceftriaxone, azithromycin, pivmecillinam, and some recent quinolones are also effective. *Shigella* infection typically does not cause life-threatening dehydration. Antimotility agents are not recommended because they are thought to prolong the systemic symptoms and may increase the risk of toxic megacolon and hemolytic-uremic syndrome. There is currently no commercially available vaccine for *Shigella* infection.

IV-130. **The answer is A.** *(Chap. 192)* This patient is suffering from classic traveler's diarrhea (of which, *Campylobacter* is a common cause). A prodrome of fever, headache, myalgia, and/or malaise often occurs 12–48 hours before the onset of diarrheal symptoms. The most common signs and symptoms of the intestinal phase are diarrhea, abdominal pain, and fever. The degree of diarrhea varies from several loose stools to grossly bloody stools; most patients presenting for medical attention have ≥10 bowel movements on the worst day of illness. Abdominal pain usually consists of cramping and may be the most prominent symptom. Pain is usually generalized but may become localized; *Campylobacter jejuni* infection may cause pseudoappendicitis. Fever may be the only initial manifestation of *C jejuni* infection, a situation mimicking the early stages of typhoid fever. Even among patients presenting for medical attention with *Campylobacter* enteritis, not all clearly benefit from specific antimicrobial therapy. Indications for therapy include high fever, bloody diarrhea, severe diarrhea, persistence for >1 week, and worsening of symptoms. Macrolides are generally the empirical treatment of choice with <10% of isolates demonstrating resistance. A single dose of azithromycin 500 mg is effective and is the regimen of choice; a 5- to 7-day course of erythromycin (250 mg orally four times daily or—for children—30–50 mg/kg/d in divided doses) is also effective. Resistance to quinolones as well as to tetracyclines is substantial; approximately 22% of U.S. isolates in 2010 were resistant to ciprofloxacin. Except in infection with *Campylobacter fetus*, bacteremia is uncommon, developing most often in immunocompromised hosts and at the extremes of age. Due to its proclivity to cause bacteremia and distant organ involvement, *C fetus* has a far worse prognosis than other subtypes. Systemic infection with *C fetus* is much more often fatal than that due to related species; this higher mortality rate reflects in part the population affected.

IV-131. **The answer is A.** *(Chap. 193)* Cholera toxin consists of a monomeric enzymatic moiety (the A subunit) and a pentameric binding moiety (the B subunit). The B pentamer binds to GM1 ganglioside, a glycolipid on the surface of epithelial cells that serves as the toxin receptor and makes possible the delivery of the A subunit to its cytosolic target. The activated A subunit (A1) irreversibly transfers adenosine diphosphate (ADP)-ribose from nicotinamide adenine dinucleotide to its specific target protein, the guanosine triphosphate (GTP)-binding regulatory component of adenylate cyclase. The ADP-ribosylated G protein upregulates the activity of adenylate cyclase; the result is the intracellular accumulation of high levels of cyclic AMP. In intestinal epithelial cells, cyclic adenosine monophosphate (AMP) inhibits the absorptive sodium transport system in villus cells and activates the secretory chloride transport system in crypt cells, and these events lead to the accumulation of sodium chloride in the intestinal lumen. Because water moves passively to maintain osmolality, isotonic fluid accumulates in the lumen. When the volume of that fluid exceeds the capacity of the rest of the gut to resorb it, watery diarrhea results. Unless the wasted fluid and electrolytes are adequately replaced, shock (due to profound dehydration) and acidosis (due to loss of bicarbonate) follow. Fever is usually absent in cases of cholera. The stool has a characteristic appearance: a nonbilious, gray, slightly cloudy fluid with flecks of mucus, no blood, and a somewhat fishy, inoffensive odor. It has been called "rice-water" stool (Figure IV-131) because of its resemblance to the water in which rice has been washed.

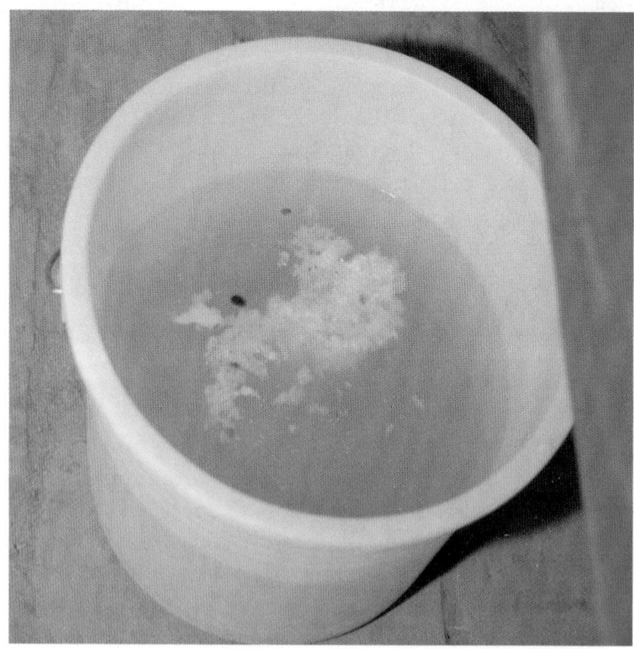

FIGURE IV-131 Courtesy of Dr. A. S. G. Faruque, International Centre for Diarrhoeal Disease Research, Dhaka; with permission.

IV-132. **The answer is D.** *(Chap. 193)* Cholera can be a devastating and rapidly deadly disease, but some patients, such as Mr. Zi, are only mildly affected. Table IV-132 describes clinical characteristics of patients with mild, moderate, or severe dehydration due to cholera. In patients with mild dehydration, antibiotics are not needed as they are not curative. In patients with moderate or severe dehydration, the use of an antibiotic to which the organism is susceptible diminishes the duration and volume of fluid loss and hastens clearance of the organism from the stool. Erythromycin is the drug of choice. For patient with mild diarrhea from cholera, oral rehydration therapy is an excellent therapeutic option. Oral rehydration solution (ORS) takes advantage of the hexose-Na^+ cotransport mechanism to move Na^+ across the gut mucosa together with an actively transported molecule such as glucose (or galactose). Cl^- and water follow. This transport mechanism remains intact even when cholera toxin is active. ORS may be made by adding safe water to prepackaged sachets containing salts and sugar or by adding 0.5 teaspoon of table salt and 6 teaspoons of table sugar to 1 L of safe water.

IV-133. **The answer is C.** *(Chap. 194e)* This patient has a classic presentation for chronic brucellosis. In endemic areas, brucellosis may be difficult to distinguish from the many other causes of fever. The true global prevalence of human brucellosis is unknown because of the imprecision of diagnosis and the inadequacy of reporting and surveillance systems in many countries. Recently, there has been increased recognition of the high incidence of brucellosis in India and parts of China and of importations to countries in Oceania, such as Fiji. However, two features recognized in the 19th century distinguish brucellosis from other tropical fevers, such as typhoid and malaria: (1) Left untreated, the fever of brucellosis shows an undulating pattern that persists for weeks before the commencement of an

TABLE IV-132 **Assessing the Degree of Dehydration in Patients with Cholera**

Degree of Dehydration	Clinical Findings
None or mild, but diarrhea	Thirst in some cases; <5% loss of total body weight
Moderate	Thirst, postural hypotension, weakness, tachycardia, decreased skin turgor, dry mouth/tongue, no tears; 5%–10% loss of total body weight
Severe	Unconsciousness, lethargy, or "floppiness"; weak or absent pulse; inability to drink; sunken eyes (and, in infants, sunken fontanelles); >10% loss of total body weight

afebrile period that may be followed by relapse. (2) The fever of brucellosis is associated with musculoskeletal symptoms and signs in about one-half of all patients. The clinical syndromes caused by the different species are similar, although *Brucella melitensis* tends to be associated with a more acute and aggressive presentation than *Brucella suis*. Vaccines based on live attenuated *Brucella* strains, such as *Brucella abortus* strain 19BA or 104M, have been used in some countries to protect high-risk populations but have displayed only short-term efficacy and high reactogenicity. The broad aims of antimicrobial therapy are to treat and relieve the symptoms of current infection and to prevent relapse. Focal disease presentations may require specific intervention in addition to more prolonged and tailored antibiotic therapy. In addition, tuberculosis must always be excluded, or—to prevent the emergence of resistance—therapy must be tailored to specifically exclude drugs active against tuberculosis (e.g., rifampin used alone) or to include a full antituberculous regimen. Serologic examination often provides the only positive laboratory findings in brucellosis. In acute infection, IgM antibodies appear early and are followed by IgG and IgA.

IV-134. **The answer is E.** *(Chap. 195)* The most likely infecting organism in this patient is *Francisella tularensis*. Gentamicin is the antibiotic of choice for the treatment of tularemia. Fluoroquinolones have shown in vitro activity against *F tularensis* and have successfully been used in a few cases of tularemia. Currently, however, it cannot be recommended as first-line therapy as data are limited in regard to its efficacy relative to gentamicin, but it can be considered if an individual is unable to tolerate gentamicin. To date, there have been no clinical trials of fluoroquinolones to definitively demonstrate equivalency with gentamicin. Third-generation cephalosporins have in vitro activity against *F tularensis*. However, use of ceftriaxone in children with tularemia resulted in almost universal failure. Likewise, tetracycline and chloramphenicol also have limited usefulness with a higher relapse rate (up to 20%) when compared to gentamicin. *F tularensis* is a small gram-negative, pleomorphic bacillus that is found both intra- and extracellularly. It is found in mud, water, and decaying animal carcasses, and ticks and wild rabbits are the source for most human infections in the southeast United States and Rocky Mountains. In western states, tabanid flies are the most common vectors. The organisms usually enter the skin through the bite of a tick or through an abrasion. On further questioning, the patient in this case reported that during the camping trip he was primarily responsible for skinning the animals and preparing dinner. He did suffer a small cut on his right hand at the site where the ulceration is apparent. The most common clinical manifestations of *F tularensis* are ulceroglandular and glandular disease, accounting for 75%–85% of cases. The ulcer appears at the site of entry of the bacteria and lasts for 1–3 weeks and may develop a black eschar at the base. The draining lymph nodes become enlarged and fluctuant. They may drain spontaneously. In a small percentage of patients, the disease becomes systemically spread, as is apparent in this case, with pneumonia, fevers, and sepsis syndrome. When this occurs, the mortality rate approaches 30% if untreated. However, with appropriate antibiotic therapy, the prognosis is very good. Diagnosis requires a high clinical suspicion because demonstration of the organism is difficult. It is rarely seen on Gram stain because the organisms stain weakly and are so small that they are difficult to distinguish from background material. On polychromatically stained tissue, they may be seen both intra- and extracellularly, singly or in clumps. Moreover, *F tularensis* is a difficult organism to culture and requires cysteine-glucose–blood agar. However, most labs do not attempt to culture the organism because of the risk of infection in laboratory workers, requiring biosafety level 2 practices. Usually the diagnosis is confirmed by agglutination testing with titers >1:160 confirming diagnosis.

IV-135. **The answer is D.** *(Chap. 196) Yersinia pestis* is the etiologic bacterial agent in the plague, a systemic zoonosis. Ancient DNA studies have confirmed that the 14th-century "Black Death" in Europe was *Y pestis* infection. Patients can present with the bubonic, septicemic, or pneumonic form of the disease. It predominantly affects small rodents in rural areas of Africa, Asia, and the Americas and is usually transmitted to humans by an arthropod vector (the flea). The oriental rat flea *Xenopsylla cheopis* is the most efficient vector for transmission of plague among rats and onward to humans. Plague can also be rarely acquired through the handling of living or dead small mammals (e.g., rabbits, hares, and prairie dogs) or wild carnivores (e.g., wildcats, coyotes, or mountain lions). Dogs and cats may bring plague-infected fleas into the home, and infected cats may transmit plague directly to humans by the respiratory route. The last recorded case of person-to-person transmission in the United States occurred in 1925.

IV-136. **The answer is E.** *(Chap. 196)* This patient has a case of bubonic plaque. Most human cases in the United States occur in two regions: "Four Corners" (the junction point of New Mexico, Arizona, Colorado, and Utah), especially northern New Mexico, northern Arizona, and southern Colorado; and further west in California, southern Oregon, and western Nevada. Prairie dogs and other small mammals serve as a reservoir. After an incubation period of 2–6 days, the onset of bubonic plague is sudden and is characterized by fever (>38°C), malaise, myalgia, dizziness, and increasing pain due to progressive lymphadenitis in the regional lymph nodes near the fleabite or other inoculation site. Lymphadenitis manifests as a tense, tender swelling (bubo) that, when palpated, has a boggy consistency with an underlying hard core. Generally, there is one painful and erythematous bubo with surrounding periganglionic edema. The bubo is most commonly inguinal but can also be crural, axillary, cervical, or submaxillary, depending on the site of the bite. There is often an eschar at the site of flea bite or inoculation. *Yersinia* species are gram-negative coccobacilli (short rods with rounded ends) 1–3 μm in length and 0.5–0.8 μm in diameter. *Y pestis* in particular appears bipolar (with a "closed safety pin" appearance) as shown in the Gram stain. The appropriate specimens for diagnosis of bubonic, pneumonic, and septicemic plague are bubo aspirate, bronchoalveolar lavage fluid or sputum, and blood, respectively. *Clostridium* and staphylococcal species are gram positive and lack the bipolar staining pattern. *Pseudomonas*, a gram-negative rod, may cause skin infections, most strikingly pyoderma gangrenosum, although this is clinically characterized by a green, foul-smelling erosion with purulent drainage as opposed to eschar and bubo formation. The filamentous fungus *Rhizopus arrhizus* is one of the most common causes of mucormycosis.

IV-137. **The answer is E.** *(Chap. 196)* This patient has presented with terminal ileitis masquerading as appendicitis ("pseudoappendicitis"), and classic clinical manifestation of *Yersinia enterocolitica*. Older children and adults are more likely than younger children to present with abdominal pain, which can be localized to the right iliac fossa—a situation that often leads to laparotomy for presumed appendicitis (pseudoappendicitis). Appendectomy is not indicated for *Yersinia* infection causing pseudoappendicitis. Thickening of the terminal ileum and cecum is seen on endoscopy and ultrasound, with elevated round or oval lesions that may overlie Peyer patches. Mesenteric lymph nodes are enlarged. Ulcerations of the mucosa are noted on endoscopy. Consumption or preparation of raw pork products (such as chitterlings) and some processed pork products is strongly linked with infection because a high percentage of pigs carry pathogenic *Y enterocolitica* strains. *Trichinella* is classically associated with consuming undercooked pork products but is associated with neuromuscular damage and inflammation as opposed to terminal ileitis. *C difficile* causes a colitis, and *E coli* can cause enteritis, although not classically associated with terminal ileitis and adenitis.

IV-138. **The answer is C.** *(Chap. 197) Bartonella* species are fastidious, facultative intracellular, low-growing, gram-negative bacteria that cause a broad spectrum of diseases in humans. *Bartonella* infections are typically transmitted by vectors such as fleas, ticks, mosquitos, or sand flies. Most *Bartonella* species have successfully adapted to survival in specific domestic or wild mammals. Prolonged intraerythrocytic infection in these animals creates a niche where the bacteria are protected from both innate and adaptive immunity and that serves as a reservoir for human infections.

IV-139. **The answer is B.** *(Chap. 197)* This patient has a history classic for typical cat-scratch disease (CSD) due to *Bartonella henselae*. In the immunocompetent, it is usually a self-limited illness. CSD has two general clinical presentations. Typical CSD, the more common, is characterized by subacute regional lymphadenopathy, whereas atypical CSD is the collective designation for numerous extranodal manifestations involving various organs. Of patients with CSD, 85%–90% have typical disease. The primary lesion, a small (0.3- to 1-cm) painless erythematous papule or pustule, develops at the inoculation site (usually the site of a scratch or a bite) within days to 2 weeks in about one-third to two-thirds of patients. Lymphadenopathy develops 1–3 weeks or longer after cat contact. The affected lymph node(s) are enlarged and usually painful, sometimes have overlying erythema, and suppurate in 10%–15% of cases. Axillary/epitrochlear nodes are most commonly involved; next in frequency are head/neck nodes and then inguinal/femoral nodes. Approximately 50% of patients have fever, malaise, and anorexia. A smaller proportion experience weight loss and night sweats mimicking the presentation of lymphoma. Fever is usually low-grade but infrequently rises to ≥39°C. Resolution is slow, requiring weeks (for fever, pain, and accompanying signs and symptoms) to months (for node shrinkage). Atypical disease includes Parinaud oculoglandular syndrome (granulomatous conjunctivitis with ipsilateral preauricular lymphadenitis), granulomatous hepatitis/splenitis, neuroretinitis (often presenting as unilateral deterioration of vision), and other ophthalmologic manifestations. In addition, neurologic involvement (encephalopathy, seizures, myelitis, radiculitis, cerebellitis, facial and other cranial or peripheral palsies), fever of unknown origin, debilitating myalgia, arthritis or arthralgia (affecting mostly women >20 years old), osteomyelitis (including multifocal disease), tendinitis, neuralgia, and dermatologic manifestations (including erythema nodosum, sometimes accompanying arthropathy) occur. For typical disease, antibiotics are not recommended. However, to rule out atypical disease, it is prudent to check laboratory studies to exclude atypical disease. For extensive lymphadenopathy (not present in this case), one may consider azithromycin 500 mg for 1 day followed by 250 mg daily for 4 days.

IV-140. **The answer is A.** *(Chap. 197)* Bacillary angiomatosis is due to infection with *B henselae* and occurs primarily in HIV-infected persons with CD4+ T-cell counts <100/μL but may also affect other immunosuppressed patients. Bacillary angiomatosis presents most commonly as one or more cutaneous lesions that are not painful and that may be tan, red, or purple in color. Subcutaneous masses or nodules, superficial ulcerated plaques, and verrucous growths are also seen. Nodular forms resemble those seen in fungal or mycobacterial infections. Subcutaneous nodules are often tender. In rare cases, other organs are involved in bacillary angiomatosis. Patients usually have constitutional symptoms, including fever, chills, malaise, headache, anorexia, weight loss, and night sweats. Kaposi sarcoma is also seen in immunocompromised individuals but is caused by human herpes virus 8 infection. Bubonic plaque is caused by *Y pestis*, whereas pyoderma gangrenosum is most often due to pseudomonal infection. Verruga peruana is due to a different *Bartonella* species, *Bartonella bacilliformis*, and is the late-onset eruptive manifestation of Carrion disease. This disease is transmitted by the phlebotomine sandfly, *Lutzomyia verrucarum*. In verruga peruana, red, hemangioma-like, cutaneous vascular lesions of various sizes appear either weeks to months after systemic illness or with no previous suggestive history. These lesions persist for months up to 1 year. Mucosal and internal lesions may also develop.

IV-141. **The answer is C.** *(Chap. 198e)* This is a classic case of donovanosis or granuloma inguinale, caused by *Klebsiella granulomatis*. Donovanosis has an unusual geographic distribution that includes Papua New Guinea, parts of southern Africa, India, the Caribbean, French Guyana, Brazil, and aboriginal communities in Australia. A lesion starts as a papule or subcutaneous nodule that later ulcerates after trauma. The incubation period is uncertain, but experimental infections in humans indicate a duration of approximately 50 days. Four types of lesions have been described: (1) the classic ulcerogranulomatous lesion (shown in Figure IV-141A), a beefy red ulcer that bleeds readily when touched; (2) a hypertrophic or verrucous ulcer with a raised irregular edge; (3) a necrotic, offensive-smelling ulcer causing tissue destruction; and (4) a sclerotic or cicatricial lesion with fibrous and scar tissue. The diagnosis is confirmed by microscopic identification of Donovan bodies (see Figure IV-141B) in tissue smears. Preparation of a good-quality smear is important. If donovanosis is suspected on clinical grounds, the smear for Donovan bodies should be taken before swab samples are collected to be tested for other causes of genital ulceration so that enough material can be collected from the ulcer. A swab should be rolled firmly over an ulcer previously cleaned with a dry swab to remove debris. Smears can be examined in a clinical setting by direct microscopy with a rapid Giemsa or Wright stain. Alternatively, a piece of granulation tissue crushed and spread between two slides can be used. Donovan bodies can be seen in large, mononuclear (Pund) cells as gram-negative intracytoplasmic cysts filled with deeply staining bodies that may have a safety-pin appearance (shown in the image). *H ducreyi* is the causative organism of chancroid, which manifests in males as sexually transmitted painful genital ulcers.

IV-142. **The answer is E.** *(Chap. 199)* This patient is chronically immunosuppressed from his antirejection prophylactic regimen, which includes both glucocorticoids and tacrolimus. The clinical presentation and microbiology are consistent with a diagnosis of nocardiosis. Nocardiosis can be caused by a number of different nocardial species. Previously it was thought that *Nocardia asteroides* caused most nocardial disease, but it has since been found that several different *Nocardia* species cause human disease including *Nocardia nova, Nocardia cyriacigeorgica, and Nocardia pseudobrasiliensis*, among others. Nocardiosis occurs worldwide and is more common among adults. The majority of cases of nocardiosis occur in patients with a host defense defect, including immunosuppression, transplantation, lymphoma, or AIDS. Pneumonia is the most common form of the disease. Patients most often have a subacute course over days to weeks, although patients who are immunosuppressed can present more acutely. Immunosuppressed patients are also more likely to produce thick sputum. Fevers, weight loss, and anorexia are common. Radiographically, single or multiple pulmonary nodules may be present and often cavitate (Figure IV-142B). Nocardiosis may spread to adjacent tissues including the pericardium and mediastinum. In half of all cases of nocardiosis, disease also spreads outside the lungs with presence of brain abscess being the most common manifestation. Other sites include skin, kidneys, bone, muscle, and eye. The characteristic Gram stain demonstrates filamentous branching gram-positive organisms. Most species of *Nocardia* are acid-fast if a weak acid is used for decolorization (e.g., modified Kinyoun method). These organisms can also be visualized by silver staining. They grow slowly in culture, and the laboratory must be alerted to the possibility of their presence on submitted specimens. A medication regimen containing a sulfonamide is the treatment of choice. The combination of trimethoprim-sulfamethoxazole is at least equivalent to a sulfonamide alone, although there is a slightly greater likelihood of hematologic toxicity with the combination drug. Prolonged treatment is required. In those with intact host defenses, treatment should be continued for 6–12 months, and for those with impaired defenses, treatment should be continued for at least 12 months. Clinical experience with other oral drugs is limited. Minocycline,

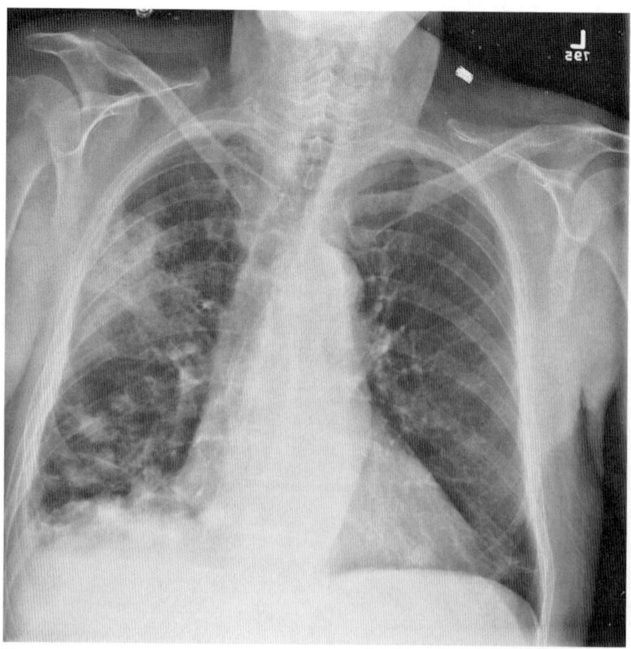

FIGURE IV-142B

linezolid, and amoxicillin-clavulanic acid generally show activity in vitro, although side effects often limit the long-term use. In addition, members of the *N nova* complex produce β-lactamases, generating resistance to amoxicillin-clavulanic acid. In severe cases, combination therapy is recommended with trimethoprim-sulfamethoxazole, amikacin, and ceftriaxone or imipenem.

IV-143 and IV-144. **The answers are D and C, respectively.** *(Chap. 200)* The patient presents with symptoms suggestive of osteonecrosis of her jaw possibly due to bisphosphonate use. Additionally, her jaw pain has progressed and now appears to be infected. *Actinomyces* is a classic oral organism with a propensity to infect the jaw, particularly when the bone is abnormal usually due to radiation or osteonecrosis. Osteonecrosis of the jaw due to bisphosphonates is an increasingly recognized risk factor for *Actinomyces* infection. Frequently, the soft tissue swelling is confused for either parotitis or a cancerous lesion. *Actinomyces* species frequently form fistulous tracts, which provide an opportunity to exam the secretions and identify either the organism itself, which is less common, or sulfur granules. Sulfur granules are an in vivo concretion of *Actinomyces* bacteria, calcium phosphate, and host material. Gram stain of *Actinomyces* infection shows intensely positive staining at the center with branching rods at the periphery. Auer rods are found in acute promyelocytic leukemia. Although head and neck cancer is in the differential diagnosis, the acuity of the presentation and fever make this less likely. Weakly acid-fast branching filaments are found in nocardial infection, which is unlikely to involve the head and neck, although both organisms frequently cause pulmonary infiltrates. Although parotitis with obstruction due to sialolith is possible, the symptoms are in the jaw and diffuse, not specifically involving the parotid gland, thus making sialolith less likely. Therapy for *Actinomyces* requires a long course of antibiotics, even though the organism is very sensitive to penicillin therapy. This is presumed to be due to the difficulty of using antibiotics to penetrate the thick-walled masses and sulfur granules. Current recommendations are for penicillin IV for 2–6 weeks followed by oral therapy for a total of 6–12 months. Surgery should be reserved for patients who are not responsive to medical therapy.

IV-145. **The answer is E.** *(Chap. 201)* The patient presents with symptoms suggestive of lung infection; his demographics suggest that an abscess might be present, and the foul-smelling breath points supports this diagnosis. His chest radiograph shows a large cavity with air-fluid level in the right lower lobe, thus confirming the diagnosis of lung abscess. Lung abscesses generally present in the dependent lobes of the lung and are often associated with aspiration of oral anaerobic bacteria that are normally found in the crevices of teeth. These organisms include *Prevotella* species, *Porphyromonas* species, non–*B fragilis* species of *Bacteroides*, and *Fusobacterium* species. Up to 60% of oral organisms produce β-lactamases, and penicillin alone is not recommended as initial therapy. Meropenem, β-lactam/β-lactamase inhibitor combinations, clindamycin, and metronidazole are all appropriate choices for initial coverage of the lung abscess. Given the difficulty with isolation and identification of anaerobic organisms, empiric therapy for suspected organisms is required, and lung abscess treatment should be continued for several weeks. However, if there is no response to therapy targeted at lung abscess for several weeks, then further testing would be warranted, generally including bronchoscopy to evaluate possible malignancy. The negative interferon-γ release assay makes tuberculosis very unlikely, and the chest x-ray did not show upper lobe infiltrates or cavities.

IV-146. **The answer is B.** *(Chap. 201)* The major reservoirs in the human body for anaerobic bacteria are the mouth, lower gastrointestinal tract, skin, and female genital tract. Generally, anaerobic infections occur proximal to these sites after the normal barrier (i.e., skin or mucous membrane) is disrupted. Thus, common infections resulting from these organisms are abdominal or lung abscess, periodontal infection, gynecologic infections such as bacterial vaginosis, or deep tissue infection. Properly obtained cultures in these circumstances generally grow a mixed population of anaerobes typical of the microenvironment of the original reservoir.

IV-147. **The answer is C.** *(Chap. 202)* Tuberculosis is most commonly transmitted from person to person by airborne droplets. Factors that affect likelihood of developing tuberculosis infection include the probability of contact with an infectious person, the intimacy and duration of contact, the degree of infectiousness of the contact, and the environment in which the contact takes place. The most infectious patients are those with cavitary pulmonary or laryngeal tuberculosis with about 10^5–10^7 tuberculous bacteria per milliliter of sputum. Individuals who have a negative acid-fast bacilli smear with a positive culture for tuberculosis are less infectious but may transmit the disease. However, individuals with only extrapulmonary (e.g., renal, skeletal) tuberculosis are considered noninfectious.

IV-148. **The answer is D.** *(Chap. 202)* Aging, chronic disease, and suppression of cellular immunity are risk factors for developing active tuberculosis in patients with latent infection. (See Table IV-148.) The greatest absolute risk factor for development of active tuberculosis is HIV positivity. The risk of developing active infection is greatest in those with the lowest CD4 counts; however, having a CD4 count above a threshold value does not negate the risk of developing an active infection. The reported incidence of developing active tuberculosis in HIV-positive individuals with a positive PPD is 10% per year, compared to a lifetime risk of 10% in immunocompetent individuals. Malnutrition and severe underweight confer a twofold greater risk of developing active tuberculosis, whereas IV drug use increases the risk 10–30 times. Patients with end-stage renal disease and who have had a solid organ transplant are also at high relative risk of developing tuberculosis. Silicosis also increases the risk of developing active tuberculosis 30-fold. Although the risk of developing active tuberculosis is greatest in the first year after exposure, the risk also increases in the elderly. Coal mining has not been associated with an increase in risk independent of other factors, such as tobacco smoking.

IV-149. **The answer is A.** *(Chap. 202)* The chest radiograph scan shows a right upper lobe infiltrate with a large cavitary lesion. In this man from an endemic area for tuberculosis, this finding should be treated as active pulmonary tuberculosis until proven otherwise. In addition, this patient's symptoms suggest a chronic illness with low-grade fevers, weight loss, and temporal wasting that would be consistent with active pulmonary tuberculosis. If a patient is suspected of having active pulmonary tuberculosis, the initial management should include documentation of disease while protecting healthcare workers and the population in general. This patient should be hospitalized in a negative-pressure room on airborne isolation until three expectorated sputum samples have been demonstrated to be negative. The samples should preferably be collected in the early morning as the burden of organisms is expected to be higher on a more concentrated sputum. The sensitivity of a single sputum for the detection of tuberculosis in confirmed cases is only 40%–60%. Thus,

TABLE IV-148 **Risk Factors for Active Tuberculosis in Persons Who Have Been Infected with Tubercle Bacilli**

Factor	Relative Risk/Odds[a]
Recent infection (<1 year)	12.9
Fibrotic lesions (spontaneously healed)	2–20
Comorbidities and iatrogenic causes	
HIV infection	21–>30
Silicosis	30
Chronic renal failure/hemodialysis	10–25
Diabetes	2–4
IV drug use	10–30
Immunosuppressive treatment	10
Tumor necrosis factor-α inhibitors	4–5
Gastrectomy	2–5
Jejunoileal bypass	30–60
Posttransplantation period (renal, cardiac)	20–70
Tobacco smoking	2–3
Malnutrition and severe underweight	2

[a]Old infection = 1.

a single sputum sample is inadequate to determine infectivity and the presence of active pulmonary tuberculosis. Skin testing with a PPD of the tuberculosis *Mycobacterium* is used to detect latent infection with tuberculosis and has no role in determining whether active disease is present. The cavitary lung lesion shown on the chest imaging could represent malignancy or a bacterial lung abscess, but given that the patient is from a high-risk area for tuberculosis, tuberculosis would be considered the most likely diagnosis until ruled out by sputum testing.

IV-150. **The answer is A.** *(Chap. 202)* The radiograph shows bilateral small (millet seed size) nodular infiltrates consistent with disseminated or miliary tuberculosis. After primary tuberculosis infection, occult hematogenous dissemination commonly occurs. However, in the absence of a sufficient acquired immune response as in patients with advanced HIV infection, which usually contains the infection, disseminated or miliary disease may result. Postprimary tuberculosis, also referred to as *reactivation* or *secondary tuberculosis*, is probably most accurately termed *adult-type tuberculosis* because it may result from endogenous reactivation of distant latent tuberculosis infection or recent infection (primary infection or reinfection). It is usually localized to the apical and posterior segments of the upper lobes, where the substantially higher mean oxygen tension (compared with that in the lower zones) favors mycobacterial growth. The superior segments of the lower lobes are also more frequently involved. The extent of lung parenchymal involvement varies greatly, from small infiltrates to extensive cavitary disease. Pleural effusion, which is found in up to two-thirds of cases of primary infection, results from the penetration of bacilli into the pleural space from an adjacent subpleural focus. It often resolves spontaneously in immunologically competent individuals. Tuberculosis is typically characterized as pulmonary or extrapulmonary. In order of frequency, the extrapulmonary sites most commonly involved in tuberculosis are the lymph nodes, pleura, genitourinary tract, bones and joints, meninges, peritoneum, and pericardium. However, virtually all organ systems may be affected. As a result of hematogenous dissemination in HIV-infected individuals, extrapulmonary tuberculosis is seen more commonly today than in the past in settings of high HIV prevalence.

Tuberculous lymphadenitis is the most common presentation of extrapulmonary tuberculosis in both HIV-seronegative and HIV-infected patients (35% of cases worldwide and more than 40% of cases in the United States in recent series); lymph node disease is particularly frequent among HIV-infected patients and among children. In the United States, besides children, women (particularly non-Caucasians) seem to be especially susceptible. Once caused mainly by *Mycobacterium bovis*, tuberculous lymphadenitis today is due largely to *M tuberculosis*. Lymph node tuberculosis presents as painless swelling of the lymph nodes, most commonly at posterior cervical and supraclavicular sites (a condition historically referred to as *scrofula*).

IV-151. **The answer is A.** *(Chap. 202)* Initial treatment of active tuberculosis associated with HIV disease does not differ from that of a non–HIV-infected person. The standard treatment regimen includes four drugs: rifampin, isoniazid, pyrazinamide, and ethambutol (RIPE). These drugs are given for a total of 2 months in combination with pyridoxine (vitamin B_6) to prevent neurotoxicity from isoniazid. Following the initial 2 months, patients continue on isoniazid and rifampin to complete a total of 6 months of therapy. These recommendations are the same as those for non–HIV-infected individuals. If the sputum culture remains positive for tuberculosis after 2 months, the total course of antimycobacterial therapy is increased from 6 to 9 months. If an individual is already on antiretroviral therapy (ART) at the time of diagnosis of tuberculosis, it may be continued, but often rifabutin is substituted for rifampin because of drug interactions between rifampin and protease inhibitors. In individuals not on ART at the time of diagnosis of tuberculosis, it is not recommended to start ART concurrently because of the risk of immune reconstitution inflammatory syndrome (IRIS) and an increased risk of medication side effects. IRIS occurs as the immune system improves with ART and causes an intense inflammatory reaction directed against the infecting organism(s). There have been fatal cases of IRIS in association with tuberculosis and initiation of ART. In addition, both ART and antituberculosis drugs have many side effects. It can be difficult for a clinician to decide which medication is the cause of the side effects and may lead unnecessarily to alterations in the antituberculosis regimen. ART should be initiated as soon as possible and preferably within 2 months. Three-drug regimens are associated with a higher relapse rate if used as a standard 6-month course of therapy and, if used, require a total of 9 months of therapy. Situations in which three-drug therapy may be used are pregnancy, intolerance to a specific drug, and in the setting of resistance. A five-drug regimen using RIPE plus streptomycin is recommended as the standard re-treatment regimen. Streptomycin and pyrazinamide are discontinued after 2 months if susceptibility testing is unavailable. If susceptibility testing is available, the treatment should be based on the susceptibility pattern. In no instance is it appropriate to withhold treatment in the setting of active tuberculosis to await susceptibility testing.

IV-152. **The answer is B.** *(Chap. 202)* The aim of treatment of latent tuberculosis is to prevent development of active disease, and the tuberculin skin test (PPD) is the most common means of identifying cases of latent tuberculosis in high-risk groups. To perform a tuberculin skin test, 5 tuberculin units of PPD are placed subcutaneously in the forearm. The degree of induration is determined after 48–72 hours. Erythema only does not count as a positive reaction to the PPD. The size of the reaction to the tuberculin skin test determines whether individuals should receive treatment for latent tuberculosis. In general, individuals in low-risk groups should not be tested. However, if tested, a reaction >15 mm is required to be considered as positive. School teachers are considered low-risk individuals. Thus, the reaction of 7 mm is not a positive result, and treatment is not required. A size of ≥10 mm is considered positive in individuals who have been infected within 2 years or those with high-risk medical conditions. The individual working in an area where tuberculosis is endemic and who has tested newly positive by skin testing should be treated as a newly infected individual. High-risk medical conditions for which treatment of latent tuberculosis is recommended include diabetes mellitus, injection drug use, end-stage renal disease, rapid weight loss, and hematologic disorders. PPD reactions ≥5 mm are considered positive for latent tuberculosis in individuals with fibrotic lesions on chest radiograph, those with close contact with an infected person, and those with HIV or who are otherwise immunosuppressed. There are two situations in which treatment for latent tuberculosis is recommended regardless of the results on skin testing. First, infants and children who have had close contact with an actively infected person should be treated. After 2 months of therapy, a skin test should be performed. Treatment can be discontinued if the skin test remains negative at that time. Also, individuals who are HIV positive and have had close contact with an infected person should be treated regardless of skin test results. (See Table IV-152.)

IV-153. **The answer is C.** *(Chap. 202)* The diagnosis of latent tuberculosis infection (LTBI) remains challenging and traditionally relied on the tuberculin skin test (TST) using PPD. Recently, two in vitro assays that measure T-cell release of interferon-γ (IFN-γ) in response to stimulation with the highly tuberculosis-specific antigens ESAT-6 and CFP-10 are available. The T-SPOT®. TB test (Oxford Immunotec, Oxford, United Kingdom) is an enzyme-linked immunospot (ELISpot) assay, and the QuantiFERON®-TB Gold test (Qiagen GmbH, Hilden, Germany) is a whole-blood enzyme-linked immunosorbent assay (ELISA) for measurement of IFN-γ. The QuantiFERON®-TB Gold In-Tube assay, which facilitates blood collection and initial incubation, also contains another specific antigen, TB7.7. These tests likely measure the response of recirculating memory T cells—normally part of a reservoir in the spleen, bone marrow, and lymph nodes—to persisting bacilli producing antigenic signals. In settings or population groups with low tuberculosis and HIV burdens, IFN-γ release assays (IGRAs) have previously been reported to be more specific than the TST as a result of less cross-reactivity due to BCG vaccination and sensitization by nontuberculous mycobacteria. Recent studies, however, suggest that IGRAs may not perform well in serial testing (e.g., among healthcare workers) and that interpretation of test results is dependent on cutoff values used to define positivity. Potential advantages of IGRAs include logistical convenience, the need for fewer patient visits to complete testing, and the avoidance of somewhat subjective measurements such as skin induration. However, IGRAs require that blood be drawn from the individual and then delivered to the laboratory in a timely fashion. IGRAs also require that testing be performed in a laboratory setting. These requirements pose challenges similar to those faced with the TST,

TABLE IV-152 **Tuberculin Reaction Size and Treatment of Latent *Mycobacterium tuberculosis* Infection**

Risk Group	Tuberculin Reaction Size, mm
HIV-infected persons	≥5
Recent contacts of a patient with tuberculosis (TB)	≥5[a]
Organ transplant recipients	≥5
Persons with fibrotic lesions consistent with old TB on chest radiography	≥5
Persons who are immunosuppressed, e.g., due to the use of glucocorticoids or tumor necrosis factor α inhibitors	≥5
Persons with high-risk medical conditions[b]	≥5
Recent immigrants (≤5 years) from high-prevalence countries	≥10
Injection drug users	≥10
Mycobacteriology laboratory personnel; residents and employees of high-risk congregate settings[c]	≥10
Children <5 years of age; children and adolescents exposed to adults in high-risk categories	≥10
Low-risk persons[d]	≥15

[a]Tuberculin-negative contacts, especially children, should receive prophylaxis for 2–3 months after contact ends and should then undergo repeat tuberculin skin testing (TST). Those whose results remain negative should discontinue prophylaxis. HIV-infected contacts should receive a full course of treatment regardless of TST results.
[b]These conditions include silicosis and end-stage renal disease managed by hemodialysis
[c]These settings include correctional facilities, nursing homes, homeless shelters, and hospitals and other healthcare facilities.
[d]Except for employment purposes where longitudinal TST screening is anticipated, TST is not indicated for these low-risk persons. A decision to treat should be based on individual risk/benefit considerations.
Source: Adapted from Centers for Disease Control and Prevention: TB elimination—treatment options for latent tuberculosis infection (2011). Available at *http://www.cdc.gov/tb/publications/factsheets/testing/skintestresults.pdf.*

including cold-chain requirements and batch-to-batch variations. Because of higher specificity and other potential advantages, IGRAs have usually replaced the TST for LTBI diagnosis in low-incidence, high-income settings. However, in high-incidence tuberculosis and HIV settings and population groups, there is limited and inconclusive evidence about the performance and usefulness of IGRAs. In view of higher costs and increased technical requirements, the WHO does not recommend the replacement of the TST by IGRAs in low- and middle-income countries. A number of national guidelines on the use of IGRAs for LTBI testing have been issued. In the United States, an IGRA is preferred to the TST for most persons over the age of 5 years who are being screened for LTBI. However, for those at high risk of progression to active tuberculosis (e.g., HIV-infected persons), either test—or, to optimize sensitivity, both tests—may be used. Because of the paucity of data on the use of IGRAs in children, the TST is preferred for LTBI testing of children under age 5. Similar to the TST, current IGRAs have only modest predictive value for incident active tuberculosis, are not useful in identifying patients with the highest risk of progression to disease, and cannot be used for diagnosis of active tuberculosis.

IV-154. **The answer is E.** *(Chap. 202)* Bacillus Calmette-Guérin (BCG) is derived from an attenuated strain of *M bovis.* It has been available since 1921. Many vaccines are available, but they vary in efficacy from 0%–80% in clinical trials. The vaccine protects infants and young children from serious forms of tuberculosis including meningitis and miliary disease. Side effects from the vaccine are rare, but BCG dissemination (BCGitis) may occur in patients with severe combined immunodeficiency or advanced HIV-induced immunosuppression. BCG will cross-react with tuberculin skin testing, but the size of the response wanes with time. BCG vaccination is currently recommended in countries with a high TB prevalence. It is not recommended in the United States because of the low prevalence of disease and cross-reactivity with tuberculin skin testing. Infants with unknown HIV infection status, infants of mothers with known HIV infection, and HIV-infected individuals should not receive BCG.

IV-155. **The answer is B.** *(Chap. 204)* The chest CT shows a "tree-in-bud" pattern in the peripheral right lung and bilateral bronchiectasis. The tree-in-bud pattern is consistent with bronchiolar inflammation and is typical of nontuberculous mycobacterial infection. Nontuberculous mycobacteria, such as *M avium* complex, may cause chronic pulmonary infections in normal hosts and those with underlying pulmonary disease immunosuppression. In normal hosts, bronchiectasis is the most common underlying condition. In immunocompetent patients without underlying disease, treatment of pulmonary infection with *M avium* complex is considered on an individual basis based on symptoms, radiographic findings, and bacteriology. Treatment should be initiated in the presence of progressive pulmonary disease or symptoms. In patients without any prior lung disease, no structural lung disease, and who do not demonstrate progressive clinical decline, *M avium* pulmonary infection can be managed conservatively. Patients with underlying lung disease, such as COPD, bronchiectasis, or cystic fibrosis, or those with a history of pulmonary tuberculosis should receive antibiotics. In the patient case, the patient has both clinical and historic reasons for antibiotic treatment. The appropriate regimen in this case is clarithromycin (or azithromycin), ethambutol, and rifampin (or rifabutin) for 12 months after culture sterilization (typically 18 months). The combination of pyrazinamide, isoniazid, rifampin, and ethambutol is effective treatment for *M tuberculosis* infection, which is not present here. Other drugs with activity against *M avium* complex include IV and aerosolized aminoglycosides, fluoroquinolones, and clofazimine.

IV-156. **The answer is A.** *(Chap. 204)* Nontuberculous mycobacteria (NTM) were originally classified as "fast-growers" and "slow-growers" based on the length of time they took to grow in culture. Although more sophisticated tests have been developed, this classification scheme is still used and is of some benefit to the clinician. Fast-growing NTMs include *Mycobacterium abscessus, Mycobacterium fortuitum*, and *Mycobacterium chelonae*. They will typically take 7 days or less to grow on standard media, allowing relatively fast identification and drug-resistance testing. Slow-growing NTM include *M avium*, *Mycobacterium marinum*, *Mycobacterium ulcerans*, and *Mycobacterium kansasii*. They often require special growth media and therefore a high pretest suspicion. The patient described in this case likely has a cutaneous infection from one of the "fast-growing" NTMs, which could be diagnosed with tissue biopsy, Gram stain, and culture.

IV-157. **The answer is C.** *(Chap. 205e)* Pyrazinamide (PZA) is first-line treatment for *M tuberculosis*. Addition of PZA for 2 months to isoniazid and rifampin allows the total duration of treatment to be shortened from 9 months to 6 months. PZA has no utility in the treatment of nontuberculous mycobacteria. Ethambutol has no serious drug interactions, but patients must be closely monitored for optic neuritis, which may manifest with decreased visual acuity, central scotoma, or difficulty seeing green (or red). All patients initiating therapy with ethambutol should have a visual and ophthalmologic examination at baseline. In the United States overall, isoniazid resistance remains uncommon. Primary isoniazid resistance is more common in patients with tuberculosis born outside the United States. Rifampin is a potent inducer of the cytochrome P450 system and has numerous drug interactions. The CDC has guidelines for managing antituberculosis drug interactions including rifampin (www.cdc.gov/tb/). Rifabutin is a less potent inducer of hepatic cytochromes. Rifabutin is recommended for HIV-infected patients who are on antiretroviral therapy with protease inhibitors or nonnucleoside reverse transcriptase inhibitors (particularly nevirapine) in place of rifampin.

IV-158. **The answer is B.** (*Chap. 206*) The image shows a diffuse maculopapular rash involving the trunk, palms, and soles. The patient's history of unprotected intercourse, a recent painless penile ulcer suspicious for a primary chancre, and the subsequent maculopapular rash involving the palms/soles is consistent with secondary syphilis. The lesion of primary syphilis is typically a painless, indurated papule that is typically located at the site of inoculation. In heterosexual men, it is typically located on the penis, although it can be variably found on the anus, rectum, lips, or oropharynx. The primary chancre typically heals spontaneously within 3–6 weeks, and because it is painless, some patients with primary syphilis do not initially seek medical attention.

Secondary syphilis is sometimes described as the "great imitator" because its manifestations are protean. Common manifestations include mucocutaneous lesions and nontender lymphadenopathy but less commonly include meningitis, hepatitis, nephropathy, gastrointestinal involvement, arthritis, periostitis, or ocular findings. The preferred therapy for patients for primary, secondary, or early latent syphilis without neurologic or ocular involvement and without confirmed penicillin allergy is a single dose of intramuscular benzathine penicillin G. For patients with late latent syphilis (or latent syphilis of unknown duration), three doses of benzathine penicillin G over 3 weeks is preferred. Two weeks of intravenous penicillin G is recommended for treatment of neurosyphilis or ocular syphilis. However, absent signs or symptoms of nervous system involvement, an RPR ≥1:32, HIV infection, CD4 ≤350/µL, or suspected treatment failure, evaluation of the CSF is not mandatory. Tetracycline and doxycycline can be considered in patients with confirmed penicillin allergy but are not preferred in patients without penicillin allergy. Due to the increasing prevalence of macrolide resistance, azithromycin is not recommended.

IV-159. **The answer is A.** *(Chap. 206)* Syphilitic involvement of the CNS can occur in both early or late syphilis and ranges from asymptomatic neurosyphilis, meningeal syphilis, meningovascular syphilis, and general paresis to tabes dorsalis. Although meningeal syphilis usually occurs within the first year after infection, general paresis or tabes dorsalis usually presents after decades of latent infection. The primary ocular finding in both general paresis and in tabes dorsalis is the Argyll Robertson pupil. Argyll Robertson pupils fail to react to light, but accommodation is preserved. Both pupils are typically involved. The pupils are typically small and do not dilate fully in dim light. However, the pupils constrict to near vision and dilate to far vision.

IV-160. **The answer is D.** *(Chap. 206)* Serologic testing for syphilis includes nontreponemal and treponemal tests. The RPR is a widely used nontreponemal antibody test that is recommended for both screening and quantification of antibody to assess syphilis activity or treatment response. Nontreponemal tests (e.g., RPR or VDRL) detect antibodies directed against the cardiolipin-cholesterol-lecithin antigen complex, and false reactions may occur in patients with autoimmune conditions, injection drug use, other active infections, or pregnancy. False-positive results increase with increasing age, approaching 10% in patients >70 years old. Treponemal-specific serologic tests detect antibodies against treponemal antigens and include the fluorescent treponemal antibody absorbed (FTA-ABS) test, the *T pallidum* particle agglutination test (TPPA), treponemal enzyme immunoassay (TP-EIA), and treponemal chemiluminescence immunoassays (TP-CIA). These tests are highly sensitive and likely remain positive after treatment. They do not distinguish current from prior infection. In early primary syphilis, treponemal tests may be more sensitive than nontreponemal tests; however, in this case, the nontreponemal test is positive and the treponemal test is negative. In a low-prevalence population, this is most consistent with a false-positive RPR.

IV-161. **The answer is A.** (*Chap. 206*) This patient's CSF profile is consistent with asymptomatic neurosyphilis. Although the CSF-VDRL is negative, this is most likely falsely negative. CSF-VDRL is a highly specific but insensitive test that may be nonreactive even in patients with symptomatic neurosyphilis. The patient's CSF studies demonstrate a pleocytosis (>5 WBC/µL) and increased protein concentration (>45 mg/dL). Therefore, treatment for neurosyphilis is warranted. Penicillin is the drug of choice for all stages of syphilis. Although early syphilis (primary syphilis, secondary syphilis without neurologic involvement, and early latent syphilis) is effectively treated with a single dose of intramuscular benzathine penicillin G, this does not produce detectable concentrations of penicillin in the CSF. It is not recommended for the treatment of neurosyphilis. Instead, aqueous crystalline penicillin G for 10–14 days is recommended for the treatment of both asymptomatic and symptomatic neurosyphilis. The dose of 18–24 MU may be administered as a continuous infusion or as 3–4 MU every 4 hours. Alternatively, if patient adherence is assured, it may be administered as a daily intramuscular injection (2.4 MU/d) with oral probenecid (500 mg PO for times a day) for 10–14 days. Three doses of benzathine penicillin G are appropriate for the treatment of late latent syphilis, not for neurosyphilis.

IV-162. **The answer is B.** *(Chap. 206)* Neurosyphilis can occur at any stage of syphilis (early or late). Although it is uncommon in the postantibiotic era, the incidence of neurosyphilis is higher in those co-infected with HIV and in those with high titer nontreponemal antibody tests.

Indications for CSF fluid examination in adults with syphilis include signs or symptoms of nervous system involvement (e.g., meningitis, hearing loss, cranial nerve palsies, altered mental status, ophthalmic disease, ataxia), RPR or VDRL titer ≥1:32, active tertiary syphilis, or suspected treatment failure. In addition, patients with HIV, especially with CD4+ T-cell count ≤350/μL, should undergo CSF examination. Otherwise, CSF examination is not routinely recommended in primary or secondary syphilis absent neurologic signs or symptoms. (See Table IV-162.)

TABLE IV-162 **Indications for Cerebrospinal Fluid Examination in Adults with All Stages of Syphilis**

All Patients
Signs or symptoms of nervous system involvement (e.g., meningitis, hearing loss, cranial nerve dysfunction, altered mental status, ophthalmic disease [e.g., uveitis, iritis, pupillary abnormalities], ataxia, loss of vibration sense), *or*
RPR or VDRL titer ≥1:32, *or*
Active tertiary syphilis, *or*
Suspected treatment failure
Additional Indications in HIV-Infected Persons
CD4+ T-cell count ≤350/μL, *or*
All HIV-infected persons (recommended by some experts)

Source: Adapted from the 2010 Sexually Transmitted Diseases Treatment Guidelines from the Centers for Disease Control and Prevention.

IV-163. **The answer is C.** *(Chap 206)* Early syphilis describes syphilis acquired within the first year and includes primary syphilis, secondary syphilis, and early latent syphilis. In contrast to late latent syphilis, patients with early syphilis are generally infectious, and their identification and treatment represent an important public health activity to interrupt the transmission of syphilis. Nearly all syphilis is transmitted by sexual contact with infectious lesions. The mucocutaneous lesions of syphilis, especially the primary chancre and condyloma lata, are teeming with spirochetes and are highly infective. The infective dose is approximately 57 organisms, and the concentration of organisms in a chancre is approximately 10^7 organisms per gram of tissue. One-third to one-half of sexual contacts of persons with infectious syphilis become infected.

IV-164. **The answer is C.** *(Chap. 208)* The clinical triad of hemorrhage, jaundice, and acute kidney injury caused by pathogenic *Leptospira* infection is eponymously known as *Weil syndrome. Leptospira* affect most mammalian species, but rats are an important reservoir. The organism may establish a symbiotic relationship with the host to persist in the urogenital tract for years. Water is a similarly important vehicle for the transmission of disease. Leptospirosis has been recognized in deteriorating inner cities with expanding rat populations. Disease ranges in severity from a mild illness that never comes to medical attention to rapidly progressive and severe illness with case fatality rates as high as 50%. In the leptospiremic phase of illness, leptospires disseminate hematogenously to vital organs. Hemorrhagic complications may involve the lungs, GI tract, urogenital tract, or skin and are often associated with thrombocytopenia. Jaundice is common, but widespread hepatic necrosis is not. The kidneys are invariably involved. Renal involvement includes acute tubular damage and interstitial nephritis, and a nonoliguric hypokalemic renal injury is characteristic of early leptospirosis. Deregulation of several transporters along the nephron (e.g., NKCC2, NHE1, Na/K ATPase, AQP1, AQP2) contribute to tubular electrolyte wasting and lead to hypokalemia and hyponatremia. Wasting of magnesium in the urine is also common in leptospiral nephropathy.

IV-165. **The answer is E.** *(Chap. 209)* Tick-borne relapsing fever (TBRF) is a spirochetal infection caused by any one of several species of *Borrelia*. The borreliae are small spirochetes that are transmitted to humans through the bite of an infected tick. The tick that transmits TBRF is *Ornithodoros* species, which feeds on a variety of squirrels and chipmunks that live near freshwater lakes. TBRF is endemic in several areas of the western United States, southern British Columbia, the Mediterranean, Africa, and the plateau regions of Mexico and South and Central America. In the United States, TBRF is rarely reported east of Montana, Colorado, New Mexico, and Texas. The general areas where TBRF is contracted is in the forested and mountainous regions of these states, although it can be contracted in the limestone caves of central Texas. Only 13 counties in the entire United States have had 50% of all cases reported in the country. After an incubation period of about 7 days, an individual infected with TBRF will begin to experience fevers that can reach as high as 106.7°F (41.5°C). Symptoms that accompany the fevers include myalgias, chills, nausea, vomiting, abdominal pain, confusion, and arthralgias. The average duration of a first episode is 3 days. If the disease is not recognized and treated, the fever will recur after a period of about 7 days. The duration of fevers is typically shorter with repeated episodes, but will continue to relapse about every 7 days until the disease is treated. Diagnosis of TBRF requires detection of the spirochetes in the blood during a febrile episode or serologic conversion. TBRF is typically treated with doxycycline or erythromycin for 7–10 days. The other options should be on the differential diagnosis for an individual with recurrent and relapsing fevers. In addition, this list would also include yellow fever, dengue fever, malaria, rat-bite fever, and infection with echovirus 9 or *Bartonella* species. Brucellosis is a bacterial infection most commonly transmitted by ingestion of contaminated milk or cheese, which this patient did not report. Colorado tick fever is a viral infection transmitted by the bite of a *Dermacentor andersoni* tick that is endemic in the western areas of the United States. The pattern of fever is slightly different from TBRF as the cycle is 2–3 days of fever followed by 2–3 days of normal temperature. Leptospirosis often has two phases of fever. The first occurs during the acute infection, lasting 7–10 days. In some individuals, the fever will recur 3–10 days later during the immune phase. The typical route of infection is prolonged contact with infected rodent droppings in wet environments. Lymphocytic choriomeningitis is a viral infection that is most commonly transmitted via contact with urine or droppings from the common house mouse. This illness usually has two phases as well. During the first phase, which occurs 8–13 days after exposure, an individual will experience fevers, malaise, and myalgias. In the second phase of illness, symptoms more typical of meningitis occur.

IV-166. **The answer is C.** *(Chap. 210)* The picture shows the characteristic rash of erythema migrans, the defining lesion of Lyme disease caused by *B burgdorferi*. Erythema migrans appears at the site of the tick bite within 3–32 days following the initial bite. It typically begins as a red macule or papule and expands slowly to form an annular lesion. As the lesion gets larger, the classic targetoid appearance develops with bright red outer ring as well as ongoing erythema at the central lesion with clearing in between. The most common sites of erythema migrans are the classic locations of tick bites, including the groin, axilla, and thigh. The presence of this lesion in an endemic area for Lyme disease is an indication for treatment and does not require serologic confirmation. *Anaplasma phagocytophilum* is the causative organism of human granulocytic anaplasmosis. This rickettsial disease is also transmitted through a tick bite and is prevalent in the upper Midwest, New England, parts of the Mid-Atlantic, and northern California. Rash occurs in about 6% of cases, although no specific rash is identified. The most common manifestations are fevers, malaise, and myalgia. *B henselae* (option B) is the organism responsible for cat-scratch fever, which can present with mild erythema near the site of the injury and markedly enlarged lymph nodes. *Ehrlichia chaffeensis* is another rickettsial organism that is transmitted by the bite of a tick and is common is in the southeast, northeast, Texas, and California. Human monocytic ehrlichiosis is the disease caused by the organism and presents with nonspecific symptoms of fever, malaise, and myalgia. Rash is also not common in ehrlichiosis. *Rickettsia rickettsii* is the rickettsial organism responsible for Rocky

Mountain spotted fever (RMSF). About 90% of individuals with RMSF have a rash during the course of the illness. The rash most commonly presents with diffuse macules beginning on the wrists and ankles and spreading to the trunk.

IV-167. **The answer is C.** *(Chap. 210)* About 8% of individuals affected by Lyme disease have cardiac involvement during the second stage of disease. Caused by *B burgdorferi*, Lyme disease is transmitted by the bite of an infected *Ixodes* tick. The first phase of the disease represents localized infection and is characterized by the presence of the erythema migrans rash. The second stage of the disease represents disseminated infection. The most common manifestations of this stage are new annular skin lesions, headache, fever, and migratory arthralgias. When cardiac involvement is present, the most common presentation is related to conduction abnormalities, including all categories of heart block. Diffuse cardiac involvement can occur with acute myopericarditis and left ventricular dysfunction. The cardiac involvement typically resolves within a few weeks, even without treatment. Acute myocardial infarction can cause complete heart block, particularly in the event of an inferior myocardial infarction. However, this patient has minimal risk factors for cardiac disease, is otherwise healthy, and has no symptoms to suggest this as a cause. Chagas disease is caused *Trypanosoma cruzi*, a parasite endemic to Mexico and Central and South America. Sarcoidosis is a systemic disease that pathologically demonstrates the diffuse presence of noncaseating granulomas in a variety of tissues. Conduction abnormalities including complete heart block and ventricular tachycardia can be the presenting symptoms of the disease. More commonly, sarcoidosis would have pulmonary manifestations. While sarcoidosis is certainly possible in this gentleman, it would be a diagnosis of exclusion as his risk factors make Lyme disease more likely. Subacute bacterial endocarditis can also result in complete heart block if the endocarditis progresses to develop a valve ring abscess. The patient with subacute bacterial endocarditis would present with a more acute illness than this gentleman, with fevers, weight loss, and most likely secondary signs of endocarditis such as Osler nodes, splinter hemorrhages, and Janeway lesions.

IV-168. **The answer is A.** *(Chap. 210)* Lyme serology tests should be done only in patients with an intermediate pretest probability of having Lyme disease. (See Table IV-168.)

TABLE IV-168 **Algorithm For Testing for and Treating Lyme Disease**

Pretest Probability	Example	Recommendation
High	Patients with erythema migrans	Empirical antibiotic treatment without serologic testing
Intermediate	Patients with oligoarticular arthritis	Serologic testing and antibiotic treatment if test results are positive
Low	Patients with nonspecific symptoms (myalgias, arthralgias, fatigue)	Neither serologic testing nor antibiotic treatment

Source: Adapted from the recommendations of the American College of Physicians (G Nichol et al: *Ann Intern Med* 128:37, 1998, with permission).

The presence of erythema migrans in both patient B and patient E is diagnostic of Lyme disease in the correct epidemiologic context. The diagnosis is entirely clinical. Patient C's clinical course sounds more consistent with systemic lupus erythematosus, and initial laboratory evaluation should focus on this diagnosis. Patients with chronic fatigue, myalgias, and cognitive change are occasionally concerned about Lyme disease as a potential etiology for their symptoms. However, the pretest probability of Lyme is low in these patients, assuming the absence of antecedent erythema migrans, and a positive serology is unlikely to be a true positive test. Lyme arthritis typically occurs months after the initial infection and occurs in approximately 60% of untreated patients. The typical attack is large joint, oligoarticular, and intermittent, lasting weeks at a time. Oligoarticular arthritis carries a broad differential diagnosis including sarcoidosis, spondyloarthropathy, rheumatoid arthritis, psoriatic arthritis, and Lyme disease. Lyme serology is appropriate in this situation. Patients with Lyme arthritis usually have the highest IgG antibody responses seen in the infection.

IV-169 and IV-170. **The answers are D and D, respectively.** *(Chap. 210)* This patient's rash is a classic erythema migrans lesion and is diagnostic for Lyme disease in her geographic region. In the United States, Lyme disease is due to *B burgdorferi*. Partial central clearing, a bright red border, and a target center are very suggestive of this lesion. The fact that multiple lesions exist implies disseminated infection, rather than a primary tick bite inoculation where only one lesion is present. Potential complications of secondary Lyme disease in the United States include migratory arthritis, meningitis, cranial neuritis, mononeuritis multiplex, myelitis, varying degrees of atrioventricular block, and, less commonly, myopericarditis, splenomegaly, and hepatitis. Third-degree or persistent Lyme disease is associated with oligoarticular arthritis of large joints and subtle encephalopathy but not frank dementia. *Borrelia garinii* infection is seen only in Europe and can cause a more pronounced encephalomyelitis.

Acute Lyme disease involving the skin and/or joints is treated with oral doxycycline unless the patient is pregnant or <9 years old. Amoxicillin and macrolides (azithromycin) are less effective therapies. Ceftriaxone is indicated for acute disease in the presence of nervous system involvement (meningitis, facial palsy, encephalopathy, radiculoneuritis) or third-degree heart block. It may also be used for treatment of patients with arthritis who do not respond to oral therapy. First-generation cephalosporins are not active against *B burgdorferi*. While the rash of erythema migrans may look like cellulitis due to staphylococci or streptococci, there is no proven efficacy of vancomycin for Lyme disease. (See Figure IV-170.)

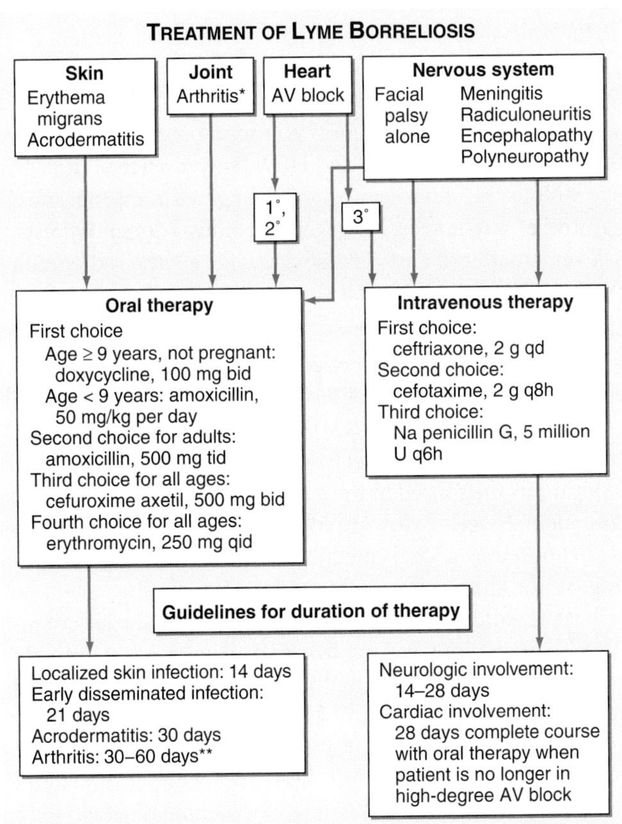

FIGURE IV-170 Algorithm for the treatment of the various early or late manifestations of Lyme borreliosis. AV, atrioventricular. *For arthritis, oral therapy should be tried first; if arthritis is unresponsive, IV therapy should be administered. **For Lyme arthritis, IV ceftriaxone (2 g given once a day for 14–28 days) also is effective and is necessary for a small percentage of patients; however, compared with oral treatment, this regimen is less convenient to administer, has more side effects, and is more expensive.

IV-171. The answer is E. *(Chap. 211)* This clinical vignette describes an individual infected with *Ehrlichia chaffeensis*, the causative agent of human monocytic ehrlichiosis (HME). This rickettsial infection is transmitted through the bite of an infected deer tick and is most common in the southeast, south-central, and mid-Atlantic states. More than 8404 cases of *E chaffeensis* infection had been reported to the CDC as of April 2013. However, active prospective surveillance has documented an incidence as high as 414 cases per 100,000 population. Most *E chaffeensis* infections are identified in the south-central, southeastern, and mid-Atlantic states, but cases have also been recognized in California and New York. All stages of the Lone Star tick (*Amblyomma americanum*) feed on white-tailed deer—a major reservoir. Dogs and coyotes also serve as reservoirs and often lack clinical signs. Tick bites and exposures are frequently reported by patients in rural areas, especially in May through July. The median age of HME patients is 52 years; however, severe and fatal infections in children also are well recognized. Of patients with HME, 60% are male. The time from incubation to symptoms of infection is about 8 days. The most prominent symptoms of HME are nonspecific and include fevers, malaise, headaches, and myalgias. Nausea, vomiting, diarrhea, cough, confusion, and rash are less common. HME can be quite severe, with 62% of all individuals requiring hospitalization and a mortality rate of approximately 3%. In severe cases, septic shock, adult respiratory distress syndrome, and meningoencephalitis can occur. Laboratory findings are helpful in suggesting possible HME. Common findings are lymphopenia, neutropenia, thrombocytopenia, and elevations in aminotransferases. If a bone marrow biopsy is done, the marrow is hypercellular, and noncaseating granulomas can be observed. Diagnosis of HME relies on PCR detection of *E chaffeensis* nucleic acids in peripheral blood. Morulae are seen only rarely (<10%) in the cytoplasm of monocytes on peripheral blood smears. Paired sera demonstrating a rise in antibody titers to >1:64 over a course of about 3 weeks can also be confirmatory. Treatment of HME is doxycycline orally or intravenously that is continued for 3–5 days after fever has resolved.

In rare instances, systemic lupus erythematosus could present with a fulminant illness that could include pancytopenia and liver function abnormalities. However, it would be more likely to have a rash and renal involvement, which this patient did not exhibit. Antibody testing for double-stranded DNA and Smith antigens would not be helpful in this case. As the patient had a normal lumbar puncture, further testing of the CSF is unlikely to yield the diagnosis. This testing is most common used to diagnose viral encephalitides or meningitis such as West Nile virus and HSV. The presence of noncaseating granulomas on bone marrow biopsy is a nondiagnostic finding. In the appropriate clinical setting, this could be suggestive of sarcoidosis. However, sarcoidosis does not present with a fulminant febrile illness over a matter of days. Moreover, while a chest radiograph may demonstrate hilar adenopathy and/or lung infiltrate, this too is a nondiagnostic finding.

IV-172. The answer is B. *(Chap. 211)* This patient demonstrates evidence of Rocky Mountain spotted fever (RMSF), which has progressed over the course of several days due to lack of initial recognition and treatment. RMSF is caused by infection with *R rickettsii* and is transmitted through the bite of an infected dog tick. RMSF has been diagnosed in 47 states and is most commonly diagnosed in the south-central and southeastern states. Symptoms typically begin about 1 week following inoculation. The initial symptoms are vague and are easily misdiagnosed as a viral infection with fever, myalgias, malaise, and headache predominating. While almost all patients with RMSF develop a rash during the course of the illness, rash is present in only 14% on the first day, and the lack of rash in a patient who is at risk for RMSF should not delay treatment. By day 3, 49% of individuals develop a rash. The rash initially is a macular rash that begins on the wrists and ankles and progresses to involve the extremities and trunk. Over time, hemorrhaging into the macules occurs and has a petechial appearance. As the illness progresses, respiratory failure and CNS manifestations can develop. Encephalitis, presenting as confusion and lethargy, is present about 25% of the time. Other manifestations can include renal failure, hepatic injury, and anemia. Treatment for RMSF is doxycycline 100 mg twice daily. It can be administered orally or intravenously. As this patient shows progressive disease with CNS involvement, hospital admission for treatment is warranted to monitor for further decompensation in the patient's condition. If the patient were more clinically stable, outpatient therapy would be appropriate. Treatment should not be delayed while awaiting confirmatory serologic testing as untreated cases of RMSF are fatal, usually within 8w15 days. Treatment with any sulfa drugs should be avoided as the drug is ineffective and can worsen the disease course. Intravenous ceftriaxone and vancomycin are appropriate agents for bacterial meningitis. Although this could be a consideration in this patient with fever, confusion, and a rash, meningococcemia would present with a more fulminant course, and the patient's risk factor (hiking in an endemic area) would make RMSF more likely.

IV-173. **The answer is D.** *(Chap. 212)* This patient presents with symptoms of atypical pneumonia, and the most common causative organism for atypical pneumonia is *M pneumoniae.* Pneumonia caused by *Mycoplasma* occurs worldwide without a specific seasonal preference. *M. pneumoniae* is a highly infectious organism and is spread by respiratory droplets. It is estimated that approximately 80% of individuals within the same family will experience the infection once one person becomes infected. Outbreaks of *M pneumoniae* also occur in institutional settings, including boarding schools and military bases. Clinical manifestations of *M pneumoniae* typically are pharyngitis, tracheobronchitis, wheezing, or nonspecific upper respiratory syndrome. While many commonly believe the organism is associated with otitis media and bullous myringitis, there are few clinical data to support this assertion. Atypical pneumonia occurs in less than 15% of individuals infected with *M pneumoniae.* The onset of pneumonia is typically gradual with preceding symptoms of upper respiratory infection. Cough is present and, although often extensive, is typically nonproductive. Examination typically demonstrates wheezing or rales in approximately 80% of patients. The most common x-ray findings are bilateral peribronchial pneumonia with increased interstitial markings. Lobar consolidation is uncommon. Definitive diagnosis requires demonstration of *M pneumoniae* nucleic acids on PCR of respiratory secretions or performance of serologic testing. (See Table IV-173.)

TABLE IV-173 **Diagnostic Tests for Respiratory *Mycoplasma pneumoniae* Infection**[a]

Test	Sensitivity, %	Specificity, %
Respiratory culture	≤60	100
Respiratory PCR	65–90	90–100
Serologic studies[b]	55–100	55–100

[a]A combination of PCR and serology is suggested for routine diagnosis. If macrolide resistance is suspected, *M pneumoniae* culture may prove useful, providing an isolate for susceptibility testing.
[b]Acute- and convalescent-phase serum samples are recommended.
Abbreviation: PCR, polymerase chain reaction.

Often, however, the patients are treating empirically without obtaining definitive diagnosis. Other causes of atypical pneumonia are *C pneumoniae* and *L pneumophila. C pneumoniae* more commonly causes pneumonia in school-aged children, although adults can become reinfected. *Legionella* pneumonia is often associated with outbreaks of disease due to contaminated water supplies. Individuals with *Legionella* pneumonia can become quite sick and develop respiratory failure. Adenovirus is a common viral cause of upper respiratory tract infection and has been associated with outbreaks of pneumonia among military recruits. *S pneumoniae* is the most common cause of community-acquired pneumonia, but typically presents with radiographic lobar or segmental consolidation.

IV-174. **The answer is D.** *(Chap. 212) M pneumoniae* is a common cause of pneumonia that is often occurs in young previously healthy individuals and is often treated empirically with standard antibiotic regimens for community-acquired pneumonia. It is spread easily person-to-person, and outbreaks in crowded conditions, such as schools or barracks, are common. Most patients develop a cough without radiographic abnormalities. When radiographic abnormalities are present, there is usually a diffuse bronchopneumonia pattern without any lobar consolidation. Pharyngitis and rhinitis are also common. *M pneumoniae* commonly induces the production of cold agglutinins, which in turn can cause an IgM- and complement-mediated intravascular hemolytic anemia. The presence of cold agglutinins is specific for *M pneumoniae* infection only in the context of a consistent clinical picture for infection, as in this patient. Cold agglutinins are more common in children. Measurement of cold agglutinins as a diagnostic test is mostly of historical interest and is not currently recommended since the development of respiratory secretion PCR testing. The blood smear shows no abnormality, which is in contrast to IgG or warm-type hemolytic anemia where spherocytes are seen.

IV-175. **The answer is C.** *(Chap. 213)* This patient is likely suffering from pneumonia due to *Chlamydia psittaci.* This organism is a relatively rare cause of pneumonia, with only about 50 confirmed cases yearly in the United States. Contrary to common belief, the organism is not limited to psittacine birds (parrots, parakeets, cockatiels, macaws), but any bird can be infected, including poultry. Most infections are seen in owners of pet birds, poultry farmers, or poultry processing workers, and outbreaks of pneumonia have been seen in poultry processing factories. Untreated psittacosis has a mortality of as high as 10%. The illness presents with nonspecific symptoms of fevers, chills, myalgias, and severe headache. Gastrointestinal symptoms with hepatosplenomegaly are also common. Severe pneumonia requiring ventilatory support can occur, and other rare manifestations include endocarditis, myocarditis, and neurologic complications. The current diagnostic tool of choice is the microimmunofluorescence test, which is a serologic test. Any titer greater than 1:16 is considered evidence of exposure to psittacosis, and paired acute and convalescent titers showing a fourfold rise in titer are consistent with psittacosis. Complement fixation tests are also used. Treatment of choice for psittacosis is tetracycline 250 mg four times daily for a minimum of 4 weeks. Public health officials should be notified to assess other workers in the factory for disease and limit exposure. While this patient has immigrated from an area endemic for tuberculosis, she had a previous negative PPD and no known tuberculosis exposures. Her chest radiograph shows diffuse consolidation, which would not be typical for reactivation of tuberculosis. Systemic infection with *S aureus* from an abscess or endocarditis could present with respiratory failure related to septic emboli. However, her chest imaging is not consistent with this, and she has no risk factors (e.g., intravenous drug use, indwelling intravenous catheter) for development of *S aureus* bloodstream infection. *L pneumophila* is associated with outbreaks of disease related to contaminated water supplies or air conditioning. It should be considered in this patient in light of her ill co-workers. However, the hepatosplenomegaly is not consistent with this diagnosis. Influenza A is also a consideration for this patient, but the time of year is not consistent for seasonal influenza. In outbreaks of pandemic influenza, this would be more likely.

IV-176. **The answer is D.** *(Chap. 213)* Congenital infection from maternal transmission can lead to severe consequences for the neonate; thus, prenatal care and screening for infection are very important. *C trachomatis* is associated with up to 25% of exposed neonates who develop inclusion conjunctivitis. It can also be associated with pneumonia and otitis media in the newborn. Pneumonia in the newborn has been associated with later development of bronchitis and asthma. Hydrocephalus can be associated with toxoplasmosis. Hutchinson triad, which is Hutchinson teeth (blunted upper incisors), interstitial keratitis, and eighth nerve deafness, is due to congenital syphilis. Sensorineural deafness can be associated with congenital rubella exposure. Treatment of *C trachomatis* in the infant consists of oral erythromycin.

IV-177. **The answer is D.** *(Chap. 213)* Urethritis in men causes dysuria with or without discharge, usually without frequency. The most common causes of urethritis in men include *N gonorrhoeae, C trachomatis, M genitalium, U urealyticum, T vaginalis,* HSV, and possibly adenovirus. *C trachomatis* accounts for 30%–50% of cases. The initial diagnosis of urethritis in men includes specific tests only for *N gonorrhoeae* and *C trachomatis.* Tenets of urethral discharge treatment include providing treatment for the most common causes of urethritis with the assumption that the patient may be lost to follow-up. Therefore, prompt empirical treatment for gonorrhea and *Chlamydia* infections with ceftriaxone and azithromycin should be given on the day of presentation to the clinic to the patient, and recent partners should be contacted for treatment. Azithromycin will also be effective for *M genitalium.* If pus can be milked from the urethra, cultures should be sent for definitive diagnosis and to allow for contact tracing by the health department, as both of the above are reportable diseases. Urine nucleic acid amplification tests are an acceptable substitute in the absence of pus. It is also critical to provide empirical treatment for at-risk sexual contacts. If symptoms do not respond to the initial empirical therapy, patients should be reevaluated for compliance with therapy, reexposure, and *T vaginalis* infection.

IV-178. **The answer is E.** *(Chap. 216)* Antibodies to HSV-2 are not routinely detected until puberty, consistent with the typical sexual transmission of the virus. Serosurveys suggest 15%–20% of American adults have HSV-2 infection. However, only 10% report a history of genital lesions. Seroprevalence is similar or higher in Central America, South America, and Africa. Recent studies in African obstetric clinics have found seroprevalence rates as high as 70%. HSV-2 infection is felt to be so pervasive in the general population because of ease of transmission, both in symptomatic and asymptomatic states. Therefore, this sexually transmitted disease (STD) is significantly more common in individuals who less frequently engage in high-risk behavior than other STDs. HSV-2 is an independent risk factor for HIV acquisition and transmission. HIV virion is shed from herpetic lesions, thus promoting transmission.

IV-179. **The answer is E.** *(Chap. 216)* Primary genital herpes due to HSV-2 is characterized by fever, headache, malaise, inguinal lymphadenopathy, and diffuse genital lesions of varying stage. The cervix and urethra are usually involved in women. While both HSV-2 and HSV-1 can involve the genitals, the recurrence rate of HSV-2 is much higher (90% in the first year) than with HSV-1 (55% in the first year). The rate of reactivation for HSV-2 is very high. Acyclovir, valacyclovir, and famciclovir are effective in shortening the duration of symptoms and lesions in genital herpes. Chronic daily therapy can reduce the frequency of recurrences in those with frequent reactivation. Valacyclovir has been shown to reduce transmission of HSV-2 between sexual partners.

IV-180. **The answer is C.** *(Chap. 216)* Herpes encephalitis accounts for 10%–20% of sporadic cases of viral encephalitis in the United States. It most commonly occurs in patients age 5–30 and >50 years old. HSV-1 accounts for >95% of cases, and most adults have clinical or serologic evidence of HSV-1 mucocutaneous infection before onset of CNS symptoms. HSV encephalitis is characterized by the acute onset of fever and focal neurologic signs, particularly in the temporal lobe. Electroencephalogram (EEG) abnormalities in the temporal lobe are common. CSF will show elevated protein, lymphocyte leukocytosis with red cells, and normal glucose. HSV PCR testing of CSF is highly sensitive and specific for diagnosis. Treatment with acyclovir reduces mortality; however, neurologic sequelae are common, particularly in older patients. Differentiation of HSV encephalitis from other viral forms is difficult. Most experts recommend initiation of empiric acyclovir in any patient with suspected encephalitis pending a confirmed or alternative diagnosis. Tuberculosis meningitis presents typically as a basilar meningitis and not encephalitis. The history, clinical findings, EEG abnormalities, and radiologic findings make fungal meningitis unlikely. CSF oligoclonal bands are typically seen in patient with multiple sclerosis.

IV-181. **The answer is C.** *(Chap. 217)* The currently available varicella-zoster virus vaccine with 18 times the viral content of the live attenuated virus vaccine used in children was shown efficacious for shingles in patients >60 years of age. The vaccine decreased the incidence of shingles by 51%, the burden of illness by 61%, and the incidence of postherpetic neuralgia by 66%. The Advisory Committee on Immunization Practices has therefore recommended that persons in this age group be offered this vaccine in order to reduce the frequency of shingles and the severity of postherpetic neuralgia. Because it is a live virus vaccine, it should not be used in immunocompromised patients.

IV-182. **The answer is E.** *(Chap. 217)* The hemorrhagic vesicles and pustules on an erythematous base grouped in a dermatomal distribution are typical of varicella-zoster virus reinfection, or shingles. Patients with herpes zoster benefit from oral antiviral therapy, as evidenced by accelerated healing of lesions and resolution of zoster-associated pain with acyclovir, valacyclovir, or famciclovir. Valacyclovir and famciclovir are superior to acyclovir in terms of pharmacokinetics and pharmacodynamics and should be used preferentially. Valacyclovir, the prodrug of acyclovir, accelerates healing and resolution of zoster-associated pain more promptly than acyclovir. The dose is 1 g by mouth three times daily for 5–7 days. Ganciclovir is used to treat disseminated infection with CMV, not varicella-zoster virus. The other agents are used to treat bacterial infections such as Lyme or *Rickettsia* (doxycycline), *Pseudomonas* (piperacillin-tazobactam), or treponemes (penicillin).

IV-183 and IV-184. **The answers are C and E, respectively.** *(Chap. 218)* EBV is the cause of heterophile-positive infectious mononucleosis (IM), which is characterized by fever, sore throat, lymphadenopathy, and atypical lymphocytosis. EBV is also associated with several human tumors, including nasopharyngeal carcinoma, Burkitt lymphoma, Hodgkin disease, and (in patients with immunodeficiencies) B-cell lymphoma. EBV infection occurs worldwide, with >90% of adults seropositive. In the developing world, most people are infected as young children and IM is uncommon, whereas in the more developed world, most are infected as adolescents or young adults and IM is more common. The virus is spread by contaminated saliva. Asymptomatic seropositive individuals shed the virus in saliva. In young children, the EBV infection causes mild disease with sore throat. Adolescents and young adults develop IM as described above plus often splenomegaly in the second to third week of disease. The WBC count is usually elevated and peaks at 10,000–20,000/μL during the second or third week of illness. Lymphocytosis is usually demonstrable, with >10% atypical lymphocytes. A morbilliform rash may occur in about 5% of patients as part of the acute illness. Most patients treated with ampicillin develop a macular rash as pictured; this rash is not predictive of future adverse reactions to penicillins. Heterophile antibody testing will be positive in up to 40% of cases of IM in the first week of illness and up to 90% by the third week. If heterophile antibody testing is negative, the more expensive testing for IgM antibodies to viral capsid antigen is more sensitive and specific. IgG antibodies to viral capsid antigen will stay present indefinitely after initial infection and are not useful for diagnosing acute disease. Treatment of uncomplicated IM is with rest, supportive measures, and reassurance. Excessive physical activity should be avoided in the first month to avoid splenic trauma. Prednisone is not indicated and may predispose to secondary infection. It has been used at high dose when IM is complicated by airway compromise due to pharyngeal swelling, autoimmune hemolytic anemia, severe thrombocytopenia, hemophagocytic syndrome, or other severe complications. Controlled trials have shown that acyclovir has no significant impact on the course of uncomplicated IM. One study showed no benefit for combined prednisone plus acyclovir.

IV-185. **The answer is D.** *(Chap 219)* CMV retinitis, a common CMV infection in HIV patients, occurs less commonly in solid organ transplant patients. CMV does affect the lung in a majority of transplant patients if either donor or recipient is CMV-seropositive before transplantation. CMV disease in transplant recipients typically develops 30–90 days after transplantation. It rarely occurs within 2 weeks of transplantation. CMV commonly causes a pneumonitis that clinically is difficult to distinguish from acute rejection. Prior CMV infection has been associated with bronchiolitis obliterans syndrome (chronic rejection) in lung transplant recipients. As with HIV, the gastrointestinal tract is commonly involved with CMV infection. Endoscopy with biopsy showing characteristic giant cells, not serum PCR, is necessary to make this diagnosis. The CMV syndrome is also common in lung transplant patients. Serum CMV PCR should be sent as part of the workup for all nonspecific fevers, worsening lung function, liver function abnormalities, or falling leukocyte counts occurring more than a couple of weeks after transplant.

IV-186. **The answer is A.** *(Chap 219)* When the transplant donor is CMV IgG positive and the recipient is negative, there is a very high risk of primary CMV infection in the recipient. However, if the recipient is IgG positive, CMV occurs as a reactivation infection. When both donor and recipient are seronegative, then the risk of any CMV infection is lowest, but not zero, as a contact with an infected host could prompt primary CMV infection. Unlike nearly all other transplant patients, many donor and recipient seronegative patients do not receive chemoprophylaxis with ganciclovir. In patients who are CMV IgG negative and who received a CMV IgG–negative transplant, transfusions should be from CMV IgG–negative donors or WBC filtered products should be administered to reduce the risk of primary CMV infection. It is not clear whether universal prophylaxis or preemptive therapy is the preferable approach in CMV-seropositive immunocompromised hosts. Both ganciclovir and valganciclovir have been used successfully for prophylaxis and preemptive therapy in transplant recipients. A CMV glycoprotein B vaccine reduced infections in a placebo-controlled trial among 464 CMV-seronegative women; this outcome raises the possibility that this experimental vaccine will reduce congenital infections, but further studies must validate this approach.

IV-187. **The answer is A.** *(Chap. 219)* Human herpesvirus (HHV)-8 or Kaposi sarcoma–associated herpesvirus (KSHV) infects B lymphocytes, macrophages, and both endothelial and epithelial cells and appears to be causally related to Kaposi sarcoma, a subgroup of AIDS-related B-cell body cavity–based lymphomas (primary effusion lymphomas), and multicentric Castleman disease. HHV-8 infection is more common in parts of Africa than in the United States. Primary HHV-8 infection in immunocompetent children may manifest as fever and maculopapular rash. Among individuals with intact immunity, chronic asymptomatic infection is the rule, and neoplastic disorders generally develop only after subsequent immunocompromise. In patients with AIDS, effective antiretroviral therapy has caused improvement in HHV-8–related disease. The virus is sensitive to ganciclovir, foscarnet, and cidofovir, but clinical benefit has not been demonstrated in trials. Invasive cervical carcinoma has been causally implicated with human papillomavirus (HPV) infection, not HHV-8.

IV-188. **The answer is C.** *(Chap. 221)* Immunocompromised patients occasionally cannot clear parvovirus infection due to lack of T-cell function. As parvovirus B19 selectively infects red cell precursors, persistent infection can lead to a prolonged red cell aplasia and persistent drop in hematocrit, with low or absent reticulocytes. Pure red cell aplasia has been reported in HIV infection, lymphoproliferative diseases, and after transplantation. Iron studies will show adequate iron but decreased utilization. The peripheral smear usually shows no abnormalities other than normocytic anemia and the absence of reticulocytes. Antibody tests are not useful in this setting as immunocompromised patients do not produce adequate antibodies against the virus. Therefore, PCR is the most useful diagnostic test. Bone marrow biopsy may be suggestive as it will show no red cell precursors, but usually a less invasive PCR test is adequate. Immediate therapy is with red cell transfusion, followed by IV immunoglobulins, which contain adequate titers of antibody against parvovirus B19.

IV-189. **The answer is D.** *(Chap. 221)* The most likely diagnosis based on her antecedent illness with a facial rash is parvovirus infection. Arthropathy is uncommon in childhood parvovirus infection but may cause a diffuse symmetric arthritis in up to 50% of adults. This corresponds to the immune phase of illness when IgM antibodies are developed. The arthropathy syndrome is more common in women than men. The distribution of affected joints is typically symmetric, most commonly in the small joints of the hands and less commonly the ankles, knees, and wrists. Occasionally, the arthritis persists over months and can mimic rheumatoid arthritis. Rheumatoid factor can be detected in serum. Parvovirus B19V infection may trigger rheumatoid disease in some patients and has been associated with juvenile idiopathic arthritis. Reactive arthritis due to *Chlamydia* or a list of other bacterial pathogens tends to affect large joints such as the sacroiliac joints and spine. It is also sometimes accompanied by uveitis and urethritis. The large number of joints involved with a symmetric distribution argues against crystal or septic arthropathy.

IV-190. **The answer is E.** *(Chap. 222)* Currently available HPV vaccines dramatically reduce rates of infection and disease produced by the HPV types in the vaccines. These products are directed against virus types that cause anogenital tract disease. Both vaccines consist of virus-like particles without any viral nucleic acid and, therefore, are not active. To date, one quadrivalent product (Gardasil, Merck) containing HPV types 6, 11, 16, and 18 and one bivalent product (Cervarix, GlaxoSmithKline) containing HPV types 16 and 18 have been licensed in the United States. HPV types 6 and 11 cause 90% of anogenital warts, whereas types 16 and 18 are responsible for 70% of cervical cancers. Efficacy has varied according to the immunologic and virologic characteristics of study populations at baseline and according to the end points evaluated. Among study participants who are shown at baseline not to be infected with a specific virus type contained in the vaccine and who adhere to the study protocol, rates of vaccine efficacy regularly exceed 90%, as measured by both infection and disease caused by that specific virus type. Study participants who are already infected at baseline with a specific virus type contained in the vaccine do not benefit from vaccination against that type but may benefit from vaccination against other virus types contained in the vaccine preparation. Thus, available HPV vaccines have potent prophylactic effects but no therapeutic effects. The CDC's Advisory Committee for Immunization Practice recommends administration of the quadrivalent HPV vaccine to all boys and girls 11–12 years of age as well as to boys/men and girls/women 13–26 years of age who have not previously been vaccinated or who have not completed the full series. For women, Papanicolaou (Pap) smear testing and screening for HPV DNA are not recommended before vaccination. After vaccination, Pap testing is recommended to detect disease caused by other oncogenic HPV types. Because 30% of cervical cancers are caused by HPV types not contained in the vaccines, no changes in cervical cancer screening programs are currently recommended. Ongoing studies are examining self-testing for HPV to replace many Pap studies in patients with no evidence of cervical infection. Recent studies implicate HPV in some forms of squamous cell carcinoma of the oropharynx. The utility of current vaccines in preventing these cancers in not yet known.

IV-191. **The answer is D.** *(Chap. 223)* This patient presents with symptoms of the common cold with a self-limited illness characterized by rhinorrhea and sore throat. The most common viruses causing the common cold are rhinoviruses, implicated in as much as 50% of common colds. Rhinoviruses are small single-stranded RNA viruses of the Picornaviridae family. There are three genetic species of rhinoviruses with 102 serotypes identified. Rhinoviruses grow preferentially at the temperature of the nasal passages (33–34°C) rather than the temperature of the lower airways (37°C). While rhinovirus infections occur year round, there are seasonal peaks of the infection in the early fall and spring in temperate climates. Overall, the rates of rhinovirus infection are highest in infants and young children and decrease with age. The virus is most often introduced into families through young children in preschool or grade school. Following the index infection, secondary infections occur in other family members 25%–70% of the time. Rhinovirus spreads through direct contact with infected secretions, which can occur through respiratory droplets or hand-to-hand contact. It can also be transmitted through large or small particle aerosols. Finally, virus can be isolated from plastic surfaces from 1–3 hours after inoculation, raising the possibility that virus can also be transmitted through environmental contact.

IV-192. **The answer is C.** *(Chap. 223)* Acute viral respiratory illnesses are the most common illness worldwide, and a wide variety of viruses have been implicated as causes. Rhinoviruses are the most common virus causing the common cold and are found in about 50% of cases. The second most commonly isolated viruses are coronaviruses. These viruses are more common in the late fall, winter, and early spring, primarily at times when rhinoviruses are less active. Adenoviruses are another cause of common cold in children, although this virus is uncommon in adults with the exception of outbreaks in individuals living in close quarters such as military recruits. Although human respiratory syncytial virus characteristically causes pneumonia and bronchiolitis in young children, the virus can cause common cold and pharyngitis in adults. Parainfluenza virus is another virus classically associated with croup in children, but causes common cold in adults. Enteroviruses most commonly cause an undifferentiated febrile illness.

IV-193. **The answer is A.** *(Chap. 223)* The common viruses causing respiratory infections often have specific associated clinical syndromes. Rhinoviruses are primarily responsible for the common cold. Coronaviruses are also commonly associated with the cold. However, in 2002–2003, there was an outbreak of a coronavirus-associated illness that originated in China and spread to 28 countries in Asia, Europe, and North and South America. This illness was named severe acute respiratory syndrome (SARS) and caused severe lower respiratory tract illness and acute respiratory distress syndrome. Overall, the case-fatality rate was 9.5%. Human respiratory syncytial virus (HRSV) is the primary agent responsible for lower respiratory disease and bronchiolitis in infants and young children. Another virus primarily associated with childhood illness is parainfluenza virus. This virus is a frequent cause of croup in young children characterized by a febrile illness with a barking cough and stridor. Adenovirus often causes a febrile illness with common cold and pharyngitis in children. In adults, it is associated with outbreaks of respiratory illness in military recruits. HSV is associated gingivostomatitis in children and pharyngotonsillitis in adults.

IV-194. **The answer is C.** *(Chap. 223)* In infants, HRSV is frequently associated with lower respiratory infections in 25%–40% of infections. This can present as pneumonia, tracheobronchitis, or bronchiolitis. In cases of lower respiratory infections, tachypnea, wheezing, and hypoxemia are common and can progress to respiratory failure. Treatment is primarily supportive, with hydration, suctioning of secretions, and administration of humidified oxygen. Bronchodilators are also used to treat wheezing and bronchospasm. In more severe cases, aerosolized ribavirin has been demonstrated to modestly improve the time to resolution of respiratory illness. The American Academy of Pediatrics states that aerosolized ribavirin "may be considered" in infants who are seriously ill or who are at high risk of complications, including those with bronchopulmonary dysplasia, those with congenital heart disease, or those who are immunosuppressed. However, no benefit has been demonstrated with use of standard intravenous immunoglobulin or HRSV-specific immunoglobulin.

IV-195. **The answer is E.** *(Chap. 224)* Pandemic strains of influenza emerge through genetic reassortment of RNA segments between viruses that affect different species, including humans, swine, and birds. This process is also called antigenic shift, during which a new strain of influenza emerges to which very few people have immunity. Antigenic shift only occurs with influenza A as it is the only influenza that crosses between species. Antigenic drift is the result of point mutations in the hemagglutinin and/or neuramidase proteins. Antigenic drift occurs frequently and is responsible for the interpandemic influenza outbreaks.

IV-196. **The answer is A.** *(Chap. 224,* www.cdc.gov/flu) This patient is presenting with an influenza-like illness during the typical flu season. Hospital infection control practices in this setting are to treat all patients presenting with an influenza-like illness as if they have influenza until proven otherwise. This would include institution of droplet precautions to prevent spread to other individuals as well as performing testing to confirm the influenza diagnosis. This is most commonly done via a nasopharyngeal swab, but can also be done on throat swab, sputum, nasotracheal aspirates, or bronchoscopic specimens if available. If influenza diagnosis is confirmed, assessment of close household contacts for individuals who may be candidates for chemoprophylaxis against influenza is important, particularly those individuals who would be at high risk of complications from influenza infection. This group includes children less than 4 years old, pregnant women, individuals age 65 years or older, individuals with heart or lung disease, individuals with abnormal immune systems, and individuals with chronic metabolic diseases or renal disease.

As far as treatment is concerned, clearly oxygen should be given to individuals who are hypoxemic. Other appropriate supportive care should also be administered including intravenous fluids and respiratory therapy support to manage secretions. In general, treatment with antiviral medications has been demonstrated to decrease the duration of symptoms by 1–1.5 days when initiated within the first 48 hours after the onset of symptoms. However, the CDC recommends treatment with antiviral medications as early as possible in patients hospitalized with severe pneumonia. There is some evidence that use of antiviral therapy might be effective in decreasing morbidity and mortality in individuals who are hospitalized with severe pneumonia even when given more than 48 hours after onset of symptoms. The preferred class of antiviral therapy is the neuraminidase inhibitors, which have efficacy against both influenza A and B. In addition, resistance is much lower among this class of medications. This class includes the drugs zanamivir, oseltamivir, and peramivir. Of these, oseltamivir is most commonly used because it is an oral medication with limited side effects. Zanamivir is given by inhalation and can cause bronchoconstriction in individuals with asthma. Peramivir is currently an investigational medication that is administered intravenously.

The adamantine agents include amantadine and rimantadine. These medications have no efficacy against influenza B and also have a high degree of antiviral resistance (>90%) in North America to H3N2 strains of influenza A. It is important to know the resistance patterns to antiviral agents during the local flu season. The CDC currently does not recommend amantadine as first-line therapy for severe influenza. Antibacterial therapy should be reserved for individuals with suspected bacterial complications of influenza.

IV-197. **The answer is D.** *(Chap. 224)* The majority of influenza infections are clinically mild and self-limited. Treatment with over-the-counter cough suppressants and analgesics such as acetaminophen is often adequate. Patients who are under the age of 18 are at risk of developing Reye syndrome if exposed to salicylates such as aspirin. The neuraminidase inhibitors oseltamivir and zanamivir have activity against influenza A and B. They can be used within 2 days of symptom onset and have been shown to reduce the duration of symptoms by a day or two. This patient has had symptoms for >48 hours; therefore, neither drug is likely to be effective. The patient's history of asthma is an additional contraindication to zanamivir, as this drug can precipitate bronchospasm. The M2 inhibitors, amantadine and rimantadine, have activity against influenza A only. However, since 2005 >90% of A/H3N2 viral isolates demonstrated resistance to amantadine, and these drugs are no longer recommended for use in influenza A.

IV-198. **The answer is B.** *(Chap. 224,* http://www.cdc.gov/flu/about/qa/nasalspray.htm) The major public health measure for prevention of influenza is vaccination. Inactivated (killed) vaccines are available and are generated from isolates of influenza A and B viruses that circulated in the previous influenza seasons and are anticipated to circulate in the upcoming season. For inactivated vaccines, 50%–80% protection against influenza is expected if the vaccine virus and the currently circulating viruses are closely related. Available inactivated vaccines have been highly purified and are associated with few reactions. Up to 5% of individuals experience low-grade fever and mild systemic symptoms 8–24 hours after vaccination, and up to one-third develop mild redness or tenderness at the vaccination site. Although the 1976 swine influenza vaccine appears to have been associated with an increased frequency of Guillain-Barré syndrome, influenza vaccines administered since 1976 generally have not been. Possible exceptions were noted during the 1992–1993 and 1993–1994 influenza seasons, when there may have been an excess risk of this syndrome (slightly more than 1 case per 1 million vaccine recipients). Large-scale studies of vaccination with the 2009 pandemic H1N1 vaccine also suggested a possible increased risk of Guillain-Barré syndrome (1 case per 1 million vaccines). However, the overall health risk following influenza substantially outweighs the potential risk associated with vaccination. Inactivated influenza vaccines have been noted to be less immunogenic in the elderly. A higher-dose trivalent vaccine containing 60 μg of each antigen and a lower-dose, intradermally administered trivalent vaccine containing 9 μg of each antigen have been approved for use in individuals ≥65 years of age and individuals 18–64 years of age, respectively.

The influenza vaccines discussed above are manufactured in eggs and should not be administered to persons with true hypersensitivity to eggs. For use in this situation, an egg-free vaccine manufactured in cells through recombinant DNA techniques (Flublok; Protein Sciences Corporation, Meriden, CT) has been approved. Active research is under way to develop vaccines with broad activity against antigenically distinct subtypes ("universal influenza vaccines").

Historically, the U.S. Public Health Service has recommended influenza vaccination for certain groups at high risk for complications of influenza on the basis of age or underlying disease or for their close contacts. Although such individuals will continue to be the focus of vaccination programs, the recommendations have been progressively expanded, and immunization of the entire population above the age of 6 months has been recommended since 2010–2011. This expanded recommendation reflects increased recognition of previously unappreciated risk factors (e.g., obesity, postpartum conditions, and racial or ethnic influences) as well as an appreciation that more widespread use of vaccine is required for influenza control. Inactivated vaccines may be administered safely to immunocompromised patients. Influenza vaccination is not associated with exacerbations of chronic nervous system diseases such as multiple sclerosis. Vaccine should be administered early in the autumn before influenza outbreaks occur and should then be given annually to maintain immunity against the most current influenza virus strains.

TABLE IV-211 **Principles of Therapy of HIV Infection**

1. Ongoing HIV replication leads to immune system damage, progression to AIDS, and systemic immune activation.
2. Plasma HIV RNA levels indicate the magnitude of HIV replication and the rate of CD4+ T-cell destruction. CD4+ T-cell counts indicate the current level of competence of the immune system.
3. Maximal suppression of viral replication is a goal of therapy; the greater the suppression, the less likely is the appearance of drug-resistant quasispecies.
4. The most effective therapeutic strategies involve the simultaneous initiation of combinations of effective anti-HIV drugs with which the patient has not been previously treated and that are not cross-resistant with antiretroviral agents that the patient has already received.
5. The antiretroviral drugs used in combination regimens should be used according to optimum schedules and dosages.
6. The number of available drugs is limited. Any decisions on antiretroviral therapy have a long-term impact on future options for the patient.
7. Women should receive optimal antiretroviral therapy regardless of pregnancy status.
8. The same principles apply to children and adults. The treatment of HIV-infected children involves unique pharmacologic, virologic, and immunologic considerations.
9. Compliance is an important part of ensuring maximal effect from a given regimen. The simpler the regimen, the easier it is for the patient to be compliant.

Source: Modified from *Principles of Therapy of HIV Infection*, U.S. Public Health Service, and the Henry J. Kaiser Family Foundation.

interruption regimens are associated with rapid increases in HIV RNA levels, rapid declines in CD4+ T-cell counts, and an increased risk of clinical progression. In clinical trials, there has been an increase in serious adverse events in the patients randomized to intermittent therapy, suggesting that some "non–AIDS-associated" serious adverse events such as heart attack and stroke may be linked to HIV replication. Given that patients can be infected with viruses that harbor drug resistance mutations, it is recommended that a viral genotype be done prior to the initiation of therapy to optimize the selection of antiretroviral agents. The three options for initial therapy most commonly in use today are three different three-drug regimens. These include tenofovir/emtricitabine/efavirenz, tenofovir/emtricitabine/atazanavir (or darunavir), and tenofovir/emtricitabine/raltegravir. There are no clear data at present on which to base distinctions between these three regimens. Following the initiation of therapy, one should expect a rapid, at least 1-log (10-fold) reduction in plasma HIV RNA levels within 1–2 months and then a slower decline in plasma HIV RNA levels to <50 copies per milliliter within 6 months. There should also be a rise in the CD4+ T-cell count of 100–150/μL that is also particularly brisk during the first month of therapy. Subsequently, one should anticipate a CD4+ T-cell count increase of 50–100 cells/year until numbers approach normal. Many clinicians feel that failure to achieve these end points is an indication for a change in therapy.

IV-213. **The answer is D.** *(Chap. 227)* Norovirus is a member of the Caliciviridae family and is a common cause of diarrhea. It is thought that noroviruses are the most common infectious agents causing mild gastroenteritis in the community. These viruses also commonly cause traveler's diarrhea and can occur in large outbreaks when individuals are confined in close quarters such as on cruise ships or in the military. It affects all age groups and is transmitted by the fecal-oral route. The virus is also present in vomitus. Inoculum with only a very few viral particles can be infectious, and the estimated case rate after exposure is 50%. Clinically, patients typically present with a sudden onset of nausea, vomiting, diarrhea, and crampy abdominal pain within 24 hours of exposure. The illness can last from 12 to 60 hours, and systemic symptoms including fever, chills, headache, and myalgias may occur. The stools are loose and watery without blood. Abdominal examination is generally benign. Death only rarely occurs and typically only in vulnerable individuals who have chronic health conditions exacerbated by dehydration. After acquiring norovirus, immunity is only short-lived, and an individual may become reinfected with a new exposure. Diagnosis is typically made on clinical grounds, although public health officials will frequently use enzyme immunoassays for assessing an acute outbreak such as the one described. Treatment is supportive only as the disease is self-limited. Rotaviruses are the leading cause of diarrheal death in children in the developing world, but generally only cause mild gastroenteritis in adults. It does not typically cause outbreaks of traveler's diarrhea. The incidence of the disease is declining in the developed world due to introduction of a rotavirus vaccine. *Bacillus cereus* and *S aureus* are both causes of food poisoning that should be included in the differential diagnosis. However, the large outbreak of illness makes norovirus more likely. Enterotoxigenic *E coli* is a frequent cause of traveler's diarrhea to tropical areas due to ingestion of contaminated foods or water. Affected patients would have been unlikely to have all been exposed during disembarkment, and the large outbreak is also not consistent with this diagnosis.

IV-214. **The answer is B.** *(Chap. 228)* The image demonstrates a child with vesicular eruptions on the hand, foo,t and mouth. This constellation of findings is characteristic of a diagnosis of hand-foot-and-mouth disease, a viral infection caused by coxsackievirus A16 or enterovirus 71. The infection has an incubation period of 4–6 days and then begins with symptoms of fever, malaise, and anorexia. Following this, vesicles appear on the buccal mucosa, tongue, and the dorsum of the hand. Only about one-third of affected individuals have a rash on the feet. The lesions are tender but nonpruritic. Lesions may also appear on the palate, uvula, or tonsillar pillars. The infection is highly contagious, with nearly 100% attack rates among exposed children. However, the disease is self-limited, with recovery within 1 week without consequence.

IV-215. **The answer is A.** *(Chap. 229)* Measles remains a common illness worldwide and continues to pose a significant health threat in the United States among individuals who are unvaccinated. Prior to the availability of the measles vaccine, an estimated 3–5 million individuals died of measles and its complications yearly. However, since the introduction of the measles vaccine in the 1960s, the number of cases of measles worldwide has declined. By 2008, the estimated number of deaths due to measles had declined to <200,000 yearly, but measles remains a common cause of death among children under the age of 5 in developing countries. Areas that continue to have a high number of measles cases include India, Pakistan, China, and Southeast Asia. Some areas of Africa also have greater numbers of measles cases. Measles is caused by a single-stranded RNA virus that is a member of the *Morbillivirus* genus. It is one of the most highly contagious directly transmitted pathogens. Outbreaks can occur in populations even if <10% of the individuals are susceptible. Susceptible household contacts have attack rates of >90%. Frequent settings for outbreaks include schools and healthcare settings. The virus is transmitted by respiratory droplets in short distances or, less commonly, by small-particle aerosols that remain suspended in the air for long periods. After exposure, there is a 10-day incubation period. During this time, the virus is replicating locally in the respiratory epithelium with development of a secondary viremia at 5–7 days. Prior to symptom onset and during viral replication, affected individuals can shed high numbers of viral particles, fostering further spread of disease. After the incubation period, initial symptoms include fever, malaise, cough, conjunctivitis, and coryza. Koplik spots (Figure IV-215) are diagnostic of measles. The bluish white dots appear initially on the buccal mucosa and are surrounded by erythema. They precede the onset of rash typically by 2 days. The rash of measles is erythematous and macular. It begins most commonly behind the ears and along the neck and hairline. It progresses to involve the face, trunk, and arms, where it may become confluent. Petechiae may be present. The rash fades in the same order of progression, and desquamation of the skin may occur. Deaths due to measles occur related to respiratory complications including bacterial pneumonia as well as encephalitis. In developed countries, the case-fatality rate of measles in children is <1 in 1000, but death rates as high as 20%–30% can occur in refugee camps. Vaccination is highly effective in measles prevention. Infants who have been vaccinated develop effective immunity by the age of 9 months in 85% and by the age of 12 months in 95%. Rates of secondary vaccine failure are low, typically around 5% or less, even 10–15 years after vaccination. Due to the misconception that measles vaccination is associated with the development of autism, there has been a rise in nonvaccination in the United States, with periodic outbreaks as a result. In this setting, the disease is most often introduced by an affected individual who recently traveled to an area where measles remains common.

IV-216. **The answer is E.** *(Chap. 229)* There is no specific antiviral therapy for measles. Treatment should include supportive measures such as hydration and management of fever. If a secondary bacterial infection is suspected based on clinical findings such as pneumonia or otitis media, then antibiotics should be initiated at that time. There is no evidence to support prophylactic use of antibiotics. Vitamin A is effective for the treatment of measles and can reduce morbidity and mortality rates. The WHO recommends administering vitamin A 200,000 units orally once per day for 2 consecutive days. A third dose is recommended 2–4 weeks later if there is documented vitamin A deficiency.

IV-217. **The answer is D.** *(Chap. 232)* The patient has been bitten by a member of a species known to carry rabies in an area in which rabies is endemic. Based on the animal vector and the facts that the skin was broken and that saliva possibly containing the rabies virus was present, postexposure rabies prophylaxis should be administered. If an animal involved in an unprovoked bite can be captured, it should be killed humanely and the head should be sent immediately to an appropriate laboratory for rabies examination by the technique of fluorescent antibody staining for viral antigen. If a healthy dog or cat bites a person in an endemic area, the animal should be captured, confined, and observed for 10 days. If the animal remains healthy for this period, the bite is highly unlikely to have transmitted rabies. Postexposure prophylactic therapy includes vigorous cleaning of the wound with a 20% soap solution to remove any virus particles that may be present. Tetanus toxoid and antibiotics should also be administered. Passive immunization with antirabies antiserum in the form of human rabies immune globulin (rather than the corresponding equine antiserum because of the risk of serum sickness) is indicated at a dose of 10 units/kg into the wound and 10 units/kg IM into the gluteal region. Second, one should actively immunize with an antirabies vaccine (either human diploid cell vaccine or rabies vaccine absorbed [RVA]) in five 1-mL doses given IM, preferably in the deltoid or anterior lateral thigh area. The five doses are given over a 28-day period. The administration of either passive or active immunization without the other modality results in a higher failure rate than does the combination therapy.

IV-218. **The answer is B.** *(Chap. 233)* This patient has a typical presentation of dengue fever. All four distinct dengue viruses (dengue 1–4) have the mosquito *Aedes aegypti* as their principal vector, and all cause a similar clinical syndrome. Thus, lifelong immunity cannot be presumed. In rare cases, second infection with a serotype of dengue virus different from that involved in the primary infection leads to dengue hemorrhagic fever with severe shock. Year-round transmission between latitudes 25°N and 25°S has been established, and seasonal forays of the viruses to points as far north as Philadelphia are thought to have taken place in the United States. Dengue fever is seen throughout Southeast Asia including Malaysia, Thailand, Vietnam, and Singapore. In the Western Hemisphere, it may be found in the Caribbean region, including Puerto Rico. With increasing spread of the vector mosquito throughout the tropics and subtropics, large areas of the world have become vulnerable to the introduction of dengue viruses, particularly through air travel by infected humans, and both dengue fever and the related dengue hemorrhagic fever are becoming increasingly common. The *A aegypti* mosquito, which is also an efficient vector of the yellow fever and chikungunya viruses, typically breeds near human habitation, using relatively fresh water from sources such as water jars, vases, discarded containers, coconut husks, and old tires. *A aegypti* usually inhabits dwellings and bites during the day. After an incubation period of 2–7 days, the typical patient experiences the symptoms described above along with the severe myalgia that gave rise to the colloquial designation "break-bone fever." There is often a macular rash on the first day as well as adenopathy, palatal vesicles, and scleral injection. The illness may last a week, with additional symptoms usually including anorexia, nausea or vomiting, marked cutaneous hypersensitivity, and—near the time of defervescence—a maculopapular rash beginning on the trunk and spreading to the extremities and the face. Laboratory findings include leukopenia, thrombocytopenia, and, in many cases, serum aminotransferase elevations. The diagnosis is made by IgM ELISA or paired serology during recovery or by antigen-detection ELISA or reverse transcriptase PCR during the acute phase. In endemic regions where specific testing is not easily available, the diagnosis is presumed in cases of a typical clinical presentation and thrombocytopenia. Given the frequency of disease and the potential for hemorrhagic fever, active investigation is pursuing an effective vaccine.

IV-219. **The answer is D.** *(Chap. 233)* Disease caused by chikungunya virus is endemic in rural areas of Africa, and more recently, cases have been reported in Europe and the Caribbean. *A aegypti* mosquitoes are the usual vectors for the disease in urban areas. In 2004, a massive epidemic began in the Indian Ocean region (in particular, on the islands of Réunion and Mauritius) and was most likely spread by travelers. Chikungunya virus poses a threat to the continental United States as suitable vector mosquitoes are present in the southern states. The disease is most common among adults, in whom the clinical presentation may be dramatic. The abrupt onset of chikungunya virus disease follows an incubation period of 2–10 days. Fever (often severe) with a saddleback pattern and severe arthralgia are accompanied by chills and constitutional symptoms and signs, such as abdominal pain, anorexia, conjunctival injection, headache, nausea, and photophobia. Migratory polyarthritis mainly affects the small joints of the ankles, feet, hands, and wrists, but the larger joints are not necessarily spared. Rash may appear at the outset or several days into the illness; its development often coincides with defervescence, which occurs around day 2 or 3 of the disease. The rash is most intense on the trunk and limbs and may desquamate. Maternal–fetal transmission has been reported and, in some cases, has led to fetal death. Recovery may require weeks, and some elderly patients may continue to experience joint pain, recurrent effusions, or stiffness for several years. This persistence of signs and symptoms may be especially common in HLA-B27–positive patients. A few patients develop leukopenia. Elevated concentrations of aspartate aminotransferase (AST) and C-reactive protein have been described, as have mildly decreased platelet counts. Treatment of chikungunya virus disease relies on nonsteroidal anti-inflammatory drugs and sometimes chloroquine for refractory arthritis. Oseltamivir is used for influenza virus infections.

IV-220. **The answer is B.** *(Chap. 234)* Several viruses of the family Filoviridae cause severe and frequently fatal viral hemorrhagic fevers in humans. The family Filoviridae includes three genera: *Cuevavirus*, *Ebolavirus*, and *Marburgvirus*. The available data suggest that the only known *Cuevavirus*, Lloviu virus (LLOV), and one *Ebolavirus*, Reston virus (RESTV), are not pathogenic for humans. The remaining four ebolaviruses—Bundibugyo virus (BDBV), Ebola virus (EBOV), Sudan virus (SUDV), and Taï Forest virus (TAFV)—cause Ebola virus disease (EVD).

Introduction of filoviruses into human populations is an extremely rare event that most likely occurs by direct or indirect contact with healthy mammalian filovirus hosts or by contact with infected, sick, or deceased nonhuman primates. Filoviruses are highly infectious but not very contagious. Natural human-to-human transmission takes place through direct person-to-person (usually skin-to-skin) contact or exposure to infected bodily fluids and tissues; there is no evidence of such transmission by aerosol or respiratory droplets. The first phase (disease onset until around day 5–7) resembles influenza and is characterized by sudden onset of fever and chills, severe headaches, cough, myalgia, pharyngitis, arthralgia of the larger joints, development of a maculopapular rash, and other systemic signs/symptoms. The second phase (approximately 5–7 days after disease onset and thereafter) typically involves the gastrointestinal tract (abdominal pain with vomiting and/or diarrhea) respiratory tract (chest pain, cough), vascular system (postural hypotension, edema), and CNS (confusion, coma, headache). Hemorrhagic manifestations such as subconjunctival injection, nosebleeds, hematemesis, hematuria, and melena are also typical. Common laboratory findings are leukopenia (with cell counts as low as 1000/μL) with a left shift prior to leukocytosis, thrombocytopenia (with counts as low as 50,000/μL), increased concentrations of liver and pancreatic enzymes, hypokalemia, hypoproteinemia, increased creatinine and urea concentrations with proteinuria, and prolonged prothrombin and partial thromboplastin times. Patients usually succumb to disease 4–14 days after infection. Patients who survive experience prolonged and sometimes incapacitating sequelae such as arthralgia, asthenia, iridocyclitis, hearing loss, myalgia, orchitis, parotitis, psychosis, recurrent hepatitis, transverse myelitis, or uveitis. Temporary hair loss and desquamation of skin areas previously affected by a typical maculopapular rash are visible consequences of the disease. Rarely, filoviruses can persist in the liver, eyes, or testicles of survivors and may cause recurrent disease months after convalescence. Any treatment of patients with suspected or confirmed filovirus infection must be administered under increased safety precautions by experienced specialists using appropriate personal protective equipment. Treatment of EVD is entirely supportive because no accepted/approved, efficacious, specific antiviral agents or vaccines are yet available.

IV-221. **The answer is D.** *(Chap. 236)* All of these pathogens are typically inhaled and cause pulmonary infection, which may resolve spontaneously or progress to active disease. Resolved infection with blastomycosis, coccidioidomycosis, *Cryptococcus*, and tuberculosis will often leave a radiographic lesion that typically looks like a solitary nodule and may be confused with potential malignancy. Latent tuberculosis is often suggested by the radiographic finding of a calcified lymph node that is typically solitary. Of the listed infections, histoplasmosis is most likely to resolve spontaneously in an immunocompetent individual leaving multiple mediastinal and splenic calcifications. These represent calcified granulomas formed after an appropriate cellular immunity response involving IL-12, TNF-α in combination with functional lymphocytes, macrophages, and epithelial cells. In endemic areas, such as the Ohio and Mississippi River Valleys in the United States, 50%–80% of adults have evidence of previous infection without clinical manifestations. In patients with impaired cellular immunity, the infection may disseminate to the bone marrow, spleen, liver, adrenal glands, and mucocutaneous membranes. Unlike tuberculosis, remote *Histoplasma* infection rarely reactivates.

IV-222. **The answer is C.** *(Chap. 236)* This silver stain shows the typical small (2–5 μm) budding yeast of *Histoplasma capsulatum* on bronchoalveolar lavage (BAL). Patients receiving infliximab and other anti-TNF therapies are at risk of developing opportunistic infection with tuberculosis, *Histoplasma*, other pathogenic fungi (including *Pneumocystis*), *Legionella*, and viruses (including CMV). These infections typically manifest after approximately 2 months of therapy, although shorter and longer durations are described. Patients with AIDS (CD4 <200), extremes of age, and prednisone therapy are also at risk of disseminated histoplasmosis. Disseminated histoplasmosis may present with shock, respiratory failure, pancytopenia, disseminated intravascular coagulation, and multiorgan failure or as a more indolent illness with focal organ dissemination, fever, and systemic symptoms. Cultures of bronchoalveolar fluid are positive in >50% of cases of acute respiratory histoplasmosis. Bone marrow and blood cultures have a high yield in disseminated cases. *Histoplasma* antigen testing of blood and BAL are also sensitive and specific. There is potential cross-reactivity with blastomycosis, coccidioidomycosis, and paracoccidioidomycosis.

IV-223. **The answer is E.** *(Chap. 236)* Patients with severe life-threatening *Histoplasma* infection should be treated with a lipid formulation of amphotericin B followed by itraconazole. In immunosuppressed patients, the degree of immunosuppression should be reduced if possible. Caspofungin (and other echinocandins) is not active against *Histoplasma* but would be used for infection with *Candida* or *Aspergillus*. Ganciclovir is recommended for CMV infection. Isoniazid/rifampin/pyrazinamide/ethambutol is recommended therapy for *M tuberculosis*. Clarithromycin/rifampin/ethambutol is recommended therapy for *M avium* complex. (See Table IV-223.)

IV-224. **The answer is C.** *(Chap. 237)* This patient likely has coccidioidomycosis with meningitis due to HIV infection as evidenced by his history, physical examination, laboratory findings, and diagnostic microbes in the CSF. Fresno is in the heart of the San Joaquin Valley, the highest endemic region for coccidioidomycosis. For reasons that are unclear, African American males and Filipino males are at highest risk of developing coccidioidal infection. Coccidioidomycosis becomes disseminated in <1% of cases, but the meninges as well as skin, bone, and joints are the most common extrapulmonary sites of invasion. Defective cellular immunity and immunosuppression increase the likelihood of dissemination and meningitis. Nuchal rigidity is mild when present, but chronic headache and confusion are typical. Untreated infection may lead to hydrocephalus. Untreated meningitis is uniformly fatal. The CSF findings in this case are typical with lymphocyte predominance, markedly low glucose, and high protein. The findings on silver stain are characteristic of spherules that are unique to coccidioidal infection and

TABLE IV-223 **Recommendations for the Treatment of Histoplasmosis**

Type of Histoplasmosis	Treatment Recommendations	Comments
Acute pulmonary, moderate to severe illness with diffuse infiltrates and/or hypoxemia	Lipid AmB (3–5 mg/kg/d) ± glucocorticoids for 1–2 weeks; then itraconazole (200 mg bid) for 12 weeks. Monitor renal and hepatic function.	Patients with mild cases usually recover without therapy, but itraconazole should be considered if the patient's condition has not improved after 1 month.
Chronic/cavitary pulmonary	Itraconazole (200 mg qd or bid) for at least 12 months. Monitor hepatic function.	Continue treatment until radiographic findings show no further improvement. Monitor for relapse after treatment is stopped.
Progressive disseminated	Lipid AmB (3–5 mg/kg/d) for 1–2 weeks; then itraconazole (200 mg bid) for at least 12 months. Monitor renal and hepatic function.	Liposomal AmB is preferred, but the AmB lipid complex may be used because of cost. Chronic maintenance therapy may be necessary if the degree of immunosuppression cannot be reduced.
Central nervous system	Liposomal AmB (5 mg/kg/d) for 4–6 weeks; then itraconazole (200 mg bid or tid) for at least 12 months. Monitor renal and hepatic function.	A longer course of lipid AmB is recommended because of the high risk of relapse. Itraconazole should be continued until cerebrospinal fluid or CT abnormalities clear.

Abbreviations: AmB, amphotericin B; CT, computed tomography.

are diagnostic when found in tissue (often in granulomas) or body fluids. Complement fixation antibodies in the CSF also indicate infection. Traditionally, amphotericin B was used for treatment of meningitis, but azole antifungals may now be used. Studies have shown itraconazole and fluconazole to be effective for coccidioidal infections. Fluconazole has excellent CSF penetration and is currently the recommended therapy. Itraconazole is likely preferred for bone and joint disease. Therapy should be lifelong because the relapse rate is >80%. While the clinical presentation and CSF findings are consistent with tuberculosis meningitis, the finding of spherules is diagnostic. Caspofungin is active against *Candida* and *Aspergillus*, not coccidioidomycosis. Penicillin G is the preferred therapy for tertiary syphilis.

IV-225. **The answer is C.** *(Chap. 237) Coccidioides immitis* is a mold that is found in the soil in the southwestern United States and Mexico. Case clusters of primary disease may appear 10–14 days after exposure, and the activities with the highest risk include archaeologic excavation, rock hunting, military maneuvers, and construction work. Only 40% of primary pulmonary infections are symptomatic. Symptoms may include those of a hypersensitivity reaction such as erythema nodosum (typically on the lower extremities), erythema multiforme (typically in a necklace distribution), arthritis, or conjunctivitis. Blood eosinophilia is common during acute infection. While pleurisy is common, significant pleural effusion only occurs in 10% of cases (typically mononuclear with negative culture). Diagnosis can be made by culture of sputum; however, when this organism is suspected, the laboratory needs to be notified as it is a biohazard level 3 fungus. Serologic tests of blood may also be helpful; however, seroconversion of primary disease may take up to 8 weeks. Skin testing is useful only for epidemiologic studies and is not done in clinical practice. Asymptomatic and most cases of focal uncomplicated pneumonia do not require therapy. (See Table IV-225.)

IV-226. **The answer is E.** *(Chap. 237)* Northern Arizona (i.e., the Grand Canyon region) is not a region of high incidence of coccidioidomycosis. Coccidioidomycosis is confined to the Western Hemisphere between the latitudes of 40°N and 40°S. In the United States, areas of high endemicity include the southern portion of the San Joaquin Valley of California and the south-central region of Arizona. However, infection may be acquired in other areas of the southwestern United States, including the southern coastal counties in California, southern Nevada, southwestern Utah, southern New Mexico, and western

TABLE IV-225 **Clinical Presentations of Coccidioidomycosis, Their Frequency, and Recommended Initial Therapy for the Immunocompetent Host**

Clinical Presentation	Frequency, %	Recommended Therapy
Asymptomatic infection	60	None
Primary pneumonia (focal)	40	In most cases, none[a]
Diffuse pneumonia	<1	Amphotericin B followed by prolonged oral triazole therapy
Pulmonary sequelae	5	
Nodule	—	None
Cavity	—	In most cases, none[b]
Chronic pneumonia	—	Prolonged triazole therapy
Disseminated disease	≤1	
Skin, bone, joint, soft tissue disease	—	Prolonged triazole therapy[c]
Meningitis	—	Lifelong triazole therapy[d]

[a]Treatment is indicated for hosts with depressed cellular immunity as well as for those with prolonged symptoms and signs of increased severity, including night sweats for >3 weeks, weight loss of >10%, a complement-fixation titer of >1:16, and extensive pulmonary involvement on chest radiography.
[b]Treatment (usually with the oral triazoles fluconazole and itraconazole) is recommended for persistent symptoms.
[c]In severe cases, some clinicians would use amphotericin B as initial therapy.
[d]Intraventricular or intrathecal amphotericin B is recommended in cases of triazole failure. Hydrocephalus may occur, requiring a CSF shunt.
Note: See text for dosages and durations.

Texas, including the Rio Grande Valley. Outside the United States, coccidioidomycosis is endemic to northern Mexico as well as to localized regions of Central America. In South America, there are endemic foci in Colombia, Venezuela, northeastern Brazil, Paraguay, Bolivia, and north-central Argentina. Eosinophilia is a common laboratory finding in acute coccidioidomycosis, and erythema nodosum is a common cutaneous clinical feature (particularly on the lower extremities in women). Mediastinal lymphadenopathy is more commonly seen on radiographs for all acute pneumonias due to endemic mycoses, including *Coccidioides*, rather than due to bacterial pneumonia. A positive complement fixation test is one method to definitively diagnose acute infection.

IV-227. **The answer is C.** *(Chap. 238)* Blastomycosis is caused by the dimorphic fungus, *Blastomyces dermatitidis*, which commonly resides in soil and is acquired through inhalation. Pulmonary infection is most common and can be acute or indolent. Extrapulmonary extension via hematogenous spread from the lungs is common, with skin lesions and osteomyelitis most common. In patients with AIDS, CNS involvement, usually as a brain abscess, has been reported in approximately 40% of cases of blastomycosis. Most cases of blastomycosis are reported from North America with the most common regions bordering the Mississippi and Ohio River basins, the upper Midwest and Canada bordering the Great Lakes, and a small area of New York and Ontario bordering the St. Lawrence River. Outside of North America, most blastomycosis cases are in Africa. Coccidioidomycosis is endemic in southern Arizona.

IV-228. **The answer is C.** *(Chap. 238)* The constellation of symptoms including chronic pneumonia with ulcerating skin lesions and soil exposure in the upper Midwest in the Great Lakes region is highly suggestive of disseminated blastomycosis infection. Sputum or skin biopsy may show broad-based budding yeast. The definitive diagnosis would be made by growth of the organism from sputum or skin biopsy. Serologic testing is of limited use due to cross-reactivity with other endemic fungi. There is a urine *Blastomyces* antigen test that appears more sensitive than serum testing. Therapy for blastomycosis in a non–life-threatening condition is with itraconazole. Lipid formulations of amphotericin are indicated in life-threatening disease or CNS disease (fluconazole can also be used for CNS disease). Blastomycosis may present with solitary pulmonary lesions that may be suggestive of malignancy and should be evaluated as such. The chronic indolent form may also be confused with pulmonary tuberculosis. The differential diagnosis of blastomycosis skin lesions includes pyoderma gangrenosum that may be associated with inflammatory bowel disease. MRSA skin lesions may be nodular and then ulcerate, but when associated with hematologic dissemination from the lung, they are usually more acute than this indolent presentation.

IV-229. **The answer is B.** *(Chap. 239)* The goal of therapy for cryptococcal meningoencephalitis in an HIV-negative patient is cure of the fungal infection, not simply control of symptoms. Therefore, lifelong therapy is not generally necessary. Pulmonary cryptococcosis in an immunocompetent host sometimes resolves without therapy. However, given the propensity of *Cryptococcus* species to disseminate from the lung, the inability to gauge the host's immune status precisely, and the availability of low-toxicity therapy in the form of fluconazole, the current recommendation is for pulmonary cryptococcosis in an immunocompetent individual to be treated with fluconazole (200–400 mg/d for 3–6 months). Extrapulmonary cryptococcosis without CNS involvement in an immunocompetent host can be treated with the same regimen, although amphotericin B (AmB; 0.5–1 mg/kg daily for 4–6 weeks) may be required for more severe cases. For CNS involvement in a host without AIDS or obvious immune impairment, most authorities recommend initial therapy with AmB (0.5–1 mg/kg daily) during an induction phase, which is followed by prolonged therapy with fluconazole (400 mg/d) during a consolidation phase. For cryptococcal meningoencephalitis without a concomitant immunosuppressive condition, the recommended regimen is AmB (0.5–1 mg/kg) plus flucytosine (100 mg/kg) daily for 6–10 weeks. Alternatively, patients can be treated with AmB (0.5–1 mg/kg) plus flucytosine (100 mg/kg) daily for 2 weeks and then with fluconazole (400 mg/d) for at least 10 weeks. Patients with immunosuppression are treated with the same initial regimens except that consolidation therapy with fluconazole is given for a prolonged period to prevent relapse. Neither caspofungin nor micafungin has activity against *Cryptococcus*. Voriconazole and posaconazole are highly active against cryptococcal strains and appear effective clinically, but clinical experience with these agents in the treatment of cryptococcosis is limited. Ceftriaxone and vancomycin are the recommended treatments for bacterial meningitis in an immunocompetent patient <50 years of age and have no role in the therapy of *Cryptococcus*.

IV-230. **The answer is A.** *(Chap. 239)* Cryptococcal meningoencephalitis presents with early manifestations of headache, nausea, gait disturbance, confusion, and visual changes. Fever and nuchal rigidity are often mild or absent. Papilledema is present in approximately 30% of cases. Asymmetric cranial nerve palsies occur in 25% of cases. Neuroimaging is often normal. If there are focal neurologic findings, magnetic resonance imaging (MRI) may be used to diagnose cryptococcomas in the basal ganglia or caudate nucleus, although they are more common in immunocompetent patients with *Cryptococcus neoformans* var. *gattii*. Imaging does not make the diagnosis. The definitive diagnosis remains CSF culture. However, capsular antigen testing in both the serum and the CSF is very sensitive and can provide a presumptive diagnosis. Approximately 90% of patients, including all with a positive CSF smear, and the majority of AIDS patients have detectable cryptococcal antigen. The result is often negative in patients with isolated pulmonary disease. However, because of a very small false-positive rate in antigen testing, CSF culture remains the definitive diagnostic test. In this condition *C neoformans* often can also be cultured from the urine; however, other testing methods are more rapid and useful. Cryptococcosis in patients with HIV infection always requires aggressive therapy and is considered incurable unless immune function improves. Therapy for cryptococcosis in the setting of AIDS has two phases: induction therapy (intended to reduce the fungal burden and alleviate symptoms) and lifelong maintenance therapy (to prevent a symptomatic clinical relapse). Pulmonary and extrapulmonary cryptococcosis without evidence of CNS involvement can be treated with fluconazole (200–400 mg/d). In patients who have more extensive disease, flucytosine (100 mg/kg/d) may be added to the fluconazole regimen for 10 weeks, with lifelong fluconazole maintenance therapy thereafter. For HIV-infected patients with evidence of CNS involvement, most authorities recommend induction therapy with AmB. An acceptable regimen is AmB (0.7–1 mg/kg) plus flucytosine (100 mg/kg) daily for 2 weeks followed by fluconazole (400 mg/d) for at least 10 weeks and then by lifelong maintenance therapy with fluconazole (200 mg/d). Lipid formulations of AmB can be substituted for AmB deoxycholate in patients with renal impairment. Cryptococcal meningoencephalitis is often associated with increased intracranial pressure, which is believed to be responsible for damage to the brain and cranial nerves. Appropriate management of CNS cryptococcosis requires careful attention to the management of intracranial pressure, including the reduction of pressure by repeated therapeutic lumbar puncture and the placement of shunts. Recent studies suggest that the addition of a short course of interferon-γ to antifungal therapy in patients with HIV infection increases clearance of cryptococci from the CSF. In HIV-infected patients with previously treated cryptococcosis who are receiving fluconazole maintenance therapy, it may be possible to discontinue antifungal drug treatment if antiretroviral therapy results in immunologic improvement. However, certain recipients of maintenance therapy who have a history of successfully treated cryptococcosis can develop an immune reconstitution syndrome when antiretroviral therapy produces a rebound in immunologic function.

IV-231. **The answer is D.** *(Chap. 240)* Many clinical conditions and risk factors have been identified that are associated with hematogenous dissemination of *Candida*. Innate immunity is the most important defense mechanism against hematogenous dissemination of the fungus, and neutrophils are the most important component of this defense. Many immunocompetent people have antibodies to *Candida*, the role of these antibodies in the defense against hematogenous spread is not clear. (See Table IV-231.)

TABLE IV-231 **Well-Recognized Factors and Conditions Predisposing to Hematogenously Disseminated Candidiasis**

Antibacterial agents	Abdominal and thoracic surgery
Indwelling intravenous catheters	Cytotoxic chemotherapy
Hyperalimentation fluids	Immunosuppressive agents for organ transplantation
Indwelling urinary catheters	Respirators
Parenteral glucocorticoids	Neutropenia
Severe burns	Low birth weight (neonates)
HIV-associated low CD4+ T-cell counts	Diabetes

Women receiving antibiotics are at risk of developing vaginal candidiasis. Patients with pulmonary alveolar proteinosis are at risk of infection with unusual organisms such as *Nocardia*, atypical mycobacteria, *Aspergillus*, and *Pneumocystis* but are not at increased risk of disseminated candidiasis in the absence of other risk factors.

IV-232. **The answer is D.** *(Chaps. 235 and 240)* This patient presents with the classic skin presentation of disseminated candidiasis. The skin lesions, severe myalgias, joint pains, and fever are typical manifestations of hematogenous spread from either a GI or skin source in a patient predisposed by neutropenia and indwelling catheters. The severe myalgias are a characteristic of this syndrome and should be taken seriously as a new complaint in a susceptible host. Blood cultures are likely to be positive, but staining of the skin lesions is positive in virtually 100% of cases. *Candida* is the only fungus that can typically be visualized on tissue Gram stain in the form of pseudohyphae and hyphae. *Aspergillus* is seen in tissue as clumps of branching (45°) septated hyphae often with angioinvasion and necrosis. *Aspergillus* may also disseminate in a prolonged neutropenic patient, usually from a lung infection, and cause rapidly progressive skin lesions, usually with a necrotic center. *Histoplasma* and *Blastomyces* can be visualized in tissue as budding yeast. Encapsulated yeasts on India ink are indicative of *Cryptococcus*. Spherules are specific to coccidioidomycosis.

IV-233. **The answer is D.** *(Chap. 240)* *Candida* species are susceptible to a number of systemic antifungal agents. Most institutions chose an agent based on their local epidemiology and resistance patterns. Fluconazole is the most commonly used agent for nonneutropenic hemodynamically stable patients, unless azole resistance is considered an issue. In a hemodynamically unstable neutropenic patient, more broad spectrum agents are typically used such as polyenes, echinocandins, or later-generation azoles such as voriconazole.

Lipid formulations of amphotericin, while not FDA approved as primary therapy, are commonly used because they are less toxic than amphotericin B deoxycholate. At present, the vast majority of isolates of *Candida albicans* are sensitive to fluconazole. *Candida glabrata* and *Candida krusei* are more sensitive to polyenes and echinocandins. Flucytosine is not used as sole therapy for *Candida*. It may be combined with amphotericin for treatment of *Candida* endophthalmitis and meningitis. (See Table IV-233.)

TABLE IV-233 **Agents for the Treatment of Disseminated Candidiasis**

Agent	Route of Administration	Dose[a]	Comment
Amphotericin B deoxycholate	IV only	0.5–1.0 mg/kg daily	Being replaced by lipid formulations
Amphotericin B lipid formulations			Not FDA approved as primary therapy, but used commonly because less toxic than amphotericin B deoxycholate
Liposomal (AmBiSome, Abelcet)	IV only	3.0–5.0 mg/kg daily	
Lipid complex (ABLC)	IV only	3.0–5.0 mg/kg daily	
Colloidal dispersion (ABCD)	IV only	3.0–5.0 mg/kg daily	Associated with frequent infusion reactions
Azoles[b]			
Fluconazole	IV and oral	400 mg/d	Most commonly used
Voriconazole	IV and oral	400 mg/d	Multiple drug interactions
			Approved for candidemia in nonneutropenic patients
Echinocandins			Broad spectrum against *Candida* species; approved for disseminated candidiasis
Caspofungin	IV only	50 mg/d	
Anidulafungin	IV only	100 mg/d	
Micafungin	IV only	100 mg/d	

[a]For loading doses and adjustments in renal failure, see Pappas PG et al: Clinical practice guidelines for the management of candidiasis: 2009 update by the Infectious Diseases Society of America. *Clin Infect Dis* 48:503, 2009. The recommended duration of therapy is 2 weeks beyond the last positive blood culture and the resolution of signs and symptoms of infection.
[b]Although ketoconazole is approved for the treatment of disseminated candidiasis, it has been replaced by the newer agents listed in this table. Posaconazole has been approved for prophylaxis in neutropenic patients and for oropharyngeal candidiasis.
Abbreviation: FDA, U.S. Food and Drug Administration.

IV-234. **The answer is B.** *(Chap. 240)* The use of antifungal agents to prevent *Candida* infections remains controversial, but some general principles have emerged in recent years. Most centers start prophylactic fluconazole in allogeneic stem cell transplant recipients. Many centers also administer them to high-risk liver transplant recipients, but not routine living related renal transplant recipients. This prophylaxis should be differentiated from the administration of empiric broad-spectrum antifungal therapy in a patient with prolonged febrile neutropenia. Voriconazole is an appropriate choice for empiric broad-spectrum therapy in an unstable patient with suspected candidemia, but it has not been shown to be superior to any other agent for prophylaxis against *Candida* in any population. Complicated postoperative surgical patients are at risk of *Candida* infection, and some centers administer prophylaxis to very high-risk patients. However, the widespread use of *Candida* prophylaxis in surgical patients is not recommended because the incidence of disseminated candidiasis is low, the cost-benefit ratio is suboptimal, and there is reasonable rationale to believe that this strategy could increase *Candida* resistance to current medications. *Candida* prophylaxis for HIV-infected patients is recommended to prevent frequent recurrent oropharyngeal or esophageal infection.

IV-235. **The answer is C.** *(Chap. 240)* Candidemia may lead to seeding of other organs. Among nonneutropenic patients, up to 10% develop retinal lesions; therefore, it is important to perform thorough funduscopy. Focal seeding can occur within 2 weeks of the onset of candidemia and may occur even if the patient is afebrile or the infection clears. The lesions may be unilateral or bilateral and are typically small white retinal exudates (see Figure IV-235). However, retinal infection may progress to retinal detachment, vitreous abscess, or extension into the anterior chamber of the eye. Patients may be asymptomatic initially but may also report blurring, ocular pain, or scotoma. Abdominal abscesses are possible but usually occur in patients recovering from profound neutropenia. Fungal endocarditis is also possible but is more common in patients who use IV drugs and may have a murmur on cardiac examination. Fungal pneumonia and pulmonary abscesses are very rare and are not likely in this patient.

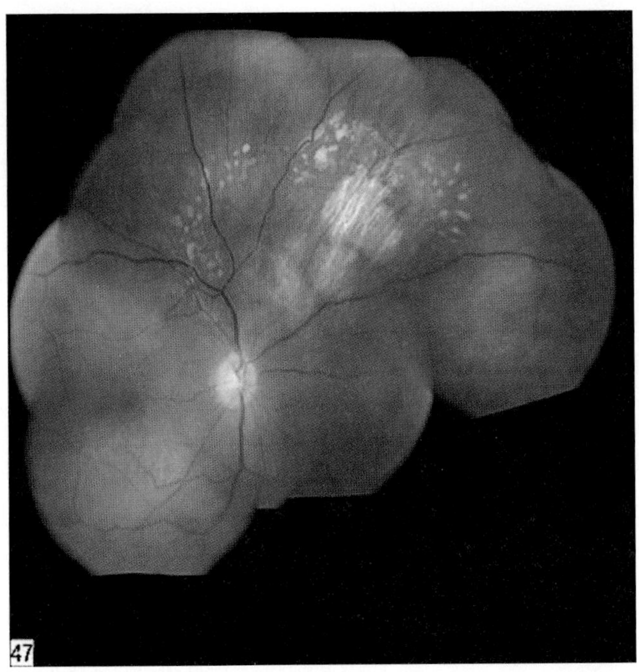

FIGURE IV-235
From Hall JB, Schmidt GA, Kress JP (eds): *Principles of Critical Care*, 4th ed. New York, McGraw-Hill, 2015.

IV-236. **The answer is A.** *(Chap. 241) Aspergillus* has a worldwide distribution, typically growing in decomposing plant materials. Immunocompetent individuals generally do not develop disease without intense exposure such as during construction or handling of moldy hay, bark, or compost. Nosocomial outbreaks are usually directly related to contaminated air source in the hospital. HEPA filtration is effective in eliminating infection from operating rooms and units with high-risk patients. Contaminated water sources are the typical reservoir of nosocomial *Legionella* outbreaks. Patient-to-patient spread in waiting rooms has been described for cystic fibrosis patients transmitting *Burkholderia* infection. Provider-to-patient transmission of MRSA and most other bacteria is reduced with effective use of alcohol-based disinfectant; however, in the case of *C difficile*, alcohol will not eliminate spores, and effective hand washing with soap/water is necessary.

IV-237. **The answer is B.** *(Chap. 241)* Diagnosis of invasive *Aspergillus* is often difficult because early therapy is essential and approximately 40% of cases are missed clinically and are diagnosed at autopsy. Sputum culture is positive in only 10%–30% of patients, and yield is higher when fungal media rather than bacterial agar is utilized. Thus, specifically requesting fungal culture is necessary. The *Aspergillus* antigen assay relies on galactomannan release during fungal growth. Antigen testing is positive days before clinical or radiologic abnormalities appear. The test may be falsely positive in patients receiving β-lactam/β-lactamase inhibitor antibiotics. The sensitivity in patients with prolonged neutropenia is likely about 80%. Prior therapeutic or empiric use of antifungal therapy lowers the sensitivity of the serum test. The test can be performed on BAL samples. The CT findings in this case are also typical of the "halo sign," which is often seen in cases of invasive pulmonary aspergillosis. The halo of ground-glass infiltrate surrounding an *Aspergillus* nodule represents hemorrhagic infarction. Other fungi may cause the halo sign, but due its tendency to be angioinvasive, *Aspergillus* is the most common. The other diagnoses in this case are much less likely given the clinical history and the radiologic signs.

IV-238. **The answer is E.** *(Chap. 241)* Intravenous voriconazole is currently the preferred therapy for invasive aspergillosis. Caspofungin, posaconazole, and lipid-based formulations of amphotericin are second-line agents. Amphotericin is not active against *Aspergillus terreus* or *Aspergillus nidulans.* Fluconazole is active against *Candida* species but not *Aspergillus.* Trimethoprim-sulfamethoxazole is used for therapy against *P jiroveci.* (See Table IV-238.)

TABLE IV-238 **Treatment of Aspergillosis**[a]

Indication	Primary Treatment	Evidence Level[b]	Precautions	Secondary Treatment	Comments
Invasive[c]	Voriconazole	AI	Drug interactions (especially with rifampin), renal failure (IV only)	AmB, caspofungin, posaconazole, micafungin	As primary therapy, voriconazole carries 20% more responses than AmB. Consider initial combination therapy with an echinocandin in nonneutropenic patients.
Prophylaxis	Posaconazole, itraconazole solution	AI	Diarrhea and vomiting with itraconazole, vincristine interaction	Micafungin, aerosolized AmB	Some centers monitor plasma levels of itraconazole and posaconazole.
Single aspergilloma	Surgery	BII	Multicavity disease: poor outcome of surgery, medical therapy preferable	Itraconazole, voriconazole, intracavity AmB	Single large cavities with an aspergilloma are best resected.
Chronic pulmonary[c]	Itraconazole, voriconazole	BII	Poor absorption of itraconazole capsules with proton pump inhibitors or H_2 blockers	Posaconazole, IV AmB, IV micafungin	Resistance may emerge during treatment, especially if plasma drug levels are subtherapeutic.
ABPA/SAFS	Itraconazole	AI	Some glucocorticoid interactions, including with inhaled formulations	Voriconazole, posaconazole	Long-term therapy is helpful in most cases. No evidence indicates whether therapy modifies progression to bronchiectasis/fibrosis.

[a]For information on duration of therapy, see text.
[b]Evidence levels are those used in treatment guidelines (TJ Walsh et al: Treatment of aspergillosis: Clinical practice guidelines of the Infectious Diseases Society of America [IDSA]. *Clin Infect Dis* 46:327, 2008).
[c]An infectious disease consultation is appropriate for these patients.
Note: The oral dose is usually 200 mg bid for voriconazole and itraconazole and 400 mg bid for posaconazole suspension. The IV dose of voriconazole for adults is 6 mg/kg twice at 12-hour intervals (loading doses) followed by 4 mg/kg q12h; a larger dose is required for children and teenagers. Plasma monitoring is helpful in optimizing the dosage. Caspofungin is given as a single loading dose of 70 mg and then at 50 mg/d; some authorities use 70 mg/d for patients weighing >80 kg, and lower doses are required with hepatic dysfunction. Micafungin is given as 50 mg/d for prophylaxis and as at least 150 mg/d for treatment; this drug has not yet been approved by the U.S. Food and Drug Administration (FDA) for this indication. AmB deoxycholate is given at a daily dose of 1 mg/kg if tolerated. Several strategies are available for minimizing renal dysfunction. Lipid-associated AmB is given at 3 mg/kg (AmBisome) or 5 mg/kg (Abelcet). Different regimens are available for aerosolized AmB, but none is FDA approved. Other considerations that may alter dose selection or route include age; concomitant medications; renal, hepatic, or intestinal dysfunction; and drug tolerability.
Abbreviations: AmB, amphotericin B; ABPA, allergic bronchopulmonary aspergillosis; SAFS, severe asthma with fungal sensitization.

IV-239. **The answer is A.** *(Chap. 241) Aspergillus* has many clinical manifestations. Invasive aspergillosis typically occurs in immunocompromised patients and presents as rapidly progressive pulmonary infiltrates. Infection progresses by direct extension across tissue planes. Cavitation may occur. Allergic bronchopulmonary aspergillosis (ABPA) is a different clinical entity. It often occurs in patients with preexisting asthma or cystic fibrosis. It is characterized by an allergic reaction to *Aspergillus* species. Clinically, it is characterized by intermittent wheezing, bilateral pulmonary infiltrates, brownish sputum, and peripheral eosinophilia. IgE may be elevated, suggesting an allergic process, and a specific reaction to *Aspergillus* species that is manifested by serum antibodies or skin testing is common. Although central bronchiectasis and fleeting infiltrates due to mucus plugging are common radiographic findings in ABPA, the presence of peripheral cavitary lung lesions is not a common feature. (See Table IV-239.)

TABLE IV-239 **Major Manifestations of Aspergillosis**

	Type of Disease			
Organ	Invasive (Acute and Subacute)	Chronic	Saprophytic	Allergic
Lung	Angioinvasive (in neutropenia), nonangioinvasive, granulomatous	Chronic cavitary, chronic fibrosing	Aspergilloma (single), airway colonization	Allergic bronchopulmonary, severe asthma with fungal sensitization, extrinsic allergic alveolitis
Sinus	Acute invasive	Chronic invasive, chronic granulomatous	Maxillary fungal ball	Allergic fungal sinusitis, eosinophilic fungal rhinosinusitis
Brain	Abscess, hemorrhagic infarction, meningitis	Granulomatous, meningitis	None	None
Skin	Acute disseminated, locally invasive (trauma, burns, IV access)	External otitis, onychomycosis	None	None
Heart	Endocarditis (native or prosthetic), pericarditis	None	None	None
Eye	Keratitis, endophthalmitis	None	None	None described

IV-240. **The answer is E.** *(Chap. 241)* Allergic bronchopulmonary aspergillosis (ABPA) is not a true infection but rather a hypersensitivity immune response to colonizing *Aspergillus* species. It occurs in ~1% of patients with asthma and in up to 15% of patients with cystic fibrosis. Patients typically have wheezing that is difficult to control with usual agents, infiltrates on chest radiographs due to mucus plugging of airways, a productive cough often with mucus casts, and bronchiectasis. Eosinophilia is common if glucocorticoids have not been administered. The total IgE is of value if >1000 IU/mL in that it represents a significant allergic response and is very suggestive of ABPA. In the proper clinical context, a positive skin test for *Aspergillus* antigen or detection of serum *Aspergillus*-specific IgG or IgE precipitating antibodies is supportive of the diagnosis. Galactomannan EIA is useful for invasive aspergillosis but has not been validated for ABPA. There is no need to try to culture an organism via BAL to make the diagnosis of ABPA. Chest CT, which may reveal bronchiectasis, or pulmonary function testing, which will reveal an obstructive defect, will not be diagnostic.

IV-241. **The answer is B.** *(Chap. 242)* Mucormycosis refers to life-threatening infection due to the Mucorales (formerly known as Zygomycetes) family of fungi. The most common fungus accounting for these infections is *Rhizopus oryzae*. The mortality of these infections approaches 50%. The Mucorales are environmentally ubiquitous; infection requires a defect in the patient's ability to kill the fungus or phagocytic function. The most common predisposing factors are diabetes, glucocorticoid therapy, neutropenia, or iron overload. Free iron supports fungal growth in serum and tissues, enhancing survival and virulence. Deferoxamine therapy predisposes to fatal infection because the chelator acts as a siderophore, directly delivering iron to the fungi. Acidosis also causes dissociation of iron from serum proteins, promoting growth of Mucorales. Patients with diabetic ketoacidosis are at particularly high risk of developing rhinocerebral mucormycosis likely due to the combination of acidosis and phagocytic defects associated with hyperglycemia. Hypoglycemia is not an identified risk factor for mucormycosis.

IV-242. **The answer is E.** *(Chap. 242)* This patient has evidence of invasive rhinocerebral mucormycosis with risk factors including acute and chronic hyperglycemia and metabolic acidosis due to chronic renal insufficiency. With a greater than 50% mortality, therapy of rhinocerebral mucormycosis requires early diagnosis, reversal of underlying predisposing conditions, surgical debridement, and immediate antifungal therapy. Insulin and hemodialysis should be initiated to correct hyperglycemia and metabolic acidosis. Amphotericin products remain the treatment of choice for mucormycosis. Liposomal amphotericin has improved CNS penetration compared to the lipid complex formations. Surgical debridement is also an important component of early therapy. If untreated, the infection quickly spreads from the ethmoid sinus to the orbit and into the cavernous sinus. Development of contralateral infection suggests cavernous sinus thrombosis and portends a very poor prognosis. Differentiation of mucormycosis from *Aspergillus* is important because *Aspergillus* species tend to infect similar hosts and are rapidly fatal. In contrast to mucormycosis species, the hyphae of *Aspergillus* species are septated, are thinner, and branch at acute angles. Voriconazole, the initial therapy for *Aspergillus*, is not indicated in mucormycosis and, in fact, has been shown to exacerbate mucormycosis in animal models. Echinocandin antifungal agents have activity against Mucorales, and animal data suggest they may have a role in combination with lipid polyene agents. (See Table IV-242.)

TABLE IV-242 **First-Line Antifungal Options for the Treatment of Mucormycosis**[a]

Drug	Recommended Dosage	Advantages and Supporting Studies	Disadvantages
Primary Antifungal Therapy			
AmB deoxycholate	1.0–1.5 mg/kg qd	• >5 decades of clinical experience	• Highly toxic
		• Inexpensive • Only licensed agent for treatment of mucormycosis	• Poor CNS penetration
LAmB	5–10 mg/kg qd	• Less nephrotoxic than AmB deoxycholate • Better CNS penetration than AmB deoxycholate or ABLC • Better outcomes than with AmB deoxycholate in murine models and a retrospective clinical review	• Expensive
ABLC	5 mg/kg qd	• Less nephrotoxic than AmB deoxycholate • Murine and retrospective clinical data suggest benefit of combination therapy with echinocandins	• Expensive • Possibly less efficacious than LAmB for CNS infection
Primary Combination Therapy[b]			
Caspofungin plus lipid polyene	70-mg IV loading dose, then 50 mg/d for ≥2 weeks 50 mg/m^2 IV in children	• Favorable toxicity profile • Synergistic in murine disseminated mucormycosis • Retrospective clinical data suggest superior outcomes for rhino-orbital-cerebral mucormycosis.	• Very limited clinical data on combination therapy
Micafungin or anidulafungin plus lipid polyene	100 mg/d for ≥2 weeks Micafungin: 4 mg/kg qd in children Micafungin: 10 mg/kg qd in low-birth-weight infants Anidulafungin: 1.5 mg/kg qd in children	• Favorable toxicity profile • Synergistic with LAmB in murine model of disseminated mucormycosis	• No clinical data

[a]Primary therapy should generally include a polyene. Non–polyene-based regimens may be appropriate for patients who refuse or are intolerant of polyene therapy or for relatively immunocompetent patients with mild disease (e.g., isolated suprafascial cutaneous infection) that can be surgically eradicated.
[b]Prospective randomized trials are necessary to confirm the suggested benefit (from animal and small retrospective human studies) of combination therapy for mucormycosis. Dose escalation of any echinocandin is not recommended because of a paradoxical loss of benefit of combination therapy at echinocandin doses of ≥3 mg/kg qd.
Abbreviations: ABLC, AmB lipid complex; AmB, amphotericin B; CNS, central nervous system; LAmB, liposomal AmB.
Source: Modified from B Spellberg et al: *Clin Infect Dis* 48:1743, 2009.

IV-243. **The answer is E.** *(Chap. 242)* The sites of infection due to Mucorales fungal infection tend to depend on specific host defense defects. The most common clinical manifestation of mucormycosis is rhinocerebral. Most cases occur in patients with diabetes or hyperglycemia due to glucocorticoid therapy (e.g., solid organ transplantation). The initial symptoms usually include facial/orbital pain or numbness, facial suffusion, and soft tissue swelling. The infection usually originates in the ethmoid sinus region and will spread rapidly to the orbit and CNS. Painful necrotic lesions may be seen in the mouth. Pulmonary mucormycosis is the second most common manifestation of Mucorales infection. Human stem cell transplantation is a common risk factor for pulmonary mucormycosis. The risk factors and presentation are similar to invasive pulmonary *Aspergillus*. Differentiation is important as antifungal therapy differs. The two diseases appear similar on chest CT, although the presence of >10 nodules, pleural effusion, or concomitant sinusitis makes mucormycosis more likely. Other sites of involvement with mucormycosis are described but less common. Cutaneous disease may result from external implantation (soil-related trauma or plant penetration) or hematogenous dissemination. Implanted cutaneous disease is also highly invasive; the development of fasciitis has a >70% mortality. Rapid surgical debridement is essential. Hematogenous dissemination has a very high mortality; involvement of the brain has a near 100% mortality. Gastrointestinal mucormycosis is most common in neonates with necrotizing enterocolitis.

IV-244. **The answer is E.** *(Chap. 243)* This patient has tinea capitis most likely caused by the dermatophytic mold, *Trichophyton*. The other dermatophytes that less frequently cause cutaneous infection include *Microsporum* and *Epidermophyton*. They are not part of the normal skin flora but can live in keratinized skin structures. Infections with these organisms are extremely common and are often called ringworm, although the causative organisms are fungi not worms. They manifest as infection of the head (tinea capitis), feet (tinea pedis), crotch (tinea cruris), and nails (tinea unguium or onychomycosis). Tinea capitis is most common in children age 3–7 but also occurs in adults. Usually, the typical appearance, as in this case, is diagnostic. Scrapings may be taken from the edge of the lesion and stained with KOH to reveal hyphae. Dermatophyte infections often respond to topical therapy. For troublesome infections, itraconazole or terbinafine for 1–2 weeks can hasten resolutions. Terbinafine is often preferred because of fewer drug interactions.

IV-245. **The answer is B.** *(Chap. 243)* Tinea versicolor is the most common superficial skin infection. It is caused by lipophilic yeasts of the genus *Malassezia*, most commonly *Malassezia furfur*. In tropical areas, the prevalence of tinea versicolor is 40%–60%, whereas in temperate areas, it is about 1%. In general, most individuals seek evaluation for cosmetic reasons as the lesions in tinea versicolor are asymptomatic or only mildly pruritic. The lesions typically appear as patches of pink or coppery-brown skin, but the areas may be hypopigmented in dark-skinned individuals. Diagnosis can be made by demonstrating the organism on potassium hydroxide preparation where a typical "spaghetti and meatballs" appearance may be seen. This is due to the presence of both spore forms and hyphal forms within the skin. Under long-wave ultraviolet A light (Wood's lamp), the affected areas fluoresce to yellow-green. The organism is sensitive to a variety of antifungals. Selenium sulfide shampoo, topical azoles, terbinafine, and ciclopirox have all been used with success. A 2-week treatment regimen typically shows good results, but the infection typically recurs within 2 years of initial treatment. *Fusarium solani* is an environmental fungus that usually causes infection in immunocompromised hosts. It can cause keratitis, onychomycosis, pneumonia, and hematogenous dissemination. *Sporothrix schenckii* is the usual etiologic agent of sporotrichosis. *Penicillium marneffei* is endemic in Vietnam, Thailand, and other Southeast Asian countries. It causes a clinical syndrome similar to disseminated histoplasmosis. *Trichophyton rubrum* is a dermatophyte that causes ringworm.

IV-246. **The answer is D.** *(Chap. 243)* *S schenckii* is a thermally dimorphic fungus found in soil, plants, and moss that most commonly affects in gardeners, farmers, florists, and forestry workers. Sporotrichosis develops after inoculation of the organism into the skin with a contaminated puncture or scratch. The disease typically presents as a fixed cutaneous lesion or with lymphocutaneous spread. The initial lesion typically ulcerates and becomes verrucous in appearance. The draining lymphatic channels become affected in up to 80% of cases. This presents as painless nodules along the lymphatic channel, which ulcerate. A definitive diagnosis is made by culturing the organism. A biopsy of the lesion may show ovoid or cigar-shaped yeast forms. Treatment for sporotrichosis is systemic therapy. Oral itraconazole continued for 2–4 weeks after the primary lesion heals is recommended therapy. Other options include saturated solution of potassium iodide and terbinafine. However, saturated solution of potassium iodide is poorly tolerated, and terbinafine has not been approved for this indication in the United States. Topical antifungals are not effective. In cases of serious systemic disease such as pulmonary sporotrichosis, amphotericin B is the treatment of choice. Caspofungin is not effective against *S schenckii.*

IV-247. **The answer is C.** *(Chap. 244)* The CT image shows bilateral symmetric ground-glass and interstitial infiltrates consistent with *P jiroveci* pneumonia (PCP). Patients receiving biologic agents, including the TNF antagonists infliximab and etanercept, are at increased risk of multiple infections including pneumocystis. Pneumocystis is thought to be a worldwide organism with most people exposed before 5 years of age. Airborne transmission has been demonstrated in animal studies, and epidemiologic studies suggest person-to-person transmission in nosocomial settings. Patients with defects in cell and humoral immunity are at risk of developing pneumonia. Most cases are in HIV-infected patients with CD4 counts <200/μL. Others at risk include patients receiving immunosuppressive agents (particularly glucocorticoids) for cancer or organ transplantation, children with immunodeficiency, premature malnourished infants, and patients receiving biologic immunomodulating agents. PCP typically presents in non–HIV-infected patients with several days of dyspnea, fever, and nonproductive cough. Often, symptoms develop during or soon after a glucocorticoid taper. *Pneumocystis* is associated with a reduced diffusing capacity on pulmonary function that will typically cause mild hypoxemia and significant oxygen desaturation with exertion. Chest radiography will often show bilateral diffuse infiltrates without pleural effusion. Early in the disease, the radiograph may be unremarkable, but chest CT will show diffuse ground-glass infiltrates as in this case. Patients receiving biologic agents are at risk of pneumonia due to tuberculosis (the patient in this case was on prophylaxis), *Aspergillus*, and *Nocardia*. *Aspergillus*, *Nocardia*, and septic emboli typically appear as nodules on chest CT. Rheumatoid nodules would be unlikely in the context of improving joint disease.

IV-248. **The answer is C.** *(Chap. 244)* Prophylaxis is effective in decreasing the risk of PCP. It is clearly indicated in HIV-infected patients with oropharyngeal candidiasis or CD4 count <200/μL and in HIV-infected or non–HIV-infected patients with a history of prior PCP. Prophylaxis may be discontinued in HIV-infected patients who respond to therapy once the CD4 count has risen to >200/μL for >3 months. For patients without HIV infection, there is no laboratory parameter, including the CD4+ T-cell count, that predicts susceptibility to PCP with adequate positive and negative accuracy. The period of susceptibility is usually estimated based on experience with the underlying disease and immunosuppressive regimen. Patients receiving a prolonged course of high-dose glucocorticoids appear to be particularly susceptible to PCP. The glucocorticoid exposure threshold that warrants chemoprophylaxis is controversial, but such preventive therapy should be strongly considered for any patient receiving more than the equivalent of 20 mg of prednisone daily for 30 days. Short courses of corticosteroids, such as during an asthma exacerbation, do not warrant PCP prophylaxis in the absence of a prior history. Trimethoprim-sulfamethoxazole remains the drug of choice for primary and secondary prophylaxis. It also provides protection from opportunistic toxoplasmosis and some bacterial infections.

IV-249. **The answer is E.** *(Chap. 244) P jiroveci* lung infection is known to worsen after initiation of treatment, likely due to lysis of organism and immune response to its intracellular contents. It is thought that adjunct administration of glucocorticoids may reduce inflammation and subsequent lung injury in patients with moderate to severe pneumonia due to *P jiroveci*. Adjunct administration of glucocorticoids in patients with moderate to severe disease as determined by a room air <70 mmHg or an A–a gradient >35 mmHg has been shown to decrease mortality. Glucocorticoids should be given for a total duration of 3 weeks. Patients often do not improve until many days into therapy and often initially worsen; steroids should be used early in the course of illness rather than waiting for lack of improvement. Pneumothoraces and adult respiratory distress syndrome (ARDS) are common feared complications of *Pneumocystis* infection. If patients present with ARDS due to PCP, they meet the criterion for adjunct glucocorticoids due to the severe nature of disease. The use of glucocorticoids as adjunctive therapy in HIV-infected patients with mild disease or in non–HIV-infected patients remains to be evaluated.

IV-250. **The answer is C.** *(Chap. 244)* Clindamycin plus primaquine is a therapeutic, not prophylactic, regimen for mild to moderate disease due to *Pneumocystis* infection. Trimethoprim-sulfamethoxazole is usually given as a first-line agent but carries a significant side effect profile including hyperkalemia, renal insufficiency, elevation of serum creatinine, granulocytopenia, hemolysis in persons with glucose-6-phosphate dehydrogenase (G6PD) insufficiency, and frequent allergic reactions, particularly in those with severe T-cell deficiency. Atovaquone is a common alternative that is given at the same dose for *Pneumocystis* prophylaxis as for therapy. Gastrointestinal symptoms are common with atovaquone. Aerosolized pentamidine can be given on a monthly basis with a risk of bronchospasm and pancreatitis. Patients who develop PCP while receiving aerosolized pentamidine often have upper lobe–predominant disease. Dapsone is commonly used for *Pneumocystis* prophylaxis; however, the physician must be aware of the possibility of methemoglobinemia, G6PD-mediated hemolysis, rare hepatotoxicity, and rare hypersensitivity reaction when using this medicine.

IV-251. **The answer is E.** *(Chap. 247)* The CT scan demonstrates a large amebic abscess in the right lobe of the liver. *E histolytica* is a common pathogen in areas of the world with poor sanitation and crowding. It is endemic in Mexico and Central America as well as in India, tropical Asia, and Africa. Transmission is oral-fecal, and the primary manifestation is colitis, which is often heme-positive. Liver abscess is a common complication, occurring after the organism crosses the colonic border and travels through the portal circulation, subsequently lodging in the liver. At the time of presentation with liver abscess, the primary gastrointestinal infection has usually cleared and organisms cannot be identified in the stool. Enzyme-linked immunosorbent assays and agar gel diffusion assays are positive in more than 90% of patients with colitis, amebomas, or liver abscess. Positive results in conjunction with the appropriate clinical syndrome suggest active disease because serologic findings usually revert to negative within 6–12 months. Up to 10% of patients with acute amebic liver abscess may have a negative serologic finding; in suspected cases with an initially negative result, testing should be repeated in 1 week. A liver biopsy is usually not necessary. Even in highly endemic areas such as South Africa, fewer than 10% of asymptomatic individuals have a positive amebic serology. The interpretation of the indirect hemagglutination test is more difficult because titers may remain positive for as long as 10 years. Treatment for amebic liver abscess is generally with metronidazole plus a luminal agent such as paromomycin or iodoquinol. *Campylobacter* is a major cause of food-borne infectious diarrhea. While usually self-limited, it may cause serious enteritis and inflammatory diarrhea, but not liver abscess.

IV-252. **The answer is A.** *(Chap. 248)* The patient presents with signs of an acute infectious illness in an endemic area for chloroquine-sensitive malaria. A thick and thin preparation of her peripheral blood is indicated to evaluate for trophozoites. The blood smear demonstrates a young trophozoite. Her neurologic findings suggest cerebral malaria, a defining feature of severe malaria. In large studies, parenteral artesunate, a water-soluble artemisinin derivative, has reduced mortality rates in severe falciparum malaria among Asian adults and children by 35% and among African children by 22.5% compared with mortality rates with quinine treatment. Artesunate is given by IV injection but can also be given by IM injection. Although the artemisinin compounds are safer than quinine and considerably safer than quinidine, only one formulation is available in the United States. IV artesunate has been approved by the FDAfor emergency use against severe malaria and can be obtained through the CDC Drug Service.

The antiarrhythmic quinidine gluconate is as effective as quinine and, because it is more readily available, has replaced quinine for the treatment of malaria in the United States. The administration of quinidine must be closely monitored if dysrhythmias and hypotension are to be avoided. If total plasma levels exceed 8 μg/mL or the QTc interval exceeds 0.6 seconds or the QRS complex widens by more than 25% of baseline, then infusion rates should be slowed or infusion stopped temporarily. If arrhythmia or saline-unresponsive hypotension develops, treatment with this drug should be discontinued. Quinine is safer than quinidine; cardiovascular monitoring is not required except when the recipient has cardiac disease. Hypoglycemia is a frequent finding in severe malaria, is associated with a poor prognosis, and may be worsened by quinidine or quinine therapy, which promotes pancreatic insulin secretion. Seizures may be due to cerebral malaria but are not a complication of quinidine. Nightmares are frequently found with mefloquine, and retinopathy is a complication of prolonged chloroquine dosing.

IV-253. **The answer is E.** *(Chap. 248)* Thick and thin smears are a critical part of the evaluation of fever in a person with recent time spent in a *Plasmodium*-endemic region. Thick smears take a longer time to process but increase sensitivity in the setting of low parasitemia. Thin smears are more likely to allow for precise morphologic evaluation to differentiate between the four different types of *Plasmodium* infection and also allow for prognostic calculation of parasitemia. The relationship between parasitemia and prognosis is complex; in general, patients with $>10^5$ parasites/μL are at increased risk of dying, but nonimmune patients may die with much lower counts, and partially immune persons may tolerate parasitemia levels many times higher with only minor symptoms. In severe malaria, a poor prognosis is indicated by a predominance of more mature *Plasmodium falciparum* parasites (i.e., >20% of parasites with visible pigment) in the peripheral blood film or by the presence of phagocytosed malarial pigment in >5% of neutrophils. If clinical suspicion is high, repeat smears should be performed if initially negative. If personnel are not available to rapidly interpret a smear, empirical therapy should be strongly considered to ward off the most severe manifestation of *P falciparum* infection. Antibody-based diagnostic tests that are sensitive and specific for *P falciparum* infection have been introduced. They will remain positive for weeks after infection and do not allow quantification of parasitemia.

IV-254. **The answer is C.** *(Chap. 248)* Malaria, while endemic in much of the world, is not endemic in Mongolia. (See Figure IV-254.) Mefloquine-resistant malaria has emerged as a problem in Southeast Asia, and there are reports of artemisinin-resistant *P falciparum* in parts of Myanmar, Thailand, Cambodia, and Vietnam. Atovaquone-proguanil (Malarone) is a fixed-combination, once-daily prophylactic agent that is very well tolerated by adults and children, with fewer adverse gastrointestinal effects than chloroquine-proguanil and fewer adverse CNS effects than mefloquine. It is effective against all types of malaria, including multidrug-resistant falciparum malaria. Atovaquone-proguanil is best taken with food or a milky drink to optimize absorption. There are insufficient data on the safety of this regimen in pregnancy. Travelers should start taking antimalarial drugs 2 days to 2 weeks before departure so that any untoward reactions can be detected and so that therapeutic antimalarial blood concentrations will be present when needed. Antimalarial prophylaxis should continue for 4 weeks after the traveler has left the endemic area, except if atovaquone-proguanil or primaquine has been taken; these drugs have significant activities against the liver stage of the infection (causal prophylaxis) and can be discontinued 1 week after departure from the endemic area.

IV-255. **The answer is C.** *(Chap. 249)* The patient is seen in an endemic area for *Babesia microti*, which includes Nantucket, Martha's Vineyard, Block Island, Shelter Island, Long Island, southeastern coastal Massachusetts, Connecticut, and Rhode Island. Her flu-like symptoms and tick bite make this disease very likely. Patients generally present with these symptoms, or occasionally neck stiffness, sore throat, abdominal pain, and weight loss. Physical examination is typically normal with the exception of fever. The presence of erythema chronicum migrans suggests concurrent Lyme disease, as rash is not a feature of babesiosis. While thick or thin preparation typically demonstrates the ring form of this protozoan, if these are negative, the 18S rRNA may be demonstrated by PCR. The ring forms are distinguished from *P falciparum* by the absence of central brownish deposit seen in malarial disease. *Babesia duncani* is typically found on the west coast of the United States, and *Babesia divergens* has been reported sporadically in Washington state, Missouri, and Kentucky. Therapy for severe *Babesia microti* disease in adults is clindamycin with additional quinine. Red blood cell exchange transfusion may be considered for *B microti*, but is not recommended as it is with *B divergens*. (See Table IV-255.)

IV-256. **The answer is C.** *(Chap. 251)* Most cases of leishmaniasis occur on the Indian subcontinent and Sudan. The most commonly used technique for diagnosis of visceral leishmaniasis

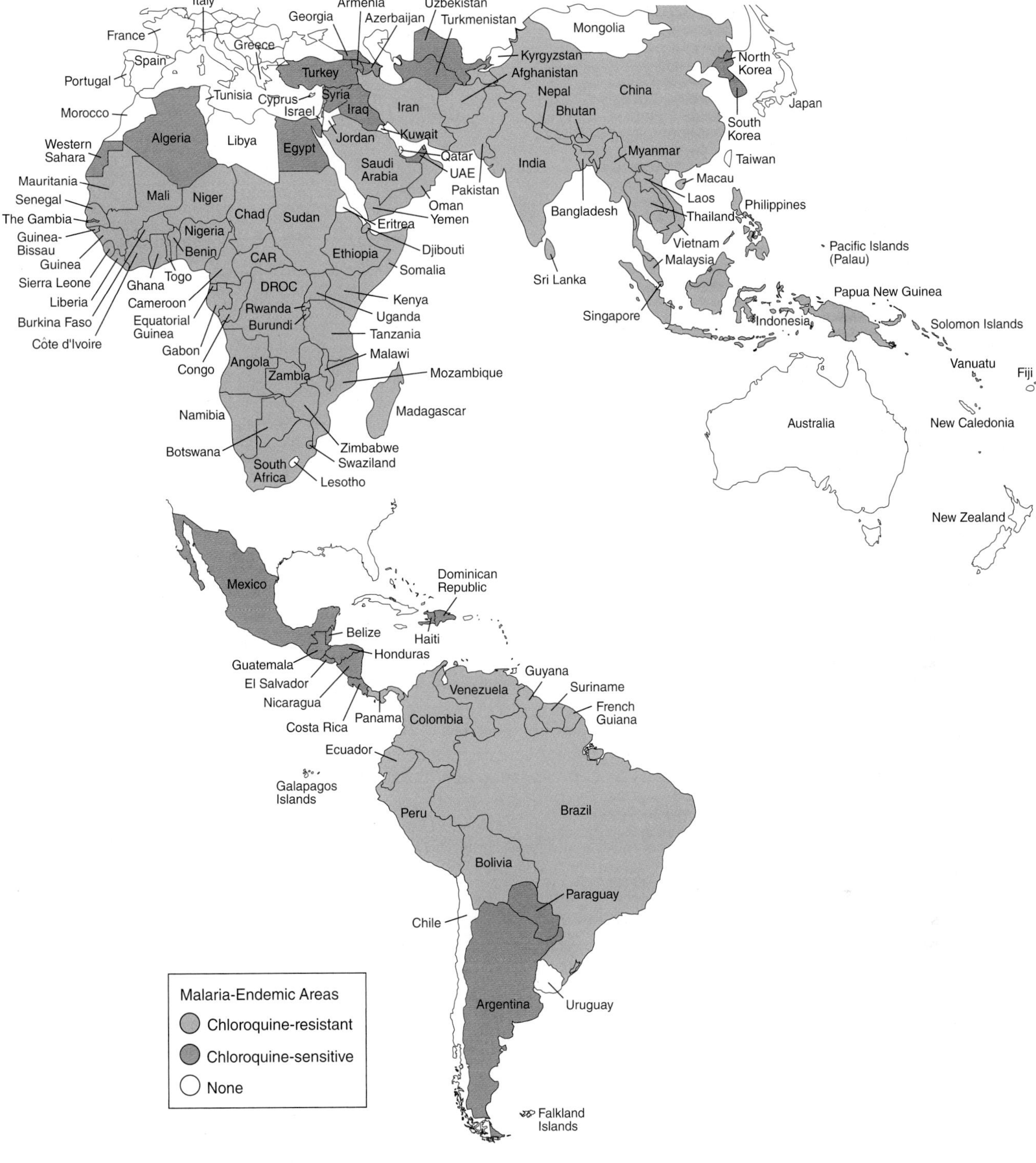

FIGURE IV-254

(kala azar) is a rapid immunochromatographic test for recombinant antigen rK39 from *Leishmania infantum.* This is widely available, rapid and safe, requiring only a fingerprick of blood with results available in approximately 15 minutes. While splenic aspiration with demonstration of amastigotes in tissue smear is the gold standard for the diagnosis of visceral leishmaniasis and culture may increase the sensitivity, the test is invasive and may be dangerous in inexperienced hands. PCR for the leishmaniasis nucleic acid is only available at specialized laboratories and is not routinely used clinically. Leishmaniasis is not diagnosed via stool analysis.

IV-257. **The answer is C.** *(Chap. 252) T cruzi* is the causative agent of Chagas disease or American trypanosomiasis, which only occurs in the Americas. The protozoa are transmitted to

TABLE IV-255 **Treatment pf Human Babesiosis**

Adults	Children
***Babesia microti* Infection (Mild to Moderate Illness[a,b])**	
Atovaquone (750 mg q12h PO) *plus* Azithromycin (500 mg/d PO on day 1, 250 mg/d PO thereafter)	Atovaquone (20 mg/kg q12h PO; maximum, 750 mg/dose) *plus* Azithromycin (10 mg/kg qd PO on day 1 [maximum, 500 mg/dose], 5 mg/kg qd PO thereafter [maximum, 250 mg/dose])
***B microti* Infection (Severe Illness[c,d])**	
Clindamycin (300–600 mg q6h IV or 600 mg q8h PO) *plus* Quinine (650 mg q6–8h PO) *plus* Consider exchange transfusion	Clindamycin (7–10 mg/kg q6–8h IV or 7–10 mg/kg q6–8h PO; maximum, 600 mg/dose) *plus* Quinine (8 mg/kg q8h PO; maximum, 650 mg/dose) *plus* Consider exchange transfusion
***Babesia divergens* Infection**	
Immediate complete exchange transfusion *plus* Clindamycin (600 mg q6–8h IV) *plus* Quinine (650 mg q8h PO)	Immediate complete exchange transfusion *plus* Clindamycin (7–10 mg/kg q6–8h IV; maximum, 600 mg/dose) *plus* Quinine (8 mg/kg q8h PO; maximum, 650 mg/dose)

[a]Treatment duration, 7–10 days.
[b]A high dose of azithromycin (600–1000 mg) combined with atovaquone has been recommended for immunocompromised hosts.
[c]Treatment typically is given for 7–10 days, but its duration may vary. In severely immunocompromised patients, therapy should be continued for at least 6 weeks, including 2 weeks after parasites are no longer detected on blood smear.
[d]Several alternative regimens have been used in a limited number of cases of *B microti* infection, and their efficacy is uncertain. These regimens include atovaquone, azithromycin, and clindamycin; atovaquone, azithromycin, and doxycycline; atovaquone, clindamycin, and doxycycline; atovaquone, doxycycline, and artemisinin; atovaquone-proguanil; azithromycin and quinine; and azithromycin, clindamycin, and doxycycline.
Sources: (1) ME Falagas, MS Klempner: *Clin Infect Dis* 22:809, 1996. (2) PJ Krause et al: *N Engl J Med* 343:1454, 2000. (3) PJ Krause et al: *Clin Infect Dis* 46:370, 2008. (4) CM Shih, CC Wang: *Am J Trop Med Hyg* 59:509, 1998. (5) CP Stowell et al: *N Engl J Med* 356:2313, 2007. (6) JM Vyas et al: *Clin Infect Dis* 45:1588, 2007. (7) GP Wormser et al: *Clin Infect Dis* 50:381, 2010.

mammalian hosts by the reduviid bugs who become infected by sucking blood from animals or humans with circulating protozoa. The infective form of *T cruzi* is excreted in the feces and infects humans through contact with breaks in the skin, mucous membranes, or conjunctiva. Infection has also been transmitted from blood transfusion, organ transplant, and ingestion of contaminated food/drink. Acute Chagas disease is typically a mild febrile illness followed by a chronic phase characterized by subpatent parasitemia, antibodies to *T cruzi*, and no symptoms. Only 10%–30% of patients with chronic Chagas disease develop symptoms, usually related to cardiac or GI lesions. Deer flies are the transmission vector of loa loa (filariasis).

IV-258. **The answer is D.** *(Chap. 252)* This patient most likely has chronic Chagas disease with cardiac involvement and biventricular systolic dysfunction. Chagas disease is a health problem in rural Mexico, Central America, and South America. Most acute cases occur in children, but the epidemiology is uncertain since most cases go undiagnosed. The heart is the organ most often involved in chronic Chagas disease with biventricular systolic dysfunction and conduction abnormalities (right bundle branch block and left anterior hemiblock). Apical aneurysms and mural thrombi may occur. Chronic Chagas disease is diagnosed by demonstration of specific IgG antibodies to *T cruzi* antigens. False-positive results may occur in patients with other parasitic infections or autoimmune disease. The WHO recommends a positive test be confirmed with a separate assay. PCR to detect

T cruzi DNA in chronically infected patients has not been shown to be superior to serology, and no commercially available PCR tests are available. Given the patient's demographics, lack of coronary artery disease risk factors, and indolent symptoms, acute myocardial infarction, ischemic cardiomyopathy, and hypertensive cardiomyopathy are less likely diagnoses. Right heart catheterization with placement of a Swan-Ganz catheter could quantify left and right heart pressures and cardiac output but would not be diagnostic.

IV-259. **The answer is A.** *(Chap. 252)* Current consensus is that all *T cruzi*–infected patients up to 18 years old and all newly infected adults be treated for acute Chagas disease. Unfortunately, the only available drugs, benznidazole and nifurtimox, lack efficacy and have notable side effects. In acute Chagas disease, nifurtimox reduces the duration of symptoms and parasitemia and decreases the acute mortality. However, only approximately 70% of acute infections are cured by a full course of treatment. Benznidazole is at least as effective as nifurtimox and is generally the treatment of choice in Latin America. The role of therapy in patient with indeterminate or chronic asymptomatic Chagas disease is controversial. Some experts recommend that therapy be offered. In contrast, randomized studies have shown benefit of treatment in children. The current antifungal azoles, including voriconazole, do not have adequate efficacy against *T cruzi*, although newer agents in this class show promise in animal studies. Serologic confirmation with *T cruzi* IgG testing is used to diagnose chronic, not acute, Chagas disease. Malaria is endemic to Honduras below 1000 m elevation, and primaquine is effective therapy in those cases. Thin and thick smears evaluated by experts should not confuse *Plasmodium* species with *T cruzi*.

IV-260. **The answer is A.** *(Chap. 242)* Human African trypanosomiasis (HAT), or sleeping sickness, is caused by the protozoan *Trypansoma brucei* complex. HAT remains a major public health problem in Africa despite its near-eradication in the 1960s. While HAT only occurs in sub-Saharan Africa, it is important to distinguish between the West African (*T b gambiense*) and East African (*T b rhodesiense*) forms. Tsetse flies are the transmission vector for both forms. Humans are the major reservoir of West African trypanosomiasis, and it occurs in rural areas, rarely affecting tourists. Antelope and cattle are the reservoir for *T b rhodesiense,* and infection has been reported in safari tourists. A primary lesion (trypanosomal chancre) typically appears a week after the bite of an infected tsetse fly. This is followed by a systemic illness with fever and lymphadenopathy (stage 1 disease). Myocarditis may occur, which can be fatal. CNS involvement follows (stage 2 disease) with CSF pleocytosis, elevated protein, and elevated pressure. During this stage, trypanosomes may be found in CSF. *T b rhodesiense* tends to be more aggressive, with CNS disease developing earlier than with *T b gambiense.* Symptoms during stage 2 disease include progressive somnolence and indifference, sometimes alternating with insomnia and nighttime restlessness. If untreated, symptoms progress to coma and death. Diagnosis requires demonstration of the protozoa from blood, CSF, lymph node material, bone marrow, or chancre fluid. There are serologic tests for *T b gambiense*, but they lack the sensitivity or specificity for treatment decisions. There are not yet commercially available PCR tests. All patients with HAT should have a lumbar puncture to evaluate for CNS involvement as that will determine therapy. Suramin is effective for stage 1 East African HAT (*T b rhodesiense).* Pentamidine is first-line treatment for stage 1 West African HAT. When CSF is involved, eflornithine is used for West African HAT and melarsoprol for East African HAT. Melarsoprol is an arsenical that is highly toxic, with a risk of encephalopathy. HAT poses complex public-health and epizootic problems in Africa. Considerable progress has been made in many areas through control programs that focus on eradication of vectors and drug treatment of infected humans. People can reduce their risk of acquiring trypanosomiasis by avoiding areas known to harbor infected insects, by wearing protective clothing, and by using insect repellent. Chemoprophylaxis is not recommended, and no vaccine is available to prevent transmission of the parasites.

IV-261. **The answer is C.** *(Chap. 253)* The MRI shows the classic lesions of encephalitis due to *T gondii* in a patient with advanced immunosuppression due to HIV infection. Cats are the definitive host for the sexual phase of *Toxoplasma*, and oocysts are shed in their feces. In the United States, up to 30% of 19-year-olds and up to 67% of >50-year-olds have serologic evidence of *Toxoplasma* exposure. Patients with HIV infection are at risk of reactivation of latent toxoplasmosis with resultant encephalitis once the CD4 T-cell count falls below 100/μL. Patients receiving immunosuppressive medication for lymphoproliferative disease or solid organ transplant are also at risk for reactivation of latent disease. While the CNS is the most common site of symptomatic reactivation disease, the lymph nodes, lung, heart, eyes, and GI tract may be involved. Toxoplasma usually causes encephalitis not meningitis; therefore, CSF findings may be unremarkable or have modest elevations of cell count and protein (with normal glucose). The treatment of choice for CNS toxoplasmosis is pyrimethamine plus sulfadiazine. Trimethoprim-sulfamethoxazole is an acceptable alternative. The differential diagnosis of encephalitis in patients with AIDS includes lymphoma, metastatic tumor, brain abscess, PML, fungal infection, and mycobacterial infection. In this case, given the classic MRI, toxoplasmosis is most likely.

IV-262. **The answer is C.** *(Chap. 254)* Of the listed protozoa, only *Giardia* can be diagnosed with stool ova and parasite examination. Stool antigen immunoassay can be utilized to diagnose *Giardia* and *Cryptosporidium*. Fecal acid-fast testing may be used to diagnose *Cryptosporidium*, *Isospora*, and *Cyclospora*. Microsporidia requires special fecal stains or tissue biopsy for diagnosis.

IV-263. **The answer is D.** *(Chap. 254)* Trichomoniasis is transmitted via sexual contact with an infected partner. Many men are asymptomatic but may have symptoms of urethritis, epididymitis, or prostatitis. Most women will have symptoms of infection that include vaginal itching, dyspareunia, and malodorous discharge. These symptoms do not distinguish *Trichomonas* infection from other forms of vaginitis, such as bacterial vaginosis. Trichomoniasis is not a self-limited infection and should be treated for symptomatic and public health reasons. Wet-mount examination for motile trichomonads has a sensitivity of 50%–60% in routine examination. Direct immunofluorescent antibody staining of secretions is more sensitive and can also be performed immediately. Culture is not widely available and takes 3–7 days. Treatment should consist of metronidazole either as a single 2-g dose or 500-mg doses twice daily for 7 days; all sexual partners should be treated. Trichomoniasis resistant to metronidazole has been reported and is managed with increased doses of metronidazole or with tinidazole.

IV-264. **The answer is E.** *(Chap. 254)* Giardiasis is diagnosed by detection of parasite antigens in the feces or by visualizing cysts or trophozoites in feces or small intestine. There is no reliable serum test for this disease. As a wide variety of pathogens are responsible for diarrheal illness, some degree of diagnostic testing beyond the history and physical examination is required for definitive diagnosis. Colonoscopy does not have a role in diagnosing *Giardia*. Giardiasis can persist in symptomatic patients and should be treated. Severe symptoms such as malabsorption, weight loss, growth retardation, and dehydration may occur in prolonged cases. Additionally, extraintestinal manifestations such as urticarial, anterior uveitis, and arthritis have been associated with potential giardiasis. A single oral 2-g dose of tinidazole is reportedly more effective than a 5-day course of metronidazole, with cure rates of >90% for both. Paromomycin, an oral poorly absorbed aminoglycoside, can be used for symptomatic patients during pregnancy, but its efficacy for eradicating infection is not known. Clindamycin and albendazole do not have a role in treatment of giardiasis. Refractory disease with persistent infection can be treated with a longer duration of metronidazole.

IV-265. **The answer is D.** *(Chap. 254)* *Cryptosporidium* typically causes a self-limited diarrheal illness in immunocompetent patients but may cause severe debilitating disease in patients with severe immunodeficiency, such as advanced HIV infection. Outbreaks in immunocompetent hosts are caused by ingestion of oocysts. Infectious oocysts are excreted in human feces causing human-to-human transmission. Waterborne transmission of oocysts accounts for disease in travelers and common-source outbreaks. Oocysts resist killing by routine chlorination of drinking and recreational water sources. Infection may be asymptomatic in immunocompetent and immunosuppressed hosts. Diarrhea is typically watery and nonbloody and may be associated with abdominal pain, nausea, fever, and anorexia. In immunocompetent hosts, symptoms usually subside in 1–2 weeks without therapy. In patients with advanced AIDS with CD4 counts <100/μL, severe symptoms may develop, leading to significant electrolyte and volume loss. Nitazoxanide is approved for treatment of *Cryptosporidium* but, to date, has not been shown to be effective in HIV-infected patients. The best available therapy for HIV patients is antiretroviral therapy to reduce immunosuppression. Tinidazole and metronidazole are used to treat giardiasis and trichomoniasis, not cryptosporidiosis.

IV-266. **The answer is D.** *(Chap. 256)* There are roughly 12 cases of trichinellosis reported each year in the United States. Since most infections are asymptomatic, this may be an underestimate. Recent outbreaks in North American have been related to ingestion of wild game, particularly bear. Heavy infections can cause enteritis, periorbital edema, myositis, and, infrequently, death. This infection, caused by ingesting *Trichinella* cysts, occurs when infected meat from pigs or other carnivorous animals is eaten. Laws that prevent feeding pigs uncooked garbage have been an important public health measure in reducing *Trichinella* infection in this country. Person-to-person spread has not been described. The majority of infections are mild and resolve spontaneously.

IV-267. **The answer is E.** *(Chap. 256)* Trichinellosis occurs when infected meat products are eaten, most frequently pork. The organism can also be transmitted through the ingestion of meat from dogs, horses, and bears. Recent outbreaks in the United States and Canada have been related to consumption of wild game, particularly bear meat. During the first week of infection, diarrhea, nausea, and vomiting are prominent features. As the parasites migrate from the GI tract, fever and eosinophilia are often present. Larvae encyst after 2–3 weeks in muscle tissue, leading to myositis and weakness. Myocarditis and maculopapular rash are less common features of this illness. In pork, larvae are killed by cooking until the meat is no longer pink or by freezing at −15°C for 3 weeks. However, arctic *Trichinella nativa* larvae in walrus or bear meat are resistant to freezing. *Giardia* and *Campylobacter* are organisms that are frequently acquired by drinking contaminated water; neither will produce this pattern of disease. While both will cause GI symptoms (and *Campylobacter* will cause fever), neither will cause eosinophilia or myositis. *Taenia solium*, or the pork tapeworm, shares a similar pathogenesis to *Trichinella* but does not cause myositis. CMV has varied presentations but none that lead to this presentation.

IV-268 and IV-269. **The answers are D and B, respectively.** *(Chap. 256)* Visceral larva migrans, caused in this case by the canine roundworm *Toxocara canis*, most commonly affects young children who are exposed to canine stool. *Toxocara* eggs are ingested and begin their life cycle in the small intestine. They migrate to many tissues in the body. Particularly characteristic of this illness are hepatosplenomegaly and profound eosinophilia, at times close to 90% of the total WBC count. Staphylococci will not typically cause eosinophilia. Trichinellosis, caused by ingesting meat from carnivorous animals that has been infected with *Trichinella* cysts, does not cause hepatosplenomegaly and is uncommon without eating a suspicious meal. Giardiasis is characterized by profuse diarrhea and abdominal pain without systemic features or eosinophilia. Cysticercosis typically causes myalgias and can spread to the brain, where it is often asymptomatic but can lead to seizures. The vast majority of *Toxocara* infections are self-limited and resolve without therapy. Rarely, severe symptoms may develop with deaths due to CNS, myocardial, or respiratory disease. Severe myocardial involvement manifests as an acute myocarditis. In these patients, glucocorticoids are administered to reduce the inflammatory complications. Antihelminthic drugs such as albendazole, mebendazole, or praziquantel have not been shown conclusively to alter the course of visceral larval migrans. Metronidazole is used for infections due to *Trichomonas*, not tissue nematodes.

IV-270. **The answer is A.** *(Chap. 256) Angiostrongylus cantonensis,* the rat lungworm, is the most common cause of human eosinophilic meningitis. The infection principally occurs in Southeast Asia and the Pacific Basin, although cases have been described in Cuba, Australia, Japan, and China. Infective larvae are excreted in rat feces and consumed by land snails and slugs. Humans acquire infection by ingesting the mollusks, vegetables contaminated by mollusk slime, or seafood (crabs, freshwater shrimp) that consumed the mollusks. The larvae migrate to the brain where they initiate a marked eosinophilic inflammatory response with hemorrhage. Clinical symptoms develop 2–35 days after ingestion of larvae, and initial presentation typically includes headache (indolent or acute), fever, nausea, vomiting, and meningismus. The CSF findings are as in this case, with an eosinophil percentage >20%. *A cantonensis* larvae are only rarely demonstrated in the CSF. The diagnosis usually relies on the presence of eosinophilic meningitis and compatible epidemiology. There is no specific chemotherapy for *A cantonensis* meningitis. Supportive care includes repeat removal of CSF to control intracranial pressure. Glucocorticoids may reduce inflammation. In most cases, cerebral angiostrongyliasis has a self-limited course with complete recovery. *Gnathostoma spinigerum* is a less common cause of eosinophilic meningoencephalitis. It also causes migratory cutaneous swellings or eye infections. It is also endemic in Southeast Asia and China and is usually transmitted by eating undercooked fish or poultry (som fak in Thailand and sashimi in Japan). *Trichinella murrelli* and *T nativa* cause trichinosis in North America and the Arctic, respectively. *Toxocara* is the cause of larval migrans.

IV-271. **The answer is B.** *(Chap. 257) Strongyloides* is the only helminth that can replicate in the human host, allowing autoinfection. Humans acquire *Strongyloides* when larvae in fecally contaminated soil penetrate the skin or mucous membranes. The larvae migrate to the lungs via the bloodstream, break through the alveolar spaces, ascend the respiratory airways, and are swallowed to reach the small intestine where they mature into adult worms. Adult worms may penetrate the mucosa of the small intestine. *Strongyloides* is endemic in Southeast Asia, sub-Saharan Africa, Brazil, and the southern United States. Many patients with *Strongyloides* are asymptomatic or have mild gastrointestinal symptoms or the characteristic cutaneous eruption, larval currens, as described in this case. Small bowel obstruction may occur with early heavy infection. Eosinophilia is common with all clinical manifestations. In patients with impaired immunity, particularly glucocorticoid therapy, hyperinfection or dissemination may occur. This may lead to colitis, enteritis, meningitis, peritonitis, and acute renal failure. Bacteremia or gram-negative sepsis may develop due to bacterial translocation through disrupted enteric mucosa. Because of the risk of hyperinfection, all patients with *Strongyloides*, even asymptomatic carriers, should be treated with ivermectin, which is more effective than albendazole. Fluconazole is used to treat candidal infections. Mebendazole is used to treat trichuriasis, enterobiasis (pinworm), ascariasis, and hookworm. Mefloquine is used for malaria prophylaxis.

IV-272. **The answer is B.** *(Chap. 257) Ascaris lumbricoides* is the longest nematode (15–40 cm) parasite of humans. It resides in tropical and subtropical regions. In the United States, it is found mostly in the rural southeast. Transmission is through fecally contaminated soil. Most commonly, the worm burden is low, and it causes no symptoms. Clinical disease is related to larval migration to the lungs or to adult worms in the gastrointestinal tract. The most common complications occur due to a high gastrointestinal adult worm burden leading to small bowel obstruction (most often in children with a narrow-caliber small bowel lumen) or migration leading to obstructive complications such as cholangitis, pancreatitis, or appendicitis. Rarely, adult worms can migrate to the esophagus and be orally expelled. During the lung phase of larval migration (9–12 days after egg ingestion), patients may develop a nonproductive cough, fever, eosinophilia, and pleuritic chest pain. Eosinophilic pneumonia syndrome (Löffler syndrome) is characterized by symptoms and lung infiltrates. Meningitis is not a known complication of ascariasis but can occur with disseminated strongyloidiasis in an immunocompromised host.

IV-273. **The answer is A.** *(Chap. 257)* Ascariasis should always be treated, even in asymptomatic cases, to prevent serious intestinal complications. Albendazole, mebendazole, and ivermectin are effective. These agents should not be administered to pregnant women. Pyrantel is safe in pregnancy. Metronidazole is used for anaerobic bacterial and *Trichomonas* infections. Fluconazole is mostly used to treat *Candida* infections. Diethylcarbamazine is first-line therapy for active lymphatic filariasis. Vancomycin has no effect on nematodes.

IV-274. **The answer is E.** *(Chap. 257)* This patient's most likely diagnosis is anisakiasis. This is a nematode infection where humans are an accidental host. It occurs hours to days after ingesting eggs that previously settled into the muscles of fish. The incidence of anisakiasis in the United States has increased as a result of the growing popularity of raw fish dishes. Most cases occur in Japan, the Netherlands, and Chile, where raw fish—sashimi, pickled green herring, and ceviche, respectively—are national culinary staples. Anisakid nematodes parasitize large sea mammals such as whales, dolphins, and seals. As part of a complex parasitic life cycle involving marine food chains, infectious larvae migrate to the musculature of a variety of fish. The main risk factor for infection is eating raw fish. Presentation mimics an acute abdomen. History is critical as upper endoscopy is both diagnostic and curative. The implicated nematodes burrow into the mucosa of the stomach causing intense pain and must be manually removed by endoscope or, on rare occasion, surgery. There is no medical agent known to cure anisakiasis. Anisakid larvae in saltwater fish are killed by cooking to 60°C, freezing at –20°C for 3 days, or commercial blast freezing, but usually not by salting, marinating, or cold smoking.

IV-275. **The answer is E.** *(Chap. 258)* This patient likely has filariasis with acute lymphadenitis due to *Wuchereria bancrofti*. It is endemic throughout the tropics and subtropics including Asia, the Pacific Islands, Africa, parts of South America, and the Caribbean. *W bancrofti* is the most widely distributed human filarial parasite and is transmitted by infected mosquitos. Lymphatic infection is common and may be acute or chronic. Chronic lower extremity lymphatic infection causes elephantiasis. Definitive diagnosis requires demonstration of the parasite. Microfilariae may be found in blood, hydrocele, or other body fluid collections by direct microscopic examination. ELISA assays for circulating antigens are available commercially and have sensitivity >93% with excellent specificity. PCR-based assays have been developed that may be as effective. In cases of acute lymphadenitis, ultrasound examination with Doppler may actually reveal motile worms in dilated lymphatics. Live worms have a distinctive movement pattern (filarial dance sign). Worms may be visualized in the spermatic cord of up to 80% of men infected with *W bancrofti*. Stool ova and parasite examination are not useful for demonstration of *W bancrofti*.

IV-276. **The answer is B.** *(Chap. 258)* Diethylcarbamazine (DEC), which has macro- and microfilaricidal properties, is first-line treatment for acute filarial lymphadenitis. Albendazole, doxycycline, and ivermectin are also used to treat microfilarial infections (not macrofilarial). There is consensus that virtually all patients with *W bancrofti* infection should be treated, even if asymptomatic, to prevent lymphatic damage. Many of these patients have microfilarial infection with subclinical hematuria, proteinuria, and so on. Albendazole and doxycycline have demonstrated macrofilaricidal efficacy. Combinations of DEC with albendazole, ivermectin, and doxycycline have efficacy in eradication programs. The WHO established a global program to eliminate lymphatic filariasis in 1997 using a single annual dose of DEC plus either albendazole (non-African regions) or ivermectin (Africa). Praziquantel is used for treatment of schistosomiasis.

IV-277. **The answer is B.** *(Chap. 258)* This patient has loiasis caused by the African eye worm *Loa loa*. It is endemic to the rain forests of Central and West Africa. Microfilaria circulate periodically in blood with macrofilaria living in subcutaneous tissues including the subconjunctiva. Loiasis is often asymptomatic in indigenous regions with recognition, as in this case, only with visualized macrofilarial migration. Angioedema and swelling may occur in affected areas. DEC is effective treatment for the macrofilarial and microfilarial stages of disease. Multiple courses may be necessary. Albendazole and ivermectin are effective in reducing microfilarial loads but are not approved by the FDA. There are reports of deaths in patients with heavy loads of microfilaria receiving ivermectin. Terbinafine is the treatment for ringworm. Voriconazole is an antifungal with no activity against worms.

IV-278. **The answer is A.** *(Chap. 259)* Human schistosomiasis is caused by five species of parasitic trematodes. *Schistosoma mansoni, Schistosoma japonicum, Schistosoma mekongi,* and *Schistosoma intercalatum* are intestinal species, whereas *Schistosoma haematobium* is a urinary species. There are reportedly up to 300 million individuals infected with *Schistosoma*. (See Figure IV-278.) *S haematobium* is not seen in South America. All forms of schistosomiasis are initiated by penetration of infective cercariae released from infected snails into fresh water. After entering skin, the schistosome migrates via venous or lymphatic

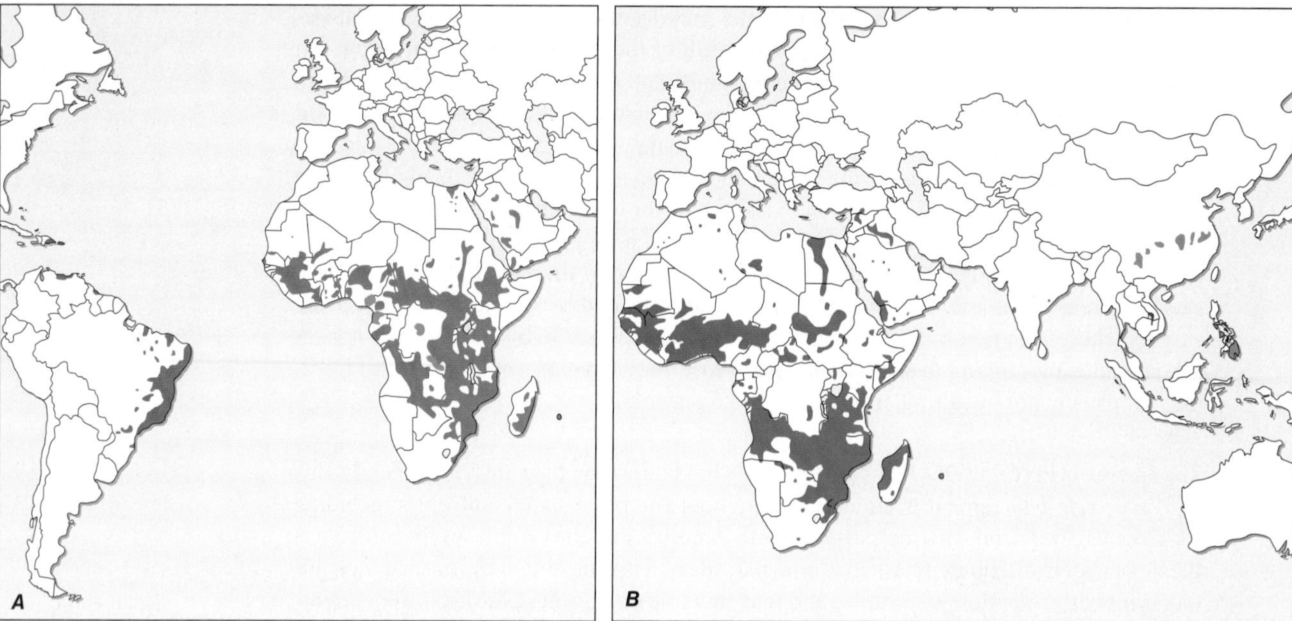

FIGURE IV-278 Global distribution of schistosomiasis. **A.** *Schistosoma mansoni* infection (*dark blue*) is endemic in Africa, the Middle East, South America, and a few Caribbean countries. *S intercalatum* infection (*green*) is endemic in sporadic foci in West and Central Africa. **B.** *S haematobium* infection (*purple*) is endemic in Africa and the Middle East. The major endemic countries for *S japonicum* infection (*green*) are China, the Philippines, and Indonesia. *S mekongi* infection (*red*) is endemic in sporadic foci in Southeast Asia.

vessels to either the intestinal or urinary venous system depending on species. Acute skin infection causes dermatitis (swimmer's itch) within 2–3 days. Katayama fever, acute schistisomal serum sickness related to migration, may develop in 4–8 weeks. Eosinophilia is common in acute infection. This has become a more common global health problem as travelers are exposed while swimming or boating in infected fresh water bodies. Chronic schistosomiasis depends on the species and the location of infection. The intestinal species are responsible for portal hypertension. *S haematobium* causes urinary symptoms and a higher risk of urinary tract carcinoma. There are immunologic tests available to diagnose schistosomiasis, and in some cases, stool or urine examination may be positive.

IV-279. **The answer is D.** *(Chap 259)* This patient has Katayama fever caused by infection with *S mansoni.* Approximately 4–8 weeks after exposure the parasite migrates through the portal and pulmonary circulations. This phase of the illness may be asymptomatic but, in some cases, evokes a hypersensitivity response and a serum sickness–type illness. Eosinophilia is usual. Since there is not a large enteric burden of parasites during this phase of the illness, stool studies may not be positive and serology may be helpful, particularly in patients from nonendemic areas. Praziquantel is the treatment of choice because Katayama fever may progress to include neurologic complications. Praziquantel remains the treatment for most helminthic infections, including schistosomiasis. Chloroquine is used for treatment of malaria; mebendazole for ascariasis, hookworm, trichinosis, and visceral larval migrans; metronidazole for amebiasis, giardiasis, and trichomoniasis; and thiabendazole for *Strongyloides*.

IV-280. **The answer is B.** *(Chap. 259) S mansoni* infection of the liver causes cirrhosis from vascular obstruction resulting from periportal fibrosis but relatively little hepatocellular injury. Hepatosplenomegaly, hypersplenism, and esophageal varices develop quite commonly, and schistosomiasis is usually associated with eosinophilia. Spider nevi, gynecomastia, jaundice, and ascites are observed less commonly than they are in alcoholic and postnecrotic fibrosis.

IV-281. **The answer is B.** *(Chap. 260)* This patient has the new onset of seizures due to neurocysticercosis due to infection with *Taenia solium* (pork tapeworm). The CT scan shows a parenchymal cysticercus with enhancement of the cyst and an internal scolex (*arrow*). The cyst represents larval oncospheres that have migrated to the CNS. Infections that cause human cysticercosis result from ingestion of *T solium* eggs, usually from close contact with a tapeworm carrier who developed intestinal infection for ingestion of undercooked pork. Autoinfection may occur if an individual ingests tapeworm eggs excreted in their own feces. Cysticeri may be found anywhere in the body, but clinical manifestations usually arise from lesions in the CNS, CSF, skeletal muscle, subcutaneous tissue, or eye. Neurologic manifestations are most common including generalized or focal seizures from surrounding inflammation, hydrocephalus from CSF outflow occlusion, or arachnoiditis. As shown in the Table IV-281, neuroradiologic demonstration of a cystic lesion

TABLE IV-281 **Diagnostic Criteria for Human Cysticercosis**[a]

1. Absolute criteria
   a. Demonstration of cysticerci by histologic or microscopic examination of biopsy material
   b. Visualization of the parasite in the eye by funduscopy
   c. Neuroradiologic demonstration of cystic lesions containing a characteristic scolex
2. Major criteria
   a. Neuroradiologic lesions suggestive of neurocysticercosis
   b. Demonstration of antibodies to cysticerci in serum by enzyme-linked immunoelectrotransfer blot
   c. Resolution of intracranial cystic lesions spontaneously or after therapy with albendazole or praziquantel alone
3. Minor criteria
   a. Lesions compatible with neurocysticercosis detected by neuroimaging studies
   b. Clinical manifestations suggestive of neurocysticercosis
   c. Demonstration of antibodies to cysticerci or cysticercal antigen in cerebrospinal fluid by enzyme-linked immunosorbent assay
   d. Evidence of cysticercosis outside the central nervous system (e.g., cigar-shaped soft-tissue calcifications)
4. Epidemiologic criteria
   a. Residence in a cysticercosis-endemic area
   b. Frequent travel to a cysticercosis-endemic area
   c. Household contact with an individual infected with *Taenia solium*

[a]Diagnosis is confirmed by either one absolute criterion or a combination of two major criteria, one minor criterion, and one epidemiologic criterion. A probable diagnosis is supported by the fulfillment of (1) one major criterion plus two minor criteria; (2) one major criterion plus one minor criterion and one epidemiologic criterion; or (3) three minor criteria plus one epidemiologic criterion.
Source: Modified from OH Del Brutto et al: *Neurology* 57:177, 2001.

containing a characteristic scolex is the absolute criterion for diagnosis of cysticercosis. Intestinal infection may be detected by fecal examination for eggs. More sensitive ELISA, PCR, and serologic testing is not currently commercially available. Treatment of neurocysticercosis after neurologic stabilization is with albendazole or praziquantel. Studies have shown faster resolution of clinical and radiologic findings compared with placebo. Initiation of therapy may be associated with worsening symptoms due to inflammation that is treated with glucocorticoids. Intestinal *T solium* infection is treated with a single dose of praziquantel. CNS cystic lesions (but without the visualized scolex) are typical of toxoplasmosis in patients with advanced HIV infection and are treated with pyrimethamine and sulfadiazine. However, in this case, the patient was documented HIV antibody negative and the CT lesion was typical for cysticercosis. Viral testing for HIV would not be helpful because toxoplasmosis is seen in advanced cases, not acute infection. Echocardiography would be indicated for suspected staphylococcal (or other bacterial) endocarditis with systemic embolization.

IV-282. **The answer is B.** *(Chap. 260)* Echinococcosis is usually caused by infection of *Echinococcus granulosus* complex or *Echinococcus multilocularis* transmitted to humans via dog feces. *E granulosus* is found on all continents with high prevalence in China, Central Asia, the Middle East, the Mediterranean region, eastern Africa, and parts of South America. *E multilocularis*, which causes multiloculated invasive lung lesions, is found in Alpine, sub-Arctic, or Arctic regions including Canada, the United States, China, Europe, and Central Asia. Echinococcal cysts, most commonly in liver followed by lung, are typically slowly enlarging and cause symptoms due to space-occupying effects. Cysts are often incidentally discovered on radiologic studies. Compression or leakage into the biliary system may cause symptoms typical for cholelithiasis or cholecystitis. Echinococcal cysts may be characterized by ultrasound. Demonstration of daughter cysts within a larger cyst is pathognomonic. Serodiagnosis may be helpful in questionable cases for diagnosis of *E granulosus*. Patients with liver cysts typically have positive serology in >90% (but not 100%) of cases. Up to 50% of patients with lung cysts may be seronegative. Biopsy is generally not recommended for cysts close to the liver edge due to the risk of leakage. Small cysts may respond to medical therapy with albendazole or praziquantel. Percutaneous aspiration, infusion of scolicidal agent, and reaspiration (PAIR) therapy is recommended for most noncomplex, nonsuperficial cysts. Surgical resection is recommended for complex cysts, superficial cysts with risk of leakage, or cysts involving the biliary system. Albendazole therapy is generally administered before and after PAIR or surgical therapy.

SECTION V

Disorders of the Cardiovascular System

QUESTIONS

DIRECTIONS: Choose the one best response to each question.

V-1. You are appointed as a cardiac epidemiologist advisor on an international committee setting global health policy. Your committee is assigned to predict health trends in a Pacific East Asian nation with a population and environment very similar to China. At this point in history, the nation is just moving from the first classic stage in the epidemiologic transition ("pestilence and famine") to the second classic stage ("receding pandemics"). In regard to the anticipated patterns of cardiovascular disease (CVD) in this nation, which of the following is true?

A. As this nation enters the stage of receding pandemics, you would expect the majority of CVD morbidity and mortality to be due to cardiomyopathies secondary to infectious agents.
B. Each nation or geographical location progresses through the five stages of epidemiologic transition identically in regard to CVD risk.
C. In this nation, when CVD mortality peaks, you would expect stroke mortality to be greater than coronary heart disease mortality.
D. One would expect a very homogeneous epidemiologic pattern of CVD risk throughout this nation over time.
E. You anticipate that CVD mortality will inexorably climb as this nation progresses through the five stages of the epidemiologic transition.

V-2. You are working in a rural health clinic in Northern India. You evaluate an 8-year-old boy who has never seen a physician. His mother tells you that he is unable to keep up with his peers in terms of physical activity. On your initial examination of his skin, you notice clubbing and cyanosis in his feet, but his hands appear normal. Without any further examination, you suspect that he has which of the following congenital abnormalities?

A. Atrial septal defect
B. Dextro-transposition of the great arteries (TGA)
C. Patent ductus arteriosus with secondary pulmonary hypertension
D. Tetralogy of Fallot
E. Ventricular septal defect

V-3. A 55-year-old African American woman with no past medical history presents precipitously to the emergency department with syncope and the electrocardiogram (ECG) noted in Figure V-3A below. You also note painful subcutaneous nodules on her legs (similar to those pictured in Figure V-3B below). You suspect that the cardiac and skin abnormalities are most likely due to:

A. Carney syndrome
B. Hypothyroidism
C. Sarcoidosis
D. Systemic lupus erythematosus
E. Tertiary syphilis

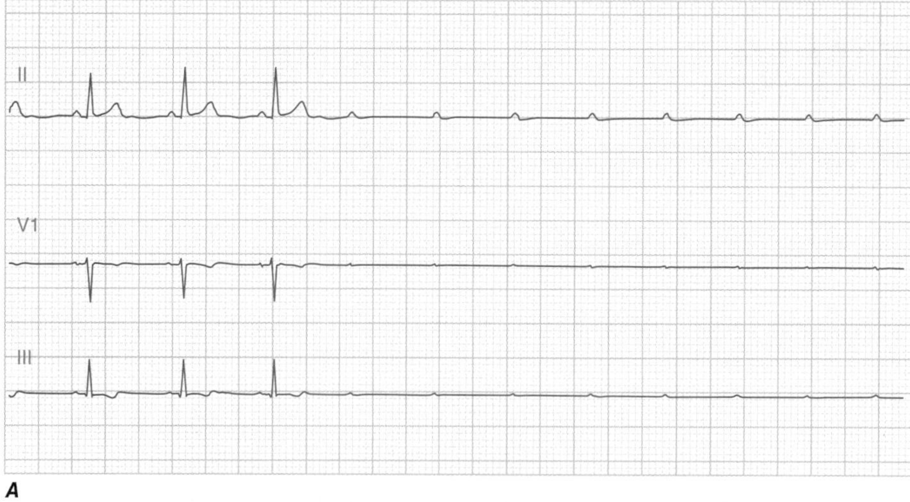

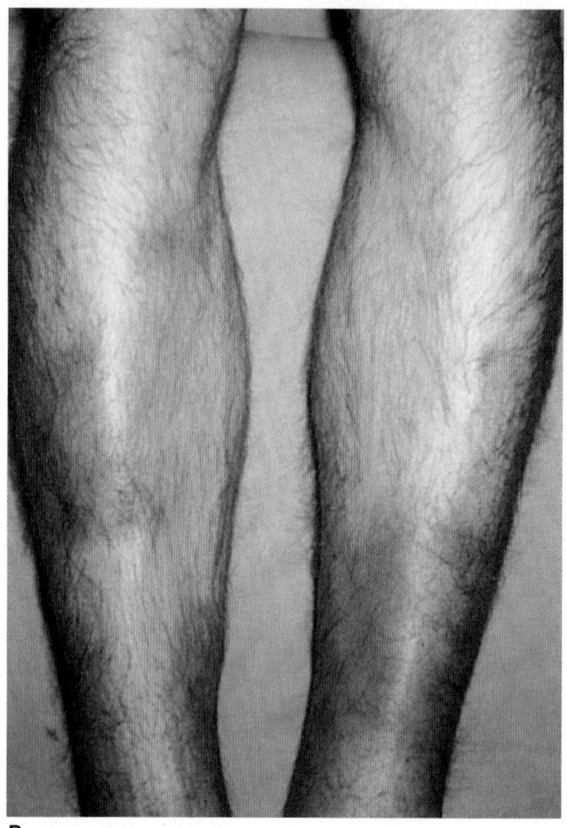

FIGURE V-3 Courtesy of Robert Swerlick, MD; with permission.

V-4. You are evaluating Mr. Estebez, a 67-year-old owner of a wildly successful chain of sushi restaurants. He complains of shortness of breath with exertion, lower extremity edema, and awakening at night feeling acutely short of breath. You wish to assess his volume status, and know that jugular venous pulse (JVP) assessment is the single most important physical examination measurement to aid you in this component of your evaluation. Which of the following statements regarding JVP measurement is true?

A. If done properly, the angle of inclination matters little to the measurement of JVP.
B. In normal patients, the JVP rises with inspiration due to the augmented volume loading of the right heart.
C. Measurement of the elevation of the top of the JVP and the sternal inflection point (angle of Louis) will provide a highly accurate measurement of central venous pressure.
D. The external jugular is preferred over the internal jugular vein due to its ease of visibility.
E. Venous pulsations above the clavicle in the sitting position are abnormal.

V-5. Which of the following statements regarding blood pressure measurements is true?

A. Systolic pressure increases and diastolic pressure decreases when measured in more distal arteries.
B. Systolic leg blood pressures are usually as much as 20 mmHg lower than arm blood pressures.
C. The concept of "white coat hypertension" (blood pressures measured in office or hospital settings significantly higher than in nonclinical settings) has been shown to be a myth.
D. The difference in blood pressure measured in both arms should be less than 20mmHg.
E. Using a blood pressure cuff that is too small will result in a marked underestimation of the true blood pressure.

V-6. A 75-year-old man presents to your emergency department appearing quite ill. His family says he has not had his normal energy for the last 6 months, and they noted he was confused and lethargic for the last day or two. As you take a history from the family, you palpate the patient's radial pulse and notice a regular beat-to-beat variability of pulse amplitude, although his rhythm is regular. Indeed, as you later take his blood pressure, you note that only every other phase I (systolic) Korotkoff sound is audible as the cuff pressure is slowly lowered and that this is independent of the respiratory cycle. Based on this, you suspect this patient has which of the following?

A. Atrial fibrillation
B. Cardiac tamponade
C. Constrictive pericarditis
D. Pulmonary embolism
E. Severe left ventricular dysfunction

V-7. A 78-year-old man is admitted to the intensive care unit with decompensated heart failure. He has longstanding ischemic cardiomyopathy. ECG shows atrial fibrillation and left bundle branch block. Chest radiograph shows cardiomegaly and bilateral alveolar infiltrates with Kerley B lines. Which of the following is least likely to be present on physical examination?

A. Fourth heart sound
B. Irregular heart rate
C. Kussmaul sign
D. Reversed splitting of the second heart sound
E. Third heart sound

V-8. A 24-year-old man is referred to cardiologist after an episode of syncope while playing basketball. He has no recollection of the event, but he was told that he collapsed while running. He awakened lying on the ground and suffered multiple contusions as a result of the fall. He has always been an active individual but recently has developed some chest pain with exertion that has caused him to restrict his activity. His father died at age 44 while rock climbing. He believes his father's cause of death was sudden cardiac death and recalls being told his father had an enlarged heart. On examination, the patient has a III/VI mid-systolic crescendo-decrescendo murmur. His ECG shows evidence of left ventricular hypertrophy. You suspect hypertrophic cardiomyopathy as the cause of the patient's heart disease. Which of the following maneuvers would be expected to cause an increase in the loudness of the murmur?

A. Handgrip exercise
B. Squatting
C. Standing
D. Valsalva maneuver
E. A and B
F. C and D

V-9. A 75-year-old woman with widely metastatic non–small-cell lung cancer is admitted to the intensive care unit with a systolic blood pressure of 73/52 mmHg. She presented complaining of fatigue and worsening dyspnea over the last 3–5 days. Her physical examination shows elevated neck veins. Chest radiograph shows a massive, water bottle–shaped heart shadow and no new pulmonary infiltrates. Which of the following additional findings is most likely present on physical examination?

A. Fall in systolic blood pressure >10 mmHg with inspiration
B. Lack of fall of the jugular venous pressure with inspiration
C. Late diastolic murmur with opening snap
D. Pulsus parvus et tardus
E. Rapid y-descent of jugular venous pressure tracing

V-10. Which of the following statements regarding normal depolarization patterns of the heart is true?

A. Each normal sinus beat is initiated by spontaneous depolarization in the atrioventricular (AV) node.
B. The normal order of depolarization is as follows: sinoatrial (SA) node – atrial myocardium – AV node – His bundle – Purkinje fibers – ventricular myocardium.
C. The right bundle branch bifurcates into an anterior and posterior fascicle.
D. The SA node is unique in its ability to spontaneously depolarize, a quality known as automaticity.
E. Within the ventricular myocardium, depolarization sweeps from epicardium to endocardium.

V-11. All of the following ECG waveforms are matched correctly to the cardiac cycle that they represent EXCEPT:

A. P wave – atrial repolarization
B. PR interval – atrial repolarization
C. QRS complex – ventricular depolarization
D. T wave – ventricular repolarization
E. U wave – ventricular repolarization

V-12. Which of the following mean QRS vectors in the frontal electrocardiographic plane is matched appropriately to its designation?

A. –20 degrees – normal axis
B. –35 degrees – right axis deviation
C. –110 degrees – left axis deviation
D. –80 degrees – extreme axis deviation
E. All of the above are incorrect.

V-13. Which of the following is represented in the ECG shown in Figure V-13?

A. First-degree heart block
B. Left bundle branch block
C. P-pulmonale
D. Right bundle branch block
E. S1Q3T3 (McGinn-White pattern) indicative of right ventricular strain

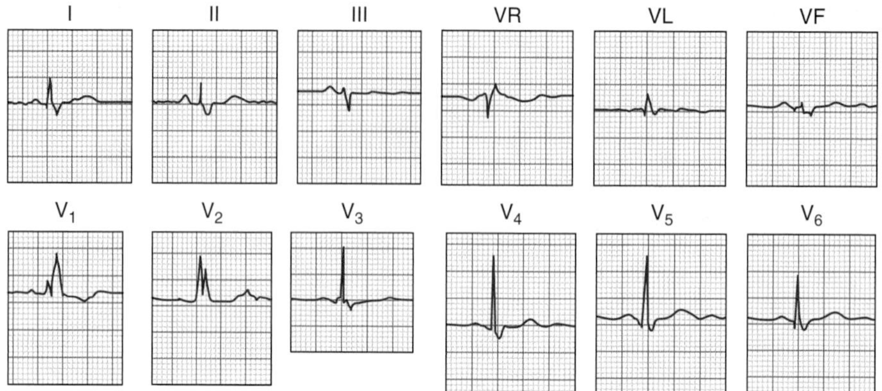

FIGURE V-13 From Fuster V, Walsh R, Harrington R, et al (eds): *Hurst's The Heart*, 13th ed. New York, NY: McGraw-Hill, 2011, Fig. 15-31B.

V-14. Which of the following options describes the primary finding in the ECG shown in Figure V-14?

A. Left ventricular hypertrophy
B. Normal ECG
C. Peaked T waves, possibly hyperkalemia
D. Sinus bradycardia
E. ST elevation in the anterior precordial leads; suspect anterior myocardial ischemia

V-15. A 56-year-old construction worker with hypertension and a prior history of tobacco abuse presents to the emergency department with 30 minutes of acute-onset nausea, dyspnea, and chest pressure. His initial ECG is presented in Figure V-15. All of the following are present in this ECG EXCEPT:

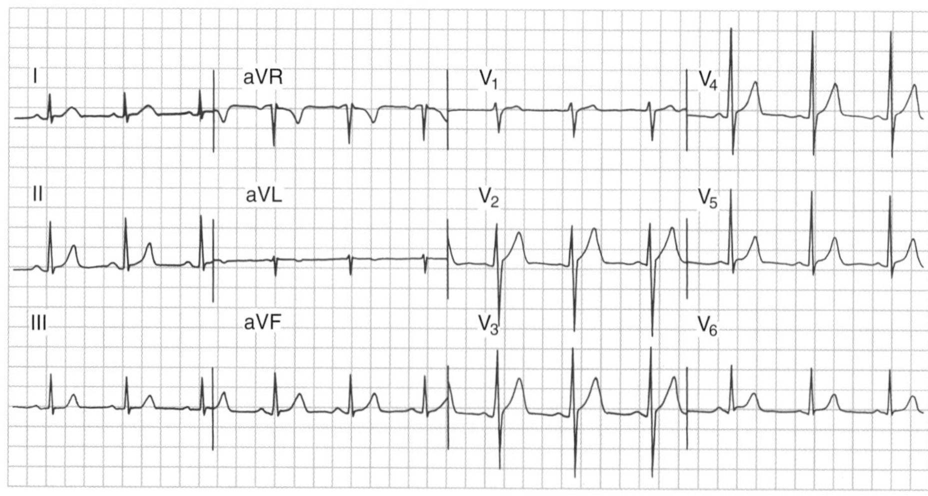

FIGURE V-14

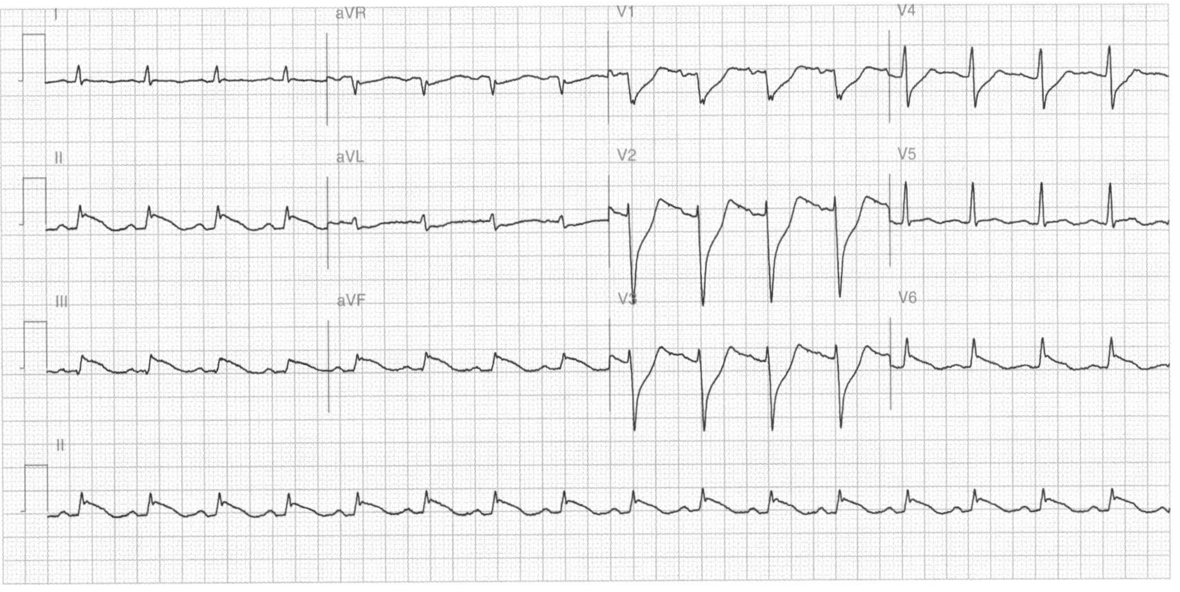

FIGURE V-15

A. Inferior myocardial ischemia
B. P waves
C. Posterior myocardial ischemia
D. Sinus tachycardia
E. Ventricular tachycardia

V-16. In the patient described in Question V-15, which of the following coronary arteries is most likely occluded?

A. First septal perforator
B. Proximal left anterior descending artery
C. Proximal left circumflex artery
D. Proximal left anterior descending and left circumflex arteries
E. Right coronary artery

V-17. A 48-year-old woman visits you in primary care clinic for initial evaluation after moving across the country. You have no past medical records, although she insists they were mailed a week prior. She states that she has had "some heart troubles," but she is not clear on the details. Also, she is on pills for "cholesterol and blood pressure." The initial ECG is shown in Figure V-17. Which of the following statements regarding this ECG is true?

A. It is likely she has suffered a prior myocardial infarction.
B. She is in normal sinus rhythm.
C. The presence of a left bundle branch block on this ECG indicates dyssynchronous mechanical contraction.
D. The presence of premature ventricular contractions and tachycardia is concerning for electrolyte imbalance.
E. The presence of anterior T-wave inversions is concerning in this ECG for acute myocardial ischemia.

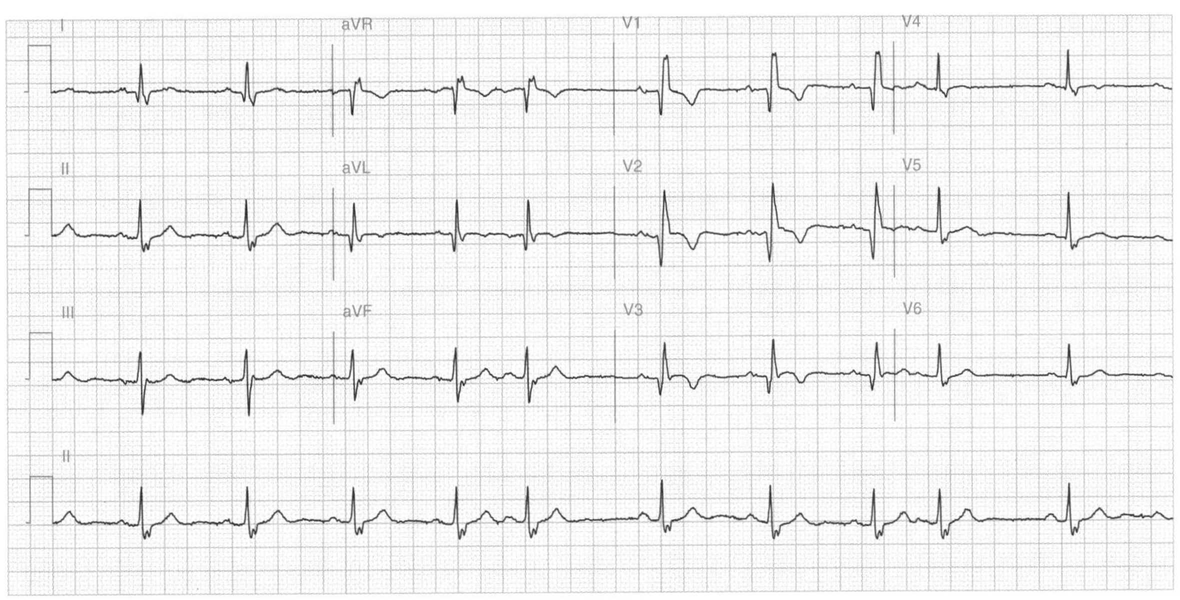

FIGURE V-17

V-18. You are asked to evaluate a 27-year-old internal medicine resident reporting 1 week of cough, coryza, and a low-grade fever. Today, he has developed rapidly escalating chest discomfort while in clinic. He notes that the pain becomes more intense when he takes a deep breath. You perform a standard 12-lead ECG (see Figure V-18). On examination, his blood pressure is normal, he is afebrile, and his jugular venous pulse is not elevated. However, he appears mildly uncomfortable from the chest pain. The next most appropriate step would be which of the following?

A. Administer aspirin, intravenous heparin, sublingual nitroglycerin, and clopidogrel.
B. Emergently obtain transthoracic echocardiogram with possible pericardiocentesis.
C. Emergently perform coronary angiography to evaluate for acute myocardial infarction.
D. Prescribe ibuprofen and colchicine.
E. Refer for treadmill stress test.

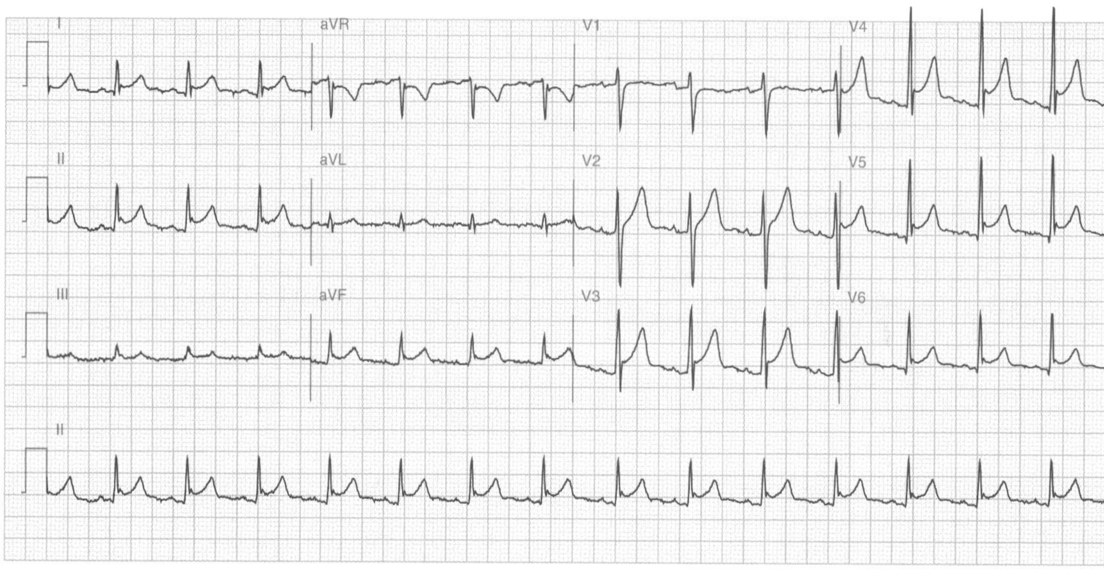

FIGURE V-18

V-19. A large snowstorm hits your area on a Thursday, and the roads are largely impassible until the following Monday. On Monday morning, a 48-year-old man is brought by emergency medical services (EMS) to the emergency department after being found with altered mental status by a neighbor. He is obtunded and unable to provide a history. You note a left brachial artery hemodialysis fistula in place. His initial ECG is shown in Figure V-19. Which of the following electrolyte abnormalities would you expect to find in this patient?

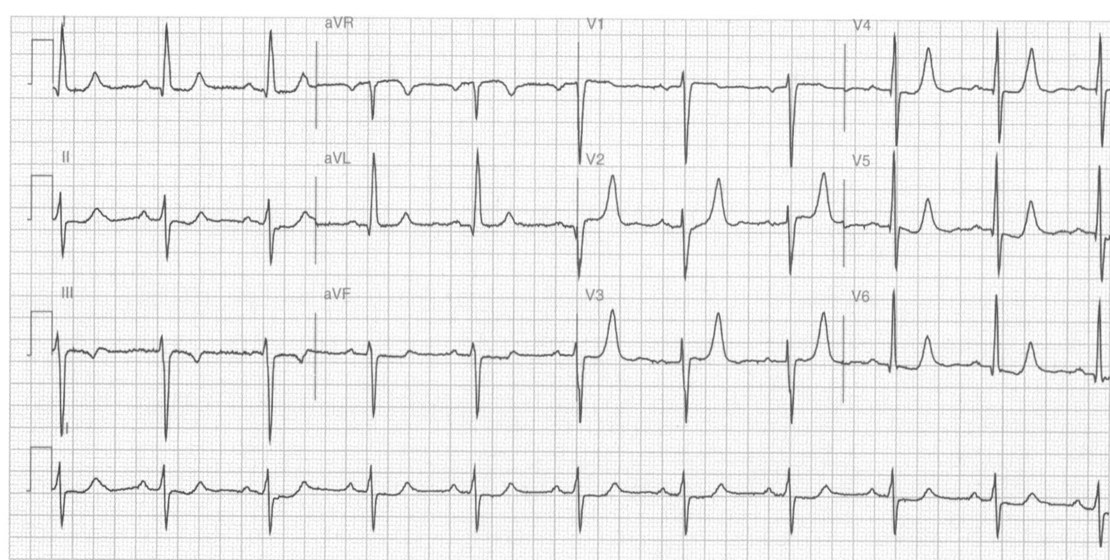

FIGURE V-19

A. Hypercalcemia
B. Hyperkalemia
C. Hypokalemia
D. Hypomagnesemia
E. Hyponatremia

V-20. A 66-year-old man is admitted to the hospital for progressive dyspnea on exertion and fatigue. He has a past medical history of tobacco abuse and is widely traveled, recently returning from a multicountry trip through South America. On presentation, his heart rate is 104 bpm and irregularly irregular. Blood pressure is 96/76 mmHg. You note an elevated jugular venous pulsation and marked lower extremity edema. Echocardiogram reveals a left ventricular ejection fraction of 55%, and still images from his echocardiogram are shown in Figure V-20. To elucidate the etiology of his heart failure, which of the following is the most appropriate diagnostic test to perform next?

A. Bone marrow biopsy
B. Genetic testing for transthyretin mutations
C. Positron emission tomography cardiac stress test
D. Serologies for *Trypanosoma cruzi*
E. Serum and urine protein electrophoresis and light chain assay

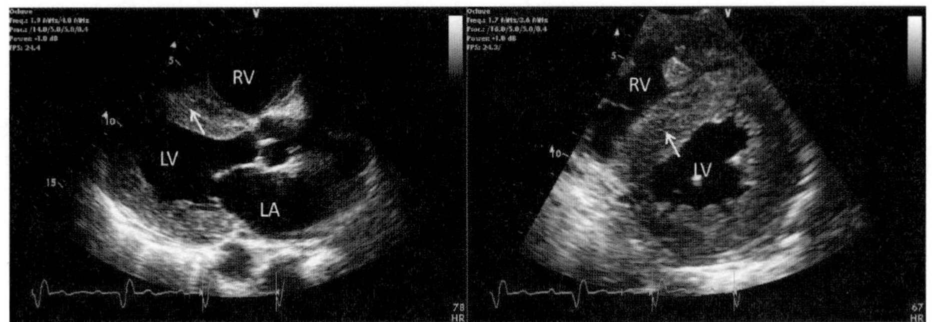

FIGURE V-20 LA, left atrium; LV, left ventricle; RV, right ventricle.

V-21. Mrs. Jackson is a 45-year-old African American woman with a history of tobacco abuse, breast cancer (status: post mastectomy and radiation), and allergy to shellfish. She presented to your general cardiology clinic 2 weeks prior reporting dyspnea while walking up a hill near her house for the past 6 months. She has never had difficulty with this hill before. Along with the dyspnea, she experiences some vague nausea and breaks out in a sweat. Resting ECG and physical examination are both unrevealing. You referred her for an exercise single-photon emission computed tomography (SPECT) myocardial perfusion technetium-99m (^{99m}Tc) sestamibi scan and received the results, pictured in Figure V-21. You quickly assess that her scan shows reversible ischemia. Which arterial territory is most likely involved in the pictured scan?

A. Left anterior descending artery
B. Left circumflex artery
C. Left main coronary artery
D. Posterior descending artery
E. Right coronary artery

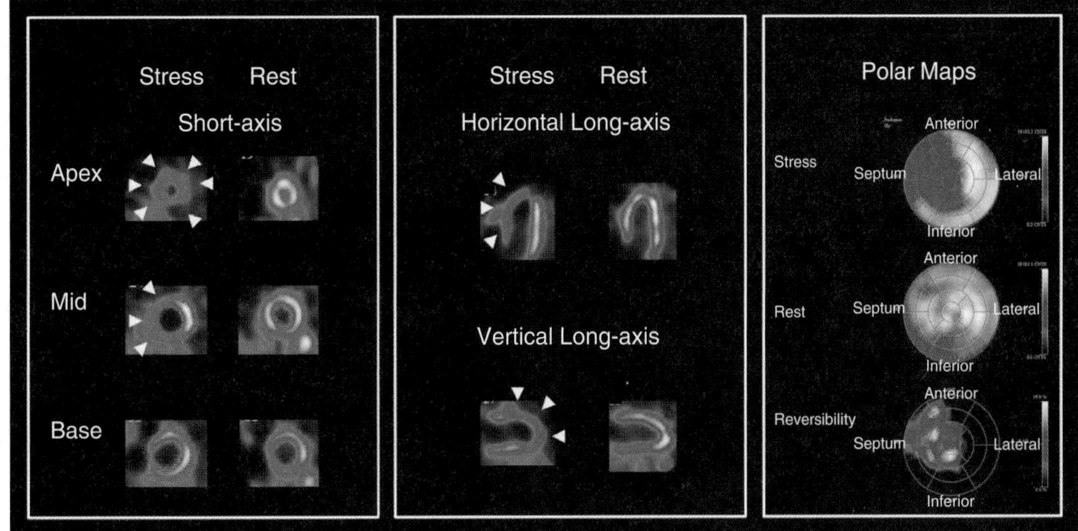

FIGURE V-21

V-22. The SA node serves as the dominant pacemaker of the heart in normal sinus rhythm. What property of SA nodal cells allows it to act at the primary pacemaker?

A. Location near the superior lateral area of the right atrium
B. More numerous intercalated discs of any other myocardial tissue
C. Most rapid phase 0 depolarization
D. Only cells with the ability to spontaneously depolarize
E. Spontaneous depolarization during phase 4 of the action potential at a more rapid rate than any other myocardial cells

V-23. Mr. Hendricks is a 21-year-old sommelier at a well-known restaurant in the city. His primary hobby is competitive bicycle racing, and he has a 150-km race coming up next weekend for which he has been training for the last 6 months. The race coordinators require every competitor to complete a comprehensive cardiovascular assessment prior to competing, and thus he comes to visit your clinic. On your assessment, you note a resting heart rate or 45 bpm with an occasional pause of up to 2 seconds. His blood pressure is 108/72 mmHg. He feels well and reports no syncopal or presyncopal episodes at rest or during exercise. Aside from the bradycardia, you note no other abnormalities on his examination. His ECG shows sinus rhythm with a PR interval of 128 msec, QRS duration of 80 msec, and occasional pauses as long as 2.2 seconds. Which of the following would be appropriate advice for Mr. Hendricks?

A. Perform electrophysiologic evaluation for consideration of a pacemaker.
B. He should not compete in the upcoming race due to concern for bradycardia and will need a tilt-table test.
C. No further follow-up is needed. Good luck with the race!
D. Obtain a 48-hour Holter monitor tracing.
E. He should undergo a treadmill stress ECG to determine the presence of chronotropic competence.

V-24. A 60-year-old man is undergoing an electrophysiology study for evaluation of syncope. After careful venous cannulation and placement of conductance and pacing catheters and after administration of 0.2 mg/kg of propranolol and 0.04 mg/kg of atropine, his heart rate is 65 bpm. After stopping the drugs and allowing adequate time for washout, his superior/lateral right atrium is paced 140 bpm. On cessation of this overdrive pacing, his next sinus beat occurs 1800 msec later. Based on these observations, this patient can be diagnosed with which of the following?

A. Amyloid cardiomyopathy
B. AV nodal disease
C. Paroxysmal atrial fibrillation
D. SA nodal disease
E. Tachy-brady syndrome

V-25. All of the following are reversible causes of SA node dysfunction EXCEPT:

A. Hypothermia
B. Hypothyroidism
C. Increased intracranial pressure
D. Lithium toxicity
E. Radiation therapy

V-26. Which of the following is a risk factor for development of thromboembolism in patients with the tachycardia-bradycardia variant of sick sinus syndrome?

A. Age >50 years
B. Atrial enlargement
C. Diabetes mellitus
D. Prothrombin 20210 mutation
E. None of the above; there is no increased risk of thromboembolism with the tachycardia-bradycardia variant of sick sinus syndrome

V-27. Normal cells within the AV node exhibit a property known as decremental conduction. If you wanted to demonstrate this property during an electrophysiology study, what maneuver could you perform?

A. Pace the right atrium at serially decreasing cycle length and measure the pace-to-His conduction time.
B. Pace the ventricle and record right atrial potentials.
C. Administer atropine 0.04 mg/kg and record AV nodal conduction time by measuring the time it takes an atrial pacing beat to reach the His bundle.
D. Administer metoprolol 10 mg intravenously and record AV nodal conduction time by measuring the time it takes an atrial pacing beat to reach the His bundle.
E. Administer adenosine 12 mg intravenously and record the AV nodal recovery time.

V-28. An 87-year-old man with a history of well-treated hypertension and aortic stenosis has become symptomatic from his aortic stenosis over the last 2 months. Yesterday, he underwent surgical aortic valve replacement with a bioprosthetic 25-mm valve with excellent intraoperative results. He was rapidly weaned from cardiopulmonary bypass and extubated within 24 hours. Per surgical protocol, he had temporary epicardial pacing wires placed on the ventricular surface and has been pacing at 90 bpm. On rounds this morning, you briefly pause his ventricular pacing to check his underlying rhythm. You note an atrial rate of 80 bpm, but a ventricular rate of 32 bpm with a wide QRS complex. There is no relationship between the P waves and QRS complexes. This patient's ventricular bradycardia is most likely due to which of the following?

A. Development of a systemic disease such as sarcoidosis or Lyme disease causing AV node dysfunction
B. Endocarditis of the new aortic bioprosthesis causing AV node block
C. SA node disease
D. Slowed AV nodal recovery after overdrive pacing
E. Surgical injury to the AV node

V-29. Mrs. Hellwig is a 25-year-old woman with systemic lupus erythematosus (SLE) complicated by nephropathy, hemolytic anemia, and pleuritis. Her disease is well controlled on therapy. She recently discovered that she is pregnant, and presents today for prenatal counseling. She specifically is concerned about the effect her autoimmune disease may have on the infant. You tell her that the most common cardiac complication in children born to mothers with SLE is:

A. AV block
B. Coronary artery disease
C. Dilated cardiomyopathy
D. Pulmonary hypertension with right ventricular (RV) failure
E. Sterile, Libman-Sacks endocarditis

V-30. Mr. Hoffman, an 82-year-old former tightrope performer, presents to your office for complaints of syncope. He states that twice in the past week, he has spontaneously passed out with no warning symptoms. Once, he struck his face, and you note that he has periorbital ecchymosis on exam. Other than this, you find nothing abnormal on examination. You request an ECG and step out of the room to begin your documentation. Shortly thereafter, your medical assistant requests your urgent presence in Mr. Hoffman's clinic room. He had another "spell" during the ECG and lost consciousness. Serendipitously, the medical assistant captured the spell on ECG, pictured in Figure V-30. What type of AV block is present and is matched to the appropriate treatment or diagnostic test?

A. Complete SA nodal block – Permanent pacemaker implantation
B. First-degree AV block – Administer atropine
C. Second-degree Mobitz type II SA nodal block – Exercise treadmill study
D. Second-degree Mobitz type I AV block: –No intervention necessary
E. Second-degree Mobitz type II AV node block – Permanent pacemaker implantation

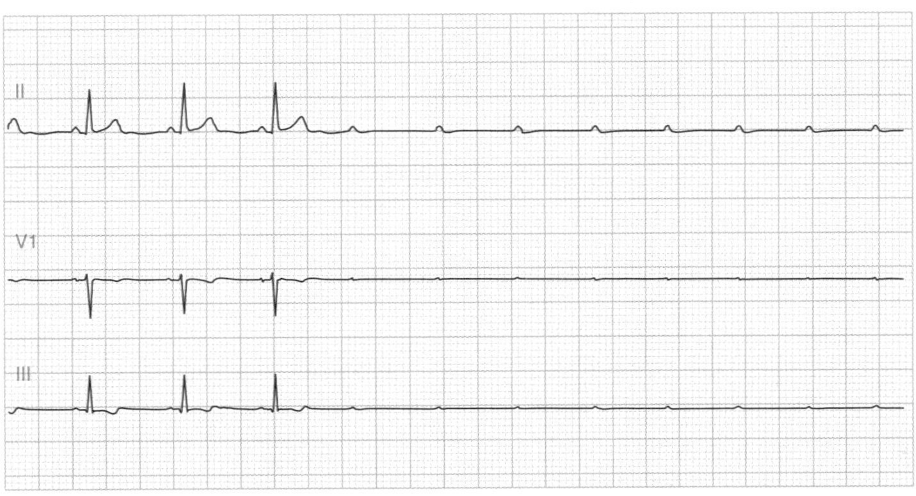

FIGURE V-30

V-31. A 19-year-old long-distance runner, who finished in the top 10 of the local marathon last year, presents for cardiac evaluation after his primary care physician ordered a Holter monitor for screening purposes. On his Holter report, several episodes of second-degree, Mobitz I (Wenckebach) AV block were noted, all occurring during sleep. The patient reports no symptoms but thinks he may have a grandfather who had a pacemaker implanted at an advanced age. What is the most appropriate next step?

A. Exercise treadmill stress ECG
B. Invasive electrophysiology study
C. Reassurance
D. Refer for pacemaker implantation
E. Serologic testing including thyroid-stimulating hormone levels

V-32. A 47-year-old woman with a history of tobacco abuse and ulcerative colitis is evaluated for intermittent palpitations. She reports that for the last 6 months, every 2–4 days she notes a sensation of her heart "flip-flopping" in her chest for approximately 5 minutes. She has not noted any precipitating factors and has not felt light headed or had chest pains with these episodes. Her physical examination is normal. A resting ECG reveals sinus rhythm and no abnormalities. Aside from checking serum electrolytes, which of the following is the most appropriate testing?

A. Abdominal computed tomography (CT) with oral and intravenous (IV) contrast
B. Event monitor
C. Holter monitor
D. Reassurance with no further testing needed
E. Referral for electrophysiology study

V-33. After further testing, the patient in Question V-32 is found to have several episodes of atrial premature contractions. Which of the following statements regarding the dysrhythmia in this patient is true?

A. Atrial premature contractions are less common that ventricular premature contractions on extended ECG monitoring.
B. Echocardiography is indicated to determine if structural heart disease is present.
C. Metoprolol should be initiated for symptom control.
D. The patient should be reassured that this is not a dangerous condition and does not require further evaluation.
E. The patient should undergo stress test to determine if ischemia is present.

V-34. Ms. Milsap is an 18-year-old high school volleyball star with a sports scholarship to the local university. As part of her admission process, she is required to undergo a full medical assessment prior to taking part in collegiate sports. Physical examination reveals no abnormalities, although she reports the rare episode of palpitations and light-headedness. ECG reveals a PR interval of 0.06 msec, QRS duration of 140 msec, and a slurred upstroke or delta wave in the initial part of the QRS. You correctly diagnose this as Wolff-Parkinson-White pattern. Which of the following findings is reassuring that Ms. Milsap will suffer no ill effects or need catheter ablation due to this abnormality?

A. Ability to increase the heart rate to 185 bpm on an exercise treadmill test
B. Electrophysiology study demonstrating that the accessory pathway has both antegrade and retrograde conduction properties
C. Electrophysiology study demonstrating that the accessory pathway is located in the posteroseptal region.
D. Exercise treadmill study demonstrating disappearance of the delta wave and wide QRS at a heart rate of 120 bpm
E. Holter monitoring demonstrating occasional runs of atrial fibrillation

V-35. An 85-year-old woman with no prior cardiac history presents to the emergency department with 2 hours of palpitations. Blood pressure, oxygen saturation, and heart rate are normal, although you note an irregularly irregular rhythm on examination. ECG shows an irregularly irregular, narrow QRS without discernable P waves at a rate of 75 bpm. Echocardiogram reveals no structural heart disease. Despite the normal heart rate, the patient is quite symptomatic with her atrial fibrillation and wants to pursue achievement of sinus rhythm. All of the following interventions may be beneficial EXCEPT:

A. Adenosine intravenously
B. Amiodarone intravenously
C. Direct current cardioversion
D. Dofetilide orally
E. Flecainide orally

V-36. A 79-year-old man with a history of coronary artery disease, ischemic cardiomyopathy with a last left ventricular (LV) ejection fraction of 30%, and hypertension presents to your office with no new complaints. Blood pressure is 108/56 mmHg, heart rate is 88 bpm, and arterial oxygen saturation is 98%. His rhythm strip is shown in Figure V-36. Based on this ECG, the patient now has a definite (class I) indication for which of the following therapies?

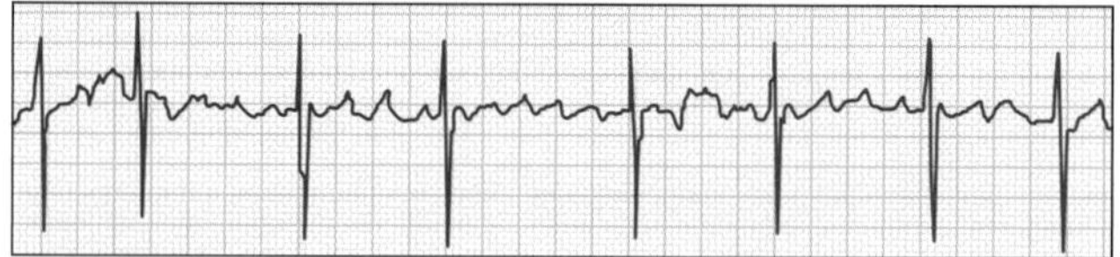

FIGURE V-36

A. Amiodarone 400 mg daily
B. Aspirin 325 mg daily
C. Flecainide 600 mg PRN palpitations
D. Systemic anticoagulation with warfarin or a novel oral anticoagulant
E. Transesophageal echocardiography followed by direct current (DC) cardioversion

V-37. A 43-year-old woman is seen in the emergency department after sudden onset of palpitations 30 minutes prior to her visit. She was seated at her work computer when the symptoms began. Aside from low back pain, she is otherwise healthy. In triage, her heart rate is 178 bpm and blood pressure is 98/56 mmHg with normal oxygen saturation. On physical examination, she has a "frog sign" in her neck and tachycardia but is otherwise normal. ECG shows a narrow complex tachycardia without identifiable P waves. Which of the following is the most appropriate first step to manage her tachycardia?

A. 5 mg metoprolol IV
B. 6 mg adenosine IV
C. 10 mg verapamil IV
D. Carotid sinus massage
E. DC cardioversion using 100 J

V-38. Which of the following statements regarding restoration of sinus rhythm after atrial fibrillation is true?

A. Dofetilide may be safely started as an outpatient.
B. In patients who are treated with pharmacotherapy and are found to be in sinus rhythm, a prolonged Holter monitor should be worn to determine if anticoagulation can be safely stopped.
C. Patients who have pharmacologically maintained sinus rhythm after atrial fibrillation have improved survival compared with patients who are treated with rate control and anticoagulation.
D. Recurrence of atrial fibrillation is uncommon when pharmacotherapy is used to maintain sinus rhythm.

V-39. A 76-year-old woman with a history of hypertension, chronic obstructive pulmonary disease (COPD), diabetes mellitus, and osteoporosis presents to the emergency department after a fall at home followed immediately by intense left hip pain. She was found by a neighbor after several hours. The patient cannot remember if she lost consciousness. She is exquisitely tender to palpation over the left hip, and her leg is shortened and externally rotated. Her mucous membranes are dry, and her skin tents easily. Blood pressure is 170/80 mmHg and heart rate is 130 bpm. Her rhythm strip is shown in Figure V-39. What is the most appropriate first step for her tachycardia?

A. Adenosine 6 mg IV
B. DC cardioversion
C. Digoxin 250 μg IV
D. Metoprolol 5 mg IV
E. Pain control and IV hydration

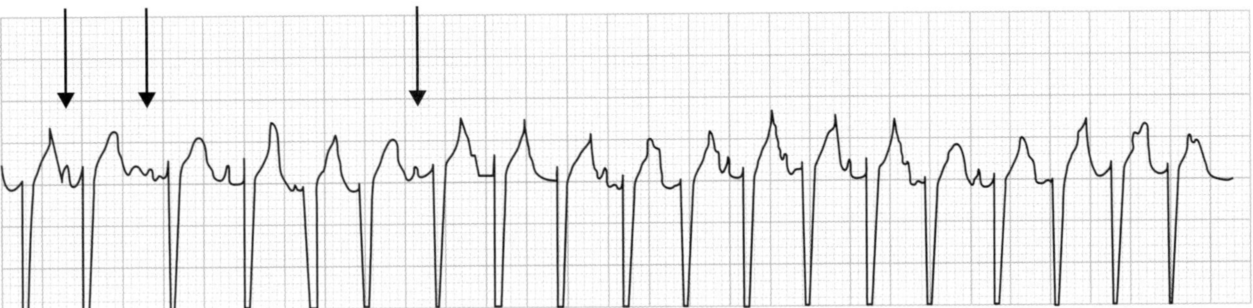

FIGURE V-39

V-40. A young woman is brought to the emergency department after witnesses observed her suddenly lose consciousness while jogging in the nearby park. She has a fractured nose and broken teeth from her fall. She does not have identification. She is nonresponsive to painful stimuli. Blood pressure is 50/palp and heart rate is close to 280 bpm. A 12-lead ECG is shown in Figure V-40. What is the next most appropriate step?

A. Amiodarone 150 mg IV stat
B. Lidocaine 1 mg IV stat
C. Metoprolol 10 mg IV
D. DC defibrillation
E. Emergent CT scan with contrast to evaluate for pulmonary embolism

V-41. What is the underlying rhythm in the patient in Question V-40?

A. Atrial fibrillation with antegrade conduction through an accessory tract
B. Atrial flutter with 1:1 conduction
C. AV reentry tachycardia
D. AV nodal reentry tachycardia
E. Ventricular tachycardia

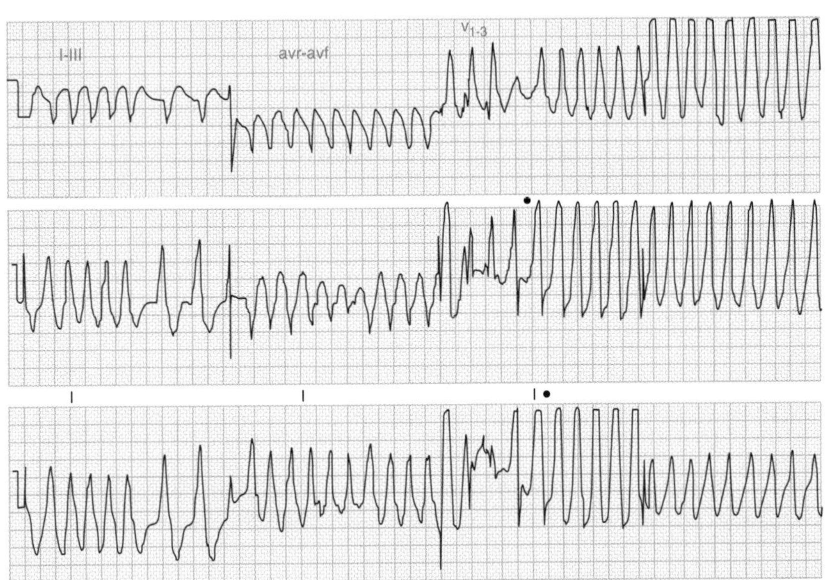

FIGURE V-40

V-42. A 67-year-old man with a history of hypertension and hyperlipidemia presented 3 hours ago to the emergency department with crushing substernal chest pain and dyspnea of acute onset. There, ST elevations were noted in the anterior and lateral leads on his ECG, and thrombolytics were administered. He was admitted to the cardiac intensive care unit. Now, his nurse calls you to his room because he is having unusual tracings on his monitor. A sample rhythm strip recorded from lead V_6 is shown in Figure V-42. What rhythm does this represent?

A. Atrial fibrillation
B. Complete heart block with a junctional escape
C. Idioventricular rhythm
D. Normal sinus rhythm with a left bundle branch block
E. Ventricular tachycardia

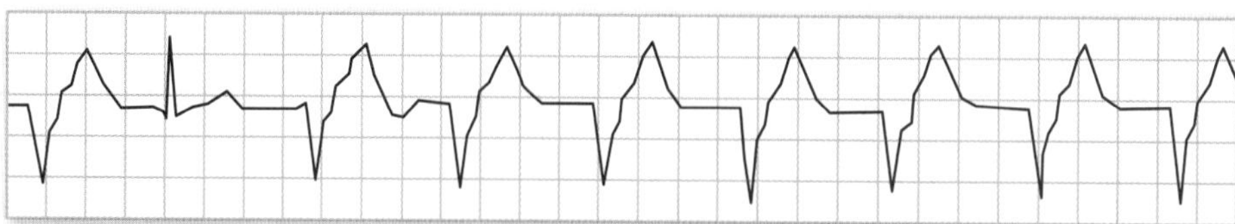

FIGURE V-42

V-43. You are having a quiet shift in the local emergency department. For the past 4 days, there has been a large snowstorm limiting traffic, and people have generally stayed indoors and out of harm's way. Suddenly, the emergency medical personnel arrive with a middle-aged woman who is obtunded. Her downstairs neighbors noted that they had not seen her for the past 4 days (since the snow started) and alerted the police who found her unconscious on her floor. On your assessment, you can barely feel a radial pulse. You note a dialysis fistula graft in her left arm. Blood pressure is 60/palp, and her ECG tracing is shown in Figure V-43. You rapidly set up for defibrillation and request a full chemistry panel. What electrolyte abnormality do you expect to find?

A. Hypercalcemia
B. Hyperkalemia
C. Hypokalemia
D. Hypomagnesemia
E. Hypophosphatemia

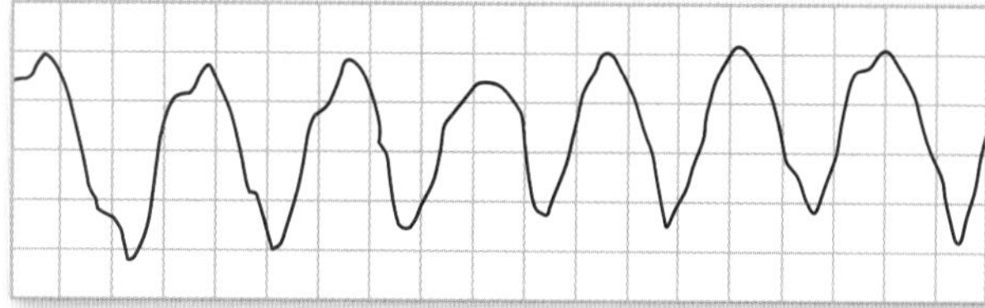

FIGURE V-43

V-44. A 71-year-old woman with ischemic cardiomyopathy and a left ventricular ejection fraction of 38% has been hospitalized for the past week with acute decompensated heart failure. After diuresis and medication optimization, she is feeling immensely better. She is on the maximally tolerated doses of an angiotensin-converting enzyme (ACE) inhibitor, β-blocker, and appropriate diuretic dose. You are planning for discharge today. On rounds, the nurse notes that the patient had several short (5–10 beats) runs of nonsustained ventricular tachycardia (NSVT) and multiple premature ventricular contractions (PVCs) overnight, although she remained asymptomatic. A medical student on the team asks if the NSVT carries any prognostic significance and if any intervention is needed. What is the most appropriate response?

A. "NSVT is common is patients with cardiomyopathy and carries no significance."
B. "NSVT is concerning in this patient. We should suppress the PVCs and NSVT with amiodarone."
C. "NSVT is associated with an increased mortality in patients with heart failure. We will refer her for an automated implantable defibrillator."
D. "NSVT is associated with an increased mortality in patients with heart failure. We should suppress the NSVT with flecainide."
E. "NSVT is associated with an increased mortality in patients with heart failure. However, suppression of PVCs and NSVT with antiarrhythmic drugs does not change this prognosis."

V-45. You are taking care of Mr. Wittstine in the cardiac intensive care unit. He is a 62-year-old man with hypertension, hyperlipidemia, and tobacco abuse who suffered a massive anterior myocardial infarction 4 days prior. He presented late to the emergency department, and thus despite expeditious primary coronary intervention with angioplasty and stent placement to his left anterior descending artery, echocardiogram today shows an ejection fraction of 25%. He has had no ventricular arrhythmias. He still feels slightly short of breath, and your examination reveals bilateral pulmonary rales and an elevated jugular venous pulse. Other than aspirin, clopidogrel, and atorvastatin, he is on no other therapy. All of the following therapies will reduce his mortality over the next 40 days EXCEPT:

A. Automated implantable defibrillator
B. Eplerenone
C. Lisinopril
D. Metoprolol
E. All of the above will reduce Mr. Wittstine's mortality

V-46. A 21-year-old college student who is studying musical education at the local university recently joined a chorus group. However, whenever she stands to sing a solo, she notes the onset of palpitations and light-headedness. While she has never lost consciousness, she occasionally has to sit down due to the dizziness. She presents to your clinic for evaluation. Her physical examination is completely normal, as is her baseline resting ECG. You ask her to sing a solo for the clinic staff and simultaneously record a 12-lead ECG (seen in Figure V-46). Her singing voice is lovely, but she quickly experiences the symptoms and has to stop. You refer her for echocardiography and cardiac MRI, which are both normal. You suspect that the patient's palpitations are due to which of the following?

A. Arrhythmogenic right ventricular dysplasia
B. Brugada syndrome
C. Hypertrophic cardiomyopathy
D. Left ventricular intrafascicular ventricular tachycardia
E. Right ventricular outflow tract ventricular tachycardia

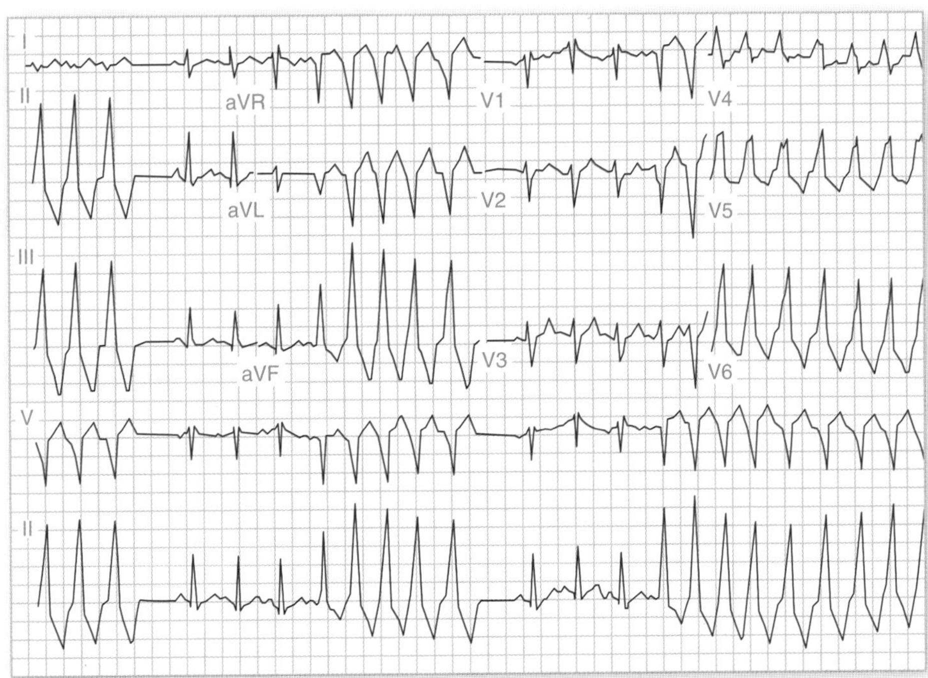

FIGURE V-46

V-47. A 47-year-old woman who is maintained on methadone for a prior history of narcotic abuse recently contracted an upper respiratory tract infection, and her friend offered her some leftover erythromycin pills. Today, she felt multiple episodes of palpitations and light-headedness, prompting presentation to the emergency department. There, rhythm strip demonstrated multiple nonsustained runs of the arrhythmia featured in Figure V-47. You administer 2 mg of IV magnesium sulfate; however, the episodes of nonsustained arrhythmia do not abate. Her laboratory examination shows a normal potassium level. What is the next most appropriate step?

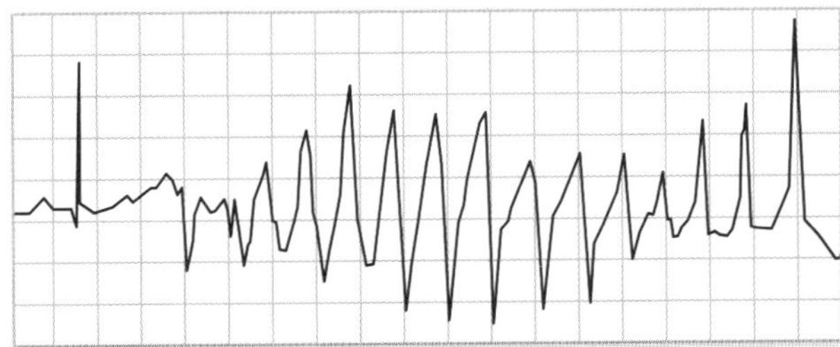

FIGURE V-47

A. Metoprolol 5 mg IV repeatedly until her resting heart rate is 60 bpm
B. Amiodarone 150 mg IV
C. Emergent referral for implantable defibrillator
D. IV isoproterenol infusion titrated to a rate of 100–120 bpm
E. Sedation and defibrillation

V-48. In an ECG with wide complex tachycardia, which of the following clues most strongly supports the diagnosis of ventricular tachycardia?

A. Atrial-ventricular dissociation
B. Classic right bundle branch block pattern
C. Irregularly irregular rhythm with changing QRS complexes
D. QRS duration >120 msec
E. Slowing of rate with carotid sinus massage

V-49. An 18-year-old man with no prior past medical history presents for his required medical assessment before beginning his freshman year at the local university. His history and examination uncover no concerning symptoms or signs. However, his ECG shows an irregular rhythm and is pictured in Figure V-49. What is the most appropriate next step?

A. Echocardiography
B. Electrophysiology study and planned ablation of an ectopic atrial focus
C. Exercise ECG stress test
D. Holter monitor to define arrhythmia burden
E. Reassurance

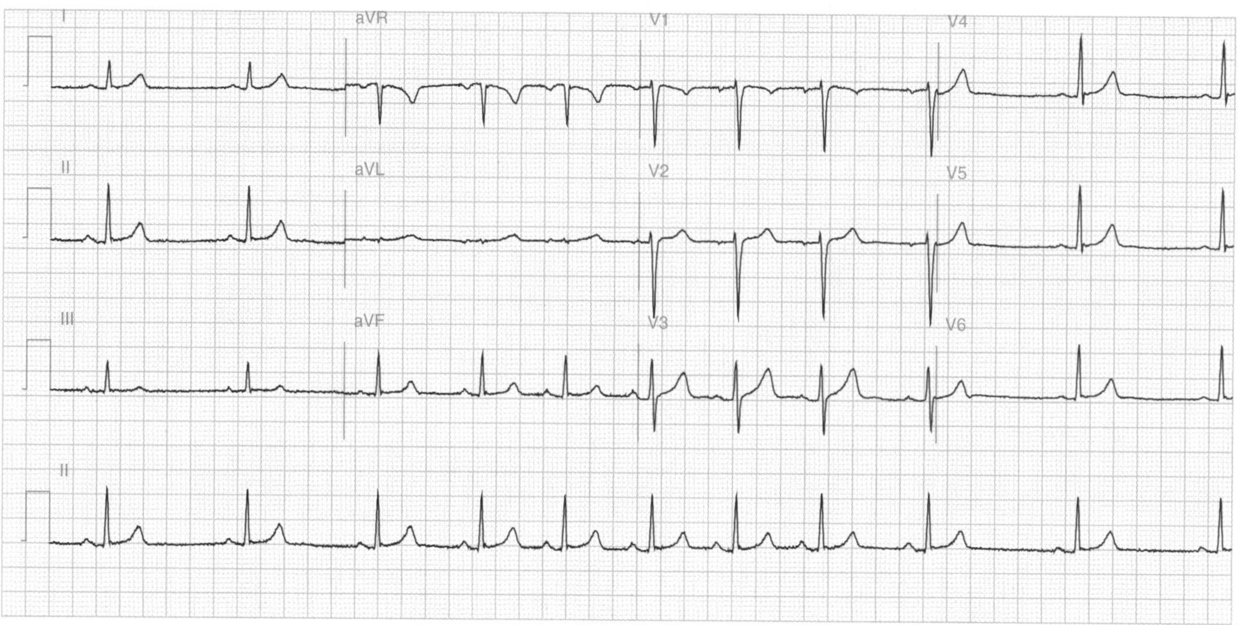

FIGURE V-49

V-50. Ms. Hardy is a 22-year-old triathlete with a history of type 1 diabetes mellitus. Unfortunately, her pharmacy provided her with an expired batch of insulin due to a clerical error, and she presented to the hospital in diabetic ketoacidotic crisis 3 days ago. With aggressive hydration, electrolyte repletion, and insulin administration, her ketoacidotic crisis was reversed. She is feeling much better and is planned for discharge tomorrow. You are called by the monitor station and told that Ms. Hardy is bradycardic. Her ECG is shown in Figure V-50. You check on her and note that she is sleeping soundly. The anatomic location of her heart block is likely where?

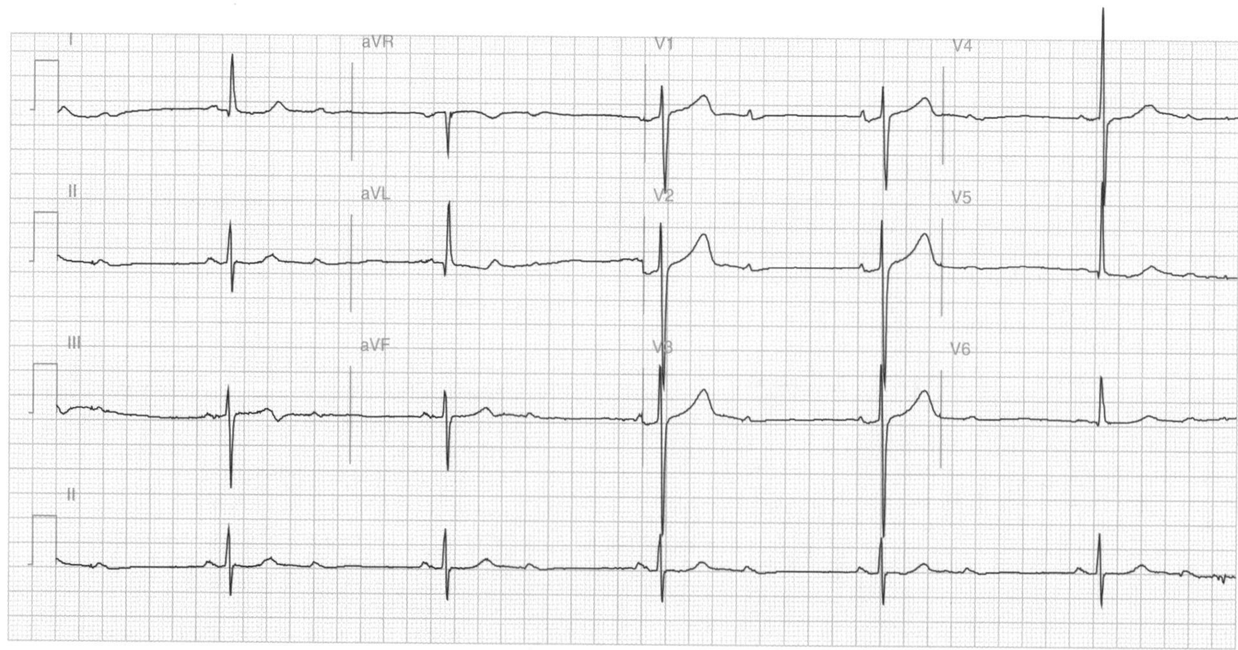

FIGURE V-50

A. AV node
B. Bachmann bundle
C. His bundle
D. Left bundle branch
E. SA node

V-51. If you were to administer atropine intravenously to Ms. Hardy, the patient in Question V-50, you would expect which of the following to occur?

A. Increase sinus rate and maintain 2:1 AV block
B. Increase sinus rate and improve heart block to 1:1 conduction
C. Increase sinus rate and worsen heart block to >2:1
D. No change in sinus rate and worsen heart block to >2:1
E. No change

V-52. An 87-year-old man with Parkinson disease takes levodopa. After running out of his medication and failing to obtain a refill, he presents to the emergency department with a parkinsonian exacerbation. On initial evaluation, he has the ECG shown in Figure V-52. Which of the following is the next most appropriate step?

A. Anticoagulation with IV heparin
B. Check serum thyroid-stimulating hormone (TSH) and obtain targeted respiratory history
C. DC cardioversion
D. Metoprolol 5 mg IV
E. No further testing or intervention

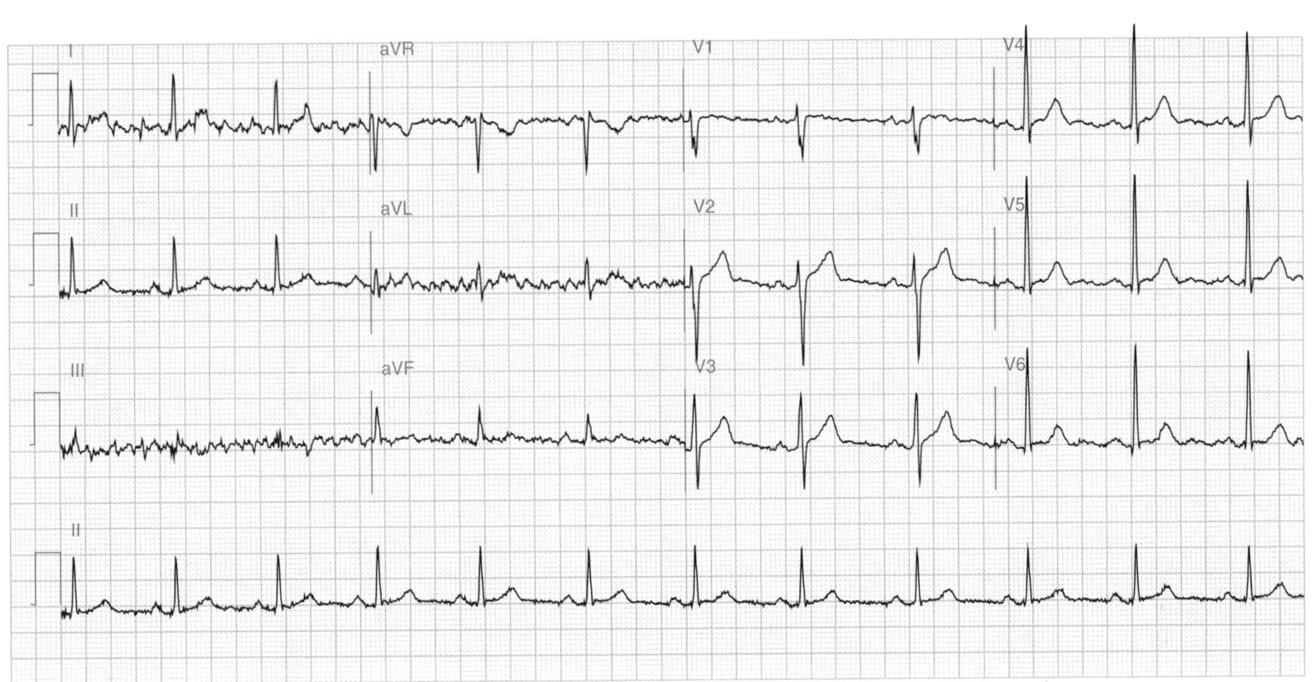

FIGURE V-52

V-53. Mr. Tillman is a 68-year-old man with a history of nonischemic cardiomyopathy, hypertension, and a transient ischemic attach 6 months ago with no obvious cause after appropriate workup. He presents to the emergency department with 5 days of not feeling well. On examination, he appears tired. Blood pressure is 110/78 mmHg, and his heart rate is 150 bpm. His jugular veins are not distended and lungs are clear. His ECG is pictured in Figure V-53. You appropriately administer 5 mg of IV metoprolol twice, which brings his heart rate down to 75 bpm. He feels much better. You consult the cardiac electrophysiologist for consideration of ablation of the etiologic arrhythmia. What is the next most appropriate step?

A. Amiodarone
B. Aspirin
C. Digoxin
D. Furosemide
E. Systemic anticoagulation

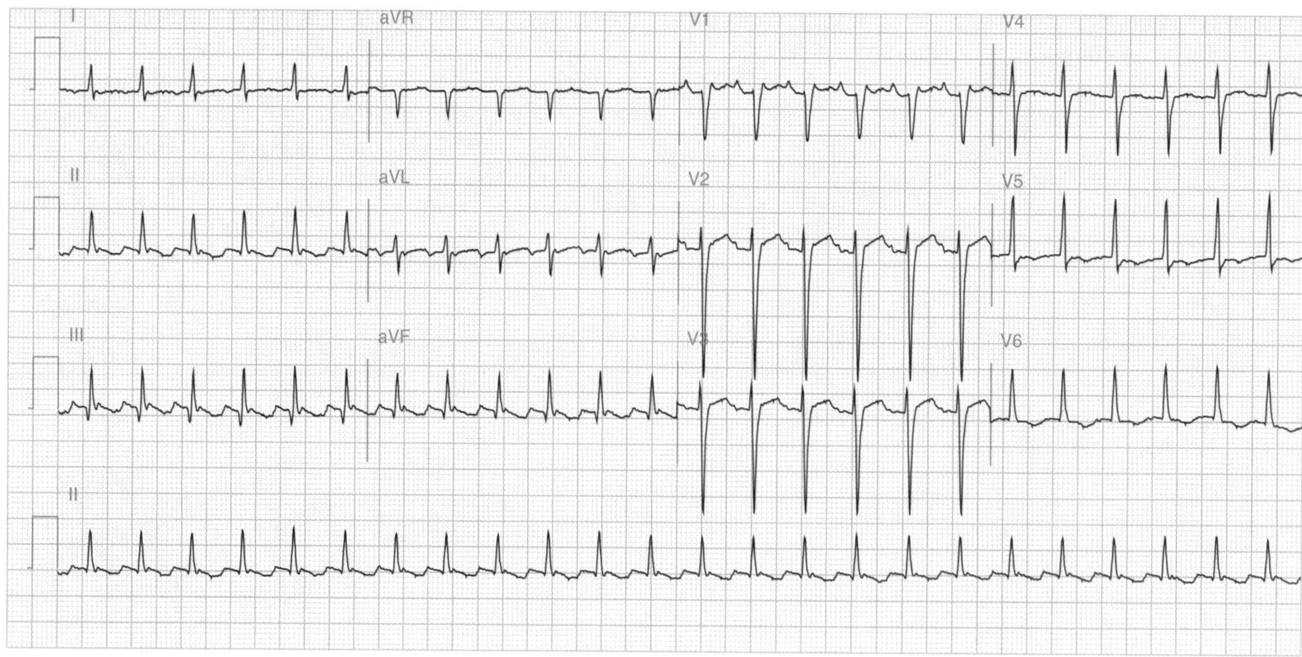

FIGURE V-53

V-54. Ms. Schoop is a 22-year-old pottery store owner who presents to you for evaluation of palpitations. Her ECG is pictured in Figure V-54. She likely has a bypass accessory tract located in the:

A. Anterior septum
B. Anterolateral left ventricle
C. Inferior left ventricle
D. Inferior septum
E. Right ventricle

V-55. A 68-year-old man with a history of myocardial infarction and congestive heart failure is comfortable at rest. However, when walking to his car, he develops dyspnea, fatigue, and sometimes palpitations. He must rest for several minutes before these symptoms resolve. Which of the following is his New York Heart Association classification?

A. Class I
B. Class II
C. Class III
D. Class IV

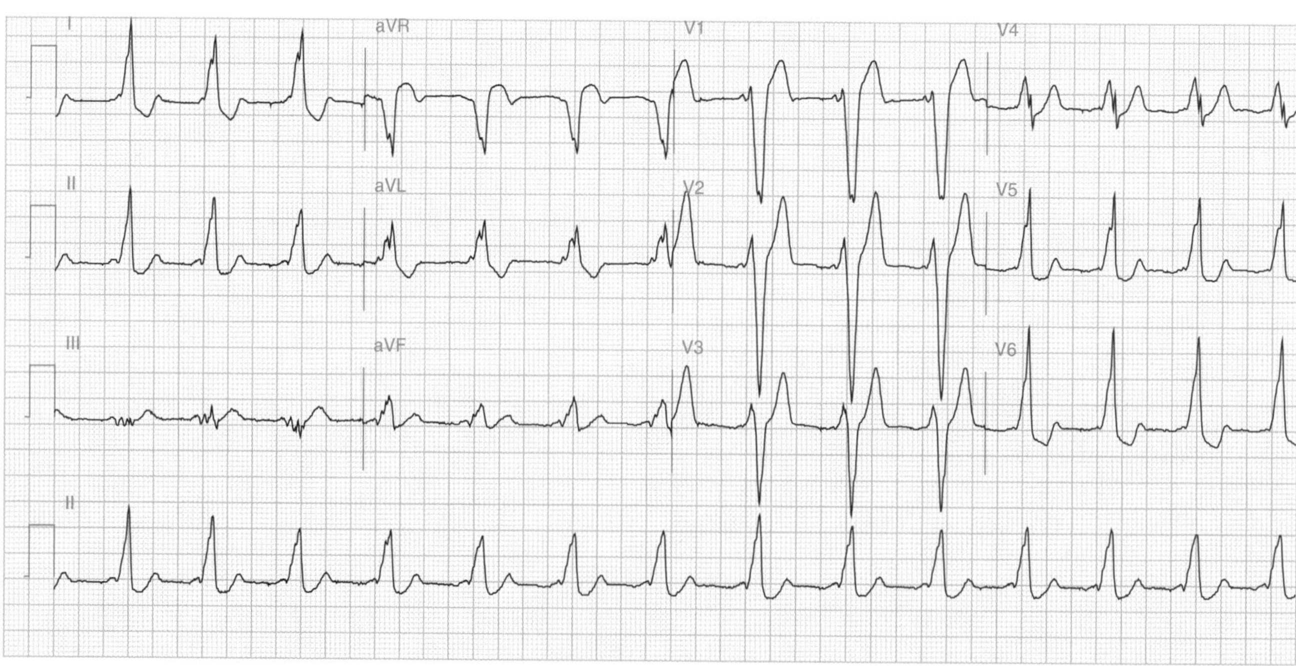

FIGURE V-54

V-56. A 47-year-old postmenopausal woman is seen for onset of severe dyspnea over the last few weeks. She reports no preceding chest pain, cough, sputum, or fever, although she does report leg swelling. Physical examination is notable for a blood pressure of 145/78 mmHg and heart rate of 123 bpm. Exophthalmos is present, as well as bilateral inspiratory crackles occupying approximately one-third of the lower chest with neck vein distention. She has a third heart sound with no murmur. Bilateral lower extremity edema is also present, with warm extremities and a fine hand tremor. Which of the following is the most likely pathophysiologic explanation for her heart failure?

A. Anemia with high-output state
B. Chronic systemic hypertension with resultant left ventricular hypertrophy and nonsystolic heart failure
C. Hemochromatosis with subsequent restrictive cardiomyopathy
D. Myocardial infarction with depressed left ventricular systolic function
E. Thyrotoxicosis with high-output state

V-57. Regarding the epidemiology and prognosis of heart failure, which of the following statements is true?

A. Among patients with heart failure with reduced ejection fraction, coronary artery disease is the most common cause.
B. Anemia is a frequent cause of heart failure among patients with a previously structurally normal heart.
C. Due to advances in medical and device therapy, the prognosis of all patients with heart failure is now excellent, with >90% surviving more than 1 year after diagnosis.
D. Familial, or genetic, cardiomyopathy is quite rare, although it should be screened for aggressively to aid diagnosis and early treatment among presymptomatic affected family members.
E. Heart failure with preserved ejection fraction makes up a minority of the total population of patients with heart failure.

V-58. From a pathophysiologic perspective, all of the following are upregulated in heart failure with reduced ejection fraction EXCEPT:

A. Angiotensin II
B. B-type natriuretic peptide (BNP)
C. Calcium uptake into the sarcoplasmic reticulum
D. Norepinephrine
E. Tumor necrosis factor

V-59. All of the following clinical conditions are associated with orthopnea EXCEPT:

A. Abdominal ascites
B. Abdominal obesity
C. Diaphragmatic weakness
D. Heart failure
E. Hepatopulmonary syndrome

V-60. A 67-year-old man presents to the emergency department with shortness of breath. He is found to have an elevated serum BNP. In addition to heart failure, all of the following may also cause an elevation in BNP EXCEPT:

A. Advanced age
B. Female sex
C. Obesity
D. Pulmonary embolism with right heart strain
E. Renal insufficiency

V-61. You are taking care of a patient with cor pulmonale in the medical intensive care unit. Unfortunately, he suffered a respiratory arrest at home and requires intubation and mechanical ventilation. Currently, with a tidal volume of 500 mL, FiO_2 of 0.4, positive end-expiratory pressure of 20 mmHg, and respiratory rate of 20, his pH is 7.40, PCO_2 is 40 mmHg, and oxygen saturation is 86%. You are concerned about the afterload experienced by his right ventricle. All of the following are likely to increase his right ventricular afterload EXCEPT:

A. Increasing FiO_2 to increase arterial oxygen saturation to 95%
B. Increasing PEEP to 35 mmHg
C. Increasing tidal volume to 750 mL
D. Reducing respiratory rate to 10

V-62. Mr. George is a 52-year-old man with longstanding hypertension and poorly controlled diabetes. He presents complaining of several months of breathlessness with exertion, acute episodes of shortness of breath when recumbent, and lower extremity edema. On examination, he has an elevated jugular venous pulse and an S_4 on auscultation. Echocardiography shows a left ventricular ejection fraction of 55% with a large left atrium. You suspect this patient has the syndrome of heart failure with preserved ejection fraction (HFpEF). Drugs targeting which of the following have convincingly demonstrated mortality reduction for patients with HFpEF?

A. Angiotensin-converting enzyme
B. Angiotensin receptor
C. Phosphodiesterase-5
D. Sodium-potassium-ATPase
E. None of the above

V-63. You are evaluating a 64-year-old woman with a history of nonischemic cardiomyopathy. She presents to the emergency department for shortness of breath. You note that she has gained 11 kg since her last cardiology appointment 2 months ago. Physical examination confirms findings associated with acute decompensated heart failure, including pulmonary rales, elevated jugular venous pulse, abdominal ascites, lower extremity edema, and a square wave blood pressure Valsalva response. Her extremities are warm, and blood pressure is 110/78 mmHg with a heart rate of 75 bpm. Her laboratory studies return with a sodium of 128 mEq/L and creatinine of 2.5 mg/dL (which is increased from her prior level of 1.2 mg/dL). Chest x-ray shows a diffuse alveolar filling pattern consistent with pulmonary edema. What is the next most appropriate step?

A. Administer digoxin 250 μg IV
B. Administer furosemide 40 mg IV
C. Insert a large-bore central IV line and prepare for ultrafiltration
D. Insertion of a pulmonary artery catheter for hemodynamic monitoring
E. Start dobutamine at 5 μg/kg/min and titrate to a urine output of 1 mL/kg/hr

V-64. Which of the following statements regarding nesiritide is true in patients with acute decompensated heart failure requiring invasive hemodynamic monitoring?

A. Nesiritide has no significant effect on blood pressure.
B. Nesiritide improves renal perfusion in states of acute decompensated heart failure.
C. Nesiritide is associated with a decreased rate of rehospitalization, but not death, from acute decompensated heart failure.
D. Nesiritide reduces pulmonary capillary wedge more rapidly than IV nitrates.
E. None of the statements are true.

V-65. Mr. Jones is a 21-year-old man who presents to the emergency department with several days of worsening shortness of breath and lethargy 1 week after a viral upper respiratory tract infection. His family brought him in after he lacked the energy to rise from the couch unassisted. His blood pressure is 88/72 mmHg, heart rate is 115 bpm, and room air oxygen saturation is 90%. Physical examination reveals pulmonary crackles, elevated jugular venous pressure, an audible S_3 gallop, and cool extremities. He is lethargic and slow to respond to questions. Laboratory analysis reveals a creatinine of 2.3 mg/dL, elevated BNP level, and mildly elevated lactate. Bedside echocardiography reveals a left ventricular ejection fraction of 15% with global hypokinesis. You start dobutamine at 5 μg/kg/min and prepare to insert a pulmonary artery catheter for hemodynamic monitoring. Which of the following hemodynamic parameters is most likely increased?

A. Cardiac output
B. Left ventricular stroke work index
C. Mixed venous oxygen saturation
D. Stroke volume
E. Systemic vascular resistance

V-66. Which of the following medications has been shown to reduce mortality in heart failure with reduced ejection fraction?

A. Bucindolol
B. Nebivolol
C. Metoprolol succinate
D. Metoprolol tartrate
E. All of the above

V-67. You are seeing a patient with newly diagnosed nonischemic cardiomyopathy with a left ventricular ejection fraction of 35%. He is euvolemic and New York Heart Association (NYHA) class I in terms of symptoms severity. His blood pressure is 120/78 mmHg, and heart rate is 80 bpm. You know that, eventually, you would like him on optimal doses of a β-blocker and an ACE inhibitor. Which of the following represents the appropriate order of initiation and dose titration of these medications?

A. Co-initiate ACE inhibitor and β-blocker at low dose. Titrate each up every 2–4 weeks to highest tolerated dose.
B. Initiate ACE inhibitor and titrate to highest tolerated dose. Then initiate β-blocker and titrate to highest tolerated dose
C. Initiate ACE inhibitor at low dose. Then initiate β-blocker at low dose. Alternate titrating the dose up for each drug to the highest tolerated dose for both.
D. Initiate β-blocker and titrate to highest tolerated dose. Then initiate ACE inhibitor and titrate to highest tolerated dose
E. The specific strategy does not matter so much as the goal of initiating both ACE inhibitor and β-blocker in a timely manner and titrating both to their optimal, highest tolerated doses.

V-68. You are seeing a 72-year-old woman with a history of ischemic cardiomyopathy and left ventricular ejection fraction of 35%. She is NYHA class II in terms of symptoms. She is on lisinopril 40 mg daily, carvedilol 25 mg twice daily, and spironolactone 25 mg daily. Her blood pressure is 102/82 mmHg, and heart rate is 60 bpm. Which of the following additional medications will further reduce her mortality?

A. Aliskiren
B. Digoxin
C. Ivabradine
D. Valsartan
E. None of the above

V-69. You are following a 57-year-old man who suffered a large anterior myocardial infarction 8 months ago. Despite a late presentation to medical care (>5 hours after chest pain onset), he underwent primary coronary intervention with excellent angiographic result. After that stay in the hospital, he has been followed by you regularly and maintains excellent medication compliance. Today, his heart rate is 65 bpm, and blood pressure is 104/82 mmHg. He looks quite well and reports absolutely no symptoms, even during a recent elk hunting trip requiring long days of hiking up and down hills. His medications are aspirin, clopidogrel, atorvastatin, carvedilol, and valsartan. His ECG shows sinus rhythm, with a right bundle branch block and QRS duration of 135 msec. Echocardiography today shows an ejection fraction of 25% with a large area of anterior dyskinesis consistent with aneurysm. Which of the following therapies is indicated to reduce this patient's mortality?

A. Implantable cardioverter defibrillator
B. Implantable cardioverter defibrillator with cardiac resynchronization capability (coronary sinus lead)
C. Ivabradine
D. Surgical ventricular remodeling
E. None of the above

V-70. You are evaluating a 25-year-old man with a history of nonischemic cardiomyopathy who underwent an orthotopic heart transplant 18 months ago. He has done very well with his course and comes today for a routine visit. You note that his blood pressure is 128/82 mmHg and heart rate is 90 bpm. His ECG appears typical for sinus rhythm with a normal PR interval and P-wave axis. On review of his chart, you note that his resting heart rate has been almost exactly 90 bpm on every visit. He feels fine. Which of the following is the most appropriate next step for his elevated resting heart rate?

A. Exercise treadmill ECG testing to evaluate for chronotropic competence
B. Initiate diltiazem 120 mg twice daily
C. Initiate metoprolol tartrate 25 mg twice daily
D. Reassurance
E. Refer for electrophysiology study to evaluate for ectopic atrial tachycardia

V-71. You are appointed to an advisory position with the government's committee on organ transplantation. The committee chairman is curious about enacting a nationwide organ-sharing strategy for heart transplant, wherein only position on the transplant list and wait time would determine organ allocation order (instead of any geographic concerns). You advise the committee chairman that this strategy is not beneficial because:

A. Blood types are grouped nonrandomly nationally, precluding true nationwide sharing
B. The different regions have highly variable criteria for severity of illness determination
C. The financial structure of reimbursement/payment nationwide would not allow it
D. There is a physiologic limit on "cold ischemic" (time out of body) time for harvested hearts that would preclude nationwide sharing
E. None of the above are true

V-72. A 28-year-old man presents to the emergency department for dyspnea on exertion. He had an orthotopic heart transplant for non-ischemic cardiomyopathy 5 years ago and, in general, has done quite well except for one cytomegalovirus reactivation within the first year. He reports that for the past 3 months, he has noticed that with decreasing amounts of exertion he has been having limiting dyspnea. He is adamant that he is experiencing no chest pain or pressure during these episodes. He has been perfectly compliant with his regimen of tacrolimus, mycophenolate mofetil, and low-dose prednisone. Echocardiography reveals a normal LV function with normal LV wall thickness. His resting ECG shows normal sinus rhythm at a rate of 80 bpm. Which of the following is the most likely cause of his symptoms?

A. Antibody-mediated rejection
B. Cellular rejection
C. Coronary artery disease
D. Endocarditis
E. Medication side effect

V-73. You are seeing Mrs. Block in the heart failure clinic. She is a 68-year-old woman with a past history of diffuse large B-cell lymphoma treated successfully with chemotherapy and eventual bone marrow transplantation 15 years previously. Unfortunately, she suffered chemotherapy-related cardiomyopathy and now has an ejection fraction of 15%. She has been hospitalized four times in the last 6 months with acute decompensated heart failure. She is currently NYHA class III to IV regarding symptoms. Recently, she underwent a cardiopulmonary exercise stress test documenting a peak oxygen consumption of 9 mL/kg/min. She is on optimal medical therapy. At a multidisciplinary transplantation meeting, she was deemed to not be a candidate for orthotopic heart transplantation due to her age and prior malignancy. She asks what other options are available for her, as her number one priority is to live 3 more years to see her grandson graduate high school. Which of the following is an appropriate response?

A. "Continuous infusion of milrinone will improve cardiac function and survival."
B. "A left ventricular assist device can improve quality of life but provides no survival benefit over optimal medical care."
C. "A left ventricular assist device can improve survival over the initial 2–5 years more than optimal medical therapy."
D. "Stem cell implantation has been shown to prolong life in patients with end-stage cardiomyopathy."
E. "There are no other options for prolonging life, and we should consider palliative measures in the future."

V-74. Which of the following statements regarding the epidemiology of congenital heart disease (CHD) in the United States is true?

A. CHD remains extremely rare, complicating 0.1% of all live births.
B. Given advances in surgical techniques and pre- and postnatal care, survival for a neonate with CHD now approaches 90%.
C. Given the declining rates of pregnancy in women with CHD, the incidence of CHD in neonates is declining.
D. The population of adults with CHD is declining given improved prenatal screening efforts.
E. Women with CHD are at no increased risk for complications during pregnancy compared with the normal population.

V-75. A 62-year-old man is being evaluated for mitral valve replacement surgery for severe mitral regurgitation. As part of his evaluation, he undergoes a transesophageal echocardiogram that demonstrates a small jet of right-to-left Doppler flow during systole across the atrial septum. The jet is located roughly in the middle of the septum and occurs when a small flap of tissue swings open <1 mm. There is no diastolic flow, nor is there a visible opening in any part of the septum during diastole. Which of the following explains the finding on echocardiography?

A. Ostium primum atrial septal defect
B. Ostium secundum atrial septal defect
C. Partial anomalous pulmonary venous return
D. Patent foramen ovale
E. Sinus venosus atrial septal defect

V-76. You are evaluating a 21-year-old man in clinic. He occasionally feels tired during his senior year of college but is otherwise asymptomatic. You first saw him 6 weeks ago and noted a harsh, holosystolic murmur at the left lower sternal border that augmented with hand grip. Suspecting a ventricular septal defect (VSD), you referred him for echocardiography, which confirmed your suspicion, visualizing a 5-mm VSD in the muscular interventricular septum. Subsequent right heart catheterization for hemodynamic assessment revealed a mean pulmonary artery pressure of 20 mmHg, pulmonary venous resistance of 2 Wood units, and systemic vascular resistance of 6 Wood units. Through meticulous serial measurements of venous oxygen saturations in the central veins and right heart, you calculate a right heart cardiac output of 7.5 L/min and systemic cardiac output of 6 L/min. Given these findings, you recommend what therapeutic course?

A. Cardiopulmonary exercise testing to define peak oxygen consumption
B. Closure with a percutaneously deployed septal occluder device
C. Consideration of heart and lung transplant
D. No intervention now; annual cardiology assessments and reimaging if any new symptoms emerge
E. Surgical correction via open heart surgery and patch repair

V-77. You are evaluating a 52-year-old patient who presented to the emergency department for chest pain and elevated cardiac enzymes. On auscultation, you can easily hear a superficial, continuous murmur at the mid-sternal level that was never documented before. Echocardiography is limited but is able to visualize all the cardiac valves, which appear completely normal. The patient undergoes a right heart catheterization. The oxygen saturation values are shown below. What is the abnormality accounting for this patient's symptoms?

Superior vena cave	58%
Right atrium	60%
Mid-coronary sinus	91%
Right ventricle	70%
Pulmonary artery	70%

A. Anomalous left coronary artery off the main pulmonary artery
B. Atrial septal defect
C. Coronary arteriovenous fistula to the coronary sinus
D. Patent ductus arteriosus
E. Ventricular septal defect

V-78. Mr. Jenson is a 40-year-old man with a congenital bicuspid aortic valve who you have been seeing for more than a decade. You obtain an echocardiogram every other year to follow the progression of his disease knowing that bicuspid valves often develop stenosis or regurgitation requiring replacement in middle age. Given his specific congenital abnormality, what other anatomic structure is important to follow on his biannual echocardiograms?

A. Aortic root size
B. Left atrial size
C. Pulmonary artery pressures
D. Pulmonic valve function
E. Tricuspid valve regurgitation

V-79. All of the following are classic definitional features of the tetralogy of Fallot EXCEPT:

A. Obstruction to RV outflow
B. Overriding aorta
C. RV hypertrophy
D. Tricuspid atresia
E. Ventricular septal defect

V-80. A 78-year-old man is evaluated for the onset of dyspnea on exertion. He has a long history of tobacco abuse, obesity, and diabetes mellitus. His current medications include metformin, aspirin, and occasional ibuprofen. On physical examination, his peripheral pulses show a delayed peak, and he has a prominent left ventricular heave. He is in a regular rhythm with a IV/VI mid-systolic murmur, loudest at the base of the heart and radiating to the carotid arteries. A fourth heart sound is present. Echocardiography confirms severe aortic stenosis without other valvular lesions. Which of the following most likely contributed to the development of his cardiac lesion?

A. Congenital bicuspid aortic valve
B. Diabetes mellitus
C. Occult rheumatic heart disease
D. Underlying connective tissue disease
E. None of the above

V-81. A 63-year-old man presents with new-onset exertional syncope and is found to have aortic stenosis. In counseling the patient, you tell him that your therapeutic recommendation is based on the observation that untreated patients with his presentation have a predicted average life span of:

A. 5 years
B. 4 years
C. 3 years
D. 2 years
E. 1 year

V-82. Mr. Belliard is an 82-year-old man who you previously followed in clinic. He was last seen 3 years ago, when he noted occasional syncope. Subsequent workup revealed severe calcific aortic stenosis, with an aortic valve area of 0.7 cm^2 and mean gradient of 45 mmHg. At that time, you recommended surgical aortic valve replacement. On the day of his operation, however, Mr. Belliard called to say he really didn't feel quite sick enough to undergo open heart surgery, and he'd be back in touch when he was ready. He missed all subsequent follow-up appointments. Today, he presents to the emergency department after several weeks of lethargy and dyspnea. His blood pressure is 82/68 mmHg and heart rate is 110 bpm, and he has an ECG showing sinus rhythm. His carotid impulse is weak and delayed, and extremities are cool to the touch. You again appreciate an S_4 on auscultation and a III/VI late-peaking systolic murmur. His renal and liver function are now impaired, and urine output is poor. The cardiothoracic surgeon on call defers emergent surgical valve replacement due to his acute renal and hepatic injury. Which of the following would be a reasonable therapeutic option to improve Mr. Belliard's short-term perfusion to permit aortic valve replacement?

A. Atorvastatin 80 mg
B. Digoxin 250 μg IV once and 125 μg orally daily thereafter
C. Metoprolol 5 mg IV serial dosing targeting a resting heart rate of 60–70 bpm
D. Percutaneous aortic balloon valvuloplasty
E. Phenylephrine continuous IV infusion titrated to a mean arterial pressure of >65

V-83. An 85-year-old former lawyer presents with several months of accelerating dyspnea on exertion and lower extremity edema. On examination, you note a laterally displaced point of maximal impulse (PMI) and an S_4 gallop. She has a III/VI systolic murmur at the base radiating to the carotid arteries. Transthoracic echocardiogram reveals a left ventricular ejection fraction of 25% with global hypokinesis. Calculated aortic valve area is 0. 8cm^2 and mean gradient is 25 mmHg. What is the next most reasonable step to determine whether this patient would benefit from aortic valve replacement?

A. Cardiac magnetic resonance imaging (MRI) to evaluate ventricular scar and aortic valve morphology
B. Cardiac positron emission tomography (PET) to determine ventricular viability
C. Coronary angiography to evaluate for the presence of obstructive coronary disease
D. Dobutamine stress echocardiography
E. Right heart catheterization to document cardiac output and filling pressures

V-84. Which of the following parameters is typically reduced in chronic severe aortic regurgitation?

A. Diastolic blood pressure
B. Left ventricular afterload
C. Left ventricular diameter
D. Left ventricular preload
E. Total left ventricular stroke volume

V-85. You are caring for a new admission to the cardiac intensive care unit, a 21-year-old woman with connective tissue disease. She presented with acute shortness of breath and a chest x-ray showing diffuse pulmonary edema. Physical examination revealed a soft, short early diastolic murmur at the right upper sternal border, and emergent echocardiography showed severe aortic regurgitation with an avulsed right coronary cusp. CT chest imaging showed no aortic dissection. On arrival to the coronary care unit, she is intubated and sedated. Blood pressure is 110/50 mmHg, and heart rate is 115 bpm. Her urine output is poor, and extremities are cool. The cardiothoracic surgical team is tied up in a heart transplant and won't be able to take this patient for at least 4 more hours. What intervention is most likely to help maintain her end-organ perfusion until surgical intervention?

A. Esmolol continuous IV infusion titrated to a heart rate of 60–70 bpm
B. Intra-aortic balloon pump
C. IV nitroprusside
D. IV norepinephrine
E. IV vasopressin

V-86. What is the most common cause of obstruction to left ventricular inflow?

A. Congenital mitral valve disease
B. Cor triatriatum
C. Infective endocarditis with large mitral valve vegetations
D. Mitral annular calcification
E. Rheumatic mitral disease

V-87. In cases of severe mitral stenosis, which of the following parameters is typically increased?

A. Cardiac output
B. Left atrial pressure
C. Left ventricular diameter
D. Left ventricular end-diastolic pressure
E. Pulmonary vascular compliance

V-88. You are caring for a 42-year-old woman with a prior history of rheumatic fever and resultant mitral stenosis. Her valvular disease is currently moderate. You know that mitral stenosis causes an elevation in left atrial pressure, which over time can cause cardiogenic pulmonary edema and pulmonary hypertension. All of the following will result in an elevation of left atrial pressure and potential worsening of lung function EXCEPT:

A. Anemia
B. Isoproterenol
C. Metoprolol
D. Pregnancy
E. Running on a treadmill

V-89. Mrs. Bream presents to the emergency department with acute worsening of shortness of breath. She is an 84-year-old woman with severe mitral stenosis who is scheduled for percutaneous mitral balloon valvotomy in 3 days. However, today while cooking chicken salad, she noted the onset of overwhelming weakness and dyspnea. On evaluation, she appears dyspneic and in mild distress. Oxygen saturation on room air is 91%, heart rate is 55 bpm, and blood pressure is 110/80 mmHg. She has rales to the mid-lung fields bilaterally. You note that her rhythm is irregularly irregular, and ECG confirms the new onset of atrial fibrillation. You suspect that she has a very high left atrial pressure causing pulmonary edema. All of the following therapeutic interventions will help lower her left atrial pressure EXCEPT:

A. IV furosemide
B. Percutaneous balloon mitral valvotomy
C. Synchronized DC cardioversion
D. Transvenous pacemaker placement and pacing at a heart rate of 90 bpm
E. All of the above will help lower left atrial pressure

V-90. A 34-year-old man with rheumatic mitral stenosis is referred to you for evaluation. He enjoys playing recreational soccer and has no limitations or symptoms. His heart rate is 65 bpm at rest. Transthoracic echocardiogram reveals a normal LV size and function, a moderately dilated left atrium, a mitral valve area of 1.7 cm^2, and relatively thin noncalcified leaflets. ECG shows left atrial enlargement and sinus rhythm. On exercise stress testing, his calculated pulmonary artery systolic pressure at peak exercise is 40 mmHg. Which of the following treatment plans do you recommend?

A. Metoprolol 25 mg orally twice daily
B. Percutaneous mitral balloon valvotomy
C. Periodic cardiology assessments and echocardiographic monitoring
D. Sildenafil 20 mg twice daily
E. Surgical mitral valve replacement

V-91. You are evaluating a 65-year-old man who has a 15-year history of nonischemic cardiomyopathy with a dilated left ventricle and an ejection fraction of 15%. Yearly echocardiograms over the past 5 years have shown severe mitral regurgitation. On optimal medical therapy, the patient has NYHA class II symptoms. Today, he specifically asks whether his valve should be fixed in order to improve his survival. You should tell him:

A. "If you were to have high pulmonary artery pressures or develop new atrial fibrillation, we would move forward with valve repair."
B. "In patients like you, valve repair has never been shown to improve survival"
C. "We should consider valve surgery only if repair is possible. Replacement would not improve your survival."
D. "While surgical methods have not shown survival benefit, percutaneous mitral valve repair has been shown to reduce mortality in patients like you."
E. "Yes, your valve should have been fixed years ago."

V-92. You are performing a right and left heart catheterization on a patient with stenosis involving two valves. Which two valves are involved based on the pressure readings listed below?

Right atrium	15 mmHg
Right ventricle	25/6 mmHg
Pulmonary artery	25/12 mmHg
Pulmonary arterial wedge pressure	12 mmHg
Left ventricle	105/6 mmHg
Aorta	105/75 mmHg

A. Aortic and mitral
B. Aortic and tricuspid
C. Mitral and pulmonic
D. Mitral and tricuspid
E. Pulmonic and tricuspid

V-93. You are evaluating a 50-year-old woman with idiopathic pulmonary arterial hypertension. Her last transthoracic echocardiogram noted severe tricuspid regurgitation in addition to a dilated hypokinetic right ventricle and estimated pulmonary artery systolic pressures exceeding 70 mmHg. On your exam, she has lower extremity edema, hepatomegaly with a pulsatile liver, jugular venous pulse elevated to the mandible with marked c-v waves and a prominent y descent, and an RV heave. She reports breathlessness with moderate exertion. What is the best treatment for her severe tricuspid regurgitation?

A. Diuretics and salt restriction accompanied by medical therapy targeting her elevated pulmonary artery pressures
B. Percutaneous balloon valvotomy
C. Percutaneous tricuspid valve repair
D. Surgical mitral valve replacement
E. Surgical tricuspid valve repair

V-94. You are seeing a 21-year-old woman for the first time today in the primary care clinic. She has never seen a physician before because her parents did not believe in Western medicine. On history, she states that she feels tired occasionally and feels like she could not quite keep up with her peers in college physical education classes. On examination, you note a systolic murmur in the left second interspace preceded by a presystolic click. Transthoracic echocardiogram confirms the presence of pulmonic stenosis with a peak gradient of 60 mmHg and doming of the pulmonic valve without any pulmonic regurgitation. What is her best treatment option?

A. Diuretics and salt restriction
B. No therapy needed
C. Percutaneous balloon valvotomy
D. Percutaneous pulmonic valve replacement
E. Surgical pulmonic valve replacement

V-95. You are taking care of a 77-year-old patient with severe aortic stenosis in the cardiac intensive care unit. Surgical aortic valve replacement is planned for tomorrow. However, suddenly, he becomes severely short of breath and manifests signs of acute pulmonary edema. On auscultation, you can now appreciate a soft, short apical systolic murmur (in addition to his previously appreciated murmur of aortic stenosis) that was not present previously. You suspect that he has suffered a ruptured mitral valve chordae and now has severe, acute mitral regurgitation. Which of the following parameters will likely increase due to his new severe mitral regurgitation?

A. Aortic valve gradient
B. Calculated aortic valve area
C. Effective stroke volume
D. Ejection fraction
E. Left ventricular afterload

V-96. Mr. Milsap is one of your longstanding clinic patients who has a history of rheumatic heart disease. His last echocardiogram noted a mean mitral valve gradient of 11 mmHg with a calculated valve area of 1.3 cm^2 at a heart rate of 60 bpm. He presents today complaining of worsening shortness of breath, and his ECG shows atrial fibrillation at a rate of 60 bpm. He has never had any bleeding episodes and had normal hematologic counts on his last check 2 weeks earlier. Which of the following options for thromboembolic prophylaxis is appropriate?

A. Apixaban
B. Dabigatran
C. Rivaroxaban
D. Warfarin
E. More information is needed prior to initiating thromboembolic prophylaxis.

V-97. All of the following are risk factors for development of peripartum cardiomyopathy EXCEPT:

A. Advanced maternal age
B. Malnutrition
C. Primiparous
D. Twin pregnancy
E. Use of tocolytics

V-98. You are evaluating a new patient in clinic. The 25-year-old patient was diagnosed with "heart failure" in another state and has since relocated. He has NYHA class II symptoms and denies angina. He presents for evaluation and management. On review of systems, the patient has been wheelchair bound for many years and has severe scoliosis. He has no family history of hyperlipidemia. His physical examination is notable for bilateral lung crackles, an S_3, and no cyanosis. An ECG is obtained in clinic and shows tall R waves in V_1 and V_2 with deep Qs in V_5 and V_6. An echocardiogram reports severe global left ventricular dysfunction with reduced ejection fraction. What is the most likely diagnosis?

A. Amyotrophic lateral sclerosis
B. Atrial septal defect
C. Chronic thromboembolic disease
D. Duchenne muscular dystrophy
E. Ischemic cardiomyopathy

V-99. Which of the following is the most common inheritance pattern for familial cardiomyopathies?

A. Autosomal dominant driven by exon duplication
B. Autosomal dominant driven by missense mutations
C. Autosomal recessive driven by exon deletion
D. Autosomal recessive driven by exon duplication
E. X-linked driven by exon deletion

V-100. A 45-year-old man with a history of obesity presents to the emergency department with dyspnea, fatigue, and a nocturnal cough that has been worsening for the past several months. He denies any chest pain or pressure at rest or with exertion. On evaluation, he has evidence of cardiomegaly with a displaced PMI and elevated filling pressures with bilateral pulmonary rales and elevated jugular venous pulse. Echocardiography reveals a globally depressed left ventricular ejection fraction of 25% with a dilated left ventricle. Which of the following tests is a Level I recommendation for further workup?

A. Cardiac MRI
B. Coronary angiography
C. Erythrocyte sedimentation rate
D. Serum iron and transferrin saturation
E. Thyroid-stimulating hormone level

V-101. A 22-year-old college student with no past medical history was seen in the urgent care clinic 3 days ago for coryza, myalgias, cough, and fever, which was typical of the viral upper respiratory illness making its way through the campus. He was given a cough suppressant and antipyretics and advised to remain hydrated. Today, he presents to the emergency department with lethargy and fatigue. He is obtunded with a heart rate of 120 bpm and blood pressure of 78/62 mmHg. His extremities are cool, and jugular venous pulse is elevated nearly to the mandible. Precordial auscultation reveals very quiet heart sounds, an S_3 gallop, and a soft murmur of mitral regurgitation. Emergent transthoracic echocardiogram shows no pericardial effusion, a nondilated left ventricle with an ejection fraction of 30%, and mild mitral regurgitation. Endomyocardial biopsy shows lymphocytic myocarditis. Which of the following statements regarding this patient's prognosis and implications for therapy are true?

A. His chance of survival is <10% without cardiac transplantation. Emergent transplant listing is warranted.
B. His chance of survival is >50%, with many similar patients having a full recovery in left ventricular function over the ensuing weeks to months. Aggressive pharmacologic and mechanical hemodynamic support is warranted.
C. Immunosuppression with high-dose systemic steroids will increase his chance of survival.
D. The presence and titer of anti-heart antibodies can help provide prognostic information for this patient.

V-102. You are evaluating a 42-year-old woman with a history of Hashimoto thyroiditis many years ago who was treated successfully with radioactive iodine. She presents to the emergency department after passing out at home and reports several days of worsening lethargy and chest discomfort. She is short of breath, with a resting heart rate of 110 bpm and blood pressure of 77/62 mmHg. Her extremities are cool, and she seems sleepy. Her whole blood lactate is elevated, and urine output for the first 2 hours of her stay is minimal. On cardiac monitor, she repeatedly has salvos of nonsustained ventricular tachycardia. Echocardiogram reveals a left ventricular ejection fraction of 15%, and emergent endomyocardial biopsy shows diffuse granulomatous lesions surrounded by extensive inflammatory infiltrate. Which of the following statements is true regarding her diagnosis?

A. Most patients with this etiology of cardiomyopathy recover with supportive care.
B. Steroids are highly effective in treating this form of cardiomyopathy.
C. The course of this cardiomyopathy is dire, often with rapid deterioration requiring urgent transplantation.
D. While seen occasionally, ventricular tachyarrhythmias are rare in this disease.
E. None of the above is true.

V-103. All of the following are associated with an elevated risk for development of cardiomyopathy during anthracycline chemotherapy EXCEPT:

A. Concomitant chest radiation
B. High total anthracycline dose
C. Preexisting cardiac disease
D. Trastuzumab administration
E. All of the above are associated with elevated risk of cardiomyopathy due to anthracyclines.

V-104. Mr. Kia is a 32-year-old bass guitarist with no past medical history. He presents with chest pain after suffering coryza, cough, fever, and muscle aches for the past week. He describes his pain as constant and radiating to his left shoulder. It is exacerbated by lying flat and during deep breaths. Examination reveals a rasping extracardiac sound present in three components per heartbeat. His ECG is pictured in Figure V-104. Troponin I levels are undetectable on presentation and 6 hours later. Blood pressure, heart rate, and oxygenation are normal. What is the most appropriate next step?

A. Aspirin 81 mg daily, metoprolol 25 mg twice daily, and atorvastatin 80 mg daily
B. Aspirin 1 g every 8 hours with omeprazole 20 mg daily
C. Heparin, aspirin, clopidogrel, and immediate coronary angiography
D. Prednisone 40 mg daily for 2 weeks followed by a taper over the ensuing 2 months
E. Transthoracic echocardiogram

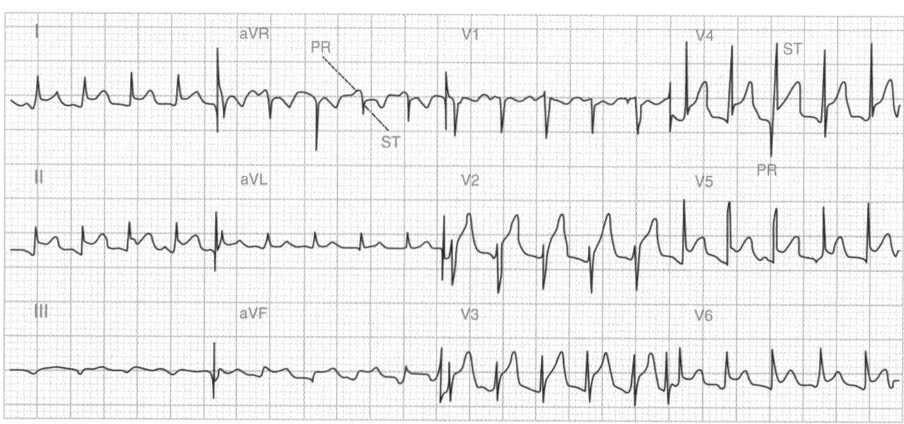

FIGURE V-104

V-105. You are caring for a 45-year-old man in the cardiac intensive care unit. He presented with chest pain and initially was thought to have acute coronary syndrome, prompting initiation of antiplatelet agents and IV heparin. After complete assessment and the return of negative serial cardiac enzymes, it became clear that he instead had acute pericarditis. Shortly after admission to the cardiac intensive care unit, he becomes hypotensive with elevated neck veins. His lungs are clear to auscultation. His extremities are cool, and you note that his brachial pulse is only palpable during expiration. What is the most likely diagnosis?

A. Aortic dissection
B. Cardiac tamponade
C. Left main coronary artery occlusion
D. Ruptured chordae tendineae
E. Ventricular septal defect

V-106. You call for emergent echocardiography in the patient described in Question V-106. In this patient, which of the following is likely to be increased during inspiration compared to expiration?

A. Left ventricular end-diastolic diameter
B. Left ventricular stroke volume
C. Mitral inflow velocity
D. Systolic blood pressure
E. Tricuspid inflow velocity

V-107. All of the following ECG characteristics will aid in differentiating acute pericarditis from acute myocardial infarction EXCEPT:

A. Absence of the development of Q waves
B. Concave shape to ST elevations
C. PR depression
D. ST elevation in V_2
E. T-wave inversions after return of the ST segments to baseline

V-108. A 35-year-old woman is admitted to the hospital with malaise, weight gain, increasing abdominal girth, and edema. The symptoms began about 3 months ago and gradually progressed. The patient reports an increase in waist size of ~15 cm. The swelling in her legs has gotten increasingly worse such that she now feels her thighs are swollen as well. She has dyspnea on exertion and two-pillow orthopnea. She has a past history of Hodgkin disease diagnosed at age 18. She was treated at that time with chemotherapy and mediastinal irradiation. On physical examination, she has temporal wasting and appears chronically ill. Her current weight is 96 kg, an increase of 11 kg over the past 3 months. Her vital signs are normal. Her jugular venous pressure is ~16 cm, and the neck veins do not collapse on inspiration. Heart sounds are distant. There is a third heart sound heard shortly after aortic valve closure. The sound is short and abrupt and is heard best at the apex. The liver is enlarged and pulsatile. Ascites is present. There is pitting edema extending throughout the lower extremities and onto the abdominal wall. Echocardiogram shows pericardial thickening, dilatation of the inferior vena cava and hepatic veins, and abrupt cessation of ventricular filling in early diastole. Ejection fraction is 65%. What is the best approach for treatment of this patient?

A. Aggressive diuresis only
B. Cardiac transplantation
C. Mitral valve replacement
D. Pericardial resection
E. Pericardiocentesis

V-109. A 45-year-old accountant with no prior past medical history has experienced occasional fevers, symmetric arthralgias, and fatigue for the past 3 months. Two weeks ago, she experienced the sudden onset of left hand weakness, which resolved within 1 hour. Multiple blood cultures have been negative. Emergent evaluation at her local emergency department included a head CT that was unrevealing. Last week, she had a transthoracic echocardiogram that showed a solitary, 2-cm mass in the left atrium arising from the interatrial septum in the vicinity of the fossa ovalis that appeared pedunculated on a fibrovascular stalk. You are seeing her back in clinic today. What is the most appropriate next step?

A. Cardiothoracic surgical removal of the mass
B. Catheter-based biopsy of the mass
C. Repeat blood cultures and inform the microbiology laboratory to plate on special media to evaluate for HACEK organisms
D. Serologies for antinuclear antibodies (ANAs), anti-DNA, and anticardiolipin antibodies
E. Whole-body PET scan to evaluate for malignancy

V-110. Which of the following malignancies carries the highest relative risk of metastasis to the heart?

A. Glioblastoma
B. Hepatocellular carcinoma
C. Malignant melanoma
D. Pancreatic adenocarcinoma
E. Small-cell lung cancer

V-111. You are attending your 12-year-old son's Little League baseball game. The score is tied 2–2 in the ninth inning, and your son's team is up to bat. On the first pitch of the inning, the batter fouls the ball directly back into the catcher's chest. The catcher immediately loses consciousness and collapses. He is pulseless with agonal respirations. You, as a physician, know that his survival depends most on which of the following?

A. Emergent transfer to a cardiac catheterization laboratory for percutaneous coronary intervention
B. Emergent transfer to a trauma center for repair of an acute aortic dissection
C. No intervention can impact this patient's survival.
D. Prompt cardiac surgery to repair an avulsed aortic valve
E. Prompt defibrillation

V-112. A 47-year-old woman with a body mass index (BMI) of 37 kg/m^2 was recently diagnosed with type 2 diabetes mellitus. As part of her patient education, you inform her that which of the following is the most common cause of death in adults with type 2 diabetes mellitus?

A. Coronary artery disease
B. Infection
C. Neuropathy
D. Renal failure
E. Stroke

V-113. Mr. Daniels is a 49-year-old man known well to your emergency department for frequent visits for alcohol intoxication. As the on-call internal medicine house officer, you are called to evaluate him for admission tonight. On arrival, he is only mildly intoxicated and able to provide a passable history. He claims that for the past 3 months, he has been increasingly short of breath with even minimal exertion and is experiencing overwhelming fatigue. He has also been awakening at night with extreme shortness of breath only alleviated by sitting on the edge of his bed. His ankles have been swollen. On examination, his blood pressure is 140/45 mmHg, and heart rate is 122 bpm. He has a bounding carotid pulse and elevated jugular venous pulse. His PMI is laterally displaced, and you clearly hear a low-pitched cardiac sound directly following the S_2. You note glossitis and find that he lacks sensation to light touch below the mid-shins bilaterally. Basic laboratory studies are notable for an albumin of 3.2 g/dL, creatinine of 1.4 mg/dL, and sodium of 134 mEq/L. Transthoracic echocardiogram reveals a left ventricular end-diastolic dimension of 6.8 cm with an ejection fraction of 70%.

You adroitly make the diagnosis and administer a substance to treat the underlying cause of Mr. Daniels's condition. Reassessment in 24 hours finds him symptomatically improved with a blood pressure of 142/76 mmHg and heart rate of 85 bpm. Repeat echocardiogram now shows his LV size to be 6.2 cm in end-diastole. Which of the following most likely caused Mr. Daniels's condition to improve so rapidly?

A. Folate
B. Penicillamine
C. Thiamine
D. Thyroxine
E. Vitamin B_{12}

V-114. A 65-year-old former factory worker with a past medical history of rheumatoid arthritis presents to your primary care clinic complaining of fatigue. She also states that she has the following symptoms: constipation, constantly feeling cold even when the thermostat is set on 80°F, brittle hair, and some lower extremity swelling. You expeditiously measure her thyroid-stimulating hormone, which is greatly elevated at 79.4 mIU/L. In regard to the present condition of her cardiovascular system, you expect a decrease in all of the following measurements EXCEPT:

A. Cardiac output
B. Heart rate
C. Pulse pressure
D. QT interval
E. Systolic blood pressure

V-115. In the current model describing the steps of atherosclerosis initiation and evolution, which of the following constitutes the first step?

A. Arterial endothelial cells overexpress adhesion receptors for leukocytes.
B. Lipoprotein particles undergo oxidative modifications.
C. Low-density lipoproteins accumulate within the arterial intima.
D. Macrophages and other leukocytes are recruited to the arterial intima.
E. Macrophages become lipid-laden foam cells via endocytosis of lipoprotein particles.

V-116. Which of the following statements regarding the pathophysiologic consequences of an atheroma is true?

A. An atheroma resulting in total vascular occlusion invariably causes infarction.
B. An enlarging atheroma does not generally encroach on the arterial lumen until the plaque exceeds 40% of the internal elastic lamina.
C. Most atheromas will eventually produce symptoms in the patient.
D. Upon initial formation, the atheromatous plaque usually grows inward toward the vessel lumen.
E. Vessels affected by atherogenesis tend to contract and get smaller in diameter.

V-117. Based on the 2013 cholesterol guidelines from the American College of Cardiology (ACC) and American Heart Association (AHA), all of the following groups are a definite statin benefit group EXCEPT:

A. All individuals who have clinical atherosclerotic cardiovascular disease (ASCVD)
B. Individuals with an elevated high-sensitivity C-reactive protein (CRP) regardless of low-density lipoprotein (LDL) cholesterol level or ASCVD risk
C. Individuals with LDL cholesterol ≥190 mg/dL without a secondary cause such as a high intake of saturated or trans fats or various drugs
D. Individuals without established ASCVD or diabetes who are 40–75 years old and who have LDL cholesterol of 70–189 mg/dL and a calculated ASCVD risk ≥7.5%
E. Patients with diabetes without established cardiovascular disease who are 40–75 years old and have LDL cholesterol of 70–189 mg/dL

V-118. A 50-year-old man presents to your clinic for his yearly check-up. Today, he is quite concerned about his future risk for heart attack and stroke after having read some concerning news articles in print and online. He has a history of vascular disease. He has gained some weight over the last decade, and his BMI today is 34 kg/m^2. His lipid panel is below:

Total cholesterol	220 mg/dL
Triglycerides	283 mg/dL
High-density lipoprotein (HDL)	29 mg/dL
LDL	132 mg/dL

You calculate his ASCVD risk as 6% with the risk calculator provided by the ACC/AHA. The patient has read that his low HDL cholesterol has been identified as correlated with his risk of future cardiovascular disease. He wants to know what you can prescribe in regard to his HDL that will definitively lower his cardiovascular risk to the largest degree. What is the correct answer?

A. An agonist of peroxisome proliferator-activated receptor α
B. An inhibitor of cholesteryl ester transfer protein
C. Fenofibrate
D. Nicotinic acid
E. Weight loss and physical activity

V-119. All of the following are major determinants of myocardial oxygen demand EXCEPT:

A. Heart rate
B. Heart rhythm
C. Myocardial contractility
D. Ventricular wall stress
E. All of the above are major determinants of myocardial oxygen demand.

V-120. Mr. Jackson is undergoing an exercise stress test. You know that as he progresses through his stress test, his myocardium will require more oxygen. How does the normal (nondiseased) heart respond to meet its higher oxygen demand?

A. Increased myocardial oxygen extraction during near-constant coronary blood flow
B. Increased oxygen extraction from the ventricular chambers
C. Relative expansion of the diastolic time period allowing increased coronary flow
D. Vasodilation of epicardial coronary arteries leading to decreased resistance and increased coronary blood flow
E. Vasodilation of intramyocardial coronary vessels leading to increased coronary blood flow

V-121. As Mr. Jackson (from Question V-120) continues on his exercise stress test, he begins to complain of a pressure-like chest pain. You suspect that he is experiencing angina due to a partially occluded coronary artery. If you were able to immediately analyze the biochemical changes occurring in his ischemic myocardium, you would note all of the following EXCEPT:

A. An increase in cytosolic calcium
B. An increase in intracellular pH
C. A shift from aerobic to anaerobic metabolism
D. Depletion of myocardial stores of high-energy phosphates
E. Leakage of potassium from myocytes

V-122. Which of the following sites is an unusual anatomic location for anginal pain radiation?

A. Back
B. Interscapular region
C. Root of the neck
D. Teeth
E. Trapezius muscle

V-123. Ms. Wilson is a 66-year-old postmenopausal U.S. postal employee. While walking her mail route over the past 9 months, she has routinely experienced chest pressure and dyspnea while climbing a certain steep hill. The pressure resolves when she rests for about 3 minutes. She has not missed any work due to these symptoms. You suspect she is experiencing angina. What term and Canadian Cardiovascular Society (CCS) Functional Class of angina is appropriate to describe her symptoms?

A. Stable angina – CCS class I
B. Stable angina – CCS class II
C. Stable angina – CCS class III
D. Stable angina – CCS class IV
E. Unstable angina

V-124. A 50-year-old accountant with a history of cigarette use completed an exercise treadmill ECG stress test. During his test, he developed upsloping ST depressions in leads II, III, and aVF. His peak heart rate achieved was 130 bpm. His blood pressure increased from 120/80 to 155/95 mmHg. What is the appropriate interpretation of this stress test?

A. Negative stress test; inappropriate hypertensive response to exercise
B. Negative stress test; nonspecific ST changes
C. Nondiagnostic stress test; normal blood pressure response
D. Positive stress test; inappropriate hypertensive response to exercise
E. Positive stress test; normal blood pressure response

V-125. A 70-year-old woman presents to the emergency department with 3 hours of acute shortness of breath and crushing substernal chest pressure. Her ECG shows 1-mm ST depression in leads II, III, and aVF without any ST elevation. Initial serum troponin level is mildly elevated. You suspect that she is having a non–ST-segment elevation myocardial infarction (NSTEMI). All of the following are causes of NSTEMI EXCEPT:

A. Coronary vasospasm
B. Increased myocardial oxygen demand produced by systemic conditions
C. Microvascular endothelial dysfunction
D. Partially occluding thrombus forming on disrupted atherothrombotic coronary plaque
E. Progressive coronary atherosclerosis leading to severe mechanical obstruction

V-126. Mr. Brian is a 57-year-old hockey team coach with a prior history of hypertension, hyperlipidemia, and tobacco abuse. He presents to the emergency department tonight after experiencing chest discomfort during a practice. He notes that he first began experiencing chest discomfort 3 weeks prior with vigorous exertion during practice. However, over the last week, it has taken less exertion to initiate the discomfort. Tonight, it occurred while he was just sitting on the bench. He describes the discomfort as a pressure, radiating to his jaw. It typically lasts about 10 minutes. His ECG shows new T-wave inversions in leads I, II, aVL, V_5, and V_6 since his last cardiogram 2 years ago at a routine physical examination. Which of the following clinical entities is an appropriate diagnosis for Mr. Brian?

A. Non–ST-segment elevation myocardial infarction
B. ST-segment elevation myocardial infarction
C. Stable angina
D. Unstable angina
E. More information is required before making a diagnosis.

V-127. Mr. Riviera is a 42-year-old man with anuric end-stage renal disease due to diabetes mellitus. Due to recent car trouble, he missed his most recent dialysis appointment and presents to the emergency department with shortness of breath. His heart rate is 105 bpm, and blood pressure is 185/100 mmHg. He has fine rales in the bilateral lower lung fields, and his jugular venous pulse is elevated. ECG shows sinus tachycardia without ST deviation. Initial troponin I assay returns at 0.14 ng/dL (normal is <0.06 ng/dL). What are the next most appropriate therapeutic and diagnostic steps?

A. Administer 80 mg of IV furosemide. Follow serial troponin I values and ECGs.
B. Administer 80 mg of aspirin. Refer for pharmacologic nuclear stress testing.
C. Initiate dual antiplatelet therapy (aspirin and clopidogrel) and heparin. Follow serial troponin I values and ECGs.
D. Initiate dual antiplatelet therapy (aspirin and clopidogrel) and heparin. Refer for urgent coronary angiography.
E. Initiate urgent hemodialysis with ultrafiltration for fluid removal. Follow serial troponin I values and ECGs.

V-128. A 67-year-old fry chef at the local Waffle Emporium presents to the emergency department with the sudden onset of crushing substernal chest pain. He has a history of hypertension, hyperlipidemia, and erectile dysfunction for which he takes daily amlodipine, simvastatin, and tadalafil. On your evaluation, his blood pressure is 145/85 mmHg, and heart rate is 90 bpm. His lungs are clear, and jugular venous pulse is not elevated. There are no murmurs or gallops on cardiac auscultation. He continues to complain of chest discomfort, rating it an 8/10. Initial troponin I result is elevated at 0.52 ng/dL (normal <0.06 ng/dL), and ECG reveals 1-mm ST depression in leads II, III, aVF, V_5, and V_6. All of the following pharmacologic therapies are reasonable to administer EXCEPT:

A. Aspirin orally
B. Clopidogrel orally
C. Heparin intravenously
D. Metoprolol intravenously
E. Nitroglycerin sublingually

V-129. Mr. Gilotra is a 57-year-old oil rig worker with a history of hypertension, tobacco abuse, and diabetes mellitus. He presents to the emergency department with 30 minutes of crushing substernal chest pain radiating to the jaw and associated with profuse sweating and shortness of breath. His blood pressure is 115/90 mmHg, and heart rate is 95 bpm. What diagnostic test will provide the most rapid method of altering therapeutic management for Mr. Gilotra?

A. 12-lead ECG
B. Coronary CT angiography
C. Echocardiogram
D. Serum creatine kinase-MB (CK-MB) band level
E. Serum troponin I level

V-130. You are evaluating a patient with chest pain in the emergency department. The ECG shows no Q waves or ST-segment changes. You wish to know whether the patient is suffering a myocardial infarction. Which of the following biomarkers is the preferred biochemical marker of myocardial infarction?

A. Creatine kinase
B. CK-MB band
C. Erythrocyte sedimentation rate
D. Lactate dehydrogenase
E. Troponin I

V-131. You are performing a diagnostic coronary angiography on Mr. Hayes. On the initial angiographic pictures, his arteries are clear of any obstructive disease. However, during a selective angiogram of the left anterior descending artery, you notice that a thrombus has formed on the tip of your catheter. During dye injection, the thrombus embolizes down the left anterior descending coronary artery causing complete obstruction to flow. Fortunately, you are able to remove the thrombus with suction thrombectomy almost immediately. If you had not been able to remove the thrombus, when would you first have expected detectable CK-MB isoform in a standard serum assay?

A. 5–10 minutes
B. 1–2 hours
C. 4–8 hours
D. 12–24 hours
E. 24–48 hours

V-132. The greatest delay between symptom onset and definitive therapy for patients with ST-segment elevation myocardial infarction usually occurs in what time interval?

A. Between onset of pain and patient's decision to call for help
B. Between patient call and emergency medical team arrival
C. Between emergency medical team arrival and arrival at the hospital
D. Between arrival at the hospital and decision to initiation reperfusion therapy
E. Between decision to initiate reperfusion therapy and the actual initiation of this therapy

V-133. All of the following medications used in the acute management of ST-segment elevation myocardial infarction are appropriately matched to their mechanism of effect EXCEPT:

A. Aspirin – reduction in thromboxane A_2
B. Abciximab – inhibition of the glycoprotein IIb/IIIa receptor
C. β-Adrenergic antagonists – reduced myocardial oxygen consumption
D. Clopidogrel – inhibition of the platelet adenosine diphosphate (ADP) receptor
E. Nitroglycerin – reduced cardiac afterload

V-134. A 61-year-old man presented to the emergency department 2 hours ago with anginal chest pain and ST-segment elevations in I, aVL, and V_1–V_3. At the time, the interventional cardiologist on call was involved in a complex case and was unable to take the patient for prompt primary percutaneous coronary intervention; thus tissue plasminogen activator (tPA) was administered. However, 120 minutes after administration of tPA, the patient continues to complain of chest pain, and his ECG shows no resolution of ST-segment elevations. What is the next most appropriate step?

A. Administer a second dose of tPA
B. Administer streptokinase 1.5 million units over 1 hour
C. Proceed with urgent coronary artery bypass grafting
D. Proceed with urgent percutaneous coronary intervention
E. Wait for 60 more minutes before pursuing any other therapeutic options

V-135. Mr. Cooper underwent tPA administration for acute ST-segment elevation myocardial infarction 1 hour previously. He had an excellent response with resolution of his ST-segment elevation and chest pain. However, the nurse pages you to evaluate a change in his rhythm. You note a wide complex ventricular rhythm with a rate of 75 bpm. Mr. Cooper continues to feel well without new symptoms, and his blood pressure is 120/80 mmHg. The next most appropriate therapeutic maneuver is which of the following?

A. Administer amiodarone 150 mg IV over 10 minutes
B. Administer flecainide 400 mg orally
C. Administer metoprolol 5 mg IV every 5 minutes × 3
D. Carotid sinus massage
E. Continue observation

V-136. An 84-year-old woman with a history of diabetes and hyperlipidemia presented to the emergency department 3 weeks ago with an ST-segment elevation myocardial infarction. She underwent emergent primary percutaneous coronary intervention to an acutely occluded left anterior descending artery. A 3.5 × 24 mm everolimus-eluting stent was placed with excellent angiographic result and complete resolution of her symptoms. She has been feeling excellent since then. Her discharge medications were metoprolol, aspirin, clopidogrel, rosuvastatin, lisinopril, and sliding scale insulin. She recently went to see her ophthalmologist who noted a right eye cataract. The ophthalmologist has contacted your office asking about your opinion on discontinuing her aspirin and/or clopidogrel to reduce bleeding risk during her cataract surgery, which has been scheduled for next week. She feels the bleeding risk on both medications is too high to perform the surgery. Which of the following should you recommend?

A. "Discontinue aspirin, continue clopidogrel, and proceed with cataract surgery."
B. "Discontinue clopidogrel, continue aspirin, and proceed with cataract surgery."
C. "Discontinue both aspirin and clopidogrel and proceed with cataract surgery."
D. "Postpone the surgery for at least 6 months, and preferably 12 months, at which time the clopidogrel can be discontinued."
E. "I advise to perform the surgery while she is on both aspirin and clopidogrel as she will never be able to stop either medication."

V-137. Ms. Constance is a 65-year-old recently retired librarian with a history of hypertension. After retirement, she began an exercise walking program but noted that she was markedly short of breath and had moderate chest pressure after only two to three blocks. She presented to your office 2 weeks ago. Given your concern that her symptoms were due to coronary artery disease, you referred her to a cardiologist for diagnostic coronary angiography. That was performed 1 week ago and revealed high-grade focal stenoses of the proximal left anterior descending artery, left circumflex artery, and right coronary artery. Other than these lesions, she did not have flow-limiting disease. The cardiologist did not perform percutaneous coronary intervention (PCI) and recommended a conversation with the local cardiothoracic surgeon to consider coronary artery bypass grafting (CABG). Ms. Constance now returns to your clinic for advice. You have the cardiologist and the cardiothoracic surgeon on conference call during the meeting. When counselling Ms. Constance about which revascularization strategy to choose, which of the following statements is true?

A. CABG has a lower mortality rate at 1 year than PCI for patients like Ms. Constance.
B. At 1 year, patients like Ms. Constance undergoing CABG have a higher risk of needing other procedures for revascularization than patients undergoing PCI.
C. PCI carries a higher risk of stroke than CABG.
D. The characteristics of coronary anatomy and the cardiologist's anticipation of success with PCI should factor into the decision.
E. PCI has a lower rate of myocardial infarction at 1 year than CABG for patients like Ms. Constance.

V-138. Mr. Gruentzig presents to your cardiology practice for shortness of breath and mild chest pressure with exertion. After a careful history and physical examination and a thorough discussion with the patient of the risks and benefits, you refer him for a technetium-99m scan, which reveals infero-apico-posterior ischemia. You promptly refer him to your colleague for coronary angiography. At angiography, he is found to have a left dominant system with a totally occluded left circumflex artery. The distal left circumflex artery is filled via collaterals from the left anterior descending artery. The interventional cardiologist is quite skilled, but she is unable to cross the total occlusion in the left circumflex using a hydrophilic wire and the antegrade approach. Which of the following statements regarding intervention on this chronic total occlusion (CTO) is true?

A. If the CTO cannot be crossed with any wire in the antegrade approach, the operator should always abandon percutaneous repair and consider referral for coronary bypass surgery.
B. Attempting to access the CTO via a retrograde approach through a collateral vessel is an option when attempting percutaneous revascularization.
C. Although the presence of a CTO is associated with a higher mortality rate, successful PCI of a CTO has never been shown to lower this mortality rate.
D. Coronary artery bypass surgery of a CTO is rarely successful due to the atretic nature of the vessel distal to the chronically occluded segment.
E. In studies, successful revascularization of chronic total coronary occlusions is associated with symptom relief but no improvement in left ventricular function.

V-139. A 67-year-old former truck driver underwent four-vessel CABG 12 years earlier with a left internal mammary artery (LIMA) graft to the left anterior descending artery (LAD), and three saphenous vein grafts (SVGs) to the first diagonal, first obtuse marginal, and right posterior descending arteries. At your visit with him today, he reports approximately 1 month of accelerating chest pain and shortness of breath with decreasing amounts of exertion. You refer him for coronary angiography, which reveals significant stenosis in the body of the SVG to the first obtuse marginal branch. Which of the following statements are true?

A. Graft failure of an SVG is almost always from thrombus embolized from the aortic anastomosis site.
B. PCI to this saphenous vein graft will require deployment of a distal protective device.
C. PCI on a saphenous vein graft is too risky to warrant proceeding. Aggressive medical management with antianginal therapy should be pursued.
D. The risk of PCI to an SVG is identical to native-vessel PCI.
E. Venous and arterial graft conduits (for example, SVG and LIMA grafts) have identical patency rate over the first 5 years following bypass grafting.

V-140. Mrs. Edwards is an 87-year-old woman with a history of extensive tobacco abuse and resultant COPD with a forced expiratory volume in 1 second (FEV_1) of 0.76 L, poorly controlled diabetes, and stage III chronic kidney disease. She was previously your patient, but has not followed up with you for the preceding 8 years. However, she comes to your clinic today complaining of chest pressure with exertion, leg swelling, shortness of breath, and accelerating fatigue with even minimal exertion. On examination, you quickly note a harsh, late-peaking systolic murmur at the right upper sternal border radiating the carotid arteries and with a musical quality at the apex. You cannot appreciate a second heart sound, and the carotid impulses are muted and arrive late compared to the PMI on palpation. You suspect severe aortic stenosis, and indeed, an echocardiogram later that day confirms aortic stenosis with a valve area of 0.59 cm^2. You refer Mrs. Edwards to a cardiothoracic surgeon who informs you that Mrs. Edwards is much too high risk for a surgical aortic valve replacement, citing a higher than 15% risk of in-hospital mortality. You are due to see Mrs. Edwards tomorrow. Which of the following statements to her would be reasonable?

A. "For this condition, medications have been shown to reduce the risk of mortality."
B. "It is okay that you are not a surgical candidate. Your condition carries a low risk of 1- and 5-year mortality, and we can control your symptoms with medications."
C. "Percutaneous aortic balloon valvotomy is a good nonsurgical treatment option and has been found to have excellent short- and long-term outcomes."
D. "Since you are not a surgical candidate, no other procedure exists for aortic valve replacement for you. We should consider hospice options."
E. "We should consider referring you for further testing to see if you are a candidate for transcatheter aortic valve replacement."

V-141. All of the following statements regarding the epidemiology of hypertension are true EXCEPT:

A. Among individuals age 60 years or older, average systolic blood pressure is higher in women.
B. Diastolic blood pressure increases steadily with age throughout life.
C. Hypertension prevalence is lower in Mexican Americans than non-Hispanic whites.
D. In industrialized nations, blood pressure increases steadily during the first two decades of life.
E. In the United States, approximately 30% of adults have hypertension.

V-142. Disease of which organ is the most common cause of mortality in hypertensive patients?

A. Brain
B. Heart
C. Kidney
D. Liver
E. Lungs

V-143. A 28-year-old woman has hypertension that is difficult to control. She was diagnosed at age 26. Since that time, she has been on increasing amounts of medication. Her current regimen consists of labetalol 1000 mg twice a day (bid), lisinopril 40 mg once a day (qd), clonidine 0.1 mg bid, and amlodipine 5 mg qd. On physical examination, she appears to be without distress. Blood pressure is 168/100 mmHg, and heart rate is 84 bpm. Cardiac examination is unremarkable, without rubs, gallops, or murmurs. She has good peripheral pulses and no edema. Her physical appearance does not reveal any hirsutism, fat maldistribution, or abnormalities of genitalia. Laboratory studies reveal a potassium of 2.8 mEq/dL and a serum bicarbonate of 32 mEq/dL. Fasting blood glucose is 114 mg/dL. What is the most likely diagnosis?

A. Congenital adrenal hyperplasia
B. Fibromuscular dysplasia
C. Cushing syndrome
D. Conn syndrome
E. Pheochromocytoma

V-144. What is the best way to diagnose the disease in the patient described in Question V-143?

A. Renal vein renin levels
B. 24-hour urine collection for metanephrines
C. MRI of the renal arteries
D. 24-hour urine collection for cortisol
E. Plasma aldosterone/renin ratio

V-145. Mr. Wilkins is a 65-year-old aeronautics engineer who has never been to the doctor and takes no medications. He is brought to the emergency department by his wife for worsening headache over the last day and confusion starting about an hour ago. His blood pressure on presentation is 230/140 mmHg, and heart rate is 90 bpm. Arterial oxygen saturation is 95%. On examination, he is moving all extremities equally, and there are no obvious deficits in his cranial nerve function, but he is clearly delirious. Cardiac examination reveals an enlarged and forceful PMI and an S_4 gallop; his lungs are clear to auscultation. Laboratory studies show a creatinine of 2.4 mg/dL, 2+ protein in his urine with hematuria, and a hematocrit of 32% with normal platelet count. You examine his peripheral blood smear and notice schistocytes. Emergent brain MRI shows old microvascular changes but no acute infarct or hemorrhage. Regarding his blood pressure management, which of the following would be the most reasonable therapeutic course?

A. 0.1 mg of clonidine orally
B. 20 mg of oral lisinopril
C. 20 mg of IV labetalol and initiation of a continuous parenteral drip for goal mean arterial pressure of 125 mmHg in the first hour
D. 90 mg of immediate-release oral nifedipine
E. Emergent plasmapheresis

V-146. Which of the following statements regarding the physiology of renal perfusion is true?

A. Due to tight precapillary regulation, the glomerular capillary endothelium is relatively shielded from pressure injury.
B. Renal cortical blood flow is less than renal medullary blood flow, and coupled with the high metabolic needs of the renal cortex, this leaves that region bordering on hypoxemia.
C. Renal perfusion is tightly regulated to the metabolic needs of the kidney.
D. Urinary albumin excretion is predictive of systemic atherosclerotic events and can present years in advance of clinical atherosclerotic disease.
E. Venous blood returning from the renal cortex has a lower oxygen content than venous blood returning from the renal medulla.

V-147. Which of the following statements regarding renal artery stenosis is true?

A. An abnormally reduced renal artery flow velocity by Doppler ultrasound is predictive of hemodynamically significant stenosis.
B. Early in the course of renal artery stenosis, elevated systemic renin levels are typical.
C. In the general population, the presence of fibromuscular dysplasia is rare (<1% prevalence).
D. Levels of renin activity observed in renal artery stenosis are predictive of response to medical therapy.
E. Usually the first clinical presentation of renal stenosis due to fibromuscular dysplasia is reduced renal function.

V-148. A 75-year-old man underwent a diagnostic coronary angiography after an abnormal stress test. Arterial access was obtained easily in the right femoral artery, and the angiography was completed with 35 mL of iodinated contrast dye. Fortunately, no significant coronary stenoses were noted. Seven days later, the man presents to the emergency department with abdominal pain and nausea. He reports that his urine output has been poor recently. Examination reveals a slight fever (38.3°C) and livedo reticularis on his lower extremities. Laboratory studies show a creatinine of 2.7 mg/dL (previously 1.1 mg/dL), white blood cell count of 10,500/mL with 21% eosinophils, and an erythrocyte sedimentation rate of 92 mm/hr. What is the mostly likely diagnosis?

A. Acute interstitial nephritis
B. Atheroembolic renal disease
C. Churg-Strauss syndrome
D. Contrast-induced nephropathy
E. Hypereosinophilic syndrome

V-149. In which of the following patients who present to an emergency department reporting acute dyspnea would a positive D-dimer result prompt additional testing for a pulmonary embolus?

A. A 24-year-old woman who is 32 weeks pregnant
B. A 48-year-old man with no past medical history who presents with calf pain following prolonged air travel; alveolar-arterial oxygen gradient is normal
C. A 56-year-old woman undergoing chemotherapy for breast cancer
D. A 62-year-old man who underwent hip replacement surgery 4 weeks previously
E. A 72-year-old man who had an acute myocardial infarction 2 weeks ago

V-150. A 42-year-old woman presents to the emergency department with acute onset of shortness of breath. She recently had been to visit her parents out of state and rode in a car for about 9 hours each way. Two days ago, she developed mild calf pain and swelling, but she thought that this was not unusual after having been sitting with her legs dependent for the recent trip. On arrival to the emergency department, she is noted to be tachypneic. Her vital signs are: blood pressure 98/60 mmHg, heart rate 114 bpm, respiratory rate 28 breaths/min, oxygen saturation 92% on room air, and weight 89 kg. The lungs are clear bilaterally. There is pain in the right calf with dorsiflexion of the foot, and the right leg is more swollen when compared to the left. An arterial blood gas measurement shows a pH of 7.52, PCO_2 of 25 mmHg, and PO_2 of 68 mmHg. Kidney and liver function are normal. A helical CT scan confirms a pulmonary embolus. All of the following agents can be used alone as initial therapy in this patient EXCEPT:

A. Enoxaparin 1 mg/kg subcutaneously (SC) twice daily
B. Fondaparinux 7.5 mg SC once daily
C. Tinzaparin 175 units/kg SC once daily
D. Unfractionated heparin IV adjusted to maintain activated partial thromboplastin time (aPTT) two to three times the upper limit of normal
E. Warfarin 7.5 mg orally once daily to maintain international normalized ratio at 2–3

V-151. Which of the following statements regarding pulmonary embolism is true?

A. Airway resistance usually decreases in the setting of an acute pulmonary embolism.
B. Almost all patients with pulmonary embolism have evidence of deep vein thrombosis at the time.
C. Alveolar hyperventilation is a typical physiologic abnormality in the presence of pulmonary embolism.
D. Hypotension in the setting of acute pulmonary embolism is often due to acute left ventricular systolic dysfunction.
E. The size of the arterial-alveolar gradient is invariably correlated with the size of the pulmonary embolism.

V-152. A 57-year-old man with a history of hypertension is admitted to the hospital with pulmonary embolism after having sudden onset of chest discomfort. His blood pressure is 132/62 mmHg, heart rate is 85 bpm, and oxygen saturation is 95% on room air. Echocardiography reveals normal right heart size and function, and cardiac troponin I is undetectable. Lower extremity Doppler ultrasound reveals an extensive deep vein thrombus from the right femoral popliteal vein. The patient is started on low-molecular-weight heparin and concomitant warfarin. On rounds the following day, he asks if insertion of an inferior vena cava (IVC) filter would be appropriate. What is the most appropriate answer?

A. "No, you would not benefit from an IVC filter at this point."
B. "No, there are currently no indications for IVC filter placement in the setting of deep vein thrombus or pulmonary embolism."
C. "We will need to go back to review your images and see how large your pulmonary embolus clot burden is before deciding whether an IVC filter is appropriate for you or not."
D. "Yes, given the presence of residual lower extremity thrombus, we will schedule you for IVC filter insertion."
E. "Yes, given your age and gender, we will schedule you for an IVC filter insertion."

V-153. Mrs. Tupulo is a 45-year-old woman with a history of morbid obesity (weight 140 kg), hypertension, and diabetes. She has been in the hospital for 4 days after having open surgical gastric bypass surgery. On postoperative day 4, she experiences sudden breathlessness, tachycardia, hypoxia, and an overwhelming sense of impending doom. Urgent chest CT angiography reveals a saddle pulmonary embolism. Her blood pressure is 70/45 mmHg, and urine output is poor. Five hundred milliliters of normal saline are administered IV, and she is initiated on dobutamine 5 μg/kg/min with a subsequent blood pressure of 82/55 mmHg. What is the next most appropriate step?

A. Enoxaparin
B. IVC filter
C. Surgical pulmonary embolectomy
D. tPA
E. Urokinase

V-154. A 67-year-old former heavy smoker is postoperative day 4 from an open aortobifemoral bypass operation for severe claudication. On routine postoperative CT scan prior to discharge, a pseudoaneurysm is noted just proximal to the aortic origin of the bypass grafts. Which of the following best defines a pseudoaneurysm?

A. A focal dilation in a vessel in which the intimal and medial layers are disrupted and the dilated segment is lined by adventitia only
B. A focal dilation of a vessel only involving one portion of the circumference
C. Apparent dilation of a vessel due to intrinsic narrowing proximal and distal to the point of apparent narrowing
D. Dilation of a vessel, though not to the size necessary to be diagnosed as a true aneurysm
E. The appearance of an aneurysmal dilation of a vessel on imaging due to the angulation of the artery and imaging technique

V-155. All of the following factors are associated with elevated risk for the development of an aortic aneurysm EXCEPT:

A. Aging
B. Cigarette smoking
C. Female sex
D. Hypercholesterolemia
E. Hypertension

V-156. You are seeing Mr. Walker in clinic for follow-up. He is a 22-year-old man with a family history of sudden death and arterial aneurysms. He is quite tall with widely spaced eyes and a bifid uvula. On his first visit, you order a transthoracic echocardiogram to investigate a diastolic murmur and note an aortic root aneurysm of 4.9 cm. He most likely has a mutation in which of the following genes?

A. Fibrillin-1
B. *SMAD3*
C. Smooth muscle–specific α-actinin
D. TGF-β receptor
E. Type III procollagen

V-157. Which of the following patients with aortic dissection or hematoma is best managed without surgical therapy?

A. A 45-year-old female with a dissection involving the aorta distal to the great vessel origin but cephalad to the renal arteries
B. A 74-year-old male with a dissection involving the root of the aorta
C. A 58-year-old male with aortic dissection involving the distal aorta and the bilateral renal arteries
D. A 69-year-old male with an intramural hematoma within the aortic root
E. All of the above patients require surgical management of their aortic disease.

V-158. A 32-year-old woman is seen in the emergency department for acute shortness of breath. A helical CT shows no evidence of pulmonary embolus, but incidental note is made of dilatation of the ascending aorta to 4.3 cm. All the following are associated with this finding EXCEPT:

A. Giant cell arteritis
B. Rheumatoid arthritis
C. Syphilis
D. Systemic lupus erythematosus
E. Takayasu arteritis

V-159. Mr. Tomazelli is a 75-year-old man with diabetes mellitus and hypertension. Despite continued counseling, he has been unable to stop smoking imported unfiltered cigarettes. At your visit today, he complains of burning pain in his bilateral calves with ambulation. It typically occurs after about two city blocks of walking on flat ground and improves with rest. He has also noted some aching calf pain during the night that improves when he sits on the side of the bed. Which of the following is likely true for Mr. Tomazelli?

A. He likely has critical aorto-iliac arterial stenosis.
B. The amplitude of his pulse volume contour will be sharp and spiked.
C. The most likely etiology of his symptoms is femoral arterial fibromuscular dysplasia.
D. The next most reasonable diagnostic test is magnetic resonance angiography.
E. The ratio of the systolic blood pressure in his ankle versus his brachial artery is likely less than 0.9.

V-160. The patient described in Question V-159 is diagnosed with symptomatic peripheral arterial disease (PAD) with bilateral ankle-brachial indices of 0.82. He asks about his prognosis and what the next step in treatment should be. Which of the following statements regarding his prognosis and therapy is true?

A. Anticoagulation with warfarin is superior to antiplatelet agents in preventing adverse cardiovascular events in patients with PAD.
B. β-Adrenergic blockers have been shown to worsen limb ischemia and should not be used in PAD.
C. He should exercise daily, walking to the point of maximal claudication before stopping to rest and allowing his symptoms to resolve.
D. His greatest risk of morbidity and mortality over the ensuing 5 years is progression to critical limb ischemia.
E. Vasodilators are first-line therapy for symptomatic PAD.

V-161. A 37-year-old woman with no significant past medical history except for a childhood murmur is evaluated for sudden-onset severe pain in her right lower extremity. Examination is notable for a young, uncomfortable woman with normal vital signs except for a heart rate of 110 bpm. The right leg has pallor distal to the right knee and is cold to the touch, and the dorsalis pedis pulse is absent. The left leg is normal. Which of the following studies is likely to diagnose the underlying reason for the patient's presentation?

A. Angiography of right lower extremity
B. Blood cultures
C. Echocardiogram with bubble study
D. Serum cytoplasmic antineutrophil cytoplasmic antibodies (c-ANCA)
E. Venous ultrasound of right upper extremity

V-162. A 32-year-old construction foreman presents with exertional pain in his bilateral forearms and hands. He smokes one pack of cigarettes per day, but otherwise has no past medical history. He has an easily palpable brachial pulse but very faint radial and ulnar pulses. A picture of his hand is shown in Figure V-162. Angiography of his upper extremity reveals smooth tapering segmental lesions in the small distal arterial vessels. Which of the following treatments has the greatest chance of success?

A. Cilostazol
B. Enoxaparin
C. Prednisone
D. Smoking cessation
E. Warfarin

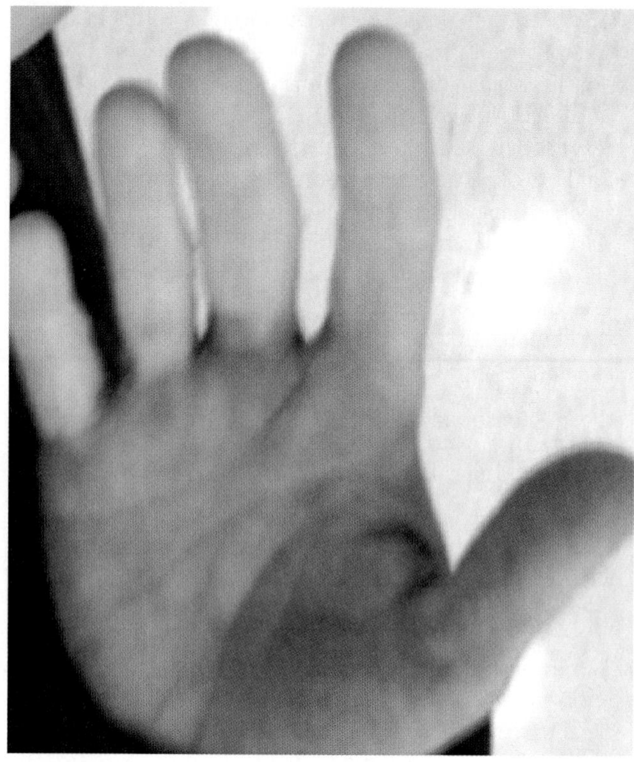

FIGURE V-162

V-163. Which of the following statements regarding chronic venous disease is true?

A. More men than women suffer from varicose veins.
B. More men than women suffer from chronic venous insufficiency with edema.
C. More than 50% of patients over 70 years old have chronic venous insufficiency.
D. Most patients with chronic venous insufficiency will develop venous ulcers.
E. All of the above are true.

V-164. Which of the following is the longest vein in the body?

A. Azygous vein
B. Greater saphenous vein
C. Inferior vena cava
D. Left common iliac vein
E. Right common femoral vein

V-165. You are evaluating a 77-year-old woman from Ohio with a history of heart failure with preserved ejection fraction, diabetes mellitus, and prior left lower extremity deep venous thrombosis status post a course of anticoagulation. For the past several months, she has complained of a cramping, burning sensation in her legs. Today she presents for evaluation of a skin ulcer, pictured in Figure V-165. On examination, you note the skin ulceration over the medial malleolus and a nonpitting woody-type edema of the bilateral ankles and shins. The skin there is darker as well. This ulcer is most likely due to which of the following?

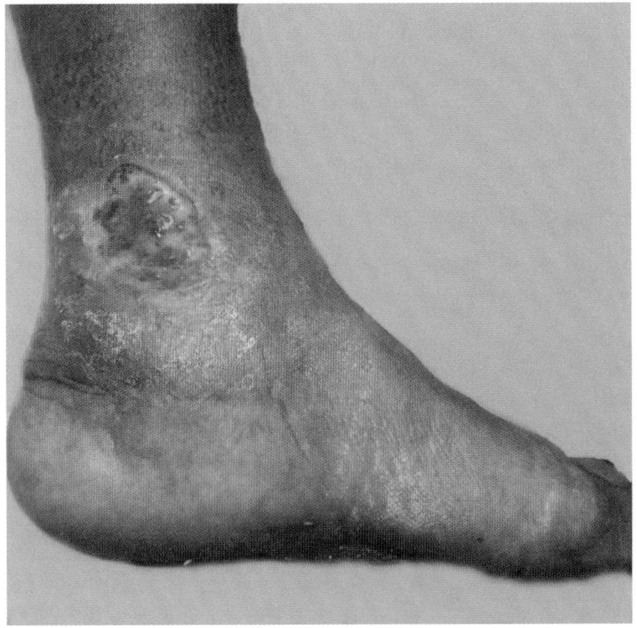

FIGURE V-165 Courtesy of Dr. Steven Dean, with permission.

A. Arachnid envenomation
B. *Bacillus anthracis* infection
C. Chronic venous insufficiency
D. Diabetic foot ulcer
E. Peripheral arterial disease

V-166. You are evaluating a 19-year-old woman in a travel clinic at your university. She complains of a nonpainful swelling of the lower extremity. On examination, the leg has thickened skin and a woody texture. A bedside ultrasound confirms patent lower extremity veins without thrombus. You suspect lymphedema and think that this is likely due to the most common cause of secondary lymphedema worldwide. What cause do you suspect?

A. Cancer involving the inguinal lymph nodes
B. Lymphogranuloma venereum
C. Lymphatic filariasis
D. Recurrent bacterial lymphangitis
E. Tuberculosis

V-167. You are taking care of a patient who suffers from chronic lymphedema due to recurrent streptococcal lymphangitis as a child. She finds her leg swelling unsightly and asks about therapeutic options. All of the following are reasonable therapeutic options for chronic lymphedema EXCEPT:

A. Decongestive physiotherapy
B. Diuretic therapy
C. Frequent leg elevation
D. Intermittent pneumatic compression devices
E. Liposuction

ANSWERS

V-1. **The answer is C.** *(Chap. 266e)* The global rise in cardiovascular disease (CVD) is the result of an unprecedented transformation in the causes of morbidity and mortality during the 20th century. Known as the epidemiologic transition, this shift is driven by industrialization, urbanization, and associated lifestyle changes and is taking place in every part of the world among all races, ethnic groups, and cultures. The transition is divided into four basic stages: pestilence and famine, receding pandemics, degenerative and man-made diseases, and delayed degenerative diseases. A fifth stage, characterized by an epidemic of inactivity and obesity, is emerging in some countries. The stages of the epidemiologic transition are shown in Table V-1.

Note that CVD mortality peaks in the third stage and then tends to decline aided by preventive strategies such as smoking cessation programs and effective blood pressure control, acute hospital management, and technologic advances, such as the availability of bypass surgery. In the stage of receding pandemics, the majority of CVD risk tends to be due to coronary heart disease, stroke, and rheumatic heart disease. Although the stages of epidemiologic transition is a useful construct to generalize expectations regarding CVD epidemiology over time, every nation experiences these stages in unique fashion due to environmental, behavioral, and genetic differences. For example, in China and Japan, stroke causes more deaths than coronary heart disease in a ratio of about three to one, as we would expect for this hypothetical nation.

TABLE V-1 Five Stages of the Epidemiologic Transition

Stage	Description	Deaths Related to CVD, %	Predominant CVD Type
Pestilence and famine	Predominance of malnutrition and infectious diseases as causes of death; high rates of infant and child mortality; low mean life expectancy	<10	Rheumatic heart disease, cardiomyopathies caused by infection and malnutrition
Receding pandemics	Improvements in nutrition and public health lead to decrease in rates of deaths related to malnutrition and infection; precipitous decline in infant and child mortality rates	10–35	Rheumatic valvular disease, hypertension, CHD, and stroke (predominantly hemorrhagic)
Degenerative and man-made diseases	Increased fat and caloric intake and decrease in physical activity lead to emergence of hypertension and atherosclerosis; with increase in life expectancy, mortality from chronic, noncommunicable diseases exceeds mortality from malnutrition and infectious disease	35–65	CHD and stroke (ischemic and hemorrhagic)
Delayed degenerative diseases	CVD and cancer are the major causes of morbidity and mortality; better treatment and prevention efforts help avoid deaths among those with disease and delay primary events; age-adjusted CVD morality declines; CVD affecting older and older individuals	40–50	CHD, stroke, and congestive heart failure
Inactivity and obesity	Overweight and obesity increase at alarming rate; diabetes and hypertension increase; decline in smoking rates levels off; a minority of the population meets physical activity recommendations	33	CHD, stroke, and congestive heart failure, peripheral vascular disease

Abbreviations: CHD, coronary heart disease; CVD, cardiovascular disease.
Source: Adapted from AR Omran: The epidemiologic transition: A theory of the epidemiology of population change. *Milbank Mem Fund Q* 49:509, 1971; and SJ Olshansky, AB Ault: The fourth stage of the epidemiologic transition: The age of delayed degenerative diseases. *Milbank Q* 64:355, 1986.

V-2. **The answer is C.** *(Chap. 267)* This patient has classic findings of differential cyanosis, or isolated cyanosis (and clubbing in this case) of the lower, but not upper, extremities. This limits the differential diagnosis to only one possibility: patent ductus arteriosus with secondary pulmonary hypertension causing right-to-left shunting at the level of the great vessels, distal to the upper extremity branches. Tetralogy of Fallot often causes central cyanosis due to right-to-left intracardiac shunting with no differential between the upper and lower extremities. Ventricular septal defect (VSD) and atrial septal defect (ASD) often have no cyanosis evident as they are most often left-to-right shunts (unless pulmonary hypertension develops resulting in Eisenmenger syndrome). Transposition of the great arteries (TGA) may exhibit varying degrees of central cyanosis, depending on the intracardiac anatomy (most often present with an ASD).

V-3. **The answer is C.** *(Chap. 267)* The electrocardiogram (ECG) shows complete heart block, and the leg lesions are consistent with erythema nodosum. This combination of findings is most likely due to sarcoidosis. Extrapulmonary sarcoidosis may manifest as cardiac conduction abnormalities (most common at the atrioventricular [AV] node), skin and joint lesions, hypercalcemia, and neurologic deficits. Hypothyroidism may cause sinus bradycardia but is usually not a cause of complete heart block. Also, the lower extremity skin finding of hypothyroidism is myxedema, a doughy, nonpitting, nonpainful edema. Carney syndrome is characterized by multiple lentigines and atrial myxomata. Systemic lupus erythematosus can be associated by erythema nodosum, although it does not often cause conduction system disease in adults. However, neonatal lupus is a common cause of complete heart block.

V-4. **The answer is E.** *(Chap. 267)* Jugular venous pulse (JVP) is the single most important physical examination measurement from which to estimate a patient's volume status. The internal jugular vein is preferred because the external jugular vein is valved and not directly in line with the superior vena cava and right atrium. Precise estimation of the central venous or right atrial pressure from bedside assessment of the jugular venous waveform has proved difficult. Venous pressure traditionally has been measured as the vertical distance between the top of the jugular venous pulsation and the sternal inflection point (angle of Louis). A distance >4.5 cm at 30 degrees of elevation is considered abnormal. However, the actual distance between the mid-right atrium and the angle of Louis varies considerably as a function of both body size and the patient angle at which the assessment is made (30, 45, or 60 degrees). The use of the sternal angle as a reference point leads to systematic underestimation of central venous pressure (CVP), and this method should be used less for semi-quantification than to distinguish a normal from an abnormally elevated CVP. Venous pulsations above the right clavicle in the sitting position are clearly abnormal, as the distance between the clavicle and the right atrium is at least 10 cm. Normally, the venous pressure should fall by at least 3 mmHg with inspiration. Kussmaul sign is defined by either a rise or a lack of fall of the JVP with inspiration and is classically associated with constrictive pericarditis, although it has been reported in patients with restrictive cardiomyopathy, massive pulmonary embolism, right ventricular infarction, and advanced left ventricular systolic heart failure. It is also a common, isolated finding in patients after cardiac surgery without other hemodynamic abnormalities.

V-5. **The answer is A.** *(Chap. 267)* The length and width of the blood pressure cuff bladder should be 80% and 40% of the arm's circumference, respectively. A common source of error in practice is to use an inappropriately small cuff, resulting in marked overestimation of true blood pressure, or an inappropriately large cuff, resulting in underestimation of true blood pressure. The cuff should be inflated to 30 mmHg above the expected systolic pressure and the pressure released at a rate of 2–3 mmHg/sec. Systolic and diastolic pressures are defined by the first and fifth Korotkoff sounds, respectively. Very low (even 0 mmHg) diastolic blood pressures may be recorded in patients with chronic, severe aortic regurgitation (AR) or a large arteriovenous fistula because of enhanced diastolic "run-off." In these instances, both the phase IV and phase V Korotkoff sounds should be recorded. Blood pressure is best assessed at the brachial artery level, although it can be measured at the radial, popliteal, or pedal pulse level. In general, measured systolic pressure increases and diastolic pressure decreases when measured in more distal arteries. Blood pressure should be measured in both arms, and the difference should be less than 10 mmHg. A blood pressure differential that exceeds this threshold may be associated with atherosclerotic or inflammatory subclavian artery disease, supravalvular aortic stenosis, aortic coarctation, or aortic dissection. Systolic leg pressures are usually as much as 20 mmHg higher than systolic arm pressures. Greater leg–arm pressure differences are seen in patients with chronic severe AR as well as patients with extensive and calcified lower extremity peripheral arterial disease. The ankle-brachial index (lower pressure in the dorsalis pedis or posterior tibial artery divided by the higher of the two brachial artery pressures) is a powerful predictor of long-term cardiovascular mortality. The blood pressure measured in an office or hospital setting may not accurately reflect the pressure in other venues. "White coat hypertension" is defined by at least three separate clinic-based measurements >140/90 mmHg and at least two non–clinic-based measurements <140/90 mmHg in the absence of any evidence of target organ damage. Individuals with white coat hypertension may not benefit from drug therapy.

V-6. **The answer is E.** *(Chap. 267)* This patient has evidence of pulsus alternans. Pulsus alternans is defined by beat-to-beat variability of pulse amplitude. It is present only when every other phase I Korotkoff sound is audible as the cuff pressure is lowered slowly, typically in a patient with a regular heart rhythm and independent of the respiratory cycle. Pulsus alternans is seen in patients with severe left ventricular systolic dysfunction and is thought to be due to cyclic changes in intracellular calcium and action potential duration. When pulsus alternans is associated with electrocardiographic T-wave alternans, the risk for an arrhythmic event appears to be increased. Cardiac tamponade or large pericardial effusions can be associated with electrical alternans (a regular variability in the QRS voltage or vector) or pulsus paradoxus, a difference between the systolic pressure at which the Korotkoff sounds are first heard (during expiration) and the systolic pressure at which the Korotkoff sounds are heard with each heartbeat, independent of the respiratory phase.

This is an exaggerated consequence of interventricular dependence. Atrial fibrillation would result in beat-to-beat variability of the pulse amplitude but also an irregularly irregular rhythm.

V-7. **The answer is A.** *(Chap. 267)* A fourth heart sound indicated left ventricular presystolic expansion and is common among patients in whom active atrial contraction is important for ventricular filling. A fourth heart sound is not found in atrial fibrillation. An irregular heart rate is characteristic of atrial fibrillation. The irregular rate is often characterized as "irregularly irregular." A third heart sound occurs during the rapid filling phase of ventricular diastole and indicates heart failure. Reversed splitting of the second heart sound occurs with left bundle branch block, as this patient demonstrates. Kussmaul sign is defined by either a rise or a lack of fall of the JVP with inspiration and is classically associated with constrictive pericarditis, although it has been reported in patients with restrictive cardiomyopathy, massive pulmonary embolism, right ventricular infarction, and advanced left ventricular systolic heart failure. It is also a common, isolated finding in patients after cardiac surgery without other hemodynamic abnormalities.

V-8. **The answer is F.** *(Chap. 267)* When a murmur of uncertain cause is identified on physical examination, a variety of physiologic maneuvers can be used to assist in the elucidation of the cause. Commonly used physiologic maneuvers include change with respiration, Valsalva maneuver, position, and exercise. In hypertrophic cardiomyopathy, there is asymmetric hypertrophy of the interventricular septum, which creates a dynamic outflow obstruction. Maneuvers that decrease left ventricular filling will cause an increase in the intensity of the murmur, whereas those that increase left ventricular filling will cause a decrease in the murmur. Of the interventions listed, both standing and a Valsalva maneuver will decrease venous return and subsequently decrease left ventricular filling, resulting in an increase in the loudness of the murmur of hypertrophic cardiomyopathy. Alternatively, squatting increases venous return and thus decreases the murmur. Maximum handgrip exercise also results in a decreased loudness of the murmur.

V-9. **The answer is A.** *(Chap. 267)* The patient is likely to have pericardial tamponade from metastatic cancer as suggested by her elevated neck veins, heart shadow shape and size, and predisposing condition. Because of the exaggerated interventricular dependence, the normal (<10 mmHg) fall in systemic blood pressure with inspiration is exaggerated (often >15 mmHg) with cardiac tamponade. This is referred to pulsus paradoxus, although it is in fact an augmentation of a normal finding. Kussmaul sign, or a lack of fall of the jugular venous pressure with inspiration, is a sign usually denoting a lack of compliance in the right ventricle, as seen most frequently in constrictive pericarditis, although it may be found in restrictive cardiomyopathy or massive pulmonary embolism. A slow y-descent, which follows the peak of the v wave, of jugular venous pressure tracing is indicative of cardiac tamponade as the restricted ventricle is slow to fill during diastole. The x-descent (systolic) may be augmented because ventricular ejection results in relative unloading of the intrapericardial pressure. Pulsus parvus et tardus, or small and slow arterial pulsation, is a late finding in aortic stenosis. Late diastolic murmur with opening snap is found in mitral stenosis.

V-10. **The answer is B.** *(Chap. 268)* The depolarization stimulus for the normal heartbeat originates in the sinoatrial (SA) node, or sinus node, a collection of pacemaker cells. These cells fire spontaneously; that is, they exhibit automaticity. Other cells exhibit automaticity, although at a slower rate, including AV nodal (junctional) cells and the Purkinje fiber cells. The first phase of cardiac electrical activation is the spread of the depolarization wave through the right and left atria, followed by atrial contraction. Next, the impulse stimulates pacemaker and specialized conduction tissues in the AV nodal and His bundle areas; together, these two regions constitute the AV junction. The bundle of His bifurcates into two main branches, the right and left bundles, which rapidly transmit depolarization wavefronts to the right and left ventricular myocardium by way of Purkinje fibers. The main left bundle bifurcates into two primary subdivisions: a left anterior fascicle and a left posterior fascicle. The depolarization wavefronts then spread through the ventricular wall, from endocardium to epicardium, triggering ventricular contraction.

V-11. **The answer is A.** *(Chap. 268)* The ECG waveforms are labeled alphabetically, beginning with the P wave, which represents atrial depolarization. The QRS complex represents ventricular depolarization, and the ST-T-U complex (ST segment, T wave, and U wave) represents ventricular repolarization. The J point is the junction between the end of the QRS complex and the beginning of the ST segment. Atrial repolarization (STa and Ta) is usually too low in amplitude to be detected, but it may become apparent in conditions such as acute pericarditis and atrial infarction.

V-12. **The answer is A.** *(Chap. 268)* Figure V-12 depicts the limb leads and respective frontal plane axis categories on the ECG. Note that normal axis extends from –30 to 90 or 100 degrees.

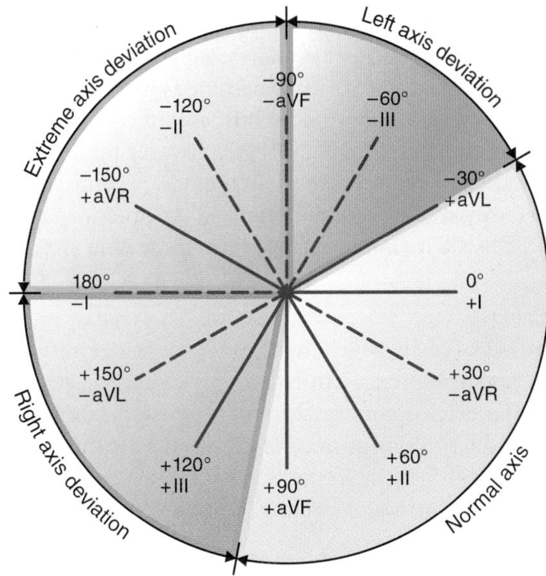

FIGURE V-12

V-13. **The answer is D.** *(Chap. 268)* This ECG exhibits classic findings of a right bundle branch block with an rSR' in V_1 and broad-based terminal S wave in I, II, and V_6. Left bundle branch block would have a similarly wide QRS, but with the terminal deflections on the QRS occurring with a leftward and posterior vector leading to a large R pattern in I and V_6 and a QS pattern in V_1. S1Q3T3 is a nonspecific ECG finding for right heart strain and is not present in this ECG. P-pulmonale is a term used to indicate right atrial abnormality or enlargement, seen on ECG as a tall P wave in lead II or V_1 (>2.5 mm). First-degree heart block is seen as a PR interval >200 msec (one large box on a standard-speed ECG).

V-14. **The answer is B.** *(Chap. 268)* This is a normal 12-lead ECG. The heart rate is about 75 bpm. The P-wave morphology and axis are normal, indicating normal atrial size and activation. The QRS axis is 70 degrees, which is normal. QRS duration is 0.08 seconds (normal), and QT interval 0.36 seconds (normal). There is no abnormal ST elevation or depression, and the T-wave morphology and size are normal.

V-15. **The answer is E.** *(Chap. 269e)* Mr. Wilson is suffering an acute inferolateral myocardial infarction (MI). Note the ST elevations in the inferior leads (II, III, aVF) and in V_6 (lateral precordial lead). Also, the striking ST depressions in the anterior precordial leads (V_1–V_4) are indicative of posterior ischemia. Here, the presence of ST depressions in an anterior lead represents the "mirror" of ST elevations in a posterior location. One can visualize the ECG pattern in the anterior leads upside down to see the reciprocal nature of the ST depressions. Although on initial glance, the QRS pattern appears wide in the anterior leads suggesting ventricular tachycardia, on further examination, there are P waves present that are associated with each QRS (seen most clearly in leads II and V_1); thus, the rhythm is sinus tachycardia. The wide appearance of the QRS is due to the striking ST deviation.

V-16. **The answer is E.** *(Chap. 269e)* This patient has an acute inferior myocardial infarction. Although it is possible that the left circumflex (LCx) arteries has coronary disease, the combination of a greater degree of ST segment elevation in lead III when compared to lead II, and the absence of ST elevation in the lateral leads (I and aVL) both make the right coronary artery (RCA) the culprit artery. The ST depressions in leads V1 through V3 indicate posterior ST elevation myocardial infarction from the occluded RCA. To further localize the lesion electrocardiographically, one should next obtain a right sided ECG, wherein the precordial leads are flipped to the right side of the chest, simply mirroring their usual left-sided position. The presence of >0.5mm of ST segment elevation in V4R would indicate a proximal right coronary artery occlusion, which carries a much higher mortality than a distal RCA occlusion.

V-17. **The answer is A.** *(Chap. 269e)* This ECG demonstrates sinus rhythm with premature atrial contractions (not normal sinus rhythm; note the fifth and ninth beats occurring early and preceded by an abnormal P wave indicating atrial origin). Also, the QRS is wide and in a right bundle branch block (RBBB) pattern as indicated by the large terminal R wave in the anterior precordial leads and broad-based terminal S wave in the lateral limb leads (I and aVL). In the presence of an RBBB, T waves in the anterior lead are often inverted and do not indicate acute ischemia. No premature ventricular contractions are present in this ECG. However, Q waves are present in the anterior precordial leads (V_1–V_3) so that the usual RBBB rsR' is simply a qR pattern, indicating a prior anterior-septal myocardial infarction.

V-18. **The answer is D.** *(Chap. 269e)* This patient has pericarditis. Often associated temporally with a viral upper respiratory infection, pericarditis is a common noncoronary cause of chest pain. The ECG is confirmatory of the history, showing diffuse, concave ST elevations with PR depressions in most leads. Lead aVR shows PR-segment elevation typical of acute pericarditis. Options A and C would be appropriate choices if the patient were having an acute myocardial infarction. Option E would *not* be appropriate in the immediate setting of myocardial infarction or pericarditis. Patients with pericarditis without signs of elevated intrapericardial pressure (elevated neck veins, tachycardia, low blood pressure, elevated pulsus paradoxus) or suspicion of purulent pericarditis (fever, sepsis) do not require an echocardiogram (option B). Treatment of acute viral or idiopathic pericarditis is with nonsteroidal anti-inflammatory drugs (NSAIDs) and colchicine.

V-19. **The answer is B.** *(Chap. 269e)* This patient likely missed a session of hemodialysis due to the impassible roads. In this setting and in combination with the tall, peaked T waves seen on the ECG, one would suspect hyperkalemia. Hyponatremia does not have a stereotypical finding on ECG. Hypercalcemia causes a shortened QT interval (usually due to a shortening specifically of the ST segment with T waves of normal duration). This patient also likely has hypocalcemia evidenced by the prolonged QT interval on ECG. The hypocalcemia in this case is due to hyperphosphatemia secondary to missed hemodialysis. Hypokalemia causes prolonged QT interval, low T-wave voltage, and often the presence of U waves. Hypomagnesemia likewise causes a prolongation of the QT interval and increases the risk of torsades de pointes.

V-20. **The answer is E.** *(Chap. 271e)* This patient demonstrates findings consistent with cardiac amyloidosis. The greatly thickened myocardium with a bright or "sparkly" appearance, left atrial enlargement, and impressive clinical heart failure in the setting of preserved systolic function all suggest infiltrative cardiomyopathy. Strain echocardiographic imaging often reveals decreased myocardial strain and strain rates with relative sparing of the apex in amyloidosis. Atrial fibrillation is common in patients with cardiac amyloidosis and carries a high risk of thromboembolic complications. The preserved ejection fraction renders ischemic disease (as evaluated by positron emission tomography [PET] stress) less likely. Although *Trypanosoma cruzi* (the etiologic agent of Chagas disease) is endemic in many South American countries, cardiac manifestations include a dilated cardiomyopathy with conduction disease as opposed to a restrictive, thickened myocardium. In the evaluation for cardiac amyloidosis, a reasonable first step is a serologic evaluation for a paraproteinemia with protein electrophoreses of the serum and urine and a light chain assay. Negative results do not rule out amyloidosis, and an endomyocardial biopsy is warranted if clinical suspicion is high enough. If a light chain paraproteinemia is confirmed, a bone marrow biopsy may be warranted later to evaluate for multiple myeloma or a plasma cell dyscrasia. Another common cause of cardiac amyloidosis is deposition of transthyretin (TTR or prealbumin) protein, either in the familial or senile forms. If amyloidosis is confirmed on biopsy and mass spectroscopy cannot be performed or suggests TTR deposition, then genetic testing for known mutations in the *TTR* gene would be warranted for prognosis and future genetic counseling should be offered to the patient and their family.

V-21. **The answer is A.** *(Chap. 271e)* This image shows reversible ischemia in all segments of the apex, the distal inferior wall, and the mid to distal septal and inferior walls. This is compatible with ischemic in the distal LAD territory. Ischemia due to significant left main coronary artery stenosis can lead to a "pseudonormal" pattern on nuclear perfusion stress tests, due to balanced ischemia and equally depressed blood flow through the entire left ventricle. Transient dilatation with stress is an important clue to the presence of balanced ischemia and may point toward left main or "triple-vessel" coronary disease. Ischemia of the left circumflex artery would spare the septum and cause reversible ischemia in the lateral and perhaps inferior walls. The right coronary artery and posterior descending artery would present with ischemia of the proximal inferior wall with variable involvement of the inferoseptal segments.

V-22. **The answer is E.** *(Chap. 274)* Many cells in the heart possess the ability to spontaneously depolarize due to slow spontaneous diastolic depolarization (phase 4). The SA node, AV node, and Purkinje cells all possess this ability. However, in normal physiologic states, the SA node possesses the "steepest" phase 4 slope and thus depolarizes more rapidly than any other potential pacemaker cells. The location does not determine the SA node's pacemaker ability, and the SA nodal cells have no intercalated discs. Phase 0 is actually slower in nodal cells than in ventricular or atrial nonnodal cells (Figure V-22).

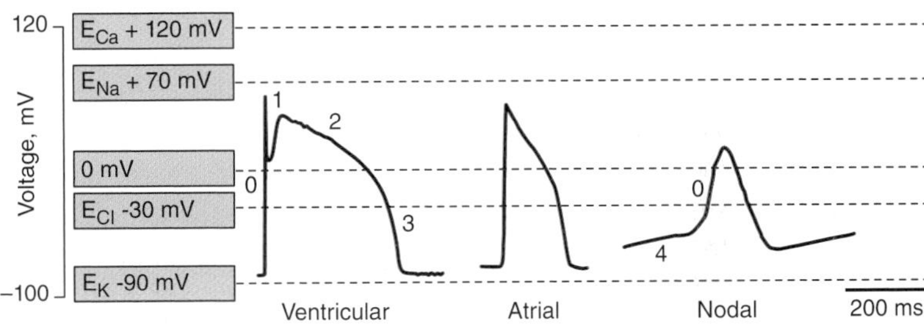

FIGURE V-22

V-23. **The answer is C.** *(Chap. 274)* Sinus bradycardia and pauses up to 3 seconds are common in young individuals, particularly in highly trained athletes. Given the normal conduction intervals on his baseline ECG, lack of symptoms, and normal physical examination, no further testing is warranted. It is clear that he has the ability to augment his heart rate if he has been training for this race.

V-24. **The answer is D.** *(Chap. 274)* Determining the intrinsic heart rate (IHR) may distinguish SA node dysfunction from slow heart rates that result from high vagal tone. The normal IHR after administration of 0.2 mg/kg of propranolol and 0.04 mg/kg of atropine is 117.2 – (0.53 × age) in bpm; a low IHR is indicative of SA disease. For this patient, his IHR should be approximately 85 bpm. Electrophysiologic testing may play a role in the assessment of patients with presumed SA node dysfunction and in the evaluation of syncope, particularly in the setting of structural heart disease. In this circumstance, electrophysiologic testing is used to rule out more malignant etiologies of syncope, such as ventricular tachyarrhythmias and AV conduction block. There are several ways to assess SA node function invasively. They include the sinus node recovery time (SNRT), which is defined as the longest pause after cessation of overdrive pacing of the right atrium near the SA node (normal: <1500 msec). This patient has no evidence of tachyarrhythmias (option E) or atrial fibrillation (option B). While amyloid cardiomyopathy might explain SA nodal dysfunction, further evidence (endomyocardial biopsy or serologic evidence of light chain disease) would be required to make this diagnosis.

V-25. **The answer is E.** *(Chap. 274)* Sinoatrial dysfunction is often divided into intrinsic disease and extrinsic disease of the node. This is a critical distinction, because extrinsic causes are often reversible and pacemaker placement is not required. Drug toxicity is a common cause of extrinsic, reversible sinoatrial dysfunction, with common culprits including β-blockers, calcium channel blockers, lithium toxicity, narcotics, pentamidine, and clonidine. Hypothyroidism, sleep apnea, hypoxia, hypothermia, and increased intracranial pressure are all also reversible forms of extrinsic dysfunction. Radiation therapy can result in permanent dysfunction of the node and therefore is an irreversible, or intrinsic, cause of SA node dysfunction. In symptomatic patients, pacemaker insertion may be indicated.

V-26. **The answer is B.** *(Chap. 274)* The tachycardia-bradycardia variant of sick sinus syndrome is associated with an increased risk of thromboembolism particularly when similar risk factors are present that increase the risk of thromboembolism in patients with atrial fibrillation. Specific risk factors associated with highest risk include age >65 years, patients with prior history of stroke, valvular heart disease, left ventricular dysfunction, or atrial enlargement. Patients with these risk factors should be treated with anticoagulation.

V-27. **The answer is A.** *(Chap. 275)* AV nodal transitional connections may exhibit decremental conduction, defined as slowing of conduction with increasingly rapid rates of stimulation. This property of the AV node is physiologically important. If a very rapid atrial arrhythmia occurs, the AV node acts as a sort of "gatekeeper" to the ventricles due to its decremental conduction. Thus, in the case of atrial fibrillation (where atrial rates often exceed 300 bpm), the ventricular rate never approaches these very rapid rates. Some accessory conduction pathways, in contrast, do not exhibit decremental conduction properties and will rapidly conduct tachycardias (such as atrial fibrillation) to the ventricles, leading to hemodynamic collapse.

V-28. **The answer is E.** *(Chap. 275)* The compact AV node (~1 × 3 × 5 mm) is situated at the apex of the triangle of Koch, which is defined by the coronary sinus ostium posteriorly, the septal tricuspid valve annulus anteriorly, and the tendon of Todaro superiorly. The compact AV node continues as the penetrating AV bundle where it immediately traverses the central fibrous body and is in close proximity to the aortic, mitral, and tricuspid valve annuli; thus, it is subject to injury in the setting of valvular heart disease or its surgical treatment. It is common for patients to experience transient AV block after valve surgery (particularly aortic valve surgery) due to the surrounding edema. Many patients will regain normal conduction as the perioperative injury and edema decrease; however, some patients will not and will require permanent pacemaker placement. It is unlikely that this patient has developed new systemic disease such as Lyme disease, sarcoidosis, or endocarditis. SA nodal disease would manifest as sinus bradycardia, which this patient does not have.

V-29. **The answer is A.** *(Chap. 275)* Congenital AV block in the setting of a structurally normal heart has been seen in children born to mothers with systemic lupus erythematosus (SLE). SLE can cause sterile endocarditis in adults but is not common in children of mothers with SLE. Similarly, early-onset coronary artery disease, pulmonary hypertension, and occasionally cardiomyopathy are described in SLE patients but not in their children just after birth.

V-30. **The answer is E.** *(Chap. 275)* This patient has Mobitz II, second-degree AV block. This particular ECG demonstrates a specific pattern of this called paroxysmal AV block. This patten and the patient's concerning symptoms of recurrent syncope indicate significant conduction disease and warrant urgent permanent pacemaker implantation. SA node block would be indicated on the surface ECG by the absence of P waves (and SA node potentials might be noted on invasive intracardiac electrograms). First-degree AV block would manifest as a prolonged PR interval (>200 msec) without any nonconducted beats. Atropine (anticholinergic) administration can sometimes help differential between Mobitz I (usually intranodal disease) and Mobitz II (usually infranodal disease) block when the ECG is not clear. Since the AV node is more heavily innervated by vagal efferents, atropine will improve the block in Mobitz I but worsen it in Mobitz II infranodal disease. The converse is largely true of maneuvers that increase vagal tone (carotid sinus massage or Valsalva).

V-31. The answer is C. *(Chap. 275)* Mobitz I (Wenckebach) AV block is a very common phenomenon in young, healthy adults, particularly during sleep and in patients with high vagal tone such as trained athletes. Given his reassuring lack of symptoms, no further testing or intervention is needed for this patient. The indications for pacemaker implantation in AV block are noted in Table V-31. Note that asymptomatic type I second-degree AV block is a class III recommendation (recommended against).

TABLE V-31 Guideline Summary for Pacemaker Implantation in Acquired AV Block

Class I

1. Third-degree or high-grade AV block at any anatomic level associated with:
   a. Symptomatic bradycardia
   b. Essential drug therapy that produces symptomatic bradycardia
   c. Periods of asystole >3 seconds or any escape rate <40 bpm while awake, or an escape rhythm originating below the AV node
   d. Postoperative AV block not expected to resolve
   e. Catheter ablation of the AV junction
   f. Neuromuscular diseases such as myotonic dystrophy, Kearns-Sayre syndrome, Erb dystrophy, and peroneal muscular atrophy, regardless of the presence of symptoms
2. Second-degree AV block with symptomatic bradycardia
3. Type II second-degree AV block with a wide QRS complex with or without symptoms
4. Exercise-induced second- or third-degree AV block in the absence of ischemia
5. Atrial fibrillation with bradycardia and pauses >5 seconds

Class IIa

1. Asymptomatic third-degree AV block regardless of level
2. Asymptomatic type II second-degree AV block with a narrow QRS complex
3. Asymptomatic type II second-degree AV block with block within or below the His at electrophysiologic study
4. First- or second-degree AV block with symptoms similar to pacemaker syndrome

Class IIb

1. AV block in the setting of drug use/toxicity, when the block is expected to recur even with drug discontinuation
2. Neuromuscular diseases such as myotonic dystrophy, Kearns-Sayre syndrome, Erb dystrophy, and peroneal muscular atrophy with any degree of AV block regardless of the presence of symptoms

Class III

1. Asymptomatic first-degree AV block
2. Asymptomatic type I second-degree AV block at the AV node level
3. AV block that is expected to resolve or is unlikely to recur (Lyme disease, drug toxicity)

Source: Modified from AE Epstein et al: *J Am Coll Cardiol* 51:e1, 2008.

V-32 and V-33. The answers are B and D, respectively. *(Chap. 276)* The patient has persistent, non–life-threatening palpitations that distress her enough to seek medical attention. A continuous Holter monitor for 24 hours is appropriate for patients in whom the symptoms happen several times over 24 hours, whereas an event monitor is triggered by the patient when symptoms occur and thus can be worn for longer period of time, which is appropriate in this patient. There is no indication of gastrointestinal triggers, so abdominal computed tomography (CT) would not be helpful. The atrial premature contractions are uncomplicated, do not require additional diagnostic evaluation at this time, and pose no additional health risk. Electrophysiology (EP) referral is indicated for patients with life-threatening or severe symptoms such as syncope.

V-34. The answer is D. *(Chap. 276)* Wolff-Parkinson-White (WPW) pattern is almost always due to accessory pathway conduction whereby electrical signals are able to propagate from atria to ventricles without first going through the AV node. As opposed to the AV node, many accessory pathways fail to exhibit decremental conduction (a slowing of conduction at increasing rates of excitation) and thus are able to rapidly conduct fast atrial rhythms to the ventricles. At exceedingly fast rates (as might be present in atrial fibrillation), this can lead to cardiovascular collapse. The observation that Ms. Milsap's delta wave disappears and QRS complex normalizes at a relatively high heart rate is reassuring. In that case, the accessory pathway cannot conduct antegrade at a rate >120 bpm and is unlikely to cause serious tachyarrhythmia. The ability to augment a rapid sinus rhythm is normal for her age and does not carry any particular prognosis. The location of the accessory pathway in a septal position makes is it somewhat more difficult to ablate with catheters, and the operator must take care to avoid the native AV node and His-Purkinje system. The ability of the accessory pathway to conduct both antegrade and retrograde makes it a substrate for atrioventricular reentrant tachycardia (AVRT).

V-35. The answer is A. *(Chap. 276)* Adenosine is a powerful "nodal-blocking agent"; that is, it blocks propagation of electrical signal through the AV node. It has a very short half-life. Administration of adenosine to a patient in atrial fibrillation will induce a transient complete heart block but will not stop the atrial fibrillation. When the adenosine wears off in a few seconds and AV conduction resumes, the ventricular rhythm will again be irregularly irregular. All the other choices have been shown to achieve sinus rhythm better than placebo in patients with atrial fibrillation.

V-36. The answer is D. *(Chap. 276)* This patient has new atrial fibrillation. When one assesses a patient with new atrial fibrillation, it is prudent to proceed through a series of decisions systematically. If the patient is hemodynamically unstable (low blood pressure, pulmonary edema, poor mentation, low urine output), then urgent direct current cardioversion is warranted. This patient is clearly stable. The next decision hinges around rate versus rhythm control. Several studies have shown clinical equipoise between rate and rhythm control strategies, with patients randomized to the rhythm control strategies undergoing far more procedures and taking more medications than patients randomized to the rate control strategies. This is also true in heart failure patients. Given the lack of symptoms and already controlled resting heart rate, rhythm control with either medications (amiodarone) or cardioversion is not a class I indication. In fact, a type I antiarrhythmic such as flecainide would be contraindicated for this patient because it has been shown to increase mortality in patients with coronary disease. The final question revolves around anticoagulation. Patients with atrial fibrillation have varying degrees of risk of thromboembolic events. Patients are stratified into risk categories by assessing set risk factors. One can remember the $CHADS_2$ mnemonic to recall each point of the risk scoring system (congestive heart failure [CHF], hypertension, age >75, diabetes, and stroke/cerebrovascular accident [which receives 2 points]). A more sensitive score includes vascular disease, age >65, and female sex (CHADS-VASc). Any combined score >1 warrants systemic anticoagulation. Patients with a score of 0 do not require systemic anticoagulation and can take full-strength aspirin. A score of 1 is intermediate and requires an in-depth discussion with the patient about their risk threshold for anticoagulation. Many experts recommend systemic anticoagulation with a $CHADS_2$ score of 1. This patient has a $CHADS_2$ score of 3 (CHF, hypertension, age) and thus warrants systemic anticoagulation.

V-37. The answer is D. *(Chap. 276)* This patient has classic symptoms for an AV nodal reentrant tachycardia. The so-called frog sign (prominent venous pulsations in the neck due to cannon A waves seen in AV dissociation) on physical examination is frequently present and suggests simultaneous atrial and ventricular contraction. First-line therapy for these reentrant narrow complex tachyarrhythmias is carotid sinus massage to increase vagal tone. Often this is all that is required to return the patient to sinus rhythm. If that is not successful, intravenous (IV) adenosine 6–12 mg may be attempted. If adenosine fails, IV β-blockers or calcium channel blockers may be used (diltiazem or verapamil). Finally, in hemodynamically compromised patients or those who have failed to respond to previous measures, direct current (DC) cardioversion with 100–200 J is indicated.

V-38. **The answer is B.** *(Chap. 276)* The AFFIRM and RACE trials compared outcomes in survival and thromboembolic events in patients with atrial fibrillation using two treatment strategies: rate control and anticoagulation versus pharmacotherapy to maintain sinus rhythm. There was no difference in events in the two groups, which was thought to be due to the inefficiencies of pharmacotherapy, with over half of patients failing drug therapy, and also the high rates of asymptomatic atrial fibrillation in the sinus rhythm group. Thus, when considering discontinuation of anticoagulation in patients who have maintained sinus rhythm, it is recommended to place a prolonged ECG monitor to ensure that asymptomatic atrial fibrillation is not present. Because of the risk of QT prolongation and polymorphic ventricular tachycardia, dofetilide and sotalol are recommended to be initiated in the hospital.

V-39. **The answer is E.** *(Chap. 276)* This rhythm is multifocal atrial tachycardia (MAT), which is easily confused with atrial fibrillation due to its irregularly irregular nature. However, MAT is distinguished by the multiple different P waves present (at least three different P-wave morphologies). MAT is classically present in patients with severe pulmonary disease and is exacerbated in the presence of acute illness. No anticoagulation is needed for MAT, and DC cardioversion is not efficacious. Some patients respond to the nondihydropyridine calcium channel blockers (diltiazem and verapamil), and amiodarone has some limited effect. In this patient, controlling the underlying cause of her tachycardia (pain and dehydration) is the most appropriate first therapy.

V-40. **The answer is D.** *(Chap. 276)* This patient is unstable with hypotension and poor cerebral perfusion due to her wide complex tachycardia. Defibrillation is the only therapy that is appropriate and should be performed immediately.

V-41. **The answer is A.** *(Chap. 276)* This ECG shows a wide complex, irregularly irregular tachycardia. Ventricular tachycardia is wide complex but is regular. Unless there is underlying conduction system disease (such as a left bundle branch block, which is unusual in a young patient), AV nodal reentry tachycardia (AVNRT), AVRT, and atrial flutter are also narrow complex and are regular. The irregularly irregular rhythm coupled with the extremely fast ventricular rate make the diagnosis of atrial fibrillation with antegrade conduction down an accessory pathway most likely. If no accessory pathway is present, the decremental conduction properties of the AV node will limit ventricular response rate. However, some accessory pathways do not have decremental conduction properties, and thus pass every atrial impulse through to the ventricle. In the setting of atrial rates above 300 (as in atrial fibrillation), this can be catastrophic.

V-42. **The answer is C.** *(Chap. 277)* This is idioventricular rhythm, which is a rhythm originating in the ventricular myocardium but with a rate <100 bpm. This rhythm, also known as accelerated idioventricular rhythm, is commonly seen after successful reperfusion and requires no specific therapy. Normal sinus rhythm is ruled out by the absence of P waves. Ventricular tachycardia requires a heart rate of >100 bpm for diagnosis. A junctional escape would likely be narrow (unless there is aberrant conduction) and much slower (40–60 bpm). Atrial fibrillation would be irregularly irregular.

V-43. **The answer is B.** *(Chap. 277)* This ECG shows a slow, sinusoidal ventricular rhythm. This bizarre rhythm is almost always due to drug effects or electrolyte disturbances. Specifically, this represents the most extreme ECG changes of hyperkalemia. Unfortunately, the scenario in this question is all too common in patients on hemodialysis who cannot or do not go to dialysis sessions. Hyperkalemia is a dreaded complication of missed dialysis and can be deadly. Hyperphosphatemia and resultant hypocalcemia can also be caused by missed hemodialysis sessions. These do not cause the observed ECG changes. Although defibrillation is appropriate, one should realize that it may not be effective until the hyperkalemia is controlled. Temporizing measures such as IV calcium, insulin and dextrose, bicarbonate, and inhaled β-agonists can be used to lower the serum potassium while emergent hemodialysis is readied.

V-44. **The answer is E.** *(Chap. 277)* Although it is true that patients with cardiomyopathy and nonsustained ventricular tachycardia (NSVT) or a high burden of premature ventricular contractions (PVCs) have a higher mortality, multiple studies have found no mortality benefit to suppressing the ventricular arrhythmias with antiarrhythmic medications. In fact, the CAST trial showed that the use of Vaughn-Williams class I drugs such as flecainide and propafenone increased mortality when used in patients with PVCs and ischemic disease. Thus, these are contraindicated in patients with any structural heart disease. Implantable defibrillator therapy is not warranted in this patient for primary prevention despite the presence of NSVT. It would be prudent to ensure that her electrolytes are normal given her recent diuresis; hypokalemia in particular is associated with an increased burden of PVCs and NSVT.

V-45. **The answer is A.** *(Chap. 277)* For survivors of an acute MI, an implantable cardioverter defibrillator (ICD) reduces mortality in certain high-risk groups: patients who have survived >40 days after the acute MI and have a left ventricular (LV) ejection fraction of ≤0.30 or who have an ejection fraction <0.35 and have symptomatic heart failure (functional class II or III). Thus, early ICD implantation is not warranted here. In patients >5 days after MI with NSVT and inducible sustained ventricular tachycardia (VT) or ventricular fibrillation (VF) on electrophysiologic studies, an automatic ICD may be considered. Angiotensin-converting enzyme (ACE) inhibitors, β-blockers, and eplerenone (aldosterone antagonists) have all been shown to reduce early mortality in patients after an anterior MI with reduced ejection fraction.

V-46. **The answer is E.** *(Chap. 277)* This patient has a subset of idiopathic VT, or VT originating in the absence of structural or inheritable cardiac disease. The presence of a normal baseline ECG, echocardiogram, and cardiac magnetic resonance imaging (MRI) essentially rule out Brugada syndrome, arrhythmogenic right ventricular dysplasia, and hypertrophic cardiomyopathy (although these are all important considerations in the patients with ventricular arrhythmias at a young age). The pictured ECG is classic for right ventricular outflow tract (RVOT) VT with a left bundle branch block pattern (indicating origin in the RV) and inferior axis (indicating origin in the cranial part, or base, of the heart). LV intrafascicular VT is another idiopathic VT, but presents with a right bundle branch block pattern. RVOT VT is often induced by scenarios with sympathetic nervous system activation, such as singing a solo in front of a crowd. This arrhythmia is not associated with sudden cardiac death and often responds to β-blockers or nondihydropyridine calcium channel blockers. Catheter ablation is an option if medical therapy fails to control the symptoms or is not desired.

V-47. **The answer is D.** *(Chap. 277)* This patients has medication-induced long QT syndrome (methadone and erythromycin are common causes) and resulting torsades de pointes (TdP). Sustained TdP is never a perfusing rhythm and can rapidly degenerate into ventricular fibrillation. For nonsustained TdP, correction of hypokalemia and expeditious administration of IV magnesium may lead to cessation of the arrhythmia. If this fails, administration of isoproterenol or pacing to a rate of 100–120 bpm will suppress PVCs and lead to rate-dependent shortening of the QT interval, thereby suppressing TdP and allowing time for the medications to washout. Inducing bradycardia (with metoprolol) or further QT prolongation with amiodarone may be harmful and lead to more TdP. Defibrillation is not warranted in NSVT. Likewise, ICD implantation is not necessary given that this is a secondary phenomenon due to drug interaction. This patient should be very cautious to avoid QT-prolonging agents in the future, however, and should consider transitioning off methadone at the earliest chance.

V-48. **The answer is A.** *(Chap. 277)* Atrial-ventricular dissociation is a classic finding in ventricular tachycardia. Physical examination may show jugular vein cannon a waves when the atria contracts against a closed tricuspid valve, and the ECG will manifest this with atrial capture and/or fusion beats. Other findings on ECG of ventricular tachycardia include QRS duration >140 msec for right bundle branch pattern in V_1 or >160 msec for left bundle morphology in lead V_1, frontal plane axis –90 to 180 degrees, delayed activation during initial phase of the QRS complex, and bizarre QRS pattern that does not mimic typical right or left bundle branch block QRS complex patterns. An irregularly irregular rhythm with changing QRS complexes suggests atrial fibrillation with ventricular preexcitation.

Carotid sinus massage, aimed at increasing vagal tone and slowing AV node conduction, is not effective at slowing ventricular tachycardia because the reentrant focus is below the AV node.

V-49. **The answer is E.** *(Chap. 278e)* This ECG demonstrates sinus arrhythmia, a normal physiologic finding particularly in young adults. During inspiration, the sinus rate speeds up to maintain cardiac output in the face of a slightly decreased left ventricular stroke volume, and vice versa during expiration. This is a normal, healthy heart rhythm and requires nor further investigation or intervention.

V-50. **The answer is A.** *(Chap. 278e)* This ECG shows 2:1 second-degree AV block; that is, there are two P waves for every QRS complex. In this type of second-degree AV block, it can be difficult to tell the difference between type I (Wenckebach) block, which is usually anatomically located at the AV node, and type II block, which is often infranodal in origin. There is no progressively prolonging or stable PR interval to distinguish. However, the presence of a narrow, normal QRS complex is sufficient to make Wenckebach block most likely, particularly in an athletic young person during sleep, a time of high vagal tone. A wide QRS complex during 2:1 conduction, particularly in a patient in whom infranodal disease would be likely, is concerning for second-degree type II block and more concerning for progression to complete or high-grade heart block.

V-51. **The answer is B.** *(Chap. 278e)* In heart block occurring at the AV node, the administration of atropine (an anticholinergic agent) will often improve the block as the AV node has a high degree of vagal efferent innervation. The SA node phase 4 action potential slope will increase as well with anticholinergic stimulation, causing faster sinus rate. In heart block occurring below the AV node, anticholinergic stimulation will often cause the appearance of a worse (3:1, 4:1, etc.) heart block as the sinus rate increases and more impulses are transmitted to the infranodal tissue during its prolonged (and unchanged with atropine) refractory period. One may use this finding to differentiate Wenckebach and type II second-degree heart block during difficult-to-interpret 2:1 conduction.

V-52. **The answer is E.** *(Chap. 278e)* This ECG illustrates tremor artifact, most notable in leads I, III, and aVL (thus making it likely that the tremor is occurring in the left arm). It is easy to confuse tremor artifact with atrial flutter or atrial fibrillation. Note the normal sinus P waves in lead II and all the precordial leads. No further testing is needed for this ECG.

V-53. **The answer is E.** *(Chap. 278e)* This ECG shows atrial flutter, with 2:1 conduction and the typical atrial rate of 300 bpm and ventricular rate of 150 bpm. The saw-tooth baseline pattern, best appreciated in the inferior leads, is a clue that this atrial flutter is "typical," or due to a macro-reentrant circuit that relies on the cavo-tricuspid isthmus. As such, it is quite amenable to ablation with a >95% success rate. However, given that Mr. Tillman's symptoms have been ongoing for >48 hours, he is at risk for development of an atrial thrombus (similar to in atrial fibrillation) and thus requires systemic anticoagulation before achievement of sinus rhythm. He will also likely require a transesophageal echocardiogram to ensure that no clot exists prior to ablation or cardioversion. Aspirin is not adequate to prevent potential embolization. Atrial flutter will generally not convert in response to amiodarone, digoxin, or other medications. Given the absence of heart failure, there is no indication for furosemide.

V-54. **The answer is E.** *(Chap. 278e)* This ECG is diagnostic of Wolff-Parkinson-White syndrome and likely explains the patient's palpitations. The presence of a left bundle–appearing delta wave/QRS complex (large R in the lateral precordial leads, I, and aVL) localizes this accessory tract to the right ventricle. Another clue is the exceedingly short PR interval; the ventricle is very preexcited as the sinus impulse arrives at the right ventricle very early because the accessory tract is so close to the SA node. Left-sided bypass tracts tend to appear slightly less preexcited (somewhat longer PR interval and slightly less wide QRS). Also, more tellingly, left-sided accessory tracts have a right bundle–like appearance with negative QRS complexes in the lateral precordial leads and lead I. Septal bypass tracts can be difficult to localize and are hallmarked by a rapid transition in QRS vector between the anterior precordial leads (V_1 and V_2 most often).

V-55. **The answer is C.** *(Chap. 279)* The New York Heart Association (NYHA) classification is a tool to define criteria that describe the functional ability and clinical manifestations of patients in heart failure. It is also used in patients with pulmonary hypertension. These criteria have been shown to have prognostic value with worsening survival as class increases. They are also useful to clinicians when reading studies to understand the entry and exclusion criteria of large clinical trials. Class I is used for patients with no limiting symptoms; class II for patients with slight or mild limitation; class III implies no symptoms at rest but dyspnea, angina, or palpitations with little exertion, and patients are moderately limited; class IV is severely limited, so that even minimal activity causes symptoms. Treatment guidelines also frequently base recommendations on these clinical stages. This patient has symptoms with mild exertion but is comfortable at rest; therefore, he is NYHA class III.

V-56. **The answer is E.** *(Chap. 279)* The patient presents with evidence of heart failure by history, and physical examination confirms this diagnosis. The warm extremities make a high-output state more likely than low cardiac output. Physical examination also shows exophthalmos and a fine tremor suggestive of hyperthyroidism. Thyrotoxicosis, along with anemia, nutritional disorders, and systemic arteriovenous shunting, can all cause high-output heart failure. The eye examination and tremor make hyperthyroidism more likely than anemia. Although systolic and diastolic dysfunction are more common causes of heart failure, disorders associated with a high-output state are often reversible, and therefore, a diagnosis should be pursued when clinical clues suggest this may be present.

V-57. **The answer is A.** *(Chap. 279)* Coronary artery disease remains the leading cause of heart failure with reduced ejection fraction, accounting for >60% of cases. Among all patients with heart failure, approximately 50% will have a preserved ejection fraction (LV ejection fraction [LVEF] >50%; option E). Although medical and device therapy has greatly advanced in the preceding decades, prognosis for heart failure patients remains grim. Community studies have shown that 30%–40% of patients die within 1 year of diagnosis and 60%–70% die within 5 years. This prognosis becomes even more dire in patients with extreme exertional limitation. NYHA class IV patients have a 50%–70% 1-year mortality (option C). Increasingly, epidemiologic data are showing that genetic cardiomyopathy (or familial cardiomyopathy) is more common than previously believed. It is now thought that >20% of all nonischemic cardiomyopathies are genetic or familial in etiology (option D). Although anemia is often an exacerbating factor in patients who already have heart failure, it is quite rare for it to cause de novo heart failure in a patient with a structurally normal heart (option B).

V-58. **The answer is C.** *(Chap. 279)* In the failing heart, multiple systems are upregulated to attempt to maintain cardiac output through augmenting sodium and water retention (angiotensin II, aldosterone, arginine vasopressin) and myocardial contractility (norepinephrine). Although initially helpful in maintaining cardiac output, these adaptations become deleterious in contributing to the development of adverse myocardial remodeling and the congestive state. Also deleterious is the upregulation of inflammatory systems (including tumor necrosis factor). Counterregulatory natriuretic peptides (such as B-type natriuretic peptide [BNP]) are also upregulated and aid in reducing systemic vascular resistance and natriuresis. In the state of heart failure, transcriptional and posttranscriptional changes in the myocyte lead to calcium leakage through the sarcoplasmic reticular membrane and, therefore, decreased calcium uptake in the sarcoplasmic reticulum.

V-59. **The answer is E.** *(Chap. 279)* Orthopnea, which is defined as dyspnea occurring in the recumbent position, is usually a later manifestation of heart failure than is exertional dyspnea. It results from redistribution of fluid from the splanchnic circulation and lower extremities into the central circulation during recumbency, with a resultant increase in pulmonary capillary pressure. Nocturnal cough is a common manifestation of this process and a frequently overlooked symptom of heart failure. Orthopnea generally is relieved by sitting upright or sleeping with additional pillows. Although orthopnea is a relatively specific symptom of heart failure, it may occur in patients with abdominal obesity or ascites and in patients with pulmonary disease whose lung mechanics favor an upright posture (such as with respiratory muscle compromise). In contrast, the hepatopulmonary syndrome is characterized by the development of pulmonary arteriovenous malformations and thus multiple shunts within the pulmonary circulation. These tend to develop in the lung bases, and thus, the patient's shunt fraction increases with an upright posture. This leads to orthodeoxia (hypoxia in the upright position) and platypnea (the sensation of shortness of breath when upright) rather than orthopnea.

V-60. **The answer is C.** *(Chap. 279)* BNP and its NT terminal fraction are increased in heart failure states and, on the population level, contribute to prognosis in heart failure states. However, it is important to recognize that natriuretic peptide levels increase with age and renal impairment, are more elevated in women, and can be elevated in right heart failure from any cause. Levels can be falsely low in obese patients. Other biomarkers such as soluble ST-2 and galectin-3 are newer biomarkers that can be used to determine the prognosis of heart failure patients.

V-61. **The answer is A.** *(Chap. 279)* The right heart is a thin-walled compliant chamber that is better suited to handle volume overload than pressure overload. In the setting of acute pressure overload (massive pulmonary embolism), the right heart quickly dilates and fails, leading to circulatory collapse. In the setting of slowly developing pulmonary hypertension (due to vascular, thrombotic, or pulmonary disease), the right heart hypertrophies in an attempt to compensate. Over time, the right ventricular (RV) contractile function becomes uncoupled from an ever-increasing afterload, and cor pulmonale or RV failure develops. In a patient with preexisting cor pulmonale, small changes in RV preload or afterload can be catastrophic. In this patient, any change leading to acidemia (reducing respiratory rate) or elevated alveolar pressures (increasing positive end-expiratory pressure, increasing tidal volume) are likely to increase RV afterload and may worsen RV stroke volume and cardiac output. Incidentally, increasing transmural pressure (plateau or end-expiratory ventilator pressures) has disparate effects on RV and LV afterload. Because the RV target vasculature is completely intrathoracic, the pressure is transmitted across the vessel walls and must be overcome by the RV. However, LV vasculature is mostly extrathoracic. Thus, the increased intrathoracic pressure is only transmitted to the LV and actually reduces afterload (transmural chamber pressure). Hypoxia causes pulmonary vasoconstriction (as opposed to the systemic circulation, where it causes vasodilation). Thus, increasing the FiO_2 in an attempt to improve the hypoxia may reduce the pulmonary vasoconstriction and lower the RV afterload.

V-62. **The answer is E.** *(Chap. 280)* While therapeutic targets in heart failure with reduced ejection fraction (HFrEF) are relatively abundant and guided by the targets of disease modification, trials in heart failure with preserved ejection fraction (HFpEF) have been largely disappointing. ACE inhibitors (option A) have been studies in many mechanistic studies and have shown no convincing mortality benefit. Similarly, angiotensin receptor blockers (option B) were studied in the CHARM-Preserved and I-PRESERVE studies and were found to have no mortality benefit. Sildenafil (a phosphodiesterase-5 inhibitor) was shown to improve filling pressures and RV function in patients with HFpEF, but did not show mortality benefit. Finally, digoxin, which inhibits sodium-potassium-ATPase, was shown to have no role in treating HFpEF in the DIG study. Overall, symptom management and blood pressure control are the goals in HFpEF treatment now. One should also remain vigilant for myocardial ischemia.

V-63. **The answer is B.** *(Chap. 280)* This patient clearly has adequate cardiac output to maintain peripheral perfusion as evidenced by her physical examination (warm extremities) and adequate blood pressure. However, her elevated creatinine is vexing and indicates that she suffers from the cardiorenal syndrome. In some cases, it truly is a depressed cardiac output causing a low glomerular filtration rate (GFR); however, these cases are typically accompanied by other signs of peripheral malperfusion. In most cases when cardiac output is not severely depressed, it is thought that a complex interplay of elevated venous pressures (reducing transglomerular perfusion pressures) and abdominal pressures leads to decreased GFR. In these cases, reducing venous pressures with diuretics is the most reasonable first option. In patients who respond poorly (rising creatinine or adverse hemodynamic effects), hemodynamic monitoring (option A) or ultrafiltration can be considered. Digoxin should be used with caution in renal insufficiency and has no real benefit acutely here. In cases where cardiac output is thought to be severely depressed and peripheral perfusion is compromised, inotropic therapy may be indicated.

V-64. **The answer is D.** *(Chap. 280)* Nesiritide is the recombinant form of human BNP. It was introduced in a fixed dose for therapy of acute decompensated heart failure after demonstration of a more rapid and greater reduction in pulmonary capillary wedge pressure than with intravenous nitrates. Enthusiasm for nesiritide waned due to concerns within the pivotal trials for development of renal insufficiency and an increase in mortality. To address these concerns, a large-scale morbidity and mortality trial, the Acute Study of Clinical Effectiveness of Nesiritide in Decompensated Heart Failure (ASCEND-HF), was completed in 2011 and randomly enrolled 7141 patients with acute decompensated heart failure to nesiritide or placebo for 24–168 hours in addition to standard care. Nesiritide was not associated with an increase or a decrease in the rates of death and rehospitalization and had a clinically insignificant benefit on dyspnea. Renal function did not worsen, but increased rates of hypotension were noted. Although this trial established the safety of nesiritide, its routine use cannot be advocated due to lack of significant efficacy.

V-65. **The answer is E.** *(Chaps. 279 and 280)* The utility of invasive hemodynamic monitoring during acute decompensated heart failure has been highly scrutinized recently. Based on several observational and randomized trials, the routine use of a pulmonary artery catheter is not recommended and should be restricted to patients who respond poorly to diuresis or experience hypotension or signs and symptoms suggestive of a low cardiac output where therapeutic targets are unclear. In this patient with hypotension and signs of low cardiac output, invasive monitoring will allow the clinician to rapidly, objectively assess any changes in hemodynamic status and respond appropriately. In states of "cold" (poor perfusion) and "wet" (elevated filling pressures, or hypervolemia) heart failure, the stroke volume and cardiac output are decreased. Left ventricular stroke work index (a calculated value that normalizes left ventricular work for the patient's body surface area and afterload) is also diminished. Mixed venous oxygen saturation is greatly diminished as well, as the Fick equation dictates that cardiac output is proportional to the venous oxygen saturation if oxygen consumption and arterial oxygen saturation are normal. Systemic vascular resistance equals the mean systemic arterial pressure minus the mean right atrial pressure divided by cardiac output. As cardiac output drops, the systemic vasculature will increase its resistance to attempt to maintain blood pressure and end-organ perfusion pressure. However, this initially compensatory action becomes deleterious because an inefficient left ventricle must work against an ever-increasing afterload. The most effective inotropic agents in acute decompensated heart failure (milrinone, and dobutamine) also have vasodilatory properties to combat this harmful systemic vascular resistance (SVR) increase.

V-66. **The answer is C.** *(Chap. 280)* β-Blockers represent the most-studied drug in the history of HFrEF. Initially avoided for their negative inotropic and chronotropic effects, they now form the foundation of neurohormonal-targeted therapy in the treatment of chronic HFrEF. However, the benefit of β-blockers is not a blanket class effect and indeed has only been demonstrated for three drugs in the numerous clinical trials: metoprolol succinate, bisoprolol, and carvedilol. Importantly, metoprolol tartrate has never been found to have mortality benefit in HFrEF, nor have β-blockers with intrinsic sympathomimetic activity (nebivolol, xamoterol).

V-67. **The answer is E.** *(Chap. 280)* Whether β-blockers or ACE inhibitors should be started first was answered by the Cardiac Insufficiency Bisoprolol Study (CIBIS) III, in which outcomes did not vary when either agent was initiated first. Thus, it matters little which agent is initiated first; what does matter is that optimally titrated doses of both ACE inhibitors and β-blockers are established in a timely manner. It should be noted that although ACE inhibitors have been shown to have a dose-dependent reduction in hospitalizations, higher tolerated doses do not materially improve survival. In contrast, β-blockers have a strong dose effect on survival. Thus, if forced to choose between a higher dose of β-blockers or ACE inhibitor due to low blood pressure, the higher dose of β-blocker may provide more survival benefit.

V-68. **The answer is E.** *(Chap. 280)* This patient is on optimal doses of the three medications forming the foundation of neurohormonal therapy for HFrEF. Digoxin was shown to reduce hospitalizations but not mortality in the DIG trial. The addition of valsartan to ACE inhibitor therapy was studied in the Val-HEFT trial and showed a trend toward worse outcomes. Similarly, aliskiren (a direct renin inhibitor) was studied in addition to ACE inhibitors in the ASTRONAUT trial and showed no mortality benefit and an abundance of side effects such as hyperkalemia and hypotension. Ivabradine, a novel heart rate–reducing agent, was studied in the SHIFT trial and showed mortality benefit, but only in patients with a heart rate >70 bpm already on βblockers. This patient's heart rate is controlled.

V-69. **The answer is A.** *(Chap. 280)* Sudden cardiac death due to ventricular arrhythmias is the mode of death in approximately half of patients with heart failure and is particularly proportionally prevalent in patients diagnosed with HFrEF in early stages of the disease. Although primary prevention of sudden cardiac death is challenging, the two most important risk markers for increased risk of death are the degree of residual left ventricular dysfunction despite optimal medical therapy (≤35%) and the underlying etiology of heart failure (post–myocardial infarction or ischemic cardiomyopathy). Currently, patients with NYHA class II to III symptoms of heart failure and an LVEF <35%, irrespective of etiology of heart failure, are appropriate candidates for implantable cardioverter defibrillator (ICD) prophylactic therapy. In patients with a history of myocardial infarction and optimal medical therapy with residual LVEF ≤30% (even when asymptomatic), placement of an ICD is appropriate. The Resynchronization–Defibrillation for Ambulatory Heart Failure Trial (RAFT) and Multicenter Automatic Defibrillator Implantation Trial with Cardiac Resynchronization Therapy (MADIT-CRT) both sought to use cardiac resynchronization therapy (CRT) in combination with an ICD. Most benefit in mildly symptomatic HFrEF patients accrues from applying this therapy in those with a QRS width of >149 msec and a left bundle branch block pattern. Attempts to further optimize risk stratification and expand indications for CRT using modalities other than electrocardiography have proven disappointing. Likewise, surgical ventricular remodeling was studied in a 1000-patient trial and found to have no disease-modifying effect. It is still used, but relegated to patients with cardioembolic strokes on anticoagulation or patients with refractory ventricular arrhythmias. Ivabradine, a novel heart rate–reducing agent, may reduce mortality in patients with HFrEF who have a resting heart rate >70 bpm while on an adequate dose of a β-blocker.

V-70. **The answer is D.** *(Chap. 281)* In patients with an orthotopic heart transplant, the donor heart is denervated during the harvest. In the absence of sympathetic or parasympathetic innervation, many patients exhibit a mild resting tachycardia or slightly elevated heart rate. Heart rate response during exercise or physiologic stress may be delayed, but is enacted by cardiac response to circulating catecholamines, primarily adrenal in origin. It is important to realize this to avoid unnecessary testing and to avoid adverse events with drug administration. In particular, atropine will have almost no effect on a patient after orthotopic heart transplant, and extreme caution should be exercised in administering adenosine because the denervated heart may have a very delayed recovery from adenosine-induced heart block.

V-71. **The answer is D.** *(Chap. 281)* In the United States, the allocation of donor organs is accomplished under the supervision of the United Network for Organ Sharing, a private organization under contract to the federal government. The United States is divided geographically into 11 regions for donor heart allocation. Allocation of donor hearts within a region is decided according to a system of priority that takes into account (1) the severity of illness, (2) the geographic distance from the donor, and (3) the patient's time on the waiting list. A physiologic limit of ~3 hours of "ischemic" (out-of-body) time for hearts precludes a national sharing of hearts. This allocation system design is reissued annually and is responsive to input from a variety of constituencies, including both donor families and transplantation professionals.

V-72. The answer is C. *(Chap. 281)* Despite usually having young donor hearts, cardiac allograft recipients are prone to develop coronary artery disease (CAD). This CAD is generally a diffuse, concentric, and longitudinal process that is quite different from "ordinary" atherosclerotic CAD, which is more focal and often eccentric. The underlying etiology most likely is primarily immunologic injury of the vascular endothelium, but a variety of risk factors influence the existence and progression of CAD, including nonimmunologic factors such as dyslipidemia, diabetes mellitus, and cytomegalovirus (CMV) infection (as in this patient). It is hoped that newer and improved immunosuppressive modalities will reduce the incidence and impact of these devastating complications, which currently account for the majority of late posttransplantation deaths. Thus far, the immunosuppressive agents mycophenolate mofetil and the mammalian target of rapamycin (mTOR) inhibitors sirolimus and everolimus have been shown to be associated with short-term lower incidence and extent of coronary intimal thickening; in anecdotal reports, institution of sirolimus was associated with some reversal of CAD. The use of statins also is associated with a reduced incidence of this vasculopathy, and these drugs are now used almost universally in transplant recipients unless contraindicated. Palliation of CAD with percutaneous interventions is probably safe and effective in the short term, although the disease often advances relentlessly. Because of the denervated status of the organ, patients rarely experience angina pectoris, even in advanced stages of disease. Antibody (humoral)–mediated rejection is exceedingly rare in a patient this far out from transplant, particularly one who fortunately has had no prior rejection episodes. While cellular rejection is possible, the presence of a normal left ventricle (and no arrhythmias) makes it less likely. Tacrolimus most commonly causes hypertension, neurologic complications, and renal insufficiency. Mycophenolate mofetil most commonly causes bone marrow suppression and diarrhea. Low-dose prednisone is generally well tolerated, although chronic steroids carry incipient risk of diabetes, obesity, skin changes, iatrogenic adrenal insufficiency, osteoporosis, and cataracts. None of these drugs classically causes dyspnea.

V-73. The answer is C. *(Chap. 281)* For patients with end-stage cardiomyopathy (NYHA class IV or peak oxygen consumption <14 mL/kg/min), the prognosis is abysmal. In the landmark REMATCH trial, the 2-year survival of the medically treated arm was only 8%. Orthotopic heart transplantation is the gold standard therapy for these patients. However, some patients are not candidates due to underlying comorbidities that would render a transplantation too dangerous. For these patients, the continuous flow left ventricular assist devices have been shown convincingly to improve mortality (2-year survival in REMATCH was approximately 60% and has improved since that study). Although it is unreasonable to predict a complication-free course (most patients have thrombotic, infectious, or neurologic complications during their course of support), the median survival for patients with left ventricular assist device support is now approaching 5 years. Stem cell therapy is currently investigational only and has never been shown to meaningfully impact survival. Similarly, milrinone or dobutamine therapy (inotropic support) can be used continuously to support quality of life as a palliative goal or as a bridge to initiation of mechanical support or transplantation. However, all studies show that the use of inotropes negatively impacts survival.

V-74. The answer is B. *(Chap 282)* The most common birth defects are cardiovascular in origin. These malformations are due to complex multifactorial genetic and environmental causes. Recognized chromosomal aberrations and mutations of single genes account for <10% of all cardiac malformations. Congenital heart disease (CHD) complicates ~1% of all live births in the general population—about 40,000 births per year—but occurs more frequently in the offspring (about 4%–10%, depending on maternal CHD type) of women with CHD. Due to the remarkable surgical advances over the last 60 years, >90% of afflicted neonates and children now reach adulthood; women with CHD may now frequently successfully bear children after competent repairs. As such, the population with CHD is steadily increasing. Women with CHD are at increased risk for peri- and postpartum complications, but maternal CHD is generally not considered an absolute contraindication to pregnancy unless the mother has certain high-risk features (e.g., cyanosis, pulmonary hypertension, decompensated heart failure, arrhythmias, aortic aneurysm).

V-75. The answer is D. *(Chap. 281)* Atrial septal defect (ASD) is a common cardiac anomaly that may be first encountered in the adult and occurs more frequently in females. Sinus venosus ASD occurs high in the atrial septum near the entry of the superior vena cava into the right atrium and is associated frequently with anomalous pulmonary venous connection from the right lung to the superior vena cava or right atrium. Ostium primum ASDs lie adjacent to the atrioventricular valves, either of which may be deformed and regurgitant. Ostium primum ASDs are common in Down syndrome, often as part of complex atrioventricular septal defects with a common atrioventricular valve and a posterior defect of the basal portion of the interventricular septum. The most common ostium secundum ASD involves the fossa ovalis and is mid-septal in location; this should not be confused with a patent foramen ovale (which is present in ~25% of healthy adults). Anatomic obliteration of the foramen ovale ordinarily follows its functional closure soon after birth, but residual "probe patency" is a common normal variant; ASD denotes a true deficiency of the atrial septum and implies functional and anatomic patency.

V-76. **The answer is D.** *(Chap. 281)* This patient has a small muscular VSD. The decision on whether to treat a VSD is complex but is based on the principle of avoiding any right ventricular and pulmonary vascular compromise. Similarly, one must avoid repairing a VSD in the setting of overt pulmonary hypertension, as this is clearly associated with worse outcomes. Closure is not recommended for patients with normal pulmonary arterial pressures with small shunts (pulmonary-to-systemic flow ratios of <1.5:1). Operative correction or transcatheter closure is indicated when there is a moderate to large left-to-right shunt with a pulmonary-to-systemic flow ratio >1.5:1, in the absence of prohibitively high levels of pulmonary vascular resistance (pulmonary arterial resistance is less than two-thirds of systemic arterial resistance). This patient has a normal pulmonary artery pressure, a pulmonary vascular resistance to SVR ratio of 0.33, and Qp:Qs of 1.25; therefore, closure is not warranted at this time, but follow-up is indicated.

V-77. **The answer is C.** *(Chap. 281)* This patient has the classic murmur and findings of myocardial ischemia associated with a spontaneous rupture of a coronary artery aneurysm to form a coronary arteriovenous fistula. In this case, the presence of an oxygenation step-up in the right heart, with near-systemic oxygenation levels in the coronary sinus (which usually has very low oxygen saturation levels), makes this diagnosis certain. An ASD would not present with such a murmur or clinical presentation. A VSD would not show such high oxygen levels in the coronary sinus. A patent ductus arteriosus can present with a similar murmur but usually causes left-to-right shunting at the level of the pulmonary artery; thus, the oxygen step-up would be there. Anomalous left coronary artery off the pulmonary artery causes myocardial ischemia, although not so precipitously and usually early in life, and is not associated with a murmur. In this condition, oxygenated blood from the aortic root flows via a dilated right coronary artery and collaterals to the left coronary artery and retrograde to the lower pressure pulmonary artery circulation via the anomalous left main coronary artery (which emerges from the pulmonary artery). Most patients die in the first year of life from myocardial ischemia and fibrosis, although a minority can live into adulthood.

V-78. **The answer is A.** *(Chap. 282)* Bicuspid aortic valve is among the most common of congenital heart cardiac abnormalities. Valvular function is often normal in early life and thus may escape detection. Due to abnormal flow dynamics through the bicuspid aortic valve, the valve leaflets can become rigid and fibrosed, leading to either stenosis or regurgitation. However, pathology in patients with bicuspid aortic valve is not limited to the valve alone. The ascending aorta is often dilated, misnamed "poststenotic" dilatation; this is due to histologic abnormalities of the aortic media and may result in aortic dissection. It is important to screen specifically for aortopathy because dissection is a common cause of sudden death in these patients.

V-79. **The answer is D.** *(Chap. 282)* The four classic components of the tetralogy of Fallot are malaligned VSD, obstruction to RV outflow, aortic override of the VSD, and RV hypertrophy (due to the RV's response to aortic pressure via the large VSD). Tricuspid atresia is associated with Ebstein anomaly and hypoplastic right heart syndrome. In these cases, a concurrent systemic-to-pulmonary connection is required to maintain early life (such as a patent ductus arteriosis). Right heart bypass operations such as the Glenn shunt or Fontan palliation can provide adequate pulmonary flow to support patients into and through early adulthood.

V-80. The answer is B. *(Chap. 283)* The patient has aortic stenosis that presented late in life. Although bicuspid aortic valve underlies nearly half of all aortic stenosis cases, this lesion typically presents earlier in life, and only 40% of patients >70 years old with aortic stenosis who undergo surgery have a bicuspid valve. Rheumatic heart disease may cause aortic stenosis, but nearly invariably, mitral stenosis is also present. Underlying connective tissue disease is not known to be associated with aortic stenosis. Modern research on development of aortic stenosis has shown that several traditional atherosclerotic risk factors are present such as diabetes mellitus, smoking, chronic kidney disease, and the metabolic syndrome. Polymorphisms of the vitamin D receptor have also been demonstrated in patients with symptomatic aortic stenosis.

V-81. The answer is C. *(Chap. 283)* Exertional syncope is a late finding in aortic stenosis and portends a poor prognosis. Patients with this symptom or with angina pectoris have an average time to death of 3 years. Patients with dyspnea have an average time to death of 2 years, and patients with heart failure have an average time to death of 1.5–2 years. Given these data, patients with severe aortic stenosis and symptoms should strongly be considered for surgical therapy.

V-82. The answer is D. *(Chap 283)* This patient is in cardiogenic shock due to his progressive aortic stenosis (AS). The natural history of symptomatic severe AS is not encouraging. Aortic valve area, on average, declines by 0.1 cm^2 per year, and gradient increases by 7 mmHg annually. The average time to death after the onset of various symptoms is as follows: angina pectoris, 3 years; syncope, 3 years; dyspnea, 2 years; and congestive heart failure, 1.5–2 years. Moreover, in >80% of patients who die with AS, symptoms had existed for <4 years. Currently, this patient has compromised organ function due to the severe LV obstruction of AS and resultant low stroke volume. Any negative inotropic or chronotropic agents may prove fatal, as reducing heart rate or stroke volume will further compromise cardiac output (option C). Digoxin is unlikely to augment stroke volume to any significant degree in the setting of severe AS and is risky in the setting of compromised renal function (option B). Although statins have been shown to slightly slow the progression of AS, they serve no role in the acute setting (option A). Phenylephrine is an α-agonist. Although it may serve to increase blood pressure, it acts via peripheral vasoconstriction, which further increases the resistance the left ventricle is working against. Percutaneous aortic balloon valvuloplasty (PABV) is a poor long-term therapeutic option because almost all patients have the recrudescence of severe AS within 6 months to a year. However, PABV can serve as bridge to definite therapy (such as surgical aortic valve replacement), temporarily improving cardiac output and end-organ perfusion to render surgical risk acceptable. Other options would be an intra-aortic balloon pump or, in rare cases, mechanical circulatory support.

V-83. The answer is D. *(Chap. 283)* This patient has evidence of the clinical entity referred to as low-gradient, low-flow AS. Conceptually, the aortic valve area during systole is dependent on two factors: (1) aortic valve morphology (e.g., calcific AS with restricted leaflet motion), and (2) ventricular contractile force. Even a normal aortic valve will open very little if the ventricle contracts very weakly. In this patient's case, the finding of a low calculated aortic valve area without a severely high gradient (severe is >40 mmHg) in the setting of reduced LV function defines the entity of low-gradient, low-flow AS. It is difficult to determine whether the valve area is low due to reason 1 or 2 during a resting echocardiography. However, dobutamine stress will accomplish two goals. First, it will assess for ventricular viability (the ability to increase stroke volume by 20%), which is shown to predict outcomes after aortic valve replacement. Second, and more importantly, as the ventricular contractility increases, it allows the clinician to differentiate between true, morphologic AS and the appearance of AS due to compromised ventricular function (termed pseudo-AS). Although the other options may aid in other facets of this patient's management, none will allow the clinician to make this differentiation.

V-84. The answer is A. *(Chap. 287)* An increase in the LV end-diastolic volume (increased preload) constitutes the major hemodynamic compensation for aortic regurgitation (AR); thus, preload is increased. The total LV stroke volume also increases to attempt to maintain effective LV stroke volume (total LV stroke volume – regurgitant volume). To do this, the LV must dilate. As the LV dilates, the wall tension to develop a given systolic blood pressure must increase as dictated by LaPlace's law, and thus, afterload is increased. During diastole, as a large volume of blood leaves the systemic circulation to regurgitate into the LV, the diastolic pressure falls, often equilibrating with the LV pressure in severe cases. Coronary perfusion occurs primarily during diastole and depends on the gradient between aortic pressure and LV pressure through the coronaries. This explains why patients with severe AR may manifest anginal symptoms.

V-85. **The answer is C.** *(Chap. 283)* This patient has severe, acute AR and indeed warrants emergent surgery. Note that her murmur is very quiet and short. In the setting of acute, severe valvular regurgitant lesions, the pressure gradient between the two chambers (in this case, the aorta and LV) quickly equilibrates during the regurgitant period. Sometimes, patients with these lesions can have no audible murmur at all, making diagnosis challenging. In this case, the goal is to reduce the regurgitant volume and thus increase effective stroke volume (total stroke volume – regurgitant volume). Interventions that increase systemic vascular resistance (vasopressin or norepinephrine) will increase regurgitant volume. Likewise, because aortic regurgitation occurs during diastole, interventions that increase diastolic time (e.g., β-blockers) will also worsen regurgitant volume. Because intra-aortic balloon pumps inflate during diastole, they will also worsen regurgitation from aorta to LV and are contraindicated in moderate or worse AR. Nitroprusside will reduce systemic vascular resistance and thus reduce the driving pressure for regurgitation. Careful administration of nitroprusside, often with concomitant invasive hemodynamic monitoring, may stabilize organ perfusion and allow surgical correction. It is important to realize that no medical therapy will correct this abnormality; surgical correction is the only definitive therapy.

V-86. **The answer is E.** *(Chap. 284)* Rheumatic fever remains the leading cause of mitral stenosis (MS). Other less common etiologies of obstruction to LV inflow include congenital mitral valve stenosis, cor triatriatum, mitral annular calcification with extension onto the leaflets, systemic lupus erythematosus, rheumatoid arthritis, left atrial myxoma, and infective endocarditis with large vegetations. Pure or predominant MS occurs in approximately 40% of all patients with rheumatic heart disease and a history of rheumatic fever. In other patients with rheumatic heart disease, lesser degrees of MS may accompany mitral regurgitation and aortic valve disease.

V-87. **The answer is B.** *(Chap 284)* In MS, the flow obstruction between the left ventricle and left atrium creates elevated left atrial pressure to maintain cardiac output. For example, once the effective mitral valve orifice reaches 1.5 cm^2, the left atrial pressure must be >25 mmHg to maintain a normal cardiac output. LV preload, diameter, and end-diastolic pressure are normal or diminished in MS. Similarly, cardiac output is normal or diminished. Due to elevated left atrial pressures, pulmonary venous pressures rise. This causes pulmonary vascular congestion and distention and reduces pulmonary vascular compliance.

V-88. **The answer is C.** *(Chap 284)* MS represents a fixed obstructive lesion between the left atrium and ventricle. Because flow across this valve occurs in diastole, any intervention that shortens diastole will cause worsened obstruction and more elevated left atrium pressures. Thus, tachycardia induced by exercise or β-agonists is detrimental in MS. Metoprolol, a β-antagonist, will not shorten diastole. Additionally, any extra volume load or higher demand for cardiac output, as in anemia, will lead to an elevated left atrial pressure. The extra blood volume of pregnancy can be particularly poorly tolerated in patients with significant MS.

V-89. **The answer is D.** *(Chap. 284)* The left atrial to left ventricular pressure gradient is highly dependent on heart rate because diastolic duration is inversely related to heart rate. In the setting of MS, a long diastolic time allows more time for the left atrium to empty and thus lower pressures. Hence, sinus bradycardia is advantageous in the setting of MS, and inducing a faster heart rate via pacemaker would be harmful. The loss of atrial systole during atrial fibrillation is often poorly tolerated in MS, and regaining sinus rhythm would undoubtedly lower atrial pressure. However, the vast majority of patients with MS are unable to maintain sinus rhythm over the long term because their atria tend to be very dilated. Diuretics and percutaneous mitral valvotomy will both lower left atrial pressure.

V-90. The answer is C. *(Chap. 284)* This patient has asymptomatic moderate MS (severe is valve area <1.5 cm^2). There is no evidence that the procedural mitral valve repair improves the prognosis of patients with slight or no functional impairment. Therefore, unless recurrent systemic embolization or severe pulmonary hypertension has occurred (pulmonary artery systolic pressures >50 mmHg at rest or >60 mmHg with exercise), valvotomy is not recommended for patients who are entirely asymptomatic and/or who have mild or moderate stenosis (mitral valve area >1.5 cm^2). Given this patient's lack of symptoms and relatively low resting heart rate, β-blockade is not warranted. Similarly, sildenafil (a pulmonary vasodilator) will not help reduce pulmonary pressures.

V-91. The answer is B. *(Chap. 284)* Mitral regurgitation (MR) occurs due to several reasons. Distinction should be drawn between primary (degenerative, organic) MR, in which the leaflets and/or chordae tendineae are primarily responsible for abnormal valve function, and functional (secondary) MR, in which the leaflets and chordae tendineae are structurally normal but the regurgitation is caused by annular enlargement, papillary muscle displacement, leaflet tethering, or their combination. This patient has functional MR due to his nonischemic dilated cardiomyopathy. In such patients, particularly those with an ejection fraction (EF) <30%, there is concern that repairing the mitral valve will lead to an overall increase in LV afterload and worsening of LV function. It is important to realize that the state of MR is one of very low afterload for the LV because it can eject easily into the low-pressure, compliant left atrium. Thus, even a slight reduction in EF (<60%) can represent significant LV dysfunction that can be unmasked after mitral valve repair. In patients with ischemic MR and significantly impaired LV systolic function (EF <30%), the risk of surgery is higher, recovery of LV performance is incomplete, and long-term survival is reduced. Referral for surgery must be individualized and made only after aggressive attempts with guideline-directed medical therapy and cardiac resynchronization therapy, when indicated. The routine performance of valve repair in patients with significant MR in the setting of severe, functional, nonischemic dilated cardiomyopathy (such as this patient) has not been shown to improve long-term survival compared with optimal medical therapy. Percutaneous therapy is currently under investigation for patients with functional MR but has not yet been shown to improve survival.

V-92. The answer is D. *(Chap 285)* Note the gradient between right atrial pressure and right ventricular end-diastolic pressure (15 and 6 mmHg, respectively) and the left atrium (represented by the pulmonary capillary wedge pressure) and left ventricular end-diastolic pressure (12 and 6 mmHg, respectively). This is diagnostic of mixed tricuspid and mitral stenosis. Also note that the gradient between the left atrium and left ventricle is not severe and that the pulmonary arterial and right ventricular pressures are not very elevated. In the presence of tricuspid stenosis, flow is decreased to the pulmonary vasculature and left heart, thus blunting the hemodynamic effects of even severe mitral stenosis. Grading the severity of mitral stenosis in this setting is quite difficult. Finally, this mix of valvular disease is essentially diagnostic of rheumatic disease. The tricuspid valve is never involved alone and is always affected only if the mitral is also involved. Radiation injury and carcinoid syndrome are two other, rarer causes of combined mitral and tricuspid valvular disease.

V-93. The answer is A. *(Chap. 285)* This patient has severe tricuspid regurgitation (TR) secondary to RV dilation and dysfunction, which is in turn secondary to her severe pulmonary arterial hypertension. In cases of functional TR, repair is relegated to instances where surgery is already being pursued for left-sided valvular lesions. Furthermore, the presence of severe pulmonary hypertension is a relative contraindication for TR repair. The RV suddenly finds itself without the "pop-off valve" of severe TR and often fails when faced with the overwhelming afterload of the abnormal pulmonary vasculature. Percutaneous tricuspid valve repair is not currently performed in clinical practice. Balloon valvotomy is a repair for tricuspid stenosis, not regurgitation. There is no indication in this patient for repair of the mitral valve. Patients with mitral valvular disease may develop significant pulmonary hypertension; however, the diagnosis of idiopathic pulmonary arterial hypertension cannot be established until significant mitral valve dysfunction has been ruled out.

V-94. The answer is C. *(Chap. 285)* Pulmonic stenosis is a rare valvular lesion encountered in adults. Fortunately, percutaneous balloon valvotomy often provides a highly efficacious, relatively low-risk therapeutic option. Diuretics can be used to treat symptoms and signs of right heart failure. Provided there is less than moderate pulmonic regurgitation, pulmonic balloon valvotomy is recommended for symptomatic patients with a domed valve and a peak gradient >50 mmHg (or mean gradient >30 mmHg) and for asymptomatic patients with a peak gradient >60 mmHg (or mean gradient >40 mmHg). Surgery may be required when the valve is dysplastic (as seen in patients with Noonan syndrome and other disorders).

V-95. The answer is D. *(Chap. 286)* This patient is in a precarious situation and likely will require emergent surgical intervention to survive. The combination of severe obstruction to LV outflow (severe AS) and acute, severe regurgitant mitral valve disorder will inevitably lead to intractable pulmonary edema and cardiogenic shock unless both structural abnormalities are corrected. At the advent of severe mitral regurgitation, the LV will be more effectively "unloaded" because now it can eject not only against the stenosed aortic valve, but also into the relatively low-pressure left atrium, and thus afterload will decline. Likewise, with more of the stroke volume going ineffectively into the left atrium, the effective stroke volume (total stroke volume – regurgitant volume) will decline. The aortic valve gradient will decline merely because there is less volume going across the aortic valve with each contraction. Likewise, because both the catheter-derived and echocardiographic-derived calculations of aortic valve area are dependent on the gradient for calculation, they will decline. Ejection fraction, however, will increase as the LV will be better able to contract in the state of relatively lower afterload. This highlights a misconception that higher ejection fraction is always better. LV ejection fraction is highly dependent not only on the contractile state of the ventricle, but also on its afterload state.

V-96. The answer is D. *(Chap. 286)* Patients with valvular atrial fibrillation are at particularly high risk for systemic thromboembolisms, including stroke. In general, unless a direct contraindication is present, these patients warrant systemic anticoagulation. It is important to remember that the novel oral anticoagulants (apixaban, dabigatran, and rivaroxaban), although easier to administer, are not approved for valvular atrial fibrillation. Warfarin remains the best "tried-and-true" option for valvular atrial fibrillation.

V-97. The answer is C. *(Chap. 287)* Peripartum cardiomyopathy is a rare complication of pregnancy and can occur during the last trimester or within the first 6 months postpartum. Risk factors include advanced age, increased parity, twin pregnancy, malnutrition, use of tocolytic therapy for premature labor, and preeclampsia.

V-98. The answer is D. *(Chap. 287)* Cardiac involvement is common in many of the neuromuscular diseases. The ECG pattern of Duchenne muscular dystrophy is unique and consists of tall R waves in the right precordial leads with an R/S ratio >1.0, often with deep Q waves in the limb and precordial leads. These patients often have a variety of supraventricular and ventricular arrhythmias and are at risk for sudden death due to the intrinsic cardiomyopathy as well as the low ejection fraction. Implantable cardioverter defibrillators should be considered in the appropriate patient. Global left ventricular dysfunction is a common finding in dilated cardiomyopathies, whereas focal wall motion abnormalities and angina are more common if there is ischemic myocardium. This patient is at risk for venous thromboembolism; however, chronic thromboembolism would not account for the severity of the left heart failure and would present with findings consistent with pulmonary hypertension. Amyotrophic lateral sclerosis is a disease of motor neurons and does not involve the heart. This patient would be young for that diagnosis. An advanced atrial septal defect would present with cyanosis and heart failure (Eisenmenger physiology).

V-99. The answer is B. *(Chap. 287)* Most familial cardiomyopathies are inherited in an autosomal dominant pattern, with occasional autosomal recessive and X-linked inheritance. Missense mutations with amino acid substitutions are the most common in cardiomyopathy. Expressed mutant proteins may interfere with function of the normal allele through a dominant negative mechanism. Mutations introducing a premature stop codon (nonsense) or shift in the reading frame (frameshift) may create a truncated or unstable protein the lack of which causes cardiomyopathy (haploinsufficiency). Deletions or duplications of an entire exon or gene are uncommon causes of cardiomyopathy, except for the dystrophinopathies.

V-100. The answer is E. *(Chap. 287)* All of the tests listed have a role in some patients with newly diagnosed cardiomyopathy. However, only a thyroid-stimulating hormone (TSH) level receives a Level I recommendation from the American College of Cardiology (ACC)/ American Heart Association (AHA) for all patients with new cardiomyopathy. All other tests listed are driven by symptoms and signs that are present. Cardiac MRI and erythrocyte sedimentation rate (ESR) levels may help diagnose inflammation in patients who are suspected to have an acute myocarditis or infiltrative disease. Coronary angiography is only recommended for patients with angina, although one must be careful to include dyspnea on exertion as an angina equivalent. Serum iron and transferrin saturation are worth checking in patients suspected of hemochromatosis. Table V-100 lists tests available for the initial evaluation of new cardiomyopathy and indicates which receive a Level I recommendation for all patients.

TABLE V-100 Initial Evaluation of Cardiomyopathy

Clinical Evaluation
Thorough history and physical examination to identify cardiac and noncardiac disorders[a]
Detailed family history of heart failure, cardiomyopathy, skeletal myopathy, conduction disorders, tachyarrhythmias, and sudden death
History of alcohol, illicit drugs, chemotherapy or radiation therapy[a]
Assessment of ability to perform routine and desired activities[a]
Assessment of volume status, orthostatic blood pressure, body mass index[a]
Laboratory Evaluation
Electrocardiogram[a]
Chest radiograph[a]
Two-dimensional and Doppler echocardiogram[a]
Magnetic resonance imaging for evidence of myocardial inflammation and fibrosis
Chemistry:
Serum sodium,[a] potassium,[a] calcium,[a] magnesium[a]
Fasting glucose (glycohemoglobin in diabetes mellitus)
Creatinine,[a] blood urea nitrogen[a]
Albumin,[a] total protein,[a] liver function tests[a]
Lipid profile
Thyroid-stimulating hormone[a]
Serum iron, transferrin saturation
Urinalysis
Creatine kinase isoforms
Cardiac troponin levels
Hematology:
Hemoglobin/hematocrit[a]
White blood cell count with differential,[a] including eosinophils
Erythrocyte sedimentation rate
Initial Evaluation When Specific Diagnoses Are Suspected
Titers for infection in the setting of clinical suspicion:
Acute viral (coxsackie, echovirus, influenza)
Human immunodeficiency virus
Chagas (*Trypanosoma cruzi*), Lyme (*Borrelia burgdorferi*), toxoplasmosis
Catheterization with coronary angiography in patients with angina who are candidates for intervention[a]
Serologies for active rheumatologic disease
Endomyocardial biopsy including sample for electron microscopy when suspecting specific diagnosis with therapeutic implications
Screening for sleep-disordered breathing

[a]Level I recommendations from ACC/AHA Practice Guidelines for Chronic Heart Failure in the Adult.

V-101. The answer is A. *(Chap. 287)* This patient presents with a classic history for fulminant viral myocarditis. A small number of patients present with fulminant myocarditis, with rapid progression from a severe febrile respiratory syndrome to cardiogenic shock that may involve multiple organ systems, leading to renal failure, hepatic failure, and coagulopathy. These patients are typically young adults who have recently been dismissed from urgent care settings with antibiotics for bronchitis or oseltamivir for viral syndromes, only to return within a few days in rapidly progressive cardiogenic shock. Prompt triage is vital to provide aggressive support with high-dose intravenous catecholamine therapy and sometimes with temporary mechanical circulatory support. Recognition of patients with this fulminant presentation is potentially lifesaving because more than half can survive, with marked improvement demonstrable within the first few weeks. The ejection fraction function of these patients often recovers to near-normal, although residual diastolic dysfunction may limit vigorous exercise for some survivors. There is no established role for measuring circulating anti-heart antibodies, which may be the result, rather than a cause, of myocardial injury and have also been found in patients with coronary artery disease and genetic cardiomyopathy. There is currently no specific therapy recommended during any stage of viral myocarditis. Large trials of immunosuppressive therapy for Dallas Criteria–positive myocarditis have been negative.

V-102. The answer is C. *(Chap. 287)* Giant cell myocarditis accounts for 10%–20% of biopsy-positive cases of myocarditis. Giant cell myocarditis typically presents with rapidly progressive heart failure and tachyarrhythmias. Diffuse granulomatous lesions are surrounded by extensive inflammatory infiltrate unlikely to be missed on endomyocardial biopsy, often with extensive eosinophilic infiltration. Associated conditions are thymomas, thyroiditis, pernicious anemia, other autoimmune diseases, and occasionally recent infections. Glucocorticoid therapy is less effective than for sarcoidosis and is sometimes combined with other immunosuppressive agents. The course is generally of rapid deterioration requiring urgent transplantation. Although the severity of presentation and myocardial histology are more fulminant than with sarcoidosis, the occasional finding of giant cell myocarditis after sarcoidosis suggests that they may, in some cases, represent different stages of the same disease spectrum.

V-103. The answer is E. *(Chap. 287)* Anthracyclines cause characteristic histologic changes of vacuolar degeneration and myofibrillar loss in the heart. Generation of reactive oxygen species involving heme compounds is currently the favored explanation for myocyte injury and fibrosis. Disruption of the large titin protein may contribute to loss of sarcomere organization. Risk for cardiotoxicity increases with higher doses, preexisting cardiac disease, and concomitant chest irradiation. There are three different presentations of anthracycline-induced cardiomyopathy. (1) Heart failure can develop acutely during administration of a single dose but may clinically resolve in a few weeks. (2) Early-onset doxorubicin cardiotoxicity develops in about 3% of patients during or shortly after a chronic course, relating closely to total dose. It may be rapidly progressive but may also resolve to good, but not normal, ventricular function. (3) The chronic presentation differs according to whether therapy was given before or after puberty. Patients who received doxorubicin while still growing may have impaired development of the heart, which leads to clinical heart failure by the time the patient reaches the early twenties. Late after adult exposure, patients may develop the gradual onset of symptoms or an acute onset precipitated by a reversible second insult, such as influenza or atrial fibrillation. Trastuzumab (Herceptin) is a monoclonal antibody that interferes with cell surface receptors crucial for some tumor growth and for cardiac adaptation. The incidence of cardiotoxicity is lower than for anthracyclines when given alone but enhanced by co-administration with them.

V-104. The answer is B. *(Chap. 288)* This patient has a classic case of acute pericarditis, likely secondary due to recent viral infection. His description of the chest pain (positional, pleuritic), examination revealing a classic three-component friction rub, ECG demonstrating diffuse ST elevation with PR depression, and negative cardiac biomarkers are all suggestive of acute pericarditis. There is no specific therapy for acute idiopathic pericarditis, but bed rest and anti-inflammatory treatment with aspirin (2–4 g/d), with gastric protection (e.g., omeprazole 20 mg/d), may be given. If this is ineffective, one of the NSAIDs, such as ibuprofen (400–600 mg tid) or indomethacin (25–50 mg tid), should be tried. In responsive patients, these doses should be continued for 1–2 weeks and then tapered over several weeks. In patients who are unresponsive, colchicine (0.5 mg bid, given for 4–8 weeks) has been found to be effective, not only in acute pericarditis, but also in reducing the risk of recurrent pericarditis. Colchicine is concentrated in and interferes with the migration of neutrophils, is contraindicated in patients with hepatic or renal dysfunction, and may cause diarrhea and other gastrointestinal side effects. Glucocorticoids (e.g., prednisone 1 mg/kg/d) usually suppress the clinical manifestations of acute pericarditis in patients who have failed therapy with the anti-inflammatory therapies described earlier but appear to increase the risk of subsequent recurrence. Therefore, full-dose corticosteroids should be given for only 2–4 days and then tapered. Anticoagulants should be avoided because their use could cause bleeding into the pericardial cavity and precipitate cardiac tamponade.

V-105 and V-106. The answers are B and E, respectively. *(Chap. 287)* This patient has physical examination findings consistent with cardiac tamponade, likely caused by bleeding into the pericardial space induced by anticoagulation in the setting of acute pericarditis. Acute myocardial infarction has been ruled out, so left main coronary artery occlusion, ruptured chordae tendineae (which would be associated with mitral regurgitation and acute pulmonary edema), and ventricular septal defect are unlikely. Acutely, a minimal amount of supranormal pericardial fluid (often ~200 mL) is required to rapidly increase intrapericardial pressure and cause cardiac tamponade. This is a medical emergency, and prompt evaluation with echocardiography and preparation for emergent pericardiocentesis are warranted. The paradoxical pulse (as noted in the question by the vanishing arterial pulse with inspiration) is an important clue to the presence of cardiac tamponade and consists of a greater than normal (10 mmHg) inspiratory decline in systolic arterial pressure. Because both ventricles share a tight incompressible covering (i.e., the pericardial sac), the inspiratory enlargement of the right ventricle in cardiac tamponade compresses and reduces left ventricular volume; leftward bulging of the interventricular septum reduces further the left ventricular cavity as the right ventricle enlarges during inspiration. Thus, in cardiac tamponade, the normal inspiratory augmentation of right ventricular volume causes an exaggerated reduction of left ventricular volume, stroke volume, and systolic pressure. Because immediate treatment of cardiac tamponade may be lifesaving, prompt measures to establish the diagnosis by echocardiography should be undertaken. When pericardial effusion causes tamponade, Doppler ultrasound shows that tricuspid and pulmonic valve flow velocities increase markedly during inspiration, whereas pulmonic vein, mitral, and aortic flow velocities diminish. In tamponade, there is late diastolic inward motion (collapse) of the right ventricular free wall and the right atrium.

V-107. The answer is D. *(Chap. 288)* The ECG in acute pericarditis without massive effusion usually displays changes secondary to acute subepicardial inflammation. It typically evolves through four stages. In stage 1, there is widespread elevation of the ST segments, often with upward concavity, involving two or three standard limb leads and V_2–V_6, with reciprocal depressions only in aVR and sometimes V_1. Also, there is depression of the PR segment below the TP segment, reflecting atrial involvement. Usually there are no significant changes in QRS complexes. After several days, the ST segments return to normal (stage 2), and only then, or even later, do the T waves become inverted (stage 3). Weeks or months after the onset of acute pericarditis, the ECG returns to normal (stage 4). In contrast, in acute myocardial infarction, ST elevations are convex, and reciprocal depression is usually more prominent; these changes may return to normal within a day or two. Q waves may develop, with loss of R-wave amplitude, and T-wave inversions are usually seen within hours before the ST segments have become isoelectric. ST-segment elevation in V_2 may be seen in either acute pericarditis or myocardial infarction.

V-108. The answer is D. *(Chap. 288)* This patient's presentation and physical examination are most consistent with the diagnosis of constrictive pericarditis. The most common cause of constrictive pericarditis worldwide is tuberculosis, but given the low incidence of tuberculosis in the United States, constrictive pericarditis is a rare condition in this country.

With the increasing ability to cure Hodgkin disease with mediastinal irradiation, many cases of constrictive pericarditis in the United States are in patients who received curative radiation therapy 10–20 years prior. These patients are also at risk for premature coronary artery disease. Risks for these complications include dose of radiation and radiation windows that include the heart. Other rare causes of constrictive pericarditis are recurrent acute pericarditis, hemorrhagic pericarditis, prior cardiac surgery, mediastinal irradiation, chronic infection, and neoplastic disease. Physiologically, constrictive pericarditis is characterized by the inability of the ventricles to fill because of the noncompliant pericardium. In early diastole, the ventricles fill rapidly, but filling stops abruptly when the elastic limit of the pericardium is reached. Clinically, patients present with generalized malaise, cachexia, and anasarca. Exertional dyspnea is common, and orthopnea is generally mild. Ascites and hepatomegaly occur because of increased venous pressure. In rare cases, cirrhosis may develop from chronic congestive hepatopathy. The jugular venous pressure is elevated, and the neck veins fail to collapse on inspiration (Kussmaul sign). Heart sounds may be muffled. A pericardial knock is frequently heard. This is a third heart sound that occurs 0.09–0.12 seconds after aortic valve closure at the cardiac apex. Right heart catheterization would show the "square root sign" characterized by an abrupt y-descent followed by a gradual rise in ventricular pressure. This finding, however, is not pathognomonic of constrictive pericarditis and can be seen in restrictive cardiomyopathy of any cause. Echocardiogram shows a thickened pericardium, dilatation of the inferior vena cava and hepatic veins, and an abrupt cessation of ventricular filling in early diastole. Pericardial resection is the only definitive treatment of constrictive pericarditis. Diuresis and sodium restriction are useful in managing volume status preoperatively, and paracentesis may be necessary. Operative mortality ranges from 5% to 10%. Underlying cardiac function is normal; thus, cardiac transplantation is not indicated. Pericardiocentesis is indicated for diagnostic removal of pericardial fluid and cardiac tamponade, which is not present on the patient's echocardiogram. Mitral valve stenosis may present similarly with anasarca, congestive hepatic failure, and ascites. However, pulmonary edema and pleural effusions are also common. Examination would be expected to demonstrate a diastolic murmur, and echocardiogram should show a normal pericardium and a thickened immobile mitral valve. Mitral valve replacement would be indicated if mitral stenosis were the cause of the patient's symptoms.

V-109. The answer is A. *(Chap. 289e)* The description of the mass is classic for an atrial myxoma, the most common primary tumor of the heart. More common in women than men and classically diagnosed in the third to sixth decades of life, myxomata can present with widely varying clinical symptoms. Most arise from the atria, and typically arise from the fossa ovalis in the left atrium. Many are asymptomatic. Myxomas typically do not metastasize distantly, and although other malignancies may metastasize to the heart, the constellation of findings and echocardiographic appearance of this lesion are most consistent with primary myxoma (option E). Some patients experience obstructive symptoms similar to mitral stenosis. Other patients will experience embolic events such as this patient. Patients may also have systemic symptoms such as fever, weight loss, cachexia, arthralgias, digital clubbing, Raynaud phenomenon, hypergammaglobulinemia, anemia, polycythemia, leukocytosis, elevated erythrocyte sedimentation rate, thrombocytopenia, and thrombocytosis. Many patients have undergone extensive rheumatologic and infectious disease workup prior to the diagnosis of their myxoma. The location of the mass would be highly unusual for endocarditis, either of the infectious or marantic varieties (options C and D). Catheter-based biopsy is generally avoided due to the high risk of provoked embolization (option B). Surgical removal of a myxoma is indicated regardless of tumor size. Myxoma recurrence rate is very low in sporadic, nonfamilial cases.

V-110. The answer is C. *(Chap. 289e)* Malignant melanoma carries the highest relative risk of cardiac metastases, followed by leukemia and lymphoma. Although the relative risk of cardiac metastases for both lung cancer and breast cancer is lower than melanoma, the absolute number of cases of cardiac metastases from these malignancies is higher due to the high incidence of these cancers. Hepatocellular carcinoma, glioblastoma, and pancreatic adenocarcinoma do not commonly metastasize to the heart. Most patients with cardiac metastases have advanced malignant disease; thus, therapy is generally palliative and consists of treatment of the primary tumor.

V-111. The answer is E. *(Chap. 289e)* This patient has suffered a commotio cordis. In this condition, blunt, nonpenetrating, often innocent-appearing injuries to the chest may trigger ventricular fibrillation even in absence of overt signs of injury. Commotio cordis occurs most often in adolescents during sporting events (e.g., baseball, hockey, football, lacrosse) and probably results from an impact to the chest wall overlying the heart during the susceptible phase of repolarization just before the peak of the T wave. Survival depends on prompt defibrillation. The described trauma in this case is not severe enough to cause aortic dissection or valvular avulsion. This 12-year-old boy is unlikely to have coronary atherosclerosis susceptible to rupture requiring percutaneous coronary intervention.

V-112. The answer is A. *(Chap. 290e)* Diabetes mellitus, both insulin- and non–insulin-dependent, is an independent risk factor for CAD and accounts for 14%–50% of new cases of cardiovascular disease. CAD is by far the most common cause of death in adults with diabetes. The incidence of CAD relates to the duration of diabetes and level of glycemic control, both motivating factors for patients to comply with therapy. Compared to their nondiabetic counterparts, diabetic patients are more likely to have a myocardial infarction, have a greater burden of CAD, have larger infarct size, and have more postinfarct complications, including heart failure, shock, and death. Importantly, diabetic patients are more likely to have atypical ischemic symptoms; nausea, dyspnea, pulmonary edema, arrhythmias, heart block, or syncope may be their anginal equivalent. Additionally, "silent ischemia," resulting from autonomic nervous system dysfunction, is more common in diabetic patients, accounting for up to 90% of their ischemic episodes.

V-113. The answer is C. *(Chaps. 290e and 96e)* Mr. Daniels has thiamine deficiency leading to high-output heart failure, a condition known as "wet beriberi." Although thiamine deficiency is most common in the developing world and in East Asia (where polished rice, which has much of the thiamine removed in processing, provides the bulk of the caloric intake), it is also seen in developed nations in patients who are alcoholics or who have chronic disease or malnutrition. Due to a reduction in vasomotor tone and resulting drop in systemic vascular resistance, these patients exhibit signs of high-output failure such as wide pulse pressure, tachycardia, bounding pulses, elevated venous filling pressures, pulmonary and peripheral edema, and dilated hearts. LV ejection fraction is often preserved or elevated. Patients with thiamine deficiency also develop glossitis, peripheral neuropathy, and anemia. Interestingly, administration of thiamine can lead to very rapid (12–48 hours) improvement in heart failure symptoms, diuretic and inotrope responsiveness, and LV size. Hypothyroidism, treated with thyroxine, leads to a reduction in cardiac output and heart rate (option D). Folate and vitamin B_{12} have been implicated in cases of hyperhomocysteinemia, a disorder associated with increased atherosclerotic risk (options A and E). The clinical benefit of normalizing homocysteine levels has not, however, been proven. Penicillamine is used to chelate copper in cases of Wilson disease, which very rarely manifests as infiltrative cardiomyopathy (option B).

V-114. The answer is D. *(Chaps. 290e and 405)* This patient clearly has symptomatic hypothyroidism confirmed by an elevated thyroid-stimulating hormone level. Cardiac manifestations of hypothyroidism include reductions in cardiac output, stroke volume, heart rate, systolic blood pressure, and pulse pressure. Pericardial effusions are present in about one-third of patients, but rarely progress to tamponade and probably result from increased capillary permeability. Other clinical signs include cardiomegaly, bradycardia, weak arterial pulses, distant heart sounds, and pleural effusions. Although the signs and symptoms of myxedema may mimic those of CHF, in the absence of other cardiac disease, myocardial failure is uncommon. The ECG generally reveals sinus bradycardia and low voltage and may show prolongation of the QT interval, decreased P-wave voltage, prolonged AV conduction time, intraventricular conduction disturbances, and nonspecific ST-T wave abnormalities.

V-115. The answer is C. *(Chap. 291e)* An integrated view of experimental results in animals and studies of human atherosclerosis suggests that the "fatty streak" represents the initial lesion of atherosclerosis. These early lesions most often seem to arise from focal increases in the content of lipoproteins within regions of the intima. In particular, the fraction of lipoproteins related to low-density lipoprotein (LDL) that bear apolipoprotein B appears causally related to atherosclerosis. This accumulation of lipoprotein particles may not result simply from increased permeability, or "leakiness," of the overlying endothelium. Rather, the lipoproteins may collect in the intima of arteries because they bind to constituents of the extracellular matrix, increasing the residence time of the lipid-rich particles within the arterial wall. Lipoproteins sequestered from (plasma) antioxidants in the extracellular space of the intima become particularly susceptible to oxidative modification, giving rise to hydroperoxides, lysophospholipids, oxysterols, and aldehydic breakdown products of fatty acids and phospholipids. Next, recruitment of leukocytes to the endothelium occurs. The inflammatory cell types typically found in the evolving atheroma include monocyte-derived macrophages. A number of adhesion molecules or receptors for leukocytes expressed on the surface of the arterial endothelial cell probably participate in the recruitment of leukocytes to the nascent atheroma. Once resident within the intima, the mononuclear phagocytes mature into macrophages and become lipid-laden foam cells, a conversion that requires the uptake of lipoprotein particles by receptor-mediated endocytosis.

V-116. The answer is B. *(Chap. 291e)* Atherosclerotic lesions occur ubiquitously in Western societies, and the prevalence of this disease is on the rise globally. Most atheromata produce no symptoms, and many never cause clinical manifestations. Numerous patients with diffuse atherosclerosis may succumb to unrelated illnesses without ever having experienced a clinically significant manifestation of atherosclerosis. Arterial remodeling during atheroma formation accounts for some of this variability in the clinical expression of atherosclerotic disease. During the initial phases of atheroma development, the plaque usually grows outward, in an abluminal direction. Vessels affected by atherogenesis tend to increase in diameter, a phenomenon known as compensatory enlargement, a type of vascular remodeling. The growing atheroma does not encroach on the arterial lumen until the burden of atherosclerotic plaque exceeds ~40% of the area encompassed by the internal elastic lamina. Flow-limiting stenoses commonly form later in the history of the plaque. Many such plaques cause stable syndromes such as demand-induced angina pectoris or intermittent claudication in the extremities. In the coronary circulation and other circulations, even total vascular occlusion by an atheroma does not invariably lead to infarction. The hypoxic stimulus of repeated bouts of ischemia characteristically induces formation of collateral vessels in the myocardium, mitigating the consequences of an acute occlusion of an epicardial coronary artery.

V-117. The answer is B. *(Chap. 291e)* The most recent 2013 ACC/AHA guidelines for cholesterol management have described only four classes of patients who derive definite benefit from statin therapy. These are described in Table V-117. While elevated high-sensitivity C-reactive protein has been shown to identify patients at increased risk for atherosclerotic

TABLE V-117 Summary of the Four Statin Benefit Groups Described in the 2013 ACC/AHA Guideline on the Treatment of Blood Cholesterol to Reduce Atherosclerotic Cardiovascular Risk in Adults

- Clinical ASCVD "secondary prevention"
- LDL-C ≥190 mg/dL without secondary cause (e.g., saturated/trans fats, drugs, certain diseases)
- Primary prevention *with* diabetes mellitus: age 40–75 years, LDL-C 70–189 mg/dL
- Primary prevention *without* diabetes mellitus: age 40–75 years, LDL-C 70–189 mg/dL, estimated ASCVD risk ≥7.5%

Abbreviations: ACC/AHA, American College of Cardiology and American Heart Association; ASCVD, atherosclerotic cardiovascular disease; LDL-C, low-density lipoprotein cholesterol.
Source: Adapted from NJ Stone et al: 2013 ACC/AHA guideline on the treatment of blood cholesterol to reduce atherosclerotic cardiovascular risk in adults. *J Am Coll Cardiol* 63:2889, 2014.

cardiovascular disease (ASCVD), the guidelines do not recommend it as an identifier of patients who are in a definite statin benefit group. However, it can be used to help decide on statin therapy for patients at intermediate risk for ASCVD.

V-118. The answer is E. *(Chap. 291e)* As the prevalence of metabolic syndrome and diabetes increases, many patients present with low concentrations of high-density lipoprotein (HDL) cholesterol (<1.0 mmol/L [<40 mg/dL]). A baseline measurement of HDL cholesterol indubitably correlates with future cardiovascular risk. Yet, the utility of therapies that raise HDL cholesterol levels in blood as effective interventions to reduce cardiovascular vascular events has come into question. Blood HDL levels vary inversely with those of triglycerides, and the independent role of HDL versus triglycerides as a cardiovascular risk factor remains unsettled. The 2013 guideline does not advocate any specific therapy for raising HDL. Indeed, multiple recent trials failed to show that raising HDL cholesterol levels improves cardiovascular outcomes, and recent genetic studies cast doubt on low HDL as a causal risk factor for atherosclerotic events. Weight loss and physical activity can raise HDL, and these lifestyle measures merit universal adoption. Nicotinic acid, particularly in combination with statins, can robustly raise HDL, but clinical trial data do not support the effectiveness of nicotinic acid in cardiovascular risk reduction. Agonists of nuclear receptors provide another potential avenue for raising HDL levels. Yet patients treated with peroxisome proliferator–activated receptor α and γ (PPAR-α and -γ) agonists have not consistently shown improved cardiovascular outcomes, and at least some PPAR agonists have been associated with worsened cardiovascular outcomes. Other agents in clinical development raise HDL levels by inhibiting cholesteryl ester transfer protein (CETP). Two such agents have undergone large-scale clinical evaluation and have not shown efficacy in improving cardiovascular outcomes.

V-119. The answer is B. *(Chap. 293)* Central to an understanding of the pathophysiology of myocardial ischemia is the concept of myocardial supply and demand. In normal conditions, for any given level of a demand for oxygen, the myocardium will control the supply of oxygen-rich blood to prevent underperfusion of myocytes and the subsequent development of ischemia and infarction. The major determinants of myocardial oxygen demand (MVO_2) are heart rate, myocardial contractility, and ventricular wall tension (stress). Heart rhythm is not a major determinant of myocardial oxygen demand.

V-120. The answer is E. *(Chap. 293)* The normal coronary circulation is dominated and controlled by the heart's requirements for oxygen. This need is met by the ability of the coronary vascular bed to vary its resistance (and, therefore, blood flow) considerably while the myocardium extracts a high and relatively fixed percentage of oxygen. Normally, intramyocardial resistance vessels demonstrate a great capacity for dilation. For example, the changing oxygen needs of the heart with exercise and emotional stress affect coronary vascular resistance and, in this manner, regulate the supply of oxygen and substrate to the myocardium. The epicardial coronary arteries, in the normal state, provide only trivial resistance to flow. Myocardial oxygen extraction is relatively fixed. During tachycardia, the diastolic time period is shortened relative to the systolic period.

V-121. The answer is B. *(Chap. 293)* A wide range of abnormalities in cell metabolism, function, and structure underlie these mechanical disturbances during ischemia. The normal myocardium metabolizes fatty acids and glucose to carbon dioxide and water. With severe oxygen deprivation, fatty acids cannot be oxidized, and glucose is converted to lactate; intracellular pH is reduced, as are the myocardial stores of high-energy phosphates (i.e., adenosine triphosphate and creatine phosphate). Impaired cell membrane function leads to the leakage of potassium and the uptake of sodium by myocytes, as well as an increase in cytosolic calcium.

V-122. The answer is E. *(Chap. 293)* Angina pain can arise in or radiate to the back, interscapular region, root of the neck, jaw, teeth, and epigastrium. Angina is rarely localized below the umbilicus or above the mandible. A useful finding in assessing a patient with chest discomfort is the fact that myocardial ischemic discomfort does not radiate to the trapezius muscles; that radiation pattern is more typical of pericarditis.

V-123. **The answer is B.** *(Chap. 293)* Many patients report a fixed threshold for angina, which occurs predictably at a certain level of activity, such as climbing two flights of stairs at a normal pace. In these patients, coronary stenosis and myocardial oxygen supply are fixed, and ischemia is precipitated by an increase in myocardial oxygen demand; they are said to have stable exertional angina. Angina can be classified by the Canadian Cardiovascular Society Functional Class as shown in Table V-123.

TABLE V-123 Cardiovascular Disease Classification Chart

Class	New York Heart Association Functional Classification	Canadian Cardiovascular Society Functional Classification
I	Patients have cardiac disease but *without* the resulting *limitations* of physical activity. Ordinary physical activity does not cause undue fatigue, palpitation, dyspnea, or anginal pain.	Ordinary physical activity, such as walking and climbing stairs, *does not cause angina*. Angina present with strenuous or rapid or prolonged exertion at work or recreation.
II	Patients have cardiac disease resulting in *slight limitation* of physical activity. They are comfortable at rest. Ordinary physical activity results in fatigue, palpitation, dyspnea, or anginal pain.	*Slight limitation* of ordinary activity. Walking or climbing stairs rapidly, walking uphill, walking or stair climbing after meals, in cold, or when under emotional stress or only during the few hours after awakening. Walking more than two blocks on the level and climbing more than one flight of stairs at a normal pace and in normal conditions.
III	Patients have cardiac disease resulting in *marked limitation* of physical activity. They are comfortable at rest. Less than ordinary physical activity causes fatigue, palpitation, dyspnea, or anginal pain.	*Marked limitation* of ordinary physical activity. Walking one to two blocks on the level and climbing more than one flight of stairs in normal conditions.
IV	Patients have cardiac disease resulting in *inability* to perform any physical activity without discomfort. Symptoms of cardiac insufficiency or of the anginal syndrome may be present even at rest. If any physical activity is undertaken, discomfort is increased.	*Inability* to perform any physical activity without discomfort—anginal syndrome *may* be present at rest.

Source: Modified from L Goldman et al: *Circulation* 64:1227, 1981.

V-124. **The answer is C.** *(Chap. 293)* The ECG exercise stress test is used to discover any limitation in exercise performance, detect typical ECG signs of myocardial ischemia, and establish their relationship to chest discomfort. The ischemic ST-segment response generally is defined as flat or downsloping depression of the ST segment >0.1 mV below baseline (i.e., the PR segment) and lasting longer than 0.08 seconds (Figure V-124). Upsloping or junctional ST-segment changes are not considered characteristic of ischemia and do not constitute a positive test. Although T-wave abnormalities, conduction disturbances, and ventricular arrhythmias that develop during exercise should be noted, they are also not diagnostic. Negative exercise tests in which the target heart rate (85% of maximal predicted heart rate [MPHR] for age and sex) is not achieved are considered nondiagnostic. This patient did not achieve 85% MPHR (220 – age = MPHR), and the ST-segment changes are described as upsloping. Finally, blood pressure increase is a normal response to exercise.

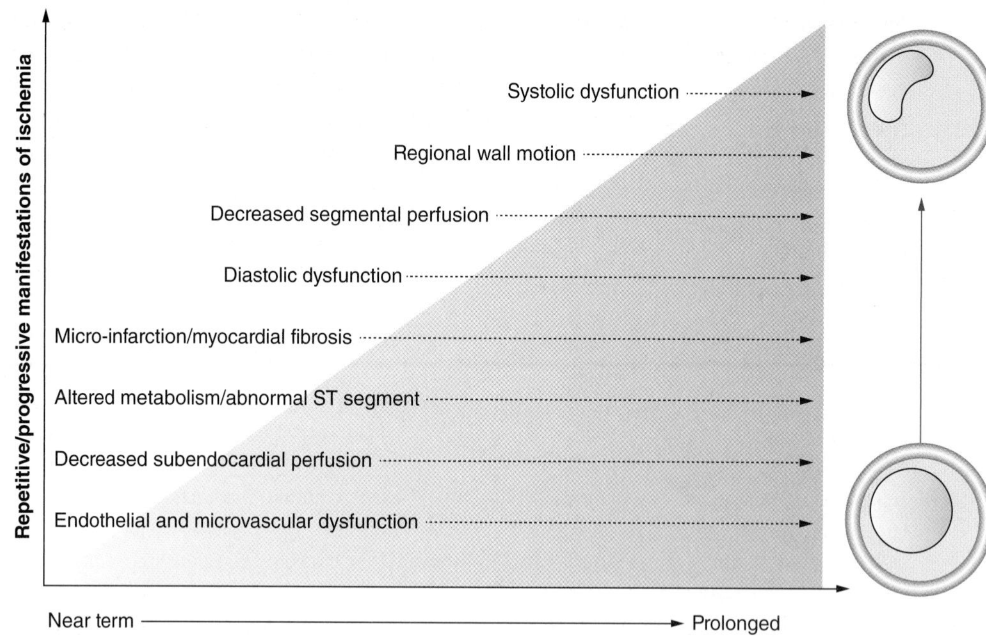

FIGURE V-124 Modified from LJ Shaw et al: *J Am Coll Cardiol* 54:1561, 2009. Original figure illustration by Rob Flewell.

V-125. The answer is C. *(Chap. 294)* Non–ST-segment elevation acute coronary syndrome (NSTE-ACS) is most commonly caused by an imbalance between oxygen supply and oxygen demand resulting from a partially occluding thrombus forming on a disrupted atherothrombotic coronary plaque or on eroded coronary artery endothelium. Severe ischemia or myocardial necrosis may occur consequent to the reduction of coronary blood flow caused by the thrombus and by downstream embolization of platelet aggregates and/or atherosclerotic debris. Other causes of NSTE-ACS include: (1) dynamic obstruction (e.g., coronary spasm, as in Prinzmetal variant angina); (2) severe mechanical obstruction due to progressive coronary atherosclerosis; and (3) increased myocardial oxygen demand produced by conditions such as fever, tachycardia, and thyrotoxicosis in the presence of fixed epicardial coronary obstruction. More than one of these processes may be involved. Although microvascular endothelial dysfunction can cause angina, it is not thought to be a cause of myocardial infarction.

V-126. The answer is E. *(Chap. 294)* The diagnosis of acute coronary syndrome (ACS) is based largely on the clinical presentation. Typically, chest discomfort is severe and has at least one of three features: (1) it occurs at rest (or with minimal exertion), lasting >10 minutes; (2) it is of relatively recent onset (i.e., within the prior 2 weeks); and/or (3) it occurs with a crescendo pattern (i.e., distinctly more severe, prolonged, or frequent than previous episodes). The diagnosis of non–ST-segment elevation myocardial infarction (NSTEMI) is established if a patient with these clinical features develops evidence of myocardial necrosis, as reflected in abnormally elevated levels of biomarkers of cardiac necrosis. Given the ECG without ST elevations, this patient does not have ST-segment elevation myocardial infarction (STEMI). Also, this clinical presentation of accelerating angina now occurring at rest obviates stable angina. However, because this patient does not yet have cardiac biomarker results, one cannot differentiate between unstable angina and NSTEMI. Further information is needed.

V-127. The answer is E. *(Chap. 294)* It is important to remember that although cardiac troponin biomarkers (troponin I or T) are quite sensitive for myocardial infarction due to coronary occlusion, they lack somewhat in specificity. In patients without a clear clinical history of myocardial ischemia, minor cardiac troponin elevations have been reported and can be caused by congestive heart failure, myocarditis, or pulmonary embolism; in addition, using high-sensitivity assays, they may occur in ostensibly normal subjects. Thus, in patients with an unclear history, small elevations of cardiac troponin, especially if they are persistent, may not be diagnostic of an ACS. In this patient, the troponin elevation is likely due to his hypertensive urgency brought on by missed hemodialysis and volume overload. Treating the proximal cause will help him. It would be prudent to continue to trend cardiac biomarkers and ECGs over time as well.

V-128. The answer is E. *(Chap. 294)* This patient is suffering from an NSTEMI. The two cornerstones of pharmacologic therapy in NSTEMI management are reduction of myocardial oxygen demand and antithrombotic therapy targeted at a presumed partially occluding thrombus forming on disrupted atherothrombotic coronary plaque. Aspirin in combination with a $P2Y_{12}$ receptor blocker (e.g., clopidogrel, ticagrelor, or prasugrel) is an appropriate antiplatelet option, and options for anticoagulants include: (1) unfractionated heparin (UFH), long the mainstay of therapy; (2) the low-molecular-weight heparin (LMWH) enoxaparin, which has been shown to be superior to UFH in reducing recurrent cardiac events, especially in patients managed by a conservative strategy but with some increase in bleeding; (3) bivalirudin, a direct thrombin inhibitor that is similar in efficacy to either UFH or LMWH but causes less bleeding and is used just prior to and/or during percutaneous coronary intervention; and (4) the indirect factor Xa inhibitor fondaparinux, which is equivalent in efficacy to enoxaparin but appears to have a lower risk of major bleeding. To reduce myocardial oxygen demand, β-blockade administration targeting a heart rate of 60 bpm is reasonable, although it should be used with caution or avoided in the presence of heart failure (not present in this patient). Likewise, nitroglycerin is a commonly used and effective antianginal therapy. However, a direct contraindication is the use of phosphodiesterase inhibitors (such as tadalafil in this patient), and co-administration can result in catastrophic hypotension.

V-129. The answer is A. *(Chap. 295)* This patient is presenting with classic ischemic chest pain by history. When present in such a classic manner, it is unmistakable. After obtaining this history, the clinical working diagnosis is ACS. The next most important step in the decision tree is to determine whether the patient is having an STEMI or non–ST-segment elevation ACS (NSTEMI or unstable angina). This can only be accomplished by the ECG. Serum biomarkers (troponin and creatine kinase [CK]-MB) take minutes to hours to return and may not be elevated in the initial several hours of an infarction. In practical terms, the high-sensitivity troponin assays are of less immediate value in patients with STEMI. Contemporary urgent reperfusion strategies necessitate making a decision (based largely on a combination of clinical and ECG findings) before the results of blood tests have returned from the laboratory. Although echocardiogram may demonstrate wall motion abnormalities in areas of ischemia, it cannot differentiate between ST-segment elevation and non–ST-segment elevation ACS. Coronary CT angiography is not warranted in a patient having active ischemic pain. Figure V-129 provides a flow chart of the decision tree facing the clinician treating a patient with ischemic discomfort.

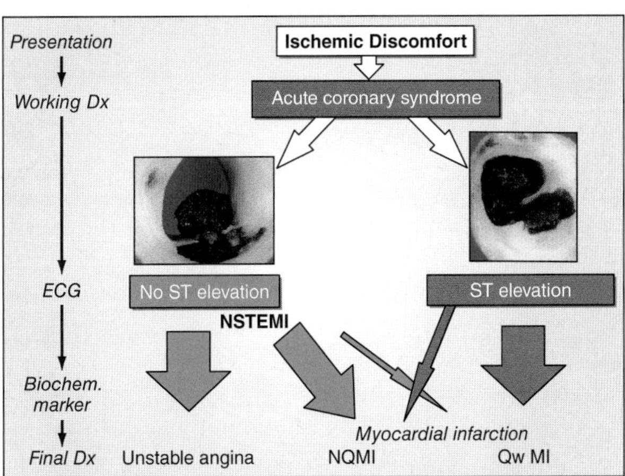

FIGURE V-129 Dx, diagnosis; ECG, electrocardiogram; NQMI, non–Q-wave myocardial infarction; NSTEMI, non–ST-segment elevation myocardial infarction; Qw MI, Q-wave myocardial infarction. Adapted from CW Hamm et al: *Lancet* 358:1533, 2001, and MJ Davies: *Heart* 83:361, 2000; with permission from the BMJ Publishing Group.

V-130. The answer is E. *(Chap. 295)* Cardiac-specific troponin T (cTnT) and cardiac-specific troponin I (cTnI) have different amino acid sequences from those of the skeletal muscle forms of these proteins. These differences permitted the development of quantitative assays for cTnT and cTnI with highly specific monoclonal antibodies. Because cTnT and cTnI are not normally detectable in the blood of healthy individuals but may increase after STEMI to levels many times higher than the upper reference limit (the highest value seen in 99% of a reference population not suffering from MI), the measurement of cTnT or cTnI is of considerable diagnostic usefulness, and they are now the preferred biochemical markers for MI. An important drawback of total creatine kinase (CK) measurement is its lack of specificity for STEMI, as CK may be elevated with skeletal muscle disease or trauma, including intramuscular injection. The MB isoenzyme of CK has the advantage over total CK that it is not present in significant concentrations in extracardiac tissue and, therefore, is considerably more specific. However, cardiac surgery, myocarditis, and electrical cardioversion often result in elevated serum levels of the MB isoenzyme. The nonspecific reaction to myocardial injury is associated with polymorphonuclear leukocytosis, which appears within a few hours after the onset of pain and persists for 3–7 days; the white blood cell count often reaches levels of 12,000–15,000/μL. The erythrocyte sedimentation rate rises more slowly than the white blood cell count, peaking during the first week and sometimes remaining elevated for 1 or 2 weeks. Similarly, the lactate dehydrogenase may rise in the setting of acute MI but is nonspecific.

V-131. The answer is C. *(Chap. 295)* CK rises within 4–8 hours and generally returns to normal by 48–72 hours. The cardiac troponin assays have a similar time frame for rise, but generally last much longer (7–10 days after STEMI). Early reperfusion will cause an earlier peak of biomarker measurements.

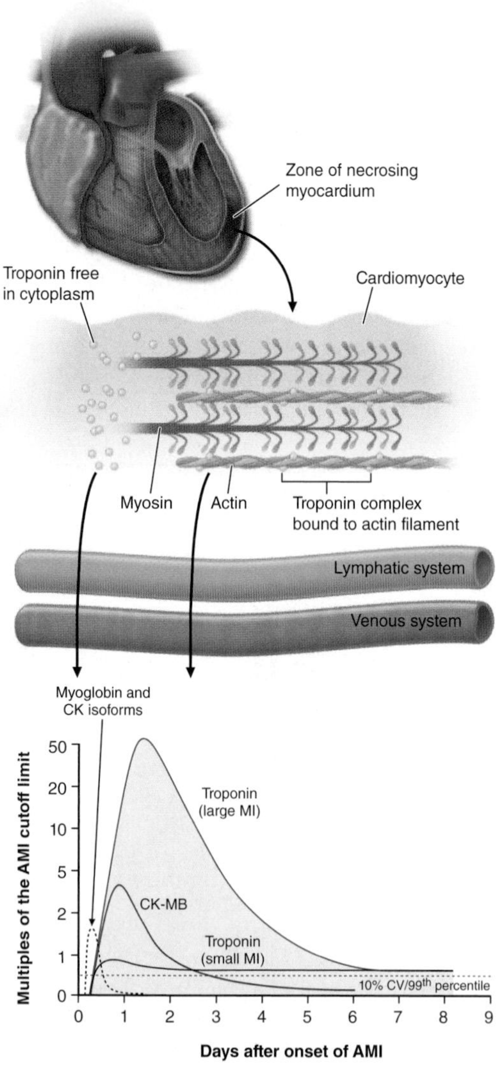

FIGURE V-131 AMI, acute myocardial infarction; CK, creatine kinase; MI, myocardial infarction. Modified from EM Antman: Decision making with cardiac troponin tests. *N Engl J Med* 346:2079, 2002 and AS Jaffe, L Babuin, FS Apple: Biomarkers in acute cardiac disease: The present and the future. *J Am Coll Cardiol* 48:1, 2006.

V-132. The answer is A. *(Chap. 295)* Most out-of-hospital deaths from STEMI are due to the sudden development of ventricular fibrillation. The vast majority of deaths due to ventricular fibrillation occur within the first 24 hours of the onset of symptoms, and of these, over half occur in the first hour. Therefore, the major elements of prehospital care of patients with suspected STEMI include: (1) recognition of symptoms by the patient and prompt seeking of medical attention; (2) rapid deployment of an emergency medical team capable of performing resuscitative maneuvers, including defibrillation; (3) expeditious transportation of the patient to a hospital facility that is continuously staffed by physicians and nurses skilled in managing arrhythmias and providing advanced cardiac life support; and (4) expeditious implementation of reperfusion therapy. The greatest delay usually occurs not during transportation to the hospital but, rather, between the onset of pain and the patient's decision to call for help. This delay can best be reduced by healthcare professionals educating the public concerning the significance of chest discomfort and the importance of seeking early medical attention. Regular office visits with patients who have a history of or are at risk for ischemic heart disease are important "teachable moments" for clinicians to review the symptoms of STEMI and the appropriate action plan.

V-133. The answer is E. *(Chap. 295)* All of these choices are appropriate therapy for patients with STEMI in certain situations. Aspirin is an irreversible cyclooxygenase inhibitor and thus inhibits the production of thromboxane A2. β-Blockers reduce myocardial oxygen demand by reducing cardiac chronotropy and inotropy. They should be used with caution in patients with myocardial infarction and any signs of delayed conduction (prolonged PR interval), heart failure, or risk for cardiogenic shock. Clopidogrel inhibits the $P2Y_{12}$ adenosine diphosphate platelet receptor to inhibit platelet aggregation. Abciximab and eptifibatide are glycoprotein IIb/IIIa inhibitors that also inhibit platelet aggregation. Although nitroglycerin is effective for antianginal effects in the setting of STEMI, it enacts those effects through decreasing preload and perhaps through some direct nitric oxide–induced coronary vasodilation. Nitroglycerin has minimal effect on systemic afterload.

V-134. The answer is D. *(Chap. 295)* This patient has evidence of failure of reperfusion with fibrinolytic therapy (persistent chest pain and ST-segment elevation >90 minutes). In this case, rescue percutaneous coronary intervention (PCI) should be pursued. Repeating a second dose of tissue plasminogen activator or a different fibrinolytic is not warranted and potentially dangerous. Coronary artery bypass grafting is not warranted prior to knowing the anatomy, and in the immediate setting after administration of fibrinolytics, it carries an exceedingly high risk of serious hemorrhage.

V-135. The answer is E. *(Chap. 295)* This patient has an accelerated idioventricular rhythm, a common finding in patients with successful reperfusion after thrombolytic therapy. This rhythm is benign and requires no further therapy. It invariably resolves on its own. Flecainide (a class I antiarrhythmic) is contraindicated in post-MI patients because it was found to increase mortality in the CAST trial. Amiodarone or metoprolol would be appropriate therapy if this was ventricular tachycardia or perhaps supraventricular tachycardia. Carotid sinus massage would be appropriate in the setting of supraventricular tachycardia.

V-136. The answer is D. *(Chap. 296e)* Percutaneous therapy of coronary artery disease underwent a paradigm shift with the introduction of coronary stents in 1994. However, metallic stents are also prone to stent thrombosis (1%–3%), either acute (<24 hours) or subacute (1–30 days), which can be ameliorated by greater attention to full initial stent deployment and the use of dual antiplatelet therapy (DAPT) (aspirin plus a platelet $P2Y_{12}$ receptor blocker [clopidogrel, prasugrel, or ticagrelor]). Late (30 days–1 year) and very late (>1 year) stent thromboses occur infrequently with stents but are slightly more common with first-generation drug-eluting stents, generally necessitating DAPT for 1 year or longer. Use of the second-generation stents (such as the everolimus-eluting stent) is associated with lower rates of late and very late stent thromboses, and shorter durations of DAPT may be possible. Premature discontinuation of DAPT, particularly in the first month after implantation, is associated with a significantly increased risk for stent thrombosis (three- to ninefold greater). Stent thrombosis results in death in 10%–20% of patients and myocardial infarction in 30%–70% of patients. Elective surgery (such as cataract removal) that requires discontinuation of antiplatelet therapy after drug-eluting stent implantation should be postponed until after 6 months and preferably after 1 year, if at all possible. At that point, clopidogrel can be reasonably discontinued if no other mitigating factors are present. If at all possible, aspirin should be continued.

V-137. The answer is D. *(Chap. 296e)* The lines between coronary artery bypass grafting (CABG) and PCI for revascularization of CAD have been shifting for the better part of two decades. As PCI technique and technology improve, it has become the dominant form of revascularization and is performed now more than twice as often as CABG. However, there remain select patients in whom CABG and PCI either exist in therapeutic equipoise or CABG is clearly a superior option. One such population is patients with multivessel disease. When revascularization is indicated, the choice of PCI or CABG depends on a number of clinical and anatomic factors. The Synergy Between Percutaneous Coronary Intervention With Taxus and Cardiac Surgery (SYNTAX) trial compared PCI with the paclitaxel drug-eluting stent to CABG in 1800 patients with three-vessel coronary disease or left main disease. The study found no difference in death or myocardial infarction at 1 year (options A and E), but repeat revascularization was significantly higher in the stent-treated group (13.5% vs. 5.9%) (option B), whereas stroke was significantly higher in the surgical group (2.2% vs. 0.6%) (option C). The combined primary end point of death, myocardial infarction, stroke, or revascularization was significantly better with CABG, particularly in those with the most extensive CAD. The 3-year results confirm these findings. The Future Revascularization Evaluation in Patients With Diabetes Mellitus: Optimal Management of Multivessel Disease (FREEDOM) trial randomized 1900 patients with diabetes and multivessel disease and showed a significantly lower primary end point of death, myocardial infarction, or stroke with CABG than PCI. These studies support CABG for those with the most severe left main and three-vessel disease or those with diabetes. Lesser degrees of multivessel disease in patients with or without diabetes have an equal outcome with PCI. The choice of PCI versus CABG is also related to the anticipated procedural success and complications of PCI and the risks of CABG (option D). For PCI, the characteristics of the coronary anatomy are critically important. The location of the lesion in the vessel (proximal or distal), the degree of tortuosity, and the size of the vessel are considered. In addition, the lesion characteristics, including the degree of the stenosis, the presence of calcium, lesion length, and presence of thrombus, are assessed.

V-138. The answer is B. *(Chap. 297e)* Chronic total occlusions (CTOs) represent one of the greatest therapeutic challenges in interventional cardiology. Proper patient and lesion selection and meticulous technique are required to successfully and safely perform PCI on a CTO. In asymptomatic high-risk patients or lesions, it is recommended to forego PCI attempts at CTO given the elevated risk profile of the procedure. However, in this symptomatic patient with a high-risk stress test, an attempt at PCI is reasonable. Incomplete revascularization due to an untreated CTO is associated with an increased mortality rate (hazard ratio = 1.36; 95% confidence interval [CI], 1.12–1.66, p <.05). Successful PCI of a CTO leads to a 3.8%–8.4% absolute reduction in mortality, symptom relief, and improved left ventricular function. Newer techniques, such as the retrograde approach to crossing total occlusions, are useful when the antegrade approach fails or is not feasible and there are well-developed collateral vessels.

V-139. The answer is B. *(Chap. 297e)* Saphenous vein grafts have a failure rate of up to 20% after 1 year and as high as 50% by 5 years. This is much higher than the failure rate of arterial conduits (e.g., left internal mammary arteries) (option D). Venous graft failure (after >1 month) results from intimal hyperplasia and atherosclerosis, rarely from embolization (option A). Saphenous vein graft PCI is associated with distal embolization of atherosclerotic debris and microthrombi leading to microvascular occlusion, reduced antegrade blood flow (the "no-reflow" phenomenon), and myocardial infarction. Although the risk of no reflow is higher in saphenous vein graft PCI than in native-vessel PCI (option D), the benefit of successful revascularization and the ability to reduce the risk with a distal protection device often warrants proceeding with PCI (option C). Embolic distal protection devices decrease the risk of distal embolization, as well as the incidence of no reflow and myocardial infarction associated with saphenous vein graft interventions (option B).

V-140. The answer is E. *(Chap. 297e)* This patient has classic findings for aortic stenosis (AS) including a late-peaking systolic murmur, pulsus parvus et tardus, and symptoms of angina and heart failure. Although some medications may reduce symptoms (e.g., diuretics for heart failure symptoms), severe AS has historically been a surgical disease; medications have no role in reducing mortality. Mortality from severe AS is high, with 1- and 5- year survival rates for nonsurgical candidates of 62% and 38%, respectively. Although percutaneous balloon valvotomy can be used for the acutely ill or "crashing" patient with severe AS, short-term complication rates are high (approximated at 10%–20%), valve area rarely exceed 1cm^2 after balloon valvotomy, most patients return to their preprocedure valve area by 6–12 months, and the procedure does not affect mortality risk. Previously, nonsurgical candidates were advised to pursue comfort measures, sometimes including hospice care. However, with the advent of transcatheter aortic valve replacement (TAVR), we are now able to offer a viable treatment option to many patients who are too high risk for surgical aortic valve replacement. TAVR has been shown to be superior to usual care in very high risk patients. Mrs. Edwards will have to undergo further testing to ensure that her anatomy is amenable to TAVR, but it remains a viable treatment option for this very ill woman.

V-141. The answer is B. *(Chap. 298)* Hypertension is present in all populations except for a small number of individuals living in developing countries. In industrialized societies, blood pressure increases steadily during the first two decades of life. In children and adolescents, blood pressure is associated with growth and maturation. Blood pressure "tracks" over time in children and between adolescence and young adulthood. In the United States, average systolic blood pressure is higher for men than for women during early adulthood, although among older individuals, the age-related rate of rise is steeper for women. Consequently, among individuals age 60 and older, systolic blood pressures of women are higher than those of men. Among adults, diastolic blood pressure also increases progressively with age until the age of 55 years, after which it tends to decrease. The consequence is a widening of pulse pressure (the difference between systolic and diastolic blood pressure) beyond age 60. In the United States, based on results of the National Health and Nutrition Examination Survey (NHANES), approximately 30% (age-adjusted prevalence) of adults, or at least 65 million individuals, have hypertension (defined as any one of the following: systolic blood pressure ≥140 mmHg, diastolic blood pressure ≥90 mmHg, or taking antihypertensive medications). Hypertension prevalence is 33.5% in non-Hispanic blacks, 28.9% in non-Hispanic whites, and 20.7% in Mexican Americans.

V-142. The answer is B. *(Chap. 298)* Heart disease is the most common cause of death in hypertensive patients. Hypertensive heart disease is the result of structural and functional adaptations leading to left ventricular hypertrophy, CHF, abnormalities of blood flow due to atherosclerotic coronary artery disease and microvascular disease, and cardiac arrhythmias. Stroke is the second most frequent cause of death in the world; it accounts for 5 million deaths each year, with an additional 15 million persons having nonfatal strokes. Elevated blood pressure is the strongest risk factor for stroke. Renal disease is a both a common effect and cause of hypertension but is not as common a cause of mortality as cardiac disease in hypertensive patients. Lung or liver dysfunction is a rarer cause of mortality in hypertensive patients.

V-143 and V-144. The answers are D and E, respectively. *(Chap. 298)* This patient presents at a young age with hypertension that is difficult to control, raising the question of secondary causes of hypertension. The most likely diagnosis in this patient is primary hyperaldosteronism, also known as Conn syndrome. The patient has no physical features that suggest congenital adrenal hyperplasia or Cushing syndrome. In addition, there is no glucose intolerance as is commonly seen in Cushing syndrome. The lack of episodic symptoms and the labile hypertension make pheochromocytoma unlikely. The findings of hypokalemia and metabolic alkalosis in the presence of difficult-to-control hypertension yield the likely diagnosis of Conn syndrome. Diagnosis of the disease can be difficult, but the preferred test is the plasma aldosterone/renin ratio. This test should be performed at 8:00 AM, and a ratio above 30 to 50 is diagnostic of primary hyperaldosteronism. Caution should be made in interpreting this test while the patient is on ACE inhibitor therapy because ACE inhibitors can falsely elevate plasma renin activity. However, a plasma renin level that is undetectable or an elevated aldosterone/renin ratio in the presence of ACE inhibitor therapy is highly suggestive of primary hyperaldosteronism. Selective adrenal vein renin sampling may be performed after the diagnosis to help determine if the process is unilateral or bilateral. Although fibromuscular dysplasia is a common secondary cause of hypertension in young females, the presence of hypokalemia and metabolic alkalosis should suggest Conn syndrome. Thus, magnetic resonance imaging of the renal arteries is unnecessary in this case. Measurement of 24-hour urine collection for potassium wasting and aldosterone secretion can be useful in the diagnosis of Conn syndrome. The measurement of metanephrines or cortisol is not indicated.

V-145. The answer is C. *(Chap. 298)* This patient is suffering from hypertensive emergency, specifically malignant hypertension. Hallmarked by rapid arterial changes and loss of cerebral autoregulation, the clinical signs include very high blood pressure, delirium due to cerebral hyperperfusion, renal failure with proteinuria and hematuria, and hemolytic anemia. Mortality in the first several hours is high with this disease state, and rapid treatment is warranted. However, most patients presenting with malignant hypertension also have longstanding chronic elevations in blood pressure and a change in the "set point" of the cerebral autoregulation. Reducing the blood pressure rapidly to normal levels for the regular population often leads to hypoperfusion and can lead to watershed cerebral infarcts. In the setting of hypertensive emergency, a reduction of mean arterial pressure in minutes to hours by 25% is recommended. Parenteral therapy has a more rapid onset and is much more easily titrated than oral therapy, which is inappropriate in the emergent setting. Immediate-release nifedipine is particularly potent and is associated with a higher risk of myocardial infarction when used in this setting. Plasmapheresis would be warranted if this were a case of thrombotic thrombocytopenic purpura (TTP), but with the normal platelets count in this case, it is unlikely TTP.

V-146. The answer is D. *(Chap. 299)* Rates of urinary albumin excretion (UAE) are predictive of systemic atherosclerotic disease events. Increased UAE may develop years before cardiovascular events. The renal vasculature is unusually complex with rich arteriolar flow to the cortex in excess of metabolic requirements, consistent with its primary function as a filtering organ. After delivering blood to cortical glomeruli, the postglomerular circulation supplies deeper medullary segments that support energy-dependent solute transport at multiple levels of the renal tubule. These postglomerular vessels carry less blood, and high oxygen consumption leaves the deeper medullary regions at the margin of hypoxemia. Thus, the venous blood from the medulla typically has much lower oxygen saturation than cortical venous blood. The glomerular capillary endothelium shares susceptibility to oxidative stress, pressure injury, and inflammation with other vascular territories.

V-147. The answer is B. *(Chap. 299)* Renal artery stenosis is common and often has only minor hemodynamic effects. The earliest finding may be an elevated systemic renin level. Fibromuscular dysplasia (FMD) is reported in 3%–5% of normal subjects presenting as potential kidney donors without hypertension. It may present clinically with hypertension in younger individuals (between age 15 and 50), most often women. FMD does not often threaten kidney function, but sometimes produces total occlusion and can be associated with renal artery aneurysms. Critical levels of stenosis lead to a reduction in perfusion pressure that activates the renin-angiotensin system, reduces sodium excretion, and activates sympathetic adrenergic pathways. These events lead to systemic hypertension characterized by angiotensin dependence in the early stages, widely varying pressures, loss of circadian blood pressure rhythms, and accelerated target organ injury, including left ventricular hypertrophy and renal fibrosis. Renovascular hypertension can be treated with agents that block the renin-angiotensin system and other drugs that modify these pressor pathways. Elevated renal artery velocities by Doppler ultrasound above 200 cm/sec generally predict hemodynamically important lesions (>60% vessel lumen occlusion). Although renin levels and activity are elevated in the state of significant renal artery stenosis, the relative level does not predict response to therapy.

V-148. The answer is B. *(Chap. 299)* This patient's clinical scenario is most consistent with atheroembolic renal disease. Atheroemboli in the kidney are strongly associated with aortic aneurysmal disease and renal artery stenosis. Most clinical cases can be linked to precipitating events, such as angiography, vascular surgery, anticoagulation with heparin, thrombolytic therapy, or trauma. Clinical manifestations of this syndrome commonly develop between 1 and 14 days after an inciting event and may continue to develop for weeks thereafter. Systemic embolic disease manifestations, such as fever, abdominal pain, and weight loss, are present in less than half of patients, although cutaneous manifestations including livedo reticularis and localized toe gangrene may be more common. Worsening hypertension and deteriorating kidney function are common. Typical laboratory findings include rising creatinine, transient eosinophilia (60%–80% of cases), elevated erythrocyte sedimentation rate (ESR), and hypocomplementemia (15% of cases). Contrast-induced nephropathy is not associated with fever, high ESR, eosinophilia, or livedo reticularis of the lower extremities. It would be unusual to develop interstitial nephritis without exposure to a new medication, and other than eosinophilia, the laboratory abnormalities are not supportive in this case. Likewise, the sudden development of hypereosinophilic syndrome in a 75-year-old man would be highly unlikely. Finally, although Churg-Strauss syndrome is a small- to medium-vessel vasculitis associated with renal dysfunction and eosinophilia, almost all patients experience atopy and asthma-like lung disease, which are absent in this patient.

V-149. The answer is B. *(Chap. 300)* The D-dimer measured by enzyme-linked immunosorbent assay (ELISA) is elevated in the setting of breakdown of fibrin by plasmin, and the presence of a positive D-dimer can prompt the need for additional imaging for deep venous thrombosis and/or pulmonary embolus in specific clinical situations where the patient would be considered to have an elevation in D-dimer. However, one must be cautious about placing value on an elevated D-dimer in other situations where there can be an alternative explanation for the elevated level. Of the scenarios listed in the question, the only patient who would be expected to have a negative D-dimer would be the patient with calf pain and recent air travel. The presence of a normal alveolar-arterial oxygen gradient cannot reliably differentiate between those with and without pulmonary embolism. In all the other scenarios, elevations in D-dimer could be related to other medical conditions and provide no diagnostic information to inform the clinician regarding the need for further evaluation. Some common clinical situations in which the D-dimer is elevated include sepsis, myocardial infarction, cancer, pneumonia, the postoperative state, and the second and third trimesters of pregnancy.

V-150. The answer is E. *(Chap. 300)* Warfarin should not be used alone as initial therapy for the treatment of venous thromboembolic disease (VTE) for two reasons. First, warfarin does not achieve full anticoagulation for at least 5 days as its mechanism of action is to decrease the production of vitamin K–dependent coagulation factors in the liver. Second, a paradoxical reaction that promotes coagulation may also occur upon initiation of warfarin as it also decreases the production of the vitamin K–dependent anticoagulants protein C and protein S, which have shorter half-lives than the procoagulant factors. For many years, unfractionated heparin delivered IV was the treatment of choice for VTE. However, it requires frequent monitoring of activated partial thromboplastin time levels and hospitalization until the therapeutic international normalized ratio is achieved with warfarin. There are now several safe and effective alternatives to unfractionated heparin that can be delivered subcutaneously. Low-molecular-weight heparins (LMWHs; enoxaparin, tinzaparin) are fragments of unfractionated heparin with a lower molecular weight. These compounds have a greater bioavailability, longer half-life, and more predictable onset of action. Their use in renal insufficiency should be considered with caution because LMWHs are renally cleared. Fondaparinux is a direct factor Xa inhibitor that, like LMWHs, requires no monitoring of anticoagulant effects and has been demonstrated to be safe and effective in treating both deep venous thrombosis and pulmonary embolism.

V-151. The answer is C. *(Chap. 300)* Many patients with pulmonary embolism (PE) have no evidence of deep venous thrombosis because the clot has already embolized to the lungs. The most common gas exchange abnormalities are arterial hypoxemia and an increased alveolar-arterial O_2 tension gradient, which represents the inefficiency of O_2 transfer across the lungs. Physiologic dead space increases because ventilation to gas exchange units exceeds blood flow through the pulmonary capillaries. Other pathophysiologic abnormalities include: (1) increased pulmonary vascular resistance due to vascular obstruction or platelet secretion of vasoconstricting neurohumoral agents, such as serotonin; release of vasoactive mediators can produce ventilation-perfusion mismatching at sites remote from the embolus, thereby accounting for discordance between a small PE and a large alveolar-arterial O_2 gradient; (2) impaired gas exchange due to increased alveolar dead space from vascular obstruction, hypoxemia from ventilation-perfusion mismatching, right-to-left shunting, or impaired carbon monoxide diffusion capacity due to loss of gas exchange surface; (3) alveolar hyperventilation due to reflex stimulation of irritant receptors; (4) increased airway resistance due to mediator-induced bronchoconstriction; and (5) decreased pulmonary compliance due to lung edema, lung hemorrhage, or loss of surfactant. In the setting of acute pulmonary embolism, pulmonary vascular resistance and thus RV pressures acutely rise. Hypotension in this setting is due to acute RV failure. The left ventricle is often contracting in a hyperdynamic fashion due to a catecholamine surge and compression from the dilated, failing RV.

V-152. The answer is A. *(Chap. 300)* In patients with PE, the two principal indications for insertion of an inferior vena cava filter are (1) active bleeding that precludes anticoagulation and (2) recurrent venous thrombosis despite intensive anticoagulation. Prevention of recurrent PE in patients with right heart failure who are not candidates for fibrinolysis and prophylaxis of extremely high-risk patients are "softer" indications for filter placement. The filter itself may fail by permitting the passage of small- to medium-size clots. Large thrombi may embolize to the pulmonary arteries via collateral veins that develop. A more common complication is caval thrombosis with marked bilateral leg swelling. Paradoxically, by providing a nidus for clot formation, filters increase the deep venous thrombosis rate, even though they usually prevent PE (over the short term). Retrievable filters can now be placed for patients with an anticipated temporary bleeding disorder or for patients at temporary high risk of PE, such as individuals undergoing bariatric surgery who have a prior history of perioperative PE. The filters can be retrieved up to several months after insertion unless thrombus forms and is trapped within the filter. The retrievable filter becomes permanent if it remains in place or if, for technical reasons such as rapid endothelialization, it cannot be removed.

V-153. The answer is C. *(Chap. 300)* This patient is suffering from massive PE as a complication of her bariatric surgery. Rather than being defined by the absolute size of clot burden of PE on imaging, massive PE is defined by the presence of hypotension due to the embolism. Usually, one would consider emergent thrombolysis (either systemic of catheter directed) for a patient with massive PE, but Ms. Tupulo has just completed a large open abdominal operation, which is a direct contraindication for thrombolytics, such as tissue plasminogen activator or urokinase, because she would be at very high risk for life-threatening hemorrhage. In this case, the goal is to alleviate right heart obstruction as soon and effectively as possible. Emergent surgical pulmonary embolectomy provides this and should be pursued before the onset of multisystem organ failure renders the surgery too high risk. Inferior vena cava filter placement could be pursued later if it is discovered that the patient has residual lower extremity thrombus. Although systemic anticoagulation will be needed after embolectomy, enoxaparin represents a poor choice given the patient's very high body weight and the only partially reversible nature of LMWHs, a consideration given the patient's high risk of bleeding.

V-154. The answer is A. *(Chap. 301)* An aneurysm is defined as a pathologic dilation of a segment of a blood vessel. A true aneurysm involves all three layers of the vessel wall and is distinguished from a pseudoaneurysm, in which the intimal and medial layers are disrupted and the dilated segment of the aorta is lined usually by adventitia only and, at times, by perivascular clot. Aneurysms also may be classified according to their gross appearance. A fusiform aneurysm affects the entire circumference of a segment of the vessel, resulting in a diffusely dilated artery. In contrast, a saccular aneurysm involves only a portion of the circumference, resulting in an outpouching of the vessel wall.

V-155. The answer is C. *(Chap. 301)* Factors associated with degenerative aortic aneurysms include aging, cigarette smoking, hypercholesterolemia, hypertension, and male sex.

V-156. The answer is D. *(Chap. 301)* This patient has a classical phenotype for Loeys-Dietz syndrome. Loeys-Dietz syndrome is caused by mutations in the genes that encode transforming growth factor (TGF)-β receptors 1 (*TGFBR1*) and 2 (*TGFBR2*). Increased signaling by TGF-β and mutations of *TGFBR1* and *TGFBR2* may cause thoracic aortic aneurysms. Mutations of the gene that encodes fibrillin-1 are present in patients with Marfan syndrome. Fibrillin-1 is an important component of extracellular microfibrils, which support the architecture of elastic fibers and other connective tissue. Deficiency of fibrillin-1 in the extracellular matrix leads to excessive signaling by TGF-β. Mutations of type III procollagen have been implicated in Ehlers-Danlos type IV syndrome. Mutations of *SMAD3*, which encodes a downstream signaling protein involved with TGF binding to its receptors, have been described in a syndrome of thoracic aortic aneurysm; craniofacial, skeletal, and cutaneous anomalies; and osteoarthritis. Mutations of the genes encoding the smooth muscle–specific alpha-actin (ACTA2), smooth muscle cell–specific myosin heavy chain 11 (MHC11), and myosin light chain kinase (MYLK) and mutations of *TGFBR2* and *SMAD3* have been reported in some patients with nonsyndromic familial thoracic aortic aneurysms.

V-157. The answer is A. *(Chap. 301)* For all patients with aortic dissection or hematoma, appropriate management includes reduction of shear stress with β-blockade and management of systemic hypertension to reduce tension on the dissection. However, emergent or urgent surgical therapy is indicated in patients with ascending aortic dissection and intramural hematomas (type A) and for complicated type B dissections (distal aorta). Complications that would warrant surgical intervention include propagation despite medical therapy, compromise of major branches, impending rupture, or continued pain. Thus, patient A has a distal dissection without evidence of complications and is the best candidate for medical therapy.

V-158. The answer is D. *(Chap. 301)* Aortitis and ascending aortic aneurysms are commonly caused by cystic medial necrosis and mesoaortitis that result in damage to the elastic fibers of the aortic wall with thinning and weakening. Many infectious, inflammatory, and inherited conditions have been associated with this finding, including syphilis, tuberculosis, mycotic aneurysm, Takayasu arteritis, giant cell arteritis, rheumatoid arthritis, and the spondyloarthropathies (ankylosing spondylitis, psoriatic arthritis, reactive arthritis, Behçet disease). In addition, it can be seen with the genetic disorders Marfan syndrome and Ehlers-Danlos syndrome. Aortic disease is not typical in systemic lupus erythematosus.

V-159. The answer is E. *(Chap. 302)* Mr. Tomazelli is describing classic symptoms of claudication due to peripheral arterial disease (PAD). By far, the most common etiology of this disease is atherosclerosis, particularly in elderly patients with hypertension, diabetes mellitus, and smoking history. The history and physical examination are often sufficient to establish the diagnosis of PAD. An objective assessment of the presence and severity of disease is obtained by noninvasive techniques. Magnetic resonance angiography, invasive catheter-based angiography, and CT angiography are not initial tests of choice but may be used to plan revascularization strategies. The initial test of choice is an ankle-brachial index (ABI). Arterial pressure can be recorded noninvasively in the legs by placement of sphygmomanometric cuffs at the ankles and the use of a Doppler device to auscultate or record blood flow from the dorsalis pedis and posterior tibial arteries. Normally, systolic blood pressure in the legs and arms is similar. Indeed, ankle pressure may be slightly higher than arm pressure due to pulse-wave amplification. Thus, the ratio of the ankle and brachial artery pressures (termed ABI) is 1.00–1.40 in normal individuals. In the presence of hemodynamically significant lower extremity stenoses, the systolic blood pressure in the leg is decreased. ABI values of 0.91–0.99 are considered "borderline," and those <0.90 are abnormal and diagnostic of PAD. One may also consider the pulse volume contour, which is blunted in cases of PAD.

V-160. The answer is D. *(Chap. 302)* The natural history of patients with PAD is influenced primarily by the extent of coexisting coronary artery and cerebrovascular disease. Patients with PAD have a 15%–30% 5-year mortality rate and a two- to sixfold increased risk of death from coronary heart disease. The likelihood of symptomatic progression of PAD is lower than the chance of succumbing to coronary artery disease (CAD). Approximately 75%–80% of nondiabetic patients who present with mild to moderate claudication remain symptomatically stable. Deterioration is likely to occur in the remainder, with approximately 1%–2% of the group ultimately developing critical limb ischemia each year. The anticoagulant warfarin is as effective as antiplatelet therapy in preventing adverse cardiovascular events but causes more major bleeding; therefore, it is not indicated to improve outcomes in patients with chronic PAD. Patients with claudication should be encouraged to exercise regularly and at progressively more strenuous levels. Supervised exercise training programs involving 30- to 45-minutes sessions, three to five times per week for at least 12 weeks, prolong walking distance. Patients also should be advised to walk until nearly maximum claudication discomfort occurs and then rest until the symptoms resolve before resuming ambulation. The beneficial effect of supervised exercise training on walking performance in patients with claudication often is similar to or greater than that realized after a revascularization procedure. Vasodilators as a class have not proved to be beneficial. During exercise, peripheral vasodilation occurs distal to sites of significant arterial stenoses. As a result, perfusion pressure falls, often to levels lower than that generated in the interstitial tissue by the exercising muscle. β-Adrenergic blockers do not worsen claudication and may be used to treat hypertension, especially in patients with coexistent CAD.

V-161. The answer is C. *(Chap. 302)* The patient presents with classic signs of arterial occlusion with limb pain and physical examination showing pallor and a pulseless, cold leg. She has no risk factors for central or peripheral atherosclerotic disease; thus, an angiogram would simply confirm the diagnosis of arterial occlusion, not demonstrate her predisposing condition. In the absence of fever or systemic symptoms, vasculitis and endocarditis are unlikely sources of arterial embolization. She likely had a paradoxical embolism in the context of an atrial septal defect, which was the source of her childhood murmur. Because many of these patients develop pulmonary hypertension with time, she is now at risk for a paradoxical embolism. Although in this context, arterial emboli frequently originate from venous thrombus, the thrombi cannot produce a paradoxical embolism in the absence of right-to-left shunt, such as in a large patent foramen ovale or an atrial septal defect, which can be demonstrated with an echocardiogram with bubble study.

V-162. The answer is D. *(Chap. 302)* This patient has a classic presentation of thromboangiitis obliterans, or Buerger disease. This is an inflammatory occlusive vascular disorder involving small- and medium-size arteries and veins in the distal upper and lower extremities. Cerebral, visceral, and coronary vessels may be affected rarely. This disorder develops most frequently in men <40 years of age who are smokers. The prevalence is higher in Asians and individuals of Eastern European descent. Although the cause of thromboangiitis obliterans is not known, there is a definite relationship to cigarette smoking in patients with this disorder. The clinical features of thromboangiitis obliterans often include a triad of claudication of the affected extremity, Raynaud phenomenon (per the figure), and migratory superficial vein thrombophlebitis. Claudication usually is confined to the calves and feet or the forearms and hands because this disorder primarily affects distal vessels. There is no specific treatment except abstention from tobacco. The prognosis is worse in individuals who continue to smoke, but results are discouraging even in those who stop smoking. Arterial bypass of the larger vessels may be used in selected instances, as well as local debridement, depending on the symptoms and severity of ischemia. Antibiotics may be useful when infection is present. Anticoagulants and glucocorticoids are not helpful. Cilostazol is a phosphodiesterase inhibitor used for intermittent claudication but has no proven role in thromboangiitis obliterans. In some cases of advanced disease, amputation may be required.

V-163. The answer is B. *(Chap. 303)* Varicose veins are dilated, bulging, tortuous superficial veins, measuring at least 3 mm in diameter. The estimated prevalence of varicose veins in the United States is approximately 15% in men and 30% in women. Chronic venous insufficiency is a consequence of incompetent veins in which there is venous hypertension and extravasation of fluid and blood elements into the tissue of the limb. It may occur in patients with varicose veins but usually is caused by disease in the deep veins. Chronic venous insufficiency with edema affects approximately 7.5% of men and 5% of women, and the prevalence increases with age, ranging from 2% among those less than 50 years old to 10% of those 70 years old. Approximately 20% of patients with chronic venous insufficiency develop venous ulcers.

V-164. The answer is B. *(Chap. 303)* Veins in the extremities can be broadly classified as either superficial or deep. The superficial veins are located between the skin and deep fascia. In the legs, these include the great and small saphenous veins and their tributaries. The great saphenous vein is the longest vein in the body. It originates on the medial side of the foot and ascends anterior to the medial malleolus and then along the medial side of the calf and thigh, and drains into the common femoral vein. The deep veins of the leg accompany the major arteries. There are usually paired peroneal, anterior tibial, and posterior tibial veins in the calf, which converge to form the popliteal vein. The popliteal vein ascends in the thigh as the femoral vein. The confluence of the femoral vein and deep femoral vein forms the common femoral vein, which ascends in the pelvis as the external iliac and then common iliac vein, which converges with the contralateral common iliac vein at the inferior vena cava. In the arms, the superficial veins include the basilic, cephalic, and median cubital veins and their tributaries. The deep veins of the arms accompany the major arteries and include the radial, ulnar, brachial, axillary, and subclavian veins. The subclavian vein converges with the internal jugular vein to form the brachiocephalic vein, which joins the contralateral brachiocephalic vein to form the superior vena cava. Bicuspid valves are present throughout the venous system to direct the flow of venous blood centrally.

V-165. The answer is C. *(Chap. 303)* This is a classic clinical picture for a chronic venous insufficiency with an active venous ulcer. Symptoms in patients with varicose veins or venous insufficiency, when they occur, include a dull ache, throbbing or heaviness, or pressure sensation in the legs typically after prolonged standing; these symptoms usually are relieved with leg elevation. Additional symptoms may include cramping, burning, pruritus, leg swelling, and skin ulceration. Edema, stasis dermatitis, and skin ulceration near the ankle may be present if there is superficial venous insufficiency and venous hypertension. Findings of deep venous insufficiency include increased leg circumference, venous varicosities, edema, and skin changes. The edema, which is usually pitting, may be confined to the ankles, extend above the ankles to the knees, or involve the thighs in severe cases. Over time, the edema may become less pitting and more indurated. Dermatologic findings associated with venous stasis include hyperpigmentation, erythema, eczema, lipodermatosclerosis, atrophie blanche, and a phlebectasia corona. Lipodermatosclerosis is the combination of induration, hemosiderin deposition, and inflammation, and typically occurs in the lower part of the leg just above the ankle. Atrophie blanche is a white patch of scar tissue, often with focal telangiectasias and a hyperpigmented border; it usually develops near the medial malleolus. A phlebectasia corona is a fan-shaped pattern of intradermal veins near the ankle or on the foot. Skin ulceration may occur near the medial and lateral malleoli. A venous ulcer is often shallow and characterized by an irregular border, a base of granulation tissue, and the presence of exudate. Ulcers due to arterial insufficiency are typically at the terminal end of a digit, since that is where flow is most limited. Diabetic ulcers are typically at pressure points such as the sides of the toes or the ball or heel of the foot. The patient's report of months of leg discomfort make *Bacillus anthracis* infection (cutaneous anthrax) and arachnid envenomation unlikely.

V-166. The answer is C. *(Chap. 303)* Secondary lymphedema is an acquired condition that results from damage to or obstruction of previously normal lymphatic channels. Recurrent episodes of bacterial lymphangitis, usually caused by streptococci, are a very common cause of lymphedema. The most common cause of secondary lymphedema worldwide is lymphatic filariasis, affecting approximately 129 million children and adults worldwide and causing lymphedema and elephantiasis in 14 million of these affected individuals. Other infectious causes include lymphogranuloma venereum and tuberculosis. In developed countries, the most common secondary cause of lymphedema is surgical excision or irradiation of axillary and inguinal lymph nodes for treatment of cancers, such as breast, cervical, endometrial, and prostate cancer, sarcomas, and malignant melanoma. Lymphedema of the arm occurs in 13% of breast cancer patients after axillary node dissection and in 22% after both surgery and radiotherapy. Lymphedema of the leg affects approximately 15% of patients with cancer after inguinal lymph node dissection. Tumors, such as prostate cancer and lymphoma, also can infiltrate and obstruct lymphatic vessels. Less common causes include contact dermatitis, rheumatoid arthritis, pregnancy, and self-induced or factitious lymphedema after application of tourniquets.

V-167. The answer is B. *(Chap. 303)* Diuretics are contraindicated in patients with lymphedema and may cause depletion of intravascular volume and metabolic abnormalities. Patients should be encouraged to participate in physical activity; frequent leg elevation can reduce the amount of edema. Psychosocial support is indicated to assist patients cope with anxiety or depression related to body image, self-esteem, functional disability, and fear of limb loss. Physical therapy, including massage to facilitate lymphatic drainage, may be helpful. The type of massage used in decongestive physiotherapy for lymphedema involves mild compression of the skin of the affected extremity to dilate the lymphatic channels and enhance lymphatic motility. Multilayered, compressive bandages are applied after each massage session to reduce recurrent edema. After optimal reduction in limb volume by decongestive physiotherapy, patients can be fitted with graduated compression hose. Occasionally, intermittent pneumatic compression devices can be applied at home to facilitate reduction of the edema. Liposuction in conjunction with decongestive physiotherapy may be considered to treat lymphedema, particularly postmastectomy lymphedema. Other surgical interventions are rarely used and are often not successful in ameliorating lymphedema. Microsurgical lymphaticovenous anastomotic procedures have been performed to rechannel lymph flow from obstructed lymphatic vessels into the venous system. Limb reduction procedures to resect subcutaneous tissue and excessive skin are performed occasionally in severe cases of lymphedema to improve mobility

SECTION VI

Disorders of the Respiratory System and Critical Care Illness

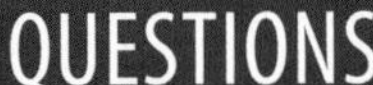

QUESTIONS

DIRECTIONS: Choose the one best response to each question.

VI-1. All of the following are typically characterized as an obstructive lung disease EXCEPT:

A. Asbestosis
B. Asthma
C. Bronchiectasis
D. Chronic bronchitis
E. Emphysema

VI-2. A 25-year-old man is brought to the emergency department by ambulance after his family found him unresponsive at home. He has a history of intravenous drug abuse and human immunodeficiency virus (HIV) with medical noncompliance. His last CD4 count was <200/μL. On initial evaluation, his blood pressure is 120/75 mmHg, heart rate is 105 bpm, respiratory rate 8 breaths/min, oxygen saturation (SaO_2) of 83%, and temperature of 36.0°C. A blood gas on room air reveals pH of 7.16, partial pressure of carbon dioxide (PCO_2) of 70 mmHg, and partial pressure of oxygen (PO_2) of 55 mmHg. Which of the following is the most likely diagnosis?

A. Asthma
B. Narcotic overdose
C. Pneumococcal pneumonia
D. Pneumocystis pneumonia
E. Pulmonary embolism

VI-3. At what lung volume does the outward recoil of the chest wall equal the inward elastic recoil of the lung?

A. Expiratory reserve volume
B. Functional residual capacity
C. Residual volume
D. Tidal volume
E. Total lung capacity

VI-4. A 65-year-old man is evaluated for progressive dyspnea on exertion that has occurred over the course of the past 3 months. His medical history is significant for an episode of necrotizing pancreatitis that resulted in multiorgan failure and acute respiratory distress syndrome. He required mechanical ventilation for 6 weeks prior to his recovery. He also has a history of 30 pack-years of tobacco, quitting 15 years previously. He is not known to have chronic obstructive pulmonary disease. On physical examination, a low-pitched inspiratory and expiratory wheeze is heard, loudest over the mid-chest area. On pulmonary function testing, the forced expiratory volume in 1 second (FEV_1) is 2.5 L (78% predicted), forced vital capacity (FVC) is 4.00 L (94% predicted), and FEV_1/FVC ratio is 62.5%. The flow-volume curve is shown in Figure VI-4A. What is the most likely cause of the patient's symptoms?

A. Aspirated foreign body
B. Chronic obstructive pulmonary disease
C. Idiopathic pulmonary fibrosis
D. Subglottic stenosis
E. Unilateral vocal cord paralysis

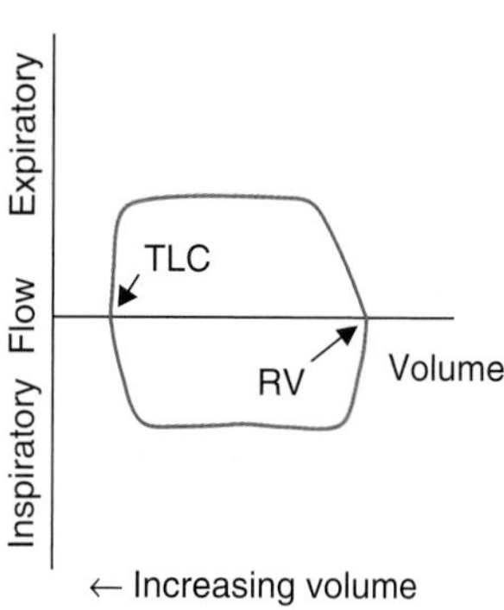

FIGURE VI-4A RV, residual volume; TLC, total lung capacity.

VI-5. A 22-year-old woman presents to the emergency department in her 23rd week of pregnancy complaining of acute dyspnea. She has had an uncomplicated pregnancy and has no other medical problems. She is taking no medications other than prenatal vitamins. On examination, she appears dyspneic. Her vital signs are as follows: blood pressure 128/78 mmHg, heart rate 126 bpm, respiratory rate 28 breaths/min, and oxygen saturation 96% on room air. She is afebrile. Her lung and cardiac examinations are normal. There is trace bilateral pitting pedal edema. A chest x-ray performed with abdominal shielding is normal, and the electrocardiogram (ECG) demonstrates sinus tachycardia. An arterial blood gas is performed. The pH is 7.52, partial pressure of arterial carbon dioxide ($PaCO_2$) is 26 mmHg, and partial pressure of arterial oxygen (PaO_2) is 85 mmHg. What is the next best step in the diagnosis and management of this patient?

A. Initiate therapy with amoxicillin for acute bronchitis.
B. Perform a computed tomography (CT) pulmonary angiogram .
C. Perform an echocardiogram.
D. Reassure the patient that dyspnea is normal during this stage of pregnancy and no abnormalities are seen on testing.
E. Treat with clonazepam for a panic attack.

VI-6 to VI-9. Match each of the following pulmonary function test results to the respiratory disorder in which it is most likely to be found.

VI-6. Myasthenia gravis

VI-7. Idiopathic pulmonary fibrosis

VI-8. Familial pulmonary hypertension

VI-9. Chronic obstructive pulmonary disease

A. Increased total lung capacity (TLC), decreased vital capacity (VC), decreased FEV_1/FVC ratio
B. Decreased TLC, decreased VC, decreased residual volume (RV), increased FEV_1/FVC ratio, normal maximum inspiratory pressure (MIP)
C. Decreased TLC, increased RV, normal FEV_1/FVC ratio, decreased MIP
D. Normal TLC, normal RV, normal FEV_1/FVC ratio, normal MIP

VI-10. A 78-year-old woman is admitted to the medical intensive care unit (ICU) with multilobar pneumonia. On initial presentation to the emergency department, her initial oxygen saturation was 60% on room air and only increased to 82% on a non-rebreather face mask. She was in marked respiratory distress and intubated in the emergency department. Upon admission to the ICU, she was sedated and paralyzed. The ventilator is set in the assist-control mode with a respiratory rate of 24 breaths/min, tidal volume of 6 mL/kg, FiO_2 of 1.0, and positive end-expiratory pressure of 12 cmH_2O. An arterial blood gas measurement is performed on these settings; the results are pH of 7.20, PCO_2 of 32 mmHg, and PO_2 of 54 mmHg. What is the cause of the hypoxemia?

A. Hypoventilation alone
B. Hypoventilation and ventilation-perfusion mismatch
C. Shunt
D. Ventilation-perfusion mismatch

VI-11. Mrs. Wittstine, a 72-year-old woman, has been complaining of low-grade fever and dyspnea for 2 weeks. She has a 10-year history of scleroderma with involvement of the digits and esophagus. She has a 30-pack-year history of cigarette smoking but quit 8 years ago. On chest radiograph, she has a nodular infiltrate in the right lower lobe. Positron emission tomography (PET)/CT shows the right lower lobe lesion to be 3 cm in diameter with nodular infiltrate characteristics and enhanced fluorodeoxyglucose (FDG) uptake. Which of the following statements about Mrs. Wittstine is most accurate?

A. Additional diagnostic studies are indicated.
B. The findings on PET/CT make infection very likely.
C. The findings on PET/CT make infection very unlikely.
D. The findings on PET/CT make malignancy very likely.
E. The findings on PET/CT make malignancy very unlikely.

VI-12. A 65-year-old man is evaluated for progressive dyspnea on exertion and dry cough that have worsened over the course of 6 months. He has not had dyspnea at rest and denies wheezing. He has not experienced chest pain. He has a history of coronary artery disease and atrial fibrillation and previously underwent a coronary artery bypass surgery 12 years previously. His medications include metoprolol, aspirin, warfarin, and enalapril. He previously smoked 1 pack of cigarettes daily for 40 years, quitting 5 years previously. His vital signs are as follows: blood pressure 122/68 mmHg, heart rate 68 bpm, respiratory rate 18 breaths/min, and oxygen saturation 92% on room air. His chest examination demonstrates bibasilar crackles present about one-third of the way up bilaterally. No wheezing is heard. He has an irregularly irregular rhythm with a II/VI holosystolic murmur at the apex. The jugular venous pressure is not elevated. No edema is present, but clubbing is noted. Pulmonary function testing reveals an FEV_1 of 65% predicted, FVC of 67% predicted, FEV_1/FVC ratio of 74%, TLC of 68% predicted, and diffusion capacity for carbon monoxide (DLCO) of 62% predicted. Which test is most likely to determine the etiology of the patient's dyspnea?

A. Bronchoscopy with transbronchial lung biopsy
B. CT pulmonary angiography
C. Echocardiography
D. High-resolution CT scan of the chest
E. Nuclear medicine stress test

VI-13. Which of the following is the major risk factor for asthma?

A. Air pollution
B. Atopy
C. Diet
D. Maternal cigarette smoking
E. Upper respiratory viral infections

VI-14. A 24-year-old woman is seen for a complaint of shortness of breath and wheezing. She notes the symptoms to be worse when she has exercised outdoors and is around cats. She has had allergic rhinitis in the spring and summer for many years and suffered from eczema as a child. On physical examination, she is noted to have expiratory wheezing. Her pulmonary function tests demonstrate an FEV_1 of 2.67 (79% predicted), FVC of 3.81 L (97% predicted), and an FEV_1/FVC ratio of 70% (86% predicted). After administration of albuterol, the FEV_1 increases to 3.0 L (12.4%). Which of the following statements regarding the patient's disease process is true?

A. Confirmation of the diagnosis will require methacholine challenge testing.
B. Mortality due to the disease has been increasing over the past decade.
C. The most common risk factor in individuals with the disorder is genetic predisposition.
D. The prevalence of the disorder has not changed in the past several decades.
E. The severity of the disease does not vary significantly within a given patient with the disease.

VI-15. A 38-year-old woman is brought to the emergency department for status asthmaticus. She rapidly deteriorates and dies of her disease. All of the following pathologic findings would likely be seen in this individual EXCEPT:

A. Infiltration of the airway mucosa with eosinophils and activated T lymphocytes
B. Infiltration of the alveolar spaces with eosinophils and neutrophils
C. Occlusion of the airway lumen by mucous plugs
D. Thickening and edema of the airway wall
E. Thickening of the basement membrane of the airways with subepithelial collagen deposition

VI-16. Which of the following patients is appropriately diagnosed with asthma?

A. A 24-year-old woman treated with inhaled corticosteroids for cough and wheezing that has persisted for 6 weeks following a viral upper respiratory infection
B. A 26-year-old man who coughs and occasionally wheezes following exercise in cold weather
C. A 34-year-old woman evaluated for chronic cough with an FEV_1/FVC ratio of 68% with an FEV_1 that increases from 1.68 L (52% predicted) to 1.98 L (61% predicted) after albuterol (18% change in FEV_1)
D. A 44-year-old man who works as a technician caring for the mice in a medical research laboratory and complains of wheezing, shortness of breath, and cough that are most severe at the end of the week
E. A 60-year-old man who has smoked two packs of cigarettes per day for 40 years who has dyspnea and cough and who has airway hyperreactivity in response to methacholine

VI-17. A 24-year-old woman was diagnosed with asthma 4 months ago and was treated with inhaled albuterol as needed. Since her last visit, she feels generally well and typically requires using her inhaler approximately four to seven times a week when around pollen or cats or when exercising in cold air. The inhaled albuterol generally helps, and she only requires a repeat round of inhalations approximately two times a week. She is on no other medications and is a nonsmoker, and her only pet is a goldfish named Puffer. Based on this information, you advise which of the following?

A. Add inhaled beclomethasone
B. Add inhaled salmeterol twice a day
C. Add inhaled tiotropium
D. Continue present therapy
E. Think of a new name for the goldfish

VI-18. A 28-year-old woman with longstanding mild persistent asthma comes to see you because she just found out that she is pregnant. Her only medications are inhaled beclomethasone twice a day and albuterol as needed. She typically uses her albuterol less than twice per week. She wants to know what to expect regarding her asthma severity and whether any medication changes should be made at this time. Which of the following statements is correct?

A. She should continue her current therapy and follow symptoms.
B. She should switch from inhaled albuterol as needed to inhaled tiotropium as needed.
C. She should switch from inhaled beclomethasone to a inhaled salmeterol.
D. There is a greater than 70% chance that her asthma symptoms will become less severe during pregnancy.
E. There is a greater than 70% chance that her asthma symptoms will become more severe during pregnancy.

VI-19. A 38-year-old woman is admitted to the medical ICU with acute hypoxemic respiratory failure. She was well and healthy until 4 days prior when she abruptly began to feel ill with fevers, chills, bilateral pleuritic chest pain, and worsening shortness of breath. She has no significant past medical history but has suffered the recent death of her father following a car accident. In coping with his loss, she began smoking cigarettes again after a 15-year period of abstinence. She has been smoking up to two packs of tobacco daily. After she began to feel ill, she started taking acetaminophen and pseudoephedrine, but otherwise takes no medications. Upon arrival in the emergency department, her oxygen saturation was 78% on room air. On a non-rebreather mask, the oxygen saturation increased to 92%. The vital signs are as follows: temperature 38.7°C (101.7°), heart rate 122 bpm, respiratory rate 28 breaths/min, and blood pressure 132/82 mmHg. She appears in moderate respiratory distress. There are bilateral diffuse crackles. The cardiovascular examination shows a regular tachycardia without murmur. The jugular venous pressure is not elevated, and no edema is present. The abdomen is soft and not tender. No hepatosplenomegaly is present. Extremity and neurology examinations are normal. Chest radiograph shows diffuse bilateral infiltrates. Her echocardiogram shows normal left heart systolic and diastolic function. She is treated with ceftriaxone 1 g intravenously (IV) daily and azithromycin 500 mg IV daily. Over the course of the first 24 hours, the patient's clinical condition continues to deteriorate. She remains febrile, and she requires intubation and mechanical ventilation. The patient's ventilator is set on assist control with a rate of 28/min, tidal volume of 330 mL, fraction of inspired oxygen (FiO_2) of 0.8, and positive end-expiratory pressure (PEEP) of 12 cmH_2O. On these settings, her arterial blood gas values are pH 7.28, $PaCO_2$ 68 mmHg, and PaO_2 62 mmHg. A bronchoalveolar lavage is performed. The cell count shows 58% neutrophils, 12% lymphocytes, and 30% eosinophils. What is the best approach to the treatment of the patient at this time?

A. Consult thoracic surgery for surgical lung biopsy.
B. Continue current IV antibiotic regimen while awaiting culture data.
C. Initiate methylprednisolone 60 mg IV every 6 hours.
D. Initiate oseltamivir 75 mg twice a day.
E. Initiate therapy with trimethoprim/sulfamethoxazole IV with prednisone 40 mg twice a day.

VI-20. A 34-year-old man is referred to clinic for evaluation of severe persistent asthma. He was diagnosed with asthma in his teenage years. At that time, he primarily noticed symptoms when he was running cross country track outdoors. He generally has been an active individual, but in the past 10 years, his asthma has become increasingly hard to control. He has been hospitalized three times for asthma exacerbations in the past 3 years. He has had to stop running and has gained 60 lb due to being on chronic oral prednisone. His current medical regimen is fluticasone/salmeterol 500/50 μg twice a day, tiotropium 18 μg daily, montelukast 10 mg daily, esomeprazole 40 mg daily, fluticasone nasal spray daily, and prednisone 10 mg daily. He uses his rescue albuterol nebulizer or metered-dose inhaler (MDI) about four times daily and awakens at night at least three times weekly. He has a chronic cough that brings up brownish mucous plugs. On examination, he has enlarged nasal turbinates but no polyps. Diffuse bilateral wheezing is heard. No crackles are present. His chest x-ray shows hyperinflation with an area of upper lung zone infiltrate in the right upper lobe. Three months ago, he had an area of atelectasis with mucous plugging in the left lower lobe. His peripheral eosinophil count is 750/μL. Which of the following tests is indicated next in the evaluation and treatment of this patient?

A. Aspirin desensitization
B. Chest CT
C. Nasal nitric oxide testing
D. Serum immunoglobulin (Ig) E level
E. Sweat chloride testing

VI-21. A 34-year-old woman seeks evaluation for a complaint of cough and dyspnea on exertion that has gradually worsened over 3 months. The patient has no past history of pulmonary complaints and has never had asthma. She started working in a pet store approximately 6 months ago. Her duties there include cleaning the reptile and bird cages. She reports occasional low-grade fevers but has had no wheezing. The cough is dry and nonproductive. Before 3 months ago, the patient had no limitation of exercise tolerance, but now she reports that she gets dyspneic climbing two flights of stairs. On physical examination, the patient appears well. She has an oxygen saturation of 95% on room air at rest but desaturates to 89% with ambulation. Temperature is 37.7°C (99.8°F). The pulmonary examination is unremarkable. No clubbing or cyanosis is present. The patient has a normal chest radiogram. A high-resolution chest CT shows diffuse ground-glass infiltrates in the lower lobes with the presence of centrilobular nodules. A transbronchial biopsy shows an interstitial alveolar infiltrate of plasma cells, lymphocytes, and occasional eosinophils. There are also several loose noncaseating granulomas. All cultures are negative for bacterial, viral, and fungal pathogens. What is the diagnosis?

A. Aspergillosis
B. Hypersensitivity pneumonitis
C. Nonspecific interstitial pneumonitis related to collagen vascular disease
D. Psittacosis
E. Sarcoidosis

VI-22. What treatment do you recommend for the patient in Question VI-21?

A. Amphotericin
B. Doxycycline
C. Glucocorticoids
D. Glucocorticoids plus azathioprine
E. Glucocorticoids plus removal of antigen

VI-23. A 75-year-old man is evaluated for a new left-sided pleural effusion and shortness of breath. He worked as an insulation worker at a shipyard for more than 30 years and did not wear protective respiratory equipment, retiring at the age of 60. He has a 50 pack-year history of tobacco with known moderate chronic obstructive pulmonary disease (COPD; FEV_1 55% predicted) and a history of myocardial infarction 10 years previously. His current medications include aspirin, atenolol, benazepril, tiotropium, and albuterol. His physical examination is consistent with a left-sided effusion with dullness to percussion and decreased breath sounds occurring over half of the hemithorax. On chest x-ray, there is a moderate left-sided pleural effusion with bilateral pleural calcifications and left apical pleural thickening. No lung mass is seen. A chest CT confirms the findings on chest x-ray and also fails to show a mass. There is compressive atelectasis of the left lower lobe. A thoracentesis is performed demonstrating an exudative effusion with 65% lymphocytes, 25% mesothelial cells, and 10% neutrophils. Cytology does not demonstrate any malignancy. Which of the following statements regarding the most likely cause of the patient's effusion or causative condition is true?

A. Cigarette smoking increases the likelihood of developing the condition.
B. Death in this disease is usually related to diffuse metastatic disease.
C. Exposure to the causative agent can be as brief as 1–2 years, and latency to expression of disease may be as great as 40 years.
D. Repeated pleural fluid cytology will most likely lead to a definitive diagnosis.
E. Therapy with a combination of surgical resection with adjuvant chemotherapy significantly improves long-term survival.

VI-24. Chronic silicosis is related to an increased risk of which of the following conditions?

A. Infection with invasive *Aspergillus*
B. Infection with *Mycobacterium tuberculosis*
C. Lung cancer
D. Rheumatoid arthritis
E. All of the above

VI-25. All of the following occupational lung diseases are correctly matched with its exposure EXCEPT:

A. Berylliosis—High-technology electronics
B. Byssinosis—Cotton milling
C. Farmer's lung—Moldy hay
D. Progressive massive fibrosis—Shipyard workers
E. Metal fume fever—Welding

VI-26. A 53-year-old man is seen in the emergency department with sudden-onset fever, chills, malaise, and shortness of breath but no wheezing. He has no significant past medical history and is a farmer. Of note, he worked earlier in the day stacking hay. Posteroanterior and lateral chest radiography shows diffuse bilateral alveolar infiltrates. Which organism is most likely to be responsible for this presentation?

A. *Nocardia asteroides*
B. *Histoplasma capsulatum*
C. *Cryptococcus neoformans*
D. *Actinomyces* species
E. *Aspergillus fumigatus*

VI-27. A 36-year-old woman is brought into intensive care after a house fire. She is obtunded but did not suffer any major burns. She is being treated for smoke inhalation. Her initial carboxyhemoglobin concentration is 25%. She is treated with 100% oxygen but remains obtunded. She subsequently develops generalized seizures. Her blood pressure rapidly declines to 60/40 mmHg. The heart rate is 150 bpm. The SaO_2 reading is 98%. There is a ruddy appearance to the patient's complexion, and a bitter almond odor is present. There is soot around the patient's nose and mouth. The pupils are dilated, and the skin is diaphoretic. Which of the following tests will yield the diagnosis?

A. Ammonia concentration
B. Blood lactate level
C. Carboxyhemoglobin level
D. Red blood cell cyanide concentration
E. Methemoglobin level

VI-28. A 51-year-old woman presents complaining of a daily cough productive of thick green sputum. The cough is worse when she first wakes in the morning. At this time, there are occasionally streaks of blood in the sputum. Her cough began about 7 years ago and has been progressively worse with production of increasing volume of sputum. She currently estimates that she brings up about half a cup of sputum daily. She reports frequently requiring antibiotics for both lower respiratory tract infections as well as sinus infections. Bilateral coarse crackles are heard in the lower lung zones. No clubbing is present. Pulmonary function tests demonstrate an FEV_1 of 1.68 L (53.3% predicted), FVC of 3.00 L (75% predicted), and FEV_1/FVC ratio of 56%. A sputum culture grows *Pseudomonas aeruginosa*. What test would you perform next in the evaluation of this patient?

A. Barium swallow study
B. Bronchoscopy
C. Chest radiography
D. High-resolution chest CT
E. Sweat chloride testing

VI-29. A 62-year-old woman is diagnosed with bronchiectasis following treatment for *Mycobacterium avium-intracellulare*, which was confirmed on two positive expectorated sputum cultures. She is treated for 24 months with clarithromycin, ethambutol, and rifampin, and her cultures have been negative for mycobacteria for the past 12 months. However, she continues to produce sputum on a daily basis, and her CT shows focal bronchiectasis in the right middle lobe. Which of the following is the best treatment for the patient at the current time?

A. Consult thoracic surgery for right middle lobectomy.
B. Continue treatment with clarithromycin, ethambutol, and rifampin.
C. Initiate airway clearance with oscillating positive expiratory pressure flutter valve.
D. Initiate treatment with dornase (DNase).
E. Initiate treatment with prednisone 20 mg daily.

VI-30. An infant is diagnosed with cystic fibrosis when a sweat chloride returns positive at 110 mmol/L after an abnormal newborn screening test. The drug ivacaftor, recently approved by the Food and Drug Administration, is indicated in patients with which of the following genetic mutations?

A. G542X
B. G551D
C. F508del
D. 621+1G>T
E. R117C

VI-31. Ivacaftor works in patients with cystic fibrosis by having which of the following actions on the cystic fibrosis transmembrane regulator (CFTR) protein?

A. Corrects protein slicing abnormalities
B. Improves conductance through the chloride ion pore
C. Increases synthesis of CFTR
D. Promotes CFTR binding at the cell membrane
E. Stabilizes CFTR protein to prolong degradation

VI-32. A 28-year-old woman is evaluated for recurrent lung and sinus infections. She recalls having at least yearly episodes of bronchitis beginning in her early teens. For the past 5 years, she states that she has been on antibiotics at least three times yearly for respiratory or sinus infections. She also reports that she has had difficulty gaining weight and has always felt short compared to her peers. On physical examination, the patient has a body mass index of 18.5 kg/m^2. Her oxygen saturation is 95% on room air at rest. Nasal polyps are present. Coarse rhonchi and crackles are heard in the bilateral upper lung zones. A chest radiograph shows bilateral upper lobe bronchiectasis with areas of mucous plugging. You are concerned about the possibility of undiagnosed cystic fibrosis. Which of the following tests would provide the strongest support for the diagnosis of cystic fibrosis in this individual?

A. DNA analysis demonstrating one copy of the F508del allele
B. Decreased baseline nasal potential difference
C. Presence of *P aeruginosa* on repeated sputum cultures
D. Sweat chloride values >40 mmol/L
E. Sweat chloride values >60 mmol/L

VI-33. A 22-year-old man with cystic fibrosis is seen for a routine follow-up. He is currently treated with recombinant human DNase and albuterol by nebulization twice daily. His primary sputum clearance technique is aerobic exercise five times weekly and autogenic drainage. He is overall feeling well, and his examination is normal. Pulmonary function testing demonstrates an FEV_1 of 4.48 L (97% predicted), FVC of 5.70 L (103% predicted), and FEV_1/FVC ratio of 79%. A routine sputum culture grows *P aeruginosa*. The only organism isolated on prior cultures has been *Staphylococcus aureus*. What do you recommend for this patient?

A. High-frequency chest wall oscillation
B. Hypertonic saline (7%) nebulized twice daily
C. Inhaled tobramycin 300 mg twice daily every other month
D. Intravenous cefepime and tobramycin for 14 days
E. Return visit in 3 months with repeat sputum cultures and treatment only if there is persistent *P aeruginosa*

VI-34. A 69-year-old man with COPD has been admitted to the hospital three times over the past year for COPD exacerbations. He has daily cough with sputum production and an FEV_1 of 45% predicted. He previously smoked a pack of cigarettes daily for 50 years, quitting 1 year ago. His oxygen saturation on room air is 91%. Which of the following treatments is most likely to decrease the frequency of his exacerbations?

A. Azithromycin 250 mg three times weekly
B. Continuous oxygen at 2 L/min
C. Nocturnal bilevel positive airway pressure with an inspiratory pressure of 18 cm H_2O and expiratory pressure of 12 cm H_2O
D. Roflumilast 500 μg daily
E. Theophylline 300 mg daily

VI-35. All of the following are risk factors for COPD EXCEPT:

A. Airway hyperresponsiveness
B. Coal dust exposure
C. Passive cigarette smoke exposure
D. Recurrent respiratory infections
E. Use of biomass fuels in poorly ventilated areas

VI-36. A 65-year-old woman is evaluated for dyspnea on exertion and chronic cough. She has a long history of tobacco use, smoking 1.5 packs of cigarettes daily since the age of 20. She is a thin woman in no obvious distress. Her oxygen saturation on room air is 93% with a respiratory rate of 22 breaths/min. The lungs are hyperexpanded on percussion with decreased breath sounds in the upper lung fields. You suspect COPD. What are the expected findings on pulmonary function testing?

	FEV_1	FVC	FEV_1/ FVC Ratio	TLC	DLCO
A.	Decreased	Normal or decreased	Decreased	Decreased	Decreased
B.	Decreased	Normal or decreased	Decreased	Increased	Decreased
C.	Decreased	Decreased	Normal	Decreased	Decreased
D.	Decreased	Normal or decreased	Decreased	Increased	Increased

VI-37. A 70-year-old man with known COPD is seen for follow-up. He has been clinically stable without an exacerbation for the past 6 months. However, he generally feels in poor health and is limited in what he can do. He reports dyspnea with usual activities. He is currently being managed with albuterol MDI twice daily and as needed. He has a 50-pack-year history of smoking and quit 5 years previously. His other medical problems include peripheral vascular disease, hypertension, and benign prostatic hyperplasia. He is managed with aspirin, lisinopril, hydrochlorothiazide, and tamsulosin. On examination, the patient has a resting oxygen saturation of 93% on room air. He is hyperinflated to percussion with decreased breath sounds at the apices and faint expiratory wheezing. His pulmonary function tests demonstrate an FEV_1 of 55% predicted, FVC of 80% predicted, and FEV_1/FVC ratio of 50%. What is the next best step in the management of this patient?

A. Initiate a trial of oral glucocorticoids for a period of 4 weeks and initiate inhaled fluticasone if there is a significant improvement in pulmonary function.
B. Initiate treatment with inhaled fluticasone 110 μg/puff twice daily.
C. Initiate treatment with inhaled fluticasone 250 μg/puff in combination with inhaled salmeterol 50 mg/puff twice daily.
D. Initiate treatment with inhaled tiotropium 18 μg/daily.
E. Perform exercise and nocturnal oximetry and initiate oxygen therapy if these demonstrate significant hypoxemia.

VI-38. A 56-year-old woman is admitted to the ICU with a 4-day history of increasing shortness of breath and cough with copious sputum production. She has known severe COPD with an FEV_1 of 42% predicted. On presentation, she has a room air blood gas with a pH of 7.26, $PaCO_2$ of 78 mmHg, and PaO_2 of 50 mmHg. She is in obvious respiratory distress with use of accessory muscles and retractions. Breath sounds are quiet with diffuse expiratory wheezing and rhonchi. No infiltrates are present on chest radiograph. Which of the following therapies has been demonstrated to have the greatest reduction in mortality rate for this patient?

A. Administration of inhaled bronchodilators
B. Administration of IV glucocorticoids
C. Early administration of broad-spectrum antibiotics with coverage of *P aeruginosa*
D. Early intubation with mechanical ventilation
E. Use of noninvasive positive-pressure ventilation

VI-39. A 63-year-old man with a long history of cigarette smoking comes to see you for a 4-month history of progressive shortness of breath and dyspnea on exertion. The symptoms have been indolent, with no recent worsening. He denies fever, chest pain, or hemoptysis. He has a daily cough of 3 to 6 tablespoons of yellow phlegm. The patient says he has not seen a physician for over 10 years. Physical examination is notable for normal vital signs, a prolonged expiratory phase, scattered rhonchi, elevated jugular venous pulsation, and moderate pedal edema. Hematocrit is 49%. Which of the following therapies is most likely to prolong his survival?

A. Atenolol
B. Enalapril
C. Oxygen
D. Prednisone
E. Theophylline

VI-40. A 62-year-old man is evaluated for dyspnea on exertion that has progressively worsened over a period of 10 months. He has a 50-pack-year history of tobacco, quitting 10 years ago. On physical examination, has a resting oxygen saturation of 94%. After ambulation of 100 m, his saturation drops to 84%. He requires oxygen at 3 L/min to maintain his saturation at greater than 90% with ambulation. His lung examination shows diffuse end-inspiratory crackles throughout both lungs. His total lung capacity is 72% predicted, residual volume is 68% predicted, and diffusing capacity is 60% predicted. The high-resolution chest CT is shown in Figure VI-40. Serologic workup for autoimmune disease is unremarkable, and thorough history yields no exposures that would lead to these findings. You suspect idiopathic pulmonary fibrosis. What is the expected finding on surgical pathology?

A. Desquamative interstitial pneumonia
B. Diffuse alveolar damage
C. Loosely organized granulomatous inflammation and fibrosis
D. Nonspecific interstitial pneumonia
E. Usual interstitial pneumonia

VI-41. What is the recommended treatment for the patient in Question VI-40?

A. Azathioprine 125 mg daily plus prednisone 60 mg daily
B. Cyclophosphamide 100 mg daily
C. Nintedanib 150 mg twice a day
D. Prednisone 60 mg daily
E. No therapy is effective for treatment of idiopathic pulmonary fibrosis.

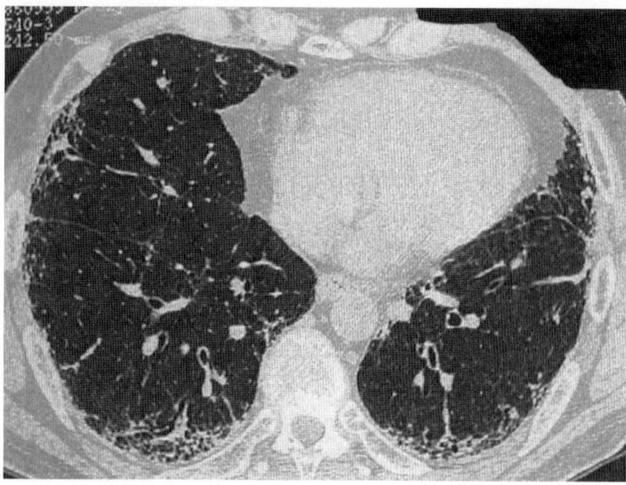

FIGURE VI-40

VI-42. What would be the expected finding on bronchoalveolar lavage in a patient with diffuse alveolar hemorrhage?

A. Atypical hyperplastic type II pneumocytes
B. Ferruginous bodies
C. Hemosiderin-laden macrophages
D. Lymphocytosis with an elevated CD4:CD8 ratio
E. Milky appearance with foamy macrophages

VI-43. A 42-year-old man presents with progressive dyspnea on exertion, low-grade fevers, and weight loss over 6 months. He also complains of a primarily dry cough, although occasionally he coughs up a thick mucoid sputum. There is no past medical history. He does not smoke cigarettes. On physical examination, the patient appears dyspneic with minimal exertion. The patient's temperature is 37.9°C (100.3°F). Oxygen saturation is 91% on room air at rest. Faint basilar crackles are heard. On laboratory studies, the patient has polyclonal hypergammaglobulinemia and a hematocrit of 52%. A CT scan reveals bilateral alveolar infiltrates that are primarily perihilar in nature with a mosaic pattern. The patient undergoes bronchoscopy with bronchoalveolar lavage. The effluent appears milky. The cytopathology shows amorphous debris with periodic acid-Schiff (PAS)–positive macrophages. What is the diagnosis?

A. Bronchiolitis obliterans organizing pneumonia
B. Desquamative interstitial pneumonitis
C. Nocardiosis
D. *Pneumocystis carinii* pneumonia
E. Pulmonary alveolar proteinosis

VI-44. For the patient in Question VI-43, what treatment is most appropriate at this time?

A. Doxycycline
B. Prednisone
C. Prednisone and cyclophosphamide
D. Trimethoprim-sulfamethoxazole
E. Whole-lung lavage

VI-45. A 56-year-old woman presents for evaluation of dyspnea and cough for 2 months. During this time, she has also had intermittent fevers, malaise, and a 5.5-kg (12-lb) weight loss. She denies having any ill contacts and has not recently traveled. She works as a nurse, and a yearly purified protein derivative test performed 3 months ago was negative. She denies any exposure to organic dusts and does not have any birds as pets. She has no other exposures and no autoimmune symptoms. She takes no medications regularly. On physical examination, diffuse inspiratory crackles and squeaks are heard. A CT scan of the chest reveals patchy alveolar infiltrates and bronchial wall thickening. Pulmonary function testing reveals mild restriction. She undergoes a surgical lung biopsy. The pathology shows granulation tissue filling the small airways, alveolar ducts, and alveoli. The alveolar interstitium has chronic inflammation and organizing pneumonia. What is the most appropriate therapy for this patient?

A. Azathioprine 100 mg daily
B. Nintedanib 150 mg twice daily
C. Pirfenidone 2403 mg daily
D. Prednisone 1 mg/kg daily
E. Referral for lung transplantation

VI-46. A 53-year-old man is admitted with fevers and right pleuritic chest pain for 5 days. He has a history of alcohol dependence. On presentation, his temperature is 39.2°C, heart rate is 112 bpm, blood pressure is 102/62 mmHg, respiratory rate is 24 breaths/min, and SaO_2 is 92% on room air. He has absent breath sounds in the right lower chest with dullness to percussion and decreased tactile fremitus. Chest radiograph confirms a right lower lobe consolidation with associated effusion. The effusion is not free flowing. Initial thoracentesis demonstrates gross pus in the pleural space, and the Gram stain is positive for gram-positive cocci in pairs and chains. A large-bore chest tube is placed. Which of the following treatments should also be recommended in this patient to improved resolution of the empyema in this individual?

A. Immediate referral for decortication
B. Intrapleural instillation of alteplase 10 mg twice daily for 3 days
C. Intrapleural instillation of alteplase 10 mg plus deoxyribonuclease 5 mg twice daily for 3 days
D. Intrapleural instillation of deoxyribonuclease 5 mg twice daily for 3 days
E. Intrapleural instillation of streptokinase 250,000 IU

VI-47. A 44-year-old woman with acquired immunodeficiency syndrome (AIDS) has acute hypoxemic respiratory failure due to *Pneumocystis jiroveci*. She is intubated and mechanically ventilated with the following settings: assist-control, tidal volume 350 mL (6 mL/kg ideal body weight), FiO_2 1.0, respiratory rate 28 breaths/min, and PEEP 12 cmH_2O. Her arterial blood gas values on these settings are as follows: pH 7.28, PaO_2 68 mmHg, and $PaCO_2$ 64 mmHg. Her inspiratory plateau pressure is 26 cmH_2O. You are called acutely to the bedside when her blood pressure abruptly drops to 70/40 mmHg. At the same time, the high-pressure alarms on the ventilator begin to alarm with peak airway pressures now registering at 55 cmH_2O. Breath sounds are inaudible on the right side and are clear on the left. What is the best course of action at this time?

A. Administer a fluid bolus to improve venous return.
B. Disconnect the patient from the ventilator to allow a full exhalation.
C. Place a large-bore needle into the right second anterior intercostal space to alleviate a tension pneumothorax.
D. Sedate the patient to achieve ventilator synchrony.
E. Suction the patient to remove obstructing mucus plugs.

VI-48. A 62-year-old woman is admitted to the hospital with a community-acquired pneumonia with a 4-day history of fever, cough, and right-sided pleuritic chest pain. The admission chest x-ray identifies a right lower and middle lobe infiltrate with an associated effusion. All of the following characteristics of the pleural effusion indicate a complicated effusion that may require tube thoracostomy EXCEPT:

A. Loculated fluid
B. Pleural fluid pH <7.20
C. Pleural fluid glucose <60 mg/dL
D. Positive Gram stain or culture of the pleural fluid
E. Recurrence of fluid following the initial thoracentesis

VI-49. A 58-year-old man is evaluated for dyspnea and found to have a moderate right-sided pleural effusion. He undergoes thoracentesis with the following characteristics.

Appearance	Serosanguineous
pH	7.48
Protein	5.8 g/dL (serum protein 7.2 g/dL)
LDH	285 IU/L (serum LDH 320 IU/L)
Glucose	66 mg/dL
WBC	3800/μL
RBC	24,000/μL
PMNs	10%
Lymphocytes	80%
Mesothelial cells	10%
Cytology	Lymphocytosis with chronic inflammation and no malignant cells or organisms identified

LDH, lactate dehydrogenase; PMNs, polymorphonuclear cells; RBC, red blood cell; WBC, white blood cell.

Which of the following is NOT likely to be a cause of the pleural effusion in this patient?

A. Cirrhosis
B. Lung cancer
C. Mesothelioma
D. Pulmonary embolism
E. Tuberculosis

VI-50. A 28-year-old man presents to the emergency department with acute-onset shortness of breath and pleuritic chest pain on the right that began 2 hours previously. He is generally healthy and has no medical history. He has smoked one pack of cigarettes daily since the age of 18. On physical examination, he is tall and thin, with a body mass index of 19.2 kg/m^2. He has a respiratory rate of 24 breaths/min with an oxygen saturation of 95% on room air. He has slightly decreased breath sounds at the right lung apex. A chest x-ray demonstrates a 20% pneumothorax on the right. Which of the following statements is true regarding pneumothorax in this patient?

A. A CT scan is likely to show emphysematous changes.
B. If the patient were to develop recurrent pneumothoraces, thoracoscopy with pleural abrasion has a success rate of near 100% for prevention of recurrence.
C. Most patients with this presentation require tube thoracostomy to resolve the pneumothorax.
D. The likelihood of recurrent pneumothorax is about 25%.
E. The primary risk factor for the development of spontaneous pneumothorax is a tall and thin body habitus.

VI-51. A 52-year-old woman from Indiana presents with worsening dyspnea on exertion and cough for a year. She denies dyspnea at rest. The cough is predominantly dry, but occasionally productive of a gritty mucus. Her past medical history is positive for hypertension and hypothyroidism. She takes benazepril and levothyroxine. She has primarily worked as a landscaper throughout her adult life. On physical examination, she appears in no distress. Her oxygen saturation is 95% on room air. Chest is clear to auscultation. Cardiovascular examination is unremarkable. She has no peripheral edema. The chest radiograph shows an old granuloma in the right lung and mediastinal calcifications. A CT scan is performed, which confirms the healed granuloma. Extensive mediastinal calcification is seen. The calcifications encase the superior vena cava and the right mainstem bronchus. An interferon-γ assay is negative. Which of the following statements regarding the patient's conditions is true?

A. A urine *Histoplasma* antigen test will be positive.
B. The most common cause of the condition is histoplasmosis or tuberculosis.
C. The patient should be referred to a surgical center specialized in the treatment of this condition.
D. Treatment with corticosteroids will improve the patient's condition.
E. Treatment with itraconazole or voriconazole will improve the patient's condition.

VI-52. A 52-year-old woman is admitted to the hospital with lethargy and marked symptoms of volume overload. She has a past medical history of morbid obesity with a body mass index of 52 kg/m^2, severe obstructive sleep apnea, hypertension, and type 1 diabetes mellitus. She is in generally poor health and has been noncompliant with her insulin as well as with continuous positive airway pressure (CPAP) as she reports claustrophobia. She cannot recall when she last used CPAP therapy. On physical examination, the patient is somnolent but arousable. Her vital signs are as follows: blood pressure 168/92 mmHg, heart rate 92 bpm, respiratory rate 14 breaths/min, afebrile, and SaO_2 82% on room air. Her SaO_2 increases to 92% on 6 L/min by nasal cannula, but her mental status becomes more lethargic. She has distant heart and lung sounds without crackles. There is 4+ edema bilaterally to the thighs and onto the abdominal wall. Chest x-ray shows low lung volumes. Initial arterial blood gas values on 6 L/min nasal oxygen are pH 7.22, $PaCO_2$ 88 mmHg, and PaO_2 72 mmHg. Which of the following statements is true regarding the patient's condition?

A. Abnormalities of the *PHOX2b* gene are associated with this condition.
B. CPAP therapy alone is adequate for treatment of this patient.
C. Initial treatment of the condition should include intubation and mechanical ventilation given the patient's known intolerance of CPAP therapy.
D. Obstructive sleep apnea coexists with the diagnosis in about 75% of cases.
E. Weight loss will lead to improvements in $PaCO_2$ over time.

VI-53. A patient with mild amyotrophic lateral sclerosis is followed by a pulmonologist for respiratory dysfunction associated with his neuromuscular disease. Which of the following symptoms in addition to $PaCO_2 \geq 45$ mmHg would necessitate therapy with noninvasive positive-pressure ventilation for hypoventilation?

A. Orthopnea
B. Poor quality sleep
C. Impaired cough
D. Dyspnea in activities of daily living
E. All of the above

VI-54. A 52-year-old man is evaluated for loud snoring and daytime fatigue. His wife urged him to come in for evaluation because his snoring has become increasingly disruptive over the past 2 years after he gained about 30 lb. She frequently sleeps in another room and reports that she has seen him stop breathing during sleep. During the day, he struggles to stay awake when he is in meetings or sitting at his computer, particularly after lunch. He has a 40-minute commute and has had to pull off the road due to feelings of sleepiness. He has a medical history of hypertension for the past 5 years and takes losartan 25 mg daily. He does not smoke and drinks one beer or glass of wine daily. His father, who is 75 years old, uses a CPAP machine for obstructive sleep apnea and has also had a myocardial infarction. On physical examination, the patient appears well. He has a body mass index of 37.1 kg/m^2. When the patient opens his mouth, you can see most of his uvula, which appears somewhat edematous. Tonsillar tissue is visible and extends just beyond tonsillar pillars. The neck circumference is 43 cm. What is the next step in the evaluation and treatment of this patient?

A. Attended in-lab polysomnogram
B. Home sleep study
C. Overnight oximetry
D. Referral for tonsillectomy
E. Treatment with autotitrating CPAP

VI-55. A 48-year-old man has recently been diagnosed with obstructive sleep apnea with an apnea-hypopnea index of 21.2/hr. He presents to the clinic for follow-up because he tried CPAP in the sleep laboratory and felt uncomfortable with it. He asks what the potential risks would be to his health if he chose to forego treatment. What advice do you give him?

A. Untreated obstructive sleep apnea has an increased risk of mortality due to cardiovascular events including myocardial infarction and stroke.
B. Untreated obstructive sleep apnea has an increased risk of depression.
C. Untreated obstructive sleep apnea is associated with a sevenfold increased risk of automobile accidents.
D. Untreated obstructive sleep apnea raises nocturnal blood pressure, and treatment with CPAP leads to a 2- to 4-mmHg drop in blood pressure.
E. All of the above is good advice to give to the patient.

VI-56. Which patient below is most likely to have the breathing pattern seen in Figure VI-56 on polysomnography?

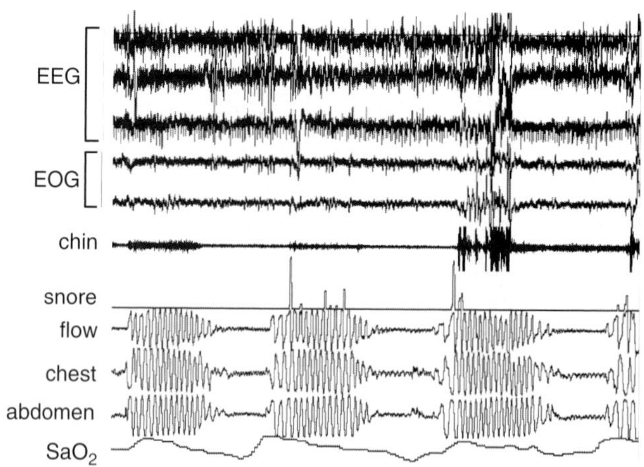

FIGURE VI-56

A. A 6-year-old boy with poor school performance, snoring, and enlarged tonsils and adenoids
B. A 36-year-old woman with a history of heroin addiction who is being treated with methadone maintenance therapy at a dose of 100 mg daily
C. A 48-year-old man evaluated for loud snoring and excessive sleepiness with a body mass index of 36.8 kg/m^2
D. A 52-year-old woman with a body mass index of 22 kg/m^2 complaining of frequent nocturnal awakenings in the setting of menopause; she does not snore
E. A 68-year-old man with atrial fibrillation and ischemic cardiomyopathy with an ejection fraction of 15%; on examination, he has elevation of the jugular venous pressure, hepatojugular reflux, and 3+ peripheral edema

VI-57. A 48-year-old man with a body mass index of 28.9 kg/m^2 is diagnosed with obstructive sleep apnea with an apnea-hypopnea index of 42/hr and a minimum oxygen saturation of 78%. What is the most appropriate initial therapy for this patient?

A. CPAP
B. Oral appliance therapy
C. Oxygen therapy
D. Uvulopalatopharyngoplasty
E. Weight loss

VI-58. A 47-year-old woman with idiopathic pulmonary arterial hypertension has failed medical therapy including IV epoprostenol. She has advanced right heart failure with severe right ventricular dysfunction on echocardiography and a cardiac index of 1.7 L/min/m^2. She is referred for lung transplantation. Which of the following statements is true?

A. She will require heart-lung transplantation for her advanced right heart failure.
B. Idiopathic pulmonary arterial hypertension patients have worse 5-year survival than other transplant recipients.
C. Single-lung transplantation is the preferred surgical procedure for idiopathic pulmonary arterial hypertension.
D. Her own right ventricular function will recover after lung transplantation.
E. She is at risk for recurrent pulmonary arterial hypertension after lung transplantation.

VI-59. A 25-year-old woman with cystic fibrosis is referred for lung transplantation. She is concerned about her long-term outcome. Which of the following is the main impediment to long-term survival after lung transplantation?

A. Bronchiolitis obliterans syndrome
B. Cytomegalovirus infection
C. Chronic kidney disease
D. Primary graft dysfunction
E. Posttransplantation lymphoproliferative disorder

VI-60. A 30-year-old man with end-stage cystic fibrosis undergoes lung transplantation. Three years later, he has a 6-month progressive decline in his renal function. Which of the following medications is the most likely etiology of this?

A. Prednisone
B. Tacrolimus
C. Albuterol
D. Mycophenolate mofetil
E. None of the above

VI-61. A 48-year-old woman is admitted to the ICU with acute respiratory distress syndrome and shock due to ascending cholangitis. Her Acute Physiology and Chronic Health Evaluation Score (APACHE II) is 19 at 24 hours. Which statement best describes the performance of severity of illness scoring systems in predicting outcomes for a patient such as the one described?

A. The APACHE II score and other severity of illness tools are useful for informing clinical research in critical illness, especially regarding severity of illness in patients enrolled in clinical trials.
B. The APACHE II score is an important predictor of individual mortality when directly applied to patient care.
C. The APACHE II score should be used to guide therapy in this patient.
D. The Simplified Acute Physiology Score (SAPS II) would perform better at predicting mortality than the APACHE II score.
E. All of the above are true.

VI-62. A 42-year-old man is admitted to the ICU after an automobile accident. He suffered a compound fracture of the femur and also had internal bleeding from a ruptured spleen and liver hematoma. He has undergone splenectomy and fixation of the femur fracture. He is intubated and sedated following surgery. His hemoglobin after surgery is 5.2 g/dL. His oxygen saturation is 92%, and his PaO_2 is 72 mmHg on FiO_2 of 0.6. A pulmonary artery catheter was placed during surgery. His cardiac output is 7.8 L/min. A lactate level is 4.8 mmol/L. Which of the following is the least important factor affecting oxygen delivery in this patient?

A. Cardiac output
B. Hemoglobin concentration
C. PaO_2
D. SaO_2

VI-63. A 67-year-old woman was admitted to the ICU with multilobar pneumonia due to *Streptococcus pneumoniae* and COPD. She requires intubation and mechanical ventilation. All of the following are appropriate interventions to prevent complications in the ICU EXCEPT:

A. Administration of enoxaparin 40 mg daily
B. Administration of omeprazole 20 mg daily
C. Aggressive blood glucose control
D. Early mobilization and physical therapy while mechanically ventilated
E. Use of a standard care bundle for insertion of central lines

VI-64. A 68-year-old man is admitted to the ICU with fevers, hypotension, and hypoxemia. He has felt ill for the past 2 to 3 days with progressive dyspnea at home. He has a history of COPD, coronary artery disease requiring three-vessel coronary artery bypass surgery, and type 2 diabetes mellitus. He continues to smoke a pack of cigarettes daily and also drinks a six-pack of beer daily. On presentation, his room air oxygen saturation is 79%. With a non-rebreather mask, his oxygen saturation remains at 87%. His blood pressure is 74/40 mmHg, and heart rate is 124 bpm. After fluid bolus, his blood pressure remains low at 86/53 mmHg. His chest radiograph is shown in Figure VI-64. Within 12 hours after admission, blood cultures are positive for *S pneumoniae.* He received his first dose of antibiotics in the emergency department and remains on treatment with ceftriaxone and moxifloxacin. He is intubated, sedated, and currently on vasopressor support. His blood gas after intubation is pH 7.28, $PaCO_2$ 52 mmHg, and PaO_2 64 mmHg on FiO_2 0.8. Which of the following best identifies the patient's diagnosis?

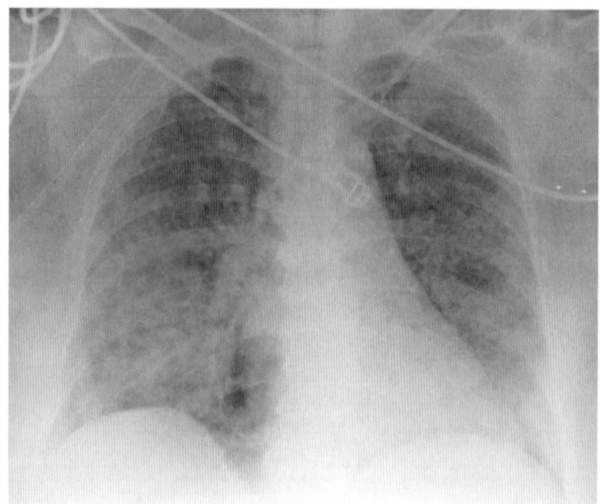

FIGURE VI-64

A. Acute interstitial pneumonia
B. Mild acute respiratory distress syndrome
C. Moderate acute respiratory distress syndrome
D. Multilobar community acquired pneumonia
E. Severe acute respiratory distress syndrome

VI-65. If a lung biopsy were to be taken 4 days after admission in the patient described in Question VI-64, which statement correctly identifies the expected findings?

A. Diffuse alveolar damage with hyaline membranes and protein-rich edema fluid in alveoli
B. Extensive eosinophil-rich infiltrate with protein-rich edema fluid
C. Extensive fibrosis of the alveolar ducts with development of bullae
D. Homogeneous infiltrate of neutrophils and leukocytes affecting all alveolar spaces
E. Proliferation of type II pneumocytes and presence of a lymphocyte-rich pulmonary infiltrate

VI-66. A 48-year-old woman is admitted to the surgical ICU following a motor vehicle accident. She has suffered a concussion, fractures of ribs 4 through 8 on the left with a hemopneumothorax, and a lacerated spleen that required splenectomy. During the surgery to remove her spleen, she required transfusion of 6 units of packed red blood cells, 6 units of platelets, and 4 units of fresh frozen plasma. Upon admission to the ICU after surgery, she remains intubated and sedated. A chest tube is in place on the left. Her chest radiograph shows diffuse bilateral infiltrates. The left lung has dense infiltrates, and there are also extensive infiltrates on the right. She is diagnosed with a left lung contusion and acute respiratory distress syndrome. She weighs 90 kg. She is 66 inches in height. Her ideal body weight is 59 kg. Her oxygen saturation on FiO_2 1.0 is 92% with an arterial blood gas showing pH of 7.28, $PaCO_2$ of 48 mmHg, and PaO_2 of 68 mmHg. What is the best initial tidal volume in this patient?

A. 236 mL
B. 354 mL
C. 472 mL
D. 540 mL
E. 590 mL

VI-67. You are managing a patient admitted to the medical ICU for severe acute respiratory distress syndrome due to necrotizing pancreatitis. The patient has an ideal body weight of 70 kg. The patient's ventilator is set on a volume control with a respiratory rate of 28 bpm, tidal volume of 420 mL, FiO_2 of 0.7, and PEEP of 8 cmH_2O. The patient is hypoxemic with an SaO_2 of 86% on these settings. You review the static pressure-volume curve for the respiratory system. The lower inflection point is at 12 cmH_2O. The upper inflection point is at 30 cmH_2O. Measured pressure with an inspiratory hold is 26 cmH_2O. Which of the following is the best choice to improve oxygenation in this patient?

A. Administer a paralytic agent
B. Decrease tidal volume to 350 mL
C. Increase FiO_2 to 0.8
D. Increase PEEP to 12 cmH_2O
E. Increase tidal volume to 560 mL

VI-68. A 75-year-old man is admitted to the ICU for sepsis in the setting of neutropenia due to chemotherapy for gastric cancer. He has severe acute respiratory distress syndrome and requires intubation. During the first 48 hours of his ICU stay, his volume status is positive 6 L. Which of the following statements regarding fluid management in acute respiratory distress syndrome is true?

A. Aggressive diuresis to maintain a low left atrial filling pressure is associated with increased risk of acute kidney injury requiring hemodialysis.
B. Maintaining a low left atrial filling pressure through diuresis improves lung compliance and improves oxygenation.
C. Maintaining a low left atrial filling pressure through diuresis shortens ICU stay and decreases mortality in the medical intensive care unit, but not the surgical ICU.
D. Placement of a pulmonary arterial catheter for accurate measurement of left atrial filling pressure improves diagnostic accuracy and provides added benefit in determining fluid management strategy.

VI-69. In which of the following situations would noninvasive mechanical ventilation be considered contraindicated?

A. Acute exacerbation of COPD
B. Acute hypoxemic respiratory failure in an individual with acute respiratory distress syndrome
C. Acute myocardial infarction
D. Decompensated systolic heart failure without acute myocardial ischemia
E. After extubation in an individual who had been intubated for COPD

VI-70. to VI-73. Match the mode of ventilation with its description.

VI-70. Assist-control ventilation

VI-71. Intermittent mandatory ventilation

VI-72. Pressure control ventilation

VI-73. Pressure support ventilation

A. This mode of ventilation is time triggered and time cycle and pressure limited. The tidal volume and inspiratory flow rate are dependent upon lung compliance.
B. This mode of ventilation provides a set minute ventilation based on respiratory rate and tidal volume. Spontaneous breaths above the set respiratory rate may be supported in a pressure mode.
C. This mode of ventilation is the most common mode of mechanical ventilation. Each breath, whether triggered by the patient or the ventilator, provides a prespecified tidal volume.
D. This mode of ventilation is patient trigged, flow cycled, and pressure limited. Use of this mode of ventilation requires a patient to be spontaneously breathing.

VI-74. A 62-year-old woman was intubated for community-acquired pneumonia and sepsis. Upon admission to the ICU, she was hypotensive and required vasopressor treatment. She was sedated with propofol to achieve comfort on the ventilator. The ICU has a daily protocol for sedation interruption. She currently has been intubated for 8 days. Which of the following is a contraindication to a spontaneous breathing trial in this patient?

A. Improving infiltrates on chest radiograph
B. FiO_2 of 0.45
C. Ongoing need for vasopressor support
D. Patient is breathing over the set respiratory rate by 8 breaths/min
E. PEEP of 8 cmH_2O

VI-75. All of the following statements regarding the pathophysiology of shock are true EXCEPT:

A. Hypotension inhibits the vasomotor center, resulting in decreased adrenergic output and increased vagal activity.
B. Metabolic changes, including glycolysis and lipolysis, raise extracellular osmolarity, leading to an osmotic gradient that increases interstitial volume at the expense of intracellular fluid volume.
C. Mitochondrial dysfunction and uncoupling of oxidative phosphorylation lead to decreased adenosine triphosphate (ATP) levels and a consequent accumulation of lactate and other reactive oxygen species.
D. Proinflammatory mediators stimulated by the innate immune system contribute significantly to multiple organ dysfunction and failure in shock.
E. Severe stress or pain causes increased release of adrenocorticotropic hormone (ACTH), subsequently increasing cortisol levels to increase gluconeogenesis, decrease peripheral uptake of glucose and amino acids, and enhance lipolysis.

VI-76. A person is admitted to the neurologic ICU with a C2-3 spinal cord transection. The patient is in shock with a blood pressure of 72/40 mmHg. What would the expected findings be on a pulmonary artery catheter?

	Central Venous Pressure and Pulmonary Capillary Wedge Pressure	Cardiac Output	Systemic Vascular Resistance	Venous O_2 Saturation
A.	↓	↓	↑	↓
B.	↑	↓	↑	↓
C.	↓↑	↑	↓	↓
D.	↓	↓↑	↓↑	↓
E.	↓	↓	↓	↓

VI-77. All of the following statements regarding the epidemiology of sepsis and septic shock are true EXCEPT:

A. Gram-positive bacteria are the most commonly isolated causative organisms in sepsis syndromes.
B. In individuals with septic shock, blood cultures are positive in 40%–70% of cases.
C. Most cases of sepsis occur in individuals with significant underlying illness.
D. Respiratory infections are the most common cause of sepsis syndromes.
E. The annual incidence of severe sepsis has increased over the past 30 years with a current incidence of approximately 3 per 1000 population.

VI-78. A 62-year-old woman presents to the emergency department for evaluation of fevers and respiratory symptoms. She began to feel ill about 2 days ago, and her symptoms have been progressively worse since that time. She has a past medical history of rheumatoid arthritis and takes adalimumab 40 mg every other week. On presentation in the emergency department, the patient appears acutely ill and dyspneic. Her oxygen saturation is 84% on room air with a respiratory rate of 25 breaths/min. Initial blood pressure is 82/44 mmHg, heart rate is 132 bpm, and temperature is 101.9°F. She has crackles over the entire lower half of her right lung. Her chest radiograph shows consolidation of the right lower and middle lobes without a pleural effusion. Blood and sputum cultures are drawn. The patient is begun on IV hydration and treatment with ceftriaxone and moxifloxacin. After 2 hours, the patient has received 2 L of normal saline. Her blood pressure is 98/70 mmHg with a heart rate of 125 bpm. She is requiring 50% oxygen by nasal mask to maintain her SaO_2 at 92%–94%. Since presentation to the emergency department, she has produced 100 mL of urine. A blood gas is performed with a pH of 7.46, $PaCO_2$ of 32 mmHg, and PaO_2 of 76 mmHg. How would this patient's presentation be classified?

A. Refractory septic shock
B. Septic shock
C. Sepsis
D. Signs of possibly harmful systemic response
E. Systemic inflammatory response syndrome

VI-79. A 68-year-old man is admitted to the ICU with septic shock. He initially presented with hypotension and fever to 102.5°F. After a 3-L normal saline bolus, he continues to be hypotensive and requires vasopressor support with norepinephrine at 10 μg/min. On presentation, no source of infection is readily apparent. Blood and urine cultures are obtained. The patient is unable to expectorate sputum. The patient's past medical history is significant for COPD, coronary artery disease, and alcohol abuse. He also was in a motor vehicle accident 20 years ago that resulted in splenectomy. He has no medication allergies. The local incidence of cephalosporin-resistant *S pneumoniae* is >1%. Which of the following is the recommended empiric antibiotic regimen for this patient?

A. Cefotaxime
B. Cefotaxime plus vancomycin
C. Levofloxacin
D. Levofloxacin plus vancomycin
E. Vancomycin

VI-80. Despite appropriate antibiotic therapy and supportive care, the mortality related to sepsis remains high with 40%–60% of patients with septic shock dying within 30 days. Multiple therapies have been attempted to improve this mortality, but many of these have been found to be ineffective after initially promising results. Examples of these include all of the following EXCEPT:

A. Activated protein C
B. Erythrocyte transfusions to maintain a hemoglobin level >7 g/dL
C. Insulin therapy to achieve tight glucose control (100–120 mg/dL)
D. Performance of adrenocorticotropin hormone stimulation tests for adrenal insufficiency
E. Tissue factor pathway inhibitor

VI-81. A 62-year-old man is brought to the emergency department for chest pain that developed while he was shoveling snow after a winter storm. The pain started abruptly 30 minutes ago and is associated with shortness of breath and nausea. The pain is rated a 10 out of 10, has an intense pressure-like quality, and is radiating down his left arm. He called for an ambulance within 10 minutes of the onset of pain. He has a history of hypertension, hyperlipidemia, tobacco use, and alcohol abuse. He has been prescribed candesartan 16 mg daily and atorvastatin 10 mg daily. However, he has not seen his doctor in more than a year. He continues to smoke 1.5 packs of tobacco daily and also drinks 6–10 beers daily. On presentation, his blood pressure is 84/50 mmHg, heart rate is 132 bpm, respiratory rate is 28 breaths/min, and SaO_2 is 91% on room air. He appears in severe distress due to pain and dyspnea. He is diaphoretic and pale. His cardiovascular examination shows a regular tachycardia with a soft S_1, and an S_3 gallop is present. There are crackles bilaterally present throughout both lungs. His pulses are thready and weak. Chest radiograph shows pulmonary edema. His ECG is shown in Figure VI-81.

He is having frequent ectopy and short runs of ventricular tachycardia. The patient is given nitroglycerin and aspirin. The cardiac catheterization laboratory is being readied for primary revascularization. However, in the meantime, the patient continues to decline. He is intubated. His blood pressure continues to fall and is most recently 76/52 mmHg with a heart rate of 122 bpm. What is the best option for initial treatment of hypotension in this patient?

A. Dopamine 5 μg/kg/min IV continuous infusion
B. Initiation of venoarterial extracorporeal membrane oxygenation
C. Nitroglycerin 10 μg/min IV continuous infusion
D. Placement of an intra-aortic balloon pump
E. Vasopressin 0.05 U/min IV continuous infusion

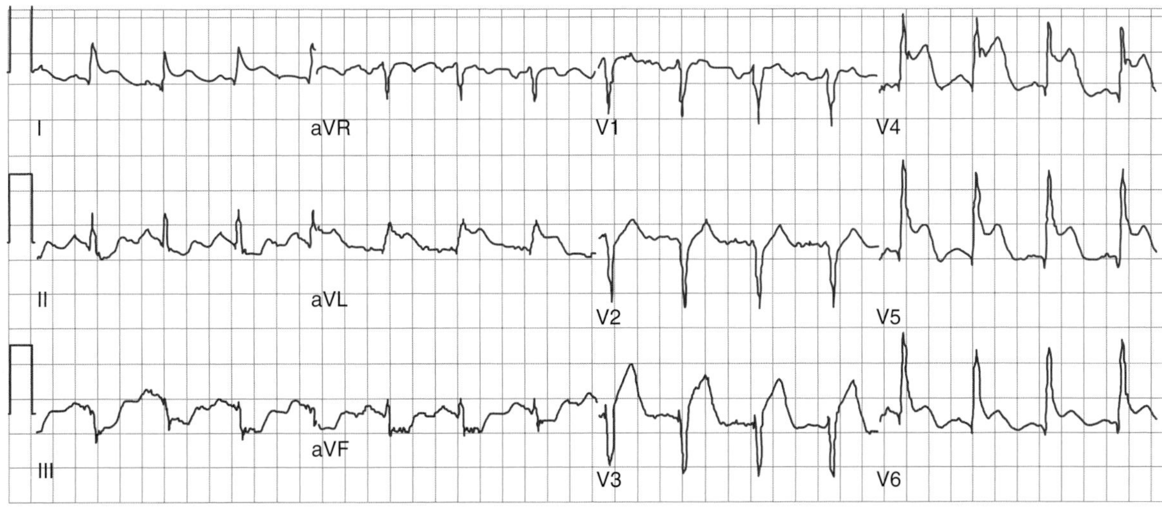

FIGURE VI-81 From Crawford MH: *Current Diagnosis & Treatment: Cardiology*, 4th ed. New York, NY: McGraw-Hill, 2009.

VI-82. A 72-year-old man with known ischemic dilated cardiomyopathy and an ejection fraction of 20% is admitted to the coronary care unit with decompensated heart failure. His blood pressure is 74/56 mmHg, and heart rate is 108 bpm. His oxygen saturation is 85% on a nonrebreather mask. His chest radiograph shows diffuse pulmonary edema and bilateral effusions. There is 4+ pitting edema bilaterally throughout both legs and in the sacrum. He has evidence of ascites. His extremities are cool to touch and cyanotic. His mental status is poor. He is lethargic and does not respond to his name. All of the following would be indicated in the initial treatment of this patient EXCEPT:

A. Dobutamine 5 μg/kg/min IV
B. Furosemide 60 mg IV
C. Initiation of mechanical ventilation
D. Morphine 2 mg IV
E. Norepinephrine 5 μg/min IV

VI-83. A 52-year-old woman is in the coronary care unit after an acute myocardial infarction in the anterior distribution. She was revascularized with a primary percutaneous angioplasty of the proximal left anterior descending artery. Twelve hours after the procedures, you are called to the bedside for an acute decline in blood pressure and dyspnea. Two hours previously, her blood pressure was 115/72 mmHg. Her current blood pressure is 90/78 mmHg. Her heart rate has increased from 88 to 120 bpm. Her oxygen saturation has declined to 86% on room air. She is diaphoretic and pale. She appears in marked distress. There is development of a new cardiac holosystolic murmur heard at the apex and radiating across the precordium into the left axilla. You suspect acute mitral regurgitation. Which of the following would be the expected findings if a pulmonary artery catheter was in place?

VI-84. All of the following statements regarding sudden cardiac death are true EXCEPT:

A. An individual can be classified as having sudden cardiac death following a resuscitated cardiac arrest if death occurs during the subsequent hospitalization or within the next 30 days.
B. Approximately 66% of individuals who experience sudden cardiac death have had prior cardiac events.
C. Asystole is the most commonly encountered rhythm in an individual with sudden cardiac death.
D. Parental history of sudden cardiac death as a first cardiac event increases the probability of a sudden cardiac event in offspring.
E. The incidence of sudden cardiac death is higher in the African American population compared to the white population.

	Right Atrial Pressure (mmHg)	**Right Ventricular Pressure (mmHg)**	**Pulmonary Artery Pressure (mmHg)**	**Pulmonary Capillary Wedge Pressure (mmHg)**	**Cardiac Index (L/min/m^2)**
A.	3	20/8	15/6	6	6.2
B.	5	20/8	22/10	11	2.8
C.	9	30/15	35/18	20 with prominent v wave	2.5
D.	14	22/15	22/10	12	2.1
E.	15	32/15	33/15	15	1.8

VI-85. Which of the following states correctly identifies a patient in a coma?

A. Akinetic mutism
B. Catatonia
C. Locked-in state
D. Metabolic encephalopathy
E. Persistent vegetative state

VI-86. A 74-year-old woman was admitted to the neurologic ICU with decreased alertness that progressed to coma following a fall on an icy sidewalk. On physical examination, the patient is minimally responsive to painful stimuli. The left pupil is enlarged. Right Babinski is upgoing, and there is apparent weakness of the right side. A magnetic resonance imaging (MRI) scan is performed (Figure VI-86). What is the etiology of the coma in this patient?

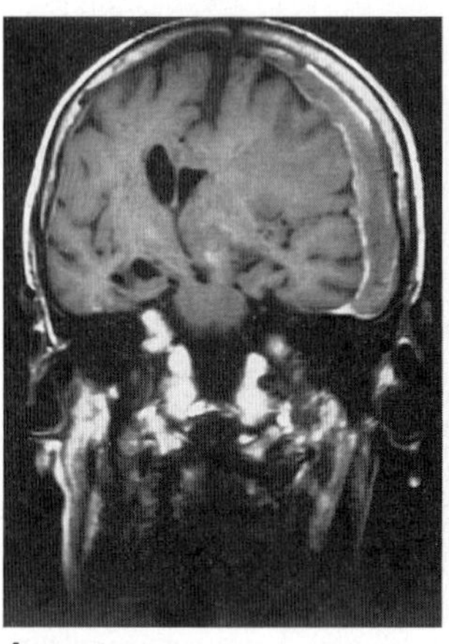

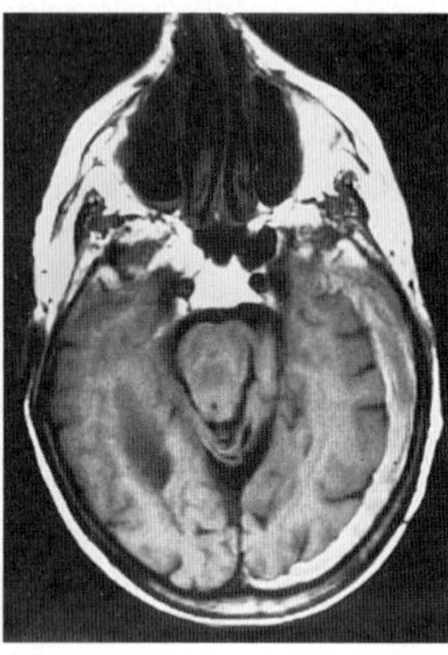

FIGURE VI-86

A. Compression of the anterior and posterior cerebral arteries
B. Compression of the midbrain against the opposite tentorial edge
C. Compression of the opposite cerebral peduncle against the tentorial edge
D. Displacement of the cerebellar tonsils into the foramen magnum
E. Entrapment of the ventricular system causing hydrocephalus

VI-87. A 44-year-old woman is admitted to the intensive care unit with decreased alertness. She was brought to the hospital after she was found unresponsive at home when she failed to show up for lunch with her mother. She has been feeling depressed after losing her job 2 months ago. She lives alone after a divorce 10 years ago. She has no pertinent past medical history, but her mother is uncertain whether the patient takes any medications. Her blood pressure on admission is 92/54 mmHg, heart rate is 112 bpm, respiratory rate is 24 breaths/min, and SaO_2 is 99% on room air. Temperature is 38.2°C. She appears flushed and has deep rapid breathing. She is unresponsive to voice, but withdraws to painful stimuli. She has intermittent muscular spasms diffusely. Her pupils are 5 mm and reactive. What is the most likely etiology of the patient's coma?

A. Concussion
B. Cortical vein thrombosis
C. Drug intoxication
D. Systemic infection
E. Meningeal infection

VI-88. A 48-year-old man was admitted to the ICU with a large intracranial bleed following a motorcycle accident. On initial CT scan, there was midline shift and evidence of uncal herniation. At the scene of the accident, the patient was initially minimally response but has been totally unresponsive to all stimuli since admission. The patient was intubated by emergency medical services en route to the hospital. He has now been admitted for 24 hours. You believe the patient is brain dead. Which of the following contributes to the diagnosis of brain death?

A. Absence of pupillary light reflex
B. Apnea
C. Loss of oculovestibular reflexes
D. Unresponsiveness to all forms of stimulation
E. All of the above are criteria for assessment of brain death.

VI-89. Intraparenchymal intracranial pressure monitoring is preferred over ventriculostomy in which of the following patients?

A. A 24-year-old man admitted with traumatic brain injury following a motor vehicle accident and a Glasgow Coma Scale score of 6
B. A 35-year-old woman with autoimmune hepatitis admitted with fulminant hepatic failure and an international normalized ratio of 3.5
C. A 48-year-old man admitted to the ICU with subarachnoid hemorrhage following a rupture of an anterior cerebral artery aneurysm
D. A 68-year-old woman admitted with a hemorrhagic stroke in the right temporal region with associated midline shift visualized on CT scan
E. All of the above are appropriate candidates for ventriculostomy.

VI-90. A 55-year-old woman is admitted to the ICU following a subarachnoid hemorrhage caused by a rupture of the posterior communicating artery. The patient is treated with intravascular placement of a coil in the aneurysm, and a ventriculostomy is placed for intracranial pressure (ICP) monitoring. Upon arrival to the ICU after surgery, she is intubated and minimally responsive to painful stimuli. She does not respond to voice. The initial ICP is 45 mmHg, and the initial blood pressure is 138/85 mmHg (mean arterial pressure, 103 mmHg) with the head of the bed elevated at 30 degrees. The ICP remains at 45 mmHg over the next 5 minutes. What would you recommend next in the management of this patient?

A. Administer 30 mL of 23.4% hypertonic saline
B. Administer dexamethasone 4 mg every 6 hours
C. Do nothing as patient has an adequate cerebral perfusion pressure
D. Drain ventriculostomy to attain an ICP <20–25 mmHg
E. Increase respiratory rate on the ventilator to decrease the $PaCO_2$ to 30 mmHg

VI-91. A 56-year-old man is admitted to the hospital following a witnessed cardiac arrest. Upon arrival of emergency medical personnel, the rhythm is ventricular fibrillation. The patient is cardioverted into sinus rhythm with return of spontaneous circulation. His estimated duration without circulation is 10 minutes. ECG demonstrated evidence of acute myocardial infarction in an anterior distribution. The patient is treated with primary angioplasty of a 100% occlusion of the proximal left anterior descending artery. He is brought to the ICU intubated and requires use of norepinephrine to maintain his mean arterial pressure greater than 60 mmHg. Initial neurologic examination shows absence of corneal and gag reflexes. When you move the head side to side, the eyes move in concert with the head movement and do not stay fixed. Intermittent myoclonus is present. You are considering use of hypothermia. Which of the following statements correctly characterizes the use of hypothermia in this patient?

A. A head CT should be performed to determine the extent of cerebral edema before deciding upon whether to employ therapeutic hypothermia.
B. Temperature management should be directed at prevention of fevers only with a target temperature of 36°C.
C. Therapeutic hypothermia is recommended to target a temperature of 32–34°C for 24 hours.
D. There is no role for therapeutic hypothermia because the patient's prognosis is very poor.
E. There is no role for therapeutic hypothermia because it does not change patient outcomes.

VI-92. A 67-year-old man has been in the ICU for 3 weeks after admission for sepsis due to pneumococcal pneumonia. He is currently on minimal ventilatory support with inspiratory pressure support of 15 cmH_2O and expiratory pressure of 5 cmH_2O. The FiO_2 is 0.4. Spontaneous tidal volumes on these settings average 450 mL. He is no longer sedated, appears alert, and is following commands. He appears weak and debilitated. He is not able to lift his arms or legs off the bed. His chest radiograph shows marked improvement in the bilateral infiltrates. For the past week, he has failed spontaneous breathing trials. When the inspiratory pressure support is dropped to less than 10 cmH_2O, the patient begins to breathe rapidly at 28 breaths/min, and the tidal volume drops to 220 mL. What is the most likely cause of the patient's inability to be liberated from the ventilator?

A. Critical illness myopathy
B. Critical illness polyneuropathy
C. Fibroproliferative progression of acute respiratory distress syndrome
D. Guillain-Barré syndrome
E. ICU-associated delirium

VI-93. A 56-year-old woman is admitted to the ICU with a thunderclap headache and a rupture of an aneurysm of the anterior cerebral artery. She is treated with endovascular coiling. On admission to the ICU, she was originally intubated and sedated. Over the course of 4 days, she is extubated but continues to demonstrate right hemiparesis and aphasia. Seven days after her presentation, she abruptly declines with alert mental status and marked worsening of her hemiparesis. A head CT is performed urgently and does not show any progression of bleeding or widening of the ventricles. She has been on nimodipine 60 mg every 4 hours since presentation. What is the most likely diagnosis for her worsened condition?

A. Cerebral edema
B. Hydrocephalus
C. Hyponatremia
D. Rerupture of the coiled aneurysm
E. Vasospasm

VI-94. What treatment would you recommend for the patient in Question VI-93 at this time?

A. Consult neurosurgery for clipping of the aneurysm
B. Free water restriction
C. Placement of a ventriculostomy
D. Intubation with hyperventilation and treatment with mannitol
E. Intravenous norepinephrine and consultation for percutaneous transluminal angioplasty

VI-95. A 64-year-old man presents to the emergency department complaining of shortness of breath and facial swelling. He smokes one pack of cigarettes daily and has done so since the age of 16. On physical examination, he appears dyspneic at an angle of 45 degrees or less. His vital signs are as follows: heart rate 124 bpm, blood pressure 164/98 mmHg, respiratory rate 28 breaths/min, temperature 37.6°C (99.6°F), and oxygen saturation 89% on room air. Pulsus paradoxus is not present. His neck veins are dilated and do not collapse with inspiration. Collateral venous dilation is noted on the upper chest wall. There is facial edema and 1+ edema of the upper extremities bilaterally. Cyanosis is present. There is dullness to percussion and decreased breath sounds over the lower half of the right lung field. Given this clinical scenario, what would be the most likely finding on CT examination of the chest?

A. A central mass lesion obstructing the right mainstem bronchus
B. A large apical mass invading the chest wall and brachial plexus
C. A large pericardial effusion
D. A massive pleural effusion leading to opacification of the right hemithorax
E. Enlarged mediastinal lymph nodes causing obstruction of the superior vena cava

VI-96. In the scenario described in Question VI-95, the initial therapy of this patient includes all of the following EXCEPT:

A. Administration of furosemide as needed to achieve diuresis
B. Elevation of the head of the bed to 45 degrees
C. Emergent radiation
D. Low-sodium diet
E. Oxygen

VI-97. A 58-year-old woman with known stage IV breast cancer presents to the emergency department with inability to move her legs. She has had lower back pain for the past 4 days and has found it difficult to lie down. There is no radiating pain. Earlier today, the patient lost the ability to move either of her legs. In addition, she has been incontinent of urine recently. She was diagnosed previously with metastatic disease to the lung and pleura from her breast cancer but was not known to have spinal or brain metastases. Her physical examination confirms absence of movement in the bilateral lower extremities associated with decreased to absent sensation below the umbilicus. There is increased tone and 3+ deep tendon reflexes in the lower extremities with crossed adduction. Anal sphincter tone is decreased, and the anal wink reflex is absent. What is the most important first step to take in the management of this patient?

A. Administration of dexamethasone 10 mg IV
B. Consult neurosurgery for emergent spinal decompression
C. Consult radiation oncology for emergent spinal radiation
D. Perform MRI of the brain
E. Perform MRI of the entire spinal cord

VI-98. A 21-year-old man is treated with induction chemotherapy for acute lymphoblastic leukemia. His initial white blood cell count prior to treatment was 156,000/μL. All of the following are expected complications during his treatment EXCEPT:

A. Acute kidney injury
B. Hypercalcemia
C. Hyperkalemia
D. Hyperphosphatemia
E. Hyperuricemia

VI-99. All of the following would be important for prevention of the complications described in Question VI-98 EXCEPT:

A. Administration of allopurinol 300 mg/m^2 daily
B. Administration of IV fluids at a minimum of 3000 mL/m^2 daily
C. Alkalinization of the urine to a pH of greater than 7.0 by administration of sodium bicarbonate
D. Frequent monitoring of serum chemistries every 4 hours
E. Prophylactic hemodialysis prior to initiating chemotherapy

ANSWERS

VI-1. The answer is A. *(Chap. 305)* The obstructive lung diseases are characterized by a reduction in the forced expiratory volume in 1 second (FEV_1)/forced vital capacity (FVC) ratio, typically below 0.70. The typical lung diseases that manifest with airways obstruction include chronic obstructive lung disease (which includes emphysema and chronic bronchitis), asthma, bronchiectasis, and bronchiolitis. Asbestosis (Chap. 311) is a lung disease caused by the inhalation of asbestos fibers. It is a fibrotic lung disease and typically manifests with a restrictive ventilator defect and gas transfer defect (reduced diffusion capacity for carbon monoxide [DLCO]) on pulmonary function testing.

VI-2. The answer is B. *(Chap. 305)* The alveolar-arterial oxygen (A-a O_2) difference can be helpful in distinguishing hypoventilation (elevated partial pressure of carbon dioxide [PCO_2]) as a cause of hypoxemia. The A-a O_2 difference on room air should be less than 15 mmHg in a young adult and typically increases slightly with age. The A-a O_2 difference cannot easily be interpreted when the fraction of inspired oxygen (FiO_2) is greater than 0.21. The A-a O_2 difference on room air is elevated in situations of hypoxemia due to ventilation-perfusion (V/Q) mismatch, shunt, or diffusion defect. It will be normal when the hypoxemia is solely due to hypoventilation. In this case, the gradient is 7.5 mmHg, consistent with hypoventilation secondary to a presumed narcotic overdose. Asthma and pulmonary embolism typically cause hypoxemia due to V/Q mismatch. Pneumococcal and pneumocystis pneumonias cause hypoxemia for multifactorial reasons, including shunt.

VI-3. **The answer is B.** *(Chap. 306e)* The functional residual capacity of the lung refers to the volume of air that remains in the lung following a normal tidal respiration. This volume of air represents the point at which the outward recoil of the chest wall is in equilibrium with the inward elastic recoil of the lungs. The lungs would remain at this volume if not for the actions of the respiratory muscles. The functional residual capacity is comprised of two lung volumes: the expiratory reserve volume and the residual volume. The expiratory reserve volume represents the additional volume of air that can be exhaled from the lungs when acted upon by the respiratory muscles of exhalation. The residual volume is the volume of air that remains in the lung following a complete exhalation and is determined by the closing pressure of the small airways.

VI-4. **The answer is D.** *(Chap. 306e)* This patient is presenting with subacute dyspnea, stridor, and airflow obstruction, which are consistent with a diagnosis of subglottic stenosis related to his prior prolonged mechanical ventilation. This is confirmed by the finding of fixed airflow obstruction on the flow-volume loop. Flow-volume loops are derived from spirometry. Following a maximum inspiratory effort from residual volume, an individual forces the maximum volume of air from their lungs, and the resultant flows are plotted against the volume. By convention, inspiration is shown on the lower portion of the curve and expiration is on the top. There are characteristic patterns of airflow obstruction that can be evaluated by examining this curve. A fixed central airflow obstruction results in flattening of the flow-volume loop in both inspiration and expiration, yielding the characteristic box-like effect, as shown in Figure VI-4B. Examples of fixed airflow obstruction include tracheal stenosis and an obstructing central airway tumor. Other patterns of large airway obstruction are a variable intrathoracic obstruction and variable extrathoracic obstruction. In these situations, flattening of the flow-volume curve occurs on only one limb of the flow-volume loop, and the pattern of flattening can be explained by the dynamic changes in pressure that affect the trachea. A variable intrathoracic obstruction causes flattening of the flow-volume curve only on expiration. During inspiration, the pleural pressure is more negative than the tracheal pressure, and the trachea remains unimpeded to flow. However, when pleural pressure rises on expiration relative to tracheal pressure, there is collapse of the trachea and flattening of flow-volume curve. An example of a variable intrathoracic obstruction is tracheomalacia. In contrast, the variable extrathoracic defect leads to flattening of the flow-volume loop on inspiration but not expiration. The relevant pressure acting on airflow in the trachea in an extrathoracic obstruction is

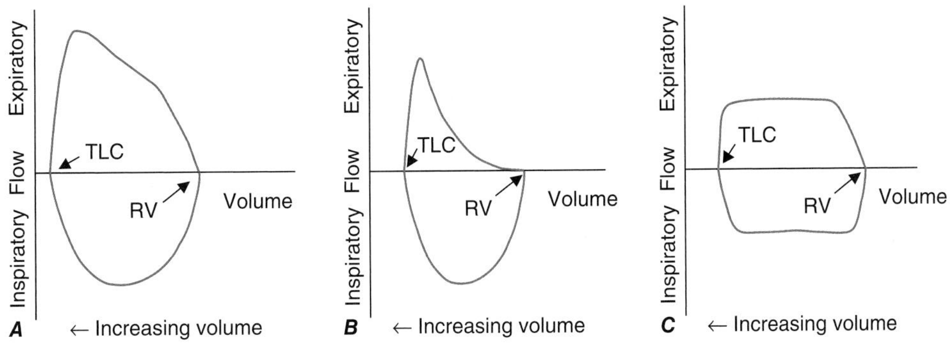

FIGURE VI-4B Flow-volume loops. *A.* Normal. *B.* Airflow obstruction. *C.* Fixed central airway obstruction. RV, residual volume; TLC, total lung capacity.

atmospheric pressure. During inspiration, the tracheal pressure drops below atmospheric pressure, leading to compromised airflow and the characteristic flattening of the flow-volume loop. However, tracheal pressure rises above atmospheric pressure during expiration, leading to a normal expiratory curve.

VI-5. **The answer is B.** *(Chap. 306e)* Pregnancy is a known risk factor for the development of venous thromboembolic disease and should be suspected in any pregnant patient presenting with acute dyspnea. Determining the need for further testing in a pregnant patient should take into account the potential risks of radiation exposure on the fetus. Unfortunately, the signs and symptoms of pulmonary embolism are often nonspecific. Most chest x-rays are normal, and sinus tachycardia may be the only finding on electrocardiogram (ECG). In addition, in the pregnant patient, dyspnea is common due to a variety of factors including the effects of progesterone as a central respiratory stimulant and increased size of the uterus later in pregnancy. The normal arterial blood gas in pregnancy shows a chronic respiratory alkalosis with a pH ranging as high as 7.47 and partial pressure of arterial carbon dioxide ($PaCO_2$) between 30 and 32 mmHg. Calculation of the alveolar-arterial gradient (A-a gradient) can be helpful in this situation. It is easy to be fooled by the presence of a normal oxygen saturation and partial pressure of oxygen on arterial blood gas, but the A-a gradient may still be elevated in the presence of respiratory alkalosis. In this case, the A-a gradient is elevated at 32 mmHg (should be <15 in a young adult in second trimester of pregnancy) and should prompt the physician to perform further workup for pulmonary embolism. The choice of test for diagnosis pulmonary embolism in pregnant patients is most commonly computed tomography (CT) pulmonary angiography, although ventilation-perfusion scanning may also be used.

VI-6. VI-7, VI-8, and VI-9. **The answers are C, B, D, and A, respectively.** *(Chap. 306e)* Ventilatory function can be easily measured with lung volume measurement and the FEV1/FVC ratio. A decreased FEV1/FVC ratio is characteristic of obstructive lung diseases. Alternatively, low lung volumes, specifically decreased total lung capacity (TLC), and occasionally decreased residual volume (RV) are characteristic of restrictive lung diseases. With extensive air trapping in obstructive lung disease, TLC is often increased, and RV may also be increased. Vital capacity (VC) is proportionally decreased. Maximal inspiratory pressure (MIP) measures respiratory muscle strength and is decreased in patients with neuromuscular disease. Thus, myasthenia gravis will produce low lung volumes and decreased MIP, whereas patients with idiopathic pulmonary fibrosis will have normal muscle strength and subsequently a normal MIP but decreased TLC and RV. In some cases of pulmonary parenchymal restrictive lung disease, the increase in elastic recoil results in an increased FEV1/FVC ratio. The hallmark of obstructive lung disease, such as chronic obstructive pulmonary disease (COPD), is a decreased FEV1/FVC ratio.

VI-10. **The answer is C.** *(Chap. 306e)* In this patient presenting with multilobar pneumonia, hypoxemia is present that does not correct with increasing the concentration of inspired oxygen. The inability to overcome hypoxemia or the lack of a notable increase in partial pressure of arterial oxygen (PaO_2) or oxygen saturation (SaO_2) with increasing fraction of inspired oxygen physiologically defines a shunt. A shunt occurs when deoxygenated blood is transported to the left heart and systemic circulation without having the capability of becoming oxygenated. Causes of shunt include alveolar collapse (atelectasis), intra-alveolar filling processes, intrapulmonary vascular malformations, or structural cardiac disease leading to right-to-left shunt. In this case, the patient has multilobar pneumonia leading to alveoli that are being perfused but unable to participate in gas exchange because they are filled with pus and inflammatory exudates. Acute respiratory distress syndrome is another common cause of shunt physiology. V/Q mismatch is the most common cause of hypoxemia and results when there are some alveolar units with low ratios (low ventilation to perfusion) that fail to fully oxygenate perfused blood. When blood is returned to the left heart, the poorly oxygenated blood admixes with blood from normal alveolar units. The resultant hypoxemia is less severe than with shunt and can be corrected with increasing the inspired oxygen concentration. Hypoventilation with or without other causes of hypoxemia is not present in this case, as the PCO_2 <40 mmHg indicates hyperventilation.

The acidosis present in this case is of a metabolic rather than a pulmonary source. Because the patient is paralyzed, she is unable to increase her respiratory rate above the set rate to compensate for the metabolic acidosis.

VI-11. The answer is A. *(Chap. 307)* This patient is at risk of infection and malignancy. The findings on positron emission tomography (PET)/CT are consistent with either diagnosis. Her risk of infection, particularly aspiration pneumonia, is related to her scleroderma-induced esophageal dysfunction, history of low-grade fever, and location. Most aspiration pneumonias involve the right lower lobe, particularly the superior segment. They may appear as consolidation or nodular infiltrates. Given her history of smoking, she is also at risk of primary lung malignancies. Fluorodeoxyglucose (FDG)-PET can often differentiate benign from malignant lesions as small as 1 cm. However, false-positive results are seen in inflammatory conditions, such as pneumonia or granulomatous diseases. False-negative findings can occur in lesions with low metabolic activity such as carcinoid tumors and bronchioloalveolar cell carcinomas.

VI-12. The answer is D. *(Chap. 307)* This patient presents with a slowly progressive illness manifested by dyspnea on exertion, dry cough, clubbing, and the presence of crackles on examination. In addition, the pulmonary function tests demonstrate restrictive lung disease. This scenario is characteristic of an individual with interstitial lung disease, most commonly idiopathic pulmonary fibrosis in individuals at this age. A more thorough history should be obtained to determine if there are any other exposures or symptoms that could identify other causes of interstitial lung disease. The next step in the evaluation of this patient is to perform a high-resolution CT scan (HRCT) of the chest. HRCT employs thinner cross-sectional images at approximately 1–2 mm rather than the usual 7–10 mm. This creates more visible details and is particularly useful for recognizing subtle changes of the interstitium and small airways including interstitial lung disease, bronchiolitis, and bronchiectasis. Bronchoscopy with transbronchial biopsy typically does not provide the detail required to adequately diagnose interstitial lung disease. It may be considered if there are specific features on HRCT that would suggest an alternative diagnosis. However, in most instances, the pathologic diagnosis of interstitial lung disease requires a surgical lung biopsy to provide definitive diagnosis. This patient's symptoms do not suggest coronary artery disease or congestive heart failure. Thus, echocardiography and nuclear stress testing are not indicated. CT scanning has evolved over the years to offer several different techniques that are useful in a variety of circumstances. Standard CT imaging is most useful for the evaluation and staging of lung masses. Helical CT scanning requires only a single breath hold and provides continuous collection of data with improved contrast enhancement and thinner collimation. Once the data are obtained, the images can be reconstructed into other views including sagittal and coronal planes as well as three-dimensional volumetric representations. A recent use of this technology is employed in the setting of virtual bronchoscopy to aid in the planning and performance of bronchoscopy. Multidectector CT scans can obtain multiple slices in a single rotation that are thinner than the usual cuts. Multidetector CT scanners are used in the performance of the CT pulmonary angiogram.

VI-13. The answer is B. *(Chap. 309)* Asthma is a heterogeneous disease with interplay between genetic and environmental factors (Table VI-13). Several risk factors that predispose to asthma have been identified. These should be distinguished from triggers, which are environmental factors that worsen asthma in a patient with established disease. Atopy is the major risk factor for asthma, and nonatopic individuals have a very low risk of developing asthma. Patients with asthma commonly suffer from other atopic diseases, particularly allergic rhinitis, which may be found in over 80% of asthmatic patients, and atopic dermatitis (eczema). The familial association of asthma and a high degree of concordance for asthma in identical twins indicate a genetic predisposition to the disease; however, whether or not the genes predisposing to asthma are similar or in addition to those predisposing to atopy is not yet clear. It now seems likely that different genes may also contribute to asthma specifically, and there is increasing evidence that the severity of asthma is also genetically determined. Although viral infections (especially rhinovirus) are common triggers of asthma exacerbations, it is uncertain whether they play a role in etiology. There is some association between respiratory syncytial virus infection in infancy and the development of asthma, but the specific pathogenesis is difficult to elucidate because this infection is very common in children. The role of dietary factors is controversial. Observational studies have shown that diets low in antioxidants such as vitamin C and vitamin A, magnesium, selenium, and omega-3 polyunsaturated fats (fish oil) or high in sodium and omega-6 polyunsaturated fats are associated with an increased risk of asthma. Vitamin D deficiency may also predispose to the development of asthma. However, interventional studies with supplementary diets have not supported an important role for these dietary factors. Obesity is also an independent risk factor for asthma, particularly in women, but the mechanisms are thus far unknown. Air pollutants, such as sulfur dioxide, ozone, and diesel particulates, may trigger asthma symptoms, but the role of different air pollutants in the etiology of the disease is much less certain. Most evidence argues against an important role for air pollution because asthma is no more prevalent in cities with a high ambient level of traffic pollution than in rural areas with low levels of pollution. There is some evidence that maternal smoking is a risk factor for asthma, but it is difficult to dissociate this association from an increased risk of respiratory infections.

TABLE VI-13 Risk Factors and Triggers Involved in Asthma

Endogenous Factors	Environmental Factors
Genetic predisposition	Indoor allergens
Atopy	Outdoor allergens
Airway hyperresponsiveness	Occupational sensitizers
Gender	Passive smoking
Ethnicity	Respiratory infections
Obesity	Diet
Early viral infections	Acetaminophen (paracetamol)
Triggers	
Allergens	
Upper respiratory tract viral infections	
Exercise and hyperventilation	
Cold air	
Sulfur dioxide and irritant gases	
Drugs (β-blockers, aspirin)	
Stress	
Irritants (household sprays, paint fumes)	

VI-14. The answer is E. *(Chap. 309)* The patient in this clinical scenario presents with symptoms typical of asthma, including shortness of breath and wheezing. She also manifests evidence of atopy, the most common risk factor for developing asthma, with sensitivity to outdoor allergens and cats. In addition, the patient has a history of allergic rhinitis and eczema, both of which are commonly seen in individuals with asthma. Indeed, over 80% of asthma patients have a concomitant diagnosis of allergic rhinitis. Atopy is present in 40%–50% of the population of affluent countries, but only a small proportion of these individuals develop asthma. Many studies have shown a genetic predisposition via family history and recent genome-wide screens, but no single genetic profile has shown high positive predictive value. Overall, the prevalence of asthma in developed countries has increased over the past 30 years, but recently has leveled off, with a prevalence of about 15% in children and 10%–12% in adults. Asthma deaths remain rare and have decreased in recent decades. In the 1960s, asthma deaths did increase with an overuse of short-acting β-agonist medications. However, since the introduction of inhaled corticosteroids as maintenance therapy, deaths have declined. Risk factors for fatal asthma include frequent use of rescue inhalers, lack of therapy with inhaled corticosteroids, and prior hospitalizations for asthma. Interestingly, the overall disease severity does not vary significantly within a given patient over the course of the disease. Individuals who have mild asthma typically continue to have mild asthma, whereas those with severe disease present with severe disease. Diagnosis of asthma can be made by demonstrating airflow obstruction with significant reversibility on bronchodilator administration. In this case, the FEV_1/FVC ratio is decreased to 70%, which is low. In addition, the FEV_1 increases by 12.4% and 230 mL. This meets the criteria for bronchodilator reversibility of increases of at least 200 mL and 12%. Bronchoprovocation testing with methacholine can be considered in individuals who have suspected asthma but have normal pulmonary function tests.

VI-15. **The answer is B.** *(Chap. 309)* The pathology of asthma has largely been determined by examining bronchial biopsies of patients with asthma as well as the lungs of individuals who die from asthma. These pathologic changes are centered around the airways with sparing of the alveolar spaces. The airways are infiltrated by eosinophils, activated T lymphocytes, and activated mucosal mast cells. However, the degree of inflammation does not correlate with the severity of asthma. Another common finding in all asthmatics and individuals with eosinophilic bronchitis is thickening of the basement membrane due to collagen deposition in the subepithelium. The airway smooth muscle is hypertrophied as well. Overall, this leads to thickening of the airway wall, which may also exhibit edematous fluid, particularly in those with fatal asthma. In cases of fatal asthma, it is also common to find multiple airways that are occluded by mucus plugs. However, the disease is limited to the airways, and infiltration of the alveolar spaces by inflammatory cells is not seen.

VI-16. **The answer is C.** *(Chap. 309)* The preferred method for diagnosing asthma is demonstration of airflow obstruction on spirometry that is at least partially reversible. This is demonstrated in option C, with a decreased FEV_1/FVC ratio, decreased FEV_1, and a significant increase in FEV_1 following administration of albuterol. For an individual to be considered responsive to a bronchodilator, the individual should experience an increase in either FEV_1 or FVC of at least 200 mL and 12%. Option A describes someone with postviral cough syndrome, which can persist for several weeks following a viral upper respiratory infection. Option B describes someone with exercise-induced bronchoconstriction (EIB), which, in absence of other symptoms to suggest asthma, should not be diagnosed as asthma. Isolated EIB lacks the characteristic airway inflammation of asthma and does not progress to asthma. Although it is estimated that 80%–90% of individuals with asthma experience EIB, many individuals who have EIB do not also have asthma. EIB is caused by hyperventilation with inhalation of cool dry air that leads to bronchospasm. Option D describes someone with occupational asthma that has occurred after working with animals in the medical laboratory for many years. Symptoms that are characteristic of occupational asthma are symptoms only while at work that improve on the weekends and during holidays. Option D describes someone with COPD. In COPD, 25%–48% of individuals can demonstrate bronchial hyperresponsive in response to methacholine.

VI-17. **The answer is A.** *(Chap. 309)* The main drugs for asthma can be divided into bronchodilators, which give rapid relief of symptoms mainly through relaxation of airway smooth muscle, and controllers, which inhibit the underlying inflammatory process (Figure VI-17). For patients with mild, intermittent asthma, a short-acting β_2-agonist is all that is required. However, use of a reliever medication more than twice a week indicates the need for regular controller therapy. This patient is using her reliever medication frequently; therefore, a controller should be added to her regimen. The treatment of choice for all patients is an inhaled corticosteroid given twice daily. It is usual to start with an intermediate dose (e.g., 200 μg twice a day of beclomethasone dipropionate or equivalent) and to decrease the dose if symptoms are controlled after 3 months. If symptoms are not controlled, a long-acting β-agonist (LABA) should be added, which is most conveniently given by switching to a combination inhaler. The dose of controller should be adjusted accordingly, as judged by the need for a rescue inhaler. Muscarinic receptor antagonists such as ipratropium bromide prevent cholinergic nerve-induced bronchoconstriction and mucus secretion. They are less effective than β_2-agonists in asthma therapy because they inhibit only the cholinergic reflex component of bronchoconstriction, whereas β_2-agonists prevent all bronchoconstrictor mechanisms. Anticholinergics, including tiotropium, may be used as additional bronchodilators in patients with asthma that is not controlled by inhaled corticosteroid and LABA combinations. Low doses of theophylline or an antileukotriene may also be considered as an add-on therapy, but these are less effective than LABA. If asthma is not controlled despite the maximal recommended dose of inhaled therapy, it is important to check compliance and inhaler technique. In these patients, maintenance treatment with an oral corticosteroid may be needed, and the lowest dose that maintains control should be used.

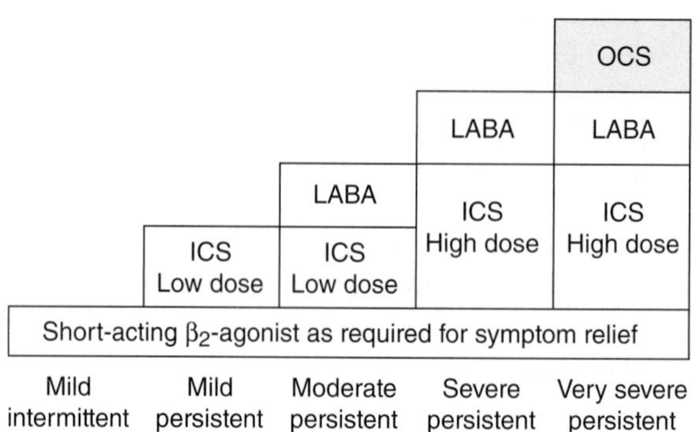

FIGURE VI-17 Stepwise approach to asthma therapy according to the severity of asthma and ability to control symptoms. ICS, inhaled corticosteroids; LABA, long-acting β_2-agonist; OCS, oral corticosteroid.

VI-18. The answer is A. *(Chap. 309)* Approximately one-third of asthmatic patients who are pregnant improve during the course of a pregnancy, one-third deteriorate, and one-third are unchanged. It is important to maintain good control of asthma because poor control may have adverse effects on fetal development. Compliance may be a problem because there is often concern about the effects of antiasthma medications on fetal development. The drugs that have been used for many years in asthma therapy have now been shown to be safe and without teratogenic potential. These drugs include short-acting β-agonists (e.g., albuterol), inhaled corticosteroids (e.g., beclomethasone), and theophylline; there is less safety information about newer classes of drugs such as LABAs (e.g., salmeterol), antileukotrienes, and anti–immunoglobulin (Ig) E. If an oral corticosteroid is needed, it is better to use prednisone rather than prednisolone because it cannot be converted to the active prednisolone by the fetal liver, thus protecting the fetus from systemic effects of the corticosteroid. There is no contraindication to breast-feeding when patients are using these drugs.

VI-19. The answer is C. *(Chap. 310)* Acute eosinophilic pneumonia is an acute respiratory syndrome that often presents with a clinical picture that is difficult to differentiate from acute lung injury or acute respiratory distress syndrome (ARDS). Clinically, patients present with a prodrome of fevers, malaise, myalgias, night sweats, dyspnea, cough, and pleuritic chest pain. Physical examination may demonstrate high fevers, bibasilar rales, and rhonchi. The clinical course is frequently marked by rapid clinical progression to hypoxemic respiratory failure that requires mechanical ventilation. Chest radiography shows bilateral pulmonary infiltrates. This clinical picture clearly overlaps with infectious causes of respiratory failure and ARDS. However, the hallmark of acute eosinophilic pneumonia is the finding of >25% eosinophils in the bronchoalveolar lavage fluid. Acute eosinophilic pneumonia most frequently presents in individuals between the ages of 20 and 40 years and is more common in men. There is no epidemiologic link between the diagnosis and a prior history of asthma. However, several case reports have linked development of acute eosinophilic pneumonia to recent initiation of cigarette smoking or exposure to other environmental stimuli including dust. A bronchoalveolar lavage showing eosinophilia >25% is sufficient to establish the diagnosis of acute eosinophilic pneumonia. A surgical lung biopsy is not necessary. If performed, it would demonstrate eosinophilic infiltration with acute and organizing diffuse alveolar damage. Peripheral eosinophilia is not present acutely at disease onset, but often becomes present between day 7 and day 30. Other organ failure is not present. The disease has a high degree of corticosteroid responsiveness and a good prognosis. Initiation of therapy with corticosteroids should not be delayed. Although there is no recommended dose of steroids for therapy, patients are often initiated on therapy with intravenous glucocorticoids with rapid improvement in the hypoxemic respiratory failure. The expected clinical course is complete resolution of clinical and radiographic features of the disease over several weeks without relapse upon tapering of steroids.

VI-20. The answer is D. *(Chap. 310)* Allergic bronchopulmonary aspergillosis (ABPA) is an eosinophilic pulmonary disorder that occurs in response to allergic sensitization to antigens from *Aspergillus* fungi. The classic presentation of an individual with ABPA is someone with an asthmatic phenotype that becomes increasingly difficult to control and may be steroid dependent. These individuals often complain of chronic cough with expectoration of thick brown mucus plugs. In addition, individuals with cystic fibrosis have an increased incidence of ABPA. ABPA can be difficult to diagnose, and many individuals have had prolonged symptoms prior to diagnosis. Initial diagnostic testing should include demonstration of elevated circulating IgE level (option D), typically >1000 IU/mL. Peripheral eosinophilia is also commonly seen. If the IgE level is elevated and suggestive of IgE, one must demonstrate sensitivity to *Aspergillus* antigens. This can be achieved by skin test reactivity, positive serum precipitins for *Aspergillus*, and/or direct measurement of circulating specific IgG and IgE to *Aspergillus*. Testing for specific IgE in the serum is most frequent accomplished via radioallergosorbent (RAST) testing. Chest CT (option B) may show central bronchiectasis as the classic manifestation of ABPA but is present in only about 30% of individuals. Other findings in ABPA including patchy infiltrates and mucus impaction. Aspirin desensitization (option A) therapy is a treatment for aspirin-sensitive asthma that characteristically presents with the Samter triad of asthma, nasal polyposis, and aspirin and/or nonsteroidal anti-inflammatory drug sensitivity. Nasal nitric oxide testing (option C) is a diagnostic test used for identification of primary ciliary dyskinesia. Sweat chloride testing (option E) is used for diagnosis of cystic fibrosis.

VI-21. and VI-22. The answers are B and E, respectively. *(Chap. 310)* The patient has a subacute presentation of hypersensitivity pneumonitis related to exposure to bird droppings and feathers at work. Hypersensitivity pneumonitis is a delayed-type hypersensitivity reaction that has a variety of presentations. Some people develop acute onset of shortness of breath, fevers, chills, and dyspnea within 6–8 hours of antigen exposure. Others may present subacutely with worsening dyspnea on exertion and dry cough over weeks to months. Chronic hypersensitivity pneumonitis presents with more severe and persistent symptoms with clubbing. Progressive worsening is common with the development of chronic hypoxemia, pulmonary hypertension, interstitial pulmonary fibrosis, and respiratory failure. The diagnosis relies on a variety of tests. Peripheral eosinophilia is not a feature of this disease as the disease is mediated through T-cell inflammation. Other nonspecific markers of inflammation may be elevated, including the erythrocyte sedimentation rate, C-reactive protein, rheumatoid factor, and serum immunoglobulins. Neutrophilia and lymphopenia can be seen. If a specific antigen is suspected, serum precipitins directed toward that antigen may be demonstrated. However, these tests are neither sensitive nor specific for the presence of disease. Chest radiography may be normal or show a diffuse reticulonodular infiltrate. Chest HRCT is the imaging modality of choice and shows ground-glass infiltrates in the lower lobes. Centrilobular infiltrates are often seen as well. In the chronic stages, patchy emphysema is the most common finding. Histopathologically, interstitial alveolar infiltrates predominate, with a variety of lymphocytes, plasma cells, and occasionally eosinophils and neutrophils seen. Loose, noncaseating granulomas are typical. Treatment requires removing the individual from exposure to the antigen. If this is not possible, the patient should wear a mask that prevents small-particle inhalation during exposure. In patients with mild disease, removal from antigen exposure alone may be sufficient to treat the disease. More severe symptoms require therapy with glucocorticoids at an equivalent prednisone dose of 1 mg/kg daily for 7 to 14 days. The steroids are then gradually tapered over 2 to 6 weeks.

VI-23. The answer is C. *(Chap. 311)* Mesothelioma is a rare malignancy of the pleura and peritoneum, with almost all cases associated with asbestos exposure. It is notable that the exposure to asbestos could seem almost minimal but still confer significant risk. Exposures of less than 1–2 years or that have occurred more than 40 years in the past have been demonstrated to confer increased risk of mesothelioma. Although tobacco smoking in association with asbestos exposure increases the risk of lung cancer several-fold, there is no additive or exponential risk of mesothelioma in those who smoke. Mesothelioma most often presents with a persistent unilateral pleural effusion that may mask the underlying pleural tumor. However, the pleura may be diffusely thickened. Typically, large pleural effusions would cause expansion of the hemithorax with mediastinal shift away from the side of the pleural effusion. However, even with large effusions, no mediastinal shift is seen on chest radiograph because the pleural thickening associated with the disease leads to a fixed chest cavity size and thoracic restriction. The most difficult diagnostic dilemma in these patients is to differentiate mesothelioma from metastatic lung carcinoma (usually adenocarcinoma) as many patients are at risk for both tumors, and lung cancer is by far the most common malignancy seen in individuals with asbestos exposure and cigarette smoking. Pleural fluid cytology is not adequate for the diagnosis of most individuals with mesothelioma, with samples being positive for the disease in less than 50% of individuals. Most often, video-assisted thoracoscopy is required to directly visualize the pleural and direct biopsy sampling. Unfortunately, there is no proven effective therapy for mesothelioma, and most patients die from local extension of the disease.

VI-24. The answer is E. *(Chap. 311)* Silicosis results from the inhalation of free silica (or crystalline quartz) and is associated with mining, stonecutting, foundry work, and quarrying. The chronic form of silicosis has been associated with an increased risk of a variety of diseases. Silica is known to be cytotoxic to alveolar macrophages and, thus, places patients at increased risk of pulmonary infections that rely on cellular immunity, including *Mycobacterium tuberculosis*, atypical mycobacteria, and fungus. In addition, silicosis is associated with the development of connective tissue disorders including rheumatoid arthritis with rheumatoid nodules (Caplan syndrome) and scleroderma. Finally, silica is listed as a probable lung carcinogen.

VI-25. The answer is D. *(Chap. 311)* Occupational lung diseases have been associated with a wide variety of organic and inorganic exposures in the workplace and clinically can range from primarily an airway disease to progressive pulmonary fibrosis. When evaluating a patient for a new pulmonary diagnosis, it is important to perform a detailed occupational history to determine if there is a possibility that the patient's profession may be causing or perpetuating the disease process. Specific clinical syndromes are associated with well-defined clinical exposures. The inorganic dusts include asbestos, silica, coal dust, beryllium, and a variety of other metals. Asbestos and silica are among the most common exposures. Asbestos exposure is associated with mining, construction, and ship repair. In areas near where asbestos mining has occurred, the general population also has shown an increased risk of asbestos-related lung disease. Clinically, asbestos exposure is associated with a range of clinical syndromes including asbestosis (interstitial lung disease), benign pleural plaques and pleural effusions, lung cancer, and mesothelioma. Silica exposure is common among miners, stone masons, and individuals involved in sand blasting or quarrying. A variety of clinical syndrome can occur with silica exposure, the most severe being progressive massive fibrosis with mass-like upper lobe consolidating nodules (>1 cm). Coal mining is also associated with a clinical picture similar to silicosis and progressive massive fibrosis. Beryllium is a lightweight metal that is highly conductive and is used in high-tech industries. The classic disease associated with beryllium exposure is a chronic granulomatous disease similar in clinical appearance to sarcoidosis. Other metals can produce any number of clinical syndromes. Welders of galvanized metal who use zinc oxide are susceptible to metal fume fever and present with an acute self-limited influenza-like illness.

Organic dusts that can lead to occupational lung disease include cotton dust, grain dust, toxic chemicals, and other agricultural dusts, among many others. Cotton milling and processing can present with a clinical syndrome known as byssinosis, which has asthma-like features. Many of the organic dust exposures also lead to hypersensitivity pneumonitis. Examples of hypersensitivity pneumonitis syndromes related to occupational exposures include farmer's lung, pigeon breeder's lung, and malt worker's lung. Typically, a specific antigen can be identified as the culprit for the development of hypersensitivity pneumonitis. In farmer's lung, the most common cause is thermophilic *Actinomyces* species found in moldy hay.

VI-26. The answer is D. *(Chap. 311)* The patient presents with acute-onset pulmonary symptoms, including wheezing, with no other medical problems. He is a farmer and was recently handling hay. The clinical presentation and radiogram are consistent with farmer's lung, a hypersensitivity pneumonitis caused by *Actinomyces*. In this disorder, moldy hay with spores of actinomycetes are inhaled and produce a hypersensitivity pneumonitis. The disorder is seen most commonly in rainy periods, when the spores multiply. Patients present generally 4–8 hours after exposure with fever, cough, and shortness of breath without wheezing. Chest radiograms often show patchy bilateral, often upper lobe infiltrates. The exposure history will differentiate this disorder from other types of pneumonia.

VI-27. The answer is D. *(Chap. 311)* Firefighters and fire victims are at risk of smoke inhalation injury, an important cause of acute cardiorespiratory failure. In addition to the risk of carbon monoxide poisoning, these individuals are also at risk from toxic inhalational injury from fumes released from the burning of synthetic materials. This patient has a carbon monoxide level that requires treatment with 100% oxygen but would not be expected to lead to significant cardiorespiratory collapse. Recently, cyanide toxicity has been recognized as a significant cause of morbidity and mortality following industrial and house fires. Cyanide toxicity can present with rapid development of neurologic and cardiorespiratory collapse. The neurologic symptoms can range from mild headache to confusion, generalized seizures, and coma. Hypotension with significant lactic acidosis is prominent. Often an elevated lactate level leads to the suspicion of concomitant cyanide toxicity in an individual with smoke inhalation injury. However to definitely make the diagnosis, one would want to assess the red blood cell cyanide concentration.

VI-28. The answer is D. *(Chap. 312)* Bronchiectasis is a common disorder that refers to an irreversible dilation of the airways that affects the lung in a focal or diffuse pattern. Historically, bronchiectasis has been characterized pathologically as cylindrical, varicose, or cystic in nature. There are numerous causes of bronchiectasis including infectious, inherited, immunologic, and idiopathic causes. The most common cause of bronchiectasis worldwide is postinfectious following tuberculosis infection. However, in developed countries, other causes are more common. The most common cause in developed countries is cystic fibrosis (CF); CF patients develop clinically significant bronchiectasis in late adolescence or early adulthood. Most children with CF are diagnosed currently through newborn screening programs, which were introduced in all states within the past decade. However, adults may continue to present with milder forms of the disease, so clinicians should continue to have a high degree of clinical suspicion for CF when an individual presents with a new diagnosis of bronchiectasis. Epidemiologically, individuals presenting with CF bronchiectasis will typically be younger than individuals with non-CF bronchiectasis. In contrast, non-CF bronchiectasis more commonly affects nonsmoking women older than 50 years. The clinical presentation of bronchiectasis is a daily cough productive of thick tenacious sputum. Physical examination demonstrates both crackles and wheezing on examination. In CF, the disease findings are more predominant in the upper lobes, whereas in certain other causes (chronic aspiration, immunoglobulin deficiency), there is a lower lobe predominance. Clubbing is variably present and generally only seen in more advance disease. The diagnosis of bronchiectasis is determined by the presence of the disease on a chest CT imaging. Chest radiography is not sensitive for the diagnosis of bronchiectasis, particularly early in the disease process. It may show "tram tracks" indicating dilated airway. Chest HRCT is the diagnostic modality of choice for confirming diagnosis. Findings include demonstration of dilated, nontapering airways that may be filled with mucus. In addition, signet-ring signs may also be seen where the airway is greater than 1.5 times the size of the adjacent blood vessel. Other findings include bronchial wall thickening, inspissated secretion with a "tree-in-bud" pattern, and cysts emanating from the bronchial wall. Once bronchiectasis has been confirmed on CT imaging, other tests may be indicated in this patient to determine the etiology of the bronchiectasis. Testing should be guided by the history and physical examination and may include sputum culture for mycobacteria and fungal organisms, immunoglobulin levels, autoimmune panel, sweat chloride testing, nasal nitric oxide testing (for primary ciliary dyskinesia), bronchoscopy, and/or tests of swallow function. Despite thorough evaluation, in as many as 25%–50% of individuals referred for workup of bronchiectasis, no specific cause is ever identified.

VI-29. The answer is C. *(Chap. 312)* Treatment of infectious bronchiectasis relies upon controlling the source of infection and maintaining good bronchial hygiene and airway clearance. The most common nontuberculous mycobacterial organism causing infection in individuals with bronchiectasis is *Mycobacterium avium-intracellculare* (MAI or MAC). The recommended treatment for MAI is a macrolide combined with ethambutol and rifampin. The recommended course of therapy is 12 months after the last positive culture. In certain instances, surgical resection can be considered for focal bronchiectasis if a patient is failing to clear the infection after a prolonged course of antibiotic therapy. However, this patient has had negative cultures for 12 months, demonstrating an appropriate response to antimicrobial therapy. Thus, options A and B are incorrect. However, the patient continues to have daily sputum expectoration related to her underlying bronchiectasis and should be instructed on appropriate bronchial hygiene and airway clearance. A variety of approaches have been used, and no one treatment has been demonstrated to be superior. Chest physiotherapy is often recommended on a daily basis to improve secretion clearance. This can be accomplished through postural drainage often combined with traditional mechanical percussion or the use of devices including high-frequency chest wall oscillation vest or oscillatory positive expiratory pressure flutter valve (option C). Regular exercise may also improve airway clearance. Mucolytic agents such as hypertonic saline are also often used. However, in contrast with CF bronchiectasis, dornase (DNase) (option D) is not used for non-CF bronchiectasis. A randomized, placebo-controlled research trial demonstrated lack of efficacy and potential harm in the non-CF population. Finally, there is no proven role for the use of daily oral corticosteroids (option E) in the absence of a disease known to respond to steroid therapy, such as allergic bronchopulmonary aspergillosis or autoimmune disease such as Sjögren syndrome.

VI-30 and VI-31. The answers are B and B, respectively. *(Chap. 313)* Cystic fibrosis is one of the most common life-shortening autosomal recessive disorders, affecting about 1 in 3300 live births in Caucasians. It is much less common in African Americans (~1 in 15,000) and Asians (~1 in 33,000). The disease is caused by an inherited defect in the cystic fibrosis transmembrane regulator (CFTR) protein, a large ion channel in the cell membrane responsible for chloride ion transport. In the absence of a functional CFTR protein, individuals with CF have a variety of disease manifestations related to impaired exocrine function. The primary disease manifestations are respiratory and pancreatic in nature with chronic sinopulmonary infections, impaired exocrine pancreatic function, and poor nutrition. The gene that encodes CFTR is located on chromosome 7, and more than 2000 mutations have been described. In understanding the genetics, it is best to categorize them according to the effect on CFTR function. Class I mutations (G542X, 621+1G>T) lead to absence of synthesis, most frequently through the presence of an abnormal stop codon. Class II mutations (F508del, the most common mutation) cause defective protein synthesis and premature degradation. Class III mutations (G551D) are gating mutations, in which the CFTR protein is present at the cell membrane but fails to function properly. Type IV mutations (R117H, R117C) are conductance mutations with impaired conductance through the ion channel pore, and Type V mutations are splice mutations that lead to a diminished number of CFTR transcripts being produced due to a promoter or splicing abnormality. One of the most exciting breakthroughs in the treatment of CF has been in the area of CFTR modulations. High-throughput screening identified small-molecule compounds that act as potentiators or correctors of CFTR and improve CFTR function. The first of these compounds to be identified was ivacaftor. This drug works as a potentiator and has been approved for individuals with gating mutations, the most common of which is G551D. Approximately 5% of the CF population has a gating mutation. In clinical trials, individuals with a G551D mutation treated with ivacaftor experienced an absolute improvement in lung function (FEV_1 percent predicted) of 10.6% and a decline in sweat chloride values to normal levels. This was sustained over the 24 weeks of the clinical trial.

Long-term data are now available that demonstrates persistent effects of ivacaftor up to 144 weeks (McKone EF et al: *Lancet Respir Med* 2014;2(11):902–910). Individuals on ivacaftor also experience an improvement in nutritional status and growth in younger individuals as well. Ivacaftor is now being combined with corrector compounds such as lumacaftor to attempt to correct the F508del processing abnormality. The combination of ivacaftor and lumacaftor was approved by the US Food and Drug Administration (FDA) in July 2015 for individuals homozygous for F508del. Other potentiator/corrector combinations are undergoing clinical trials.

VI-32. **The answer is E.** *(Chap. 313 and J Pediatr 2008;153(2):S4–S14)* CF is a common autosomal recessive disorder that affects 1 out of every 3300 live births in the Caucasian population of North America and Europe. There have been more than 2000 mutations identified in the gene for the CFTR protein—the abnormal protein identified in CF. This protein is a large transmembrane protein involved in the transport of chloride and other ions, and abnormalities of the CFTR lead to abnormalities of salt and water transport. The primary clinical manifestations of CF are due to the effects of the mutated CFTR in the lungs, gastrointestinal tract, and pancreas. In the lungs, abnormal CFTR leads to thick, sticky mucus with abnormal mucociliary clearance. A patient will have recurrent respiratory infections with development of cystic bronchiectasis over time. The presenting manifestation in infancy is often meconium ileus and can lead to constipation and distal intestinal obstruction in adults. Failure of the CFTR in the pancreas prevents appropriate release of pancreatic enzymes to allow for proper digestion of food, especially fatty foods, with resultant malnutrition and steatorrhea. While most patients with CF present in infancy or childhood, about 5% of all individuals with CF will not be diagnosed until adulthood. Presenting symptoms in adulthood can be myriad and often result from minor mutations of the *CFTR* gene. These symptoms can include recurrent lung and sinus infections, malnutrition, sinus disease, and infertility, especially absence of the vas deferens in men. The standard test for the diagnosis of CF is the sweat chloride test. Elevated values are pathognomonic for CF, with a cutoff of >60 mmol/L in adults being diagnostic. Values greater than 40 mmol/L fall within the indeterminate range. Given the large number of mutations that can cause CF, genetic testing can be expensive and is not the first test performed when CF is suspected. A screening CF genetic panel often only identifies between approximately 20 and 80 of the common CF mutations. If only one mutation is identified, then this may represent the carrier state, or it could represent CF with a more rare mutation requiring more detailed genetic analysis, including full gene sequencing. In such cases, referral to a tertiary CF care center is helpful for data interpretation. In some instances, nasal potential difference testing can be helpful because CF patients demonstrate an elevated baseline nasal potential difference with failure to respond to stimulation with β-agonists. Presence of *Pseudomonas aeruginosa* is common in adults with CF but is not specific for the diagnosis of the disease because bronchiectasis from any cause can lead to *P aeruginosa* colonization.

VI-33. **The answer is C.** *(Chap. 313 and Ann Am Thorac Soc 2014;11(10):1640–1650)* Individuals with CF experience recurrent pulmonary and sinus infections. In childhood, the most commonly isolated organisms are *Haemophilus influenzae* and *Staphylococcus aureus*. However, over time, most adults demonstrate *P aeruginosa*. It is now recognized that chronic colonization with *Pseudomonas*, especially multidrug-resistant organisms, is associated with a more rapid decline in lung function. The Cystic Fibrosis Foundation recommends quarterly office visits with a physician with assessment of respiratory cultures at each visit. When *Pseudomonas* is initially detected, attempts to eradicate the organism should be undertaken. The recommended regimen for eradication is an inhaled antibiotic with the aminoglycoside antibiotic tobramycin as the preferred agent. This will be continued every other month until the next office visit to determine if therapy should be continued. For all patients chronically colonized with *Pseudomonas*, inhaled tobramycin every other month should be continued on an indefinite basis. In addition, azithromycin 500 mg three times weekly or 250 mg daily is also used. Whether azithromycin primarily exerts its beneficial effect through anti-inflammatory or antimicrobial actions is not definitively known at the present time. Because the patient is clinically well without any symptoms of acute exacerbation, the use of intravenous antibiotics is not required. Chest wall oscillation and hypertonic saline are both mechanisms to improve airway clearance. While the patient may need to improve airway clearance in the future, the most important component of his care at present is to eradicate new growth of *Pseudomonas*. His current exercise regimen and autogenic drainage provide a component of airway clearance in his maintenance care plan.

VI-34. **The answer is D.** *(Chap. 314)* Acute exacerbations of COPD are a frequent cause of morbidity and mortality in COPD, contributing to >70% of healthcare expenditures for COPD. Risk factors for development of acute exacerbation include severity of airflow obstruction (FEV_1 <50% predicted), history of prior exacerbations, and elevated ratio of pulmonary artery to aorta on chest CT. Acute exacerbations of COPD cost over $10 billion to the healthcare system in the United States annually. Thus, determining the causes of exacerbations and prevention of future exacerbations have been important targets in the care of COPD patients. Most acute exacerbations are associated with airway inflammation or infection, including acquiring a new strain of bacteria or a viral respiratory infection. Therefore, strategies for prevention have been primarily focused on decreasing inflammatory responses and preventing infections. The selective phosphodiesterase-4 inhibitor roflumilast has been demonstrated to decrease exacerbation frequency in individuals with COPD who have symptoms of chronic bronchitis and frequent exacerbations. However, it has limited effects of pulmonary function and chronic respiratory symptoms. The macrolide antibiotic azithromycin has both anti-inflammatory and antibiotic properties. In a randomized controlled trial, it has been shown to decrease exacerbation frequency and increase time to first exacerbation when administered at a dose of 500 mg daily, not 250 mg three times weekly. Other interventions that also decrease exacerbation frequency include use of inhaled glucocorticoids in individuals with frequent exacerbations or asthmatic symptoms and influenza vaccination. Long-acting anticholinergic medications and long-acting β-agonists decrease exacerbations as well. Oxygen therapy and nocturnal ventilation are not indicated for prevention of exacerbations. Theophylline yields modest improvements in lung function but has no proven effect on exacerbations.

VI-35. **The answer is D.** *(Chap. 314)* COPD affects more than 10 million Americans and is currently the fourth leading cause of death in the United States. Worldwide, COPD is also increasing as cigarette smoking, the primary risk factor for the development of COPD, is increasing in prevalence throughout the world. While cigarette smoking is clearly identified as a risk factor for COPD, other factors have also been identified to contribute to the risk of COPD. In many developing countries, the prevalence of smoking among women remains low. However, the incidence of COPD is increasing in women as well as men. In many developing countries, this increased incidence of COPD in women is attributable to the use of biomass fuels in poorly ventilated areas for heat and cooking. In addition, passive cigarette smoke exposure may also contribute. Occupational exposures also lead to an increased risk of COPD. Although some exposures such as cotton textile dust and gold mining have not been definitively associated with COPD, coal dust exposure is a risk factor for emphysema in both smokers and nonsmokers. Inherent properties of the airways also affect the risk of COPD. Airway hyperresponsiveness increases the risk of lung function decline and is a risk factor for COPD. Although there is much interest in the role of chronic or recurrent infections as a risk factor for COPD, there has been no proven link.

VI-36. **The answer is B.** *(Chap. 314)* COPD is a disease process encompassing the clinical entities of emphysema and chronic bronchitis. COPD is defined pathophysiologically by the presence of irreversible airflow obstruction with hyperinflation and impaired gas exchange. The airflow obstruction occurs for several reasons including decreased elastic recoil of the lungs, increased airway inflammation, and increased closure of small airways due to loss of tethering in emphysematous lungs. This leads to early closure of airways in expiration with air trapping and hyperinflation. Finally, the loss of alveoli in emphysematous lungs leads to a progressive decline in gas exchange with alterations of ventilation-perfusion relationships. On pulmonary function testing, these pathophysiologic changes result in a typical pattern with the primary characteristic of COPD being a decrease in the FEV_1/FVC ratio and FEV_1. The severity of airflow obstruction is graded by the degree of decline in the percent predicted FEV_1. The FVC may or may not be decreased. With hyperinflation, the TLC increases with a concomitant increase in RV. Finally, the DLCO is also characteristically decreased in most cases of COPD. Some patients with pure chronic bronchitis without any emphysematous component may have a preserved DLCO, although this is a rare presentation for COPD. This same pattern of pulmonary function testing can be seen in asthma with the exception of the DLCO, which is typically normal asthma. A decrease in TLC is characteristic in restrictive ventilator disorders, such as pulmonary fibrosis, but not in obstructive disorders such as COPD.

VI-37. The answer is D. *(Chap. 314)* This patient has a known diagnosis of COPD, with worsening symptoms and pulmonary function testing consistent with a moderate degree of disease. By the Global Initiative for Lung Disease (GOLD) criteria, the patient would have stage II disease. He is currently undermanaged with a short-acting β-agonist only in the setting of limiting symptoms. Unfortunately, there is no medical therapy that alters mortality or definitively decreases rate of decline in lung function in COPD with the exception of smoking cessation, oxygen for chronic hypoxemia, and lung volume reduction surgery in a small subset of highly selected patients. Therefore, the goal of therapy in COPD is to improve symptoms and quality of life. The best initial medication for this patient would be to add a long-acting bronchodilator in the form of the antimuscarinic agent tiotropium. In large randomized controlled trials, tiotropium has been demonstrated to improve symptoms and decrease exacerbations in COPD. Ipratropium, a short-acting anticholinergic medication, also improves symptoms but has not been similarly shown to decrease exacerbation rate. Combinations of long-acting β-agonists and inhaled glucocorticoids have also been shown to decrease exacerbations and improve quality of life in COPD. The largest trial of these medications to date has demonstrated a trend toward improved mortality. Currently, the recommendation for initiation of long-acting β-agonist and inhaled glucocorticoid combinations is to consider starting the medication if the patient has two or more exacerbations yearly or demonstrates significant acute bronchodilator reactivity on pulmonary function testing. At one time, physicians considered prescribing long-term oral glucocorticoids if a patient demonstrated significant improvement in lung function in response to a trial of oral steroids. However, long-term treatment with steroids has an unfavorable risk-benefit ratio including weight gain, osteoporosis, and increased risk of infection, especially pneumonia. Oxygen therapy improves outcomes in individuals who are hypoxemic at rest or have borderline hypoxemia with evidence of end-organ damage (e.g., pulmonary hypertension, polycythemia). Although oxygen may be prescribed for individuals with isolated exercise or nocturnal hypoxemia, research to date has not demonstrated any change in outcomes with oxygen in these settings.

VI-38. The answer is E. *(Chap. 314)* Acute exacerbations of COPD are marked by an increase in dyspnea, an increase in sputum, and a change in sputum color. Acute exacerbations of COPD account for more than $10 billion in healthcare expenditures annually in the United States, with significant morbidity and mortality associated with these exacerbations. Prompt treatment can improve symptoms and decrease hospitalizations and mortality in this setting. In patients presenting with hypercarbic respiratory failure in the setting of an acute exacerbation, the treatment that has demonstrated the strongest reduction in mortality, when compared to traditional mechanical ventilation, is noninvasive positive-pressure ventilation (NIPPV). NIPPV also decreases the need for endotracheal intubation, complications, and length of stay in the hospital. Antibiotics, bronchodilators, and glucocorticoids are all cornerstones of therapy in the treatment of acute exacerbations in COPD but have not been demonstrated in clinical trials to have similar mortality benefits in the situation of acute hypercarbic respiratory failure. Specifically, no benefit is demonstrated for intravenous versus oral corticosteroids. Likewise, the choice of antibiotic should be made based on local susceptibility patterns, and need for broad-spectrum antibiotics that cover for *Pseudomonas* is not typically indicated. Recent studies have demonstrated that high-flow nasal oxygen may be an effective alternative to NIPPV, with improved outcomes (need for mechanical ventilation) and improved patient comfort.

VI-39. The answer is C. *(Chap. 314)* The only therapies that have been proven to improve survival in patients with COPD are smoking cessation, oxygen in patients with resting hypoxemia, and lung volume reduction surgery in a very small subset of highly selected patients. This patient probably has resting hypoxemia resulting from the presence of an elevated jugular venous pulse, pedal edema, and elevated hematocrit. Theophylline has been shown to increase exercise tolerance in patients with COPD through a mechanism other than bronchodilation. Oral glucocorticoids are not indicated in the absence of an acute exacerbation and may lead to complications if they are used indiscriminately. Atenolol and enalapril have no specific role in therapy for COPD but are often used when there is concomitant hypertension or cardiovascular disease.

VI-40 and VI-41. The answers are E and C, respectively. *(Chap. 315 and Am J Respir Crit Care Med 2015;192(2):238–248)* Idiopathic pulmonary fibrosis (IPF) is the most common cause of idiopathic interstitial pneumonia. The disease typically presents with progressive dyspnea on exertion and dry cough in an older individual. IPF is rare in individuals younger than age 50 years. On physical examination, inspiratory crackles and clubbing are common. Pulmonary function tests demonstrate restrictive ventilatory defect (low TLC, low RV, low VC) with a low DLCO. As in the chest HRCT shown, there is typically interstitial fibrosis that is worse in the bases and begins in the subpleural areas, often associated with traction bronchiectasis and honeycombing. Atypical findings that should cause one to consider an alternative diagnosis include the presence of ground-glass infiltrates, nodular opacities, an upper lobe predominance of disease, and prominent hilar or mediastinal lymphadenopathy. Bronchoscopic biopsy is insufficient for histologic confirmation, and a surgical lung biopsy is required for definitive diagnosis. The histologic hallmark of IPF is usual interstitial pneumonia, but can also occur in rheumatologic diseases or due to secondary exposures. In these cases, the prognosis is better than when the diagnosis is IPF. If no other secondary cause is identified, the diagnosis of IPF is given. The natural history of IPF is one of continued progression of disease and a high mortality rate. Acute exacerbations also occur with a rapid progression of symptoms associated with a pattern of diffuse ground-glass opacities on CT. These are associated with a high mortality. Until recently, no treatment had been demonstrated to slow progression of disease. Recently, two therapies have been approved by the FDA for treatment of IPF—nintedanib and pirfenidone (*Am J Respir Crit Care Med* 2015;192(2):238–248). Nintedanib is an intracellular tyrosine kinase inhibitor that inhibits several growth factors including vascular endothelial growth factor, fibroblast growth factor, and platelet-derived growth factor. A recent trial demonstrated that use of this medication slowed the rate of decline in FVC and could potentially decrease mortality. Pirfenidone is an oral antifibrotic medication that has been demonstrated to decrease fibroblast proliferation and collagen synthesis. It too has also been shown to decrease decline in FVC and potentially decrease mortality. Therapies that have been shown to not benefit in IPF include glucocorticoids, immunosuppressant agents, and *N*-acetylcysteine. Referral for lung CT should be considered in all patients with a diagnosis of IPF due to the unpredictability of the diagnosis.

VI-42. The answer is C. *(Chap. 315)* In many cases of interstitial lung disease, bronchoscopy can offer some clues to the cause of the disease. Diffuse alveolar hemorrhage is a pathologic process that can occur in many diseases including vasculitis, Goodpasture syndrome, systemic lupus erythematosus, crack cocaine use, mitral stenosis, and idiopathic pulmonary hemosiderosis, among many others. On bronchoscopy, one would expect to see a progressively greater blood return on sequential aliquots of lavage fluid. Microscopic examination would show hemosiderin-laden macrophages and red blood cells. Atypical hyperplastic type II pneumocytes are seen in diffuse alveolar damage or cases of drug toxicity. Ferruginous bodies and dust particles are found in asbestos-related pulmonary disease. Lymphocytosis is common in hypersensitivity pneumonitis and sarcoidosis. Hypersensitivity pneumonitis has a low CD4:CD8 ratio, whereas sarcoidosis has an elevated CD4:CD8 ratio. The bronchoalveolar lavage fluid in pulmonary alveolar proteinosis has a milky appearance with foamy macrophages.

VI-43 and VI-44. The answers are E and E, respectively. *(Chap. 315)* Pulmonary alveolar proteinosis is a rare disorder that usually presents between ages 30 and 50 years. It is slightly more common in men. Three distinct subtypes have been described: congenital, acquired, and secondary (most frequently caused by acute silicosis or hematologic malignancies). Interestingly, the pathogenesis of the disease has been associated with antibodies to granulocyte-macrophage colony-stimulating factor (GM-CSF) in most cases of acquired disease in adults. The pathobiology of the disease is failure of clearance of pulmonary surfactant. These patients typically present with subacute dyspnea on exertion with fatigue and low-grade fevers. Associated laboratory abnormalities include polycythemia, hypergammaglobulinemia, and increased lactate dehydrogenase levels. Elevated serum levels of lung surfactant proteins A and D have been described, and autoantibodies to GM-CSF can be found in both the serum and bronchoalveolar lavage fluid. Classically, the CT appearance is described as "crazy pavement" with ground-glass alveolar infiltrates in a perihilar distribution and intervening areas of normal lung. Bronchoalveolar lavage is diagnostic, with large amounts of amorphous proteinaceous material seen. Macrophages filled with periodic acid-Schiff–positive material are also frequently seen. The treatment of choice is whole-lung lavage through a double-lumen endotracheal tube. Survival at 5 years is higher than 95%, although some patients will need a repeat whole-lung lavage. Treatment of pulmonary alveolar proteinosis with GM-CSF remains experimental.

VI-45. **The answer is D.** *(Chap. 315)* This patient is presenting with subacute pulmonary symptoms, intermittent fevers, myalgias, and malaise. The biopsy shows a pattern of cryptogenic organizing pneumonia (COP). COP (formerly bronchiolitis obliterans organizing pneumonia) usually presents in the fifth or sixth decades with a flulike illness. Symptoms include fevers, malaise, weight loss, cough, and dyspnea. Inspiratory crackles are common, and late inspiratory squeaks may also be heard. Pulmonary function testing reveals restrictive lung disease. The typical pattern on chest HRCT is patchy areas of airspace consolidation, nodular opacities, and ground-glass opacities that occur more frequently in the lower lung zones. Pathology shows the presence of granulation tissue plugging airways, alveolar ducts, and alveoli. There is frequently chronic inflammation in the alveolar interstitium. Treatment with high-dose steroids is effective in two-thirds of individuals, with most individuals being able to be tapered to lower doses over the first year. Azathioprine is an immunosuppressive therapy that is commonly used in interstitial lung disease due to usual interstitial pneumonitis. While it may be considered in COP unresponsive to glucocorticoids, it would not be a first-line agent used without concomitant steroid therapy. Because most patients with COP respond to corticosteroids, referral for lung transplantation is not required unless there is a failure to respond to therapy. Nintedanib and pirfenidone are treatments for idiopathic pulmonary fibrosis.

VI-46. **The answer is C.** *(Chap. 316)* Empyema refers to the presence of a grossly purulent pleural effusion, which is present in this clinical scenario. The management of an empyema requires placement of a chest tube for drainage, and a recent randomized, placebo-controlled clinical trial demonstrated improved outcomes with use of both alteplase (tissue plasminogen activator) and deoxyribonuclease (DNase) twice daily for 3 days beginning within the first day after chest tube placement. The trial was conducted using a factorial design comparing the combination therapy to placebo and to either therapy alone. The combination of alteplase and DNase showed improved resolution of pleural fluid, shorter duration of hospital stay, and lesser need for surgical intervention when compared to placebo or either therapy alone (Rahman NM et al: *N Engl J Med* 2011;365:518–526).

VI-47. **The answer is C.** *(Chap. 316)* Tension pneumothorax is a life-threatening complication that must be rapidly recognized and alleviated. If undetected, it will rapidly progress to cardiovascular collapse and death. Tension pneumothorax most commonly occurs during mechanical ventilation and during resuscitative efforts. An initial sign during mechanical ventilation is high peak inspiratory pressures or difficulty with ventilation. Hypotension and hypoxemia are signs of impending cardiovascular collapse and are caused by decreased venous return to the heart and reduced cardiac output. The physical examination may show absence of breath sounds on the affected side with enlargement of the hemithorax, hyperresonance to percussion, and mediastinal shift to the contralateral side. A chest radiograph would be confirmatory, but in an acute setting, there may not be time to obtain the testing. If clinical suspicion is high, treatment should not be delayed as tension pneumothorax is a medical emergency and the patient is likely to die if the tension is not relieved. A large-bore needle should be placed into the pleural space through the second anterior intercostal space. If a large amount of air escapes after the needle is inserted, the diagnosis is confirmed. The needle should remain in place until definitive treatment with a tube thoracostomy can be performed.

VI-48. **The answer is E.** *(Chap. 316)* Parapneumonic effusions are one of the most common causes of the exudative pleural effusion. When an effusion is identified in association with pneumonia, it is prudent to perform a thoracentesis if the fluid can be safely accessed. One way to know whether there is enough fluid for thoracentesis is to perform a lateral decubitus film and observe if there is free-flowing fluid at a volume of >10 mm from the chest wall. However, if the fluid does not layer, this may indicate a complex loculated fluid. A loculated effusion often indicates an infected effusion and may require chest tube drainage or surgical intervention. Other factors that are associated with the need for more invasive procedures include pleural fluid pH <7.20, pleural fluid glucose <60 mg/dL (<3.3 mmol/L), positive Gram stain or culture of the pleural fluid, and presence of gross pus in the pleural space (empyema). Fluid recurrence following initial thoracentesis does indicate a complicated pleural effusion, but a repeat thoracentesis should be performed to ensure no concerning features have developed.

VI-49. **The answer is A.** *(Chap. 316)* The characteristics of the pleural fluid in this patient are consistent with an exudate by Light's criteria. These criteria are as follows: pleural fluid protein/serum protein ratio >0.5, pleural fluid lactate dehydrogenase (LDH)/serum LDH ratio >0.6, and pleural fluid LDH more than two-thirds of the upper limit of normal serum values. If one of the criteria is met, then the effusion would be classified as an exudate. This patient clearly meets the criteria for an exudate. Exudative pleural effusions occur when there are alterations in the local environment that change the formation and absorption of pleural fluid. The most common causes of exudative pleural effusion are infection and malignancy. Other less common causes include pulmonary embolism, chylothorax, autoimmune diseases, asbestos exposure, drug reactions, hemothorax, and following cardiac surgery or other cardiac injury, among others. Unfortunately, 25% of transudative effusions can be incorrectly identified as exudates by these criteria. Most often, this occurs when the effusion has an increased number of cells to cause an elevation in the LDH or has been treated with diuretics to cause an increase in pleural fluid protein. Transudative effusions are most often caused by heart failure, but can also be seen in cirrhosis, nephrotic syndrome, and myxedema.

VI-50. **The answer is B.** *(Chap. 316)* A primary spontaneous pneumothorax occurs in the absence of trauma to the thorax. Most individuals who present with a primary spontaneous pneumothorax are young, and primary spontaneous pneumothorax occurs almost exclusively in cigarette smokers, the primary risk factor. Primary spontaneous pneumothorax is also more common in men and has been associated with a tall, thin body habitus. The primary cause is the rupture of small apical pleural blebs or cysts, and the CT scan of the chest is often normal. About half of individuals will experience more than one primary spontaneous pneumothorax. The initial treatment is simple needle aspiration, which is most commonly done with ultrasound or CT guidance. Oxygen is given simultaneously to speed resorption of the residual air in the pleural space. If conservative treatment fails, tube thoracostomy can be performed. Pneumothoraces that fail to resolve or are recurrent often require thoracoscopy with stapling of blebs and pleural abrasion, a treatment that is effective in almost 100% of cases.

VI-51. **The answer is B.** *(Chap. 317)* Chronic fibrosing mediastinitis most commonly occurs after granulomatous inflammation in the lymph nodes in the mediastinum that leads to an exuberant calcification response. Over time, the inflammation can cause significant disruption to the vital structures that course through the mediastinum and lead to the clinical symptoms of fibrosing mediastinitis. The most common causes of fibrosing mediastinitis are histoplasmosis and tuberculosis. Other causes include sarcoidosis, silicosis, or other fungal diseases. Symptoms are related to compression of mediastinal structures including the superior vena cava, pulmonary arteries or veins, or large airway compression. The phrenic or recurrent laryngeal nerves may also become paralyzed. The most common symptom is dyspnea on exertion. Patients may also develop chronic cough with lithoptysis or hemoptysis due to erosion of the calcific lymph nodes into airways. Patients may describe lithoptysis as gritty or sandy sputum. Hemoptysis can be large volume and may necessitate surgical intervention for control. However, other than antituberculous therapy for tuberculous mediastinitis, no medical or surgical therapy has any effectiveness on the treatment of fibrosing mediastinitis. This patient most likely has histoplasmosis as the cause of her disease because histoplasmosis is endemic in Indiana. Because the fibrosing mediastinitis is a sequela of an old infection, the urine *Histoplasma* antigen test would not yield a positive result.

VI-52. The answer is E. *(Chap. 318)* Obesity hypoventilation syndrome (OHS) is a disorder of chronic hypoventilation that has an unknown prevalence as no large population studies have been conducted. However, the prevalence is expected to increase as the prevalence of obesity is rising worldwide. OHS requires a body mass index >30 kg/m^2 and the presence of chronic alveolar hypoventilation for diagnosis, with a daytime awake $PaCO_2$ ≥45 mmHg. In more than 90% of cases, concomitant obstructive sleep apnea (OSA) is also present. The pathogenesis of OHS is not fully understood, although it is known that there is a downregulation of the central respiratory drive in response to carbon dioxide. Multiple physiologic factors acting together likely lead to this including OSA, increased work of breathing, respiratory muscle impairment, V/Q mismatching, and depressed central chemo-responsiveness to hypoxemia and hypercarbia. Most patients present with daytime sleepiness, headaches, and symptoms typical of OSA. These patients should be treated with weight loss and positive airway pressure therapy. Sustained weight loss will lead to improvements in $PaCO_2$ over time. Continuous positive airway pressure (CPAP) therapy does lead to improvement in daytime hypercapnia and hypoxemia in more than half of patients with OHS and OSA but is not recommended for use if patients have sustained hypoxemia after resolution of obstructive apneic events. In these individuals bilevel positive airway pressure (BiPAP) therapy is used. BiPAP is also used if a patient cannot tolerate the typically high levels of CPAP required for treatment. Some patients with OHS may present acutely with decompensated symptoms of right heart failure and respiratory failure as in this scenario. When a patient presents in acute decompensated OHS, BiPAP is the treatment of choice acutely as well. Even in patients who have previously failed home noninvasive therapy, this remains the treatment of choice for their acute condition and may prevent intubation and mechanical ventilation. The *PHOX2b* gene mutation plays no role in OHS but is associated with congenital central hypoventilation syndromes.

VI-53. The answer is E. *(Chap. 318)* Patients with amyotrophic lateral sclerosis (ALS) often develop hypoventilation due to involvement of their respiratory pump muscles (e.g., diaphragm, intercostal muscles, sternocleidomastoids). NIPPV has been used successfully in the therapy of patients with hypoventilation such as ALS. Nocturnal NIPPV can improve daytime hypercapnia, prolong survival, and improve health-related quality of life. Current ALS guidelines are to institute NIPPV if symptoms of hypoventilation exist and $PaCO_2$ is ≥45 mmHg, nocturnal desaturation to <89% is documented for 5 consecutive minutes, maximal inspiratory pressure is <60 cmH_2O, or FVC is <50% predicted. Symptoms of hypoventilation are not particular to ALS and may include the following: dyspnea during activities of daily living, orthopnea in diseases that affect diaphragm function, poor-quality sleep, daytime hypersomnolence, early morning headaches, anxiety, and impaired cough in neuromuscular disease.

VI-54. The answer is B. *(Chap. 319)* Obstructive sleep apnea/hypopnea syndrome (OSAHS) is a common condition estimated to affect up to 2%–15% of middle-aged individuals and >20% of elderly individuals and is associated with repeated collapse of the upper airway during sleep. This patient exhibits multiple risk factors and gives a strong history to support a diagnosis of OSAHS, placing him at high risk to have moderate to severe OSAHS. The greatest risk factor the patient has that places him at high risk for disease is obesity.

Approximately 40%–60% of cases of OSAHS are attributable to excess body weight. The second major risk factor for OSAHS is male sex because men are two to four times more likely to have OSAHS than women. The reasons men develop more OSAHS include greater central obesity and relatively longer pharyngeal length, which in turn contribute to greater upper airway collapsibility. In addition, female sex hormones provide a stabilizing effect on the upper airway and stimulate ventilatory drive. Thus, premenopausal women are relatively protected from OSAHS at comparable levels of obesity when compared to men. Other risk factors that this patient has include a positive family history of the disease and hypertension. Other common risk factors for OSAHS in the general population include craniofacial abnormalities, adenotonsillar hypertrophy, various endocrine syndromes (acromegaly, hypothyroidism), increasing age, and some ethnic groups. For instance, individuals of Asian descent often develop OSAHS at a lower range of body mass index, most likely due to ethnic difference in craniofacial structure. In addition, individuals of African American race are at higher risk of OSAHS when compared to whites. This patient also gives many symptoms that are concerning for OSAHS including loud snoring, witnessed apneas, and daytime sleepiness. Given that there is a high clinical suspicion of disease, home sleep testing will likely be adequate for diagnosis of disease in this patient. Home sleep tests can be performed in a variety of ways, but most will record respiratory effort, nasal flow, and oxygen saturation. In a patient with a high suspicion of disease, these tests can be a cost-efficient means of diagnosis. However, the home tests may yield false-negative results because these tests do not measure the electroencephalogram, and thus, no accurate measure of sleep time is obtained. Therefore, the respiratory events are determined based on total recording time rather than total sleep time. If a patient is awake during much of the recording time, this could cause a false-negative result. An attended in-lab polysomnogram remains the gold standard for diagnosis OSAHS but is significantly more expensive. In this individual with a high pretest suspicion of disease, the cost would not be justified. An overnight oximetry provides only oxygen levels and heart rate and is not adequate for diagnosis of OSAHS. Treatment with a CPAP device may be recommended after a diagnosis is confirmed, but this would not be the next step in the treatment of the patient. The patient has only minimally enlarged tonsils. A tonsillectomy would not be expected to alleviate his symptoms.

VI-55. The answer is E. *(Chap. 319)* There are numerous benefits to treating OSAHS, and the consequences of untreated OSAHS are numerous and can be severe. They primarily fall in one of three categories: neurocognitive, cardiovascular, and metabolic. The neurocognitive effects are the ones most readily identified by the patient and include daytime sleepiness and inability to concentrate. In addition, individuals with untreated OSAHS have an increased risk of depression, particularly somatic depression with irritability, fatigue, and lack of energy. Moreover, untreated OSAHS increases the risk of occupational accidents by more than twofold and automobile accidents by as much as sevenfold. In addition to the neurocognitive effects, untreated OSA leads to increased sympathetic nervous system activity and increased systemic inflammatory responses. This leads to a loss of the normal nocturnal fall in blood pressure. However, treatment with CPAP can reduce 24-hour ambulatory blood pressure, although the overall effect on blood pressure is modest, decreasing the blood pressure about by 2–4 mmHg. Other cardiovascular and metabolic effects include an increased risk of coronary artery disease, heart failure with and without reduced ejection fraction, atrial and ventricular arrhythmias, atherosclerosis, stroke, and diabetes. Treatment with CPAP yields improvements in insulin resistance, decreases the recurrence rate of atrial fibrillation, and reduces several biomarkers of cardiovascular disease.

VI-56. The answer is E. *(Chap. 319)* Cheyne-Stokes respiration is a type of central sleep apnea associated with hypocapnia and demonstrates a crescendo-decrescendo pattern of breathing. Pathophysiologically, this occurs because the baseline carbon dioxide during wakefulness is below the apneic threshold during sleep. Thus, at sleep onset, a central apneic event occurs allowing carbon dioxide to rise. When this rise in carbon dioxide is detected centrally, there is an exaggerated respiratory response that leads to hyperpnea and hyperventilation, driving the carbon dioxide levels below the apneic threshold again, creating a self-perpetuating cycle of apnea and hyperpnea. It occurs more commonly in individuals with heart failure or atrial fibrillation due to a delay in circulation time. This prolonged circulation delay between the pulmonary capillaries and the central carbon dioxide–sensing chemoreceptors contributes to these ongoing cycles of hyperpnea and apnea. In many individuals with Cheyne-Stokes respiration, it has been observed that the pattern of breathing may worsen over the course of the night and the fluid is redistributed centrally, further prolonging circulation time.

VI-57. **The answer is A.** *(Chap. 319)* The treatment of choice for most adults with OSAHS is nasal CPAP. CPAP delivers a set pressure that is sufficient to overcome the tendency of the posterior oropharynx to collapse. This pressure ranges generally from 5–15 cmH_2O, although pressures as high as 20 cmH_2O can be used. However, the rates of adherence to CPAP therapy are highly variable. Many patients complain of claustrophobia, nasal congestion, aerophagia, or facial pain. If tolerated, there is a large body of data demonstrating beneficial effects of CPAP on blood pressure, alertness, mood, and insulin sensitivity, and likely improvement in cardiovascular outcomes. Oral appliance therapy is generally considered second-line therapy in mild to moderate OSA if the patient fails to tolerate CPAP. It can be prescribed as initial therapy if the patient prefers. In most studies, the improvement in the apnea-hypopnea index with oral appliance is ≥50% in about two-thirds of individuals. Side effects of oral appliances include temporomandibular joint pain and tooth movement. Surgical interventions for OSAHS in adults have provided less than desired benefits, and it can be difficult to determine which patients will derive the greatest benefits in the absence of a known anatomic abnormality. Uvulopalatopharyngoplasty is the most common surgical procedure over the past two decades and is associated with a success rate similar to oral appliance therapy. Weight loss is generally recommended for all patients with OSAHS but should not be the only therapy recommended for an individual with this degree of OSAHS. Supplemental oxygen can improve oxygen saturation, but there is little evidence that it improves OSAHS symptoms and the apnea-hypopnea index.

VI-58. **The answer is D.** *(Chap. 320e)* Common indications for lung transplantation include COPD, idiopathic pulmonary fibrosis, CF, emphysema, and pulmonary arterial hypertension (Table VI-58). Five-year survival is similar for all indications for lung transplantation at approximately 50%. For most indications, double lung transplantation is the preferred procedure, and it is mandatory for patients with suppurative lung disease like CF. In general, in patients with idiopathic pulmonary arterial hypertension, double lung transplantation is preferred because of concern of overcirculation in the low-resistance vascular bed transplanted lung when a native lung is present with markedly elevated pulmonary vascular resistance. It is rare for the primary disease to recur after transplantation, and this has not been described in idiopathic pulmonary arterial hypertension. The right ventricle is highly plastic and will generally recover function after elevated pulmonary vascular resistance is removed by lung transplantation. Subsequently, it is rare to perform heart-lung transplantation in pulmonary arterial hypertension patients unless there is concomitant complex congenital heart disease that cannot be repaired at the time of lung transplantation.

VI-59. **The answer is A.** *(Chap. 320e)* The long-term complications of lung transplantation are multisystem and range from the diseases that affect the lung and are complications of a foreign body in the chest to distant organ disease, either due to infections or complications of immunosuppressive therapy. Although osteoporosis, posttransplantation lymphoproliferative disorders, and chronic kidney disease are important complications of steroids, calcineurin inhibitors, and other agents used for immunosuppression, the major complications after transplantation are in the lung. Primary graft dysfunction is a form of acute lung injury immediately after lung transplantation that is relatively rare, with severe disease occurring in only 10%–20% of cases. Airway complications such as anastomotic dehiscence or stenosis have similar occurrence rates, but can usually be managed bronchoscopically with good survival. Rejection of transplanted organ is very common and is the main limitation to better medium- and long-term outcomes. Rejection occurs as acute cellular rejection often presenting with cough, low-grade fever, dyspnea, infiltrates on radiographs, and declining lung function. In contrast, chronic rejection typically presents with advancing obstruction on pulmonary function testing, no infiltrates,

TABLE VI-58 Disease-Specific Guidelines for Referral and Transplantation

Chronic Obstructive Pulmonary Disease
Referral
BODE index >5
Transplantation
BODE index 7–10
or
Any of the following criteria:
Hospitalization for exacerbation, with $PaCO_2$ >50 mmHg
Pulmonary hypertension or cor pulmonale, despite oxygen therapy
FEV_1 <20% with either DLCO <20% or diffuse emphysema
Cystic Fibrosis/Bronchiectasis
Referral
FEV_1 <30% or rapidly declining FEV_1
Hospitalization in ICU for exacerbation
Increasing frequency of exacerbations
Refractory or recurrent pneumothorax
Recurrent hemoptysis not controlled by bronchial artery embolization
Transplantation
Oxygen-dependent respiratory failure
Hypercapnia
Pulmonary hypertension
Idiopathic Pulmonary Fibrosis
Referral
Pathologic or radiographic evidence of UIP, regardless of vital capacity
Transplantation
Pathologic or radiographic evidence of UIP
and
Any of the following criteria:
DLCO <39%
Decrement in FVC ≥10% during 6 months of follow-up
Decrease in SpO_2 to <88% during a 6-min walk test
Honeycombing on HRCT (fibrosis score >2)
Idiopathic Pulmonary Arterial Hypertension
Referral
NYHA functional class III or IV, regardless of therapy
Rapidly progressive disease
Transplantation
Failure of therapy with IV epoprostenol (or equivalent drug)
Persistent NYHA functional class III or IV during maximal medical therapy
Low (<350 m) or declining 6-min walk test
Cardiac index <2 L/min per m^2
Right atrial pressure >15 mmHg

Abbreviations: BODE, body mass index (B), airflow obstruction (O), dyspnea (D), exercise capacity (E); DLCO, diffusing capacity for carbon monoxide; FEV_1, forced expiratory volume in 1 second; FVC, forced vital capacity; HRCT, high-resolution computed tomography; ICU, intensive care unit; NYHA, New York Heart Association; $PaCO_2$, partial pressure of carbon dioxide in arterial blood; SpO_2, arterial oxygen saturation by pulse oximetry; UIP, usual interstitial pneumonitis.
Source: Summarized from JB Orens et al: J Heart Lung Transplant 25:745, 2006. For BODE index, BR Celli et al: N Engl J Med 350:1005, 2004.

and worsening dyspnea on exertion. This constellation in posttransplantation patients is termed bronchiolitis obliterans syndrome. Fifty percent of lung transplant patients have some degree of bronchiolitis obliterans syndrome, and it is the main impediment to better long-term survival. Therapy often involves augmented immunosuppression, although there is no consensus of how to do this or the duration of this augmentation.

VI-60. The answer is B. *(Chap. 320e)* Chronic kidney disease is a common finding in patients after lung transplantation and is associated with poorer outcomes. Although rarely patients may have hemolytic-uremic syndrome underlying the kidney disease, it is usually acute, and the most common etiology of gradually progressive decline in renal function is calcineurin inhibitor neuropathy. Cyclosporine and tacrolimus are calcineurin inhibitors commonly used in immunosuppressive regimens after lung transplantation. The exact mechanism of this toxicity is unclear but may include a direct toxicity of inhibition of the calcineurin-NFAT system within the kidney, alteration in glomerular blood flow, and host-environment interactions within the kidney with calcineurin inhibitors. Prednisone, albuterol, and mycophenolate mofetil are not known to be nephrotoxic.

VI-61. The answer is A. *(Chap. 321)* Several different severity of illness (SOI) scores have been developed for use in critically ill populations. Two of the most common systems are the Acute Physiology and Chronic Health Evaluation (APACHE II) score and the Simplified Acute Physiology (SAPS II) score. SOI scores are primarily useful as tools to assess populations of critically ill individuals, but the scores do not perform well at predicting individual patient outcomes. These scores are used primarily in clinical trials to compare SOI between groups of patients enrolled in trials. These scores are also used by hospital administrations to assess quality of intensive care unit (ICU) care over time and also to help determine appropriate nursing and ancillary support staffing levels. No SOI score should be used to direct an individual patient's care, although decision support tools based on SOI scores are being investigated. The APACHE II score is the most commonly used SOI score. This score assigns values based on a variety of demographic, medical history, and clinical values taking the worst value in the first 24 hours after admission. Population mortality ranges based on published values range from <5%–10% for scores between 0 and 4 and as high as 80%–90% for scores ≥35 points. Updated versions of the APACHE score (APACHE III and IV) have been published. The SAPS II score is more frequently used in Europe. This score is not disease specific, although it does add higher values for AIDS, metastatic cancer, or hematologic malignancy. Both scores are used in a similar manner.

VI-62. The answer is C. *(Chap. 321)* Oxygen delivery (Q_{O2}) is a function of both cardiac output (CO) and the oxygen content of the blood (Ca_{O2}) and can be expressed by the following equation:

$$Q_{O2} = CO \times [1.39 \times \text{hemoglobin} \times SaO_2 + (0.003 \times PaO_2)]$$

From this equation, the effect of PaO_2 on overall oxygen delivery is negligible. Nearly all oxygen delivered to the tissues is bound to hemoglobin. One can improve oxygen delivery by increasing cardiac output, increasing hemoglobin, or improving oxygen saturation.

VI-63. The answer is C. *(Chap. 321)* In patients admitted to the ICU, one of the most important aspects of care is to prevent complications that may occur during the process of care. One of the most common complications is nosocomial infections, including hospital- or ventilator-acquired pneumonia, catheter-related bloodstream infections, urinary tract infections, and *Clostridium difficile* infection. It is important to remove indwelling devices such as central lines, urinary catheters, and endotracheal tubes as soon as clinically possible. Another important preventative measure to decrease nosocomial infections includes ensuring appropriate sterile procedures for device insertion. Using care bundles and emphasizing good hand washing protocols are important strategies for decreasing nosocomial infections. Individuals in the ICU are also at increased risk of deep venous thrombosis due to immobility and often have factors that increase hypercoagulability. Standard interventions to prevent deep venous thrombosis include use of low-molecular-weight heparin or low-dose heparin along with sequential compression devices. Protection against development of stress ulcers is accomplished with histamine-2 blockers or proton pump inhibitors. The patients who benefit most from stress ulcer prophylaxis are those with coagulopathy, shock, or respiratory failure. Enteral nutrition is preferred over parenteral nutrition, although no definitive data demonstrate that early use of enteral nutrition provides benefit. ICU-acquired weakness is also a common complication of ICU care. The mechanisms are poorly understood. Interventions that may improve functional outcomes in critical illness include early physical and occupational therapy. Use of tight glucose control with intensive insulin therapy was thought to improve ICU outcomes, but further study has demonstrated no benefits on nosocomial infection and increased hypoglycemia with this mode of therapy.

VI-64 and VI-65. The answers are E and A, respectively. *(Chap. 322)* This patient has evidence of severe ARDS. The annual incidence of ARDS is 60 cases per 100,000 population. In individuals admitted to the ICU with respiratory failure, approximately 20% of these will meet the criteria for ARDS, although it is generally underrecognized in the ICU population. ARDS is a clinical syndrome of severe dyspnea of rapid onset, hypoxemia, and diffuse pulmonary infiltrates that may lead to respiratory failure. There are myriad causes of ARDS, including sepsis, pneumonia, aspiration pneumonitis, trauma, acute pancreatitis, multiple transfusions, and toxic inhalation injury among others. The most common causes of ARDS are sepsis and pneumonia, which cause about 40%–50% of all cases of ARDS. Clinically, ARDS is diagnosed in the presence of acute bilateral pulmonary infiltrates and hypoxemia without evidence of increased left atrial filling pressure. A consensus panel has recently revised the definition of ARDS into three categories of mild, moderate, and severe based on degree of hypoxemia as determined by the ratio of PaO_2 to FiO_2, commonly called P:F ratio. Mild ARDS is present if PaO_2/FiO_2 is ≤300 mmHg, but >200 mm Hg. Moderate ARDS is diagnosed when PaO_2/FiO_2 is ≤200 mmHg and >100 mmHg. Severe ARDS is diagnosed when PaO_2/FiO_2 is ≤100 mmHg. In this case, the ratio of PaO_2 to FiO_2 is 80 mmHg, placing the patient in the category of severe ARDS. The natural history of ARDS is three stages: exudative, proliferative, and fibrotic. In the early exudative stage of ARDS, there is an acute injury to alveolar capillary endothelial cells and type I pneumocytes. This results in loss of the normal alveolar barrier with subsequent leakage of protein-rich fluid into the alveoli (noncardiogenic pulmonary edema). In the early phase, the inflammatory cell infiltrate is predominantly neutrophils. Pathologically, the finding is described as diffuse alveolar damage. Hyaline membranes and loss of type I pneumocytes are seen. The exudative phase of ARDS lasts for approximately the first 7 days of illness. The second phase of ARDS is the proliferative phase, which begins around day 7 and continues through day 21. Most patients recover during this phase and are able to be liberated from mechanical ventilation. Histologically, early signs of repair can be seen in this phase with shift to a lymphocyte-predominant infiltrate, proliferation of type II pneumocytes, and organization of the alveolar edema. Only a few individuals who develop ARDS fail to recover during the proliferative phase and continue into the fibrotic stage of the disease. Pathologically, individuals who develop fibrotic ARDS demonstrate extensive alveolar and interstitial fibrosis at sites of prior alveolar edema. The acinar architecture frequently becomes distorted, leading to development of emphysematous changes with large bullae. Fibrotic proliferation may also occur in the intima of pulmonary vasculature, leading to development of pulmonary hypertension. Given the timing of the presentation, this patient would be expected to be in the exudative phase of ARDS and exhibit diffuse alveolar damage, loss of type I pneumocytes, and hyaline membranes.

VI-66. The answer is B. *(Chap. 322)* This individual has severe ARDS due to trauma, a pulmonary contusion, and possible transfusion-related lung injury. Mechanical ventilation is frequently necessary for individuals suffering from ARDS and has been essential for prolonging life and improving mortality from this disorder. However, appropriate ventilator management is necessary to prevent further morbidity from ventilator-associated lung injury. ARDS is not experienced uniformly across the lung tissue. The dependent portions of the lungs are typically the most affected, while other areas of the lung may be spared. The portions of the lung that are most affected are poorly compliant and are prone to alveolar collapse. Alternatively, the more normal portions of the lungs have better lung compliance. With positive-pressure ventilation, ventilator-associated lung injury may occur as a result of overdistention of the more normal areas of the lung with resultant perpetuation of alveolar damage and capillary leak in these areas. In the poorly compliant areas, respirations initiated by the ventilator can lead to repetitive opening and closure of alveoli, causing further damage in these areas. Because of this, a strategy that employs low tidal volumes to prevent alveolar overdistention and recurrent alveolar collapse is recommended. The ARDS Network conducted a clinical trial that compared low tidal volume ventilation to conventional ventilation and demonstrated improved mortality with the low tidal volume strategy (31% vs. 40%). The recommended initial tidal volume setting is 6 mL/kg of ideal body weight. This strategy is recommended in all patients with ARDS, and the improvement in outcomes is not affected by obesity.

VI-67. **The answer is D.** *(Chap. 322)* Hypoxemia in ARDS results in shunt physiology with the presence of alveolar and interstitial fluid and loss of surfactant. In turn, there is significant loss of lung compliance and development of alveolar collapse that is worse in the dependent portions of the lungs. During mechanical ventilation, the goal is to minimize overdistention of less affected areas of the lungs while maximizing alveolar recruitment. Positive end-expiratory pressure (PEEP) is used to prevent alveolar collapse at end-expiration. Trials of mechanical ventilation with high-PEEP compared to low-PEEP strategies did not show any differences in outcomes when a low tidal volume ventilation strategy was used. More recently, a trial used a strategy that involved constructing static pressure-volume curves of the lung on the mechanical ventilator. With this strategy, a lower inflection point can be calculated. This point identifies the pressure at which the alveoli open. In ARDS, this point is typically 12–15 cmH_2O. In theory, setting the PEEP to this pressure will maximize oxygenation and prevent lung injury. Trials of this mode of ventilation improve lung function and may have an effect on mortality. More recently, strategies employing esophageal pressure catheters to estimate optimal transpulmonary pressure are being studied to determine the effects on oxygenation, duration of mechanical ventilation, and mortality.

VI-68. **The answer is B.** *(Chap. 322 and N Engl J Med 2006;354:2564–2575)* Optimal fluid management in ARDS is felt to be important to minimize extravasation of fluid into the interstitium and alveolar spaces. However, in individuals with septic shock or other causes of hypotension, expansion of fluid volume to optimal levels is important in the management of hypotension. Whether an aggressive or conservative fluid management strategy was most important in acute lung injury was not known as there were concerns that a conservative fluid management strategy would increase the likelihood of end-organ failure, especially acute kidney injury. A trial sponsored by the ARDS Network attempted to answer this question by randomizing individuals with acute lung injury to a conservative versus liberal fluid management strategy. This trial demonstrated that a conservative fluid management strategy to maintain low left atrial pressure improved pulmonary mechanics and oxygenation while decreasing the duration of mechanical ventilation, ICU stay, and mortality. At the same time, there was no increased incidence of acute kidney injury.

VI-69. **The answer is C.** *(Chap. 323)* Noninvasive ventilation (NIV) refers to respiratory support that is provided through a tight-fitting face mask or nasal mask. NIV can be administered with bilevel positive expiratory pressure ventilation or pressure support ventilation. Both modes of ventilation provide a higher positive pressure with inspiration and decrease to a lower pressure with expiration to decrease work of breathing and provide assisted ventilation. The major difficulty with using NIV clinically is poor patient tolerance due to the use of a tight-fitting mask and psychological discomfort and anxiety. The primary group of individuals who have benefited from the use of NIV are those with acute exacerbations of COPD. In those with COPD, several randomized trials have shown low failure rates in individuals with pH of 7.25 to 7.35, along with decreased need for invasive ventilation, decreased length of ICU stay, and decreased mortality in some studies. In those with pH >7.35, NIV confers no benefit over standard therapy. In those with pH <7.25, use of NIV has a higher failure rate that is inversely proportional to the degree of acidosis. Another group of individuals who may benefit from NIV are those with decompensated systolic heart failure with respiratory acidosis. In these individuals, a large clinical trial demonstrated a decreased need for invasive mechanical ventilation. NIV in these individuals decreased both preload and afterload and can provide assistance to the failing heart (Gray A, et al: *N Engl J Med* 2008;359(2):142–151). A last group for which NIV has shown promise is in individuals immediately after extubation, especially individuals with COPD or hypercapnic respiratory failure. NIV is associated with higher failure rates in individuals with acute hypoxemic respiratory failure and ARDS. Invasive mechanical ventilation is the ventilatory method of choice in these individuals, although not strictly contraindicated. Contraindications to mechanical ventilation include absence of spontaneous respirations, cardiac or respiratory arrest, severe encephalopathy, severe gastrointestinal bleed, hemodynamic instability, unstable angina or acute myocardial infarction, facial surgery or trauma, upper airway obstruction, inability to protect airway, and inability to clear secretions.

VI-70, VI-71, VI-72, and VI-73. The answers are C, B, A, and D, respectively. *(Chap. 323)* Mechanical ventilation can be delivered in many different modes, which refers to the manner in which the breaths are triggered, cycled, and delivered. The most common mode of mechanical ventilation is assist-control. This mode is volume cycled and flow limited. An inspiratory cycle may be triggered by patient effort or, if there is no patient effort within a specific time, by a timer within the ventilator. Each breath, whether triggered by patient effort or the ventilator, delivers an operator-specified tidal volume. This mode is frequently the initial mode of mechanical ventilation when a patient is intubated as it ensures a known minute ventilation in the absence of respiratory effort. Common difficulties with the use of assist-control ventilation are asynchrony with the ventilator and tachypnea, which can lead to respiratory alkalosis and/or generation of dynamic hyperinflation. This occurs when a patient triggers an inspiratory cycle before a full exhalation occurs. Commonly known as auto-PEEP, dynamic hyperinflation can lead to decreased venous return and a fall in cardiac output. It may also lead to barotrauma, including pneumothorax and pneumomediastinum. Intermittent mandatory ventilation (IMV) is a mixed mode of ventilation. IMV is primarily a volume-cycled and flow-limited mode of ventilation and is most often delivered in a synchronized mode (SIMV). The ventilator will deliver a mandatory number of breaths at a specified tidal volume. If a patient breathes only at the set respiratory rate, SIMV is essentially the same as assist-control ventilation. When a patient breathes above the set respiratory rate, the spontaneous breaths may be unassisted or assisted with a pressure support mode of ventilation. SIMV was commonly used as a weaning mode of ventilation, but clinical trials have shown that trials of spontaneous breathing lead to a shorter duration of mechanical ventilation and more rapid extubation. Pressure control ventilation (PCV) is time triggered, time cycled, and pressure limited. This mode is often used in individuals who have preexisting barotrauma or for postoperative thoracic surgery patients. It is also used in ARDS to limit ventilator-induced lung injury. In PCV, there is no prespecified minimum tidal volume or minute ventilation. Rather, a specified pressure is set during inspiration by the operator, and the tidal volume and inspiratory flow rate are dependent upon lung compliance. Pressure support ventilation (PSV) is patient triggered, flow cycled, and pressure limited. PSV requires a patient to spontaneously initiate respiration because no machine-delivered breaths are given. PSV provides graded assistance through application of an inspiratory pressure that augments spontaneous respiration. The pressure support falls to a specified expiratory pressure when the flow falls below a certain rate. PSV is often combined with SIMV to augment the spontaneously generated breaths. PSV also is used in ventilator weaning as it is generally well tolerated.

VI-74. The answer is C. *(Chap. 323)* Spontaneous breathing trials (SBTs) have been determined to be the best way to assess whether a patient has recovered sufficiently from respiratory failure to be extubated. An SBT can be implemented via T-piece, CPAP at low levels of pressure (1–5 cmH_2O), or pressure support ventilation applied to offset the resistance of the endotracheal tube. A patient will undergo an SBT from 30 minutes to 2 hours to determine if respiration can be maintained to support liberation from mechanical ventilation. It is important to recognize which patients are appropriate to undergo SBT. The following conditions predict patients who are ready for weaning attempts: (1) lung injury is stable or resolving; (2) gas exchange is adequate, with PEEP generally <8 cmH_2O and FiO_2 <0.5; (3) hemodynamic parameters are stable without need for ongoing vasopressor support; and (4) the patient has spontaneous respiratory activity.

VI-75. The answer is A. *(Chap. 324)* Shock is a complex pathophysiologic process that occurs in response to a decline in tissue perfusion. Clinically, shock states manifest with a mean arterial pressure <60 mmHg. This nonspecific term can be caused by many different etiologies including sepsis, hypovolemia, trauma, hypoadrenal states, neurologic causes, and cardiac causes. Shock states result in a decrease in tissue oxygen delivery. In turn, this creates a multifaceted response that can become a self-perpetuating process that leads to further tissue injury. Hypotension disinhibits the vasomotor center, leading to increased adrenergic output and decreased vagal tone. Norepinephrine leads to significant splanchnic and peripheral vasoconstriction in an attempt to maintain cerebral and cardiac blood flow. Other constrictor substances are secreted as well including angiotensin II, vasopressin, endothelin-1, and thromboxane A_2. In addition, there is pressure to maintain intravascular fluid volume through alterations in hydrostatic pressure and osmolarity. However, constriction of arterioles leads to reduction in capillary hydrostatic pressure and the number of capillary beds perfused. This limits the capillary surface area available for perfusion with the resultant increase in vascular oncotic pressure. This in turn leads to a net reabsorption of fluid into the vascular bed. Metabolic changes including glycolysis, lipolysis, and proteolysis further increase interstitial and intravascular volume at the expense of intracellular volume due to their effects on raising extracellular osmolarity. Within the cells, there is rapid depletion of high-energy phosphate stores. This leads to mitochondrial dysfunction with uncoupling of oxidative phosphorylation with accumulation of reactive oxygen species, lactate, and hydrogen ions. The byproducts of anaerobic metabolism can overcome the compensatory vasoconstrictor mechanisms and lead to further hypotension. Extensive proinflammatory pathways are activated in shock and contribute to the development of multiple organ dysfunction and failure. After the initial insult, a counterregulatory process should be initiated to balance the proinflammatory response. In individuals who have an excessive proinflammatory response that cannot be effectively regulated, the inflammatory process may continue unregulated and lead to further organ injury and failure. At the system level, shock affects a variety of endocrine, cardiac, pulmonary, and renal processes, among others. In addition to increases in norepinephrine, the stress associated with shock increases adrenocorticotropic hormone (ACTH) to increase cortisol secretion. Renin is also released in response to adrenergic discharge and decreased renal perfusion. Renin induces the formation of angiotensin I, which is converted to the active angiotensin II, which is a potent vasoconstrictor. Angiotensin II also stimulates release of aldosterone and vasopressin. The cardiac response to shock is to initially compensate by increasing heart rate. Many causes of shock, however, are associated with depression of myocardial contractility such that stroke volume is decreased for any given filling pressure. The pulmonary response may lead to development of noncardiogenic pulmonary edema, ARDS, and decreased lung compliance. Finally, the kidney responds to shock by conserving salt and water.

VI-76. The answer is E. *(Chap. 324)* Different causes of shock are associated with different physiologic findings throughout the vascular system. Although rarely used in most cases of shock, a pulmonary artery catheter can be used to measure these values. However, it is important to understand pathologically what occurs in the vascular system. The typical measured variables include cardiac output (CO), systemic vascular resistance (SVR), mixed venous oxygen saturation (S_VO_2), central venous pressure (CVP), and pulmonary capillary wedge pressure (PCWP). Patients who have interruption of sympathetic vasomotor input after high cervical cord injury or major head injury may experience neurogenic shock. In neurogenic shock, there is arteriolar dilation and venodilation. The result is a fall in all variables measured (CO, SVR, S_VO_2, CVP, and PCWP) (option E). Hypovolemia is the most common cause of shock and occurs due to acute blood loss or significant loss of plasma volume due to extravascular fluid sequestration. Gastrointestinal or renal fluid losses may also lead to hypovolemic shock. In hypovolemic shock, CO is low; SVR is elevated; and S_VO_2, CVP, and PCWP are low (option A). Cardiogenic shock (option B) has similarly low CO, elevated SVR, and low S_VO_2. However, CVP and PCWP are elevated. Septic shock can be hyperdynamic or hypodynamic. Early in the septic shock, the hyperdynamic state predominates and is associated with increased CO, low SVR, and low S_VO_2. CVP and PCWP are variable and may be low, normal, or elevated (option C). The hypodynamic state of septic shock is associated with low CO and high SVR with variable effect of CVP, PCWP, and S_VO_2. Shock following trauma is most often due to hypovolemia. However, after intravascular volume is restored, some individuals will continue to experience hypotension due to loss of plasma volume into the interstitium and injured tissues.

This type of shock will be associated with variable effects on CO and SVR with low S_VO_2, CVP, and PCWP. Finally, hypoadrenalism is a rare cause of shock associated with unrecognized adrenal insufficiency. Hypoadrenal shock presents with a low CO, low S_VO_2, low CVP, low PCWP, and normal to low SVR.

VI-77. **The answer is A.** *(Chap. 325)* Sepsis and septic shock represent a harmful host response to infection and are contributing factors to more than 200,000 deaths in the United States each year. Over the past 30 years, the incidence of sepsis has risen along with our aging population. Annually, there are more than 750,000 cases of sepsis yearly with an incidence of 3 per 1000 population. Most cases of sepsis occur in individuals with underlying illness. The incidence also increases with age and increasing comorbidities. Other risk factors for sepsis include immunocompromised state and indwelling vascular or mechanical devices. The most common source of infection in individuals with sepsis is the lungs, accounting for 64% of cases of sepsis. Microbial invasion of the bloodstream is not required for an individual to develop the systemic response that leads to multiorgan dysfunction in sepsis. Blood cultures are only positive in 40%–70% of cases of septic shock and approximately 20%–40% of cases of severe sepsis. When a culture is positive from any site, the most common organisms are gram-negative bacteria (62%), with *P aeruginosa* and *Escherichia coli* being the most common. Gram-positive bacteria are present in approximately 47% of cases, and 19% occurred in people infected with fungi. Because the numbers add up to >100%, it should be noted that multiple bacteria may be implicated in sepsis.

VI-78. **The answer is C.** *(Chap. 325 and JAMA 2016;315:801–810)* Sepsis represents a dysregulated host response to infection, and severity can range broadly from a mild inflammatory response to refractory septic shock (Table VI-78). Multiple professional medical societies have attempted to create a standardized definition of sepsis and septic shock over the years to aid in early identification of sepsis with the goal of improving patient outcomes. The most recent definition of sepsis simplifies diagnosis into two categories: sepsis and

TABLE VI-78 Definitions Used to Describe the Condition of Septic Patients

Bacteremia	Presence of bacteria in blood, as evidenced by positive blood cultures
Signs of possibly harmful systemic response	Two or more of the following conditions: (1) fever (oral temperature >38°C [>100.4°F]) or hypothermia (<36°C [<96.8°F]); (2) tachypnea (>24 breaths/min); (3) tachycardia (heart rate >90 bpm); (4) leukocytosis (>12,000/μL), leukopenia (<4000/μL), or >10% bands
Sepsis (or severe sepsis)	The harmful host response to infection; systemic response to proven or suspected infection plus some degree of organ hypofunction, i.e.:
	1. *Cardiovascular:* Arterial systolic blood pressure ≤90 mmHg or mean arterial pressure ≤70 mmHg that responds to administration of IV fluid
	2. *Renal:* Urine output <0.5 mL/kg/hr for 1 hr despite adequate fluid resuscitation
	3. *Respiratory:* PaO_2/FiO_2 ≤250 or, if the lung is the only dysfunctional organ, ≤200
	4. *Hematologic:* Platelet count <80,000/μL or 50% decrease in platelet count from highest value recorded over previous 3 days
	5. *Unexplained metabolic acidosis:* A pH ≤7.30 or a base deficit ≥5.0 mEq/L and a plasma lactate level >1.5 times upper limit of normal for reporting lab
Septic shock	Sepsis with hypotension (arterial blood pressure <90 mmHg systolic, or 40 mmHg less than patient's normal blood pressure) for at least 1 hr despite adequate fluid resuscitation[a]
	Or
	Need for vasopressors to maintain systolic blood pressure ≥90 mmHg *or* mean arterial pressure ≥70 mmHg
Refractory septic shock	Septic shock that lasts for >1 hr and does not respond to fluid or pressor administration

[a]Fluid resuscitation is considered adequate when the pulmonary artery wedge pressure is ≥12 mmHg or the central venous pressure is ≥8 mmHg.

septic shock. This eliminates prior categories included in the continuum of sepsis including systemic inflammatory response syndrome (SIRS) and severe sepsis. SIRS criteria may be present in many individuals with infection who do not develop progressive symptoms of sepsis. The symptoms that may indicate a harmful systemic response to infection are many of those previously included in the SIRS definition, including fever or hypothermia, tachypnea, tachycardia, and leukocytosis. However, SIRS can be present due to systemic inflammatory responses with other stresses such as trauma or acute pancreatitis that are not caused by infection. Thus, the term SIRS is neither sensitive nor specific for identifying patients at risk of developing sepsis. Severe sepsis was also a term with limited specificity and did not provide additional risk stratification. In the simplified definition, there is greater reliance on use of the Sequential Organ Failure Assessment (SOFA) score. Sepsis is thus defined as a suspected or documented infection with an acute increase of ≥2 points, whereas septic shock is clinically defined as sepsis with need for vasopressor support and elevated lactate (>2 mmol/L) despite adequate fluid resuscitation. The SOFA score incorporates a variety of measures to determine the magnitude of multiorgan dysfunction. Variables include PaO_2/FiO_2 ratio, platelet count, bilirubin, Glasgow Coma Scale score, creatinine, urine output, and blood pressure/vasopressor support. Sepsis is identified as evidence of infection with evidence of organ dysfunction. Using the SOFA score as a determinant of organ dysfunction creates a more standard measure for identifying sepsis. A patient may be considered in refractory septic shock if the mean arterial pressure remains low for >1 hour despite fluid resuscitation and vasopressors. Refractory septic shock is not included in the guidelines.

VI-79. **The answer is B.** *(Chap. 325)* Blood cultures are positive in only 40%–70% of cases of sepsis, although in most individuals, a source of infection can be identified through examination of infected material (e.g., sputum, abscess fluid, urine) or through the identification of RNA or DNA in blood or tissue samples. In some individuals, the immediate source of infection is not apparent. In cases of sepsis and septic shock, it is important to initiate antibiotic therapy immediately while awaiting culture data to become available. A delay in antibiotic therapy as little as 1 hour has been associated with lower survival rates. In addition, use of "inappropriate" antibiotics defined on the basis of local susceptibility patterns and published guidelines for empiric antibiotic therapy is associated with a fivefold increase in mortality. This patient has evidence of septic shock and has had a prior splenectomy. Patients who have had splenectomy are at risk for sepsis due to encapsulated organisms. In these individuals, sepsis is most commonly caused by *Streptococcus pneumoniae*, but *Haemophilus influenzae* and *Neisseria meningitidis* may also be implicated. In an asplenic patient with sepsis, the patient should be empirically treated with cefotaxime or ceftriaxone. In areas where there is significant resistance of *S pneumoniae* to cephalosporins, vancomycin should be added. In most areas, the cephalosporin resistance is only 1%. If a patient is allergic to cephalosporins, fluoroquinolones should be used as an alternative medication.

VI-80. **The answer is B.** *(Chap. 325)* Mortality in sepsis remains high, with approximately 20%–35% of individuals dying when severe sepsis is present and up to 60% dying due to septic shock. Mortality increases with increasing age and number of comorbidities. Numerous interventions have been attempted to try to decrease mortality by providing better supportive care or targeting the underlying pathophysiologic mechanisms that lead to organ failure in sepsis. An example of a supportive measure that has been proven ineffective in sepsis is insulin therapy to achieve tight glucose control. The rationale for lower blood glucose in sepsis was that hyperglycemia was associated with poorer outcomes in critical illness. After initial enthusiasm from data generated by a single-center trial in a surgical ICU, the benefits were not demonstrated in a medically ill population. Meta-analyses have concluded that intensive insulin therapy does not affect survival and may lead to harm, particularly from hypoglycemia. Anemia also frequently develops in individuals with critical illness. The target hemoglobin necessary to maintain oxygen-carrying capacity has to be balanced against potential harm from transfusion therapy, including infection and transfusion-associated acute lung injury. A randomized trial demonstrated that patients were not harmed by a lower hemoglobin threshold for transfusion (7 g/dL) compared to a higher hemoglobin goal (9 g/dL). Patients with refractory hypotension in sepsis have been shown to have a relative deficiency of cortisol in the face of profound metabolic stress. This so-called critical illness–related corticosteroid insufficiency may lead to worse outcomes in critical illness. Trials to determine which patients would most benefit from corticosteroid replacement used adrenocorticotropin hormone stimulation to assess adrenal response to stimulus. However, this approach did not lead to improved outcomes, and most practitioners favor a more empiric approach to corticosteroid replacement. Hydrocortisone should be considered at a dose of 50 mg every 6 hours in patients with septic shock on vasopressors. If clinical improvement occurs with use of hydrocortisone over 24–48 hours, then a course of therapy for 5–7 days is indicated. Other interventions that have been trialed but failed for septic shock include endotoxin-neutralizing proteins, inhibitors of cyclooxygenase or nitric oxide synthase, anticoagulants, polyclonal antibodies, and inhibitors of tumor necrosis factor-α, interleukin-1, platelet-activating factor, and tissue factor pathway. One of the most widely known medications used for sepsis was recombinant activated protein C (APC). This medication was approved by the FDA for severe sepsis and septic shock based on the outcome of a randomized controlled trial that showed a mortality benefit in patients who were more severely ill. Subsequent trials showed no benefit in patients with less severe illness and in children. A subsequent confirmatory trial showed no benefit to APC, and it was removed from the market 10 years after being approved.

VI-81. The answer is D. *(Chap. 326)* The ECG shows ST-segment elevation in leads I, aVL, and V_3-V_6. This patient is presenting in cardiogenic shock in the setting of acute anterior myocardial infarction (MI), likely due to occlusion of the left anterior descending coronary artery. Cardiogenic shock is characterized by systemic hypoperfusion due to depression of the cardiac index and sustained arterial hypotension despite an elevated filling pressure. The incidence of cardiogenic shock was as high as 20% in the 1960s. Over time, this has decreased to about 5%–7% in the setting of early reperfusion therapy for acute myocardial infarction (MI). The cause of cardiogenic shock in acute MI is primarily due to left ventricular pump failure in approximately 80% of cases but can be associated with acute mitral regurgitation in the setting of papillary muscle dysfunction, ventricular septal rupture, right ventricular failure in inferior MI, or free wall rupture. Only 25% of patients who develop cardiogenic shock in the setting of acute MI will present already in shock. Another 25% will develop it within the first 6 hours after presentation. The other 50% of individuals who develop cardiogenic shock in acute MI will develop it after this time point. Rapid recognition and treatment of the underlying myocardial ischemia are the most important tools in the management of patients with acute MI and cardiogenic shock. Supportive measures include providing adequate volume to maintain left ventricular filling pressure and treatment of pain while avoiding medications that have negative inotropic effects. Mechanical ventilation is commonly required to prevent hypoxemia. Augmentation of blood pressure to maintain cardiac perfusion is often required. No vasopressor agent has been shown to change the outcome of patients in established cardiogenic shock. Norepinephrine is a potent vasoconstrictor and inotropic agent. In a trial comparing norepinephrine with dopamine, norepinephrine was associated with fewer adverse events, including arrhythmias. Given the relative safety compared to dopamine, norepinephrine is the preferred initial agent for blood pressure support. Dopamine should be a second-line agent in this patient given the presence of ventricular ectopy and tachycardia because dopamine is associated with the development of tachyarrhythmias. Vasopressin is a potent vasoconstrictor and may be considered in only low doses in the treatment of shock. Doses greater than 0.03 U/min have been associated with coronary and mesenteric ischemia. Nitroglycerin as a continuous drip may be considered for venodilation and management of the patient's pain. However, it would be expected to decrease blood pressure and should not be used in the absence of other means of circulatory support. Of the options listed, the best choice for circulatory support in this patient is the placement of an intra-aortic balloon pump. This temporary percutaneous device is inserted into the aorta via the femoral artery, and the balloon is expanded during ventricular diastole to maintain coronary artery perfusion pressure. During systole, the rapid deflation of the blood provides effective afterload reduction to support a failing heart. Venoarterial extracorporeal membrane oxygenation is rarely used for acute MI but may be considered when respiratory failure complicates cardiogenic shock.

VI-82. The answer is A. *(Chap. 326)* The patient has evidence of decompensated ischemic cardiomyopathy with marked volume overload, pulmonary edema, and cardiogenic shock. Initial management of this patient includes maintenance of adequate oxygenation and circulatory support while initiating diuresis. Figure VI-82 outlines the optimal treatment for acute pulmonary edema. Oxygenation should be maintained, and intubation with mechanical ventilation is frequently required. The combination of nitroglycerin and morphine provides venodilation and decreases venous return and, in turn, decreases the work of breathing. Morphine further provides symptomatic relief of dyspnea and anxiety. Furosemide or other loop diuretics should be administered at the equivalent furosemide dose of 0.5–1.0 mg/kg. Norepinephrine may be required when the systolic blood pressure is less than 100 mmHg to maintain a mean arterial pressure of 60 mmHg. Dobutamine is a positive inotropic agent that is often used for cardiogenic shock but may acutely cause a decline in blood pressure. It should be considered when the systolic blood pressure is 70–100 mmHg without signs and symptoms of shock.

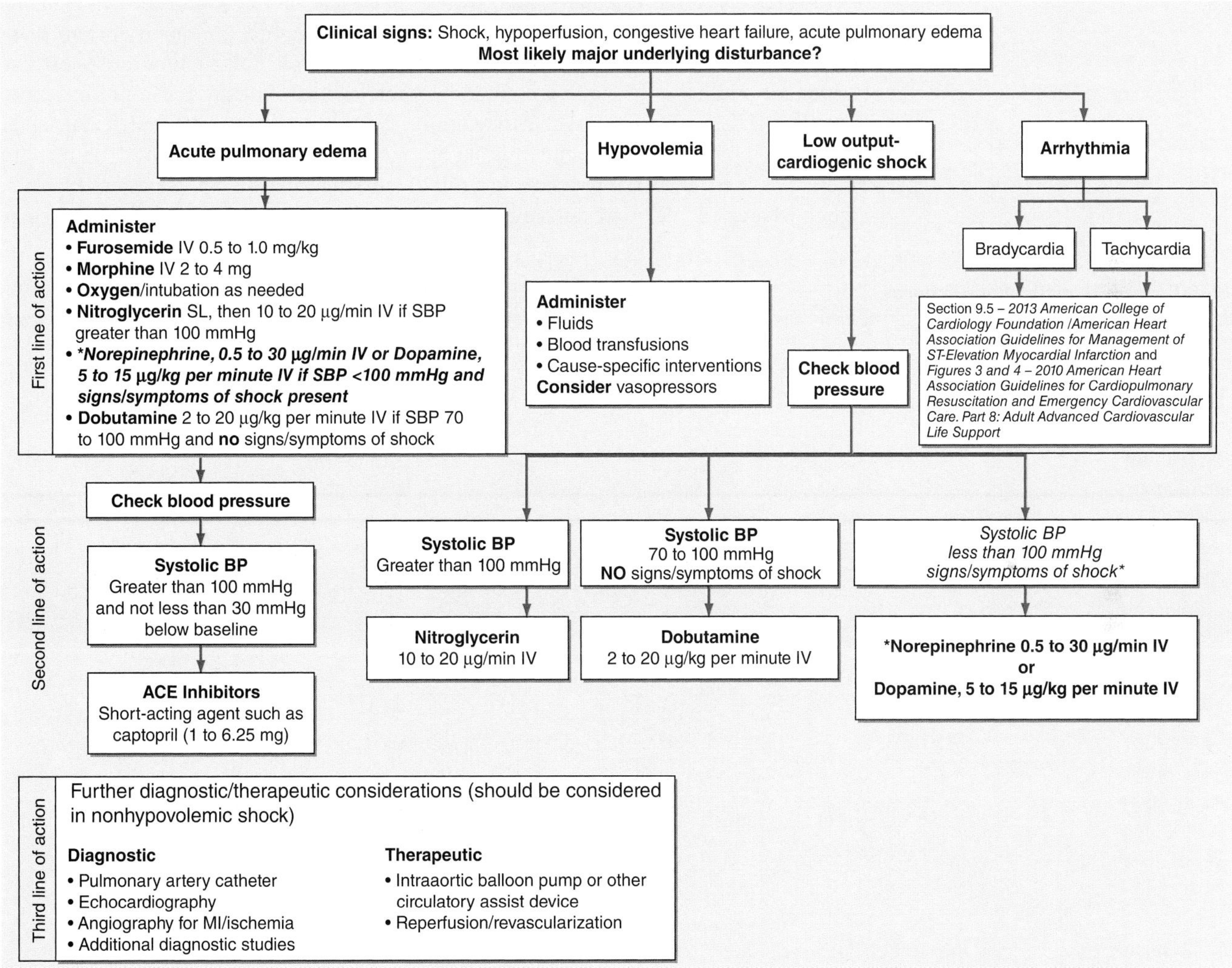

FIGURE VI-82 ACE, angiotensin-converting enzyme inhibitors; BP, blood pressure; IV, intravenous; SBP, systolic blood pressure; SL, sublingual. Modified from Guidelines 2000 for Cardiopulmonary Resuscitation and Emergency Cardiovascular Care. Part 7: The era of reperfusion: Section 1: Acute coronary syndromes [acute myocardial infarction]. The American Heart Association in collaboration with the International Liaison Committee on Resuscitation. *Circulation* 102:I172, 2000.

VI-83. The answer is C. *(Chap. 326)* Table VI-83 outlines the hemodynamic patterns that can be seen in various forms of shock, including shock caused by a variety of complications of acute MI. This patient presents with acute hypotension following a coronary revascularization procedure for acute anterior MI. Acute severe mitral regurgitation can occur following acute MI due to papillary muscle dysfunction and rupture, resulting in cardiogenic shock and/or pulmonary edema. This complication most often occurs within the first day after an MI, although there is a second peak of occurrence several days after MI. Other complications that can occur after MI resulting in rapid development of hypotension and cardiogenic shock include ventricular septal rupture, cardiac tamponade, and free wall rupture. It is important to understand the hemodynamics of these complications as well as other causes of shock, although clinically, pulmonary artery catheters are used less frequently these days because their use has not been associated with improvements in care. Normal values (option B) are shown in the top most portion of the table and are important for general knowledge regarding the circulatory system. A patient with acute mitral regurgitation (option C) would have normal to elevated right atrial pressure and elevations in the right ventricular systolic pressure and pulmonary artery pressures, although right ventricular diastolic pressure may be normal or elevated. The most characteristic finding is an elevation in the pulmonary capillary wedge pressure (PCWP) with a prominent v wave. The large v wave represents the pressure generated during systole across the regurgitant mitral valve. Cardiac index would be low normal to low, with normal to elevated systemic vascular resistance. Individuals with cardiac tamponade demonstrate equalization of pressures across the vascular system with a low cardiac index (option E). This is manifest as right atrial pressure, right ventricular diastolic pressure, pulmonary artery diastolic pressure, and PCWP all manifesting similar values. Free wall rupture causes cardiac tamponade and has a dramatic presentation, often leading to death. It can present more subacutely if the pericardium is able to temporarily seal the rupture site. Ventricular septal rupture presents similarly to acute mitral regurgitation. However, the hemodynamics are different as the right atrial pressure and right ventricular diastolic pressure are typically higher, whereas PCWP may not be as elevated. Cardiogenic shock with right ventricular

TABLE VI-83 Hemodynamic Patterns[a]

	RA, mmHg	RVS, mmHg	RVD, mmHg	PAS, mmHg	PAD, mmHg	PCW, mmHg	CI, (L/min)/m^2	SVR, (dyn · s)/cm^5
Normal values	<6	<25	0–12	<25	0–12	<6–12	≥2.5	(800–1600)
MI without pulmonary edema[b]	–	–	–	–	–	~13 (5–18)	~2.7 (2.2–4.3)	–
Pulmonary edema	↔↑	↔↑	↔↑	↑	↑	↑	↔↓	↑
Cardiogenic shock								
LV failure	↔↑	↔↑	↔↑	↔↑	↑	↑	↓	↔↑
RV failure[c]	↑	↓↔↑[d]	↑	↓↔↑[d]	↔↓↑[d]	↓↔↑[d]	↓	↑
Cardiac tamponade	↑	↔↑	↑	↔↑	↔↑	↔↑	↓	↑
Acute mitral regurgitation	↔↑	↑	↔↑	↑	↑	↑	↔↓	↔↑
Ventricular septal rupture	↑	↔↑	↑	↔↑	↔↑	↔↑	↑PBF ↓SBF	↔↑
Hypovolemic shock	↓	↔↓	↔↓	↓	↓	↓	↓	↑
Septic shock	↓	↔↓	↔↓	↓	↓	↓	↑	↓

[a]There is significant patient-to-patient variation. Pressure may be normalized if cardiac output is low.
[b]Forrester et al classified nonreperfused MI patients into four hemodynamic subsets. (From JS Forrester et al: *N Engl J Med* 295:1356, 1976.) PCW pressure and CI in clinically stable subset 1 patients are shown. Values in parentheses represent range.
[c]"Isolated" or predominant RV failure.
[d]PCW and pulmonary artery pressures may rise in RV failure after volume loading due to RV dilation and right-to-left shift of the interventricular septum, resulting in impaired LV filling. When biventricular failure is present, the patterns are similar to those shown for LV failure.
Abbreviations: CI, cardiac index; MI, myocardial infarction; P/SBF, pulmonary/systemic blood flow; PAS/D, pulmonary artery systolic/diastolic; PCW, pulmonary capillary wedge; RA, right atrium; RVS/D, right ventricular systolic/diastolic; SVR, systemic vascular resistance.
Source: Table prepared with the assistance of Krishnan Ramanathan, MD.

failure that can occur following inferior MI or pulmonary embolus will demonstrate a low cardiac index and elevated right atrial and right ventricular diastolic pressures with a wedge pressure that may be low, normal, or elevated (option D). The patient presenting with elevated cardiac output and low right atrial and ventricular pressures as well as low PCWP is most typical of a patient with septic shock.

VI-84. The answer is B. *(Chap. 327)* Sudden cardiac death (SCD) is responsible for between 200,000 and 450,000 deaths yearly in the United States. SCD is defined as natural death due to cardiac causes with presentation within 1 hour or less from a change heralding the onset of the terminal clinical event and the onset of cardiac arrest. In an individual who experiences an unwitnessed death, pathologists may expand the definition to up to 24 hours after the individual was last seen to be alive and stable. If an individual is successfully resuscitated from SCD, he or she would still be classified as SCD if death occurs during the initial hospitalization or within 30 days of the resuscitated cardiac event. In two-thirds of individuals, SCD is the first clinical expression of underlying cardiac disease, and up to half of all cardiac deaths are sudden and unexpected. SCD can occur due to primary arrhythmia, arrhythmia induced following an acute cardiac event, a structural abnormality following a prior cardiac event, or acute low-output states that may occur due to acute pulmonary embolism, ruptured aortic aneurysm, anaphylaxis, and cardiac tamponade, among other causes. There is a peak in sudden, unexpected deaths between birth and 6 months of age (sudden infant death syndrome), with a second peak that occurs between the ages of 45 and 75 years with an incidence of 1–2 per 1000 per year. Individuals of African American descent have a higher incidence of SCD compared to the white population. Young and middle-aged men have a higher risk of SCD compared to women, but with advancing age, the gender differences in SCD disappear. Genetic factors also play a role in the risk for SCD because having a parental history of SCD as an initial presentation of cardiac disease increases the likelihood of a similar event in offspring. Other risk factors include those of cardiac disease, including smoking, diabetes, hyperlipidemia, and hypertension. In the past, ventricular fibrillation and ventricular tachycardia were the most common arrhythmias seen in patients experiencing SCD. However, asystole currently accounts for about 50% of all cases of SCD. Prognosis and outcome depend on the underlying etiology of the event. Ventricular tachycardia and ventricular fibrillation have significantly better outcomes when compared to individuals who present with asystole or pulseless electrical activity.

VI-85. The answer is D. *(Chap. 328)* Coma is a surprisingly common medical condition that is responsible for a large number of admissions to emergency and critical care units. Coma refers to a deep sleeplike state from which a patient cannot be aroused. It occurs on a continuum of disorders of decreased alertness that includes stupor, in which a patient can be transiently aroused with vigorous stimulation and with generally purposeful response to painful stimuli. Drowsiness is a light state of decreased alertness that is similar to light sleep. A patient can be aroused easily, and alertness typically persists for a period after arousal. There are multiple etiologies of coma and several disorders that can cause unresponsiveness that can be confused with coma. Some of the common causes of coma include drug intoxications, metabolic derangements, severe systemic infections, shock, seizures, hypertensive encephalopathy, concussion, meningitis, encephalitis, intracranial hemorrhage, and intracranial mass lesions, among others. One condition that is often confused with coma is the persistent vegetative state. A vegetative state refers to someone who has emerged from coma with an awake appearance but is unresponsive. There are few, if any, meaningful responses to stimuli from the environment. Persistent vegetative state occurs following significant damage to both cerebral hemispheres with preservation of brainstem function. It occurs most commonly following cardiac arrest or traumatic brain injury. A minimally conscious state is similar to the persistent vegetative state but less severe. The patient appears awake, can make rudimentary vocalizations, and may have some purposeful motor behaviors, occasionally in response to commands. Other syndromes that can mimic coma include akinetic mutism, catatonia, and locked-in state. Akinetic mutism occurs due to extreme hydrocephalus or damage to the medial thalamic nuclei or frontal lobes. In akinetic mutism, the patient appears awake and is able to think and form memories but is unable to move or speak. Upon recovery, the patient can recount events from the period of the mutism. Catatonia usually occurs in individuals with severe psychiatric illness. Patients make few voluntary or responsive movements, although they do not appear distressed. On careful examination, it usually becomes apparent the patient is responsive. Eyes will move with head rotation, and the patient will blink with a visual threat. Other subtle signs may be present as well. Locked-in syndrome occurs following an injury to the ventral pons. In this setting, the patient has normal cerebral function but has no means to produce speech or movement. The only movements a patient will have are voluntary vertical movement of the eyes and lid elevation.

VI-86. **The answer is B.** *(Chap. 328)* Figure VI-86 shows a large left-sided subdural hematoma with compression of the upper midbrain and lower thalamic regions. The regions are displaced away from the mass, and there is transtentorial uncal herniation of the medial temporal lobe. Cerebral herniation occurs when brain is displaced by an adjacent mass into a contiguous compartment that it does not occupy. There are several types of brain herniation: uncal, central, transfalcical, and foraminal. The most common type is uncal herniation, which occurs when brain is displaced across the tentorium from the supratentorial to infratentorial compartment. The uncus (anterior medial temporal gyrus) moves into the tentorial opening just anterior and adjacent to the midbrain. This causes compression of the ipsilateral third nerve with subsequent enlargement of the ipsilateral pupil. Coma is caused by compression of the midbrain against the opposite tentorial edge. Lateral displacement of the midbrain may also cause compression of the opposite cerebral peduncle causing a contralateral hemiparesis and Babinski sign. Central transtentorial herniation causes a symmetric displacement of the thalamic structures through the tentorial opening, compressing the midbrain. Miotic pupils and decreased alertness occur as opposed to enlargement of a single pupil with uncal herniation. As both central and uncal herniation progress, there is a similar progression of clinical signs with progressive dysfunction of the midbrain, pons, and finally, the medulla. Transfalcical herniation occurs when cingulate gyrus is displaced under the falx and across the midline. Foraminal herniation occurs when the cerebellar tonsils are forced into the foramen magnum and results in rapid death due to compression of the respiratory center.

VI-87. **The answer is C.** *(Chap. 328)* The coma in this patient is caused by drug intoxication, most likely tricyclic antidepressant overdose. Coma is commonly caused by drug intoxications and compounded by the resulting metabolic derangements. Because the patient is unresponsive, it is not possible to obtain a medical history, but family members and friends should be queried to assist with determining a possible cause. This patient has had recent depression, which could potentially indicate use of antidepressant medications and also increased suicide risk. Tricyclic antidepressants exert an anticholinergic effect. Common symptoms include an alerted level of consciousness, cardiac conduction abnormalities, arrhythmias, and evidence of anticholinergic activity including elevated temperature, flushing, and dilated pupils. If cardiac conduction delays are present, sodium bicarbonate should be given. Other supportive care includes use of intravenous fluids and management of agitation.

VI-88. **The answer is E.** *(Chap. 328)* Brain death refers to the irreversible loss of all cerebral and brainstem function. Cardiac activity is preserved, and respiration is maintained only by artificial means. In Western society, brain death is considered equivalent to death, and the respirator can be disconnected to allow cardiac death to occur. Careful examination of a patient needs to be performed to assess when brain death has occurred. At the time of examination, the patient needs to be normothermic and have been without treatment with sedative medications for at least 6–24 hours. Patients should also be maintaining a systolic blood pressure >100 mmHg and be euvolemic. Ideal criteria are simple, can be assessed at the bedside, and should have no chance of diagnostic error. Three essential elements of brain death include:

1. Widespread cortical destruction identified by coma and unresponsiveness to all stimuli.
2. Global brainstem damage evidenced by absent pupillary light reflexes and loss of oculovestibular and corneal reflexes
3. Loss of medullary function with complete and irreversible apnea

The pupils are usually mid-sized, but can be enlarged. However, they should not be miotic. Deep tendon reflexes may be present, and Babinski response is usually absent or flexor. The apnea test is performed by preoxygenating a patient with 100% FiO_2 for up to 10 minutes, with oxygen delivered via transtracheal cannula throughout the test. The patient remains off the ventilator for 8–10 minutes, and signs of respiration are observed. At the end of the test, an arterial blood gas is performed to demonstrate that $PaCO_2$ has risen to 50–60 mmHg. Apnea is confirmed if there is no evidence of respiration when the $PaCO_2$ has risen to a level that should have stimulated respiration. The apnea test should be terminated if the patient develops cardiovascular instability. Other ancillary tests are sometimes performed in patients who cannot undergo clinical testing of brain death. Examples of scenarios in which ancillary tests may be useful include patients who are hemodynamically unstable, patients with diseases causing baseline carbon dioxide retention, and in the presence of prior sedation or neuromuscular blocking agents. The purpose of ancillary testing is to demonstrate lack of cerebral blood flow, and ancillary testing can include radionuclide brain imaging, cerebral angiography, and/or transcranial Doppler measurements.

VI-89. The answer is B. *(Chap. 330)* Monitoring intracranial pressure (ICP) is an important tool in the care of selected critically ill patients due to neurologic injury or disease. ICP can be monitored by ventriculostomy, intraparenchymal transducer, epidural catheter, or subarachnoid catheters. Epidural or subarachnoid catheters are less reliable and are less frequently used. Ventriculostomy is considered the "gold standard" for ICP monitoring because it offers the advantage of providing a means of cerebrospinal fluid drainage in the event of elevated ICP. In addition, ventriculostomy monitoring also provides greater accuracy because it has the ability to be recalibrated, whereas the intraparenchymal monitor does not. Patients who are most likely to be considered for ICP monitoring are those with severe primary neurologic disorders, including severe traumatic brain injury (Glasgow Coma Scale ≤8), large tissue shifts from supratentorial ischemic or hemorrhagic stroke, intraventricular hemorrhage, or posterior fossa stroke. Individuals with fulminant hepatic failure are also at risk for severe cerebral edema leading to herniation. ICP monitoring is recommended for these individuals, although intraparenchymal monitoring is often more appropriate than ventriculostomy due to the presence of coagulopathy. These patients are at particularly high risk of bleeding. In addition, individuals with diffuse cerebral edema, such as in fulminant hepatic failure, typically have small ventricles leading to difficulty in placement.

VI-90. The answer is D. *(Chap. 330)* The primary goal of ICP monitoring in patients with severe neurologic injury and elevated ICP is to maintain adequate cerebral perfusion pressure (CPP). CPP is calculated as mean arterial pressure minus the ICP, and the goal CPP is ≥60 mmHg. Normal ICP is <20 mmHg. Thus, this patient is showing evidence of marked elevations in ICP with a CPP of 58 mmHg. When ICP remains elevated for more than 5 minutes, therapy should be undertaken to decrease the ICP. It is important to consider the underlying cause of ICP in an individual when determining treatment plan. In patients with hydrocephalus or subarachnoid hemorrhage, draining cerebrospinal fluid via the ventriculostomy will decrease the ICP. In patients with more diffuse cerebral edema from head trauma or stroke, medical approaches are more appropriate. This patient has hydrocephalus due to subarachnoid bleeding. Therefore, the first line of treatment should be to drain the ventriculostomy. If this fails to adequately alleviate the elevations in ICP, other treatment modalities including osmolar therapy, sedation, hyperventilation, or vasopressors to increase mean arterial pressure can be considered. There are two osmolar therapies that are frequently used: mannitol or 23.4% saline bolus. Deep sedation may be required, and a variety of agents may be used. Neuromuscular blockade may be used as well. Hyperventilation to drop the $PaCO_2$ to 30–35 mmHg works acutely to drop the ICP, but the effect is limited. Vasopressors can be considered to increase the mean arterial pressure and thus ensure an improved CPP. Glucocorticoids are best used in individuals with vasogenic edema from tumor or abscess. In those with refractory elevations in ICP, decompressive craniectomy, high-dose barbiturate therapy, or hypothermia may also be employed.

VI-91. The answer is C. *(Chap. 330)* Therapeutic hypothermia refers to the purposeful induction of hypothermia to temperatures of 32–34°C, and it is primarily used following cardiac arrest. The rationale for use of therapeutic hypothermia is to provide a neuroprotective effect to limit neuronal cell injury and death following a substantial hypoxic insult. Initially, two trials suggested that use of therapeutic hypothermia would improve functional outcomes in patients who remained comatose after resuscitation from cardiac arrest. Subsequent trials showed no significant difference in neurologic outcomes if the temperature was maintained at 32°C or 36°C so long as development of fever was prevented. Treatment guidelines currently support therapeutic hypothermia for 12–24 hours when the initial rhythm was ventricular fibrillation. While cerebral edema is a common complication of cardiac arrest and a leading cause of death, there is no recommendation to perform head imaging prior to initiating therapeutic hypothermia. Complications of therapeutic hypothermia include coagulopathy and increased risk of infection.

VI-92. The answer is B. *(Chap. 330)* Critical illness polyneuropathy is the most common peripheral nervous system complication of critical illness. Prior studies have shown that as many as 70% of individuals hospitalized in intensive care units with sepsis develop critical illness polyneuropathy. The clinical presentation of critical illness polyneuropathy is diffuse weakness with decreased deep tendon reflexes and distal sensory loss. On electrophysiologic testing, a diffuse, symmetric distal axonal sensorimotor neuropathy is seen. The cause of critical illness polyneuropathy is not known but is postulated to be due to circulating inflammatory cytokines that are commonly elevated is sepsis and other critical illness. Risk factors for development of the syndrome include sepsis, prolonged critical illness, and multiorgan system failure. In severe cases, critical illness polyneuropathy can lead to decreased respiratory muscle strength and can contribute to prolonged ventilator dependence. Treatment is supportive, and recovery is spontaneous, although it may take weeks to months for full recovery.

Critical illness myopathy is a term used to describe several discrete muscular disorders in critically ill individuals. It is less common than critical illness polyneuropathy and may have elevated levels of serum creatine kinase. As disease progresses, electromyography can show abnormal spontaneous activity. Muscle biopsy is variable, with results ranging from type II atrophy to panfascicular necrosis. This patient does not show evidence of fibroproliferative progression of acute respiratory distress syndrome as the chest radiograph shows clearing of infiltrates. The patient also requires minimal ventilatory support with good tidal volumes. Guillain-Barré syndrome is an acute demyelinating polyneuropathy that presents as a cause of respiratory failure and is not present in this case. ICU delirium is a common complication of ICU care but should not result in low tidal volumes when ventilatory support is decreased.

VI-93 and VI-94. The answers are E and E, respectively. *(Chap. 330)* Nontraumatic subarachnoid hemorrhage (SAH) occurs most commonly following rupture of a saccular, or berry, aneurysm. Autopsy and angiography studies have identified aneurysms in 2% of the adult population, affecting 4 million individuals. The yearly incidence of SAH due to aneurysmal rupture is 20,000–30,000 cases. Many patients die before reaching the hospital. If a patient survives to hospital admission, the 28-day mortality rate is 45%. More than half of individuals who survive have significant neurologic injury with lingering manifestations. The patient with SAH should be admitted to a critical care unit with expertise in managing SAH. Initial treatment of SAH includes early aneurysmal repair while managing intracranial hypertension. Repair of the aneurysm may be accomplished via neurosurgical clipping or endovascular coiling of the aneurysm. Generally coiling has shown improved functional outcomes in those undergoing endovascular procedures. Medical management is complex. Intracranial hypertension is common and frequently requires management with ventriculostomy. Medical management of elevated intracranial pressures is also often required. If a patient survives the initial period following SAH, the patient is vulnerable to several causes of delayed neurologic deficits that typically present within 1–2 weeks after the event. Vasospasm refers to the narrowing of the arteries at the base of the brain following SAH and is the most common cause of delayed morbidity and mortality in SAH. Signs of ischemic injury and change in neurologic exam herald the development of vasospasm. Nimodipine is typically prescribed at a dose of 60 mg every 4 hours upon admission to the ICU to attempt to prevent vasospasm. Vasospasm can be detected by x-ray angiography or transcranial Doppler ultrasound. Surveillance for vasospasm is often performed via transcranial Doppler ultrasound on a daily or every-other-day basis.

In addition to nimodipine, management of acute vasospasm includes raising cerebral perfusion pressure and volume expansion. Phenylephrine and norepinephrine are the most frequently used vasopressors. If vasospasm is refractory to these treatments, intra-arterial vasodilators and/or percutaneous transluminal angioplasty should be considered. Other causes of delayed neurologic deficits following SAH include rerupture of the aneurysm, hydrocephalus, and hyponatremia. The incidence of rerupture of an aneurysm is ~30% in the first month after presentation, with a peak incidence within the first 7 days. Mortality associated with rerupture is 60%. Early endovascular coiling or surgical clipping of the aneurysm decreases the incidence of rerupture. Hydrocephalus can occur acutely or subacutely after SAH. Subacute development of hydrocephalus is more common and presents over a few days or weeks with progressive drowsiness, incontinence, and slowed mentation. The patient in this scenario had a CT scan that did not show increasing blood, cerebral edema, or development of hydrocephalus. Hyponatremia occurs following SAH due to natriuresis and volume depletion. Electrolytes are typically assessed at least twice daily following SAH as hyponatremia can develop fairly acutely.

VI-95 and VI-96. **The answers are E and C, respectively.** *(Chap. 331)* This clinical scenario describes an individual with superior vena cava (SVC) syndrome, which is an oncologic emergency. Eighty-five percent of cases of SVC syndrome are caused by either small-cell or squamous cell cancer of the lung. Other causes of SVC syndrome include lymphoma, aortic aneurysm, thyromegaly, fibrosing mediastinitis, thrombosis, histoplasmosis, and Behcet syndrome. The typical clinical presentation is dyspnea, cough, and facial and neck swelling. Symptoms are worsened by lying flat or bending forward. As the swelling progresses, it can lead to glossal and laryngeal edema with symptoms of hoarseness and dysphagia. Other symptoms can include headaches, nasal congestion, pain, dizziness, and syncope. In rare cases, seizures can occur from cerebral edema, although this is more commonly associated with brain metastases. On physical examination, dilated neck veins with collateralization on the anterior chest wall are frequently seen. There is also facial and upper extremity edema associated with cyanosis. The diagnosis of SVC syndrome is a clinical diagnosis. A pleural effusion is seen in about 25% of cases, more commonly on the right. A chest CT would demonstrate decreased or absent contrast in the central veins with prominent collateral circulation and would help elucidate the cause. Most commonly, this would be mediastinal adenopathy or a large central tumor obstructing venous flow. The immediate treatment of SVC syndrome includes oxygen, elevation of the head of the bed, and administration of diuretics in combination with a low-sodium diet. Conservative treatment alone often provides adequate relief of symptoms and allows determination of the underlying cause of the obstruction. In this case, this would include histologic confirmation of cell type of the tumor to provide more definitive therapy. Radiation therapy is the most common treatment modality and can be used in an emergent situation if conservative treatment fails to provide relief to the patient.

VI-97. **The answer is A.** *(Chap. 331)* This patient presents with symptoms of spinal cord compression in the setting of known stage IV breast cancer. This represents an oncologic emergency as only 10% of patients presenting with paraplegia regain the ability to walk. Most commonly, patients develop symptoms of localized back pain and tenderness days to months before developing paraplegia. The pain is worsened by movement, cough, or sneezing. In contrast to radicular pain, the pain related to spinal cord metastases is worse with lying down. Patients presenting with back pain alone should have a careful examination to attempt to localize the lesion prior to development of more severe neurologic symptoms. In this patient with paraplegia, there is a definitive level at which sensation is diminished. This level is typically one to two vertebrae below the site of compression. Other findings include spasticity, weakness, and increased deep tendon reflexes. In those with autonomic dysfunction, bowel and bladder incontinence will occur with decreased anal tone, absence of the anal wink and bulbocavernosus reflexes, and bladder distention. The most important initial step is the administration of high-dose intravenous corticosteroids to minimize associated swelling around the lesion and prevent paraplegia while allowing further evaluation and treatment. Magnetic resonance imaging (MRI) should be performed of the entire spinal cord to evaluate for other metastatic disease that may require therapy. Although a brain MRI may be indicated in the future to evaluate for brain metastases, it is not required in the initial evaluation because the bilateral nature of the patient's symptoms and sensory level clearly indicate the spinal cord as the site of the injury. Once an MRI is performed, a definitive treatment plan can be made. Most commonly, radiation therapy is used with or without surgical decompression.

VI-98 and VI-99. The answers are B and E, respectively. *(Chap. 331)* Tumor lysis syndrome occurs most commonly in individuals undergoing chemotherapy for rapidly proliferating malignancies, including acute leukemias and Burkitt lymphoma. In rare instances, it can be seen in chronic lymphoma or solid tumors. As the chemotherapeutic agents act on these cells, there is massive tumor lysis that results in release of intracellular ions and nucleic acids. This leads to a characteristic metabolic syndrome of hyperuricemia, hyperphosphatemia, hyperkalemia, and hypocalcemia. Acute kidney injury is frequent and can lead to renal failure requiring hemodialysis if uric acid crystallizes within the renal tubules. Lactic acidosis and dehydration increase the risk of acute kidney injury. Hyperphosphatemia occurs due to the release of intracellular phosphate ions and causes a reciprocal reduction in serum calcium. This hypocalcemia can be profound, leading to neuromuscular irritability and tetany. Hyperkalemia can become rapidly life-threatening and cause ventricular arrhythmia. Knowing the characteristics of tumor lysis syndrome, one can attempt to prevent the known complications from occurring. It is important to monitor serum electrolytes frequently during treatment. Laboratory studies should be obtained no less than three times daily, but more frequent monitoring is often needed. Allopurinol should be administered prophylactically at high doses. If allopurinol fails to control uric acid to less than 8 mg/dL, rasburicase, a recombinant urate oxidase, can be added at a dose of 0.2 mg/kg. Throughout this period, the patient should be well hydrated with alkalinization of the urine to a pH of greater than 7.0. This is accomplished by administration of intravenous normal or half-normal saline at a dose of 3000 mL/m^2 daily with sodium bicarbonate. Prophylactic hemodialysis is not performed unless there is underlying renal failure prior to starting chemotherapy.

SECTION VII

Disorders of the Kidney and Urinary Tract

QUESTIONS

DIRECTIONS: Choose the one best response to each question.

VII-1. Which of the following is a potential etiology for ischemic acute renal failure?

A. Apoptosis and necrosis of tubular cells
B. Decreased glomerular vasodilation in response to nitric oxide
C. Increased glomerular vasoconstriction in response to elevated endothelin levels
D. Increased leukocyte adhesion within the glomerulus
E. All of the above

VII-2. All of the following are risk factors for postoperative acute kidney injury EXCEPT:

A. Cardiac surgery with cardiopulmonary bypass
B. Diabetes mellitus
C. Female sex
D. Intraoperative hypotension
E. Significant operative blood loss

VII-3. A 57-year-old man with a history of diabetes mellitus and chronic kidney disease with a baseline creatinine of 1.8 mg/dL underwent cardiac catheterization for acute myocardial infarction. He is subsequently diagnosed with acute kidney injury related to iodinated contrast. All of the following statements are true regarding his acute kidney injury EXCEPT:

A. Fractional excretion of sodium will be low.
B. His creatinine is likely to peak within 3–5 days.
C. His diabetes mellitus predisposed him to develop contrast nephropathy.
D. Transient tubule obstruction with precipitated iodinated contrast contributed to development of his acute kidney injury.
E. White blood cell casts are likely on microscopic examination of urinary sediment.

VII-4. Which of the following acute kidney injury patients is most likely to have evidence of bilateral hydronephrosis on ultrasound evaluation of the kidneys?

A. A 19-year-old man with purpura fulminans associated with gonococcal sepsis
B. A 37-year-old woman undergoing chemotherapy and radiation for advanced cervical cancer
C. A 48-year-old man with chronic renal insufficiency due to hypertension that received iodinated contrast for an abdominal angiogram
D. A 53-year-old man with *Escherichia coli* 0157:H7 associated thrombotic thrombocytopenic purpura
E. An 85-year-old woman who resides in a nursing home with pyelonephritis and sepsis

VII-5. In evaluation for acute kidney injury in a patient who has recently undergone cardiopulmonary bypass during mitral valve replacement, which of the following findings on urine microscopy is most suggestive of cholesterol emboli as the source of renal failure?

A. Calcium oxalate crystals
B. Eosinophiluria
C. Granular casts
D. Normal sediment
E. White blood cell casts

VII-6. A 54-year-old man is admitted to the medical intensive care unit with sepsis associated with pneumococcal pneumonia. He requires mechanical ventilation as well as norepinephrine to maintain a mean arterial pressure >60 mmHg. Invasive hemodynamics show adequate left heart filling pressures, and he is not known to have left ventricular dysfunction. On the third hospital day, his urine output drops and creatinine increases to 3.4 mg/dL. Acute tubular injury is diagnosed. Which of the following agents has been shown to improve outcomes associated with his acute tubular injury?

A. Furosemide
B. Bosentan
C. Low-dose dopamine
D. Insulin-like growth factor
E. None of the above

VII-7. It is hospital day 5 for a 65-year-old patient with prerenal azotemia secondary to dehydration. His creatinine was initially 3.6 mg/dL on admission, but it has improved today to 2.1 mg/dL. He complains of mild lower back pain, and you prescribe naproxen to be taken intermittently. By what mechanism might this drug further impair his renal function?

A. Afferent arteriolar vasoconstriction
B. Afferent arteriolar vasodilatation
C. Efferent arteriolar vasoconstriction
D. Proximal tubular toxicity
E. Ureteral obstruction

VII-8. Which of the following tissue injury biomarkers has been shown to predict the onset of acute kidney injury after an ischemic or hypotensive event?

A. Blood urea nitrogen (BUN)
B. Interleukin-18
C. Kidney injury molecule-1 (KIM-1)
D. Neutrophil gelatinase-associated lipocalin (NGAL)
E. None of the above

VII-9. Which of the following patients has the greatest risk of progression to chronic kidney disease?

A. A 30-year-old man with an estimated glomerular filtration rate (GFR) of 50 mL/min/1.73 m^2 and 350 mg/g of persistent albuminuria
B. A 45-year-old man with an estimated GFR of 90 mL/min/1.73 m^2 and <30 mg/g of persistent albuminuria
C. A 55-year-old man with an estimated GFR of 70 mL/min/1.73 m^2 and 100 mg/g of persistent albuminuria
D. A 65-year-old woman with an estimated GFR of 65 mL/min/1.73 m^2 and <30 mg/g of persistent albuminuria
E. A 75-year-old man with an estimated GFR of 35 mL/min/1.73 m^2 and <30 mg/g of persistent albuminuria

VII-10. In stage V chronic kidney disease, glomerular filtration rate is below which of the following levels?

A. 90 mL/min/1.73 m^2
B. 60 mL/min/1.73 m^2
C. 25 mL/min/1.73 m^2
D. 15 mL/min/1.73 m^2
E. 0 mL/min/1.73 m^2 (anuria)

VII-11. What is the leading cause of death in patients with chronic kidney disease?

A. Cardiovascular disease
B. Hyperkalemia
C. Infection
D. Malignancy
E. Uremia

VII-12. All of the following statements regarding the use of exogenous erythropoietin in patients with chronic kidney disease are true EXCEPT:

A. Exogenous erythropoietin should be administered with a target hemoglobin concentration of 100–115 g/L.
B. Use of exogenous erythropoietin is associated with improved cardiovascular outcomes.
C. Use of exogenous erythropoietin is associated with increased risk of stroke in patients with concomitant type 2 diabetes mellitus.
D. Use of exogenous erythropoietin may be associated with faster progression to the need for dialysis.
E. Use of exogenous erythropoietin is associated with increased incidence of thromboembolic events.

VII-13. A 63-year-old woman with chronic kidney disease is maintained on daily peritoneal dialysis. Her past medical history is notable for hypertension and atrial fibrillation. Her medications include losartan and warfarin. Two days ago, she noticed a small painful nodule on her abdomen that has progressed to involve skin necrosis and ulceration of the abdominal wall (Figure VII-13). All of the following statements regarding her condition are true EXCEPT:

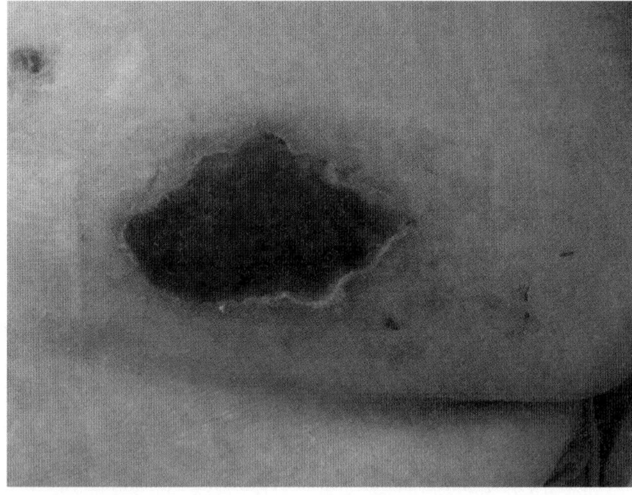

FIGURE VII-13

A. Oral calcium supplement may be a risk factor.
B. Pathologically, there is vascular occlusion.
C. *Pseudomonas* co-infection is typical.
D. Severe hyperparathyroidism may not be present.
E. Warfarin is a risk factor for development of the lesion.

VII-14. A patient is followed closely by her nephrologist for stage IV chronic kidney disease associated with focal segmental glomerulosclerosis. Which of the following is an indication for initiation of maintenance hemodialysis?

A. Acidosis controlled with daily bicarbonate administration
B. Bleeding diathesis
C. BUN >110 mg/dL without symptoms
D. Creatinine >5 mg/dL without symptoms
E. Hyperkalemia controlled with sodium polystyrene

VII-15. A 27-year-old woman with chronic kidney disease is undergoing hemodialysis and is found to be hypotensive during her treatment. Which of the following is a potential mechanism for hypotension during hemodialysis?

A. Antihypertensive agents
B. Excessive ultrafiltration
C. Impaired autonomic responses
D. Osmolar shifts
E. All of the above

VII-16. A 35-year-old woman with hypertensive kidney disease progresses to end-stage renal disease. She was initiated on peritoneal dialysis 1 year ago and has done well with relief of her uremic symptoms. She is brought to the emergency department with fever, altered mental status, diffuse abdominal pain, and cloudy dialysate. Her peritoneal fluid is withdrawn through her catheter and sent to the laboratory for analysis. The fluid white blood cell count is 125/μL with 85% polymorphonuclear neutrophils. Which organism is most likely to be found on culture of the peritoneal fluid?

A. *Candida albicans*
B. *E coli*
C. *Mycobacterium tuberculosis*
D. *Pseudomonas aeruginosa*
E. *Staphylococcus epidermidis*

VII-17. A 45-year-old woman begins hemodialysis for end-stage renal disease associated with diabetes mellitus. Which of the following is her most likely eventual cause of death?

A. Dementia
B. Major bleeding episode
C. Myocardial infarction
D. Progressive uremia
E. Sepsis

VII-18. The "dose" of dialysis is currently defined as which of the following?

A. The counter-current flow rate of the dialysate
B. The fractional urea clearance
C. The hours per week of dialysis
D. The number of sessions actually completed in a month

VII-19. Your patient with end-stage renal disease on hemodialysis has persistent hyperkalemia. He has a history of total bilateral renal artery stenosis, which is why he is on hemodialysis. He only has electrocardiogram changes when his potassium rises above 6.0 mEq/L, which occurs a few times per week. You admit him to the hospital for further evaluation. Your laboratory evaluation, nutrition counseling, and medication adjustments have not impacted his serum potassium. What is the next reasonable step to undertake for this patient?

A. Adjust the dialysate.
B. Administer a daily dose of furosemide.
C. Perform "sodium modeling."
D. Implant an automatic defibrillator.
E. Perform bilateral nephrectomy.

VII-20. Which of the following statements is true regarding kidney transplantation?

A. Five-year survival rates are similar between recipients of living donor kidneys and deceased donor kidneys.
B. Deceased donor age does not influence graft survival.
C. Renal transplantation offers no cost benefit compared to hemodialysis.
D. When first-degree relatives are donors, graft survival rate at 1 year is 5%–7% greater than deceased donors.
E. When followed for >20 years, renal complication rates in single kidney donors are common.

VII-21. All of the following are considered expanded donor criteria for renal transplantation EXCEPT:

A. Deceased donor >60 years
B. Deceased donor >50 years, hypertension, and creatinine >1.5 mg/dL
C. Deceased donor >50 years, hypertension, and death caused by cerebrovascular accident (CVA)
D. Deceased donor >50 years, death caused by CVA, and creatinine >1.5 mg/dL
E. Presence of antibodies against the donor kidney in the recipient at the time of the anticipated transplantation

VII-22. All of the following are likely causes of glomerular damage leading to renal failure EXCEPT:

A. Diabetes mellitus
B. Fanconi syndrome
C. Lupus nephritis
D. Malignant hypertension
E. Mutation of *TRPC6* cation channel

VII-23. A 21-year-old man is diagnosed with poststreptococcal glomerulonephritis. Which of the following is likely to be found in his urine?

A. >3 g/24 hr proteinuria without hematuria
B. Macroscopic hematuria and 24-hour urinary albumin of 227 mg
C. Microscopic hematuria with leukocytes and 24-hour urinary albumin of 227 mg
D. Positive urine culture for *Streptococcus*
E. Sterile pyuria without proteinuria

VII-24. A 50-year-old obese female with a 5-year history of mild hypertension controlled by a thiazide diuretic is being evaluated because proteinuria was noted on a urine dipstick during her routine yearly medical visit. Physical examination discloses a height of 167.6 cm (66 in), weight of 91 kg (202 lb), blood pressure of 130/80 mmHg, elevated jugular venous pressure, a fourth heart sound, and trace pedal edema. Laboratory values are as follows:

Serum creatinine: 106 μmol/L (1.2 mg/dL)
BUN: 6.4 mmol/L (18 mg/dL)
Creatinine clearance: 87 mL/min
Urinalysis: pH 5.0; specific gravity 1.018; protein 3+; no glucose; occasional coarse granular cast
Urine protein excretion: 5.9 g/d

A renal biopsy demonstrates that 60% of the glomeruli, mostly in the corticomedullary junction, have segmental scarring by light microscopy, with the remainder of the glomeruli appearing unremarkable. (See Figure VII-24.) What is the most likely diagnosis?

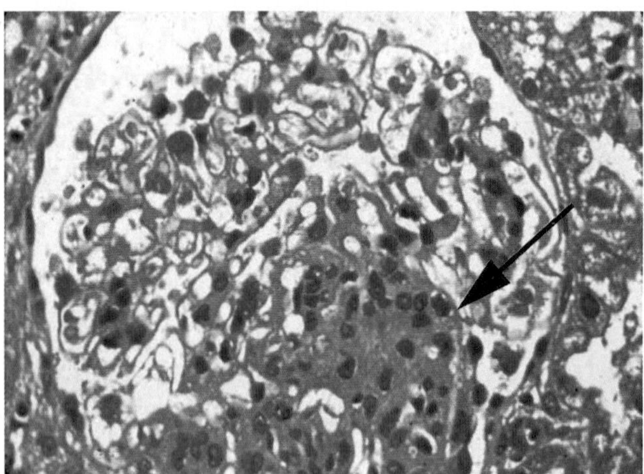

Figure VII-24 EGN/UPenn Collection.

A. Focal segmental sclerosis
B. Hypertensive nephrosclerosis
C. Minimal change (nil) disease
D. Membranous glomerulopathy
E. Crescentic glomerulonephritis

VII-25. All of the following statements regarding diabetic nephropathy are true EXCEPT:

A. Approximately 40% of patients with type 1 or type 2 diabetes will develop nephropathy.
B. Diabetic nephropathy is the single most common cause of chronic renal failure in the United States.
C. In patients with type I diabetes, control of blood sugar concentration impacts the development and progression of nephropathy.
D. Pathologic changes are predominantly in the distal tubule and loop of Henle.
E. The earliest clinically detectable indicator of diabetic nephropathy is albuminuria.

VII-26. Which of the following is an extrarenal manifestations of autosomal dominant polycystic kidney disease?

A. Aortic regurgitation
B. Aortic root dilation
C. Colonic diverticula
D. Intracranial aneurysm
E. All of the above

VII-27. A 28-year-old woman was recently diagnosed with autosomal dominant polycystic kidney disease after an episode of hematuria. She is concerned about intracranial aneurysm risk. Which of the following statements is true regarding this risk?

A. Family history of ruptured intracranial aneurysms does not increase risk of rupture.
B. Prior intracranial hemorrhage does not increase risk of subsequent hemorrhage.
C. The size of the aneurysm does not correlate with its risk of spontaneous rupture.
D. There is no increased risk of intracranial aneurysm in this condition.
E. Uncontrolled hypertension augments the risk of spontaneous rupture.

VII-28. A 21-year-old male college student is evaluated for profound fatigue that has been present for several years but has recently become debilitating. He also reports several foot spasms and cramps and occasionally sustained muscle contractions that are uncontrollable. He is otherwise healthy, takes no medications, and denies tobacco or alcohol use. On examination, he is well developed with normal vital signs including blood pressure. The remainder of the examination is normal. Laboratory evaluation shows a sodium of 138 mEq/L, potassium of 2.8 mEq/L, chloride of 90 mEq/L, and bicarbonate of 30 mmol/L. Magnesium level is normal. Urine screen for diuretics is negative, and urine chloride is elevated. Which of the following is the most likely diagnosis?

A. Bulimia nervosa
B. Diuretic abuse
C. Gitelman syndrome
D. Liddle syndrome
E. Type 1 pseudohypoaldosteronism

VII-29. A patient with a history of Sjögren syndrome has the following laboratory findings: plasma sodium 139 mEq/L, chloride 112 mEq/L, bicarbonate 15 mEq/L, and potassium 3.0 mEq/L. Urine studies show a pH of 6.0, sodium of 15 mEq/L, potassium of 10 mEq/L, and chloride of 12 mEq/L. What is the most likely diagnosis?

A. Chronic diarrhea
B. Type I renal tubular acidosis (RTA)
C. Type II RTA
D. Type III RTA
E. Type IV RTA

VII-30. A 16-year-old female star gymnast presents to your office complaining of fatigue, diffuse weakness, and muscle cramps. She has no previous medical history and denies tobacco, alcohol, or illicit drug use. There is no significant family history. Examination shows a thin female with normal blood pressure. Body mass index (BMI) is 18 kg/m^2. Oral examination shows poor dentition. Muscle tone is normal, and neurologic examination is normal. Laboratory studies show hematocrit of 38.5%, creatinine of 0.6 mg/dL, serum bicarbonate of 30 mEq/L, and potassium of 2.7 mEq/L. Further evaluation should include which of the following?

A. Plasma renin and aldosterone levels
B. Serum magnesium level
C. Urinalysis and urine culture
D. Urine toxicology screen for diuretics
E. Urine toxicology screen for opiates

VII-31. In which of the following cases would treatment with corticosteroids for biopsy-proven interstitial nephritis be most likely to impact long-term renal recovery?

A. A 37-year-old woman with sarcoidosis
B. A 48-year-old man with slowly progressing interstitial nephritis over 2 months with fibrosis found on biopsy
C. A 54-year-old man with diabetes mellitus and recent *Salmonella* infection
D. A 63-year-old man with allergic interstitial nephritis after cephalosporin antibiotic use
E. None of the above

VII-32. A 58-year-old woman undergoes a hysterectomy and postoperatively develops acute respiratory distress syndrome. She is treated with mechanical ventilation and broad-spectrum antibiotics. Aside from hypothyroidism, she has no underlying medical conditions. On day 5 of her hospitalization, her urine output is noted to fall, and her serum creatinine rises from 1.2 to 2.5 mg/dL. Allergic interstitial nephritis from cephalosporin antibiotics is suspected. Which of the following findings will confirm this diagnosis?

A. Hematuria
B. Peripheral blood eosinophilia
C. Urinary eosinophils on urine microscopy
D. White blood cell casts on urine microscopy
E. None of the above

VII-33. A 63-year-old man is admitted to the hospital with acute renal failure. He has a history of diabetes that has been well controlled for the past 10 years with diet, exercise, and metformin. Over the last 4 months, he has complained of progressive fatigue, anorexia, and diffuse bone pain. He has taken ibuprofen intermittently for the bone pain with minimal relief. His physical examination reveals normal vital signs, clear lungs, normal cardiac and abdominal examination, and diffuse bony tenderness over his hips, long bones, and spine. Laboratory examination is notable for the following results: BUN 68 mg/dL, creatine 5.8 mg/dL, potassium 4.7 mEq/L, calcium 13.4 mg/dL, hemoglobin 8 g/dL, serum protein 9.0 g/dL, and albumin 2.8 g/dL. Renal function was normal 1 year ago. A renal biopsy is performed (hematoxylin and eosin stain; Figure VII-33.) Which of the following is the most likely diagnosis?

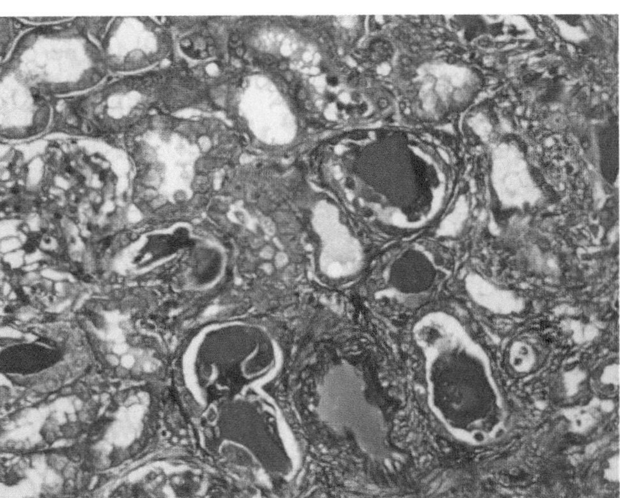

FIGURE VII-33 Courtesy of Dr. Michael N. Koss, University of Southern California Keck School of Medicine; with permission.

A. Diabetic nephropathy
B. Focal segmental glomerulosclerosis
C. Goodpasture syndrome
D. Light chain cast nephropathy
E. Lupus nephritis

VII-34. A 44-year-old obese woman undergoes elective cholecystectomy for cholelithiasis. Postoperatively she does well and is discharged after 3 days. Two days after discharge, she develops altered mental status and fever and is brought to the emergency department by her family. She takes an antidepressant but is otherwise healthy. Her temperature is 103°F, pulse is 127 bpm, blood pressure is 110/78 mmHg, and she has a normal respiratory rate and oxygen saturation. Examination is notable for confusion and a well-healed surgical incision. Routine chemistries are drawn and show normal electrolytes, BUN of 80 mg/dL, creatinine of 2.5 mg/dL, white blood cell count of 17.3 × 10^3/μL, hematocrit of 30%, and platelet count of 25 × 10^3/μL. A peripheral blood smear shows schistocytes and confirms low platelets without clumping. Which of the following statements regarding her condition is true?

A. Low activity of the metalloprotease ADAMTS13 is likely present in her peripheral blood.
B. Plasma exchange is unlikely to be helpful.
C. Her condition was likely caused by an occult *E coli* 0157:H7 infection.
D. Her condition is more common in men than women.
E. Untreated mortality from this condition is low.

VII-35. A 35-year-old woman presents with complaints of bilateral lower extremity edema, polyuria, and moderate left-sided flank pain that began approximately 2 weeks ago. There is no past medical history. She is taking no medications and denies tobacco, alcohol, or illicit drug use. Examination shows normal vital signs, including normal blood pressure. There is 2+ edema in bilateral lower extremities. The 24-hour urine collection is significant for 3.5 g of protein. Urinalysis is bland except for the proteinuria. Serum creatinine is 0.7 mg/dL, and ultrasound examination shows the left kidney measuring 13 cm and the right kidney measuring 11.5 cm. You are concerned about renal vein thrombosis. What test do you choose for the evaluation?

A. Computed tomography of the renal veins
B. Contrast venography
C. Magnetic resonance venography
D. ^{99}Tc-labeled pentetic acid (DTPA) imaging
E. Ultrasound with Doppler evaluation of the renal veins

VII-36. A 28-year-old woman who is in her 30th week of her second pregnancy has been followed closely because of mild hypertension. Her first pregnancy was complicated by preeclampsia. She now complains of worsening fatigue over the last day. Her blood pressure is 140/90 mmHg, and she has a heart rate of 84 bpm and room air oxygen saturation of 95%. Fetal monitoring shows no distress. Laboratory studies are notable for a hemoglobin of 6 g/dL (10 g/dL 1 week ago) and platelet count of 80,000/dL (180,000/dL 1 week ago). A peripheral blood smear shows schistocytes. All of the following statements are true about her condition EXCEPT:

A. Glucocorticoids are effective in reducing morbidity and mortality.
B. Her liver function enzymes are likely elevated.
C. Preeclampsia predisposes to the condition.
D. Renal failure is common.
E. The condition will likely resolve after delivery of the fetus.

VII-37. A 48-year-old man with diabetes mellitus, hyperlipidemia, and atrial fibrillation presents to the emergency department for evaluation of left flank pain and groin pain that has been severe and present for approximately 3 hours. His medications include metformin, atorvastatin, and warfarin. He is uncomfortable and has a temperature of 37°C, heart rate of 105 bpm, blood pressure of 145/95 mmHg, respiratory rate of 21 breaths/min, and room air oxygen saturation of 98%. His physical examination is notable for left flank pain but no abdominal organomegaly or focal tenderness. An electrocardiogram shows sinus tachycardia with nonspecific ST-T wave changes. International normalized ratio is 2.0. His renal function is normal, and urine analysis shows many red blood cells, few white blood cells, no bacteria, and no crystals. Which of the following is the preferred diagnostic study?

A. 24-Hour urine collection
B. Cystoscopy
C. Magnetic resonance imaging
D. Noncontrast computed tomography (CT) scan
E. Ultrasound

VII-38. A noncontrast abdominal CT is performed. (See Figure VII-38.) Which of the following is the most likely diagnosis?

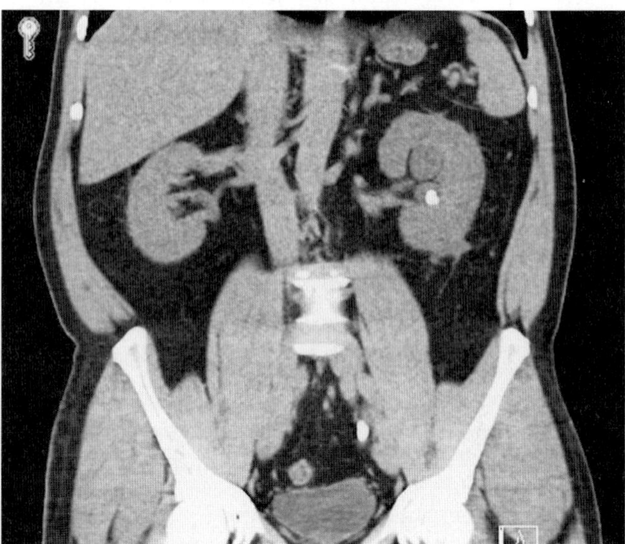

FIGURE VII-38 Image courtesy of Dr. Stuart Silverman, Brigham and Women's Hospital.

A. Appendicitis
B. Nephrolithiasis
C. Renal cell carcinoma
D. Pyelonephritis
E. Retroperitoneal hematoma

VII-39. Which of the following is the most common type of kidney stone?

A. Calcium
B. Cysteine
C. Oxalic acid
D. struvite
E. Uric acid

VII-40. A 54-year-old woman with a history of colon cancer treated with resection and chemotherapy 2 years earlier is admitted to the hospital after routine lab work at her primary care physician's office showed a BUN of 65 mg/dL and a creatinine of 4.5 mg/dL. She reports mild fatigue and recent lower back pain, but otherwise feels well. She does admit to recent nonsteroidal anti-inflammatory drug (NSAID) use but has not taken more than the recommended quantity. Aside from stopping the NSAID and avoidance of nephrotoxins, which of the following studies should be the next step?

A. CT of the abdomen/pelvis with oral contrast
B. Postvoid residual volume of bladder
C. Retrograde urography
D. Ultrasound of the abdomen/kidney
E. Urinary fractional excretion of sodium

VII-41. A 67-year-old man presents to the emergency department with severe abdominal distention and pain. He is found to have a palpable bladder, and after Foley catheter placement, 1.5 L of urine passes. His prostate-specific antigen is not elevated, but he does report that he has had difficulty passing his urine for several weeks, culminating in no urination for 2 days. His BUN is 89 mg/dL, and creatinine is 6.4 mg/dL. Over the next 4 days of hospitalization, his BUN and creatinine fall, but his urine output is found to be rising. He is not receiving intravenous fluids. He passes 6 L of urine on the third and fourth hospital days. Which of the following is the most likely explanation for the increased urine output?

A. Cerebral salt wasting
B. Decreased medullary osmolarity
C. Increased activation of the renin-angiotensin-aldosterone system
D. Increased tubule pressure
E. Postobstructive diuresis

VII-42. The patient described in Question VII-41 is at risk for which of the following complications?

A. Erythrocytosis
B. Hyperchloremic metabolic acidosis
C. Hyperkalemia
D. Prerenal azotemia
E. Systemic hypertension

VII-43. The pain associated with acute urinary tract obstruction is a result of which of the following?

A. Compensatory natriuresis
B. Decreased medullary blood flow
C. Increased renal blood flow
D. Vasodilatory prostaglandins

ANSWERS

VII-1. The answer is E. *(Chap. 334)* Ischemic acute renal failure has many potential etiologies. Microvascular disorders include increased vasoconstriction from endothelin and other mediators, decreased nitric oxide, prostaglandin- or bradykinin-mediated vasodilation, increased endothelial and vascular smooth muscle cell damage, and increased leukocyte adhesion. Tubular factors include cytoskeletal breakdown, loss of polarity, apoptosis and necrosis, desquamation of viable and necrotic cells, tubular obstruction, and backleak. Inflammatory and vasoactive mediators may affect both tubular and microvascular pathophysiologic mechanisms. (See Figure VII-1.)

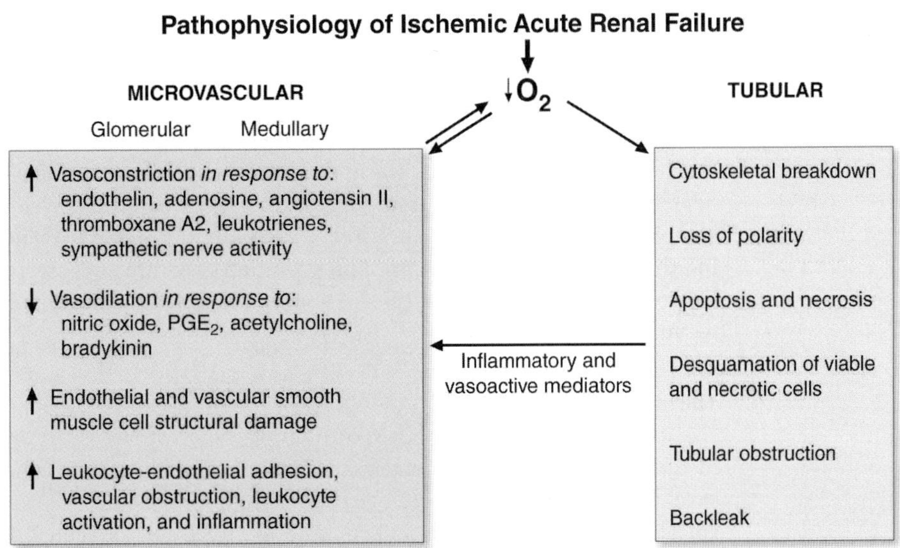

FIGURE VII-1 PGE_2, prostaglandin E_2.
From JV Bonventre, JM Weinberg: *J Am Soc Nephrol* 14:2199, 2003.

VII-2. **The answer is C.** *(Chap. 334)* Ischemia-associated acute kidney injury (AKI) is a serious complication in the postoperative period, especially after major operations involving significant blood loss and intraoperative hypotension. The procedures most commonly associated with AKI are cardiac surgery with cardiopulmonary bypass (particularly for combined valve and bypass procedures), vascular procedures with aortic cross-clamping, and intraperitoneal procedures. Severe AKI requiring dialysis occurs in approximately 1% of cardiac and vascular surgery procedures. The risk of severe AKI has been less well studied for major intraperitoneal procedures but appears to be of comparable magnitude. Common risk factors for postoperative AKI include underlying chronic kidney disease, older age, diabetes mellitus, congestive heart failure, and emergency procedures. Gender is not a known risk factor independent of the other factors listed above. The use of nephrotoxic agents including iodinated contrast for cardiac imaging prior to surgery may increase the risk of AKI.

VII-3. **The answer is E.** *(Chap. 334)* Iodinated contrast agents that are commonly used in cardiovascular and computed tomography (CT) imaging are a major cause of AKI. Underlying mechanisms leading to kidney injury include transient tubular obstruction by contrast material, hypoxia in the other renal medulla due to alterations in renal microcirculation and occlusion of small vessels, and cytotoxic damage to the tubules directly or through the generation of free radicals by contrast material. Risk factors for contrast-associated nephropathy include diabetes mellitus, congestive heart failure, preexisting chronic kidney disease, and multiple myeloma–associated renal failure. Serum creatinine begins to rise at 24–48 hours and will peak at 3–5 days, usually with resolution within a week. Urinary sediment is bland, without casts. The fractional excretion of sodium is low in many cases, particularly early before tubular injury is extensive because of the microvascular source of injury. Other diagnostic agents implicated as a cause of AKI are high-dose gadolinium used for magnetic resonance imaging (MRI) and oral sodium phosphate solutions used as bowel purgatives.

VII-4. **The answer is B.** *(Chap. 334)* Postrenal obstruction is an important and potentially reversible cause of AKI. Ultrasound evaluation of the kidneys classically demonstrates bilateral hydronephrosis, because unilateral obstruction is unlikely to cause kidney injury unless a single functioning kidney is present, chronic kidney disease preexists, or, rarely, reflex vasospasm of the unobstructed kidney is present. Advanced cervical cancer with invasion into the urinary system or retroperitoneum is a common cause of obstructive uropathy. Thrombotic thrombocytopenia purpura, disseminated gonococcus with sepsis, and pyelonephritis are intrinsic causes of acute kidney failure and will not cause bilateral hydronephrosis. Neither chronic hypertensive nephropathy nor contrast-induced nephropathy will cause bilateral hydronephrosis.

VII-5. **The answer is B.** *(Chap. 334)* Cholesterol emboli are an important cause of AKI in patients who have undergone cardiac procedures that may disrupt aortic atherosclerotic disease and shower cholesterol emboli. Livedo reticularis is a common finding on physical examination, and peripheral blood eosinophilia may be present. When found, eosinophiluria is highly suggestive. The other major cause of eosinophiluria is acute interstitial nephritis. White blood cell casts suggest interstitial nephritis, pyelonephritis, glomerulonephritis, or malignant infiltration of the kidney. Calcium oxalate crystals are found in ethylene glycol intoxication, and granular casts are suggestive of acute ischemic kidney injury (acute tubular necrosis, glomerulonephritis, vasculitis, and tubulointerstitial nephritis).

VII-6. **The answer is E.** *(Chap. 334)* AKI is a poor prognostic indicator in patients in the intensive care unit, as has been shown in multiple types of intensive care units for multiple medical conditions. Unfortunately, care of critically ill patients with AKI is supportive, because no specific therapy has been shown to improve outcomes. Agents that have specifically been shown to have no benefit in the treatment of acute tubular injury include atrial natriuretic peptide, low-dose dopamine, endothelin antagonists, loop diuretics, calcium channel blockers, α-adrenergic receptor blockers, prostaglandin analogs, antioxidants, insulin-like growth factor, and antibodies against leukocyte adhesion molecules. Volume repletion is critical to ensure adequate perfusion, and diuretics are only indicated in patients with replete fluid status and low urinary flow rates.

VII-7. **The answer is A.** *(Chap. 334)* Nonsteroidal anti-inflammatory drugs (NSAIDs) do not alter glomerular filtration rate in normal individuals. However, in states of mild to moderate hypoperfusion (as in prerenal azotemia) or in the presence of chronic kidney disease, glomerular perfusion and filtration fraction are preserved through several compensatory mechanisms. In response to a reduction in perfusion pressures, stretch receptors in afferent arterioles trigger a cascade of events that lead to afferent arteriolar dilatation and efferent arteriolar vasoconstriction, thereby preserving glomerular filtration fraction. These mechanisms are partly mediated by the vasodilators prostaglandin E_2 and prostacyclin. NSAIDs can impair the kidney's ability to compensate for a low perfusion pressure by interfering with local prostaglandin synthesis and inhibiting these protective responses. Ureteral obstruction is not the mechanism by which the NSAID impairs renal function in this scenario. NSAIDs are not known to be proximal tubule toxins.

VII-8. **The answer is E.** *(Chap. 334)* The optimal use of AKI biomarkers as diagnostic, therapeutic, or prognostic tools is an area of active investigation. None have yet been shown to be useful. Blood urea nitrogen (BUN) and creatinine are functional biomarkers of glomerular filtration rather than tissue injury biomarkers and, therefore, may be suboptimal for the diagnosis of actual parenchymal kidney damage. BUN and creatinine are also relatively slow to rise after kidney injury. Kidney injury molecule-1 (KIM-1) is a type 1 transmembrane protein that is abundantly expressed in proximal tubular cells injured by ischemia or nephrotoxins such as cisplatin. KIM-1 is not expressed in appreciable quantities in the absence of tubular injury or in extrarenal tissues. KIM-1 can be detected shortly after ischemic or nephrotoxic injury in the urine and, therefore, may be an easily tested biomarker in the clinical setting. Neutrophil gelatinase-associated lipocalin (NGAL; also known as lipocalin-2 or siderocalin) is another novel biomarker of AKI. NGAL was first discovered as a protein in granules of human neutrophils. NGAL can bind to iron siderophore complexes and may have tissue-protective effects in the proximal tubule. NGAL is highly upregulated after inflammation and kidney injury and can be detected in the plasma and urine within 2 hours of cardiopulmonary bypass–associated AKI. Other candidate biomarkers of AKI include interleukin (IL)-18, a proinflammatory cytokine of the IL-1 superfamily that may mediate ischemic proximal tubular injury, and L-type fatty acid–binding protein, which is expressed in ischemic proximal tubule cells and may be renoprotective by binding free fatty acids and lipid peroxidation products.

VII-9 and VII-10. **The answers are A and D, respectively.** *(Chap. 335)* Chronic kidney disease (CKD) encompasses a spectrum of different pathophysiologic processes associated with abnormal kidney function and a progressive decline in glomerular filtration rate (GFR). Stages of CKD are stratified by both estimated GFR and the degree of albuminuria in order to predict risk of progression of CKD. Previously, CKD had been staged solely by the GFR. However, the risk of worsening of kidney function is closely linked to the amount of albuminuria, and so it has been incorporated into the classification. Note that although age impacts GFR, it is not an independent criterion for risk of progression to CKD. CKD is still staged by GFR. GFR is ≥90 mL/min/1.73 m^2 in stage I, 60–89 mL/min/1.73 m^2 in stage II, 30–59 mL/min/1.73 m^2 in stage III, 15–29 mL/min/1.73 m^2 in stage IV, and <15 mL/min/1.73 m^2 in stage V. (See Figure VII-10.)

Prognosis of CKD by GFR and albuminuria categories: KDIGO 2012				Persistent albuminuria categories description and range		
				A1	A2	A3
				Normal to mildly increased	Moderately increased	Severely increased
				<30 mg/g <3 mg/mmol	30–300 mg/g 3–30 mg/mmol	>300 mg/g >30 mg/mmol
GFR categories (ml/min/1.73 m^2) description and range	G1	Normal or high	≥90			
	G2	Mildly decreased	60–89			
	G3a	Mildly to moderately decreased	45–59			
	G3b	Moderately to severely decreased	30–44			
	G4	Severely decreased	15–29			
	G5	Kidney failure	<15			

FIGURE VII-10 Reproduced with permission from *Kidney Int Suppl* 3:5–14, 2013.

VII-11. The answer is A. *(Chap. 335)* The leading cause of morbidity and mortality in patients with CKD regardless of stage is cardiovascular disease. The presence of CKD is a major risk factor for ischemic heart disease; in addition to traditional cardiovascular risk factors, patients with CKD have additional risk factors including anemia, hyperphosphatemia, hyperparathyroidism, sleep apnea, and systemic inflammation. Left ventricular hypertrophy and dilated cardiomyopathy are also frequently present in CKD and strongly associated with cardiovascular morbidity and mortality.

VII-12. The answer is B. *(Chap. 335)* Anemia is a common consequence of CKD and may be multifactorial, with etiologies including relative erythropoietin deficiency, iron deficiency, chronic inflammation, diminished red cell survival, and bleeding diathesis. Several trials of erythropoietin supplementation in patients with CKD have failed to show improved cardiovascular outcomes with this therapy. Indeed, these trials have shown a higher incidence of thromboembolic events and stroke in type 2 diabetics and potentially faster progression to need for dialysis. Because of these concerning findings, erythropoietin use has been altered from prior recommendations, and current practice is to target a hemoglobin concentration of 100–115 g/L.

VII-13. The answer is C. *(Chap. 335)* This patient has calciphylaxis. Calciphylaxis (calcific uremic arteriolopathy) is a devastating condition seen almost exclusively in patients with advanced CKD. It is heralded by livedo reticularis and advances to patches of ischemic necrosis, especially on the legs, thighs, abdomen, and breasts. Pathologically, there is evidence of vascular occlusion in association with extensive vascular and soft tissue calcification. It appears that this condition is increasing in incidence. Originally, it was ascribed to severe abnormalities in calcium and phosphorus control in dialysis patients, usually associated with advanced hyperparathyroidism. However, more recently, calciphylaxis has been seen with increasing frequency in the absence of severe hyperparathyroidism. Other etiologies have been suggested, including the increased use of oral calcium as a phosphate binder. Warfarin is commonly used in hemodialysis patients, and one of the effects of warfarin therapy is to decrease the vitamin K- dependent regeneration of matrix GLA protein. The GLA protein is important in preventing vascular calcification. Thus, warfarin treatment is considered a risk factor for calciphylaxis, and if a patient develops this syndrome, this medication should be discontinued and replaced with alternative forms of anticoagulation. *Pseudomonas* bacteremia may cause ecthyma gangrenosum, which may have a necrotic plaque, typically in neutropenic patients. This patient was treated with hyperbaric oxygen, intravenous thiosulfate, and discontinuation of warfarin with slow resolution of the ulceration.

VII-14. The answer is B. *(Chap. 336)* The commonly accepted criteria for initiating patients on maintenance dialysis include the presence of uremic symptoms, the presence of hyperkalemia unresponsive to conservative management, persistent extracellular volume expansion despite diuretics, acidosis refractory to medical therapy, bleeding diathesis, or a creatinine clearance or estimated GFR below 10 mL/min/1.73 m^2. Single BUN or creatinine values alone are inadequate to initiate maintenance dialysis.

VII-15. The answer is E. *(Chap. 336)* Hypotension is the most common complication of hemodialysis. There are many potential etiologies of hypotension including antihypertensive use, excessive ultrafiltration, impaired vasoactive or autonomic responses, impaired cardiac reserve, and osmolar shifts. Less common causes include dialyzer reactions and high-output heart failure related to large arteriovenous fistulas. Manipulation of buffer for dialysate, alterations of timing of ultrafiltration, and midodrine may be used to improve hemodynamic tolerance to hemodialysis. Patients with unexpected or new hypotension during stable dialysis should also be evaluated for graft infection and bacteremia.

VII-16. The answer is E. *(Chap. 336)* The major complication of peritoneal dialysis therapy is peritonitis, although other complications include catheter-associated nonperitonitis infections, weight gain, metabolic derangements, and residual uremia. Peritonitis is usually a result of a failure of sterile technique during the exchange procedure. Transvisceral infection from the bowel is much less common. Because of the high dextrose used in dialysate, there is a conducive environment for development of bacterial infection. This can be diagnosed by the presence of >100/μL leukocytes with >50% polymorphonuclear cells on microscopy. Cloudy dialysate and abdominal pain are the most common symptoms. The most commonly isolated bacteria are skin flora such as *Staphylococcus*. Gram-negative organisms, fungi, and mycobacteria have also been described. A Cochrane review (Wiggins KJ et al: *Cochrane Database Syst Rev* 1:CD005284, 2008) concluded that intraperitoneal administration of antibiotics was more effective than intravenous administration and that adjunctive treatment with urokinase or peritoneal lavage offers no advantage. Intraperitoneal vancomycin is common initial empiric therapy. In cases where peritonitis is due to hydrophilic gram-negative rods (e.g., *Pseudomonas* spp.) or yeast, antimicrobial therapy is usually not sufficient, and catheter removal is required to ensure complete eradication of infection.

VII-17. The answer is C. *(Chap. 336)* The most common cause of mortality in patients with end-stage renal disease is cardiovascular disease (stroke and myocardial infarction). Although the underlying mechanisms driving this association are under active investigation, the shared risk factors of diabetes, hypertension, and dyslipidemia, in addition to specific risks such as increased inflammation, hyperhomocysteinemia, anemia, and altered vascular function, are thought to play an important role. Inefficient or inadequate dialysis is a risk for patients with difficult vascular access or poor adherence to therapy. Patients receiving hemodialysis are at risk and often develop neurologic, hematologic, and infectious complications. Nevertheless, the biggest risk to survival in these patients is also the most common cause of death in the general population.

VII-18. The answer is B. *(Chap. 336)* Although the dose is classically defined as a derivation of the fractional urea clearance, factors that are also important include patient size, residual kidney function, dietary protein intake, comorbid conditions, and the degree of anabolism/catabolism. Since the landmark studies of Sargent and Gotch relating the measurement of the dose of dialysis using urea concentrations with morbidity in the National Cooperative Dialysis Study, the *delivered* dose of dialysis has been measured and considered as a quality assurance and improvement tool. Although the fractional removal of urea nitrogen and derivations thereof are considered to be the standard methods by which "adequacy of dialysis" is measured, a large, multicenter, randomized clinical trial (the HEMO Study) failed to show a difference in mortality associated with a large difference in urea clearance. Current targets include a urea reduction ratio (the fractional reduction in BUN per hemodialysis session) of >65%–70% and a body water– indexed clearance × time product (KT/V) above 1.2 or 1.05, depending on whether urea concentrations are "equilibrated." For the majority of patients with end-stage renal disease, between 9 and 12 hours of dialysis are required each week, usually divided into three equal sessions. Several studies have suggested that longer hemodialysis session lengths may be beneficial (independent of urea clearance), although these studies are confounded by a variety of patient characteristics, including body size and nutritional status. Hemodialysis "dose" should be individualized, and factors other than the urea nitrogen should be considered, including the adequacy of ultrafiltration or fluid removal and control of hyperkalemia, hyperphosphatemia, and metabolic acidosis. A recent randomized clinical trial (the Frequent Hemodialysis Network Trial) demonstrated improved control of hypertension and hyperphosphatemia, reduced left ventricular mass, and improved self-reported physical health with hemodialysis given six times per week compared to the usual three times per week. A companion trial in which frequent nocturnal hemodialysis was compared to conventional hemodialysis at home showed no significant effect on left ventricular mass or self-reported physical health. Finally, an evaluation of the U.S. Renal Data System registry showed a significant increase in mortality and hospitalization for heart failure after the longer interdialytic interval that occurs over the dialysis "weekend."

VII-19. The answer is A. *(Chap. 336)* The potassium concentration of dialysate is usually 2.5 mEq/L but may be varied depending on the predialysis serum potassium. This patient may need a lower dialysate potassium concentration. Sodium modeling is an adjustment of the dialysate sodium that may lessen the incidence of hypotension at the end of a dialysis session. Aldosterone defects, if present, are not likely to play a role in this patient since his kidneys are not being perfused. Therefore, nephrectomy is not likely to control his potassium. Similarly, since the patient is likely anuric, there is no efficacy in using loop diuretics to effect kaluresis. This patient has no approved indications for implantation of a defibrillator.

VII-20. The answer is D. *(Chap. 337)* Both deceased and living donor kidney transplantation is highly successful. When compared to hemodialysis, there are substantial cost-benefit advantages to individuals and society related to decreased morbidity, subsequent hospitalizations, and mortality. Currently, deceased-donor grafts have a 92% 1-year survival and living-donor grafts have a 96% 1-year survival. Although there has been improvement in long-term survival, it has not been as impressive as the short-term survival, and currently, the "average" life expectancy of a living-donor graft is around 20 years, whereas that of a deceased-donor graft is close to 14 years. When first-degree relatives are donors, the graft survival rates are higher than those with grafts from deceased donors by 5%–7% at 1 year. This difference persists for up to 10 years. The loss of kidney transplant due to acute rejection is rare. Most allografts succumb at varying rates to a chronic process consisting of interstitial fibrosis, tubular atrophy, vasculopathy, and glomerulopathy, the pathogenesis of which is incompletely understood. There are few reported complications for donors, particularly in the absence of hypertension or diabetes mellitus. For deceased donors, older age and presence of preexisiting renal damage or prolonged ischemia decrease the longevity of the graft. (See Table VII-20.)

TABLE VII-20 Mean Rates of Graft and Patient Survival for Kidneys Transplanted in the United States from 1998 to 2008[a]

	1-Year Follow-Up		5-Year Follow-Up		10-Year Follow-Up	
	Grafts, %	Patients, %	Grafts, %	Patients, %	Grafts, %	Patients, %
Deceased donor	92	96	72	84	46	64
Living donor	96	99	81	91	59	77

[a]All patients transplanted are included, and the follow-up unadjusted survival data from the 1-, 5-, and 10-year periods are presented to show the attrition rates over time within the two types of organ donors.
Source: Data from Summary Tables, 2009 Annual Reports, Scientific Registry of Transplant Recipients.

VII-21. The answer is E. *(Chap. 337)* The number of patients with end-stage renal disease has been increasing every year, and it is always greater than] the number of available donors. As the number of patients with end-stage kidney disease increases, the demand for kidney transplantations continues to increase. In 2011, there were 55,371 active adult candidates on the waiting list, and less than 18,000 patients were transplanted. This imbalance is set to worsen over the coming years with the predicted increased rates of obesity and diabetes worldwide. In an attempt to increase utilization of deceased-donor kidneys and reduce discard rates of organs, criteria for the use of so-called expanded criteria donor (ECD) kidneys and kidneys from donors after cardiac death (DCD) have been developed. ECD kidneys are usually used for older patients who are expected to fare less well on dialysis. At the 1-year mark, graft survival is higher for living-donor recipients, most likely because those grafts are not subject to as much ischemic injury. At 5 and 10 years, however, there is a steeper decline in survival of those with deceased-donor kidneys. Among the few absolute immunologic contraindications to transplantation is the presence of antibodies against the donor kidney at the time of the anticipated transplantation that can cause hyperacute rejection. Those harmful antibodies include natural antibodies against the ABO blood group antigens and antibodies against human leukocyte antigen (HLA) class I (A, B, C) or class II (DR) antigens. These antibodies are routinely excluded by proper screening of the candidate's ABO compatibility and direct cytotoxic cross-matching of candidate serum with lymphocytes of the donor. (See Table VII-21.)

TABLE VII-21 Definition of an Expanded Criteria Donor and a Non–Heart-Beating Donor (Donation After Cardiac Death)

Expanded Criteria Donor (ECD)
Deceased donor >60 years Deceased donor >50 years and hypertension and creatinine >1.5 mg/dL Deceased donor >50 years and hypertension and death caused by cerebrovascular accident (CVA) Deceased donor >50 years and death caused by CVA and creatinine >1.5 mg/dL
Donation After Cardiac Death[a] (DCD)
I. Brought in dead II. Unsuccessful resuscitation III. Awaiting cardiac arrest IV. Cardiac arrest after brainstem death V. Cardiac arrest in a hospital patient

[a]Kidneys can be used for transplantation from categories II–V but are commonly only used from categories III and IV. The survival of these kidneys has not been shown to be inferior to that of deceased-donor kidneys.

Note: Kidneys can be both ECD and DCD. ECD kidneys have been shown to have a poorer survival, and there is a separate shorter waiting list for ECD kidneys. They are generally used for patients for whom the benefits of being transplanted earlier outweigh the associated risks of using an ECD kidney.

VII-22. The answer is B. *(Chap. 338)* There are a wide variety of diseases that can cause glomerular injury to the kidney, ranging from genetic conditions such as *TRPC6* mutation causing cation channel dysfunction and associated focal segmental glomerulosclerosis to glomerular stress from systemic hypertension and/or diabetes mellitus. Inflammatory disease, such as lupus nephritis, Wegener granulomatosis, and poststreptococcal glomerulonephritis, may also cause glomerular disease. Fanconi syndrome is a classic disease of tubular dysfunction with associated aminoaciduria, type 2 renal tubular acidosis, and rickets, not glomerular disease.

VII-23. The answer is C. *(Chap. 338)* The hallmark of glomerular renal disease is microscopic hematuria and proteinuria. Immunoglobulin A (IgA) nephropathy and sickle cell disease are the exception to this, when gross hematuria may be present. Proteinuria may be heavy (>3 g/24 hr) or lighter with microalbuminuria (30–300 mg/24 hr) depending on the underlying disease or site of the immune lesion. Patients with poststreptococcal glomerulonephritis often have pyuria, but cultures are not expected to be positive because the infection is usually a skin or mucosal infection, and it is the immune reaction that drives the renal lesion. (See Table VII-23.)

TABLE VII-23 Patterns of Clinical Glomerulonephritis

Glomerular Syndromes	Proteinuria	Hematuria	Vascular Injury
Acute Nephritic Syndromes			
Poststreptococcal glomerulonephritis[a]	+/++	++/+++	–
Subacute bacterial endocarditis[a]	+/++	++	–
Lupus nephritis[a]	+/++	++/+++	+
Antiglomerular basement membrane disease[a]	++	++/+++	–
IgA nephropathy[a]	+/++	+++[c]	–
ANCA small-vessel vasculitis[a]			
Granulomatosis with polyangiitis (Wegener)	+/++	++/+++	++++
Microscopic polyangiitis	+/++	++/+++	++++
Churg-Strauss syndrome	+/++	++/+++	++++
Henoch-Schönlein purpura[a]	+/++	++/+++	++++
Cryoglobulinemia[a]	+/++	++/+++	++++
Membranoproliferative glomerulonephritis[a]	++	++/+++	–
Mesangioproliferative glomerulonephritis	+	+/++	–
Pulmonary-Renal Syndromes			
Goodpasture syndrome[a]	++	++/+++	–
ANCA small-vessel vasculitis[a]			
Granulomatosis with polyangiitis (Wegener)	+/++	++/+++	++++
Microscopic polyangiitis	+/++	++/+++	++++
Churg-Strauss syndrome	+/++	++/+++	++++
Henoch-Schönlein purpura[a]	+/++	++/+++	++++
Cryoglobulinemia[a]	+/++	++/+++	++++
Nephrotic Syndromes			
Minimal change disease	++++	–	–
Focal segmental glomerulosclerosis	+++/++++	+	–
Membranous glomerulonephritis	++++	+	–
Diabetic nephropathy	++/++++	–/+	–
AL and AA amyloidosis	+++/++++	+	+/++
Light-chain deposition disease	+++	+	–
Fibrillary-immunotactoid disease	+++/++++	+	+
Fabry disease	+	+	–
Basement Membrane Syndromes			
Anti-GBM disease[a]	++	++/+++	–
Alport syndrome	++	++	–
Thin basement membrane disease	+	++	–
Nail-patella syndrome	++/+++	++	–
Glomerular Vascular Syndromes			
Atherosclerotic nephropathy	+	+	+++
Hypertensive nephropathy[b]	+/++	+/++	++
Cholesterol emboli	+/++	++	+++
Sickle cell disease	+/++	+++[c]	+++
Thrombotic microangiopathies	++	++	+++
Antiphospholipid syndrome	++	++	+++
ANCA small-vessel vasculitis[a]			
Granulomatosis with polyangiitis (Wegener)	+/++	++/+++	++++
Microscopic polyangiitis	+/++	++/+++	++++
Churg-Strauss syndrome	+++	++/+++	++++
Henoch-Schönlein purpura[a]	+/++	++/+++	++++
Cryoglobulinemia[a]	+/++	++/+++	++++
AL and AA amyloidosis	+++/++++	+	+/++
Infectious Disease–Associated Syndromes			
Poststreptococcal glomerulonephritis[a]	+/++	++/+++	–
Subacute bacterial endocarditis[a]	+/++	++	–
Human immunodeficiency virus	+++	+/++	–
Hepatitis B and C	+++	+/++	–
Syphilis	+++	+	–
Leprosy	+++	+	–
Malaria	+++	+/++	–
Schistosomiasis	+++	+/++	–

[a]Can present as rapidly progressive glomerulonephritis (RPGN); sometimes called crescentic glomerulonephritis.
[b]Can present as a malignant hypertensive crisis producing an aggressive fibrinoid necrosis in arterioles and small arteries with microangiopathic hemolytic anemia.
[c]Can present with gross hematuria.
Abbreviations: AA, amyloid A; AL, amyloid L; ANCA, antineutrophil cytoplasmic antibodies; GBM, glomerular basement membrane.

VII-24. The answer is A. *(Chap. 338)* Focal segmental glomerulosclerosis (FSGS) refers to a pattern of renal injury characterized by segmental glomerular scars that involve some but not all glomeruli; the clinical findings of FSGS largely manifest as proteinuria. When the secondary causes of FSGS are eliminated, the remaining patients are considered to have primary FSGS. Secondary causes of FSGS include viral infection (human immunodeficiency virus (HIV), hepatitis B, parvovirus), hypertensive nephropathy, reflux nephropathy, cholesterol emboli, drugs (heroin, analgesics, pamidronate), oligomeganephronia, renal dysgenesis, Alport syndrome, sickle cell disease, lymphoma, radiation nephritis, and a number of familial podocytopathies. The incidence of FSGS is increasing, and it now represents up to one-third of cases of nephrotic syndrome in adults and one-half of cases of nephrotic syndrome in African Americans, in whom it is seen more commonly. FSGS can present with hematuria, hypertension, any level of proteinuria, or renal insufficiency. Nephrotic-range proteinuria, African American race, and renal insufficiency are associated with a poor outcome, with 50% of patients reaching renal failure in 6–8 years. FSGS rarely remits spontaneously, but treatment-induced remission of proteinuria significantly improves prognosis. Treatment of patients with *primary FSGS* should include inhibitors of the renin-angiotensin system. The treatment of *secondary FSGS* typically involves treating the underlying cause and controlling proteinuria. There is no role for steroids or other immunosuppressive agents in secondary FSGS. Hypertensive nephrosclerosis exhibits more prominent vascular changes and patchy, ischemic, totally sclerosed glomeruli. In addition, nephrosclerosis seldom is associated with nephrotic-range proteinuria. Minimal change disease usually is associated with symptomatic edema and normal-appearing glomeruli as demonstrated on light microscopy. This patient's presentation is consistent with that of membranous nephropathy, but the biopsy is not. With membranous glomerular nephritis, all glomeruli are uniformly involved with subepithelial dense deposits. There are no features of crescentic glomerulonephritis present.

The characteristic pattern of focal (not all glomeruli) and segmental (not the entire glomerulus) glomerular scarring is shown in the figure. The history and laboratory features are also consistent with this lesion: some associated hypertension, diminution in creatinine clearance, and a relatively inactive urine sediment. The "nephropathy of obesity" may be associated with this lesion secondary to hyperfiltration; this condition may be more likely to occur in obese patients with hypoxemia, obstructive sleep apnea, and right-sided heart failure.

VII-25. The answer is D. *(Chap. 338)* Diabetic nephropathy is the single most common cause of chronic renal failure in the United States, accounting for 45% of patients receiving renal replacement therapy, and is a rapidly growing problem worldwide. Approximately 40% of patients with type 1 or 2 diabetes develop nephropathy, but due to the higher prevalence of type 2 diabetes (90%) compared to type 1 (10%), the majority of patients with diabetic nephropathy have type 2 disease. Renal lesions are more common in African American, Native American, Polynesian, and Maori populations. Risk factors for the development of diabetic nephropathy include hyperglycemia, hypertension, dyslipidemia, smoking, a family history of diabetic nephropathy, and gene polymorphisms affecting the activity of the renin-angiotensin-aldosterone axis. Thickening of the glomerular basement membrane is a sensitive indicator for the presence of diabetes but correlates poorly with the presence or absence of clinically significant nephropathy. Immunofluorescence microscopy often reveals the nonspecific deposition of IgG (at times in a linear pattern) or complement staining without immune deposits on electron microscopy. Prominent vascular changes are frequently seen with hyaline and hypertensive arteriosclerosis. This is associated with varying degrees of chronic glomerulosclerosis and tubulointerstitial changes. Renal biopsies from patients with types 1 and 2 diabetes are largely indistinguishable. Multiple lines of evidence support an important role for increases in glomerular capillary pressure (intraglomerular hypertension) in alterations in renal structure and function. The natural history of diabetic nephropathy in patients with type 1 or 2 diabetes is similar. However, because the onset of type 1 diabetes is readily identifiable and the onset of type 2 diabetes is not, a patient newly diagnosed with type 2 diabetes may present with *advanced diabetic nephropathy*. At the onset of diabetes, renal hypertrophy and glomerular hyperfiltration are present. The degree of glomerular hyperfiltration correlates with the subsequent risk of clinically significant nephropathy. In the approximately 40% of patients with diabetes who develop diabetic nephropathy, the earliest manifestation is an increase in albuminuria detected by sensitive radioimmunoassay. Albuminuria in the range of 30–300 mg/24 hr is called *microalbuminuria*. Microalbuminuria appears 5–10 years after the onset of diabetes. It is currently recommended to test patients with type 1 disease for microalbuminuria 5 years after diagnosis of diabetes and yearly thereafter and, because the time of onset of type 2 diabetes is often unknown, to test type 2 patients at the time of diagnosis of diabetes and yearly thereafter.

Microalbuminuria is a potent risk factor for cardiovascular events and death in patients with type 2 diabetes. Proteinuria in frank diabetic nephropathy can be variable, ranging from 500 mg to 25 g/24 hr, and is often associated with nephrotic syndrome. Also, characteristically, patients with advanced diabetic nephropathy have normal to enlarged kidneys, in contrast to other glomerular diseases where kidney size is usually decreased. After the onset of proteinuria, renal function inexorably declines, with 50% of patients reaching renal failure over another 5–10 years; thus, from the earliest stages of microalbuminuria, it usually takes 10–20 years to reach end-stage renal disease. Once renal failure appears, however, survival on dialysis is shorter for patients with diabetes compared to other dialysis patients. Good evidence supports the benefits of blood sugar and blood pressure control as well as inhibition of the renin-angiotensin system in retarding the progression of diabetic nephropathy. In patients with type 1 diabetes, intensive control of blood sugar clearly prevents the development or progression of diabetic nephropathy. The evidence for benefit of intensive blood glucose control in patients with type 2 diabetes is less certain, with current studies reporting conflicting results. Controlling systemic blood pressure decreases renal and cardiovascular adverse events in this high-risk population. Drugs that inhibit the renin-angiotensin system, independent of their effects on systemic blood pressure, have been shown in numerous large clinical trials to slow the progression of diabetic nephropathy at early (microalbuminuria) and late (proteinuria with reduced glomerular filtration) stages, independent of any effect they may have on systemic blood pressure. Patients with type 1 diabetes for 5 years who develop albuminuria or declining renal function should be treated with angiotensin-converting enzyme (ACE) inhibitors. Patients with type 2 diabetes and microalbuminuria or proteinuria may be treated with ACE inhibitors or angiotensin receptor blocker (ARBs). Evidence suggests increased risk for cardiovascular adverse events in some patients with a combination of two drugs (ACE inhibitors, ARBs, renin inhibitors, or aldosterone antagonists) that suppress several components of the renin-angiotensin system.

VII-26. The answer is E. *(Chap. 339)* Autosomal polycystic kidney disease is a common genetic disorder accounting for up to 4% of end-stage renal disease cases in the United States. Although the most common manifestations of this condition are renal cysts, hematuria, urinary tract infection, and occasionally nephrolithiasis, there are several common extrarenal manifestations including intracranial aneurysm, aortic root and annulus dilatation, valvular heart disease including aortic regurgitation and mitral valve prolapse, hepatic cysts, hernias, and colonic diverticulae with a high propensity to perforate.

VII-27. The answer is E. *(Chap. 339)* Patients with autosomal dominant polycystic kidney disease have a two- to fourfold increased risk of subarachnoid or cerebral hemorrhage compared to the general population. Hemorrhage tends to occur before age 50 in patients with a family history of intracranial hemorrhage, with a personal history of intracranial hemorrhage, with aneurysms >10 mm, or with uncontrolled hypertension.

VII-28. The answer is C. *(Chaps. 66 and 339)* The patient presents with hypokalemia and hypochloremic metabolic alkalosis in the absence of hypertension. This is most commonly due to surreptitious vomiting or diuretic abuse, but in this case, the urine diuretic screen was negative. In patients with surreptitious vomiting, urine chloride levels are low to preserve intravascular volume, and this was not present in this patient. Bartter syndrome and Gitelman syndrome have hypokalemia and hypochloremic metabolic alkalosis with inappropriately elevated urine chloride levels. Gitelman syndrome is less severe and presents later in life than Bartter syndrome, which is commonly found in childhood due to failure to thrive. Additionally, Gitelman syndrome has more prominent fatigue and muscle cramping. Most forms of Bartter syndrome also have associated hypomagnesemia and hypocalciuria. Patients with type 1 pseudohypoaldosteronism have severe renal salt wasting and hyperkalemia. Liddle syndrome presents with apparent aldosterone excess with severe hypertension, hypokalemia, and metabolic alkalosis.

VII-29. The answer is B. *(Chaps. 63 and 340)* This patient has a normal anion gap metabolic acidosis (anion gap, 12). The calculated urine anion gap ($Na^+ + K^+ - Cl^-$) is +3; thus, the acidosis is unlikely to be due to gastrointestinal bicarbonate loss. In this patient, the diagnosis is type I renal tubular acidosis (RTA), or distal RTA. This is a disorder in which the distal nephron does not lower pH normally. It is associated with a urine pH >5.5, hypokalemia, and lack of bicarbonaturia. Sjögren syndrome is one of the autoimmune diseases (along with systemic lupus erythematosus, granulomatous interstitial nephritis, IgG4-related systemic disease, and idiopathic autoimmune interstitial nephritis) that may be associated with acute interstitial nephritis and tubular dysfunction. Sjögren-associated type I RTA may be associated with calcium phosphate stones and nephrocalcinosis. Type II RTA, or proximal RTA, includes a pH <5.5, hypokalemia, a positive urine anion gap, bicarbonaturia, hypophosphatemia, and hypercalciuria. This condition results from defective resorption of bicarbonate. Type III RTA is rare and most commonly is seen in children. Type IV RTA is also referred to as hyperkalemic distal RTA. Hyporeninemic hypoaldosteronism is the most common cause of type IV RTA and is usually associated with diabetic nephropathy.

VII-30. The answer is D. *(Chaps. 63 and 340)* In any patient with hypokalemia, the use of diuretics must be excluded. Diuretics or chronic hypokalemia may cause an acute interstitial nephritis with tubular injury. This patient has multiple warning signs for the use of agents to alter her weight, including her age, gender, and participation in competitive sports. Her body mass index is low, and the oral examination may suggest chronic vomiting. Chronic vomiting may be associated with a low urine chloride level. Once diuretic use and vomiting are excluded, the differential diagnosis of hypokalemia and metabolic alkalosis includes magnesium deficiency, Liddle syndrome, Bartter syndrome, and Gitelman syndrome. Liddle syndrome is associated with hypertension and undetectable aldosterone and renin levels. It is a rare autosomal dominant disorder. Classic Bartter syndrome has a presentation similar to that of this patient. It may also include polyuria and nocturia because of hypokalemia-induced diabetes insipidus. Gitelman syndrome can be distinguished from Bartter syndrome by hypomagnesemia and hypocalciuria.

VII-31. The answer is A. *(Chap. 340)* Acute interstitial nephritis is a common cause of both acute and chronic kidney dysfunction. Many causes of interstitial nephritis are successfully treated with glucocorticoids with improved rates of long-term renal recovery, including Sjögren syndrome, sarcoidosis, systemic lupus erythematosus, adult tubulointerstitial nephritis with uveitis, and idiopathic or other granulomatous interstitial nephritis (Table VII-31). In patients with gradually progressive disease or fibrosis on biopsy, the benefit is less clear. Additionally, allergic interstitial nephritis recovery may be accelerated with glucocorticoid therapy, but long-term renal recovery is not proven to be improved. Postinfectious interstitial nephritis has been associated with many bacterial and viral pathogens but generally resolves with treatment of the underlying condition.

TABLE VII-31 Indications for Corticosteroids and Immunosuppressives in Interstitial Nephritis

Absolute Indications
• Sjögren syndrome • Sarcoidosis • SLE interstitial nephritis • Adults with TINU • Idiopathic and other granulomatous interstitial nephritis
Relative Indications
• Drug-induced or idiopathic AIN with: Rapid progression of renal failure Diffuse infiltrates on biopsy Impending need for dialysis Delayed recovery • Children with TINU • Postinfectious AIN with delayed recovery (?)

Abbreviations: AIN, acute interstitial nephritis; SLE, systemic lupus erythematosus; TINU, tubulointerstitial nephritis with uveitis.
Source: Modified from S Reddy, DJ Salant: *Ren Fail* 20:829, 1998.

VII-32. The answer is E. *(Chap. 340)* Allergic interstitial nephritis is a common cause of unexplained acute renal failure. This is generally a clinical diagnosis with acute renal failure in the context of exposure to a potential offending agent (often NSAIDs, antibiotics, anticonvulsants, proton pump inhibitors) and improvement in renal function with withdrawal of the agent. Peripheral blood eosinophilia supports the diagnosis but is rarely found. Urine microscopy often shows white blood cell casts and hematuria, but these are not specific findings. Urine eosinophils are neither sensitive nor specific for allergic interstitial nephritis. A renal biopsy is generally not required, but may show extensive tubulointerstitial infiltration of white cells including eosinophils. Discontinuation of the offending agent often leads to reversal of the renal injury. However, depending on the duration of exposure and degree of tubular atrophy and interstitial fibrosis that has occurred, the renal damage may not be completely reversible. Glucocorticoid therapy may accelerate renal recovery but does not appear to impact long-term renal survival. It is best reserved for patients with severe renal failure in which dialysis is imminent or if renal function continues to deteriorate despite stopping the offending drug.

VII-33. The answer is D. *(Chap. 340)* The biopsy shows many atrophic tubules filled with eosinophilic casts surrounded by giant cell reactions. This finding is diagnostic of light chain nephropathy due to multiple myeloma. The eosinophilic casts consist of filtered Bence-Jones protein aggregating in tubules. Patients with multiple myeloma may develop acute renal failure in the setting of hypovolemia, infection, or hypercalcemia or after exposure to NSAIDs or radiographic contrast media. The diagnosis of light chain cast nephropathy (LCCN), commonly known as myeloma kidney, should be considered in patients who fail to recover when the precipitating factor is corrected or in any elderly patient with otherwise unexplained acute renal failure. Filtered monoclonal light chains may also cause less pronounced renal manifestations in the absence of obstruction, due to direct toxicity to proximal tubular cells and intracellular crystal formation. This may result in isolated tubular disorders such as renal tubular acidosis or full Fanconi syndrome. The goals of treatment are to correct precipitating factors such as hypovolemia and hypercalcemia, discontinue potential nephrotoxic agents, and treat the underlying plasma cell dyscrasia. Plasmapheresis to remove light chains is of questionable value for LCCN.

VII-34. The answer is A. *(Chap. 341)* The patient presents with the classic pentad for thrombotic thrombocytopenic purpura (TTP), including fever, neurologic findings, renal failure, hemolytic anemia, and thrombocytopenia. This condition is more common in women than men and black than white patients and may be triggered by a number of factors including pregnancy, infection, surgery, and pancreatitis. Several drugs have been implicated in the pathogenesis of TTP such as immunosuppressive agents, chemotherapeutic agents, and antiplatelet drugs. TTP may be differentiated from hemolytic uremic syndrome (HUS) by demographics, with HUS typically affecting young children and TTP being more common in middle-aged persons. Additionally, HUS is generally triggered by a diarrheal illness, which is much less common in TTP. On a molecular level, the metalloprotease ADAMTS13 specific for von Willebrand factor is generally low if not absent in activity in TTP. Development of HUS is likely driven by bacterial toxins such as shiga toxin or shiga-like toxin, often from *Escherichia coli* 0157:H7. Because TTP is associated with low protein levels that may be driven by autoantibodies, plasma exchange serves the dual purpose of removing the aberrant antibody and repleting protein levels. With appropriate therapy, 1-month mortality is approximately 20%. Mortality in patients who do not receive treatment is close to 90%, primarily from microvascular thrombosis and multiorgan failure.

VII-35. The answer is C. *(Chap. 341)* Renal vein thrombosis occurs in 10%–15% of patients with nephrotic syndrome accompanying membranous glomerulopathy and oncologic disease. The clinical manifestations can be variable but may be characterized by fever, lumbar tenderness, leukocytosis, and hematuria. Magnetic resonance venography is the most sensitive and specific noninvasive form of imaging to make the diagnosis of renal vein thrombosis. Ultrasound with Doppler is operator-dependent and therefore may be less sensitive. Contrast venography is the gold standard for diagnosis, but it exposes the patient to a more invasive procedure and contrast load. Nuclear medicine screening is not performed to make this diagnosis.

VII-36. The answer is A. *(Chap. 341)* HELLP (hemolysis, elevated liver enzymes, low platelets) syndrome is a dangerous complication of pregnancy associated with microvascular injury. Occurring in 0.2%–0.9% of all pregnancies and in 10%–20% of women with severe preeclampsia, this syndrome carries a mortality rate of 7.4%–34%. Most commonly developing in the third trimester, 10% of cases occur before week 27, and 30% occur postpartum. Although a strong association exists between HELLP syndrome and preeclampsia, nearly 20% of cases are not preceded by recognized preeclampsia. Risk factors include abnormal placentation, family history, and elevated levels of fetal mRNA for FLT1 (vascular endothelial growth factor receptor 1) and endoglin. Patients with HELLP syndrome have higher levels of inflammatory markers (C-reactive protein, IL-1Ra, and IL-6) and soluble HLA-DR than do those with preeclampsia alone. Renal failure occurs in half of patients with HELLP syndrome, although the etiology is not well understood. Although renal failure is common, the organ that defines this syndrome is the liver. Subcapsular hepatic hematomas sometimes produce spontaneous rupture of the liver and can be life-threatening. Neurologic complications such as cerebral infarction, cerebral and brainstem hemorrhage, and cerebral edema are other potentially life-threatening complications. Many features are shared by HELLP syndrome, atypical HUS (aHUS), and TTP. Diagnosis of HELLP syndrome is complicated by the fact that aHUS and TTP also can be triggered by pregnancy. Serum levels of ADAMTS13 activity are reduced (by 30%–60%) in HELLP syndrome but not to the levels seen in TTP (<5%). Other markers, such as antithrombin III (decreased in HELLP syndrome but not in TTP) and D-dimer (elevated in HELLP syndrome but not in TTP), may also be useful. HELLP syndrome usually resolves spontaneously after delivery, although some HELLP cases occur postpartum. Glucocorticoids may decrease inflammatory markers, although two randomized controlled trials failed to show much benefit. Plasma exchange should be considered if hemolysis is refractory to glucocorticoids and/or delivery, especially if TTP has not been ruled out.

VII-37 and VII-38. The answers are D and B, respectively. *(Chap. 342)* This patient has a typical clinical, laboratory, and radiologic presentation of nephrolithiasis. The CT shows a 10-mm obstructing calculus in the distal left ureter at the level of S1 and another 6-mm stone in the interpolar region of the left kidney. There is also left hydronephrosis and perinephric fat stranding. At present, there are no widely accepted, evidence-based guidelines for the evaluation and treatment of nephrolithiasis. The diagnosis is often made based on the history, physical examination, and urinalysis. Thus, it may not be necessary to wait for radiographic confirmation before treating the symptoms. The diagnosis is confirmed by an appropriate imaging study, preferably helical CT, which is highly sensitive, allows visualization of uric acid stones (traditionally considered "radiolucent"), and is able to avoid radiocontrast. Helical CT detects stones as small as 1 mm that may be missed by other imaging modalities. Typically, helical CT reveals a ureteral stone or evidence of recent passage (e.g., perinephric stranding or hydronephrosis), whereas a plain abdominal radiograph (kidney/ureter/bladder, or KUB) can miss a stone in the ureter or kidney, even if it is radiopaque, and does not provide information on obstruction. Abdominal ultrasound offers the advantage of avoiding radiation and provides information on hydronephrosis, but it is not as sensitive as CT and images only the kidney and possibly the proximal segment of the ureter; thus most ureteral stones are not detectable by ultrasound. Urologic intervention, such as cystoscopy, should be postponed unless there is evidence of a urinary tract infection (UTI), a low probability of spontaneous stone passage (e.g., a stone measuring ≥6 mm or an anatomic abnormality), or intractable pain. A ureteral stent may be placed cystoscopically, but this procedure typically requires general anesthesia, and the stent can be quite uncomfortable, may cause gross hematuria, and may increase the risk of UTI. Many patients who experience their first episode of colic seek emergent medical care. Randomized trials have demonstrated that parenterally administered NSAIDs (such as ketorolac) are just as effective as opioids in relieving symptoms and have fewer side effects. Excessive fluid administration has not been shown to be beneficial; therefore, the goal should be to maintain euvolemia. Use of an α-blocker may increase the rate of spontaneous stone passage.

VII-39. The answer is A. *(Chap. 342)* It is clinically important to identify the stone type, which informs prognosis and selection of the optimal preventive regimen. Calcium stones account for 75%–85% of all kidney stones. Although they are most commonly caused by idiopathic hypercalciuria, hypocitraturia, hyperuricosuria, and primary hyperparathyroidism are also causes. Uric acid stones are the next most common stone, followed by cysteine and struvite. Oxalic acid does not form stones without complexing with a positive cation, such as calcium. Struvite stones are precipitated by bacterial infections, such as *Proteus*, that promote conversion of urea to ammonium and raise urinary pH. General management for calcium stones includes increasing consumption of water and following a low-protein diet. If this is ineffective, thiazide diuretics may be used.

VII-40. The answer is D. *(Chap. 343)* Urinary tract obstruction is an important and potentially reversible cause of kidney failure. This patient is at risk for urinary obstruction based on her history of colon cancer. Although recent NSAID use may be contributing to the rapidity of her kidney damage, routine dosing is less likely to cause AKI in the absence of preexisiting renal dysfunction. Ultrasound of the kidneys is the best screening test for obstruction. Hydroureter and/or hydronephrosis may be found and suggest presence of obstruction. Although obstruction may be unilateral, it rarely causes clinically significant renal failure in the absence of underlying renal disease. CT of the abdomen is useful after ultrasound to evaluate the site and etiology of obstruction. Postvoid residual is useful if functional causes of obstruction are suspected, such as urinary retention. After the obstruction site is located, retrograde urography with stent placement may be indicated, but only after defining the presence or absence of obstruction.

VII-41 and VII-42. The answers are E and D, respectively. *(Chap. 343)* The patient has relief of recent urinary obstruction and is now making an inappropriately large amount of urine. This is likely due to postobstructive diuresis, which results from release of obstruction, increase in GFR over the course of days, decreased tubule pressure, and increased solute load per nephron, resulting in increased urine output. Decreased medullary osmolarity is a feature of chronic obstruction and persistent obstruction. The patient has not had recent head trauma or neurosurgical procedure and is unlikely to have cerebral salt wasting. Increased activation of the renin-angiotensin-aldosterone system is associated with chronic, unrelieved obstruction. Patients with postobstructive diuresis are at risk for volume depletion with possible development of prerenal azotemia and resultant AKI as well as electrolyte imbalance, particularly due to losses of sodium, potassium, phosphate, magnesium, and free water. Erythrocytosis may be seen in patients with obstruction, but is a rare feature and not associated with postobstructive diuresis. Systemic hypotension is more common than hypertension due to volume depletion.

VII-43. The answer is C. *(Chap. 343)* In acute urinary tract obstruction, pain is due to distention of the collecting system or renal capsule. Acutely, there is a compensatory increase in renal blood flow when kidney function is impaired by obstruction, which further exacerbates capsular stretch. Eventually, vasodilatory prostaglandins act to preserve renal function when GFR has decreased. Medullary blood flow decreases as the pressure of the obstruction further inhibits the renal parenchyma from perfusing; however, the ensuing chronic renal destruction may occur without substantial pain. When an obstruction has been relieved, there is a postobstructive diuresis that is mediated by relief of tubular pressure, increased solute load (per nephron), and natriuretic factors. There can be an extreme amount of diuresis, but this is not painful.

SECTION VIII

Disorders of the Gastrointestinal System

QUESTIONS

DIRECTIONS: Choose the one best response to each question.

VIII-1. The advantages of endoscopy over barium radiography in the evaluation of dysphagia include all of the following EXCEPT:

A. Ability to assess function and morphology
B. Ability to intervene as well as diagnose
C. Ability to obtain biopsy specimens
D. Increased sensitivity for the detection of abnormalities identified by color, e.g. Barrett metaplasia
E. Increased sensitivity for the detection of mucosal lesions

VIII-2. A 47-year-old man is evaluated in the emergency department for chest pain that developed at a restaurant after swallowing a piece of steak. He reports intermittent episodes of meat getting stuck in his lower chest over the past 3 years, but none as severe as this event. He denies food regurgitation outside of these episodes or heartburn symptoms. He is able to swallow liquids without difficulty and has not had any weight loss. Which of the following is the most likely diagnosis?

A. Achalasia
B. Adenocarcinoma of the esophagus
C. Esophageal diverticula
D. Plummer-Vinson syndrome
E. Schatzki ring

VIII-3. Which of the following has a well-established association with gastroesophageal reflux?

A. Chronic sinusitis
B. Dental erosion
C. Pulmonary fibrosis
D. Recurrent aspiration pneumonia
E. Sleep apnea

VIII-4. A 36-year-old woman with acquired immunodeficiency syndrome (AIDS) and a CD4 count of 35/μL presents with odynophagia and progressive dysphagia. The patient reports daily fevers and a 20-lb weight loss. The patient has been treated with clotrimazole troches without relief. On physical examination, the patient is cachectic with a body mass index (BMI) of 16 and a weight of 86 lb. The patient has a temperature of 38.2°C (100.8°F). She is noted to be orthostatic by blood pressure and pulse. Examination of the oropharynx reveals no evidence of thrush. The patient undergoes esophagogastroduodenoscopy (EGD), which reveals serpiginous ulcers in the distal esophagus without vesicles. No yellow plaques are noted. Multiple biopsies are taken that show intranuclear and intracytoplasmic inclusions in large endothelial cells and fibroblasts. What is the best treatment for this patient's esophagitis?

A. Ganciclovir
B. Glucocorticoids
C. Fluconazole
D. Foscarnet
E. Thalidomide

VIII-5. A 43-year-old man presents with 6 months of worsening dysphagia and postprandial regurgitation. He reports difficulty and pain with swallowing both liquids and solids, he has no difficulty with the initial components of swallowing but reports pain in the mid-chest region. He will frequently regurgitate undigested food 20–60 minutes after eating or drinking. In the past 2 months, he has lost 15 lb. He also has had one episode of presumed pneumonia 4 months ago notable for a right lower lobe infiltrate. He has no significant past medical history, takes no medications, and does not smoke cigarettes. He works as a service representative at a major electronics store and has never left the United States. Other than signs of recent weight loss, his physical examination is unremarkable. A barium swallow is performed and shown in Figure VIII-5 below. Which of the following is the most likely cause of his disease?

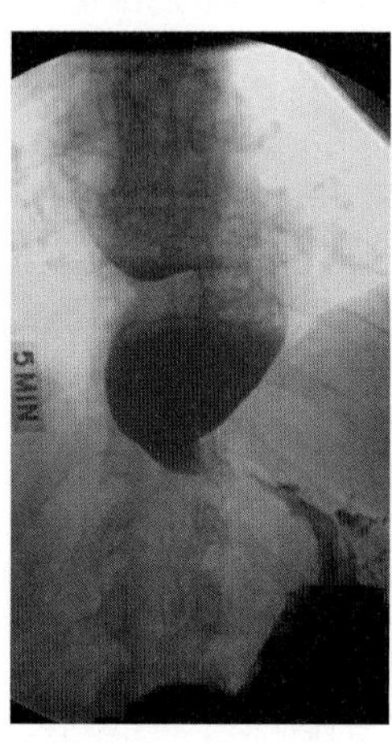

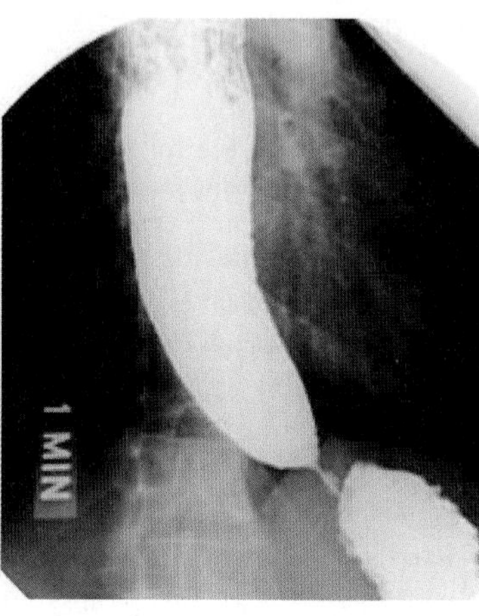

FIGURE VIII-5

A. Autoimmune reaction to latent herpes virus
B. Diffuse spasm on smooth muscle
C. Infection by *Trypanosoma cruzi*
D. Malignant growth of columnar epithelial cells
E. Malignant growth squamous epithelial cells

VIII-6. In the patient described in Question VIII-5, which of the following is the most efficacious therapy?

A. Botulinum toxin
B. Calcium channel blocker
C. Esophagectomy
D. Nitroglycerine
E. Radiation therapy

VIII-7. A 64-year-old man with a long history of abdominal pain, heartburn, and dyspepsia has an EGD to evaluate for peptic ulcer disease. No gastric or duodenal ulcers are found, but there are tongues of reddish mucosa extending proximally from the gastroesophageal junction into the esophagus. Biopsies of these areas demonstrate columnar metaplasia. All of the following statements regarding this diagnosis are true EXCEPT:

A. Finding high-grade dysplasia mandates further intervention.
B. High-dose proton pump inhibitor therapy will likely cause regression of the mucosal abnormalities.
C. The incidence of these lesions has increased in the era of potent acid suppression.
D. The patient has a high risk of coexisting cancer.
E. The patient is at significant risk of esophageal adenocarcinoma.

VIII-8. A 57-year-old man is evaluated with an EGD after an episode of hematemesis. The patient reports a history of tobacco use and hypercholesterolemia but is otherwise healthy. He has had lower back pain for the past month and has been intermittently using acetaminophen 1000 mg for relief. His endoscopy shows a 3-cm duodenal ulcer. Which of the following statements is correct regarding this finding?

A. The lesion should be biopsied because duodenal ulcers have an elevated risk of being due to carcinoma.
B. First-line therapy should be discontinuation of acetaminophen use.
C. The patient is not at risk for any associated cancers.
D. Poor socioeconomic status is a risk factor for development of this condition.
E. Antral gastritis is rarely found with this condition.

VIII-9. A 58-year-old man is evaluated for abdominal pain by his primary care physician. He reports severe stress at the job for the last 3 months and has since noted that he has epigastric pain that is relieved by eating and drinking milk. He has not had food regurgitation, dysphagia, or bloody emesis or bowel movements. He denies any symptoms in his chest. Peptic ulcer disease is suspected. Which of the following statements regarding noninvasive testing for *Helicobacter pylori* is true?

A. There is no reliable noninvasive method to detect *H pylori*.
B. Stool antigen testing is not appropriate for either diagnosis of or proof of cure after therapy for *H pylori*.
C. Plasma antibodies to *H pylori* offer the greatest sensitivity for diagnosis of infection.
D. Expose to low-dose radiation is a limitation to urea breath test.
E. False-negative test results using the urea breath test may occur with recent use of nonsteroidal anti-inflammatory drugs (NSAIDs).

VIII-10. A 44-year-old woman complains of 6 months of epigastric pain that is worst between meals. She also reports symptoms of heartburn. The pain is typically relieved by over-the-counter antacid medications. She comes to clinic after noting her stools darkening. She has no significant past medical history and takes no medications. Her physical examination is normal except for diffuse mid-epigastric pain. Her stools are heme positive. She undergoes EGD, which demonstrates a well-circumscribed, 2-cm duodenal ulcer that is positive for *H pylori*. Which of the following is the recommended initial therapy given these findings?

A. Lansoprazole, clarithromycin, and metronidazole for 14 days
B. Pantoprazole and amoxicillin for 21 days
C. Pantoprazole and clarithromycin for 14 days
D. Omeprazole, bismuth, tetracycline, and metronidazole for 14 days
E. Omeprazole, metronidazole, and clarithromycin for 7 days

VIII-11. A 57-year-old man with peptic ulcer disease experiences transient improvement with *H pylori* eradication. However, 3 months later, symptoms recur despite acid-suppressing therapy. He does not take NSAIDs. Stool analysis for *H pylori* antigen is negative. Upper gastrointestinal (GI) endoscopy reveals prominent gastric folds together with the persistent ulceration in the duodenal bulb previously detected and the beginning of a new ulceration 4 cm proximal to the initial ulcer. Fasting gastrin levels are elevated, and basal acid secretion is 15 mEq/hr. What is the best test to perform to make the diagnosis?

A. No additional testing is necessary.
B. Blood sampling for gastrin levels following a meal
C. Blood sampling for gastrin levels following secretin administration
D. Endoscopic ultrasonography of the pancreas
E. Genetic testing for mutations in the *MEN1* gene

VIII-12. A 65-year-old man presented to the hospital 2 weeks ago with an acute abdomen, hypotension, anemia, and respiratory failure. His past medical history was notable for hypertension and hypercholesterolemia for which he took enalapril and atorvastatin. At laparotomy, he was found to have a perforated duodenal ulcer with peritonitis and hemoperitoneum. A vagotomy and Billroth I anastomosis were performed. He has improved gradually and is increasing his oral intake and ambulation. His white blood cell (WBC) count and hemoglobin are normal. This afternoon approximately 3 hours after lunch, he reported the acute onset of lightheadedness, confusion, palpitations, and diaphoresis. His temperature is 36.0°C, heart rate is 110 bpm, blood pressure is 120/70 mmHg, and oxygen saturation is 95% on room air. Which of the following is most likely present?

A. Anemia
B. Hypoglycemia
C. Pulmonary embolism on helical chest computed tomography (CT)
D. Seizure focus on electroencephalogram (EEG)
E. ST elevation on electrocardiogram (ECG)

VIII-13. In the patient described in Question VIII-12, which of the following is the most likely diagnosis?

A. Acute GI bleed
B. Diabetes mellitus
C. Dumping syndrome
D. Inferior wall myocardial infarction
E. Pulmonary embolism

VIII-14. A 23-year-old woman is evaluated by her primary care physician for diffuse, crampy abdominal pain. She reports that she has had abdominal pain for the last several years, but it is getting worse and now associated with intermittent diarrhea without flatulence. This does not waken her at night. Stools do not float and are not hard to flush. She has not noted any worsening with specific foods, but she does have occasional rashes on her lower legs. She has lost about 10 lb over the last year. She is otherwise healthy and takes no medications. Which of the following is the most appropriate recommendation at this point?

A. Increased dietary fiber intake
B. Measurement of antiendomysial antibody
C. Measurement of 24-hour fecal fat
D. Referral to gastroenterologist for endoscopy
E. Trial of lactose-free diet

VIII-15. All of the following are direct complications of short bowel syndrome EXCEPT:

A. Cholesterol gallstones
B. Coronary artery disease
C. Gastric acid hypersecretion
D. Renal calcium oxalate calculi
E. Steatorrhea

VIII-16. A 54-year-old man is evaluated by a gastroenterologist for diarrhea that has been present for approximately 1 month. He reports stools that float and are difficult to flush down the toilet; these can occur at any time of day or night but seem worsened by fatty meals. In addition, he reports pain in many joints lasting days to weeks and not relieved by ibuprofen. His wife notes that the patient has had difficulty with memory for the last few months. He has lost 30 pounds and reports intermittent low-grade fevers. He takes no medications and is otherwise healthy. Endoscopy is recommended. Which of the following is the most likely finding on small bowel biopsy?

A. Dilated lymphatics
B. Flat villi with crypt hyperplasia
C. Mononuclear cell infiltrate in the lamina propria
D. Normal small bowel biopsy
E. Periodic acid–Schiff (PAS)–positive macrophages containing small bacilli

VIII-17. A 54-year-old man presents with 1 month of diarrhea. He states that he has 8–10 loose bowel movements a day. He has lost 8 lb during this time. Vital signs and physical examination are normal. Serum laboratory studies are normal. A 24-hour stool collection reveals 500 g of stool with a measured stool osmolality of 200 mOsmol/L and a calculated stool osmolality of 210 mOsmol/L. Based on these findings, what is the most likely cause of this patient's diarrhea?

A. Celiac sprue
B. Chronic pancreatitis
C. Lactase deficiency
D. Vasoactive intestinal peptide tumor
E. Whipple disease

VIII-18. Which of the following GI disorders is characterized by increased absorption from the GI tract into the portal circulation?

A. Celiac disease
B. Crohn disease
C. Hemochromatosis
D. Pernicious anemia
E. Whipple disease

VIII-19. Which of the following statements regarding the epidemiology of inflammatory bowel disease is correct?

A. Monozygotic twins are highly concordant for ulcerative colitis.
B. Oral contraceptive use decreases the incidence of Crohn disease.
C. Persons of Asian descent have the highest rates of ulcerative colitis and Crohn disease.
D. Smoking may decrease the incidence of ulcerative colitis.
E. Typical age of onset for Crohn disease is 40–50 years old.

VIII-20. A 24-year-old woman is admitted to the hospital with a 1-year history of severe abdominal pain and chronic diarrhea that has been bloody for the past 2 months. She reports a 20-lb weight loss, frequent fevers, and night sweats. She denies vomiting. Her abdominal pain is crampy and primary involves her right lower quadrant. She is otherwise healthy. Examination is concerning for an acute abdomen with rebound and guarding present. CT shows free air in the peritoneum. She is urgently taken to the operating room for surgical exploration, where she is found to have multiple strictures and a perforation of her bowel in the terminal ileum. The rectum was spared, and a fissure from the duodenum to the jejunum is found. The perforated area is resected and adhesions lysed. Which of the following findings on pathology of her resected area confirms her diagnosis?

A. Crypt abscesses
B. Flat villi
C. Noncaseating granuloma throughout the bowel wall
D. Special stain for *Clostridium difficile* toxin
E. Transmural acute and chronic inflammation

VIII-21. A 45-year-old man with ulcerative colitis has been treated for the past 5 years with infliximab with excellent resolution of his bowel symptoms and endoscopic evidence of normal colonic mucosa. He is otherwise healthy. He is evaluated by a dermatologist for a lesion that initially was a pustule over his right lower extremity but has since progressed in size with ulceration. The ulcer is moderately painful. He does not recall any trauma to the area. On examination, the ulcer measures 15 × 7 cm, and central necrosis is present. The edges of the ulcer are violaceous. No other lesions are identified. Which of the following is the most likely diagnosis?

A. Erythema nodosum
B. Metastatic Crohn disease
C. Psoriasis
D. Pyoderma gangrenosum
E. Pyoderma vegetans

VIII-22. Inflammatory bowel disease (IBD) may be caused by exogenous factors. GI flora may promote an inflammatory response or may inhibit inflammation. Probiotics have been used to treat IBD. Which of the following organisms has been used in the treatment of IBD?

A. *Campylobacter* spp.
B. *C difficile*
C. *Escherichia* spp.
D. *Lactobacillus* spp.
E. *Shigella* spp.

VIII-23. Your 33-year-old patient with Crohn disease has had a disappointing disease response to glucocorticoids and 5-aminosalicylic acid (5-ASA) agents. He is interested in steroid-sparing agents. He has no liver or renal disease. You prescribe once-weekly methotrexate injections. In addition to monitoring hepatic function and complete blood count, what other complication of methotrexate therapy do you advise the patient of?

A. Disseminated histoplasmosis
B. Lymphoma
C. Pancreatitis
D. Pneumonitis
E. Primary sclerosing cholangitis

VIII-24. All of the following statements regarding the risk of cancer in patients with IBD are correct EXCEPT:

A. Patients with Crohn disease are at greater risk for hematologic malignancies than the general population.
B. Patients with Crohn disease are at lower risk of GI malignancies than patients with ulcerative colitis.
C. Patients with long-standing ulcerative colitis are at increased risk of developing carcinoma of the colon.
D. Screening colonoscopy is recommended every 1–2 years in patients with a >8- to 10-year history of extensive ulcerative colitis regardless of age.
E. Ulcerative colitis patients with high-grade dysplasia found on colonoscopy should undergo immediate colectomy.

VIII-25. Which of the following patients requires no further testing before making the diagnosis of irritable bowel syndrome and initiating treatment?

A. A 76-year-old woman with 6 months of intermittent crampy abdominal pain that is worse with stress and associated with bloating and diarrhea.
B. A 25-year-old woman with 6 months of abdominal pain, bloating, and diarrhea that has worsened steadily and who now awakes from sleep at night to move her bowels.
C. A 30-year-old man with 6 months of lower abdominal crampy pain relieved with bowel movements, usually loose. Symptoms are worse during the daytime at work and better on the weekend. Weight loss is not present.
D. A 19-year-old female college student with 2 months of diarrhea and worsening abdominal pain with occasional blood in her stool.
E. A 27-year-old woman with 6 months of intermittent abdominal pain, bloating, and diarrhea without associated weight loss. Crampy pain and diarrhea persist after a 48-hour fast.

VIII-26. A 29-year-old woman comes to see you in clinic because of abdominal discomfort. She feels abdominal discomfort on most days of the week, and the pain varies in location and intensity. She notes constipation as well as diarrhea, but diarrhea predominates. Compared to 6 months ago, she has more bloating and flatulence than she has had before. She identifies eating and stress as aggravating factors, and her pain is relieved by defecation. You suspect irritable bowel syndrome. Laboratory data include: WBC count 8000/μL, hematocrit 32%, platelets 210,000/μL, and erythrocyte sedimentation rate (ESR) 44 mm/hr. Stool studies show the presence of lactoferrin but no blood. Which intervention is appropriate at this time?

A. Antidepressants
B. Ciprofloxacin
C. Colonoscopy
D. Reassurance and patient counseling
E. Stool bulking agents

VIII-27. After a careful history and physical and a cost-effective workup, you have diagnosed a 24-year-old woman patient with irritable bowel syndrome. What other condition would you reasonably expect to find in this patient?

A. Abnormal brain anatomy
B. Autoimmune disease
C. History of sexually transmitted diseases
D. Psychiatric diagnosis
E. Sensory hypersensitivity to peripheral stimuli

VIII-28. A 24-year-old woman has had 2 years of abdominal complaints characterized by episodic abdominal pain that is relieved by stooling. She reports that she has frequent small stools often soon after eating. She does not wake at night to use the bathroom. She has treated herself with various over-the-counter medications. She reports that she has tried a variety of diets recommended by daytime television that have occasionally but not consistently helped her symptoms. Her past medical history is notable for mild depression for which she takes fluoxetine. Her physical examination is completely normal, as are her basic metabolic panel, thyroid function, and complete blood count. A diet low in which of the following has been shown to be beneficial in patients such as her?

A. Animal protein
B. Capsaicin
C. Fermentable oligosaccharides, disaccharides, monosaccharides, and polyols
D. Rice and rice products
E. Vegetable protein

VIII-29. A 78-year-old woman is admitted to the hospital with fever, loss of appetite, and left lower quadrant pain. She is not constipated but has not moved her bowels recently. Laboratory examination is notable for an elevated WBC count. These symptoms began approximately 3 days ago and have steadily worsened. Which of the following statements regarding the use of radiologic imaging to evaluate her condition is true?

A. Air-fluid levels are commonly seen on plain abdominal films.
B. Less than 25% of patients present with peritoneal signs.
C. Lower GI bleeding will likely be visualized on CT angiography.
D. Thickened colonic wall is not required on CT for the diagnosis of her likely condition.
E. Ultrasound of the pelvis is the best modality to visualize the likely pathologic process.

VIII-30. Which of the following patients is MOST appropriate for surgical management of the their acute diverticulitis?

A. A 45-year-old woman with rheumatoid arthritis treated with infliximab and prednisone.
B. A 63-year-old woman with diverticulitis in the descending colon and a distal stricture.
C. A 70-year-old woman with end-stage renal disease and colonic wall thickening of 8 mm on CT scan.
D. A 77-year-old man with two episodes of diverticulitis in the past 2 years.
E. None of the above patients requires surgical management.

VIII-31. A 67-year-old man is evaluated by the emergency department for blood in the toilet bowel after moving his bowels. Blood was also present on the toilet paper after wiping. He does report straining and recent constipation. He has a history of systemic hypertension and hyperlipidemia. Vital signs are normal, and he is not orthostatic. Anoscopy shows external hemorrhoids, hematocrit is normal, and bleeding does not recur during his 6-hour emergency department stay. Which of the following is the most appropriate management?

A. Ciprofloxacin and metronidazole
B. Cortisone suppositories and fiber supplementation
C. Hemorrhoidal banding
D. Operative hemorrhoidectomy
E. Upper endoscopy

VIII-32. Which of the following statements regarding anorectal abscess is true?

A. Anorectal abscess is more common in diabetic patients.
B. Anorectal abscess is more common in women.
C. Difficulty voiding is uncommon and should prompt further evaluation of anorectal abscess.
D. Examination in the operating room under anesthesia is required for adequate exploration in most cases.
E. The peak incidence is in the seventh decade of life.

VIII-33. An 88-year-old woman is brought to your clinic by her family because she has become increasingly socially withdrawn. The patient lives alone and has been reluctant to visit or be visited by her family. Family members, including seven children, also note a foul odor in her apartment and on her person. She has not had any weight loss. Alone in the examining room, she only complains of hemorrhoids. On mental status examination, she does have signs of depression. Which of the following interventions is most appropriate at this time?

A. Head CT scan
B. Treatment with an antidepressant medication
C. Physical examination including genitourinary and rectal examination
D. Screening for occult malignancy
E. Serum thyroid-stimulating hormone

VIII-34. An 85-year-old woman is brought to a local emergency department by her family. She has been complaining of abdominal pain off and on for several days, but this morning, she states that this is the worst pain of her life. She is able to describe a sharp, stabbing pain in her abdomen. Her family reports that she has not been eating and seems to have no appetite. She has a past medical history of atrial fibrillation and hypercholesterolemia. She has had two episodes of vomiting and, in the emergency department, experiences diarrhea that is hemoccult positive. On examination, she is afebrile, with a heart rate of 105 bpm and blood pressure of 111/69 mmHg. Her abdomen is mildly distended, and she has hypoactive bowel sounds. She does not exhibit rebound tenderness or guarding. She is admitted for further management. Several hours after admission, she becomes unresponsive. Blood pressure is difficult to obtain and at best approximation is 60/40 mmHg. She has a rigid abdomen. Surgery is called, and the patient is taken for emergent laparotomy. She is found to have acute mesenteric ischemia. Which of the following statements is true regarding this diagnosis?

A. Mortality for this condition is >50%.
B. Risk factors include low-fiber diet and obesity.
C. The "gold standard" for diagnosis is CT scan of the abdomen.
D. The lack of acute abdominal signs in this case is unusual for mesenteric ischemia.
E. The splanchnic circulation is poorly collateralized.

VIII-35. A 63-year-old man with a history of diabetes and myocardial infarction was admitted to the medical intensive care unit (ICU) 1 day ago with sepsis due to pneumococcal pneumonia with bacteremia. He was started on antibiotics immediately but initially required high doses of noradrenaline and fluids to stabilize his blood pressure. The noradrenaline was weaned off approximately 12 hours ago. Over the past 2 hours, he has had increasing abdominal pain, distension, and bloody stools. His physical examination is notable for blood pressure of 100/50 mmHg, regular heart rate of 100 bpm, respiratory rate of 22 breaths/min, and oxygen saturation of 93% on high-flow nasal oxygen. He has a diffusely tender abdomen with no audible bowel sounds. An abdominal radiograph shows multiple small bowel air-fluid levels. Which of the following is the most likely diagnosis?

A. Arterial embolus
B. *C difficile* colitis
C. Inflammatory bowel disease
D. Nonocclusive mesenteric ischemia
E. Venous thrombosis

VIII-36. A 74-year-old woman is 2 days status post hip surgery for a fracture after a fall. Her only medication prior to admission was a calcium supplement, and she has no prior surgical history. Over the past 24 hours, she has had increasing abdominal discomfort and distension. She received a dose of cefazolin prior to surgery but no other antibiotics. On physical examination, she is afebrile with blood pressure of 140/80 mmHg, heart rate of 110 bpm, respiratory rate of 16 breaths/min, and oxygen saturation of 100% on 2 L of nasal oxygen. She has a distended tympanic abdomen with absent bowel sounds. There is no rebound tenderness. Her upright abdominal film is shown in Figure VIII-36. Which of the following is the most likely diagnosis?

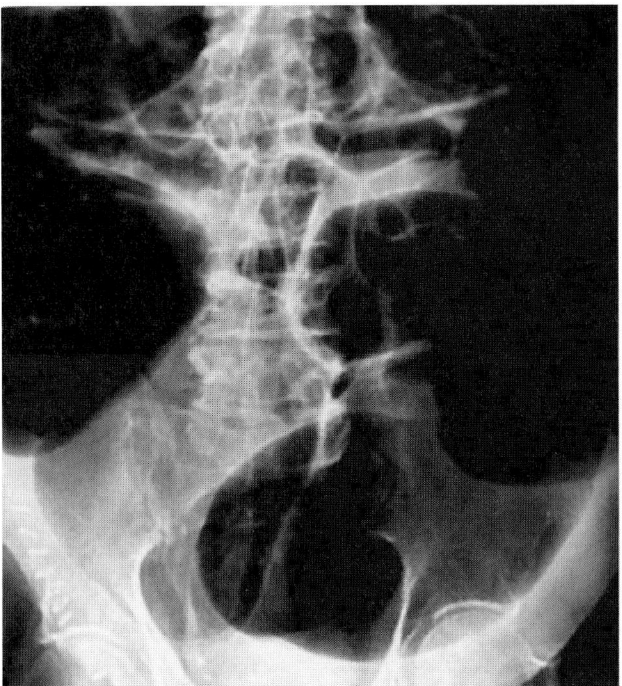

FIGURE VIII-36 (Reproduced, with permission, from Bongard FS, Sue DY [eds]. *Current Critical Care Diagnosis & Treatment.* Originally published by Appleton & Lange. Copyright (c) 1994 by The McGraw-Hill Companies, Inc., Fig. 13-18A.)

A. Acalculous cholecystitis
B. Colonic pseudo-obstruction
C. Perforated duodenal ulcer
D. Small bowel obstruction
E. Small bowel ileus

VIII-37. Which of the following is the next recommended therapy for the patient described in Question VIII-36?

A. Atropine
B. Laparotomy
C. Morphine
D. Neostigmine
E. Vancomycin

VIII-38. All of the following are potential causes of appendix obstruction and appendicitis EXCEPT:

A. *Ascaris* infection
B. Carcinoid tumor
C. Cholelithiasis
D. Fecalith
E. Measles infection

VIII-39. A 32-year-old woman is evaluated in the emergency department for abdominal pain. She reports a vague loss of appetite for the past day and has had progressively severe abdominal pain, initially at her umbilicus, but now localized to her right lower quadrant. The pain is crampy. She has not moved her bowels or vomited. She reports that she is otherwise healthy and has had no sick contact. Exam is notable for a temperature of 100.7°F and heart rate of 105 bpm, but otherwise, vital signs are normal. Her abdomen is tender in the right lower quadrant, and pelvic examination is normal. Urine pregnancy test is negative. Which of the following imaging modalities is most likely to confirm her diagnosis?

A. CT of the abdomen without contrast
B. Colonoscopy
C. Pelvic ultrasound
D. Plain film of the abdomen
E. Ultrasound of the abdomen

VIII-40. A 38-year-old man is seen in the urgent care center with several hours of severe abdominal pain. His symptoms began suddenly, but he reports several months of pain in the epigastrium after eating, with a resultant 10-lb weight loss. He takes no medications besides over-the-counter antacids and has no other medical problems or habits. On physical examination, temperature is 38.0°C (100.4°F), pulse is 130 bpm, respiratory rate is 24 breaths/min, and blood pressure is 110/50 mmHg. His abdomen has absent bowel sounds and is rigid with involuntary guarding diffusely. A plain film of the abdomen is obtained and shows free air under the diaphragm. Which of the following is most likely to be found in the operating room?

A. Necrotic bowel
B. Necrotic pancreas
C. Perforated duodenal ulcer
D. Perforated gallbladder
E. Perforated gastric ulcer

VIII-41. Which of the following is the mostly likely source of peritonitis in the patient in Question VIII-40?

A. Bile
B. Blood
C. Foreign body
D. Gastric contents
E. Pancreatic enzymes

VIII-42. A 61-year-old man is admitted to your service for swelling of the abdomen. You detect ascites on clinical examination and perform a paracentesis. The results show a WBC count of 300 leukocytes/μL with 35% polymorphonuclear cells. The peritoneal albumin level is 1.2 g/dL, protein is 2.0 g/dL, and triglycerides are 320 mg/dL. Peritoneal cultures are pending. Serum albumin is 2.6 g/dL. Which of the following is the most likely diagnosis?

A. Congestive heart failure
B. Peritoneal tuberculosis
C. Peritoneal carcinomatosis
D. Chylous ascites
E. Bacterial peritonitis

VIII-43. Which of the following is the most common symptom or sign of liver disease?

A. Fatigue
B. Itching
C. Jaundice
D. Nausea
E. Right upper quadrant pain

VIII-44. In women, what is the average amount of reported daily alcohol intake that is associated with the development of chronic liver disease?

A. 1 drink
B. 2 drinks
C. 3 drinks
D. 6 drinks
E. 12 drinks

VIII-45. All of the following are CAGE questions, which should be a component of the medical history focusing on alcohol abuse and dependence, EXCEPT:

A. Do you feel like you have a greater tolerance for alcohol than your friends?
B. Have you ever felt you ought to cut down on your drinking?
C. Have people annoyed you by criticizing your drinking?
D. Have you ever felt guilty or bad about your drinking?
E. Have you ever had a drink first thing in the morning to steady your nerves or get rid of a hangover?

VIII-46. Elevation in all of the following laboratory studies would be indicative of liver disease EXCEPT:

A. 5′-Nucleotidase
B. Aspartate aminotransferase
C. Conjugated bilirubin
D. Unconjugated bilirubin
E. Urine bilirubin

VIII-47. All of the following statements regarding liver function tests are true EXCEPT:

A. Alanine aminotransferase (ALT) is found in liver, cardiac muscle, skeletal muscle, and kidney.
B. Elevation of aspartate aminotransferase (AST) and ALT to >1000 IU/L is typical of ischemic hepatitis.
C. Elevation of AST is more specific for liver dysfunction than elevation of ALT.
D. Increased AST and ALT with an AST:ALT ratio of >3 is typical of acute viral hepatitis.
E. The magnitude of elevated AST and ALT has important prognostic significance in acute hepatitis.

VIII-48. A 26-year-old male resident is noticed by his attending physician to have yellow eyes after his 24-hour call period. When asked, the resident states he has no medical history, but on occasion, he has thought he might have mild jaundice when he is stressed or has more than four to five alcoholic drinks. He never sought medical treatment because he was uncertain, and his eyes would return fully to normal within 2 days. He denies nausea, abdominal pain, dark urine, light-colored stools, pruritus, or weight loss. On examination, he has a BMI of 20.1 kg/m^2, and his vital signs are normal. Scleral icterus is present. There are no stigmata of chronic liver disease. The patient's abdomen is soft and nontender. The liver span is 8 cm to percussion. The liver edge is smooth and palpable only with deep inspiration. The spleen is not palpable. Laboratory examinations are normal except for a total bilirubin of 3.0 mg/dL. Direct bilirubin is 0.2 mg/dL. AST, ALT, and alkaline phosphatase are normal. Hematocrit, lactate dehydrogenase, and haptoglobin are normal. Which of the following is the most likely diagnosis?

A. Autoimmune hemolytic anemia
B. Crigler-Najjar syndrome type 1
C. Choledocholithiasis
D. Dubin-Johnson syndrome
E. Gilbert syndrome

VIII-49. What is the next step in the evaluation and management of the patient in Question VIII-48?

A. Genotype studies
B. Peripheral blood smear
C. Prednisone
D. Reassurance
E. Right upper quadrant ultrasound

VIII-50. Which of the following statements regarding the hyperbilirubinemia seen in patients with significant intravascular hemolysis is true?

A. Bilirubin values <4 mg/dL imply concomitant gallbladder or biliary dysfunction.
B. Bilirubin values >4 mg/dL (68 μmol/L) imply concomitant liver dysfunction.
C. It is typically composed of 50% conjugated and 50% unconjugated bilirubin.
D. Prolonged hemolysis may result in the development of nephrolithiasis due to bile pigment stones.

VIII-51. A 34-year-old man presents to the physician complaining of yellow eyes. For the past week, he has felt ill, with decreased oral intake, low-grade fevers (~100°F), fatigue, nausea, and occasional vomiting. With the onset of jaundice, he has noticed pain in his right upper quadrant. He currently uses marijuana and ecstasy and has a prior history of injection drug use with cocaine. He has no other past medical history, but he was unable to donate blood for reasons that he cannot recall 4 years previously. His social history is remarkable for working as a veterinary assistant. On sexual history, he reports five male sexual partners over the past 6 months. He does not consistently use condoms. On physical examination, he appears ill and has obvious jaundice with scleral icterus. His liver is 15 cm to percussion, palpable 6 cm below the right costal margin. The edge is smooth and tender to palpation. The spleen is not enlarged. There are no stigmata of chronic liver disease. His AST is 1232 IU/L, ALT is 1560 IU/L, alkaline phosphatase is 394 IU/L, total bilirubin is 13.4 mg/dL, and direct bilirubin is 12.2 mg/dL. His international normalized ratio (INR) is 2.3, and activated partial thromboplastin time (aPTT) is 52 seconds. Hepatitis serologies are sent and reveal the following

Hepatitis A IgM	negative
Hepatitis A IgG	negative
Hepatitis B core IgM	positive
Hepatitis B core IgG	negative
Hepatitis B surface antigen	positive
Hepatitis B surface antibody	negative
Hepatitis B e antigen	positive
Hepatitis B e antibody	negative
Hepatitis C antibody	positive

What is the cause of the patient's current clinical presentation?

A. Acute hepatitis A infection
B. Acute hepatitis B infection
C. Acute hepatitis C infection
D. Chronic hepatitis B infection
E. Drug-induced hepatitis

VIII-52. In the patient described in Question VIII-51, what would be the best approach to prevent development of chronic hepatitis?

A. Administration of anti-hepatitis A virus immunoglobulin (Ig) G
B. Administration of lamivudine
C. Administration of pegylated interferon-α plus ribavirin
D. Administration of prednisone beginning at a dose of 1 mg/kg daily
E. Do nothing and observe as 99% of individuals with this disease recover

VIII-53 Which of the following viral causes of acute hepatitis is most likely to cause fulminant hepatitis in a pregnant woman?

A. Hepatitis A
B. Hepatitis B
C. Hepatitis C
D. Hepatitis D
E. Hepatitis E

VIII-54. A 16-year-old girl had visited your clinic 1 month ago with jaundice, vomiting, malaise, and anorexia. Two other family members were ill with similar symptoms. Based on viral serologies, including a positive anti-hepatitis A virus IgM, a diagnosis of hepatitis A was made. The patient was treated conservatively, and 1 week after first presenting, she appeared to have made a full recovery. She returns to your clinic today complaining of the same symptoms she had 1 month ago. She is jaundiced, and an initial panel of laboratory tests returns elevated transaminases. Which of the following offers the best explanation of what has occurred in this patient?

A. Co-infection with hepatitis C
B. Inappropriate treatment of initial infection
C. Incorrect initial diagnosis; this patient likely has hepatitis B
D. Reinfection with hepatitis A
E. Relapse of hepatitis A

VIII-55. A 26-year-old woman presents to your clinic and is interested in getting pregnant. She seeks your advice regarding vaccines she should obtain, and in particular asks about the hepatitis B vaccine. She works as a receptionist for a local business, denies alcohol or illicit drug use, and is in a monogamous relationship. Which of the following is true regarding hepatitis B vaccination?

A. Hepatitis B vaccine consists of two intramuscular doses 1 month apart.
B. Only patients with defined risk factors need to be vaccinated.
C. Pregnancy is not a contraindication to the hepatitis B vaccine.
D. This patient's hepatitis serologies should be checked prior to vaccination.
E. Vaccination should not be administered to children under 2 years old.

VIII-56. An 18-year-old man presents to a rural clinic with nausea, vomiting, anorexia, abdominal discomfort, myalgias, and jaundice. He describes occasional alcohol use and is sexually active. He describes using heroin and cocaine "a few times in the past." He works as a short-order cook in a local restaurant. He has lost 15.5 kg (34 lb) since his last visit to clinic and appears emaciated and ill. On examination, he is noted to have icteric sclerae and a palpable, tender liver below the right costal margin. In regard to acute hepatitis, which of the following is true?

A. A distinction between viral etiologies cannot be made using clinical criteria alone.
B. Based on age and risk factors, he is likely to have hepatitis B infection.
C. He does not have hepatitis E virus, as this infects only pregnant women.
D. This patient cannot have hepatitis C because his presentation is too acute.
E. This patient does not have hepatitis A because his presentation is too fulminant.

VIII-57. A 36-year-old man presents with fatigue and tea-colored urine for 5 days. Physical examination reveals jaundice and tender hepatomegaly but is otherwise unremarkable. Laboratories are remarkable for an AST of 2400 IU/L and an ALT of 2640 IU/L. Alkaline phosphatase is 210 IU/L. Total bilirubin is 8.6 mg/dL. Which of the following diagnoses is least likely to cause this clinical picture and these laboratory abnormalities?

A. Acute hepatitis A infection
B. Acute hepatitis B infection
C. Acute hepatitis C infection
D. Acetaminophen ingestion
E. Budd-Chiari syndrome

VIII-58. Which of the following drugs has a direct toxic effect on hepatocytes?

A. Acetaminophen
B. Chlorpromazine
C. Halothane
D. Isoniazid
E. Rosuvastatin

VIII-59. A 32-year-old woman is admitted to the ICU following an overdose of acetaminophen with co-ingestion of alcohol. She was known to be alert and interactive about 4 hours prior to her presentation when she had a fight with her boyfriend who then left the home. When he returned 6 hours later, he found an empty bottle of acetaminophen 500-mg capsules as well as an empty vodka bottle. The exact number of pills in the bottle is unknown, but the full bottle held as much as 50 capsules. The patient was unresponsive and had vomited, so her boyfriend called 911. Upon arrival to the emergency department, the patient is stuporous. Her vital signs are: pulse 109 bpm, respiratory rate 20 breaths/min, blood pressure 96/52 mmHg, and oxygen saturation 95% on room air. Her examination shows mild nonspecific abdominal pain with palpation. The liver is not enlarged. Her initial laboratory values show a normal complete blood count, normal electrolytes, and kidney function. The AST is 68 IU/L, ALT is 46 IU/L, alkaline phosphatase is 110 IU/L, and total bilirubin is 1.2 mg/dL. Glucose and coagulation studies are normal. The serum alcohol level is 210 g/dL. The acetaminophen level is 350 μg/mL. What is the most appropriate next step in the treatment of this patient?

A. Administration of activated charcoal or cholestyramine
B. Administration of *N*-acetylcysteine 140 mg/kg followed by 70 mg/kg every 4 hours for a total of 15–20 doses
C. Continued monitoring of liver function, glucose, and coagulation studies every 4 hours with administration of *N*-acetylcysteine if these begin to change
D. Do nothing as normal liver function tests and coagulation studies are indicative of only a minor ingestion
E. Initiate hemodialysis for toxin clearance

VIII-60. A 31-year-old healthcare worker is found to have a newly positive tuberculin skin test 6 weeks after an exposure to a patient with active pulmonary tuberculosis. He is asymptomatic and has a normal chest radiograph. Which of the following statements regarding initiation of isoniazid (INH) prophylactic therapy is true?

A. Acute hepatocellular injury due to INH is an idiosyncratic reaction that will manifest within the first 2 months of initiation of therapy.
B. Controlled trials have demonstrated that monthly monitoring of aminotransferase levels reduces morbidity in U.S. healthcare workers receiving INH prophylaxis.
C. Elevation of aminotransferase levels in the first 2 months of therapy is an indication to stop INH and switch to another drug.
D. The patient has a 50%–70% chance of transient elevation of his aminotransferase levels in the first 2 months of treatment.
E. The frequency of acute hepatocellular injury due to INH is age-dependent, increasing in patients >35 years of age.

VIII-61. You are caring for a 48-year-old former drug user with chronic hepatitis C who is currently on no medications and whose most recent cardiovascular risk profile suggests he would benefit from initiation of statin therapy. His most recent liver function tests reveal high normal AST and ALT, normal alkaline phosphatase, and normal INR. He has not initiated antiviral therapy because of insurance issues with the new expensive curative therapies. Which of the following statements regarding statin therapy is true?

A. Monitoring of aminotransferase levels should be initiated in patients starting statin therapy.
B. Overall, between 5% and 10% of patients receiving statins develop mild reversible elevations in aminotransferase levels.
C. Statins are not contraindicated in patients with chronic hepatitis C.
D. Statins should be discontinued in asymptomatic patients who develop an isolated elevation in aminotransferase activity.

VIII-62. All of the following are likely causes of chronic hepatitis EXCEPT:

A. Autoimmune hepatitis
B. Hepatitis A virus
C. Hepatitis B virus
D. Hepatitis C virus
E. Hepatitis D virus

VIII-63. A 38-year-old woman is evaluated for elevated transaminase levels that were identified during routine laboratory testing for life insurance. She is originally from Thailand and immigrated to the United States 10 years previously. She has been married to an American for the past 12 years, meeting him while he was living abroad for business. She previously worked in Thailand as a deputy tourism minister for the government but is not currently employed. She has no significant past medical history. She had one uncomplicated pregnancy at the age of 22. When queried about risk factors for liver disease, she denies alcohol intake or drug abuse. She has never had a blood transfusion. She recalls an episode of jaundice that she did not seek evaluation for about 15 years ago. It resolved spontaneously. She currently feels well, and her husband wished to have her added to his life insurance policy. There is no stigmata of chronic liver disease. Her laboratory studies reveal an AST of 346 IU/L, ALT of 412 IU/L, alkaline phosphatase of 98 IU/L, and total bilirubin 1.5 of mg/dL. Further workup includes the following viral studies: hepatitis A IgG positive, hepatitis B surface antigen positive, hepatitis B e antigen positive, anti-hepatitis B virus core IgG positive, and hepatitis C IgG negative. The HBV DNA level is 4.8×10^4 IU/mL. Which of the following medications is indicated for this patient?

A. Acyclovir
B. Entecavir
C. Ritonavir
D. Simeprevir
E. No treatment is necessary

VIII-64. A 46-year-old man is known to have chronic hepatitis C virus (HCV) infection. He is a former intravenous drug user for more than 20 years who has been abstinent from drug use for 1 year. He was treated for tricuspid valve endocarditis 3 years previously. He does not know when he acquired HCV. His laboratory studies show a positive HCV IgG antibody with a viral load of greater than 1 million copies. The virus is genotype 2. His AST is 82 IU/L, and his ALT is 74 IU/L. He undergoes liver biopsy, which demonstrates a moderate degree of bridging fibrosis. Which of the following is the most predictive of the development of cirrhosis?

A. Abnormal transaminases
B. Bridging fibrosis on liver biopsy
C. Genotype 2
D. History of bacterial endocarditis
E. History of intravenous drug use

VIII-65. A 34-year-old woman is evaluated for fatigue, malaise, arthralgias, and a 10-lb weight loss over the past 6–8 weeks. She has no past medical history. Since feeling poorly, she has taken approximately one or two tablets of acetaminophen 500 mg daily. On physical examination, her temperature is 100.2°F, respiratory rate is 18 breaths/min, blood pressure is 100/48 mmHg, heart rate is 92 bpm, and oxygen saturation is 96% on room air. She has scleral icterus. Her liver edge is palpable 3 cm below the right costal margin. It is smooth and tender. The spleen is not enlarged. She has mild synovitis in the small joints of her hands. Her AST is 542 IU/L, ALT is 657 IU/L, alkaline phosphatase is 102 IU/L, total bilirubin is 5.3 mg/dL, and direct bilirubin is 4.8 mg/dL. Which of the following tests would be LEAST likely to be positive in this diagnosis?

A. Antinuclear antibodies in a homogeneous pattern
B. Anti-liver/kidney microsomal antibodies
C. Antimitochondrial antibodies
D. Hypergammaglobulinemia
E. Rheumatoid factor

VIII-66. In chronic hepatitis B virus infection, presence of hepatitis B e antigen signifies which of the following?

A. Development of liver fibrosis leading to cirrhosis
B. Dominant viral population is less virulent and less transmissible
C. Increased likelihood of an acute flare in the next 1–2 weeks
D. Ongoing viral replication
E. Resolving infection

VIII-67. All of the following statements regarding alcoholic liver disease are true EXCEPT:

A. Fatty liver is present in >90% of daily and binge drinkers.
B. Hepatitis C infection worsens the prognosis of alcoholic liver disease.
C. Over 50% of alcoholics will develop alcoholic hepatitis.
D. Quantity and duration of alcohol consumption are the most important risk factors for the development of alcoholic liver disease.
E. The pathologic hallmarks of alcoholic liver disease are fatty liver, hepatitis, and cirrhosis.

VIII-68. A 32-year-old woman is admitted to the hospital with fever, abdominal pain, and jaundice. She drinks approximately 6 beers daily and has recently increased her alcohol intake to more than 12 beers daily. She has no other substance abuse history and has no prior history of alcoholic liver disease or pancreatitis. She is not taking any medications. On physical examination, she appears ill and disheveled with a fruity odor to her breath. Her vital signs are: heart rate 122 bpm, blood pressure 95/56 mmHg, respiratory rate 22 breaths/min, temperature 101.2°F, and oxygen saturation 98% on room air. She has scleral icterus, and spider angiomata are present on the trunk. The liver edge is palpable 10 cm below the right costal margin. The liver is smooth and tender to palpation. The spleen is not palpable. No ascites or lower extremity edema is present. Laboratory studies demonstrate as AST of 431 IU/L, ALT of 198 IU/L, bilirubin of 8.6 mg/dL, alkaline phosphatase of 201 IU/L, amylase of 88 U/L, and lipase of 50 U/L. Total protein is 6.2 g/dL, and albumin is 2.8 g/dL. The prothrombin time is 29 seconds (control, 13 seconds) with INR of 2.2. What is the best approach to treatment of this patient?

A. Administer intravenous fluids, thiamine, and folate and observe for improvement in laboratory tests and clinical condition.
B. Administer intravenous fluids, thiamine, folate, and imipenem while awaiting blood culture results.
C. Administer prednisone 40 mg daily for 4 weeks before beginning a taper.
D. Consult surgery for management of acute cholecystitis.
E. Perform an abdominal CT with intravenous contrast to assess for necrotizing pancreatitis.

VIII-69. Which of the following statements regarding nonalcoholic fatty liver disease (NAFLD) is true?

A. Imaging studies suggest that fatty liver is present to some degree in 10% of adult Americans.
B. NAFLD does not occur in lean individuals.
C. NAFLD is more common in African Americans than Hispanic Americans.
D. NAFLD is strongly associated with obesity and insulin resistance.
E. While common in the United States, NAFLD is uncommon in other countries.

VIII-70. A 44-year-old man seeks evaluation for an abnormal finding on ultrasonography. He has a history of type 2 diabetes mellitus and is on insulin therapy. Last week, he was evaluated in the emergency department for mid-epigastric pain likely due to NSAID therapy for muscle aches (he recently started exercising because his wife told him to lose weight). During the evaluation, an abdominal ultrasound showed marked fatty infiltration of the liver. Laboratory studies show his transaminases are 2× normal with normal alkaline phosphatase, bilirubin, and prothrombin time. Other than insulin, he takes no medications, does not consume alcohol or illicit drugs, and has no family history of liver disease. On physical examination, he is obese (BMI, 32 kg/m^2) with normal vital signs and no other abnormalities. You think he likely has NAFLD. All of the following statements regarding his potential therapy are true EXCEPT:

A. Bariatric surgery is safe in patients with NAFLD.
B. Exercise may reduce hepatic steatosis.
C. Statins may worsen inflammation in NAFLD.
D. There are no Food and Drug Administration–approved therapies for NAFLD.
E. Vitamin E may reduce aminotransferase levels and hepatic steatosis.

VIII-71. All of the following statements regarding alcohol-induced liver disease are true EXCEPT:

A. Alcohol-induced cirrhosis is characterized by predominantly large (>2 cm) nodules.
B. Alcohol use is the most common cause of cirrhosis in the United States.
C. Chronic alcohol use can cause liver fibrosis in the absence of accompanying inflammation.
D. Excessive alcohol use can cause acute hepatitis.
E. Excessive alcohol use can worsen liver disease due to hemochromatosis.

VIII-72. A 64-year-old man is admitted to the ICU with a large GI bleed. EGD reveals esophageal varices. He is confused and unable to provide any history. His physical examination is notable for abnormal hand findings as shown in Figures VIII-72A and VIII-72B. Ultrasound demonstrates a small liver consistent with cirrhosis. Which of the following is the most likely cause of his cirrhosis?

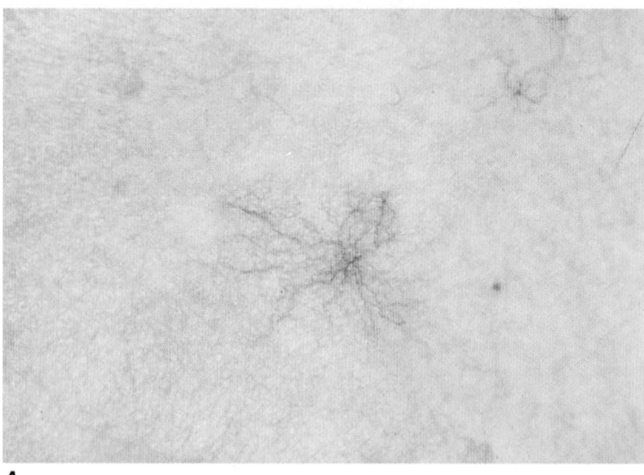

A

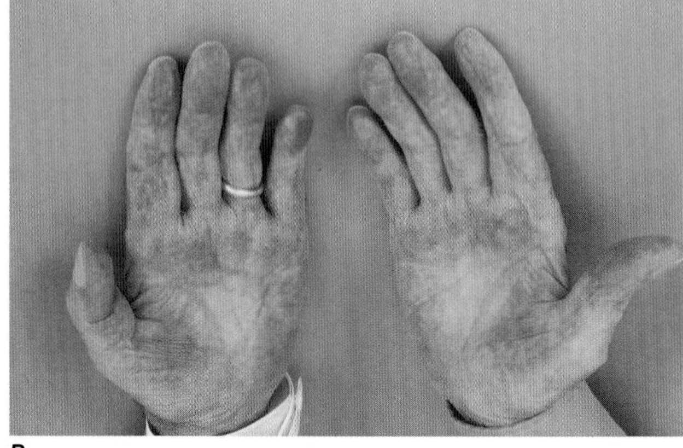

B

FIGURE VIII-72

A. Alcoholism
B. Autoimmune hepatitis
C. Chronic hepatitis C infection
D. Hemochromatosis
E. Primary biliary cirrhosis

VIII-73. In the patient described in Question VIII-72, all of the following may be used to control his variceal bleeding EXCEPT:

A. Endoscopic sclerotherapy
B. Endoscopic variceal ligation
C. Octreotide
D. Propranolol
E. Transjugular intrahepatic portosystemic shunt

VIII-74. You are following a 44-year-old woman with cirrhosis due to chronic hepatitis C infection. To date, she has no evidence of portal hypertension, and her disease is well controlled on her current medical regimen. All of the following new findings on a diagnostic study are suggestive of the development of portal hypertension EXCEPT:

A. 15-cmHg gradient between wedged and free hepatic vein pressures
B. Ascites on ultrasound
C. Enlarged spleen on physical examination
D. Left atrial dilation on echocardiogram
E. Thrombocytopenia

VIII-75. A 63-year-old man with cirrhosis and portal hypertension due to hemochromatosis presents with altered mental status. He has chronic ascites controlled with diet and spironolactone. He has a history of one esophageal bleed but none since starting propranolol. His family reports that over the last 2 days, he has become more confused, but he has had no melena or hematemesis. He is afebrile with normal vital signs, and physical examination is notable for ascites, asterixis, and being oriented only to person. His laboratory examination is notable for a hemoglobin of 10.1 (baseline, 9.5), creatinine of 1.4 (baseline, 1.4), and blood urea nitrogen of 45 (baseline, 18). A paracentesis is performed that yields reveals clear fluid with 800 WBC (40% neutrophils). Which of the following is the most indicated therapy?

A. Ampicillin, ceftriaxone, vancomycin
B. Cefotaxime
C. EGD with banding
D. Hemodialysis
E. Lactulose

VIII-76. A 48-year-old woman presents complaining of fatigue and itching. She has been tired for the past 6 months and recently has developed itching diffusely. It is worse in the evening hours but is intermittent. She does not note it to be worse following hot baths or showers. Her past medical history is significant only for hypothyroidism for which she takes levothyroxine 125 μg daily. On physical examination, she has mild jaundice and scleral icterus. The liver is enlarged to 15 cm on palpation and is palpable 5 cm below the right costal margin. Xanthomas are seen on both elbows. Hyperpigmentation is noticeable on the trunk and arms where the patient has excoriations. Laboratory studies demonstrate the following: WBC 8,900/μL, hemoglobin 13.3 g/dL, hematocrit 41.6%, and platelets 160,000/μL. The creatinine is 1.2 mg/dL. The AST is 52 IU/L, ALT is 62 IU/L, alkaline phosphatase is 216 IU/L, total bilirubin is 3.2 mg/dL, and direct bilirubin is 2.9 mg/dL. The total protein is 8.2 g/dL, and albumin is 3.9 U/L. The thyroid-stimulating hormone is 4.5 U/mL. Antimitochondrial antibodies are positive. Perinuclear antineutrophil cytoplasmic antibodies (ANCA) and cytoplasmic ANCA are negative. What is the most likely cause of the patient's symptoms?

A. Lymphoma
B. Polycythemia vera
C. Primary biliary cirrhosis
D. Primary sclerosis cholangitis
E. Uncontrolled hypothyroidism

VIII-77. A 42-year-old man with cirrhosis related to hepatitis C and alcohol abuse has ascites requiring frequent large-volume paracentesis. All of the following therapies would be indicated for this patient EXCEPT:

A. Fluid restriction to less than 2 L daily
B. Furosemide 40 mg daily
C. Sodium restriction to less than 2 g daily
D. Spironolactone 100 mg daily
E. Transjugular intrahepatic portosystemic shunt if medical therapy fails

VIII-78. Which of the following statements about cardiac cirrhosis is true?

A. AST and ALT levels may mimic the very high levels seen in acute viral hepatitis.
B. Budd-Chiari syndrome cannot be distinguished clinically from cardiac cirrhosis.
C. Echocardiography is the gold standard for diagnosing constrictive pericarditis as a cause of cirrhosis.
D. Prolonged passive congestion from right-sided heart failure results in congestion and necrosis of portal triads, resulting in subsequent fibrosis.
E. Veno-occlusive disease can be confused with cardiac cirrhosis and is a major cause of morbidity and mortality in patients undergoing liver transplantation.

VIII-79. You are asked to consult on a 62-year-old white woman with pruritus for 4 months. She has noted progressive fatigue and a 5-lb weight loss. She has intermittent nausea but no vomiting and denies changes in her bowel habits. There is no history of prior alcohol use, blood transfusions, or illicit drug use. The patient is widowed and had two heterosexual partners in her lifetime. Her past medical history is significant only for hypothyroidism, for which she takes levothyroxine. Her family history is unremarkable. On examination, she is mildly icteric. She has spider angiomata on her torso. You palpate a nodular liver edge 2 cm below the right costal margin. The remainder of the examination is unremarkable. A right upper quadrant ultrasound confirms your suspicion of cirrhosis. You order a complete blood count and a comprehensive metabolic panel. What is the most appropriate next test?

A. 24-Hour urine copper
B. Antimitochondrial antibodies
C. Endoscopic retrograde cholangiopancreatography
D. Hepatitis B serologies
E. Serum ferritin

VIII-80. All of the following are potential indications for liver transplantation EXCEPT:

A. Autoimmune hepatitis
B. Cholangiocarcinoma
C. Primary biliary cirrhosis
D. Primary hepatocellular carcinoma
E. Primary sclerosing cholangitis

VIII-81. Which of the following patients is highest priority for liver transplantation?

A. A 24-year-old woman with cirrhosis due to autoimmune hepatitis. She has been on the transplant list for 2 months and now has an elevated bilirubin, INR, and creatinine.
B. A 38-year-old woman with chronic hepatitis C and normal bilirubin and INR.
C. A 49-year-old man with alcoholic cirrhosis who has been on the transplant list for 6 months. He has had two esophageal variceal bleeds.
D. A 59-year-old man with a history of hyperlipidemia who was admitted to the ICU 2 days ago with fulminant hepatic failure due to mistakenly ingesting *Amanita* mushrooms from his lawn.
E. A 64-year-old woman with primary hepatocellular carcinoma admitted to the hospital with acute renal failure.

VIII-82. A 44-year-old woman is evaluated for complaints of abdominal pain. She describes the pain as a postprandial burning pain. It is worse with spicy or fatty foods and is relieved with antacids. She is diagnosed with a gastric ulcer and is treated appropriately for *H pylori*. During the course of her evaluation for her abdominal pain, the patient had a right upper quadrant ultrasound that demonstrated the presence of gallstones. Following treatment of *H pylori*, her symptoms have resolved. She is requesting your opinion regarding whether treatment is required for the finding of gallstone disease. Upon review of the ultrasound report, there were numerous stones in the gallbladder, including in the neck of the gallbladder. The largest stone measures 2.8 cm. What is your advice to the patient regarding the risk of complications and the need for definitive treatment?

A. Given the size and number of stones, prophylactic cholecystectomy is recommended.
B. No treatment is necessary unless the patient develops symptoms of biliary colic frequent and severe enough to interfere with the patient's life.
C. The only reason to proceed with cholecystectomy is development of gallstone pancreatitis or cholangitis.
D. The risk of developing acute cholecystitis is about 5%–10% per year.
E. Ursodeoxycholic acid should be given at a dose of 10–15 mg/kg daily for a minimum of 6 months to dissolve the stones.

VIII-83. A 62-year-old man has been hospitalized in intensive care for the past 3 weeks following an automobile accident resulting in multiple long bone fractures and acute respiratory distress syndrome. He has been slowly improving but remains on mechanical ventilation. He is now febrile and hypotensive requiring vasopressors. He is being treated empirically with cefepime and vancomycin. Multiple blood cultures are negative. He has no new infiltrates or increasing secretions on chest radiograph. His laboratory studies demonstrated a rise in his liver function tests, bilirubin, and alkaline phosphatase. Amylase and lipase are normal. A right upper quadrant ultrasound shows sludge in the gallbladder but no stones. The bile duct is not dilated. What is the next best step in the evaluation and treatment of this patient?

A. Discontinue cefepime
B. Initiate treatment with clindamycin
C. Initiate treatment with metronidazole
D. Perform hepatobiliary scintigraphy
E. Refer for exploratory laparotomy

VIII-84. All the following are associated with an increased risk for cholesterol stone cholelithiasis EXCEPT:

A. Gallbladder sludge on ultrasound
B. High-protein diet
C. Oral contraceptives
D. Pregnancy
E. Rapid weight loss

VIII-85. All of the following conditions are associated with an increased risk of pigment stone cholelithiasis EXCEPT:

A. Alcoholic cirrhosis
B. Chronic biliary tract infection
C. Chronic hemolytic anemia
D. Cystic fibrosis
E. Primary biliary cirrhosis

VIII-86. A 41-year-old woman presents to your clinic with a week of jaundice. She notes pruritus, icterus, and dark urine. She denies fever, abdominal pain, or weight loss. The examination is unremarkable except for yellow discoloration of the skin. Total bilirubin is 6.0 mg/dL, and direct bilirubin is 5.1 mg/dL. AST is 84 IU/L, and ALT is 92 IU/L. Alkaline phosphatase is 662 IU/L. CT scan of the abdomen is unremarkable. Right upper quadrant ultrasound shows a normal gallbladder but does not visualize the common bile duct. What is the most appropriate next management step?

A. Antibiotics and observation
B. Endoscopic retrograde cholangiopancreatography
C. Hepatitis serologies
D. Hepatobiliary iminodiacetic acid (HIDA) scan
E. Serologies for antimitochondrial antibodies

VIII-87. A 32-year-old woman is being evaluated for her second episode of acute-onset right upper quadrant pain and jaundice. She's noticed worsening jaundice over the last 2 weeks and now complains of diffused itchiness. She has a 10-year history of ulcerative colitis treated with sulfasalazine. She is found to have a markedly elevated serum bilirubin and alkaline phosphatase. Her aminotransferases and prothrombin time are normal. Ultrasound shows no gallstones. Magnetic resonance cholangiopancreatography reveals a beaded appearance of her intrahepatic and extrahepatic bile ducts due to multiple discrete strictures. All of the following statements regarding her diagnosis are true EXCEPT:

A. Cyclosporine A is the most effective medical therapy.
B. Median survival with medical therapy is approximately 10 years.
C. She may be a candidate for liver transplantation.
D. Surgical therapy is rarely indicated.
E. The biliary disease is associated with her ulcerative colitis.

VIII-88. Which of the following is the most important ion secreted by the pancreas?

A. Bicarbonate
B. Chloride
C. Magnesium
D. Potassium
E. Sodium

VIII-89. A 45-year-old woman with known history of cholelithiasis is admitted to the hospital with severe mid-epigastric pain, fever to 38.5°C, tachycardia to 110 bpm, and a blood pressure of 100/50 mmHg. Her examination shows a diffusely tender abdomen with guarding. Radiographs show an abdominal ileus with no free air. Laboratories are notable for a hemoglobin of 15 g/dL and elevations or amylase and lipase. Which of the following statements regarding this patient's likely diagnosis is true?

A. Elevated lipase is more specific than elevated amylase for the diagnosis of acute pancreatitis.
B. Hypercalcemia occurs in >75% of cases of acute pancreatitis.
C. Magnitude of lipase elevation above normal is correlated with the severity of acute pancreatitis.
D. Serum amylase levels will remain elevated for up to 30 days after the resolution of acute pancreatitis.
E. The combination of elevated serum amylase and metabolic acidosis (pH <7.32) has a >90% positive predictive value for acute pancreatitis.

VIII-90. A 27-year-old woman is admitted to the hospital with acute-onset severe right upper quadrant pain that radiates to the back. The pain is constant and not relieved with eating or bowel movements. Her labs show marked elevation in amylase and lipase, and acute pancreatitis is diagnosed. Which of the following is the best first test to demonstrate the etiology of her pancreatitis?

A. Right upper quadrant ultrasound
B. Serum alcohol level
C. Serum triglyceride level
D. Technetium HIDA scan
E. Urine drug screen

VIII-91. A 58-year-old man with severe alcoholism is admitted to the hospital with acute pancreatitis. His symptoms have been present for 3 days, and he has persisted to drink heavily. He now has persistent vomiting and feels dizzy upon standing. On examination, he has severe epigastric and right upper quadrant tenderness and decreased bowel sounds, and he appears uncomfortable. A faint blue discoloration is present around the umbilicus. What is the significance of this finding?

A. A CT of the abdomen is likely to show severe necrotizing pancreatitis.
B. Abdominal plain film is likely to show pancreatic calcification.
C. Concomitant appendicitis should be ruled out.
D. He likely has a pancreatico-aortic fistula.
E. Pancreatic pseudocyst is likely present.

VIII-92. A 36-year-old man is admitted to the hospital with acute pancreatitis. In order to determine the severity of disease and risk of mortality, the Bedside Index of Severity in Acute Pancreatitis (BISAP) is calculated. All of the following variables are used to calculate this score EXCEPT:

A. Age >60 years
B. Blood urea nitrogen >35
C. Impaired mental status
D. Pleural effusion
E. Serum lipase >3× normal

VIII-93. A 54-year-old man is admitted to the ICU with severe pancreatitis. His BMI is ≥30 kg/m^2, and he has a prior history of diabetes mellitus. A CT of the abdomen is obtained and shows severe necrotizing pancreatitis. He is presently afebrile. Which of the following medications has been shown to be effective in the treatment of acute necrotizing pancreatitis?

A. Calcitonin
B. Cimetidine
C. Glucagon
D. Imipenem
E. None of the above

VIII-94. Which of the following statements regarding enteral feeding in acute pancreatitis is true?

A. A patient with persistent evidence of pancreatic necrosis on CT 2 weeks after acute presentation should be maintained on bowel rest.
B. All patients with elevations of amylase and lipase and CT evidence of pancreatitis should be fasted until amylase and lipase normalize.
C. Enteral feeding has been demonstrated to have fewer infectious complications than total parenteral nutrition in the management of patients with acute pancreatitis.
D. Patients requiring surgical removal of infected pancreatic pseudocysts should be treated with total parental nutrition.
E. Total parenteral nutrition has been shown to maintain integrity of the intestinal tract in acute pancreatitis.

VIII-95. A 47-year-old woman presents to the emergency department with severe mid-abdominal pain radiating to her back. The pain began acutely and is sharp. She denies cramping or flatulence. She has had two episodes of emesis of bilious material since the pain began, but this has not lessened the pain. She currently rates the pain as a 10 out of 10 and feels the pain is worse in the supine position. For the past few months, she has had intermittent episodes of right upper and mid-epigastric pain that occur after eating but subside over a few hours. These are associated with a feeling of excess gas. She denies any history of alcohol abuse. She has no medical history of hypertension or hyperlipidemia. On physical examination, she is writhing in distress and slightly diaphoretic. Vital signs are: heart rate 127 bpm, blood pressure 92/50 mmHg, respiratory rate 20 breaths/min, temperature 37.9°C, oxygen saturation 88% on room air. Her BMI is 29 kg/m^2. The cardiovascular examination reveals a regular tachycardia. The chest examination shows dullness to percussion at bilateral bases with a few scattered crackles. On abdominal examination, bowel sounds are hypoactive. There is no rash or bruising evident on inspection of the abdomen. There is voluntary guarding on palpation. The pain with palpation is greatest in the periumbilical and epigastric area without rebound tenderness. There is no evidence of jaundice, and the liver span is about 10 cm to percussion. Amylase level is 750 IU/L, and lipase level is 1129 IU/L. Other laboratory values include: AST 168 IU/L, ALT 196 IU/L, total bilirubin 2.3 mg/dL, alkaline phosphatase 268 IU/L, lactate dehydrogenase 300 U/L, and creatinine 1.9 mg/dL. The hematocrit is 43%, and WBC count is 11,500/μL with 89% neutrophils. An arterial blood gas shows a pH of 7.32, PCO2 of 32 mmHg, and PO2 of 56 mmHg. An ultrasound confirms a dilated common bile duct with evidence of pancreatitis manifested as an edematous and enlarged pancreas. A CT scan shows no evidence of necrosis. After 3 L of normal saline, her blood pressure comes up to 110/60 mmHg with a heart rate of 105 bpm. Which of the following best describes the pathophysiology of this disease?

A. Intrapancreatic activation of digestive enzymes with autodigestion and acinar cell injury
B. Chemoattraction of neutrophils with subsequent infiltration and inflammation
C. Distant organ involvement and systemic inflammatory response syndrome related to release of activated pancreatic enzymes and cytokines
D. All of the above

VIII-96. A 25-year-old woman with cystic fibrosis is diagnosed with chronic pancreatitis. She is at risk for all of the following complications EXCEPT:

A. Vitamin B_{12} deficiency
B. Vitamin A deficiency
C. Pancreatic carcinoma
D. Niacin deficiency
E. Steatorrhea

VIII-97. A 64-year-old man seeks evaluation from his primary care physician because of chronic diarrhea. He reports that he has two or three large loose bowel movements daily. He describes them as markedly foul smelling, and they often leave an oily ring in the toilet. He also notes that the bowel movements often follow heavy meals, but if he fasts or eats low-fat foods, the stools are more formed. Over the past 6 months, he has lost about 18 kg (40 lb). In this setting, he reports intermittent episodes of abdominal pain that can be quite severe. He describes the pain as sharp and in a mid-epigastric location. He has not sought evaluation of the pain previously, but when it occurs, he will limit his oral intake and treat the pain with nonsteroidal anti-inflammatory drugs. He notes the pain has not lasted for >48 hours and is not associated with meals. His past medical history is remarkable for peripheral vascular disease and tobacco use. He currently smokes one pack of cigarettes daily. In addition, he drinks two to six beers daily. He has stopped all alcohol intake for up to a week at a time in the past without withdrawal symptoms. His current medications are aspirin 81 mg daily and albuterol metered-dose inhaler on an as-needed basis. On physical examination, the patient is thin but appears well. His BMI is 18.2 kg/m^2. Vital signs are normal. Cardiac and pulmonary examinations are normal. The abdominal examination shows mild epigastric tenderness without rebound or guarding. The liver span is 12 cm to percussion and palpable 2 cm below the right costal margin. There is no splenomegaly or ascites present. There are decreased pulses in the lower extremities bilaterally. An abdominal radiograph demonstrates calcifications in the epigastric area, and CT scan confirms that these calcifications are located within the body of the pancreas. No pancreatic ductal dilatation is noted. An amylase level is 32 U/L, and lipase level is 22 U/L. What is the next most appropriate step in diagnosing and managing this patient's primary complaint?

A. Advise the patient to stop all alcohol use and prescribe pancreatic enzymes.
B. Advise the patient to stop all alcohol use and prescribe narcotic analgesia and pancreatic enzymes.
C. Perform angiography to assess for ischemic bowel disease.
D. Prescribe prokinetic agents to improve gastric emptying.
E. Refer the patient for endoscopic retrograde cholangiopancreatography for sphincterotomy.

ANSWERS

VIII-1. **The answer is A.** *(Chap. 347)* Endoscopy, also known as esophagogastroduodenoscopy (EGD) is the best test for evaluation of the proximal gastrointestinal tract. Because of high-quality images, disorders of color such as Barrett metaplasia and mucosal irregularities are easily demonstrated. Sensitivity of endoscopy is superior to that of barium radiography for mucosal lesions. Because the endoscope has an instrumentation channel, biopsy specimens are easily obtained, and dilation of strictures can also be performed. The sensitivity of radiography compared with endoscopy for detecting reflux esophagitis reportedly ranges from 22%–95%, with higher grades of esophagitis (i.e., ulceration or stricture) exhibiting greater detection rates. Conversely, the sensitivity of barium radiography for detecting esophageal strictures is greater than that of endoscopy, especially when the study is done in conjunction with barium-soaked bread or a 13-mm barium tablet. Barium studies also provide an assessment of esophageal function and morphology that may be undetected on endoscopy. The major shortcoming of barium radiography is that it rarely obviates the need for endoscopy. Barium radiography does not require sedation, which in some populations at risk for conscious sedation is an important consideration.

VIII-2. **The answer is E.** *(Chap. 347)* Intermittent solid food dysphagia is a classic symptom in Schatzki ring in which a distal esophageal ring occurs at the squamocolumnar mucosal junction. The origin of these rings is unknown, and smaller rings with a lumen of greater than 13 mm are common in the general population (up to 15%). When the lumen is less than 13 mm, dysphagia may occur. Schatzki rings typically occur in persons older than 40 years and often cause "steakhouse syndrome" from meat getting stuck at the ring. The rings are easily treated with dilation. Plummer-Vinson syndrome also includes esophageal rings, but typically, the rings occur in the proximal esophagus, are associated with iron-deficiency anemia, and occur in middle-aged women. Achalasia involves both solid and liquid dysphagia often with regurgitation. Adenocarcinoma often includes solid and liquid dysphagia at later stages. Most esophageal diverticulae are asymptomatic.

VIII-3. **The answer is B.** *(Chap. 347)* Aside from the discomfort and local complications of gastroesophageal reflux disease (GERD), a number of other, non–gastrointestinal (GI)-related sites may have complications related to GERD. Syndromes with well-established association with GERD include chronic cough, laryngitis, asthma, and dental erosions. Other diseases have implicated GERD as potentially contributory, but the role of GERD is less well established. These include pharyngitis, pulmonary fibrosis, chronic sinusitis, cardiac arrhythmias, sleep apnea, and recurrent aspiration pneumonia.

VIII-4. **The answer is A.** *(Chap. 347)* This patient has symptoms of esophagitis. In patients with human immunodeficiency virus (HIV), various infections can cause this disease, including herpes simplex virus (HSV), cytomegalovirus (CMV), varicella-zoster virus (VZV), *Candida*, and HIV itself. The lack of thrush does not rule out *Candida* as a cause of esophagitis, and EGD is necessary for diagnosis. CMV classically causes serpiginous ulcers in the distal esophagus that may coalesce to form large ulcers. Brushings alone are insufficient for diagnosis, and biopsies must be performed. Biopsies reveal intranuclear and intracytoplasmic inclusions with enlarged nuclei in large fibroblasts and endothelial cells. Given this patient's notable swallowing symptoms, intravenous ganciclovir is the treatment of choice. Valganciclovir is an effective oral preparation. Foscarnet is useful in treating ganciclovir-resistant CMV. HSV manifests as vesicles and punched-out lesions in the esophagus with the characteristic finding on biopsy of ballooning degeneration with ground-glass changes in the nuclei. It can be treated with acyclovir or foscarnet in resistant cases. Candida esophagitis has the appearance of yellow nodular plaques with surrounding erythema. Treatment usually requires fluconazole therapy. Finally, HIV alone can cause esophagitis that can be quite resistant to therapy. On EGD, these ulcers appear deep and linear. Treatment with thalidomide or oral glucocorticoids is employed, and highly active antiretroviral therapy should be considered.

VIII-5 and VIII-6. **The answers are A and A, respectively.** *(Chap. 347)* The barium swallow image demonstrates achalasia with esophageal dilation narrowing at the gastroesophageal junction and an air-fluid level in the mid-esophagus. Achalasia is a rare disease caused by loss of ganglion cells within the esophageal myenteric plexus with a population incidence of about 1:100,000; it usually presents between age 25 and 60. With long-standing disease, aganglionosis is noted. The disease involves both excitatory (cholinergic) and inhibitory (nitric oxide) ganglionic neurons. This leads to impaired deglutitive lower esophageal sphincter (LES) relaxation and absent peristalsis. Increasing evidence suggests that the ultimate cause of ganglion cell degeneration in achalasia is an autoimmune process attributable to a latent infection with human HSV-1 combined with genetic susceptibility. Long-standing achalasia is characterized by progressive dilatation and sigmoid deformity of the esophagus with hypertrophy of the LES. Clinical manifestations may include dysphagia, regurgitation, chest pain, and weight loss. Most patients report solid and liquid food dysphagia. Regurgitation occurs when food, fluid, and secretions are retained in the dilated esophagus. Patients with advanced achalasia are at risk for bronchitis, pneumonia, or lung abscess from chronic regurgitation and aspiration. The differential diagnosis of achalasia includes diffuse esophageal spasm, Chagas disease, and pseudoachalasia. Chagas disease is endemic in areas of central Brazil, Venezuela, and northern Argentina and spread by the bite of the reduviid (kissing) bug that transmits the protozoan *Trypanosoma cruzi*. The chronic phase of the disease develops years after infection and results from destruction of autonomic ganglion cells throughout the body, including the heart, gut, urinary tract, and respiratory tract. Tumor infiltration, most commonly seen with carcinoma in the gastric fundus or distal esophagus, can mimic idiopathic achalasia. The resultant "pseudoachalasia" accounts for up to 5% of suspected cases and is more likely with advanced age, abrupt onset of symptoms (<1 year), and weight loss. Hence, endoscopy is a necessary part of the evaluation of achalasia. When the clinical suspicion for pseudoachalasia is high and endoscopy nondiagnostic, computed tomography (CT) scanning or endoscopic ultrasound may be of value. There is no known way of preventing or reversing achalasia. Therapy is directed at reducing LES pressure so that gravity and esophageal pressurization promote esophageal emptying. Peristalsis rarely, if ever, recovers. Botulinum toxin, injected into the LES under endoscopic guidance, inhibits acetylcholine release from nerve endings and improves dysphagia in about 66% of cases for at least 6 months. The only durable therapies for achalasia are pneumatic dilatation and Heller myotomy. Pneumatic dilatation, with a reported efficacy ranging from 32%–98%, is an endoscopic technique using a noncompliant, cylindrical balloon dilator positioned across the LES and inflated to a diameter of 3–4 cm. The major complication is perforation, with a reported incidence of 0.5%–5%.

VIII-7. **The answer is B.** *(Chap. 347)* Barrett metaplasia is the most serious complication of GERD. It has a strong association with the subsequent development of esophageal adenocarcinoma. The incidence of these lesions has increased, not decreased, in the era of potent acid suppression. Barrett metaplasia is endoscopically recognized by tongues of reddish mucosa extending proximally from the gastroesophageal junction or histopathologically identified by the finding of specialized columnar metaplasia. Barrett metaplasia can progress to adenocarcinoma through the intermediate stages of low- and high-grade dysplasia. Due to this risk, areas of Barrett metaplasia and especially any included areas of mucosal irregularity should be extensively biopsied. No high-level evidence confirms that aggressive antisecretory therapy or antireflux surgery causes regression of Barrett esophagus or prevents adenocarcinoma. Although the management of Barrett esophagus remains controversial, the finding of dysplasia in Barrett esophagus, particularly high-grade dysplasia, mandates further intervention. In addition to the high rate of progression to adenocarcinoma, there is also a high prevalence of unrecognized coexisting cancer with high-grade dysplasia. Nonetheless, treatment remains controversial. Esophagectomy, intensive endoscopic surveillance, and mucosal ablation have all been advocated. Currently, esophagectomy is the gold standard treatment for high-grade dysplasia in an otherwise healthy patient with minimal surgical risk. However, esophagectomy has a mortality ranging from 3%–10%, along with substantial morbidity. As a result of these factors and the increasing evidence of the effectiveness of endoscopic therapy with purpose-built radiofrequency ablation devices, many now favor this therapy as a preferable management strategy.

VIII-8. **The answer is D.** *(Chap. 348)* The patient has a duodenal ulcer, which is almost universally due to *Helicobacter pylori* infection, although in a minority of cases, nonsteroidal anti-inflammatory drug (NSAID) use may either facilitate development or be the only identified cause. The patient was taking acetaminophen and not a traditional NSAID, making *H pylori*–associated peptic ulcer disease the most likely cause of the findings. *H pylori* infection is closely correlated with advancing age, low socioeconomic status, and low education levels. After initial infection, antral gastritis is common, and in a portion of patients, duodenal or gastric ulcers form. Associated with these conditions is the development of gastric cancer or mucosa-associated lymphoid tissue (MALT) lymphoma. Duodenal ulcers are rarely cancerous, whereas this is a not an uncommon finding in gastric ulcers. After discovery of the ulcer, first-line therapy is eradication of *H pylori* in addition to acid suppression.

VIII-9. **The answer is D.** *(Chap. 348)* Noninvasive testing for *H pylori* infection is recommended in patients with suggestive symptoms and no other indication for endoscopy (e.g., GI bleeding, atypical symptoms). Several tests have good sensitivity and specificity, including plasma serology for *H pylori*, ^{14}C- or ^{13}C-urea breath test, and the fecal *H pylori* antigen test (Table VIII-9). Sensitivity and specificity are >80% and >90%, respectively, for serology, whereas the sensitivity and specificity of the urea breath test and fecal antigen testing are >90% for both. Serology is not useful for early follow-up after therapy completion because antibody titers will take several weeks to months to fall. The urea breath test, which relies on the presence of urease secreted by *H pylori* to digest the swallowed radioactive urea and liberate ^{14}C or ^{13}C as part of ammonia, is simple and rapid. It is useful for early follow-up because it requires living bacteria to secrete urease and produce a positive test. The limitations to the test include requirement for ingestion of radioactive materials, albeit low dose, and false-negative results with recent use of proton pump inhibitors, antibiotics, or bismuth compounds.

TABLE VIII-9 **Tests for Detection of *H pylori***

Test	Sensitivity/ Specificity, %	Comments
Invasive (Endoscopy/Biopsy Required)		
Rapid urease	80–95/95–100	Simple, false negative with recent use of PPIs, antibiotics, or bismuth compounds
Histology	80–90/>95	Requires pathology processing and staining; provides histologic information
Culture	—/—	Time-consuming, expensive, dependent on experience; allows determination of antibiotic susceptibility
Noninvasive		
Serology	>80/>90	Inexpensive, convenient; not useful for early follow-up
Urea breath test	>90/>90	Simple, rapid; useful for early follow-up; false negatives with recent therapy (see rapid urease test); exposure to low-dose radiation with ^{14}C test
Stool antigen	>90/>90	Inexpensive, convenient

Abbreviation: PPIs, proton pump inhibitors.

VIII-10. **The answer is A.** *(Chap. 348)* Documented eradication of *H pylori* in patients with peptic ulcer disease (PUD) is associated with a dramatic decrease in ulcer recurrence to <10%–20% as compared to 59% in gastric ulcer patients and 67% in duodenal ulcer patients when the organism is not eliminated. Eradication of the organism may lead to diminished recurrent ulcer bleeding. The effect of its eradication on ulcer perforation is unclear. Extensive effort has been made in determining who of the many individuals with *H pylori* infection should be treated. The common conclusion arrived at by multiple consensus conferences around the world is that *H pylori* should be eradicated in patients with documented PUD. This holds true independent of time of presentation (first episode or not), severity of symptoms, presence of confounding factors such as ingestion of NSAIDs, or whether the ulcer is in remission. Multiple drugs have been evaluated in the therapy of *H pylori*. No single agent is effective in eradicating the organism. Combination therapy for 14 days provides the greatest efficacy, although regimens based on sequential administration of antibiotics also appear promising. A shorter administration course (7–10 days), although attractive, has not proved as successful as the 14-day regimens. Suggested treatment regimens for *H pylori* are outlined in Table VIII-10. Choice of a particular regimen will be influenced by several factors, including efficacy, patient tolerance, existing antibiotic resistance, and cost of the drugs. The aim for initial eradication rates should be 85%–90%. Dual therapy (proton pump inhibitor [PPI] plus amoxicillin, PPI plus clarithromycin, ranitidine bismuth citrate [Tritec] plus clarithromycin) is not recommended in view of studies demonstrating eradication rates of <80%–85%. Addition of acid suppression assists in providing early symptom relief and enhances bacterial eradication. Triple therapy, although effective, has several drawbacks, including the potential for poor patient compliance and drug-induced side effects. Compliance is being addressed by simplifying the regimens so that patients can take the medications twice a day. Simpler (dual therapy) and shorter regimens (7 and 10 days) are not as effective as triple therapy for 14 days. Two anti–*H pylori* regimens are available in prepackaged formulation: Prevpac (lansoprazole, clarithromycin, and amoxicillin) and Helidac (bismuth subsalicylate, tetracycline, and metronidazole). The contents of the Prevpac are to be taken twice per day for 14 days, whereas Helidac constituents are taken four times per day with an antisecretory agent (PPI or H_2 blocker), also taken for at least 14 days. Clarithromycin-based triple therapy should be avoided in settings where *H pylori* resistance to this agent exceeds 15%–20%. Quadruple therapy should be reserved for patients with failure to eradicate *H pylori* after an effective initial course.

TABLE VIII-10 **Regimens Recommended for Eradication of *H pylori* Infection**

Drug	Dose
Triple Therapy	
1. Bismuth subsalicylate *plus*	2 tablets qid
Metronidazole *plus*	250 mg qid
Tetracycline[a]	500 mg qid
2. Ranitidine bismuth citrate *plus*	400 mg bid
Tetracycline *plus*	500 mg bid
Clarithromycin or metronidazole	500 mg bid
3. Omeprazole (lansoprazole) *plus*	20 mg bid (30 mg bid)
Clarithromycin *plus*	250 or 500 mg bid
Metronidazole[b] *or*	500 mg bid
Amoxicillin[c]	1 g bid
Quadruple Therapy	
Omeprazole (lansoprazole)	20 mg (30 mg) daily
Bismuth subsalicylate	2 tablets qid
Metronidazole	250 mg qid
Tetracycline	500 mg qid

[a]Alternative: use *prepacked* Helidac (see text).
[b]Alternative: use prepacked Prevpac (see text).
[c]Use either metronidazole or amoxicillin, not both.

VIII-11. **The answer is C.** *(Chap. 348)* Fasting gastrin levels can be elevated in a variety of conditions, including atrophic gastritis with or without pernicious anemia, G-cell hyperplasia, and acid suppressive therapy (gastrin levels increase as a consequence of loss of negative feedback). The diagnostic concern in a patient with persistent ulcers following optimal therapy is Zollinger-Ellison syndrome (ZES). The result is not sufficient to make a diagnosis because gastrin levels may be elevated in a variety of conditions. Elevated basal acid secretion also is consistent with ZES, but up to 12% of patients with PUD may have basal acid secretion as high as 15 mEq/hr. Thus, additional testing is necessary. Gastrin levels may go up with a meal (>200%), but this test does not distinguish G-cell hyperfunction from ZES. The best test in this setting is the secretin stimulation test. An increase in gastrin levels >200 pg within 15 minutes of administering 2 μg/kg of secretin by intravenous bolus has a sensitivity and specificity of >90% for ZES. Endoscopic ultrasonography is useful in locating the gastrin-secreting tumor once the positive secretin test is obtained. Genetic testing for mutations in the gene that encodes the menin protein can detect the fraction of patients with gastrinomas that are a manifestation of multiple endocrine neoplasia type 1 (Wermer syndrome). Gastrinoma is the second most common tumor in this syndrome after parathyroid adenoma, but its peak incidence is generally in the third decade.

VIII-12 and VIII-13. **The answers are B and C, respectively.** *(Chap. 348)* Surgical intervention in PUD can be viewed as being either elective, for treatment of medically refractory disease, or as urgent/emergent, for the treatment of an ulcer-related complication. The development of pharmacologic and endoscopic approaches for the treatment of PUD and its complications has led to a substantial decrease in the number of operations needed for this disorder, with a decrease of over 90% for elective ulcer surgery over the last four decades. Refractory ulcers are an exceedingly rare occurrence. Surgery is more often required for treatment of an ulcer-related complication. Free peritoneal perforation occurs in ~2%–3% of DU patients. As in the case of bleeding, up to 10% of these patients will not have antecedent ulcer symptoms. Concomitant bleeding may occur in up to 10% of patients with perforation, with mortality being increased substantially. The procedure that provides the lowest rates of ulcer recurrence (1%) but has the highest complication rate is vagotomy (truncal or selective) in combination with antrectomy. Antrectomy is aimed at eliminating an additional stimulant of gastric acid secretion, gastrin. Two principal types of reanastomoses are used after antrectomy: gastroduodenostomy (Billroth I) and gastrojejunostomy (Billroth II). Dumping syndrome consists of a series of vasomotor and GI signs and symptoms and occurs in patients who have undergone vagotomy and drainage (especially Billroth procedures). Two phases of dumping, early and late, can occur. Early dumping takes place 15–30 minutes after meals and consists of crampy abdominal discomfort, nausea, diarrhea, belching, tachycardia, palpitations, diaphoresis, light-headedness, and, rarely, syncope. These signs and symptoms arise from the rapid emptying of hyperosmolar gastric contents into the small intestine, resulting in a fluid shift into the gut lumen with plasma volume contraction and acute intestinal distention. Release of vasoactive GI hormones (vasoactive intestinal polypeptide, neurotensin, motilin) is also theorized to play a role in early dumping. The late phase of dumping typically occurs 90 minutes to 3 hours after meals. Vasomotor symptoms (light-headedness, diaphoresis, palpitations, tachycardia, and syncope) predominate during this phase. This component of dumping is thought to be secondary to hypoglycemia from excessive insulin release. Dumping syndrome is most noticeable after meals rich in simple carbohydrates (especially sucrose) and high osmolarity. Ingestion of large amounts of fluids may also contribute. Up to 50% of postvagotomy and drainage patients will experience dumping syndrome to some degree early on. Signs and symptoms often improve with time, but a severe protracted picture can occur in up to 1% of patients. Although this patient is certainly at risk of pulmonary embolism and myocardial infarction, his symptoms are typical of hypoglycemia due to dumping syndrome.

VIII-14. **The answer is B.** *(Chap. 349)* The patient presents with nonspecific GI symptoms, but the presence of weight loss does suggest malabsorption syndrome. Patients with lactose intolerance are usually able to relate symptoms to consumption of milk-based products and also report a strong history of crampy pain and flatulence. Therefore, a lactose-free diet is unlikely to be helpful. The patient does not have nocturnal diarrhea, which is commonly a feature of steatorrhea along with floating stools. In the absence of symptoms suggesting fat malabsorption, the first test should not be fecal fat measurement. Because the patient has weight loss, irritable bowel syndrome is less likely, and increased dietary fiber is unlikely to be useful. Finally, the patient's symptoms may be consistent with celiac disease. The widespread availability of antibodies to gliadin, endomysium, and tissue transglutaminase can be easily measured in peripheral blood. Antiendomysial antibody has a 90%–95% sensitivity and equal specificity, making it a reasonable first test in symptomatic individuals. The presence of the antibody is not diagnostic, however, and duodenal biopsy is recommended. Duodenal biopsy will show villous atrophy, absence or reduced height of villi, cuboidal appearance of surface epithelial cells, and increased lymphocytes and plasma cells in the lamina propria. These changes regress with complete removal of gluten from the diet.

VIII-15. **The answer is B.** *(Chap. 349)* Short bowel syndrome is a descriptive term referring to the many clinical complications that may occur after resection of varying lengths of the small bowel. Rarely, these complications may be due to congenital abnormalities of the small bowel. Most commonly, in adults, short bowel syndrome occurs in mesenteric vascular disease, primary mucosal or submucosal disease (Crohn disease), and operations without preexisting small bowel disease such as trauma. Multiple factors contribute to diarrhea and steatorrhea including gastric acid hypersecretion, increased bile acids in the colon due to absent or decreased reabsorption in the small bowel, and lactose intolerance due to increased gastric acid secretion. Nonintestinal symptoms may include renal calcium oxalate calculi due to an increase in oxalate absorption by the large intestine with subsequent hyperoxaluria. This may be due to increased fatty acids in the colon that bind calcium, and therefore, calcium in the gut is not free to bind oxalate and free oxalate is thus absorbed in the large intestine. Increased bile acid pool size results in the generation of cholesterol gallstones from supersaturation in gallbladder bile. Gastric hypersecretion of acid is well described and thought to be due to loss of inhibition of gastric acid secretion because of absent short bowel, which secretes inhibitory hormones. Coronary artery disease is not described as a complication of short bowel syndrome.

VIII-16. **The answer is E.** *(Chap. 349)* The patient presents with symptoms suggestive of Whipple disease, a chronic multisystem disease often including diarrhea/steatorrhea, migratory arthralgias, weight loss, and central nervous system (CNS) or cardiac problems. Generally the presentation is of insidious onset, and dementia is a late finding and poor prognostic sign. The disease primarily occurs in middle-aged white males. The diagnosis requires small bowel biopsy and demonstration of periodic acid–Schiff (PAS)–positive macrophages within the small bowel. Small bacilli are often present and suggest the diagnosis of Whipple disease. Similar macrophages may be found in other affected organs (e.g., the CNS). Dilated lymphatics are present in patients with intestinal lymphangiectasia. Mononuclear cell infiltrate in the lamina propria is often demonstrated in patients with tropical sprue, and flat villi with crypt hyperplasia is the hallmark of celiac disease.

VIII-17. **The answer is D.** *(Chap. 349)* This patient has a stool osmolality gap (measured stool osmolality – calculated stool osmolality) of 10 mOsmol/L, suggesting a secretory rather than an osmotic cause for diarrhea. Secretory causes of diarrhea include toxin-mediated diarrhea (cholera, enterotoxigenic *Escherichia coli*) and intestinal peptide–mediated diarrhea in which the major pathophysiology is a luminal or circulating secretagogue. The distinction between secretory diarrhea and osmotic diarrhea aids in forming a differential diagnosis. Secretory diarrhea will not decrease substantially during a fast and has a low osmolality gap. Osmotic diarrhea will generally decrease during a fast and has a high (>50 mOsmol/L) osmolality gap. Celiac sprue, chronic pancreatitis, lactase deficiency, and Whipple disease all cause an osmotic diarrhea. A low stool osmolality (<290 mOsmol/kg H_2O) reflects the addition of either dilute urine or water, indicating either collection of urine and stool together or so-called factitious diarrhea, a form of Münchausen syndrome.

VIII-18. **The answer is C.** *(Chap. 349)* Almost all GI malabsorption clinical problems are associated with *diminished* intestinal absorption of one or more dietary nutrients and are often referred to as the malabsorption syndrome. Most malabsorption syndromes are associated with steatorrhea, an increase in stool fat excretion to >6% of dietary fat intake. The only clinical conditions in which absorption is *increased* are hemochromatosis and Wilson disease, in which absorption of iron and copper, respectively, is elevated. Celiac disease may cause significant malabsorption of multiple nutrients, with diarrhea, steatorrhea, weight loss, and the consequences of nutrient depletion (i.e., anemia and metabolic bone disease) or depletion of a single nutrient (e.g., iron or folate deficiency, osteomalacia, edema from protein loss). Malabsorption of bile salts and vitamins is common in Crohn disease due to ileal involvement. The magnitude of malabsorption is dependent on the extent of disease. Whipple disease is a chronic multisystemic disease associated with diarrhea, steatorrhea, weight loss, arthralgia, and CNS and cardiac problems; it is caused by the bacterium *Tropheryma whipplei*.

VIII-19. **The answer is D.** *(Chap. 351)* The incidence of inflammatory bowel disease is highly influenced by ethnicity, location, and environmental factors. Both conditions have their highest incidence in the United Kingdom and North America, and the peak incidence has a bimodal distribution of age of presentation: 15–30 years and 60–80 years of age. Incidence of both ulcerative colitis and Crohn disease is highest among persons of Ashkenazi Jewish population. Prevalence decreases progressively in non-Jewish white, African American, Hispanic, and Asian populations. Cigarette smoking is associated with a decreased incidence of ulcerative colitis but may cause Crohn disease. Oral contraceptive use is associated with a slightly higher incidence of Crohn disease but not ulcerative colitis. Monozygotic twins are highly concordant for Crohn disease but not ulcerative colitis.

VIII-20. **The answer is C.** *(Chap. 351)* Chronic, bloody diarrhea associated with weight loss and systemic symptoms in a young person is highly suggestive of inflammatory bowel disease. The patient's surgical findings suggest discontinuous lesions, which is typical of Crohn disease. Ulcerative colitis, in contrast, typically affects the rectum and proceeds caudally from there without normal mucosa until the area of inflammation terminates. The presence of strictures and fissures further supports the diagnosis of Crohn disease, as these are not features of ulcerative colitis. Microscopically, both ulcerative colitis and Crohn disease may have crypt abscess, and although Crohn disease is more often transmural, full-thickness disease may be present in ulcerative colitis. The hallmark of Crohn disease is granulomas that may be present throughout the bowel wall and involve the lymph nodes, mesentery, peritoneum, liver, and pancreas. Although pathognomonic for Crohn disease, granulomas are only found in about half of surgical resections. Flat villi are not always present in either disease and are more commonly found in isolation with celiac disease.

VIII-21. **The answer is D.** *(Chap. 351)* There are a number of dermatologic manifestations of inflammatory bowel disease (IBD), and each type of IBD has a particular predilection for different dermatologic conditions. This patient has pyoderma gangrenosum. Pyoderma gangrenosum can occur in up to 12% of patients with ulcerative colitis and is characterized by a lesion that begins as a pustule and progresses concentrically to surrounding normal skin. The lesions ulcerate with violaceous, heaped margins and surrounding erythema. They are typically found on the lower extremities. Often the lesions are difficult to treat and respond poorly to colectomy; similarly, pyoderma gangrenosum is not prevented by colectomy. Treatment commonly includes intravenous antibiotics, glucocorticoids, dapsone, infliximab, and other immunomodulatory agents. Erythema nodosum is more common in Crohn disease and attacks correlate with bowel symptoms. The lesions are typically multiple, red hot, tender nodules measuring 1–5 cm and are found on the lower legs and arms. Psoriasis is more common in ulcerative colitis. Finally, pyoderma vegetans is a rare disorder in intertriginous areas reported to be a manifestation of IBD in the skin.

VIII-22. **The answer is D.** (*Chap. 351 and Cochrane Database Syst Rev 2007 Oct 17; [4]*) Despite being described as a clinical entity for over a century, the etiology of IBD remains cryptic. Current theory is related to an interplay between inflammatory stimuli in genetically predisposed individuals. Recent studies have identified a group of genes or polymorphisms that confer risk of IBD. Multiple microbiologic agents, including some that reside as "normal" flora, may initiate IBD by triggering an inflammatory response. Anaerobic organisms (e.g., *Bacteroides* and *Clostridia* spp.) may be responsible for the induction of inflammation. Other organisms, for unclear reasons, may have the opposite effect. These "probiotic" organisms include *Lactobacillus* spp., *Bifidobacterium* spp., *Taenia suis*, and *Saccharomyces boulardii*. *Shigella*, *Escherichia*, and *Campylobacter* spp. are known to promote inflammation. Studies of probiotic therapy in adults and children with IBD have shown potential benefit for reducing disease activity.

VIII-23. **The answer is D.** *(Chap. 295)* Methotrexate, azathioprine, cyclosporine, tacrolimus, and anti–tumor necrosis factor (TNF) antibody are reasonable options for patients with Crohn disease, depending on the extent of macroscopic disease. Pneumonitis is a rare but serious complication of methotrexate therapy. Primary sclerosing cholangitis is an extraintestinal manifestation of IBD. Pancreatitis is an uncommon complication of azathioprine, and IBD patients treated with azathioprine are at fourfold increased risk of developing a lymphoma. Anti-TNF antibody therapy is associated with an increased risk of tuberculosis, disseminated histoplasmosis, and a number of other infections.

VIII-24. **The answer is B.** *(Chap. 351)* Patients with long-standing ulcerative colitis (UC) are at increased risk for developing colonic epithelial dysplasia and carcinoma. The risk of neoplasia in chronic UC increases with duration and extent of disease. From one large meta-analysis, the risk of cancer in patients with UC is estimated at 2% after 10 years, 8% after 20 years, and 18% after 30 years of disease. Data from a 30-year surveillance program in the United Kingdom calculated the risk of colorectal cancer to be 7.7% at 20 years and 15.8% at 30 years of disease. The rates of colon cancer are higher than in the general population, and colonoscopic surveillance is the standard of care. Annual or biennial colonoscopy with multiple biopsies is recommended for patients with >8–10 years of extensive colitis (greater than one-third of the colon involved) or 12–15 years of proctosigmoiditis (less than one-third but more than just the rectum). The cancer risks in Crohn disease and UC are probably equivalent for similar extent and duration of disease. Thus, the same endoscopic surveillance strategy used for UC is recommended for patients with chronic Crohn colitis. If flat high-grade dysplasia is encountered on colonoscopic surveillance, the usual treatment is colectomy for UC and either colectomy or segmental resection for Crohn disease. If flat low-grade dysplasia is found, most investigators recommend immediate colectomy. Patients with Crohn disease may have an increased risk of non-Hodgkin lymphoma, leukemia, and myelodysplastic syndromes.

VIII-25. **The answer is C.** *(Chap. 352)* Irritable bowel syndrome (IBS) is characterized by the following: recurrence of lower abdominal pain with altered bowel habits over a period of time without progressive deterioration, onset of symptoms during periods of stress or emotional upset, absence of other systemic symptoms such as fever and weight loss, and small-volume stool without evidence of blood. Warning signs that the symptoms may be due to something other than IBS include presentation for the first time in old age, progressive course from the time of onset, persistent diarrhea after a 48-hour fast, and presence of nocturnal diarrhea or steatorrheal stools. Each patient, except for patient C, has "warning" symptoms that should prompt further evaluation.

VIII-26. **The answer is C.** *(Chap. 352)* Although this patient has signs and symptoms consistent with IBS, the differential diagnosis is large. Few tests are required for patients who have typical IBS symptoms and no alarm features. In this patient, alarm features include anemia, an elevated erythrocyte sedimentation rate, and evidence of white blood cells in the stool. Alarm features warrant further investigation to rule out other GI disorders such as colonic pathology including diverticular disease or IBD. In this case, colonoscopy to evaluate for luminal lesions and mucosal characteristics would be the logical first step. At this point, with the warning signs, empiric therapy for IBS is premature. Reassurance, stool-bulking agents, and antidepressants are all therapies to consider if a patient does indeed have IBS.

VIII-27. **The answer is D.** *(Chap. 352)* Up to 80% of patients with IBS also have abnormal psychiatric features; however, no single psychiatric diagnosis predominates. The mechanism is not well understood but may involve altered pain thresholds. Although these patients are hypersensitive to colonic stimuli, this does not carry over to the peripheral nervous system. Functional brain imaging shows disparate activation in, for example, the mid-cingulate cortex, but brain anatomy does not discriminate IBS patients from those without IBS. An association between a history of sexual abuse and IBS has been reported. There is no reported association with sexually transmitted diseases. Patients with IBS do not have an increased risk of autoimmunity.

VIII-28. **The answer is C.** *(Chap. 352)* This patient has a diarrhea-predominant form of IBS. Alteration in bowel habits is the most consistent clinical feature in IBS. The most common pattern is constipation alternating with diarrhea, usually with one of these symptoms predominating. At first, constipation may be episodic, but eventually, it becomes continuous and increasingly intractable to treatment with laxatives. Patients whose predominant symptom is constipation may have weeks or months of constipation interrupted with brief periods of diarrhea. In other patients, diarrhea may be the predominant symptom. Diarrhea resulting from IBS usually consists of small volumes of loose stools. Most patients have stool volumes of <200 mL. Nocturnal diarrhea does not occur in IBS. Diarrhea may be aggravated by emotional stress or eating. Stool may be accompanied by passage of large amounts of mucus. Bleeding is not a feature of IBS unless hemorrhoids are present, and malabsorption or weight loss does not occur.

Bowel pattern subtypes are highly unstable, with patients frequently alternating between constipation, diarrhea, or a mixed pattern. A diet low in fermentable oligosaccharides, disaccharides, monosaccharides, and polyols (FODMAPs) has been shown to be helpful in IBS patients (Table VIII-28). FODMAPs are poorly absorbed by the small intestine and fermented by bacteria in the colon to produce gas and osmotically active carbohydrates. A randomized controlled study showed that a diet low in FODMAPs reduced symptoms in IBS patients.

TABLE VIII-28 **Some Common Food Sources of FODMAPs**

Food Type	Free Fructose	Lactose	Fructans	Galacto-oligosaccharides	Polyols
Fruits	Apple, cherry, mango, pear, watermelon		Peach, persimmon, watermelon		Apple, apricot, pear, avocado, blackberries, cherry, nectarine, plum, prune
Vegetables	Asparagus, artichokes, sugar snap peas		Artichokes, beetroot, Brussels sprout, chicory, fennel, garlic, leek, onion, peas		Cauliflower, mushroom, snow peas
Grains and cereals			Wheat, rye, barley		
Nuts and seeds			Pistachios		
Milk and milk products		Milk, yogurt, ice cream, custard, soft cheeses			
Legumes			Legumes, lentils, chickpeas	Legumes, chickpeas, lentils	
Other	Honey, high-fructose corn syrup		Chicory drinks		
Food additives			Inulin, FOS		Sorbitol, mannitol, maltitol, xylitol, isomalt

Abbreviations: FODMAPs, fermentable oligosaccharides, disaccharides, monosaccharides, and polyols; FOS, fructo-oligosaccharides.
Source: Adapted from PR Gibson et al: *Am J Gastroenterol* 107:657, 2012.

VIII-29. **The answer is B.** *(Chap. 353)* The patient presents with classic signs of diverticulitis with fever, abdominal pain that is usually left lower quadrant, anorexia or obstipation, and leukocytosis. This most commonly occurs in older individuals. Patients may present with acute abdomen due to perforation, although this occurs in <25% of cases. Plain radiographs of the abdomen are seldom helpful but may show the presence of an air-fluid level in the left lower quadrant indicating a giant diverticulum with impending perforation. CT with oral contrast is the diagnostic modality of choice with the following findings: sigmoid diverticula, thickened colonic wall >4 mm, and inflammation within the pericolic space with or without the collection of contrast material or fluid. In 16% of patients, an abdominal abscess may be present. Symptoms of IBS may mimic those of diverticulitis. Therefore, suspected diverticulitis that does not meet CT criteria or is not associated with a leukocytosis or fever is not diverticular disease. Other conditions that can mimic diverticular disease include an ovarian cyst, endometriosis, acute appendicitis, and pelvic inflammatory disease. Although the benefit of colonoscopy in the evaluation of patients with diverticular disease has been called into question, its use is still considered important in the exclusion of colorectal cancer. The parallel epidemiology of colorectal cancer and diverticular disease provides enough concern for an endoscopic evaluation before operative management. Therefore, a colonoscopy should be performed ~6 weeks after an attack of diverticular disease. Although diverticular disease may result in hematochezia, these are generally not temporally linked to diverticulitis.

VIII-30. **The answer is B.** *(Chap. 353)* Medical management is appropriate for many patients with uncomplicated diverticular disease. Uncomplicated disease involves fever, abdominal pain, leukocytosis, and anorexia/obstipation, whereas complicated disease is characterized by abscess formation, perforation, strictures, or fistulae. Uncomplicated disease accounts for at least 75% of cases. Medical therapy generally involves bowel rest and antibiotics, usually trimethoprim/sulfamethoxazole or ciprofloxacin and metronidazole targeting aerobic gram-negative rods and anaerobic bacteria. Patients with more than two attacks of diverticulitis were previously thought to require surgical therapy, but newer data suggest that these patients do not have an increased risk of perforation and can continue medical management. Patients with immunosuppressive therapy, chronic renal failure, or collagen vascular disease have a fivefold higher risk of perforation during recurrent attacks. Surgical therapy is indicated for surgical low-risk patients with complicated disease, such as a stricture.

VIII-31. **The answer is B.** *(Chap. 353)* Hemorrhoids can be internal or external; however, they are normally internal and may prolapse to the external position. Hemorrhoids are staged in the following manner: stage I, enlargement with bleeding; stage II, protrusion with spontaneous reduction; stage III, protrusion requiring manual reduction; and stage IV, irreducible protrusion. Stage I, which this patient has, is treated with fiber supplementation, cortisone suppositories, and/or sclerotherapy. Stage II is treated with fiber and cortisone suppositories. Stage III is offered the prior three therapies and banding or operative hemorrhoidectomy. Stage IV patients benefit from fiber and cortisone therapy as well as operative hemorrhoidectomy. Although substantial upper GI bleeding may result in hematochezia, the absence of suggestive signs/symptoms and the consistent findings of hemorrhoids do not indicate the need for upper endoscopy.

VIII-32. **The answer is A.** *(Chap. 353)* An anorectal abscess is an abnormal fluid-containing cavity in the anorectal region. Anorectal abscess results from an infection involving the glands surrounding the anorectal canal. The disease is more common in males, with a peak incidence in the third to fifth decades. Patients with diabetes, with IBD, or who are immunocompromised are at increased risk for this condition. Perianal pain with defecation and fever are common presenting symptoms.

VIII-33. **The answer is C.** *(Chap. 353)* This patient has symptoms (social isolation), signs (foul odor), and risk factors (multiparity) for procidentia (rectal prolapse) and fecal incontinence. Procidentia is far more common in women than men and is often associated with pelvic floor disorders. It is not uncommon for these patients to become socially withdrawn and suffer from depression because of the associated fecal incontinence. The foul odor is a result of poor perianal hygiene due to the prolapsed rectum. Although depression in the elderly is an important medical problem, it is too premature in the evaluation to initiate medical therapy for depression. Occult malignancy and thyroid abnormalities may cause fecal incontinence and depression, but a physical examination would be diagnostic and avoid costly tests. Often patients are concerned they have a rectal mass or carcinoma. Examination after an enema often makes the prolapse apparent. Medical therapy is limited to stool-bulking agents or fiber. Surgical correction is the mainstay of therapy.

VIII-34. **The answer is A.** *(Chap. 354)* Mesenteric ischemia is a relatively uncommon and highly morbid illness. Acute mesenteric ischemia is usually due to arterial embolus (usually from the heart) or to thrombosis in a diseased vascular bed. Major risk factors include age, atrial fibrillation, valvular disease, recent arterial catheterization, and recent myocardial infarction. Ischemia occurs when the intestines are inadequately perfused by the splanchnic circulation. This blood supply has extensive collateralization and can receive up to 30% of the cardiac output, making poor perfusion an uncommon event. Patients with acute mesenteric ischemia will frequently present with pain out of proportion to their initial physical examination. As ischemia persists, peritoneal signs and cardiovascular collapse will follow. Mortality is >50%. While radiographic imaging can suggest ischemia, the gold standard for diagnosis is laparotomy.

VIII-35. **The answer is D.** *(Chap. 354)* This patient with a history of atherosclerotic cardiovascular disease and diabetes is at high risk for nonocclusive mesenteric ischemia in the setting of sepsis, hypotension, and administered vasoconstrictors. Intestinal ischemia is further classified based on etiology, which dictates management (Table VIII-35): (1) arteria-occlusive mesenteric ischemia, (2) nonocclusive mesenteric ischemia, and (3) mesenteric venous thrombosis. Risk factors for arteria-occlusive mesenteric ischemia are generally acute in onset and include atrial fibrillation, recent myocardial infarction, valvular heart disease, and recent cardiac or vascular catheterization, all of which result in embolic clots reaching the mesenteric circulation. Nonocclusive mesenteric ischemia, also known as "intestinal angina," is generally more insidious and most often seen in the aging population affected by atherosclerotic disease. Nonocclusive mesenteric ischemia is also seen in patients receiving high-dose vasopressor infusions, patients with cardiogenic or septic shock, and patients with cocaine overdose. Nonocclusive mesenteric ischemia is the most prevalent GI disease complicating cardiovascular surgery. Mesenteric venous thrombosis is less common and is associated with the presence of a hypercoagulable state including protein C or S deficiency, anti–thrombin III deficiency, polycythemia vera, and carcinoma. In the absence of atrial fibrillation, nonocclusive mesenteric ischemia is more likely in this patient. There is no reason to suspect IBD as a cause of the bloody stools in this critically ill patient with known bacteremic sepsis, and the patient has only been on antibiotics for 1 day and is unlikely to have *Clostridium difficile* colitis at this point.

TABLE VIII-35 **Overview of the Management of Acute Intestinal Ischemia**

Condition	Key to Early Diagnosis	Treatment of Underlying Cause	Treatment of Specific Lesion	Treatment of Systemic Consequence
Arterio-occlusive mesenteric ischemia				
1. Arterial embolus	Computed tomography (CT) angiography Early laparotomy	Anticoagulation Cardioversion Proximal thrombectomy	Laparotomy Embolectomy Vascular bypass Assess viability and resect dead bowel	Ensure hydration Give antibiotics Reverse acidosis Optimize oxygen delivery Avoid vasoconstrictors
2. Arterial thrombosis	Duplex ultrasound Angiography	Anticoagulation Hydration	Endovascular approach: thrombolysis, angioplasty, and stenting Endarterectomy/thrombectomy or vascular bypass Assess viability and resect dead bowel	Give antibiotics Reverse acidosis Optimize oxygen delivery Support cardiac output Avoid vasoconstrictors
Mesenteric venous thrombosis Venous thrombosis	Spiral CT Angiography with venous phase	Anticoagulation Massive hydration	Anticoagulation ± laparotomy/thrombectomy/catheter-directed thrombolysis Assess viability and resect dead bowel	Give antibiotics Reverse acidosis Optimize oxygen delivery Support cardiac output Avoid vasoconstrictors
Nonocclusive mesenteric ischemia	Vasospasm: Angiography Hypoperfusion: Spiral CT or colonoscopy	Ensure hydration Support cardiac output Avoid vasoconstrictors	Vasospasm: Intra-arterial vasodilators Hypoperfusion: Delayed laparotomy Assess viability and resect dead bowel	Ensure hydration Give antibiotics Reverse acidosis Optimize oxygen delivery Support cardiac output Avoid vasoconstrictors

Source: Modified from GB Bulkley, in JL Cameron (ed): *Current Surgical Therapy*, 2nd ed. Toronto: BC Decker, 1986.

VIII-36 and VIII-37. **The answers are B and D, respectively.** *(Chap. 355)* The radiograph shows massively dilated colon extending to the rectum. This radiograph is consistent with colonic pseudo-obstruction or Ogilvie syndrome. Ogilvie syndrome may be seen in elderly patients after nonabdominal surgery or in patients with underlying autonomic dysfunction. The presence of gas in the colon makes small bowel obstruction unlikely. There is no extraintestinal air that would be suggestive of small or large bowel perforation. Small bowel ileus is characterized by multiple small bowel air-fluid levels on radiograph. The differential for extensive colonic dilation includes toxic megacolon due to *C difficile* infection. In this case, that is less likely given the recent surgery and lack of antibiotic treatment. Neostigmine is an acetylcholinesterase inhibitor that increases cholinergic (parasympathetic) activity and can stimulate colonic motility. Some studies have shown it to be moderately effective in alleviating acute colonic pseudo-obstruction. It is the most common therapeutic approach and can be used once it is certain that there is no mechanical obstruction. Cardiac monitoring is required, and atropine should be immediately available for symptomatic bradycardia. Intravenous administration induces defecation and flatus within 10 minutes in the majority of patients who will respond. Surgical therapy may be necessary in cases of bowel perforation or impending perforation. Morphine, with its anticholinergic side effects, may worsen small or large bowel pseudo-obstruction. Oral vancomycin is the treatment for *C difficile* infection.

VIII-38. **The answer is C.** *(Chap. 356)* Obstruction of the appendiceal lumen is believed to typically result in appendicitis. Although obstruction is most commonly caused by fecalith, which results from accumulation and inspissation of fecal matter around vegetable fibers, other causes have been described. These other potential causes include enlarged lymphoid follicles associated with viral infection (e.g., measles), inspissated barium, worms (e.g., pinworms, *Ascaris*, and *Taenia*), and tumors such as carcinoma or carcinoid. Cholelithiasis is a common cause of acute pancreatitis.

VIII-39. **The answer is A.** *(Chap. 356)* The patient presents with typical findings for acute appendicitis with anorexia, progressing to vague periumbilical pain, followed by localization to the right lower quadrant. Low-grade fever and leukocytosis are frequently present. Although acute appendicitis is primarily a clinical diagnosis, imaging modalities are frequently employed because the symptoms are not always classic. Plain radiographs are rarely helpful except when an opaque fecalith is found in the right lower quadrant (<5% of cases). Ultrasound may demonstrate an enlarged appendix with a thick wall but is most useful to rule out ovarian pathology, tubo-ovarian abscess, or ectopic pregnancy. The effectiveness of ultrasonography as a tool to diagnose appendicitis is highly operator dependent. Even in very skilled hands, the appendix may not be visualized. Its overall sensitivity is 0.86, with a specificity of 0.81. Nonenhanced and contrast-enhanced CT are superior to ultrasound or plain radiograph in the diagnosis of acute appendicitis with sensitivity of 0.94 and specificity of 0.95. Findings often include a thickened appendix with periappendiceal stranding and often the presence of a fecalith (Figure VIII-39). Free air is uncommon, even in the case of a perforated appendix. Nonvisualization of the appendix on CT is associated with surgical findings of a normal appendix 98% of the time. Colonoscopy has no role in the diagnosis of acute appendicitis.

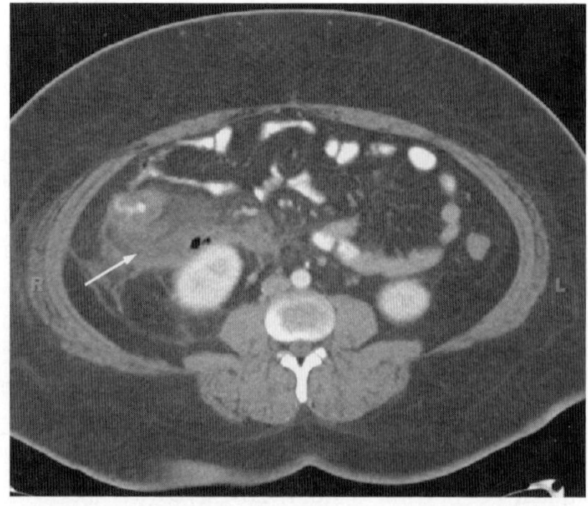

FIGURE VIII-39

VIII-40 and VIII-41. The answers are C and D, respectively. *(Chap. 356)* The patient presents with several months of epigastric abdominal pain that is worse after eating. His symptoms are highly suggestive of peptic ulcer disease, with the worsening pain after eating suggesting a duodenal ulcer. The current presentation with acute abdomen and free air under the diaphragm points to a diagnosis of perforated viscus. Perforated gallbladder is less likely in light of the duration of symptoms and the absence of the significant systemic symptoms that often accompany this condition. Because the patient is relatively young with no risk factors for mesenteric ischemia, necrotic bowel from an infarction is highly unlikely. Pancreatitis can have a similar presentation, but a pancreas cannot perforate and liberate free air. Peritonitis is most commonly associated with bacterial infection, but it can be caused by the abnormal presence of physiologic fluids, for example, gastric contents, bile, pancreatic enzymes, blood, or urine, or by foreign bodies. In this case, peritonitis is most likely due to the presence of gastric juice in the peritoneal cavity after perforation of a duodenal ulcer has allowed these juices to leave the gut lumen.

VIII-42. The answer is A. *(Chaps. 59 and 357)* Diagnostic paracentesis is part of the routine evaluation in a patient with ascites. Fluid should be examined for its gross appearance, protein content, cell count and differential, and albumin. Cytologic and culture studies should be performed when one suspects infection or malignancy. The serum-ascites albumin gradient (SAG) offers the best correlation with portal pressure. A high gradient (>1.1 g/dL) is characteristic of uncomplicated cirrhotic ascites and differentiates ascites caused by portal hypertension from ascites not caused by portal hypertension in more than 95% of cases. Conditions that cause a low gradient include more "exudative" processes such as infection, malignancy, and inflammatory processes. Similarly, congestive heart failure and nephrotic syndrome cause high gradients. In this patient, the SAG is 1.5 g/dL, indicating a high gradient. The low number of leukocytes and polymorphonuclear cells makes bacterial or tubercular infection unlikely. Chylous ascites often is characterized by an opaque milky fluid with a triglyceride level greater than 1000 mg/dL in addition to a low SAG.

VIII-43. The answer is A. *(Chap. 357)* The most common and most characteristic symptom of liver disease is fatigue. Unfortunately, it is also very nonspecific, with little specific diagnostic utility. The fatigue in liver disease seems to improve in the morning and worsen throughout the day, but it can be intermittent. Jaundice is the hallmark of liver disease and is much more specific. Jaundice, however, is typically a sign of more advanced disease. Itching is also typically a symptom of more advanced disease and is more common in cholestatic causes of liver disease. Nausea often occurs in severe disease and can be accompanied by vomiting. Right upper quadrant pain is a less common symptom and indicates stretching of the liver capsule.

VIII-44. The answer is B. *(Chap. 357)* Women are more susceptible to the effects of alcohol on the liver. On average, drinking about two drinks daily can lead to chronic liver disease in women, whereas men report drinking about three drinks daily. However, in individuals with alcoholic cirrhosis, the average daily alcohol intake is usually much higher, and heavy levels of drinking for more than 10 years are typical prior to the onset of liver disease.

VIII-45. The answer is A. *(Chap. 357)* In assessing alcohol intake, the history should also focus on whether alcohol abuse or dependence is present. Alcoholism is usually defined by the behavioral patterns and consequences of alcohol intake, not by the amount. *Abuse* is defined by a repetitive pattern of drinking alcohol that has adverse effects on social, family, occupational, or health status. *Dependence* is defined by alcohol-seeking behavior, despite its adverse effects. Many alcoholics demonstrate both dependence and abuse, and dependence is considered the more serious and advanced form of alcoholism. A clinically helpful approach to diagnosis of alcohol dependence and abuse is the use of the CAGE questionnaire, which is recommended for all medical history taking. One "yes" response should raise suspicion of an alcohol use problem, and more than one "yes" response is a strong indication of abuse or dependence.

VIII-46. The answer is D. *(Chap. 358)* It is important to understand the patterns of laboratory abnormalities that indicate liver disease is present. One way to consider laboratory evaluation of liver disease is to consider three general categories of tests: tests based on excretory function of the liver, tests of biosynthetic activity of the liver, and coagulation factors. The most common tests of liver function fall under the category of tests based on the detoxification and excretory function of the liver. These include serum bilirubin, urine bilirubin, ammonia, and enzyme levels. Bilirubin can exist as a conjugated and an unconjugated form. The unconjugated form is often referred to as the indirect fraction. Isolated elevation in the unconjugated form of bilirubin is typically not related to liver disease but is most commonly seen in hemolysis and a number of benign genetic conditions such as Gilbert syndrome. In contrast, conjugated hyperbilirubinemia almost always indicates disease of the liver or biliary tract. Conjugated bilirubin is water soluble and excreted in the urine, but unconjugated bilirubin is not. Rather, it binds to albumin in the blood. Therefore, bilirubinuria implies liver disease as well. Among the serum enzymes, it is useful to consider enzymes as those that are associated with hepatocellular injury or those that reflect cholestasis. Alanine and aspartate aminotransferases are the primary enzymes that indicate hepatocyte injury. Alkaline phosphatase is the most common enzyme elevated in cholestasis, but bone disease also causes increased alkaline phosphatase. In some cases, one needs additional information to determine whether the alkaline phosphatase is liver or bone in origin. Other tests that would be elevated in cholestatic liver disease are 5′-nucleotidase and γ-glutamyl transferase. The primary test of synthetic function is measurement of serum albumin. Coagulation factors can be directly measured, but impaired production of coagulation factors in liver disease is primarily inferred from elevations in prothrombin time.

VIII-47. **The answer is B.** *(Chap. 358)* The aminotransferases are sensitive indicators of liver cell injury and are most helpful in recognizing acute hepatocellular diseases such as hepatitis. They include aspartate aminotransferase (AST) and alanine aminotransferase (ALT). AST is found in the liver, cardiac muscle, skeletal muscle, kidneys, brain, pancreas, lungs, leukocytes, and erythrocytes in decreasing order of concentration. ALT is found primarily in the liver and is therefore a more specific indicator of liver injury. The aminotransferases are normally present in the serum in low concentrations. These enzymes are released into the blood in greater amounts when there is damage to the liver cell membrane, resulting in increased permeability. Liver cell necrosis is not required for the release of the aminotransferases, and there is a poor correlation between the degree of liver cell damage and the level of the aminotransferases. Thus, the absolute elevation of the aminotransferases is of no prognostic significance in acute hepatocellular disorders.

Any type of liver cell injury can cause modest elevations in the serum aminotransferases. Levels of up to 300 IU/L are nonspecific and may be found in any type of liver disorder. Minimal ALT elevations in asymptomatic blood donors rarely indicate severe liver disease; studies have shown that fatty liver disease is the most likely explanation. Striking elevations—i.e., aminotransferases >1000 IU/L—occur almost exclusively in disorders associated with extensive hepatocellular injury such as viral hepatitis, ischemic liver injury (prolonged hypotension or acute heart failure), or toxin- or drug-induced liver injury.

The pattern of the aminotransferase elevation can be helpful diagnostically. In most acute hepatocellular disorders, the ALT is higher than or equal to the AST. Whereas the AST:ALT ratio is typically <1 in patients with chronic viral hepatitis and nonalcoholic fatty liver disease, a number of groups have noted that as cirrhosis develops, this ratio rises to >1. An AST:ALT ratio >2:1 is suggestive, whereas a ratio >3:1 is highly suggestive, of alcoholic liver disease. The AST in alcoholic liver disease is rarely >300 IU/L, and the ALT is often normal. The aminotransferases are usually not greatly elevated in obstructive jaundice.

VIII-48 and VIII-49. **The answers are E and D, respectively.** *(Chap. 359)* This patient is presenting with an asymptomatic and mild elevation in unconjugated hyperbilirubinemia that has occurred during a time of increased stress, fatigue, and likely decreased caloric intake. This presentation is characteristic of Gilbert syndrome, an inherited disorder of bilirubin conjugation. In Gilbert syndrome, there is a mutation of the *UGT1A1* gene that encodes bilirubin UDP-glucuronosyltransferase, which leads to a reduction in activity on the enzyme to 10%–35% of normal. This enzyme is of critical importance in the conjugation of bilirubin. Most of the time, there is no apparent jaundice because the reduced ability to conjugate bilirubin is not reduced to a degree that leads to an elevation of bilirubin. However, during times of stress, fatigue, alcohol use, decreased caloric intake, or intercurrent illness, the enzyme can become overwhelmed, leading to a mild hyperbilirubinemia. Typical bilirubin levels are less than 4.0 mg/dL unless the individual is ill or fasting. Diagnosis usually occurs during young adulthood, and episodes are self-limited and benign. If a liver biopsy were to be performed, hepatic histology would be normal. No treatment is necessary because there are no long-term consequences of Gilbert syndrome, and patient reassurance is recommended. Other inherited disorders of bilirubin conjugation are Crigler-Najjar syndromes types 1 and 2. Crigler-Najjar syndrome type 1 is a congenital disease characterized by more dramatic elevations in bilirubin as high as 20–45 mg/dL that is first diagnosed in the neonatal period and is present throughout life. This rare disorder was once fatal in early childhood due to the development of kernicterus. However, with phototherapy, individuals are now able to survive into adulthood, although neurologic deficits are common. Crigler-Najjar syndrome type 2 is similar to type 1, but the elevations in bilirubin are not as great. Kernicterus is rare. This is due to the fact that there is some residual function of the bilirubin UDP-glucuronosyltransferase enzyme (<10%) that is totally absent in type 1 disease. Hemolysis is another frequent cause of elevated unconjugated bilirubin. Hemolysis can be caused by many factors including medications, autoimmune disorders, and inherited disorders, among others. However, the normal hematocrit, lactate dehydrogenase, and haptoglobin eliminate hemolysis as a possibility. Dubin-Johnson syndrome is another congenital hyperbilirubinemia. However, it is a predominantly conjugated hyperbilirubinemia caused by a defect in biliary excretion from hepatocytes. Obstructive choledocholithiasis is characterized by right upper quadrant pain that is often exacerbated by fatty meals. The absence of symptoms or elevation in other liver function tests, especially alkaline phosphatase, also makes this diagnosis unlikely.

VIII-50. **The answer is B.** *(Chap. 359)* Increased destruction of erythrocytes leads to increased bilirubin turnover and unconjugated hyperbilirubinemia; the hyperbilirubinemia is usually modest in the presence of normal liver function. Hemolysis alone cannot result in a sustained hyperbilirubinemia of more than 4 mg/dL (~68 μmol). Higher values imply concomitant hepatic dysfunction. When hemolysis is the only abnormality in an otherwise healthy individual, the result is a purely unconjugated hyperbilirubinemia, with the direct-reacting fraction as measured in a typical clinical laboratory being ≤15% of the total serum bilirubin. In the presence of systemic disease, which may include a degree of hepatic dysfunction, hemolysis may produce a component of conjugated hyperbilirubinemia in addition to an elevated unconjugated bilirubin concentration. Prolonged hemolysis may lead to the precipitation of bilirubin salts within the gallbladder or biliary tree, resulting in the formation of gallstones in which bilirubin, rather than cholesterol, is the major component. Such pigment stones may lead to acute or chronic cholecystitis, biliary obstruction, or any other biliary tract consequence of calculous disease.

VIII-51. **The answer is B.** *(Chap. 360)* This patient presents with acute hepatitis, which has numerous etiologies. These include viruses, toxins/drugs, autoimmune diseases, metabolic disease, alcohol, ischemia, pregnancy, and other infectious etiologies including rickettsial diseases and leptospirosis. In this clinical scenario, the patient does have risk factors for hepatitis A, B, and C infection, including being a man who has sex with men and a prior history of injection drug use. All acute viral hepatitis presents with a similar clinical pattern, although incubation periods vary after exposure. The most common initial symptoms are fatigue, anorexia, nausea, vomiting, myalgias, and headache. These symptoms precede the onset of jaundice by about 1–2 weeks. Once jaundice develops, the prodromal symptoms regress. On physical examination, there is usually obvious icterus with an enlarged and tender liver. Splenomegaly can occur. AST and ALT are elevated with peak levels that are quite variable between 400 and 4000 IU/L, and alkaline phosphatase levels are increased to a much lesser degree. Hyperbilirubinemia (levels 5–20 mg/dL) occurs with primarily increased levels of conjugated bilirubin. Thus, it is important to recognize the patterns of antibody production in the viral hepatitides. Hepatitis A is an RNA virus that presents with acute hepatitis and is transmitted by the fecal-oral route. In the acute state, the immunoglobulin (Ig) M would be elevated, which is not seen in this scenario. Hepatitis B virus is a DNA virus with three common antigens that are tested serologically to determine the time course of the illness. These antigens are the surface antigen, the core antigen, and the e antigen, which is a nucleocapsid protein produced from the same gene as the core antigen but immunologically distinct. Several distinct patterns can be observed. In acute hepatitis B, the core IgM, surface antigen, and e antigen are all positive, which is what is seen in this case. At this point, the patient is highly infectious, with viral shedding in body fluids, including saliva. In a late acute infection, core IgG may be positive at the same time as surface and e antigen positivity. In chronic hepatitis B, this same pattern of serologies is seen. If a patient has a prior infection without development of chronic hepatitis, the core IgG and surface antibody is positive. However, when immunity is obtained via vaccination, only the surface antibody (SAb) is positive, the e antigen and surface antigen will be negative since the patient was never infected. The variety of antigen-antibody positivities that can result are outlined in Table VIII-51 below. Acute

TABLE VIII-51 **Antigen and Antibody Profiles in Viral Hepatitis**

Hepatitis Type	Virus Particle, nm	Morphology	Genome[a]	Classification	Antigen(s)	Antibodies	Remarks
HAV	27	Icosahedral nonenveloped	7.5-kb RNA, linear, ss, +	Hepatovirus	HAV	Anti-HAV	Early fecal shedding Diagnosis: IgM anti-HAV Previous infection: IgG anti-HAV
HBV	42	Double-shelled virion (surface and core) spherical	3.2-kb DNA, circular, ss/ds	Hepadnavirus	HBsAg HBcAg HBeAg	Anti-HBs Anti-HBc Anti-HBe	Bloodborne virus; carrier state Acute diagnosis: HBsAg, IgM anti-HBc Chronic diagnosis: IgG anti-HBc, HBsAg
	27	Nucleocapsid core			HBcAg HBeAg	Anti-HBc Anti-HBe	Markers of replication: HBeAg, HBV DNA
	22	Spherical and filamentous; represents excess virus coat material			HBsAg	Anti-HBs	Liver, lymphocytes, other organs Nucleocapsid contains DNA and DNA polymerase; present in hepatocyte nucleus; HBcAg does not circulate; HBeAg (soluble, nonparticulate) and HBV DNA circulate—correlate with infectivity and complete virions HBsAg detectable in >95% of patients with acute hepatitis B; found in serum, body fluids, hepatocyte cytoplasm; anti-HBs appears following infection—protective antibody
HCV	Approximately 50–80	Enveloped	9.4-kb RNA, linear, ss, +	Hepacivirus	HCV C100-3 C33c C22-3 NS5	Anti-HCV	Bloodborne agent, formerly labeled non-A, non-B hepatitis Acute diagnosis: anti-HCV (C33c, C22-3, NS5), HCV RNA Chronic diagnosis: anti-HCV (C100-3, C33c, C22-3, NS5) and HCV RNA; cytoplasmic location in hepatocytes
HDV	35–37	Enveloped hybrid particle with HBsAg coat and HDV core	1.7-kb RNA, circular, ss, –	Resembles viroids and plant satellite viruses (genus *Deltavirus*)	HBsAg HDAg	Anti-HBs Anti-HDV	Defective RNA virus, requires helper function of HBV (hepadnaviruses); HDV antigen (HDAg) present in hepatocyte nucleus Diagnosis: anti-HDV, HDV RNA; HBV/HDV co-infection—IgM anti-HBc and anti-HDV; HDV superinfection—IgG anti-HBc and anti-HDV
HEV	32–34	Nonenveloped icosahedral	7.6-kb RNA, linear, ss, +	Hepevirus	HEV antigen	Anti-HEV	Agent of enterically transmitted hepatitis; rare in United States; occurs in Asia, Mediterranean countries, Central America Diagnosis: IgM/IgG anti-HEV (assays not routinely available); virus in stool, bile, hepatocyte cytoplasm

[a]ss, single-strand; ss/ds, partially single-strand, partially double-strand; –, minus-strand; +, plus-strand.

Abbreviations: HAV, hepatitis A virus; HBV, hepatitis B virus; HCV, hepatitis C virus; HDV, hepatitis D virus; HEV, hepatitis E virus; Ig, immunoglobulin.

hepatitis C often is detectable with contemporary immunoassays early during the disease when the aminotransferases are positive. Thus, a positive HCV antibody could indicate acute hepatitis C in this individual. However, given his clinical history of prior injection drug use and inability to donate blood, this likely indicates chronic hepatitis C infection. In some instances, ecstasy has been reported to cause drug-induced hepatitis, but given the viral serologies in this patient, this would be unlikely.

VIII-52. **The answer is E.** *(Chap. 360)* No treatment is recommended for acute hepatitis B in most individuals because 99% of infected individual recover without assistance. Therefore, it would not be expected that an individual would derive any particular benefit from treatment. In severe acute hepatitis B, nucleoside analogues, including lamivudine, have been used successfully, although there are no clinical trial data to support such an approach. Hepatitis A is an acute and self-limited illness that does not progress to chronic liver disease. Thus, no treatment is required. Anti–hepatitis A virus immunoglobulin can be give prophylactically following a known exposure to prevent development of disease, but it is not helpful in established disease. There is no role for oral or intravenous corticosteroids in the treatment of acute viral hepatitis of any etiology. It has demonstrated no clinical benefit and may increase the risk of developing chronic disease.

VIII-53. **The answer is E.** *(Chap. 360)* In most instances, patients with any form of acute viral hepatitis do not succumb to fulminant liver failure. However, pregnant women are highly susceptible to fulminant hepatic failure in the setting of acute hepatitis E infection. This RNA virus is an enteric virus that is endemic in India, Asia, Africa, the Middle East, and Central America and is spread via contaminated water supplies. Person-to-person spread is rare. Generally, the clinical course of hepatitis E infection is mild and the rate of fulminant hepatitis is only 1%–2%. However, in pregnant women, this is as high as 10%–20%. For hepatitis A and C, the rate of fulminant hepatic failure is about 0.1% or less. It is slightly higher for hepatitis B, at around 0.1%–1%. Hepatitis D occurs as a coinfection with hepatitis B virus. When the two viruses are acquired simultaneously, the rate of fulminant hepatitis is about 5% or less. When hepatitis D is acquired in the setting of chronic hepatitis B infection, this number rises to 20%.

VIII-54. **The answer is E.** *(Chap. 360)* Hepatitis A virus (HAV) is an acute, self-limited virus that is acquired almost exclusively via the fecal-oral route. It is classically a disease of poor hygiene and overcrowding. Outbreaks have been traced to contaminated water, milk, frozen raspberries and strawberries, green onions, and shellfish. Infection occurs mostly in children and young adults. It almost invariably resolves spontaneously and results in lifelong immunity. Fulminant disease occurs in ≤0.1% of cases, and there is no chronic form (in contrast to hepatitis B and C). Diagnosis is made by demonstrating a positive IgM antibody to HAV, as described earlier. An IgG antibody to HAV indicates immunity, obtained by previous infection or vaccination. A small proportion of patients will experience relapsing hepatitis weeks to months after a full recovery from HAV infection. This too is self-limited. There is no approved antiviral therapy for HAV. An inactivated vaccine has decreased the incidence of the disease, and it is recommended for all U.S. children, for high-risk adults, and for travelers to endemic areas. Passive immunization with immunoglobulin is also available, and it is effective in preventing clinical disease before exposure or during the early incubation period.

VIII-55. **The answer is C.** *(Chap. 360)* The current hepatitis B vaccine is a recombinant vaccine consisting of yeast-derived hepatitis B surface antigen particles. A strategy of vaccinating only high-risk individuals in the United States has been shown to be ineffective, and universal vaccination against hepatitis B is now recommended. Pregnancy is not a contraindication to vaccination. Vaccination should ideally be performed in infancy. Routine evaluation of hepatitis serologies is not cost-effective and is not recommended. The vaccine is given in three divided intramuscular doses at 0, 1, and 6 months.

VIII-56. **The answer is A.** *(Chap. 360)* A clear distinction between viral etiologies of acute hepatitis cannot be made on clinical or epidemiologic features alone. This patient is at risk of many forms of hepatitis due to his lifestyle. Given his occupation in food services, from a public health perspective, it is important to make an accurate diagnosis. Serologies must be obtained to make a diagnosis. Although hepatitis C virus typically does not present as an acute hepatitis, this is not absolute. Hepatitis E virus infects men and women equally and resembles hepatitis A virus in clinical presentation. This patient should be questioned regarding IV drug use, and in addition to hepatitis serologies, an HIV test should be performed.

VIII-57. **The answer is C.** *(Chaps. 358 and 360)* Causes of extreme elevations in serum transaminases generally fall into a few major categories, including viral infections, toxic ingestions, and vascular/hemodynamic causes. Both acute hepatitis A and hepatitis B infections may be characterized by high transaminases. Fulminant hepatic failure may occur, particularly in situations in which acute hepatitis A occurs on top of chronic hepatitis C infection or if hepatitis B and hepatitis D are co-transmitted. Most cases of acute hepatitis A or B infection in adults are self-limited. Hepatitis C is an RNA virus that does not typically cause acute hepatitis. However, it is associated with a high probability of chronic infection. Therefore, progression to cirrhosis and hepatoma is increased in patients with chronic hepatitis C infection. Extreme transaminitis is highly unlikely with acute hepatitis C infection. Acetaminophen remains one of the major causes of fulminant hepatic failure and is managed by prompt administration of *N*-acetylcysteine. Budd-Chiari syndrome is characterized by posthepatic thrombus formation. It often presents with jaundice, painful hepatomegaly, ascites, and elevated transaminases.

VIII-58. **The answer is A.** *(Chap. 361)* The liver is the primary site for metabolism of many drugs and, as such, is susceptible to injury related to drugs and toxins. Indeed, the most common cause of acute hepatic failure is drug-induced liver injury. In general, it is useful to think of chemical hepatotoxicity within two broad categories: direct toxic effects or idiosyncratic reactions. Drugs or toxins that cause a direct toxic effect on liver are either poisons themselves or are metabolized to toxic substances. With agents that cause a direct toxic effect on hepatocytes, there is a predictable, dose-related pattern of injury, and the time to effect is relatively short. The most common drug or toxin causing direct hepatocyte toxicity is acetaminophen. In therapeutic doses, acetaminophen does not cause liver injury. However, in higher doses, one of the metabolites of acetaminophen, *N*-acetyl-*p*-benzoquinone imine (NAPQI), can overwhelm the glutathione stores of the liver that are necessary to convert NAPQI to a nontoxic metabolite and lead to hepatocyte necrosis. Other medications or toxins that cause direct hepatocyte injury are carbon tetrachloride, trichloroethylene, tetracycline, and the *Amanita phalloides* mushroom. More commonly known as the death cap mushroom, ingestion of a single *A phalloides* mushroom can contain enough hepatotoxin to be lethal. Idiosyncratic reactions are infrequent and unpredictable. There is no dose dependency, and the timing of hepatic injury has little association with the duration of drug treatment. Many drugs produce idiosyncratic reactions, and often, it is difficult to know when an idiosyncratic reaction will lead to more serious liver failure. Often, mild increases in transaminase levels will occur, but over time, adaptation leads to a return of liver enzymes to normal levels. In other instances, idiosyncratic reactions can lead to fulminant hepatic failure. Although rare, serious hepatic reactions can lead to medications being removed from the market. It is now recognized that many idiosyncratic reactions are related to metabolites that cause liver injury. However, it is likely that individual genetic variations in liver metabolism are the primary cause, and these are not predictable effects of the drug given our current state of knowledge. Common medications that can lead to idiosyncratic drug reactions include halothane, isothane, isoniazid, 3-hydroxy-3-methylglutaryl–coenzyme A (HMG-CoA) reductase inhibitors, and chlorpromazine.

VIII-59. **The answer is B.** *(Chap. 305)* Acetaminophen overdose is the most common cause of acute liver failure and the most common cause of drug-induced liver failure that leads to transplantation. Acetaminophen is metabolized in the liver through two pathways. The primary pathway is a phase II reaction that produces nontoxic sulfate and glucuronide metabolites. The minor pathway occurs through a phase I reaction leading to production of NAPQI. This metabolite is directly toxic to liver cells and can lead to hepatocyte necrosis. With therapeutic use of acetaminophen, glutathione in the liver rapidly converts

NAPQI to a nontoxic metabolite that is excreted in the urine. However, glutathione stores can become depleted in the setting of a large acute ingestion, chronic alcoholism, or chronic ingestion of increased acetaminophen. In addition, alcohol upregulates the first enzyme in the metabolic pathway, causing NAPQI to accumulate more quickly in alcoholics. Given the known hepatotoxicity of acetaminophen, the U.S. Food and Drug Administration has recommended a maximum daily dose of no more than 3.25 g, with lower doses in individuals with chronic alcohol use. Acute ingestions of 10–15 g of acetaminophen are sufficient to cause clinical evidence of liver injury, and doses higher than 25 g can lead to fatal hepatic necrosis. The course of illness with acute acetaminophen ingestion follows a predictable pattern. Nausea, vomiting, abdominal pain, and shock occur within 4–12 hours after ingestion. Liver enzymes and synthetic function are normal at this time. Within 24–48 hours, these symptoms subside and are followed by evidence of hepatic injury. Maximal levels of aminotransferases can reach more than 10,000 IU/L and may not occur until 4–6 days after ingestion. These patients must be followed carefully for fulminant hepatic failure with serious complications including encephalopathy, cerebral edema, marked coagulopathy, renal failure, metabolic acidosis, electrolyte abnormalities, and refractory shock. Levels of acetaminophen are predictive of the development of hepatotoxicity. The first level should be measured no sooner than 4 hours after a known ingestion. Levels should be plotted on a nomogram that relates levels to the time after ingestion. If, at 4 hours, the acetaminophen level is greater than 300 μg/mL, significant hepatotoxicity is likely. In the setting of overdose, it may be difficult to know the exact quantity and timing of an ingestion. For the patient presenting in the clinical scenario in this question, her level of greater than 300 μg/mL is quite concerning for a large ingestion, and treatment should be initiated immediately. The primary treatment for acetaminophen overdose is *N*-acetylcysteine. *N*-Acetylcysteine acts to replete glutathione levels in the liver and also provides a reservoir of sulfhydryl groups to bind to the toxic metabolites. The typical regimen of *N*-acetylcysteine is 140 mg/kg given as a loading dose, followed by 70 mg/kg every 4 hours for a total of 15–20 doses. This drug can also be given by continuous infusion. Activated charcoal or cholestyramine should only be given if the patient presents within 30 minutes after ingestion. Hemodialysis will not accelerate clearance of acetaminophen and will not protect the liver. Most patients with fulminant hepatic failure develop acute renal failure, often requiring hemodialysis. If a patient survives an acetaminophen overdose, there is usually no chronic liver injury.

VIII-60. **The answer is E.** *(Chap. 361)* Isoniazid (INH) remains central to most antituberculous prophylactic and therapeutic regimens, despite its long-standing recognition as a hepatotoxin. In 10% of patients treated with INH, elevated serum aminotransferase levels develop during the first few weeks of therapy; however, these elevations in most cases are self-limited, mild (values for ALT <200 IU/L), and resolve despite continued drug use. This adaptive response allows continuation of the agent if symptoms and progressive enzyme elevations do not follow the initial elevations. Acute hepatocellular drug-induced liver injury secondary to INH is evident with a variable latency period up to 6 months and is more frequent in alcoholics and patients taking certain other medications, such as barbiturates, rifampin, and pyrazinamide. If the clinical threshold of encephalopathy is reached, severe hepatic injury is likely to be fatal or to require liver transplantation. Liver biopsy reveals morphologic changes similar to those of viral hepatitis or bridging hepatic necrosis. Substantial liver injury appears to be age-related, increasing substantially after age 35; the highest frequency is in patients over age 50. Even for patients >50 years of age monitored carefully during therapy, hepatotoxicity occurs in only ~2%, well below the risk estimate derived from earlier experiences. Many public health programs that require INH prophylaxis for a positive tuberculin skin test or Quantiferon test include monthly monitoring of aminotransferase levels, although this practice has been called into question. Even more effective in limiting serious outcomes may be encouraging patients to be alert for symptoms such as nausea, fatigue, or jaundice, because most fatalities occur in the setting of continued INH use despite clinically apparent illness.

VIII-61. **The answer is C.** *(Chap. 361)* HMG-COA reductase inhibitors, or statins, may cause an idiosyncratic mixed hepatocellular and cholestatic reaction. Between 1% and 2% of patients taking lovastatin, simvastatin, pravastatin, fluvastatin, or one of the newer statin drugs for the treatment of hypercholesterolemia experience asymptomatic, reversible elevations (greater than threefold) of aminotransferase activity. Acute hepatitis-like histologic changes, centrilobular necrosis, and centrilobular cholestasis have been described in a very small number of cases. In a larger proportion, minor aminotransferase elevations appear during the first several weeks of therapy. Careful laboratory monitoring can distinguish between patients with minor, transitory changes, who may continue therapy, and those with more profound and sustained abnormalities, who should discontinue therapy. Because clinically meaningful aminotransferase elevations are so rare after statin use and do not differ in meta-analyses from the frequency of such laboratory abnormalities in placebo recipients, the National Lipid Association's Safety Task Force concluded that liver test monitoring was not necessary in patients treated with statins and that statin therapy need not be discontinued in patients found to have asymptomatic isolated aminotransferase elevations during therapy. Statin hepatotoxicity is not increased in patients with chronic hepatitis C, hepatic steatosis, or other underlying liver diseases, and statins can be used safely in these patients.

VIII-62. **The answer is B.** *(Chap. 362)* Chronic hepatitis represents a series of liver disorders of varying causes and severity in which hepatic inflammation and necrosis continue for at least 6 months. Milder forms are nonprogressive or only slowly progressive, whereas more severe forms may be associated with scarring and architectural reorganization, which, when advanced, lead ultimately to cirrhosis. Several categories of chronic hepatitis have been recognized. These include chronic viral hepatitis, drug-induced chronic hepatitis, and autoimmune chronic hepatitis. In many cases, clinical and laboratory features are insufficient to allow assignment into one of these three categories; these "idiopathic" cases are also believed to represent autoimmune chronic hepatitis (Table VIII-62). Finally, clinical and laboratory features of chronic hepatitis are observed occasionally in patients with such hereditary/metabolic disorders as Wilson disease (copper overload), α_1-antitrypsin deficiency (Chaps. 365 and 429), and nonalcoholic fatty liver disease (Chap. 367e), and even occasionally in patients with alcoholic liver injury (Chap. 363). Both of the enterically transmitted forms of viral hepatitis, hepatitis A and E, are self-limited and do not cause chronic hepatitis.

TABLE VIII-62 **Clinical and Laboratory Features of Chronic Hepatitis**

Type of Hepatitis	Diagnostic Test(s)	Autoantibodies	Therapy
Chronic hepatitis B	HBsAg, IgG anti-HBc, HBeAg, HBV DNA	Uncommon	IFN-α, PEG IFN-α Oral agents: First-line: entecavir, tenofovir Second-line: lamivudine, adefovir, telbivudine
Chronic hepatitis C	Anti-HCV, HCV RNA	Anti-LKM1[a]	PEG IFN-α plus ribavirin Telaprevir[b] Boceprevir[b]
Chronic hepatitis D	Anti-HDV, HDV RNA, HBsAg, IgG anti-HBc	Anti-LKM3	IFN-α, PEG IFN-α[c]
Autoimmune hepatitis	ANA[d] (homogeneous), anti-LKM1 (±) Hyperglobulinemia	ANA, anti-LKM1, anti-SLA[e]	Prednisone, azathioprine
Drug-associated	—	Uncommon	Withdraw drug
Cryptogenic	All negative	None	Prednisone (?), azathioprine (?)

[a]Antibodies to liver-kidney microsomes type 1 (autoimmune hepatitis type II and some cases of hepatitis C).
[b]Administered as a triple-drug combination with PEG IFN and ribavirin. Recently, two additional drugs were approved for hepatitis C, simeprevir and sofosbuvir (see *www.hcvguidelines.org*).
[c]Early clinical trials suggested benefit of IFN-α therapy; PEG IFN-α is as effective, if not more so, and has supplanted standard IFN-α.
[d]Antinuclear antibody (autoimmune hepatitis type I).
[e]Antibodies to soluble liver antigen (autoimmune hepatitis type III).
Abbreviations: HBc, hepatitis B core; HBeAg, hepatitis B e antigen; HBsAg, hepatitis B surface antigen; HBV, hepatitis B virus; HCV, hepatitis C virus; HDV, hepatitis D virus; IFN-α, interferon-α; IgG, immunoglobulin G; LKM, liver-kidney microsome; PEG IFN-α, pegylated interferon-α; SLA, soluble liver antigen.

VIII-63. **The answer is B.** *(Chap. 362)* The patient in this scenario has evidence of chronic active hepatitis B virus (HBV) infection. The presence of hepatitis B e antigen (HBeAg) is indicative of ongoing viral replication, and individuals with HBeAg positivity typically have high levels of HBV DNA on testing. The spectrum of clinical infection in chronic hepatitis B is quite variable, and often, individuals are asymptomatic with elevated liver enzymes identified on testing for other reasons. Thus, the decision to treat chronic HBV infection should not be based on clinical features. Most experts recommend treatment of HBeAg-positive chronic HBV infection with HBV DNA levels $>2 \times 10^4$ IU/mL if the ALT is elevated greater than twice the upper limit of normal (Table VIII-63). To date, seven drugs have been approved for treatment of chronic HBV: injectable interferon (IFN) α; pegylated IFN (long-acting IFN bound to polyethylene glycol [PEG IFN]); and the oral agents lamivudine, adefovir dipivoxil, entecavir, telbivudine, and tenofovir. PEG IFN, entecavir, or tenofovir is recommended as first-line therapy. Simeprevir is a protease inhibitor that is approved for the treatment of hepatitis C virus infection. Acyclovir is used to treat herpes simplex viral infections, and ritonavir is a protease inhibitor used to treat HIV infection. The patient's husband should also be screened for HBV given the continued viremia.

TABLE VIII-63 **Recommendations for Treatment of Chronic Hepatitis B**[a]

HBeAg Status	Clinical	HBV DNA (IU/mL)	ALT	Recommendation
HBeAg-reactive	[b]	$>2 \times 10^4$	$\leq 2 \times$ ULN[c,d]	No treatment; monitor. In patients >40,
	Chronic hepatitis	$>2 \times 10^4$[d]	$>2 \times$ ULN[d]	with family history of hepatocellular carci-
	Cirrhosis compensated	$>2 \times 10^3$	< or > ULN	noma, and/or ALT persistently at the high
	Cirrhosis decompensated	$<2 \times 10^3$	>ULN	end of the twofold range, liver biopsy may
		Detectable	< or > ULN	help in decision to treat
		Undetectable	< or > ULN	Treat[e]
				Treat[e] with oral agents, not PEG IFN
				Consider treatment[f]
				Treat[e] with oral agents[g], not PEG IFN;
				refer for liver transplantation
				Observe; refer for liver transplantation
HBeAg-negative	[b]	$\leq 2 \times 10^3$	≤ULN	Inactive carrier; treatment not necessary
	Chronic hepatitis	$>10^3$	1 to $>2 \times$ ULN[d]	Consider liver biopsy; treat[h] if biopsy
	Chronic hepatitis	$>10^4$	$>2 \times$ ULN[d]	shows moderate to severe inflammation
	Cirrhosis compensated	$>2 \times 10^3$	< or > ULN	or fibrosis
	Cirrhosis decompensated	$<2 \times 10^3$	>ULN	Treat[h,i]
		Detectable	< or > ULN	Treat[e] with oral agents, not PEG IFN
		Undetectable	< or > ULN	Consider treatment[f]
				Treat[h] with oral agents[g], not PEG IFN;
				refer for liver transplantation
				Observe; refer for liver transplantation

[a]Based on practice guidelines of the American Association for the Study of Liver Diseases (AASLD). Except as indicated in footnotes, these guidelines are similar to those issued by the European Association for the Study of the Liver (EASL).
[b]Liver disease tends to be mild or inactive clinically; most such patients do not undergo liver biopsy.
[c]This pattern is common during the early decades of life in Asian patients infected at birth.
[d]According to the EASL guidelines, treat if HBV DNA is $>2 \times 10^3$ IU/mL and ALT is >ULN.
[e]One of the potent oral drugs with a high barrier to resistance (entecavir or tenofovir) or PEG IFN can be used as first-line therapy (see text). These oral agents, but not PEG IFN, should be used for IFN-refractory/intolerant and immunocompromised patients. PEG IFN is administered weekly by subcutaneous injection for a year; the oral agents are administered daily for at least a year and continued indefinitely or until at least 6 months after HBeAg seroconversion.
[f]According to EASL guidelines, patients with compensated cirrhosis and detectable HBV DNA at any level, even with normal ALT, are candidates for therapy. Most authorities would treat indefinitely, even in HBeAg-positive disease after HBeAg seroconversion.
[g]Because the emergence of resistance can lead to loss of antiviral benefit and further deterioration in decompensated cirrhosis, a low-resistance regimen is recommended—entecavir or tenofovir monotherapy or combination therapy with the more resistance-prone lamivudine (or telbivudine) plus adefovir. Therapy should be instituted urgently.
[h]Because HBeAg seroconversion is not an option, the goal of therapy is to suppress HBV DNA and maintain a normal ALT. PEG IFN is administered by subcutaneous injection weekly for a year; caution is warranted in relying on a 6-month posttreatment interval to define a sustained response, because the majority of such responses are lost thereafter. Oral agents, entecavir or tenofovir, are administered daily, usually indefinitely or until, as very rarely occurs, virologic and biochemical responses are accompanied by HBsAg seroconversion.
[i]For older patients and those with advanced fibrosis, consider lowering the HBV DNA threshold to $>2 \times 10^3$ IU/mL.
Abbreviations: AASLD, American Association for the Study of Liver Diseases; ALT, alanine aminotransferase; EASL, European Association for the Study of the Liver; HBeAg, hepatitis B e antigen; HBsAg, hepatitis B surface antigen; HBV, hepatitis B virus; PEG IFN, pegylated interferon; ULN, upper limit of normal.

VIII-64. **The answer is B.** *(Chap. 362)* Chronic hepatitis develops in about 85% of all individuals affected with hepatitis C virus (HCV), and 20%–25% of these individuals will progress to cirrhosis over about 20 years. Among those infected with HCV, about one-third of individuals will have normal or near-normal levels of aminotransferases, although liver biopsy demonstrates active hepatitis in an many as one-half of patients. Moreover, about 25% of individuals with normal aminotransferase levels at one point in time will develop elevations in these enzymes later and can develop progressive liver disease. Thus, normal aminotransferase levels at a single point in time do not definitively rule out the possibility that cirrhosis can develop. Progression to end-stage liver disease in individuals with chronic HCV hepatitis is more likely in older individuals and in patients with longer duration of infection, advanced histologic stage and grade, genotype 1 infection, more complex quasi-species diversity, concomitant other liver disease, HIV infection, and obesity. Among these factors, the best prognostic indicator for the development of progressive liver disease is liver histology. Specifically, patients who have moderate to severe inflammation or necrosis, including septal or bridging fibrosis, have the greatest risk of developing cirrhosis over the course of 10–20 years.

VIII-65. **The answer is C.** *(Chap. 362)* Three types of autoimmune hepatitis have been identified based on clinical and laboratory characteristics. Type I autoimmune hepatitis is typically a disorder seen in young women. The clinical characteristics can be variable from those of chronic hepatitis to fulminant hepatic failure, and many of the features are difficult to distinguish from other causes of chronic hepatitis. In some individuals, extrahepatic manifestations, including fatigue, malaise, weight loss, anorexia, and arthralgias, can be quite prominent. Liver enzymes are elevated but may not correlate with the clinical severity of disease. In more severe cases, elevations in serum bilirubin between 3 and 10 mg/dL can be seen. Hypoalbuminemia occurs in advanced disease, and hypergammaglobulinemia (>2.5 g/dL) is common. The circulating antibody profile in autoimmune hepatitis depends to some extent on the type of hepatitis. Antinuclear antibodies are positive in a homogeneous staining pattern almost invariably in the disease, and rheumatoid factor is also common. Perinuclear antineutrophilic cytoplasmic antibody may be positive, but in an atypical fashion. Anti–smooth muscle antibodies and anti-liver/kidney microsomal antibodies are frequently seen, but these are nonspecific because other causes of chronic hepatitis can lead to positivity of these enzymes. Because of the lack of a specific autoimmune profile, the diagnostic criteria for autoimmune hepatitis incorporate a variety of clinical and laboratory features. Specific features that argue against this diagnosis include prominent alkaline phosphatase elevation, presence of mitochondrial antibodies, markers of viral hepatitis, history of hepatotoxic drugs or excess alcohol intake, histologic evidence of bile duct injury, or atypical biopsy features including excess hepatic iron, fatty infiltration, and viral inclusions. Antimitochondrial antibodies are typically seen in primary biliary cirrhosis.

VIII-66. **The answer is D.** *(Chaps. 360 and 362)* In the course of acute hepatitis B, HBeAg positivity is common and usually transient. Persistence of HBeAg in the serum for >3 months indicates an increased likelihood of development of chronic hepatitis B. In chronic hepatitis B, presence of HBeAg in the serum indicates ongoing viral replication and increased infectivity. It is also a surrogate for inflammatory liver injury but not fibrosis. The development of antibody to HBeAg (anti-HBe) is indicative of the nonreplicative phase of HBV infection. During this phase, intact virions do not circulate and infectivity is less. Currently, quantification of HBV DNA with polymerase chain reaction allows risk stratification because $<10^3$ virions/μL is the approximate threshold for liver injury and infectivity.

VIII-67. **The answer is C.** *(Chap. 363)* The pathology of alcoholic liver disease consists of three major lesions, with the progressive injury rarely existing in a pure form: (1) fatty liver, (2) alcoholic hepatitis, and (3) cirrhosis. Fatty liver is present in >90% of daily as well as binge drinkers. A much smaller percentage of heavy drinkers will progress to alcoholic hepatitis, thought to be a precursor to cirrhosis. The prognosis of severe alcoholic liver disease is dismal; the mortality of patients with alcoholic hepatitis concurrent with cirrhosis is nearly 60% at 4 years. Although alcohol is considered a direct hepatotoxin, only between 10% and 20% of alcoholics will develop alcoholic hepatitis. The explanation for this apparent paradox is unclear but involves the complex interaction of facilitating factors, such as drinking patterns, diet, obesity, and gender. There are no diagnostic tools that can predict individual susceptibility to alcoholic liver disease. Quantity and duration of alcohol intake are the most important risk factors involved in the development of alcoholic liver disease. The roles of beverage type(s) (i.e., wine, beer, or spirits) and pattern of drinking (daily versus binge drinking) are less clear. Chronic infection with hepatitis C virus (HCV) is an important comorbidity in the progression of alcoholic liver disease to cirrhosis. Even moderate alcohol intake of 20–50 g/d increases the risk of cirrhosis and hepatocellular cancer in HCV-infected individuals. Patients with both alcoholic liver injury and HCV infection develop decompensated liver disease at a younger age and have poorer overall survival.

TABLE VIII-67 **Risk Factors for Alcoholic Liver Disease**

Risk Factor	Comment
Quantity	In men, 40–80 g/d of ethanol produces fatty liver; 160 g/d for 10–20 years causes hepatitis or cirrhosis. Only 15% of alcoholics develop alcoholic liver disease.
Gender	Women exhibit increased susceptibility to alcoholic liver disease at amounts >20 g/d; two drinks per day is probably safe.
Hepatitis C	HCV infection concurrent with alcoholic liver disease is associated with younger age for severity, more advanced histology, and decreased survival.
Genetics	Patatin-like phospholipase domain-containing protein 3 (PNPLA3) has been associated with alcoholic cirrhosis.
Fatty liver	Alcohol injury does not require malnutrition, but obesity and nonalcoholic fatty liver are risk factors. Patients should receive vigorous attention to nutritional support.

VIII-68. **The answer is C.** *(Chap. 363)* This patient presents with severe acute alcoholic hepatitis. In its earliest form, alcoholic liver disease is marked by fatty infiltration of the liver. In more acute alcoholic hepatitis, there is hepatocyte injury with balloon degeneration and necrosis. Many cases of alcoholic hepatitis are asymptomatic. However, as in this case, the severe manifestations can include fever, jaundice, spider nevi, and abdominal pain that can mimic an acute abdomen in its severity. On laboratory examination, the AST is typically elevated more than the ALT, although the total transaminase levels are rarely greater than 400 IU/L. Hyperbilirubinemia can be quite marked with lesser elevation in alkaline phosphatase. Hypoalbuminemia and coagulopathy are poor prognostic indicators. A discriminate function (DF) can be calculated as follows: (4.6 × the prolongation of prothrombin time above control) + serum bilirubin. A DF >32 is associated with poor prognosis and is an indication for treatment of acute alcoholic hepatitis. The Model for End-Stage Liver Disease (MELD) score can also be used for prognostication in acute alcoholic hepatitis, with a score greater than 21 being an indication for treatment as well. This patient has a DF of >80, indicating very severe disease and a poor prognosis. Complete abstinence from alcohol is imperative. Treatment with prednisone 40 mg daily (or prednisolone 32 mg daily) for 4 weeks should be initiated. Following the initial period, a taper should be achieved over a period of 4 weeks. The role of tumor necrosis factor (TNF)-α expression and receptor activity in alcoholic liver injury has led to an examination of TNF inhibition as an alternative to glucocorticoids for severe alcoholic hepatitis. The nonspecific TNF inhibitor pentoxifylline (400 mg three times daily for 4 weeks) demonstrated improved survival in the therapy of severe alcoholic hepatitis, primarily due to a decrease in hepatorenal syndrome. Monoclonal antibodies that neutralize serum TNF-α should not be used in alcoholic hepatitis because of studies reporting increased deaths secondary to infection and renal failure. Liver transplantation is an accepted indication for treatment in selected and motivated patients with end-stage cirrhosis. Outcomes are equal or superior to other indications for transplantation.

VIII-69. The answer is D. *(Chap. 364)* Nonalcoholic fatty liver disease (NAFLD) is the most common chronic liver disease in many parts of the world, including the United States. Population-based abdominal imaging studies have demonstrated fatty liver in at least 25% of American adults. Because the vast majority of these subjects deny hazardous levels of alcohol consumption (defined as greater than one drink per day in women or two drinks per day in men), they are considered to have NAFLD. NAFLD is strongly associated with overweight/obesity and insulin resistance. However, it can also occur in lean individuals and is particularly common in those with a paucity of adipose depots (i.e., lipodystrophy). Ethnic/racial factors also appear to influence liver fat accumulation; the documented prevalence of NAFLD is lowest in African Americans (~25%), highest in Americans of Hispanic ancestry (~50%), and intermediate in American whites (~33%).

VIII-70. The answer is C. *(Chap. 364)* At present, there are no Food and Drug Administration–approved therapies for the treatment of NAFLD. Thus, the current approach to NAFLD management focuses on treatment to improve the risk factors for nonalcoholic steatohepatitis (NASH; i.e., obesity, insulin resistance, metabolic syndrome, dyslipidemia). Based on our understanding of the natural history of NAFLD, only patients with NASH or those with features of hepatic fibrosis on liver biopsy are considered currently for targeted pharmacologic therapies. Lifestyle changes and dietary modification are the foundation for NAFLD treatment. Many studies indicate that lifestyle modification can improve serum aminotransferases and hepatic steatosis, with loss of at least 3%–5% of body weight improving steatosis, but greater weight loss (up to 10%) necessary to improve steatohepatitis. The benefits of different dietary macronutrient contents (e.g., low-carbohydrate vs. low-fat diets, saturated vs. unsaturated fat diets) and different intensities of calorie restriction appear to be comparable. In adults with NAFLD, exercise regimens that improve fitness may be sufficient to reduce hepatic steatosis, but their impact on other aspects of liver histology remains unknown. Antioxidants have also been evaluated for the treatment of NAFLD because oxidant stress is thought to contribute to the pathogenesis of NASH. Vitamin E, an inexpensive yet potent antioxidant, has been examined in several small pediatric and adult studies with varying results. In all of those studies, vitamin E was well tolerated, and most showed modest improvements in aminotransferase levels, radiographic features of hepatic steatosis, and/or histologic features of NASH. Statins are an important class of agents to treat dyslipidemia and decrease cardiovascular risk. There is no evidence to suggest that statins cause liver failure in patients with any chronic liver disease, including NAFLD. The incidence of liver enzyme elevations in NAFLD patients taking statins is also no different than that of healthy controls or patients with other chronic liver diseases. Moreover, several studies have suggested that statins may improve aminotransferases and histology in patients with NASH. However, there is continued reluctance to use statins in patients with NAFLD. The lack of evidence that statins harm the liver in NAFLD patients, combined with the increased risk for cardiovascular morbidity and mortality in NAFLD patients, warrants the use of statins to treat dyslipidemia in patients with NAFLD/NASH. Although interest in bariatric surgery as a treatment for NAFLD exists, a recently published Cochrane review concluded that lack of randomized clinical trials or adequate clinical studies prevents definitive assessment of benefits and harms of bariatric surgery as a treatment for NASH. Most studies of bariatric surgery have shown that it is generally safe in individuals with well-compensated chronic liver disease and improves hepatic steatosis and necroinflammation (i.e., features of NAFLD/NASH); however, effects on hepatic fibrosis have been variable.

VIII-71. The answer is A. *(Chap. 365)* Alcohol is the most commonly used drug in the United States, and more than two-thirds of adults drink alcohol each year. Thirty percent have had a binge within the past month, and over 7% of adults regularly consume more than two drinks per day. Unfortunately, more than 14 million adults in the United States meet the diagnostic criteria for alcohol abuse or dependence. In the United States, chronic liver disease is the 10th most common cause of death in adults, and alcoholic cirrhosis accounts for approximately 40% of deaths due to cirrhosis. Excessive chronic alcohol use can cause several different types of chronic liver disease, including alcoholic fatty liver, alcoholic hepatitis, and alcoholic cirrhosis. Furthermore, use of excessive alcohol can contribute to liver damage in patients with other liver diseases, such as hepatitis C, hemochromatosis, and fatty liver disease related to obesity. Chronic alcohol use can produce fibrosis in the absence of accompanying inflammation and/or necrosis. Fibrosis can be centrilobular, pericellular, or periportal. When fibrosis reaches a certain degree, there is disruption of the normal liver architecture and replacement of liver cells by regenerative nodules. In alcoholic cirrhosis, the nodules are usually <3 mm in diameter; this form of cirrhosis is referred to as micronodular. With cessation of alcohol use, larger nodules may form, resulting in a mixed micronodular and macronodular cirrhosis.

VIII-72. **The answer is A.** *(Chap. 365)* The patient's hands show palmar erythema typical of alcoholic cirrhosis. This finding and the gynecomastia and testicular atrophy make alcoholic cirrhosis the most likely diagnosis. The testicular atrophy may be due to either a direct toxic effect of alcohol or hormonal effects. All of the other items may also cause liver cirrhosis (Table VIII-72).

TABLE VIII-72 **Causes of Cirrhosis**

Alcoholism	Cardiac cirrhosis
Chronic viral hepatitis	Inherited metabolic liver disease
Hepatitis B	Hemochromatosis
Hepatitis C	Wilson disease
Autoimmune hepatitis	α_1-Antitrypsin deficiency
Nonalcoholic steatohepatitis	Cystic fibrosis
Biliary cirrhosis	Cryptogenic cirrhosis
Primary biliary cirrhosis	
Primary sclerosing cholangitis	
Autoimmune cholangiopathy	

VIII-73. **The answer is D.** *(Chap. 365)* The approach to patients once they have had a variceal bleed is first to treat the acute bleed, which can be life-threatening, and then to prevent further bleeding. The medical management of acute variceal hemorrhage includes the use of vasoconstricting agents, usually somatostatin or octreotide. Balloon tamponade (Sengstaken-Blakemore tube or Minnesota tube) can be used in patients who cannot receive endoscopic therapy immediately or who need stabilization prior to endoscopic therapy. Endoscopic intervention is used as first-line treatment to control bleeding acutely. Some endoscopists will use variceal injection therapy (sclerotherapy) as initial therapy, particularly when bleeding is vigorous. Variceal band ligation is used to control acute bleeding in over 90% of cases and should be repeated until obliteration of all varices is accomplished. When esophageal varices extend into the proximal stomach, band ligation is less successful. In these situations, when bleeding continues from gastric varices, consideration for a transjugular intrahepatic portosystemic shunt (TIPS) should be made. This offers an alternative to surgery for acute decompression of portal hypertension. Encephalopathy can occur in as many as 20% of patients after TIPS and is particularly problematic in elderly patients and in patients with preexisting encephalopathy. TIPS should be reserved for individuals who fail endoscopic or medical management or who are poor surgical risks. TIPS can sometimes be used as a bridge to transplantation. Prevention of further bleeding is usually accomplished with repeated variceal band ligation until varices are obliterated. B-Blockers, such as propranolol and nadolol, have been shown to decrease the risk of recurrent variceal bleeding and reduce mortality from a subsequent bleed but should not be used in the setting of the acutely bleeding patient.

VIII-74. **The answer is D.** *(Chap. 365)* In patients with cirrhosis who are being followed chronically, the development of portal hypertension is usually revealed by the presence of thrombocytopenia; the appearance of an enlarged spleen; or the development of ascites, encephalopathy, and/or esophageal varices with or without bleeding. In previously undiagnosed patients, any of these features should prompt further evaluation to determine the presence of portal hypertension and liver disease. Varices should be identified by endoscopy. Abdominal imaging, either by CT or magnetic resonance imaging (MRI), can be helpful in demonstrating a nodular liver and in finding changes of portal hypertension with intra-abdominal collateral circulation. If necessary, interventional radiologic procedures can be performed to determine wedged and free hepatic vein pressures that will allow for the calculation of a wedged-to-free gradient, which is equivalent to the portal pressure. The average normal wedged-to-free gradient is 5 mmHg, and patients with a gradient >12 mmHg are at risk for variceal hemorrhage. While dilation of the right atrium may be found in cases of cardiac cirrhosis, dilation of the left atrium is characteristic of left ventricular failure.

VIII-75. **The answer is B.** *(Chap. 365)* Spontaneous bacterial peritonitis (SBP) is a common and severe complication of ascites characterized by spontaneous infection of the ascitic fluid without an intra-abdominal source. In patients with cirrhosis and ascites severe enough for hospitalization, SBP can occur in up to 30% of individuals and can have a 25% in-hospital mortality rate. Bacterial translocation is the presumed mechanism for development of SBP, with gut flora traversing the intestine into mesenteric lymph nodes, leading to bacteremia and seeding of the ascitic fluid. The most common organisms are *E coli* and other gut bacteria; however, gram-positive bacteria, including *Streptococcus viridans*, *Staphylococcus aureus*, and *Enterococcus* spp., can also be found. If more than two organisms are identified, secondary bacterial peritonitis due to a perforated viscus should be considered. The diagnosis of SBP is made when the fluid sample has an absolute neutrophil count >250/μL. In this case, the patient has an absolute neutrophil count of 320/μL (800 × 0.4). Patients with ascites may present with fever, altered mental status, elevated white blood cell count, and abdominal pain or discomfort, or they may present without any of these features. Therefore, it is necessary to have a high degree of clinical suspicion, and peritoneal taps are important for making the diagnosis. Treatment is with a second-generation cephalosporin, with cefotaxime being the most commonly used antibiotic. In patients with variceal hemorrhage, the frequency of SBP is significantly increased, and prophylaxis against SBP is recommended when a patient presents with upper GI bleeding. Furthermore, in patients who have had an episode(s) of SBP and recovered, once-weekly administration of antibiotics is used as prophylaxis for recurrent SBP. There is no indication for hemodialysis with the normal serum creatine or EGD with no history of bleeding and a stable hemoglobin. Blood urea nitrogen (BUN) may increase as a result of the infection. Similarly, although the BUN is elevated and the patient has altered mental status, lactulose would not treat the primary disorder causing the altered mental status. Given the likely diagnosis of SBP, empiric therapy for meningitis is not warranted at this time.

VIII-76. **The answer is C.** *(Chap. 365)* The clinical presentation is consistent with a cholestatic picture, which can present with painless jaundice and pruritus. The pruritus can be prominent and is present in 50% of individuals at the time of diagnosis. The pruritus is typically intermittent and worse in the evening. There is no other prominent association, such as following hot baths or showers, which occurs in polycythemia vera. Other causes of pruritus outside of cholestasis include lymphoma and uncontrolled hypo- or hyperthyroidism. However, the laboratory studies in this patient clearly represent cholestasis with an elevation in alkaline phosphatase and bilirubin. The clinical characteristics are more commonly seen in primary biliary cirrhosis compared to primary sclerosis cholangitis as the patient is a middle-aged female with positive antimitochondrial antibodies. In contrast, primary sclerosing cholangitis is associated with positive perinuclear antineutrophil cytoplasmic antibodies in 65% of patients, and 50% of individuals with primary sclerosing cholangitis have a history of ulcerative colitis.

VIII-77. **The answer is A.** *(Chap. 365)* The cornerstone of the management of ascites is sodium restriction to less than 2 g daily. A common misconception is to institute a fluid restriction as well. However, this is neither effective nor necessary. With a sodium restriction to 2 g daily, most mild ascites can be managed quite well. If sodium restriction alone fails to correct ascites, then initiation of diuretics is required. Spironolactone at a dose of 100–200 mg daily is the initial diuretic used for ascites and can be titrated as high as 400–600 mg daily if tolerated. Loop diuretics can be added to spironolactone. The typical agent is furosemide beginning at 40–80 mg daily with maximum doses of about 120–160 mg daily. Care must be taken to avoid renal dysfunction with loop diuretics, and higher doses may not be tolerated. If ascites is refractory to these treatments, TIPS can be considered. This procedure creates a direct portocaval shunt by introducing an expandable metal stent from the hepatic veins through the substance of the liver into the portal veins. Thus, TIPS decreases portal pressures, which in turn decrease ascites and the risk of variceal bleeding. However, hepatic encephalopathy typically worsens following TIPS.

VIII-78. **The answer is A.** *(Chap. 365)* Severe right-sided heart failure may lead to chronic liver injury and cardiac cirrhosis. Elevated venous pressure leads to congestion of the hepatic sinusoids and of the central vein and centrilobular hepatocytes. Centrilobular fibrosis develops, and fibrosis extends outward from the central vein, not the portal triads. Gross examination of the liver shows a pattern of "nutmeg liver." Although transaminases are typically mildly elevated, severe congestion, particularly associated with hypotension, may result in dramatic elevation of AST and ALT 50- to 100-fold above normal. Budd-Chiari syndrome, or occlusion of the hepatic veins or inferior vena cava, may be confused with congestive hepatopathy. However, the signs and symptoms of congestive heart failure are absent in patients with Budd-Chiari syndrome, and these patients can be easily distinguished clinically from those with heart failure. Veno-occlusive disease may result from hepatic irradiation and high-dose chemotherapy in preparation for hematopoietic stem cell transplantation. It is not a typical complication of liver transplantation. Although echocardiography is a useful tool for assessing left and right ventricular function, findings may be unimpressive in patients with constrictive pericarditis. A high index of suspicion for constrictive pericarditis (e.g., prior episodes of pericarditis, mediastinal irradiation) should lead to a right-sided heart catheterization with demonstration of the "square root sign," limitation of right heart filling pressure in diastole that is suggestive of restrictive cardiomyopathy. Cardiac MRI may also be helpful in determining which patients should proceed to cardiac surgery.

VIII-79. **The answer is B.** *(Chap. 365)* The presence of cirrhosis in an elderly woman with no prior risk factors for viral or alcoholic cirrhosis should raise the possibility of primary biliary cirrhosis (PBC). PBC is characterized by chronic inflammation and fibrous obliteration of intrahepatic ductules. The cause is unknown, but autoimmunity is assumed because there is an association with other autoimmune disorders, such as autoimmune thyroiditis, CREST syndrome, and sicca syndrome. The vast majority of patients with symptomatic disease are women. The antimitochondrial antibody (AMA) test is positive in over 90% of patients with PBC and only rarely is positive in other conditions. This makes it the most useful initial test in the diagnosis of PBC. Because there are false-positive results, if AMA is positive, a liver biopsy is performed to confirm the diagnosis. The 24-hour urine copper collection is useful in the diagnosis of Wilson disease. Hepatic failure from Wilson disease typically occurs before age 50 years. Hemochromatosis may result in cirrhosis. It is associated with lethargy, fatigue, loss of libido, discoloration of the skin, arthralgias, diabetes, and cardiomyopathy. Ferritin levels are usually increased, and the most suggestive laboratory abnormality is an elevated transferrin saturation percentage. Although hemochromatosis is a possible diagnosis in this case, PBC is more likely in light of the clinical scenario. Although chronic hepatitis B and hepatitis C are certainly in the differential diagnosis and must be ruled out, they are unlikely because of the patient's history and lack of risk factors.

VIII-80. **The answer is B.** *(Chap. 368)* Liver transplantation is indicated in adults for end-stage cirrhosis of all causes. Routine candidates for liver transplantation are patients with alcoholic cirrhosis, chronic viral hepatitis, and primary hepatocellular malignancies. Although all three of these categories are considered to be high risk, liver transplantation can be offered to carefully selected patients. Currently, chronic hepatitis C and alcoholic liver disease are the most common indications for liver transplantation, accounting for over 40% of all adult candidates who undergo the procedure. Patients with alcoholic cirrhosis can be considered as candidates for transplantation if they meet strict criteria for abstinence and reform; however, these criteria still do not prevent recidivism in up to a quarter of cases. In sclerosing cholangitis and Caroli disease (multiple cystic dilatations of the intrahepatic biliary tree), recurrent infections and sepsis associated with inflammatory and fibrotic obstruction of the biliary tree may be an indication for transplantation. Because prior biliary surgery complicates and is a relative contraindication for liver transplantation, surgical diversion of the biliary tree has been all but abandoned for patients with sclerosing cholangitis. Patients with chronic hepatitis C have early allograft and patient survival comparable to those of other subsets of patients after transplantation; however, reinfection in the donor organ is universal, recurrent hepatitis C is insidiously progressive, allograft cirrhosis develops in 20%–30% at 5 years, and cirrhosis and late organ failure occur at a higher frequency beyond 5 years. With the introduction of highly effective direct-acting antiviral agents targeting hepatitis C, it is expected that allograft outcomes will improve significantly in the coming years. In patients with chronic hepatitis B, in the absence of measures to prevent recurrent hepatitis B, survival after transplantation is reduced by approximately 10%–20%; however, prophylactic use of hepatitis B immune globulin (HBIg) during and after transplantation increases the success of transplantation to a level comparable to that seen in patients with nonviral causes of liver decompensation. Specific oral antiviral drugs can be used both for prophylaxis against and for treatment of recurrent hepatitis B. Patients with primary hepatocellular carcinoma with a single tumor <5 cm or three or fewer tumors of <3 cm have 5-year recurrence-free survival rates similar to those with nonmalignant disease. Because of the high rate of recurrent disease after transplantation, patients with cholangiocarcinoma are not transplantation candidates.

VIII-81. **The answer is D.** *(Chap. 368)* Currently in the United States, all donor livers are distributed through a nationwide organ-sharing network (United Network for Organ Sharing [UNOS]) designed to allocate available organs based on regional considerations and recipient acuity. Recipients who have the highest disease severity generally have the highest priority, but allocation strategies that balance highest urgency against best outcomes continue to evolve to distribute cadaver organs most effectively. Allocation is based on the MELD score, which is based on a mathematical model that includes bilirubin, creatinine, and international normalized ratio. Neither waiting time (except as a tie breaker between two potential recipients with the same MELD scores) nor posttransplantation outcome is taken into account. Use of the MELD score has been shown to reduce waiting list mortality, to reduce waiting time prior to transplantation, and to be the best predictor of pretransplantation mortality. The highest priority (status 1) for liver transplantation continues to be reserved for patients with fulminant hepatic failure or primary graft nonfunction.

VIII-82. **The answer is B.** *(Chap. 369)* In the National Health and Nutrition Examination Survey, the prevalence of gallstone disease in the United States was 7.9% in men and 16.6% in women. Although the disease is quite prevalent, not all patients with gallstone disease require cholecystectomy. It is estimated that 1%–2% of patients with asymptomatic gallstone disease will develop complications that will require surgery yearly. Therefore, it is important to know which patients with asymptomatic gallstones require referral for surgery. The first factor to consider is whether the patient has symptoms that are caused by gallstones and are frequent enough and severe enough to necessitate surgery. Commonly called biliary colic, the classic symptoms of gallstone disease are right upper quadrant pain and fullness that begins suddenly and can last as long as 5 hours. Nausea and vomiting can accompany the episode. Vague symptoms of epigastric fullness, dyspepsia, and bloating following meals should not be considered biliary colic. A second factor that would be considered in recommending a patient for cholecystectomy is whether the patient has a prior history of complications of gallstone disease such as pancreatitis or acute cholecystitis. A final factor that would lead to the recommendation for cholecystectomy is the presence of anatomical factors that would increase the likelihood of complications such as a porcelain gallbladder or congenital abnormalities of the biliary tract. Individuals with very large stones (>3 cm) would also need to be considered carefully for cholecystectomy. Ursodeoxycholic acid can be used in some instances to dissolve gallstones. It acts to decrease the cholesterol saturation of bile and also allows dispersion of cholesterol from stones by producing a lamellar crystalline phase. However, it is only effective in individuals with radiolucent stones measuring less than 10 mm.

VIII-83. The answer is D. *(Chap. 369)* A practitioner needs to have a high index of suspicion for acalculous cholecystitis in critically ill patients who develop decompensation during the course of treatment for the underlying disease and have no other apparent source of infection. Some predisposing conditions for the development of acalculous cholecystitis include serious trauma or burns, postpartum following prolonged labor, prolonged parenteral hyperalimentation, and during the postoperative period following orthopedic and other major surgical procedures. The clinical manifestations of acalculous cholecystitis are identical to calculous disease, but the disease is more difficult to diagnose. Ultrasonography and CT scanning typically only show biliary sludge, but they may demonstrate large and tense gallbladders. Hepatobiliary scintigraphy often shows delayed or absent gallbladder emptying. Successful management relies on accurate and early diagnosis. In critically ill patients, a percutaneous cholecystostomy may be the safest immediate procedure to decompress an infected gallbladder. Once the patient is stabilized, early elective cholecystectomy should be considered. Metronidazole to provide anaerobic coverage should be added, but this would not elucidate or adequately treat the underlying condition.

VIII-84. The answer is B. *(Chap. 369)* Gallstones are very common, particularly in Western countries, with cholesterol stones being responsible for >90% of cases of cholelithiasis and pigment stones account for the remaining <10%. Cholesterol is essentially water-insoluble. Stone formation occurs in the setting of factors that upset cholesterol balance. Obesity, cholesterol-rich diets, high-calorie diets, and certain medications affect biliary secretion of cholesterol. Intrinsic genetic mutations in certain populations may affect the processing and secretion of cholesterol in the liver. Pregnancy results in both an increase in cholesterol saturation during the third trimester and changes in gallbladder contractility. Although rapid weight loss and low-calorie diets are associated with gallstones, there is no evidence that a high-protein diet confers an added risk of cholelithiasis.

VIII-85. The answer is E. *(Chap. 369)* Pigment stone cholelithiasis may be black or brown stones. Black pigment stones are composed of either pure calcium bilirubinate or polymer-like complexes with calcium and mucin glycoproteins. They are more common in patients who have chronic hemolytic states (with increased conjugated bilirubin in bile), liver cirrhosis, Gilbert syndrome, or cystic fibrosis. Gallbladder stones in patients with ileal diseases, ileal resection, or ileal bypass generally are also black pigment stones. Enterohepatic recycling of bilirubin in ileal disease states contributes to their pathogenesis. Brown pigment stones are composed of calcium salts of unconjugated bilirubin with varying amounts of cholesterol and protein. They are caused by the presence of increased amounts of unconjugated, insoluble bilirubin in bile that precipitates to form stones. Sometimes, the enzyme is also produced when bile is chronically infected by bacteria, and such stones are brown. Pigment stone formation is frequent in Asia and is often associated with infections in the gallbladder and biliary tree, including parasitic infections. Primary biliary cirrhosis is associated with cholesterol stones because of decreased bile acid secretion.

VIII-86. The answer is B. *(Chaps. 58 and 369)* The clinical presentation is consistent with a cholestatic picture. Painless jaundice always requires an extensive workup, as many of the underlying pathologies are ominous and early detection and intervention often offers the only hope for a good outcome. The gallbladder showed no evidence of stones, and the patient shows no evidence of clinical cholecystitis, and so a hepatobiliary iminodiacetic acid (HIDA) scan is not indicated. Similarly, antibiotics are not necessary at this point. The cholestatic picture without significant elevation of the transaminases on the liver function tests makes acute hepatitis unlikely. Antimitochondrial antibodies are elevated in cases of PBC, which may present in a similar fashion. However, PBC is far more common in women than in men, and the average age of onset is the fifth or sixth decade. The lack of an obvious lesion on CT scan does not rule out a source of the cholestasis in the biliary tree. Malignant causes, such as cholangiocarcinoma and tumor of the ampulla of Vater, and nonmalignant causes, such as sclerosing cholangitis and Caroli disease, may be detected only by direct visualization with endoscopic retrograde cholangiopancreatography (ERCP). ERCP is useful both diagnostically and therapeutically as stenting procedures may be done to alleviate the obstruction.

VIII-87. **The answer is A.** *(Chap. 369)* Primary or idiopathic sclerosing cholangitis (PSC) is characterized by a progressive, inflammatory, sclerosing, and obliterative process affecting the extrahepatic and/or the intrahepatic bile ducts. The disorder occurs in up to 75% of patients with inflammatory bowel disease, especially ulcerative colitis. It may also be associated with autoimmune pancreatitis; multifocal fibrosclerosis syndromes such as retroperitoneal, mediastinal, and/or periureteral fibrosis; Riedel struma; or pseudotumor of the orbit. Immunoglobulin G4 (IgG4)–associated cholangitis is a recently described biliary disease of unknown etiology that presents with biochemical and cholangiographic features indistinguishable from PSC, is often associated with autoimmune pancreatitis and other fibrosing conditions, and is characterized by elevated serum IgG4 and infiltration of IgG4-positive plasma cells in bile ducts and liver tissue. In contrast to PSC, it is not associated with inflammatory bowel disease and should be suspected if associated with increased serum IgG4 and unexplained pancreatic disease. Patients with PSC often present with signs and symptoms of chronic or intermittent biliary obstruction: right upper quadrant abdominal pain, pruritus, jaundice, or acute cholangitis. Late in the course, complete biliary obstruction, secondary biliary cirrhosis, hepatic failure, or portal hypertension with bleeding varices may occur. The diagnosis is usually established by finding multifocal, diffusely distributed strictures with intervening segments of normal or dilated ducts, producing a beaded appearance on cholangiography. Patients are at higher risk of cholangiocarcinoma. Therapy with cholestyramine may help control symptoms of pruritus, and antibiotics are useful when cholangitis complicates the clinical picture. Glucocorticoids, methotrexate, and cyclosporine have not been shown to be efficacious in PSC. In cases where high-grade biliary obstruction (dominant strictures) has occurred, balloon dilatation or stenting may be appropriate. Only rarely is surgical intervention indicated. The prognosis is unfavorable, with a median survival of 9–12 years following the diagnosis, regardless of therapy. Four variables (age, serum bilirubin level, histologic stage, and splenomegaly) predict survival in patients with PSC and serve as the basis for a risk score. PSC is a common indication for liver transplantation.

VIII-88. **The answer is A.** *(Chap. 371)* Bicarbonate is the ion of primary physiologic importance within pancreatic secretion. The ductal cells secrete bicarbonate predominantly derived from plasma (93%) more than from intracellular metabolism (7%). Bicarbonate enters the duct lumen through the sodium bicarbonate cotransporter with depolarization caused by chloride efflux through the cystic fibrosis transmembrane conductance regulator (CFTR). Secretin and vasoactive intestinal peptide bind at the basolateral surface and cause an increase in secondary messenger intracellular cyclic adenosine monophosphate, and act on the apical surface of the ductal cells, opening the CFTR and promoting secretion. CCK, acting as a neuromodulator, markedly potentiates the stimulatory effects of secretin. Acetylcholine also plays an important role in ductal cell secretion. Intraluminal bicarbonate secreted from the ductal cells helps neutralize gastric acid and creates the appropriate pH for the activity of pancreatic enzymes and bile salts on ingested food.

VIII-89. **The answer is A.** *(Chap. 371)* In combination with a consistent clinical story and radiographic findings, serum amylase and lipase values threefold or more above normal virtually clinch the diagnosis of acute pancreatitis. Gut perforation, ischemia, and infarction should be excluded. Serum lipase is the preferred test and has a higher specificity than serum amylase. There is no correlation between the severity of pancreatitis and the degree of serum lipase and amylase elevations. After 3–7 days, even with continuing evidence of pancreatitis, total serum amylase values tend to return toward normal. However, pancreatic isoamylase and lipase levels may remain elevated for 7–14 days. Elevation of serum amylase is not specific for acute pancreatitis; notably, patients with metabolic academia (e.g., diabetic ketoacidosis) may have spurious elevation of serum amylase without pancreatitis. Hypocalcemia occurs in approximately 25% of cases of acute pancreatitis, whereas hypercalcemia is not a feature.

VIII-90. **The answer is A.** (*Chap. 371*) The most common cause of acute pancreatitis in the United States is gallstones causing common bile duct obstruction. Although bile duct obstruction may be demonstrated on technetium HIDA scan, right upper quadrant ultrasound is preferred for ease, demonstration of gallstones in the gallbladder, and demonstration of obstructed bile duct. Alcohol is the second most common cause, followed by complications of ERCP. Hypertriglyceridemia accounts for 1%–4% of cases with triglyceride levels usually >1000 mg/dL. Other potential common causes include trauma, surgery, drugs such as valproic acid, anti-HIV medications, estrogens, and sphincter of Oddi dysfunction. Additionally, a number of rare causes have been described. The most judicious first step in evaluation is to test for gallstones and pursue more rare causes after the most common cause has been ruled out.

VIII-91. **The answer is A.** *(Chap. 371)* Physical examination in acute pancreatitis commonly shows an uncomfortable patient, often with low-grade fever, tachycardia, and hypotension. Abdominal tenderness and muscle rigidity are often present to varying degrees. Cullen sign is a faint blue discoloration around the umbilicus that may occur as the result of hemoperitoneum. Turner sign is blue-red-purple or green-brown discoloration of the flanks from tissue catabolism of hemoglobin. Both of these signs indicate the presence of severe necrotizing pancreatitis.

VIII-92. **The answer is E.** *(Chap. 313)* The BISAP (Bedside Index of Severity in Acute Pancreatitis) score has recently replaced Ranson's criteria and Acute Physiology and Chronic Health Evaluation II (APACHE II) severity scores as the recommended modality to assess severity of pancreatitis due to the cumbersome nature of the prior scores and the requirement of prior scores to collect a large amount of clinical and laboratory data over time. Severity of acute pancreatitis should be determined in the emergency department to assist in patient triage to a regular hospital ward or step-down unit or direct admission to an intensive care unit. BISAP incorporates five clinical and laboratory parameters obtained within the first 24 hours of hospitalization—BUN >25 mg/dL, impaired mental status (Glasgow coma score <15), systemic inflammatory response syndrome, age >60 years, and pleural effusion on radiography—that can be useful in assessing severity (Table VIII-92). The

TABLE VIII-92 **Severe Acute Pancreatitis**

Risk Factors for Severity
- Age >60 years
- Obesity, BMI >30
- Comorbid disease (Charlson comorbidity index)

Markers of Severity at Admission or Within 24 Hours
- SIRS—defined by presence of 2 or more criteria:
  - Core temperature <36°C or >38°C
  - Heart rate >90 bpm
  - Respirations >20/min or PCO_2 <32 mmHg
  - White blood cell count >12,000/μL, <4000/μL, or 10% bands
- APACHE II
- Hemoconcentration (hematocrit >44%)
- Admission BUN (>22 mg/dL)
- BISAP Score
  - (B) BUN >25 mg/dL
  - (I) Impaired mental status
  - (S) SIRS: ≥2 of 4 present
  - (A) Age >60 years
  - (P) Pleural effusion
- Organ failure (Modified Marshall Score)
- Cardiovascular: systolic BP <90 mmHg, heart rate >130 bpm
- Pulmonary: PaO_2 <60 mmHg
- Renal: serum creatinine >2.0 mg/dL

Markers of Severity During Hospitalization
- Persistent organ failure
- Pancreatic necrosis

Abbreviations: APACHE II, Acute Physiology and Chronic Health Evaluation II; BMI, body mass index; BISAP, Bedside Index of Severity in Acute Pancreatitis; BP, blood pressure; BUN, blood urea nitrogen; SIRS, systemic inflammatory response syndrome.

presence of three or more of these factors was associated with substantially increased risk for in-hospital mortality among patients with acute pancreatitis. In addition, an elevated hematocrit >44% and admission BUN >22 mg/dL are also associated with more severe acute pancreatitis. Incorporating these indices with the overall patient response to initial fluid resuscitation in the emergency ward can be useful at triaging patients to the appropriate hospital acute care setting. Elevation of serum lipase is important for establishing the diagnosis of acute pancreatitis, but the degree of elevation is not correlated with severity of disease.

VIII-93. **The answer is E.** *(Chap. 371)* Several trials over the last several decades have demonstrated that there is no role for prophylactic antibiotics in the management of either interstitial or necrotizing pancreatitis. Antibiotics are only recommended for patients who appear septic at presentation while awaiting the results of culture data. If cultures are negative, antibiotics should be discontinued to decrease the risk of development of fungal superinfection. Similarly, several drugs have been evaluated in the treatment of acute pancreatitis and found to be of no benefit. These drugs include H^2 blockers, glucagon, protease inhibitors such as aprotinin, glucocorticoids, calcitonin, nonsteroidal anti-inflamatory drugs, and lexipafant, a platelet-activating factor inhibitor. A recent meta-analysis of somatostatin, octreotide, and the antiprotease gabexate mesylate in the therapy of acute pancreatitis suggested reduced mortality rate but no change in complications with octreotide and no effect on mortality but reduced pancreatic damage with gabexate.

VIII-94. **The answer is C.** *(Chap. 371)* A low-fat solid diet can be administered to subjects with mild acute pancreatitis after the abdominal pain has resolved. Persistent inflammatory changes in the pancreas may remain for weeks to months after an episode of acute pancreatitis. Similarly, there may be prolonged elevation of amylase and lipase. In this regard, persistent changes on CT or persistent pancreatic enzyme elevation should not discourage clinicians from feeding hungry patients with acute pancreatitis. Although there had been prior concern that feeding patients with pancreatitis may exacerbate pancreatic inflammation, this has not been demonstrated. Enteral feeding maintains gut barrier integrity, limits bacterial translocation, is less expensive, and has fewer com- plications than total parenteral nutrition. The choice of gastric versus nasojejunal enteral feeding is currently under investigation.

VIII-95. **The answer is D.** *(Chap. 371)* The pathophysiology of acute pancreatitis evolves in three phases. During the initial phase, pancreatic injury leads to intrapancreatic activation of digestive enzymes with subsequent autodigestion and acinar cell injury. Acinar injury is primarily attributed to activation of zymogens (proenzymes), particularly trypsinogen, by lysosomal hydrolases. Once trypsinogen is converted to trypsin, the activated trypsin further perpetuates the process by activating other zymogens to further autodigestion. The inflammation initiated by intrapancreatic activation of zymogens leads to the second phase of acute pancreatitis, with local production of chemokines that causes activation and sequestration of neutrophils in the pancreas. Experimental evidence suggests that neutrophilic inflammation can also cause further activation of trypsinogen, leading to a cascade of increasing acinar injury. The third phase of acute pancreatitis reflects the systemic processes that are caused by release of inflammatory cytokines and activated proenzymes into the systemic circulation. This process can lead to the systemic inflammatory response syndrome with acute respiratory distress syndrome, extensive third-spacing of fluids, and multiorgan failure. The morphologic features of acute pancreatitis are provided in Table VIII-95.

VIII-96. **The answer is D.** *(Chap. 371)* Chronic pancreatitis is a common disorder in any patient population with relapsing acute pancreatitis, especially patients with alcohol dependence, pancreas divisum, and cystic fibrosis. The disorder is notable for both endocrine and exocrine dysfunction of the pancreas. Often, diabetes ensues as a result of loss of islet cell function; although insulin-dependent, it is generally not as prone to diabetic ketoacidosis or coma as are other forms of diabetes mellitus. Because pancreatic enzymes are essential to fat digestion, their absence leads to fat malabsorption and steatorrhea. In addition, the

TABLE VIII-95 **Revised Atlanta Definitions of Morphologic Features of Acute Pancreatitis**

Morphologic Feature	Definition	Computed Tomography Criteria
Interstitial pancreatitis	Acute inflammation of the pancreatic parenchyma and peripancreatic tissues, but without recognizable tissue necrosis	Pancreatic parenchyma enhancement by IV contrast agent No findings of peripancreatic necrosis
Necrotizing pancreatitis	Inflammation associated with pancreatic parenchymal necrosis and/or peripancreatic necrosis	Lack of pancreatic parenchymal enhancement by IV contrast agent and/or presence of findings of peripancreatic necrosis (see below—ANC and WON)
Acute pancreatic fluid collection	Peripancreatic fluid associated with interstitial edematous pancreatitis with no associated peripancreatic necrosis. This term applies only to areas of peripancreatic fluid seen within the first 4 weeks after onset of interstitial edematous pancreatitis and without the features of a pseudocyst.	Occurs in the setting of interstitial edematous pancreatitis Homogeneous collection with fluid density Confined by normal peripancreatic fascial planes No definable wall encapsulating the collection Adjacent to pancreas (no intrapancreatic extension)
Pancreatic pseudocyst	An encapsulated collection of fluid with a well-defined inflammatory wall usually outside the pancreas with minimal or no necrosis. This entity usually occurs >4 weeks after onset of interstitial edematous pancreatitis.	Well circumscribed, usually round or oval Homogeneous fluid density No nonliquid component Well-defined wall; i.e., completely encapsulated Maturation usually requires >4 weeks after onset of acute pancreatitis; occurs after interstitial edematous pancreatitis
Acute necrotic collection (ANC)	A collection containing variable amounts of both fluid and necrosis associated with necrotizing pancreatitis; the necrosis can involve the pancreatic parenchyma and/or the peripancreatic tissues.	Occurs only in the setting of acute necrotizing pancreatitis Heterogeneous and nonliquid density of varying degrees in different locations (some appear homogeneous early in their course) No definable wall encapsulating the collection Location—intrapancreatic and/or extrapancreatic
Walled-off necrosis (WON)	A mature, encapsulated collection of pancreatic and/or peripancreatic necrosis that has developed a well-defined inflammatory wall. WON usually occurs >4 weeks after onset of necrotizing pancreatitis.	Heterogeneous with liquid and nonliquid density with varying degrees of loculations (some may appear homogeneous) Well-defined wall; i.e., completely encapsulated Location—intrapancreatic and/or extrapancreatic Maturation usually requires 4 weeks after onset of acute necrotizing pancreatitis

Source: Modified from P Banks et al: Gut 62:102, 2013.

fat-soluble vitamins (A, D, E, and K) are not absorbed. Vitamin A deficiency can lead to neuropathy. Vitamin B_{12}, or cobalamin, is often deficient. This deficiency is hypothesized to be due to excessive binding of cobalamin by cobalamin-binding proteins other than intrinsic factor that are normally digested by pancreatic enzymes. Replacement of pancreatic enzymes orally with meals will correct the vitamin deficiencies and steatorrhea. The incidence of pancreatic adenocarcinoma is increased in patients with chronic pancreatitis, with a 20-year cumulative incidence of 4%. Chronic abdominal pain is nearly ubiquitous in this disorder, and narcotic dependence is common. Niacin is a water-soluble vitamin, and absorption is not affected by pancreatic exocrine dysfunction.

VIII-97. **The answer is A.** *(Chap. 371)* This patient likely has chronic pancreatitis related to longstanding alcohol use, which is the most common cause of chronic pancreatitis in adults in the United States. Chronic pancreatitis can develop in individuals who consume as little as 50 g of alcohol daily (equivalent to ~30–40 ounces of beer). The patient's description of his loose stools is consistent with steatorrhea, and the recurrent bouts of abdominal pain are likely related to his pancreatitis. In most patients, abdominal pain is the most prominent symptom. However, up to 20% of individuals with chronic pancreatitis present with symptoms of maldigestion alone. The evaluation for chronic pancreatitis should allow one to characterize the pancreatitis as large- versus small-duct disease. Large-duct disease is more common in men and is more likely to be associated with steatorrhea. In addition, large-duct disease is associated with the appearance of pancreatic calcifications and abnormal tests of pancreatic exocrine function. Women are more likely to have small-duct disease, with normal tests of pancreatic exocrine function and normal abdominal radiography. In small-duct disease, the progression to steatorrhea is rare, and the pain is responsive to treatment with pancreatic enzymes. The findings on CT and abdominal radiograph of this patient are characteristic of chronic pancreatitis, and no further workup should delay treatment with pancreatic enzymes. Treatment with pancreatic enzymes orally will improve maldigestion and lead to weight gain, but they are unlikely to fully resolve maldigestive symptoms. Narcotic dependence can frequently develop in individuals with chronic pancreatitis due to recurrent and severe bouts of pain. However, because this individual's pain is mild, it is not necessary to prescribe narcotics at this point in time. An ERCP or magnetic resonance cholangiopancreatography (MRCP) may be considered to evaluate for a possible stricture that is amenable to therapy. However, sphincterotomy is a procedure performed via ERCP that may be useful in treating pain related to chronic pancreatitis and is not indicated in the patient. Angiography to assess for ischemic bowel disease is not indicated because the patient's symptoms are not consistent with intestinal angina. Certainly, weight loss can occur in this setting, but the patient usually presents with complaints of abdominal pain after eating and pain that is out of proportion with the clinical examination. Prokinetic agents would likely only worsen the patient's malabsorptive symptoms and are not indicated.

SECTION IX

Rheumatology and Immunology

QUESTIONS

DIRECTIONS: Choose the one best response to each question.

IX-1. All of the following are key features of the innate immune system EXCEPT:

A. Exclusively a feature of vertebrate animals
B. Important cells include macrophages and natural killer lymphocytes
C. Nonrecognition of benign foreign molecules or microbes
D. Recognition by germline-encoded host molecules
E. Recognition of key microbe virulence factors but no recognition of self-molecules

IX-2. A 29-year-old man with episodic abdominal pain and stress-induced edema of the lips, tongue, and occasionally larynx is likely to have low functional or absolute levels of which of the following proteins?

A. C1 esterase inhibitor
B. C5A (complement cascade)
C. Cyclooxygenase
D. Immunoglobulin (Ig) E
E. T-cell receptor, α chain

IX-3. Which of the following statements best describes the function of proteins encoded by the human major histocompatibility complex (MHC) I and II genes?

A. Activation of the complement system
B. Binding to cell surface receptors on granulocytes and macrophages to initiate phagocytosis
C. Nonspecific binding of antigen for presentation to T cells
D. Specific antigen binding in response to B-cell activation to promote neutralization and precipitation

IX-4. All of the following statements regarding primary immunodeficiency disorders are true EXCEPT:

A. Infections of the upper or lower respiratory tract suggest a defective antibody response.
B. Most are diagnosed by the presence of recurrent or unusually severe infections.
C. Recurrent infections due to *Candida* species suggest impaired T-cell immunity.
D. They are typically genetic diseases with Mendelian inheritance.
E. While most aspects of the immune system may be involved, innate immunity is not affected by these disorders.

IX-5. A 19-year-old college freshman comes to the university clinic complaining of tender, painful skin lesions in his axilla. (See Figure IX-5.) He reports that he has had similar episodes throughout his life for which he receives antibiotics. He has a lab printout from his last episode that reports a positive culture for *Serratia marcescens*. All of the following statements regarding this patient and his likely diagnosis are true EXCEPT:

A. Human stem cell transplantation is curative.
B. Infections with catalase-negative organisms are typical.
C. Prophylactic use of trimethoprim/sulfamethoxazole is effective in reducing risk of bacterial infections.
D. The disease is caused by defective production of reactive oxygen species in phagolysosomes.
E. The disease is most likely transmitted by X-linked recessive inheritance.

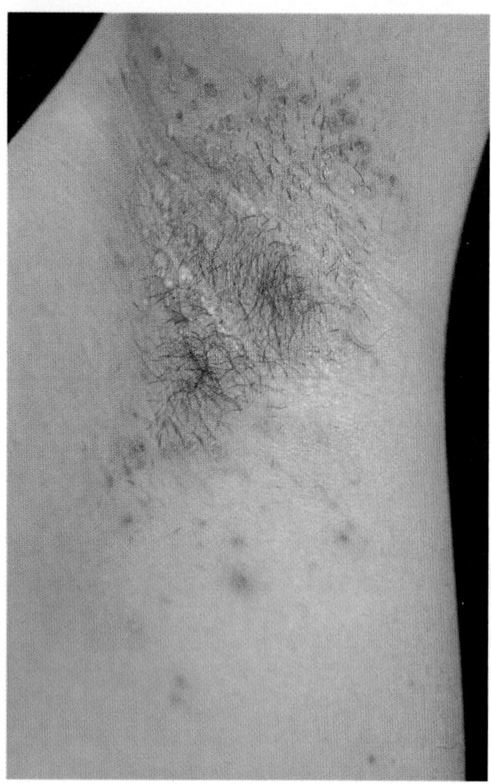

FIGURE IX-5 From Wolff W, Johnson RA, Saavedra AP: *Fitzpatrick's Color Atlas & Synopsis of Clinical Dermatology*, 7th ed. New York, NY: McGraw-Hill, 2013, Fig. 31-25.

IX-6. A 37-year-old man has recently been diagnosed with systemic hypertension. He is prescribed lisinopril as initial monotherapy. He takes this medication as prescribed for 3 days and, on the third day, notes that his right hand is swollen, mildly itching, and tingling. Later that evening, his lips become swollen and he has difficulty breathing. Which of the following statements accurately describes this condition?

A. His symptoms are due to direct activation of mast cells by lisinopril.
B. His symptoms are due to impaired bradykinin degradation by lisinopril.
C. His symptoms are unlikely to recur if he is switched to enalapril.
D. Peripheral blood analysis will show deficiency of C1 inhibitor.
E. Plasma IgE levels are likely to be elevated.

IX-7. A 28-year-old woman seeks evaluation from her primary care doctor for recurrent episodes of hives and states that she is "allergic to cold weather." She reports that for more than 10 years she would develop areas of hives when exposed to cold temperatures, usually on her arms and legs. She has never sought evaluation previously and states that, over the past several years, the occurrence of the hives has become more frequent. Other than cold exposure, she can identify no other triggers for development of hives. She has no history of asthma or atopy. She denies food intolerance. Her only medication is oral contraceptive pills, which she has taken for 5 years. She lives in a single-family home that was built 2 years ago. On examination, she develops a linear wheal after being stroked along her forearm with a tongue depressor. Upon placing her hand in cold water, her hand becomes red and swollen. In addition, there are several areas with a wheal and flare reaction on the arm above the area of cold exposure. What is the next step in the management of this patient?

A. Assess for the presence of antithyroglobulin and antimicrosomal antibodies.
B. Check C1 inhibitor levels.
C. Discontinue the oral contraceptive pills.
D. Treat with cetirizine 10 mg daily.
E. Treat with cyproheptadine 8 mg daily.

IX-8. A 23-year-old woman seeks evaluation for seasonal rhinitis. She reports that she develops symptoms yearly in the spring and fall. During this time, she develops rhinitis with postnasal drip and cough that disrupts her sleep. In addition, she will also note itchy and watery eyes. When the symptoms occur, she takes nonprescription loratadine, 10 mg daily, with significant improvement in her symptoms. What is the most likely allergen(s) causing this patient's symptoms?

A. Grass
B. Ragweed
C. Trees
D. A and B
E. B and C
F. All of the above

IX-9. You are working in the emergency department when a 3-year-old boy arrives by ambulance. He was eating tonight when he suddenly starting wheezing, coughing, and then became progressively less responsive. His parents are certain he did not aspirate. On arrival, his blood pressure is low, and he is working hard to breath. You auscultate a tight wheeze bilaterally. You accurately diagnose him with anaphylaxis and initiate appropriate therapy. Which of the following is true regarding anaphylaxis?

A. An atopic history is a risk factor for anaphylaxis to penicillin therapy.
B. Anaphylaxis most often onsets 1–2 hours after antigen exposure.
C. Older age is associated with improved outcomes in anaphylaxis.
D. The failure to use epinephrine within the first 20 minutes of symptoms is a risk factor for death due to anaphylaxis.
E. Intravenous glucocorticoids are effective for acute anaphylaxis.

IX-10. Rheumatic fever develops due to an autoimmune process. Which of the following mechanisms of autoimmunity is primarily responsible for the development of rheumatic fever?

A. Endocrine abnormalities
B. Increased B-cell function
C. Intrinsic cytokine imbalance
D. Increased T-cell help due to cytokine stimulation
E. Molecular mimicry

IX-11. Which of the following describes the pathophysiologic autoimmune mechanism responsible for Graves disease?

A. Antibody-dependent cellular cytotoxicity
B. Complement-activating autoantibody
C. Inactivating autoantibody
D. Stimulating autoantibody
E. T-cell–mediated cellular cytotoxicity

IX-12. Which of the following autoantibodies is least likely to be present in a patient with systemic lupus erythematosus?

A. Anti-dsDNA
B. Antinuclear antibodies
C. Anti-La (SS-B)
D. Antiphospholipid
E. Antierythrocyte

IX-13. A 23-year-old woman is evaluated by her primary care physician because she is concerned that she may have systemic lupus erythematosus after hearing a public health announcement on the radio. She has no significant past medical history, and her only medication is occasional ibuprofen. She is not sexually active and works in a grocery store. She reports that she has had intermittent oral ulcers and right knee pain. Physical examination shows no evidence of alopecia, skin rash, or joint swelling/inflammation. Her blood work shows that she has a positive antinuclear antibody (ANA) at a titer of 1:40, but no other abnormalities. Which of the following statements is true?

A. Four diagnostic criteria are required to be diagnosed with systemic lupus erythematosus; this patient has three.
B. Four diagnostic criteria are required to be diagnosed with systemic lupus erythematosus; this patient has two.
C. If a urinalysis shows proteinuria, she will meet criteria for systemic lupus erythematosus.
D. She meets criteria for systemic lupus erythematosus because she has three criteria for disease.
E. The demonstration of a positive ANA alone is adequate to diagnose systemic lupus erythematosus.

IX-14. A 32-year-old woman with long-standing diagnosis of systemic lupus erythematosus is evaluated by her rheumatologist as routine follow-up. A new cardiac murmur is heard, and an echocardiogram is ordered. She is feeling well and has no fevers, weight loss, or preexisting cardiac disease. A vegetation on the mitral valve is demonstrated. Which of the following statements is true?

A. Blood cultures are unlikely to be positive.
B. Glucocorticoid therapy has been proven to lead to improvement in this condition.
C. Pericarditis is frequently present concomitantly.
D. The lesion has a low risk of embolization.
E. The patient has been surreptitiously using injection drugs.

IX-15. A 24-year-old woman is newly diagnosed with systemic lupus erythematosus. Which of the following organ system complications is she most likely to have over the course of her lifetime?

A. Cardiopulmonary
B. Cutaneous
C. Hematologic
D. Musculoskeletal
E. Renal

IX-16. A 45-year-old African American woman with systemic lupus erythematosus (SLE) presents to the emergency department with complaints of headache and fatigue. Her prior manifestations of SLE have been arthralgias, hemolytic anemia, malar rash, and mouth ulcers, and she is known to have high titers of antibodies to double-stranded DNA. She currently is taking prednisone, 5 mg daily, and hydroxychloroquine, 200 mg daily. On presentation, she is found to have a blood pressure of 190/110 mmHg with a heart rate of 98 bpm. A urinalysis shows 25 red blood cells (RBCs) per high-power field with 2+ proteinuria. No RBC casts are identified. Her blood urea nitrogen is 88 mg/dL, and creatinine is 2.6 mg/dL (baseline 0.8 mg/dL). She has not previously had renal disease related to SLE and is not taking nonsteroidal anti-inflammatory drugs. She denies any recent illness, decreased oral intake, or diarrhea. What is the most appropriate next step in the management of this patient?

A. Initiate cyclophosphamide, 500 mg/m^2 body surface area intravenously (IV), and plan to repeat monthly for 3–6 months.
B. Initiate hemodialysis.
C. Initiate high-dose steroid therapy (IV methylprednisolone, 1000 mg daily for 3 doses, followed by oral prednisone, 1 mg/kg daily) and mycophenolate mofetil, 2 g daily.
D. Initiate plasmapheresis.
E. Withhold all therapy until renal biopsy is performed.

IX-17. A 27-year-old woman is admitted to the intensive care unit after recent delivery of a full-term infant 3 days prior. The patient was found to have right hemiparesis and a blue left hand. Physical examination is also notable for livedo reticularis. Her laboratories were notable for a white blood cell (WBC) count of 10.2/μL, hematocrit of 35%, and platelet count of 13,000/μL. Her blood urea nitrogen (BUN) is 36 mg/dL, and her creatinine is 2.3 mg/dL. Although this pregnancy was uneventful, the three prior pregnancies resulted in early losses. A peripheral smear shows no evidence of schistocytes. Which of the following laboratory studies will best confirm the underlying etiology of her presentation?

A. Anticardiolipin antibody panel
B. Antinuclear antibody
C. Doppler examination of her left arm arterial tree
D. Echocardiography
E. Magnetic resonance imaging (MRI) of her brain

IX-18. A 28-year-old woman comes to the emergency department complaining of 1 day of worsening right leg pain and swelling. She drove in a car 8 hours back from a hiking trip 2 days ago and then noticed some pain in the leg. At first she thought it was due to exertion, but it has worsened over the day. Her only past medical history is related to difficulty getting pregnant, with two prior spontaneous abortions. Her physical examination is notable for normal vital signs, heart, and lung examination. Her right leg is swollen from the mid-thigh down and is tender. Doppler studies demonstrate a large deep venous thrombosis in the femoral and ileac veins extending into the pelvis. Laboratory studies on admission prior to therapy show normal electrolytes, normal WBC and platelet counts, normal prothrombin time, and an activated partial thromboplastin time 3× normal. Her pregnancy test is negative. Low-molecular-weight heparin therapy is initiated in the emergency department. Subsequent therapy should include which of the following?

A. Rituximab 375 mg/m^2 per week for 4 weeks
B. Warfarin with international normalized ratio (INR) goal of 2.0–3.0 for 3 months
C. Warfarin with INR goal of 2.0–3.0 for 12 months
D. Warfarin with INR goal of 2.5–3.5 for life
E. Warfarin with an INR goal of 2.5–3.5 for 12 months followed by daily aspirin for life

IX-19. Patients with antiphospholipid syndrome will often falsely test positive for which of the following infectious diseases?

A. Malaria
B. Human immunodeficiency virus (HIV)
C. Schistosomiasis
D. Hepatitis C
E. Syphilis

IX-20. Which of the following is the most frequent site of joint involvement in established rheumatoid arthritis?

A. Distal interphalangeal joint
B. Hip
C. Knee
D. Spine
E. Wrist

IX-21. In patients with established rheumatoid arthritis, all of the following pulmonary radiographic findings may be explained by their rheumatologic condition EXCEPT:

A. Bilateral interstitial infiltrates
B. Bronchiectasis
C. Lobar infiltrate
D. Solitary pulmonary nodule
E. Unilateral pleural effusion

IX-22. Which of the following is the earliest plain radiographic finding of rheumatoid arthritis?

A. Juxta-articular osteopenia
B. No abnormality
C. Soft tissue swelling
D. Subchondral erosions
E. Symmetric joint space loss

IX-23. All of the following are characteristic extra-articular manifestations of rheumatoid arthritis EXCEPT:

A. Anemia
B. Cutaneous vasculitis
C. Pericarditis
D. Secondary Sjögren syndrome
E. Thrombocytopenia

IX-24. All of the following agents have been shown to have disease-modifying antirheumatic drug (DMARD) efficacy in patients with rheumatoid arthritis EXCEPT:

A. Infliximab
B. Leflunomide
C. Methotrexate
D. Naproxen
E. Rituximab

IX-25. All of the following are characteristics of Felty syndrome EXCEPT:

A. Neutropenia
B. Nodular rheumatoid arthritis
C. Occurs in the late stages of rheumatoid arthritis
D. Splenomegaly
E. Thrombocytopenia

IX-26. Which of the following malignancies are patients with rheumatoid arthritis specifically at higher risk for?

A. Colon cancer
B. Lung cancer
C. Lymphoma
D. Melanoma
E. Glioblastoma multiforme

IX-27. Which of the following is the most common clinical presentation of acute rheumatic fever?

A. Carditis
B. Chorea
C. Erythema marginatum
D. Polyarthritis
E. Subcutaneous nodules

IX-28. A 19-year-old recent immigrant from Ethiopia comes to your clinic to establish primary care. She currently feels well. Her past medical history is notable for a recent admission to the hospital for new-onset atrial fibrillation. As a child in Ethiopia, she developed an illness that caused uncontrolled flailing of her limbs and tongue lasting approximately 1 month. She also has had three episodes of migratory large-joint arthritis during her adolescence that resolved with pills that she received from the pharmacy. She is currently taking metoprolol and warfarin and has no known drug allergies. Physical examination reveals an irregularly irregular heart beat with normal blood pressure. Her point of maximal impulse (PMI) is most prominent at the midclavicular line and is normal in size. An early diastolic rumble and 3/6 holosystolic murmur are heard at the apex. A soft early diastolic murmur is also heard at the left third intercostal space. You refer her to a cardiologist for evaluation of valve replacement and echocardiography. What other intervention might you consider at this time?

A. Daily aspirin
B. Daily doxycycline
C. Low-dose corticosteroids
D. Monthly penicillin G injections
E. Penicillin G injections as needed for all sore throats

IX-29. Most of the manifestations of acute rheumatic fever present approximately 3 weeks after the precipitating group A streptococcal infection. Which manifestation may present several months after the precipitating infection?

A. Chorea
B. Erythema marginatum
C. Fever
D. Polyarthritis
E. Subcutaneous nodules

IX-30. A patient with a diagnosis of scleroderma who has diffuse cutaneous involvement presents with malignant hypertension, oliguria, edema, hemolytic anemia, and renal failure. You make a diagnosis of scleroderma renal crisis. Which of the following is the recommended treatment?

A. Captopril
B. Carvedilol
C. Clonidine
D. Diltiazem
E. Nitroprusside

IX-31. Which of the following is nearly twice as common in patients with diffuse cutaneous systemic sclerosis than in limited cutaneous systemic sclerosis?

A. Esophageal involvement
B. Pulmonary arterial hypertension
C. Pulmonary fibrosis
D. Raynaud phenomenon
E. Skin involvement

IX-32. Which of the following autoantibodies is typically present in high titers in patients with mixed connective tissue disease?

A. Anti-centromere
B. Anti-La
C. Anti-Ro
D. Anti–Scl-70
E. Anti–U1-RNP

IX-33. A 57-year-old woman with depression and chronic migraine headaches reports several years of dry mouth and dry eyes. Her primary complaint is that she can no longer eat her favorite crackers, although she does report photosensitivity and eye burning on further questioning. She has no other associated symptoms. Examination shows dry, erythematous, sticky oral mucosa. All of the following tests are likely to be positive in this patient EXCEPT:

A. La/SS-B antibody
B. Ro/SS-A antibody
C. Schirmer I test
D. Scl-70 antibody
E. Sialometry

IX-34. A patient with primary Sjögren syndrome that was diagnosed 6 years ago and treated with tear replacement for symptomatic relief notes continued parotid swelling for the last 3 months. She has also noted enlarging posterior cervical lymph nodes. Evaluation shows leukopenia and low C4 complement levels. What is the most likely diagnosis?

A. Amyloidosis
B. Chronic pancreatitis
C. HIV infection
D. Lymphoma
E. Secondary Sjögren syndrome

IX-35. Which of the following is the most common extraglandular manifestation of primary Sjögren syndrome?

A. Arthralgias/arthritis
B. Lymphoma
C. Peripheral neuropathy
D. Raynaud phenomenon
E. Vasculitis

IX-36. A 43-year-old Japanese woman presents to your clinic with 6 months of dry irritated eyes, dry mouth, and cheek swelling. On examination, she has parotic gland enlargement bilaterally. Sialometry is abnormal. Biopsy of the minor salivary glands in the lip shows granulomatous inflammation. Serologies show a negative SS-A and SS-B antibodies. Which of the following is the most likely diagnosis?

A. Systemic sclerosis
B. Sarcoidosis
C. Sjögren syndrome
D. HIV-associated sicca syndrome
E. Eosinophilic granulomatosis with polyangiitis

IX-37. Histocompatibility antigen HLA-B27 is present in what percentage of North American patients with ankylosing spondylitis?

A. 10%
B. 30%
C. 50%
D. 90%
E. 100%

IX-38. Which of the following is the most common extra-articular manifestation of ankylosing spondylitis?

A. Anterior uveitis
B. Aortic insufficiency
C. Inflammatory bower disease
D. Pulmonary fibrosis
E. Third-degree heart block

IX-39. Mr. Charleston is a 25-year-old man seeing his primary care physician for evaluation of low back pain. The pain is severe, worse in the morning, improved with exercise, and worse with rest; in particular, nighttime sleeping is difficult. He does feel quite stiff in the morning for at least 30 minutes. An MRI of his lower back is obtained and shows active inflammation in the sacroiliac joint. On further questioning, he reports a history of unilateral eye redness treated with corticosteroids about 2 years ago. A test for HLA-B27 is positive. Which of the following is first-line therapy for his condition?

A. Infliximab
B. Naproxen
C. Prednisone
D. Rituximab
E. Tramadol

IX-40. Mr. Husten is a 27-year-old man seen at his primary care physician's office for evaluation of painful arthritis involving the right knee associated with diffuse bilateral finger swelling. He is otherwise healthy but does recall a severe bout of diarrheal illness about 3–4 weeks prior that spontaneously resolved. He works as a recreation supervisor at a daycare center and said many of the children had a similar diarrheal illness. He takes no medications and reports rare marijuana use. On review of systems, he reports painful urination. Examination shows inflammatory arthritis of the right knee, dactylitis, and normal genitourinary examination. He is diagnosed with reactive arthritis. Which of the following was the most likely etiologic agent of his diarrhea?

A. *Campylobacter jejuni*
B. *Clostridium difficile*
C. *Escherichia coli*
D. *Helicobacter pylori*
E. *Shigella flexneri*

IX-41. Which of the following statements regarding the arthritis of Whipple disease is true?

A. Arthritis is a rare finding in Whipple disease.
B. Joint manifestations are usually concurrent with gastrointestinal symptoms and malabsorption.
C. Radiography frequently shows joint erosions.
D. Synovial fluid examination is unlikely to show polymorphonuclear cells.
E. None of the above

IX-42. Which of the following definitions best fits the term *enthesitis*?

A. A palpable vibratory or crackling sensation elicited with joint motion
B. Alteration of joint alignment so that articulating surfaces incompletely approximate each other
C. Inflammation at the site of tendinous or ligamentous insertion into bone
D. Inflammation of the periarticular membrane lining the joint capsule
E. Inflammation of a saclike cavity near a joint that decreases friction

IX-43. All of the following help distinguish psoriatic arthritis from other joint disorders EXCEPT:

A. Dactylitis
B. Enthesitis
C. Nail pitting
D. Presence of diarrhea
E. Shortening of digits

IX-44. Which cardiac valvular lesion is most common in patients with ankylosing spondylitis?

A. Aortic regurgitation
B. Mitral regurgitation
C. Mitral stenosis
D. Pulmonic stenosis
E. Tricuspid regurgitation

IX-45. All of the following vasculitic syndromes are thought to be due to immune complex deposition EXCEPT:

A. Cryoglobulinemic vasculitis
B. Granulomatosis with polyangiitis
C. Henoch-Schönlein purpura
D. Polyarteritis nodosa associated with hepatitis B
E. Serum sickness

IX-46. A 40-year-old male presents to the emergency department with 2 days of low-volume hemoptysis. He reports that he has been coughing up 2–5 tablespoons of blood each day. He does report mild chest pain, low-grade fevers, and weight loss. In addition, he has had about 1 year of severe upper respiratory symptoms including frequent epistaxis and purulent discharge treated with several courses of antibiotics. Aside from mild hyperlipidemia, he is otherwise healthy. His only medications are daily aspirin and lovastatin. On physical examination, he has normal vital signs, and upper airway is notable for saddle nose deformity and clear lungs. A computed tomography (CT) of the chest shows multiple cavitating nodules, and urinalysis shows red blood cells. Which of the following tests offers the highest diagnostic yield to make the appropriate diagnosis?

A. Deep skin biopsy
B. Percutaneous kidney biopsy
C. Pulmonary angiogram
D. Surgical lung biopsy
E. Upper airway biopsy

IX-47. An 84-year-old woman is seen by her primary care physician for evaluation of severe headaches. She noted these several weeks ago, and they have been getting worse. Although she has not had any visual aura, she is concerned that she has been intermittently losing vision in her left eye for the last few days. She denies new weakness or numbness, but she does report jaw pain with eating. Her past medical history includes coronary artery disease requiring a bypass grafting 10 years prior, diabetes mellitus, hyperlipidemia, and mild depression. Full review of symptoms is notable for night sweats and mild low back pain particularly prominent in the morning. Which of the following is the next most appropriate step?

A. Aspirin 975 mg orally daily
B. Measurement of erythrocyte sedimentation rate
C. Immediate initiatinon of glucocorticoid
D. Referral for temporal artery biopsy
E. Referral for ultrasound of temporal artery

IX-48. A 54-year-old man is evaluated for cutaneous vasculitis and peripheral nephropathy. Because of concomitant renal dysfunction, he undergoes kidney biopsy that shows glomerulonephritis. Cryoglobulins are demonstrated in the peripheral blood. Which of the following laboratory studies should be sent to determine the etiology?

A. Hepatitis B surface antigen
B. Antineutrophil cytoplasmic antibody (ANCA)
C. Hepatitis C polymerase chain reaction
D. HIV antibody
E. Rheumatoid factor

IX-49. An 18-year-old man is admitted to the hospital with acute onset of crushing substernal chest pain that began abruptly 30 minutes ago. He reports the pain radiating to his neck and right arm. He has otherwise been in good health. He currently plays trumpet in his high school marching band but does not participate regularly in aerobic activities. On physical examination, he is diaphoretic and tachypneic. His blood pressure is 100/48 mmHg and heart rate is 110 bpm. His cardiovascular examination has a regular rhythm but is tachycardic. A 2/6 holosystolic murmur is heard best at the apex and radiates to the axilla. His lungs have bilateral rales at the bases. The electrocardiogram demonstrates 4 mm of ST elevation in the anterior leads. On further questioning regarding his past medical history, he recalls having been told that he was hospitalized for some problem with his heart when he was 2 years old. His mother, who accompanies him, reports that he received aspirin and γ-globulin as treatment. Since that time, he has required intermittent follow-up with echocardiography. What is the most likely cause of this patient's acute coronary syndrome?

A. Dissection of the aortic root and left coronary ostia
B. Presence of a myocardial bridge overlying the left anterior descending artery
C. Thrombosis of a coronary artery aneurysm
D. Vasospasm following cocaine ingestion
E. Vasculitis involving the left anterior descending artery

IX-50. You are seeing in follow-up a 46-year-old man who, 6 months ago, presented to the hospital acutely with hemoptysis, diffuse nodular pulmonary infiltrates, and glomerulonephritis. Workup revealed a positive serologic study for antibodies against cytoplasmic ANCA, and he was eventually diagnosed with granulomatosis with polyangiitis. Treatment was initiated with high-dose glucocorticoids and daily cyclophosphamide with excellent clinical response. You are ready today to have the patient transition from induction therapy with cyclophosphamide to maintenance therapy with azathioprine. What blood test should you check before starting azathioprine?

A. ANCA titers
B. Cryoglobulins
C. CYP3A4 genotyping
D. Glucose-6-phosphate dehydrogenase enzyme levels
E. Thiopurine methyltransferase enzyme activity

IX-51. All of the following vascular beds are typically affected by polyarteritis nodosa EXCEPT:

A. Cerebral arteries
B. Coronary arteries
C. Pulmonary arteries
D. Renal arteries
E. Splanchnic arteries

IX-52. Lung biopsy has the greatest diagnostic yield in which of the following vasculitic syndromes?

A. Cryoglobulinemic vasculitis
B. Cutaneous vasculitis
C. Granulomatosis with polyangiitis (Wegener)
D. IgA vasculitis (Henoch-Schönlein)
E. Polyarteritis nodosa

IX-53. In a patient with suspected granulomatosis with polyangiitis (Wegener), which of the following lung radiologic findings is least likely?

A. Bronchiectasis
B. Endobronchial stenosis
C. Multiple cavitating nodules
D. Nodular infiltrates
E. Solitary cavitating nodule

IX-54. Which of the following is required for the diagnosis of Behçet disease?

A. Large-vessel vasculitis
B. Pathergy test
C. Recurrent oral ulceration
D. Recurrent genital ulceration
E. Uveitis

IX-55. A 25-year-old woman presents with a complaint of painful mouth ulcerations. She describes these lesions as shallow ulcers that last for 1 or 2 weeks. The ulcers have been appearing for the last 6 months. For the last 2 days, the patient has had a painful red eye. She has had no genital ulcerations, arthritis, skin rashes, or photosensitivity. On physical examination, the patient appears well developed and in no distress. She has a temperature of 37.6°C (99.7°F), heart rate of 86 bpm, blood pressure of 126/72 mmHg, and respiratory rate of 16 breaths/min. Examination of the oral mucosa reveals two shallow ulcers with a yellow base on the buccal mucosa. The ophthalmologic examination is consistent with anterior uveitis. The cardiopulmonary examination is normal. She has no arthritis, but medially on the right thigh, there is a palpable cord in the saphenous vein. Laboratory studies reveal an erythrocyte sedimentation rate of 68 seconds. WBC count is 10,230/μL with a differential of 68% polymorphonuclear cells, 28% lymphocytes, and 4% monocytes. The antinuclear antibody and anti-dsDNA antibody are negative. C3 is 89 mg/dL, and C4 is 24 mg/dL. What is the most likely diagnosis?

A. Behçet syndrome
B. Bullous pemphigoid
C. Discoid lupus erythematosus
D. Sjögren syndrome
E. Systemic lupus erythematosus

IX-56. All of the following are known complications of Behçet syndrome EXCEPT:

A. Arterial thrombosis
B. Central nervous system involvement
C. Deep vein thrombosis
D. Pulmonary artery vasculitis
E. All of the above are known complications of Behçet's syndrome.

IX-57. An elevation in which of the following serum enzymes is the most *sensitive* indicator of myositis?

A. Aldolase
B. Creatinine kinase
C. Glutamic-oxaloacetic transaminase
D. Glutamate pyruvate transaminase
E. Lactate dehydrogenase

IX-58. A 64-year-old woman is evaluated for weakness. She has had several weeks of difficulty brushing her teeth and combing her hair. She has also noted a rash on her face. Examination is notable for a heliotrope rash and proximal muscle weakness. Serum creatinine kinase (CK) is elevated, and she is diagnosed with dermatomyositis. After evaluation by a rheumatologist, she is found to have anti-Jo-1 antibodies. She is also likely to have which of the following findings?

A. Ankylosing spondylitis
B. Inflammatory bowel disease
C. Interstitial lung disease
D. Primary biliary cirrhosis
E. Psoriasis

IX-59. A 63-year-old woman is evaluated for a rash on her eyes and fatigue for 1 month. She reports difficulty with arm and leg strength and constant fatigue, but no fevers or sweats. She also has noted that she has a red discoloration around her eyes. She has hypothyroidism but is otherwise well. On examination, she has a heliotrope rash and proximal muscle weakness. A diagnosis of dermatomyositis is made after demonstration of elevated serum creatinine kinase and confirmatory electromyograms. Which of the following studies should be performed as well to look for associated conditions?

A. Mammogram
B. Serum antinuclear antibody measurement
C. Stool examination for ova and parasites
D. Thyroid-stimulating immunoglobulins
E. Titers of antibodies to varicella-zoster

IX-60. You are seeing Mr. Blumenthal today, who has been your long-term patient. He has a history of coronary artery disease, suffering a lateral myocardial infarction 1 year ago. At that time, he was started on simvastatin, aspirin, metoprolol, and lisinopril. About 2 months ago, he started noting thigh and shoulder soreness. One month after onset, his muscle pain had increased and he was noticing weakness. His CK was elevated to 8× the upper limit of normal. His simvastatin was discontinued 3 weeks ago. Today, he reports that his pain has continued and, if anything, is worse than a month ago. His CK is 12× the upper limit of normal. What is the next best test to establish a diagnosis?

A. Antibody against 3-hydroxy-3-methylglutaryl–coenzyme A reductase (HMGCR)
B. Antinuclear antibody (ANA)
C. Anti-Jo-1 antibody
D. Antibody against signal recognition particle (SRP)
E. Aldolase levels

IX-61. A 47-year-old man is evaluated for 1 year of recurrent episodes of bilateral ear swelling. The ear is painful during these events, and the right ear has become floppy. He is otherwise healthy and reports no illicit habits. He works in an office, and his only sport is tennis. On examination, the left ear has a beefy red color and the pinna is tender and swollen; the earlobe appears minimally swollen but is neither red nor tender. Which of the following is the most likely explanation for this finding?

A. Behçet syndrome
B. Cogan syndrome
C. Hemoglobinopathy
D. Recurrent trauma
E. Relapsing polychondritis

IX-62. All of the following have been implicated in the proposed pathogenesis of sarcoidosis EXCEPT:

A. Exposure to mold
B. Genetic susceptibility
C. Immune response to mycobacterial proteins
D. Infection with *Propionibacterium acnes*
E. Malignant expansion of helper T cells

IX-63. Which of the following statements regarding pulmonary sarcoidosis is true?

A. Lung involvement is the second most common manifestation of sarcoidosis, behind only cutaneous involvement.
B. Obstructive disease is a rare manifestation of pulmonary sarcoidosis.
C. Pulmonary hypertension never responds to therapy in sarcoidosis patients.
D. Pulmonary infiltrates in sarcoidosis tend to be predominantly an upper lobe process.
E. The presence of cough should prompt evaluation for a cause other than pulmonary sarcoidosis.

IX-64. You are seeing Mr. Blanko, a 55-year-old white man with a history of sarcoidosis. He ran out of prednisone about 2 months prior to seeing you and, except for some constipation, feels well. A metabolic panel reveals a calcium of 12.2 mg/dL (normal up to 10.5 mg/dL). You know that sarcoidosis can be associated with hypercalcemia. Which of the following is the correct mechanism for sarcoidosis-associated hypercalcemia?

A. Direct granulomatous involvement of the axial skeleton causing calcium release from bones
B. Direct stimulation of increased intestinal calcium absorption
C. Increased parathyroid hormone production
D. Increased production of 1,25-dihydroxyvitamin D
E. Increased production of 25-hydroxyvitamin D

IX-65. In which population is cardiac sarcoidosis most common?

A. African American
B. East European
C. Japanese
D. South American
E. Australian

IX-66. Which of the following is a potential cardiac manifestation of sarcoidosis?

A. Dilated cardiomyopathy
B. Heart block
C. Valvular stenosis
D. Ventricular tachyarrhythmias
E. All of the above

IX-67. You are rounding on Mr. Spareti today. He is a 34-year-old man who presented to you with unexplained pancreatitis 2 weeks ago. Imaging of his pancreas showed diffuse pancreatic enlargement. He denies any alcohol intake and did not have any gallstones on imaging. Interestingly, on examination, he also has marked lacrimal gland and submandibular gland enlargement. Biopsy of his submandibular gland is pictured in Figure IX-67. The cells pictured in the figure stained strongly positive for IgG4, CD19, and CD138. Which of the following is the appropriate therapy?

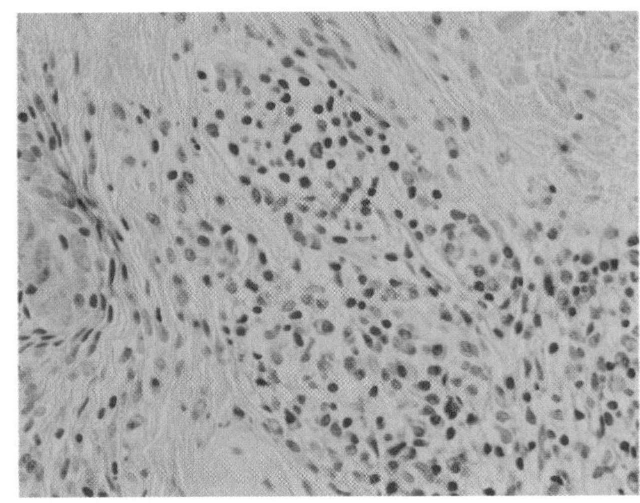

FIGURE IX-67

A. Thalidomide and dexamethasone
B. Cytomegalovirus (CMV) immunoglobulin and ganciclovir
C. Systemic chemotherapy
D. Prednisone
E. Anakinra

IX-68. You are seeing a 19-year-old woman today in consultation for recurrent fevers. She reports several years of fevers, occurring on average every 2–3 months. These episodes are unpredictable, although she thinks they may occur in times of psychological stress. Each febrile episode lasts 2–3 days. She also has recurrent episodes of abdominal pain. Repeated blood cultures have been negative, even during acute febrile episodes. Similarly, abdominal CT scans have shown no obvious etiology for her pain. During one episode, she underwent an exploratory laparotomy, which showed peritoneal adhesions and a sterile neutrophilic peritoneal exudate. She also notes that when she exercises, she develops intense muscle pains that last for days. An extensive serologic search for autoantibodies returned negative, including antinuclear antibodies. Which of the following is the most likely diagnosis?

A. Familial Mediterranean fever
B. Lymphoma
C. Relapsing fever
D. Subacute bacterial endocarditis
E. Systemic lupus erythematosus

IX-69. You are seeing a 19-year-old woman whom you just diagnosed with familial Mediterranean fever. Which of the following medications would you prescribe to reduce attacks and help prevent the development of systemic amyloidosis?

A. Colchicine
B. Cyclosporine
C. Diflunisal
D. Prednisone
E. Thalidomide

IX-70. Which of the following joints is often spared by osteoarthritis?

A. Cervical spine
B. Distal interphalangeal joint
C. Hip
D. Proximal interphalangeal joint
E. Wrist

IX-71. Which of the following statements regarding osteoarthritis is true?

A. During the diagnostic workup of a suspected osteoarthritic joint, MRI is warranted to evaluate for any other causes.
B. Loss of cartilage causes pain due to direct stimulation of pain receptors in joint cartilage itself.
C. Osteoarthritis is the second most common cause of arthritis, behind rheumatoid arthritis.
D. Synovial fluid white blood cell count is usually <1000 cells/μL in osteoarthritis.
E. The severity of radiographic changes in osteoarthritis correlates well with symptoms.

IX-72. You are seeing Mrs. Hudson today, a 60-year-old obese woman with bilateral knee osteoarthritis. Mrs. Hudson describes pain most days and limiting pain at least 2 days per week. She has tried activity modification (walking less) without success. All of the following therapies have been shown to be efficacious in treating osteoarthritis symptoms EXCEPT:

A. Acetaminophen
B. Glucocorticoid steroid intra-articular injections
C. Glucosamine-chondroitin
D. Naproxen
E. Total joint arthroplasty

IX-73. You are seeing Mr. Hinsley, a 72-year-old man with only a history of hypertension on hydrochlorothiazide. He presents today with acute, excruciating knee pain. On examination, his knee is warm, mildly erythematous, swollen, and tender to the touch or passive movement. Microscopic examination of joint fluid is shown in Figure IX-73A. What is Mr. Hinsley's most likely metabolic derangement?

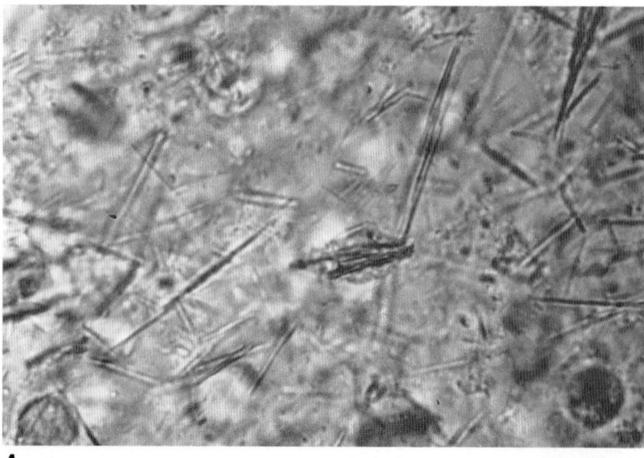

FIGURE IX-73A

A. Acute bacterial joint infection
B. Antibodies to antinuclear antigens
C. Hyaline cartilage degeneration
D. Increased production of inorganic pyrophosphate
E. Uric acid overproduction

IX-74. You are planning on starting allopurinol for Ms. Maggy for a new diagnosis of gouty arthritis. Which of the following best describes appropriate dosing strategies for allopurinol?

A. Allopurinol and azathioprine are commonly used together in the treatment of gout.
B. Allopurinol dosing should be adjusted for liver function.
C. Allopurinol dosing should be titrated to achieve a serum uric acid level <6 mg/dL.
D. Allopurinol should be avoided when patients are taking colchicine.
E. Allopurinol toxicity is more common in patients expressing HLA-B27.

IX-75. A 42-year-old woman is seen in her primary care doctor's office complaining of diffuse pains and fatigue. She has a difficult time localizing the pain to any particular joint or location, but reports it affects her upper and lower extremities, neck, and hips. It is described as achy and 10 out of 10 in intensity. She feels that her joints are stiff but does not notice that it is worse in the morning. The pain has been present for the past 6 months and is increasing in intensity. She has tried both over-the-counter ibuprofen and acetaminophen without significant relief. The patient feels as if the pain is interfering with her ability to get restful sleep and is making it difficult for her to concentrate. She has missed multiple days of work as a waitress and fears that she will lose her job. There is a medical history of depression and obesity. The patient currently is taking venlafaxine sustained release 150 mg daily. She has a family history of rheumatoid arthritis in her mother. She smokes one pack of cigarettes daily. On physical examination, vital signs are normal. Body mass index is 36 kg/m^2. Joint examination demonstrates no erythema, swelling, or effusions. There is diffuse pain with palpation at the insertion points of the suboccipital muscles, at the midpoint of the upper border of the trapezius muscle, along the second costochondral junction, at the lateral epicondyles, and along the medial fat pad of the knees. All of the following statements regarding the cause of this patient's diffuse pain syndrome are true EXCEPT:

A. Cognitive dysfunction, sleep disturbance, anxiety, and depression are common comorbid neuropsychological conditions.
B. Pain in this syndrome is associated with increased evoked pain sensitivity.
C. Pain in this syndrome is often localized to specific joints.
D. This syndrome is present in 2%–5% of the general population, but increases in prevalence to 20% or more of patients with degenerative or inflammatory rheumatic disorders.
E. Women are nine times more likely than men to be affected by this syndrome.

IX-76. A 36-year-old woman presents to your office with diffuse pain throughout her body associated with fatigue, insomnia, and difficulty concentrating. She finds the pain difficult to localize but reports that it is 7–8 out of 10 in intensity and not relieved by nonsteroidal anti-inflammatory medications. She has a long-standing history of generalized anxiety disorder and is treated with sertraline 100 mg daily as well as clonazepam 1 mg twice daily. On examination, she has pain with palpation at several musculoskeletal sites. Her laboratory examination demonstrates a normal complete blood count, basic metabolic panel, erythrocyte sedimentation rate, and rheumatoid factor. You diagnose her with fibromyalgia. All of the following therapies are recommended as part of the treatment plan for fibromyalgia EXCEPT:

A. An exercise program that includes strength training, aerobic exercise, and yoga
B. Cognitive-behavioral therapy for insomnia
C. Milnacipran
D. Oxycodone
E. Pregabalin

IX-77. A 53-year-old woman presents to your clinic complaining of fatigue and generalized pain that have worsened over 2 years. She also describes irritability and poor sleep and is concerned that she is depressed. She reveals that she was recently separated from her husband and has been stressed at work. Which of the following elements in her history and physical examination would meet American College of Rheumatology criteria for diagnosis of fibromyalgia?

A. Diffuse chronic pain and abnormal sleep
B. Diffuse pain without other etiology and evidence of major depression
C. Major depression, life stressor, chronic pain, and female sex
D. Major depression and pain on palpation at 6 of 18 tender point sites
E. Widespread chronic pain and pain on palpation at 11 of 18 tender point sites

IX-78. A 42-year-old man is found to have the following finding on a physical examination (Figure IX-78). All of the following conditions are associated with this finding EXCEPT:

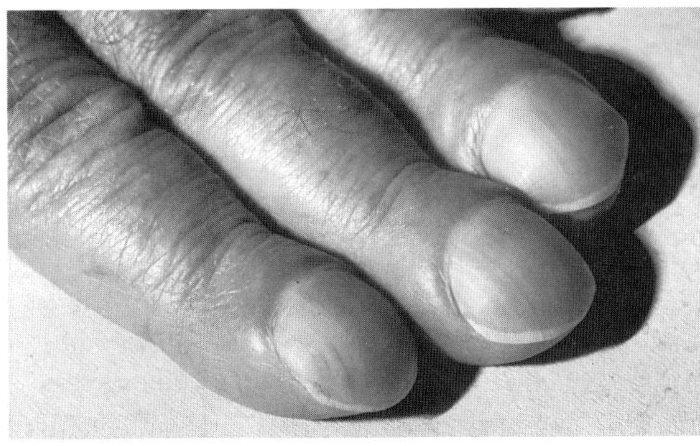

FIGURE IX-78 Reprinted from the Clinical Slide Collection on the Rheumatic Diseases, © 1991, 1995. Used by permission of the American College of Rheumatology.

A. Chronic obstructive pulmonary disease
B. Cyanotic congenital heart disease
C. Cystic fibrosis
D. Hepatocellular carcinoma
E. Hyperthyroidism

IX-79. A 52-year-old man presented to his primary care physician complaining of new-onset pain in the knuckles of his index and middle fingers of both hands. On examination, the second and third metacarpophalangeal (MCP) joints of both hands are swollen and tender. The rest of his physical examination is normal. His past medical history is only notable for hyperlipidemia controlled with atorvastatin. His laboratory studies are notable for an elevated ferritin, and after demonstration of a mutation of the *HFE* gene, he is diagnosed with hemochromatosis. Which of the following statements regarding his joint abnormalities is true?

A. The second and third finger MCPs are also typically involved in osteoarthritis.
B. Arthropathy is unlikely related to hemochromatosis.
C. Arthropathy may progress with phlebotomy.
D. Arthropathy occurs in less than 20% of patients with hemochromatosis.
E. Radiographs are likely to show erosions in the MCPs.

IX-80. A 64-year-old woman is seen by her primary care physician complaining of hip pain for about 1 week. She localizes the pain to the lateral aspect of her right hip and describes it as sharp. It is worse with movement, and she finds it difficult to lie on her right side. The pain began soon after the patient was planting her garden. She has a medical history of obesity, osteoarthritis of the knees, and hypertension. Her medications include losartan 50 mg daily and hydrochlorothiazide 25 mg daily. For the pain, she has taken ibuprofen 600 mg as needed with mild to moderate relief of pain. On physical examination, the patient is not febrile and her vital signs are unremarkable. On examination of the hip, pain is elicited with external rotation and resisted abduction of the hip. Direct palpation over the lateral aspect of the upper portion of the femur near the hip joint reproduces the pain. What is the most likely diagnosis in this patient?

A. Avascular necrosis of the hip
B. Iliotibial band syndrome
C. Meralgia paresthetica
D. Septic arthritis
E. Trochanteric bursitis

IX-81. A 32-year-old woman is seen in clinic with a complaint of left knee pain. She enjoys running long distances and is currently training for a marathon. She is running on average 30–40 miles weekly. She currently is experiencing an aching pain on the lateral aspect of her left knee. There is a burning sensation that also continues up the lateral aspect of her thigh. She denies any injury to her knee, and she has not felt that it was hot or swollen. She is otherwise healthy and takes no medications other than herbal supplements. Physical examination of the knee reveals point tenderness over the lateral femoral condyle that is worse with flexing the knee. The patient is asked to lie on her right side with her right knee and hip flexed at 90 degrees. Her left leg is extended at the hip and slowly lowered into adduction behind the bottom leg, reproducing the patient's left knee pain. All of the following treatments can be recommended for this patient EXCEPT:

A. Assessment of the patient's running shoes to ensure a proper fit
B. Glucocorticoid injection so as not to interfere with the patient's continued preparation for the upcoming marathon
C. Ibuprofen 600–800 mg every 6 hours as needed for pain
D. Referral for physical therapy
E. Referral for surgical release if conservative therapy fails

IX-82. A 58-year-old woman presents complaining of right shoulder pain. She does not recall any prior injury but notes that she feels that the shoulder has been getting progressively more stiff over the last several months. She previously had several episodes of bursitis of the right shoulder that were treated successfully with nonsteroidal anti-inflammatory drugs and steroid injections. The patient's past medical history is also significant for diabetes mellitus, for which she takes metformin and glyburide. On physical examination, the right shoulder is not warm or red but is tender to touch. Passive and active range of motion are limited in flexion, extension, and abduction. A right shoulder radiogram shows osteopenia without evidence of joint erosion or osteophytes. What is the most likely diagnosis?

A. Adhesive capsulitis
B. Avascular necrosis
C. Bicipital tendinitis
D. Osteoarthritis
E. Rotator cuff tear

IX-83. A 32-year-old woman presents to clinic with right thumb and wrist pain that has worsened over several weeks. She has pain when she pinches her thumb against her other fingers. Her only other history is that she is a new mother with an 8-week-old infant at home. On physical examination, she has mild swelling and tenderness over the radial styloid process, and pain is elicited when she places her thumb in her palm and grasps it with her fingers. A Phalen maneuver is negative. Which condition is most likely?

A. Carpal tunnel syndrome
B. De Quervain tenosynovitis
C. Gouty arthritis of the first metacarpophalangeal joint
D. Palmar fasciitis
E. Rheumatoid arthritis

IX-84. You are evaluating Ms. Rumpulo, a 42-year-old woman who complains of pain on the underside of her right heel that is excruciating in the morning when she first walks from bed to the bathroom. The pain improves somewhat during the morning but again worsens mid-day particularly when climbing stairs. She has a past medical history of hypertension, smokes one pack per day of cigarettes, and works as a waitress at a diner. Medications include hydrochlorothiazide and oral contraceptives. Physical examination is unremarkable except for flat feet and focal tenderness on the bottom of the right heel. There is no tenderness at the ankle or calf, and the diameters of the lower legs are equivalent. A radiograph of the right heel and ankle shows only heel spurs. All of the following statements regarding Ms. Rumpulo's condition are true EXCEPT:

A. Heel spurs are not diagnostic.
B. Local glucocorticoid injection incurs a risk of plantar facial rupture.
C. Oral contraceptives and smoking are risk factors.
D. Orthotic shoe implants may be beneficial.
E. The prognosis for improvement is good.

ANSWERS

IX-1. The answer is A. *(Chap. 372e)* The innate immune system is phylogenetically the oldest form of immunologic defense system, inherited from invertebrates. This defense system uses germline-encoded proteins to recognize pathogen-associated molecular patterns. Cells of the innate immune system include macrophages, dendritic cells, and natural killer lymphocytes. The critical components of the innate immune system include recognition by germline-encoded host molecules and recognition of key microbe virulence factors, but no recognition of self-molecules and of benign foreign molecules or microbes. Adaptive immunity is found only in vertebrate animals and is based on generation of antigen receptors on T and B lymphocytes by gene rearrangements, such that individual T or B cells express unique antigen receptors on their surface capable of recognizing diverse environmental antigens.

IX-2. The answer is A. *(Chap. 372e)* Complement activity, which results from the sequential interaction of a large number of plasma and cell membrane proteins, plays an important role in the inflammatory response. The classic pathway of complement activation is initiated by an antibody-antigen interaction. The first complement component (C1, a complex composed of three proteins) binds to immune complexes with activation mediated by C1q. Active C1 then initiates the cleavage and concomitant activation of components C4 and C2. The activated C1 is destroyed by a plasma protease inhibitor termed *C1 esterase inhibitor*. This molecule also regulates clotting factor XI and kallikrein. Patients with a deficiency of C1 esterase inhibitor may develop angioedema, sometimes leading to death by asphyxia. Attacks may be precipitated by stress or trauma. In addition to low antigenic or functional levels of C1 esterase inhibitor, patients with this autosomal dominant condition may have normal levels of C1 and C3 but low levels of C4 and C2. Danazol therapy produces a striking increase in the level of this important inhibitor and alleviates the symptoms in many patients. An acquired form of angioedema caused by a deficiency of C1 esterase inhibitor has been described in patients with autoimmune or malignant disease.

IX-3. The answer is C. *(Chap. 373e)* The human major histocompatibility complex (MHC) genes are located on a 4-megabase region on chromosome 6. The major function of the MHC complex genes is to produce proteins that are important in developing immunologic specificity through their role in binding antigen for presentation to T cells. This process is nonspecific, and the ability of a human leukocyte antigen (HLA) molecule to bind to a particular protein depends on the molecular fit between the amino acid sequence of a particular protein and the corresponding domain on the MHC molecule. Once a peptide has bound, the MHC-peptide complex binds to the T-cell receptor, after which the T cell must determine if an immune response should be generated. If an antigen is similar to an endogenous protein, the potential antigen will be recognized as a self-peptide, and tolerance to the antigen will be continued. The MHC I and II complexes have been implicated in the development of many autoimmune diseases, which occur when T cells fail to recognize a peptide as a self-peptide and an immune response is allowed to develop. MHC I and II genes also play a major role in tissue compatibility for transplantation and are important in generating immune-mediated rejection. The other options listed as answers refer to functions of immunoglobulins. The variable region of the immunoglobulin is a B-cell–specific response to an antigen to promote neutralization of the antigen through agglutination and precipitation. The constant region of the immunoglobulin is able to nonspecifically activate the immune system through complement activation and promotion of phagocytosis by neutrophils and macrophages.

IX-4. The answer is E. *(Chap. 374)* Hundreds of gene products have been characterized as effectors or mediators of the immune system *(Chap. 372e)*. Whenever the expression or function of one of these products is genetically impaired (provided the function is nonredundant), a primary immunodeficiency (PID) occurs. PIDs are genetic diseases with primarily Mendelian inheritance. More than 250 conditions have now been described, and deleterious mutations in approximately 210 genes have been identified. The overall prevalence of PIDs has been estimated in various countries at 5 per 100,000 individuals; however, given the difficulty in diagnosing these rare and complex diseases, this figure is probably an underestimate. PIDs can involve all possible aspects of immune responses, from innate through adaptive, cell differentiation, and effector function and regulation. For the sake of clarity, PIDs should be classified (see Table IX-4) according to (1) the arm of the immune system that is defective and (2) the mechanism of the defect (when known). The consequences of PIDs vary widely as a function of the molecules that are defective. This concept translates into multiple levels of vulnerability to infection by pathogenic and opportunistic microorganisms, ranging from extremely broad (as in severe combined immunodeficiency [SCID]) to narrowly restricted to a single microorganism (as in Mendelian susceptibility to mycobacterial disease [MSMD]). The locations of the sites of infection and the causal microorganisms involved will thus help physicians arrive at proper diagnoses. PIDs can also lead to immunopathologic responses such as allergy (as in Wiskott-Aldrich syndrome), lymphoproliferation, and autoimmunity. A combination of recurrent infections, inflammation, and autoimmunity can be observed in a number of PIDs, thus creating obvious therapeutic challenges. The most frequent symptom prompting the

TABLE IX-4 Classification of Primary Immune Deficiency Diseases

Deficiencies of the Innate Immune System	
• Phagocytic cells:	
- Impaired production: severe congenital neutropenia (SCN)	
- Asplenia	
- Impaired adhesion: leukocyte adhesion deficiency (LAD)	
- Impaired killing: chronic granulomatous disease (CGD)	
• Innate immunity receptors and signal transduction:	
- Defects in Toll-like receptor signaling	
- Mendelian susceptibility to mycobacterial disease	
• Complement deficiencies:	
- Classical, alternative, and lectin pathways	
- Lytic phase	
Deficiencies of the Adaptive Immune System	
• T lymphocytes:	
- Impaired development	Severe combined immune deficiencies (SCIDs)
- Impaired survival, migration, function	DiGeorge syndrome Combined immunodeficiencies Hyper-IgE syndrome (autosomal dominant) DOCK8 deficiency CD40 ligand deficiency Wiskott-Aldrich syndrome Ataxia-telangiectasia and other DNA repair deficiencies
• B lymphocytes:	
- Impaired development	XL and AR agammaglobulinemia
- Impaired function	Hyper-IgM syndrome Common variable immunodeficiency (CVID) IgA deficiency
Regulatory Defects	
• Innate immunity	Autoinflammatory syndromes (outside the scope of this chapter) Severe colitis
• Adaptive immunity	Hemophagocytic lymphohistiocytosis (HLH) Autoimmune lymphoproliferation syndrome (ALPS) Autoimmunity and inflammatory diseases (IPEX, APECED)

Abbreviations: APECED, autoimmune polyendocrinopathy candidiasis ectodermal dysplasia; AR, autosomal recessive; IPEX, immunodysregulation polyendocrinopathy enteropathy X-linked syndrome; XL, X-linked.

diagnosis of a PID is the presence of recurrent or unusually severe infections. Infections of the respiratory tract (bronchi, sinuses) mostly suggest a defective antibody response. In general, invasive bacterial infections can result from complement deficiencies, signaling defects of innate immune responses, asplenia, or defective antibody responses. Viral infections, recurrent *Candida* infections, and opportunistic infections are generally suggestive of impaired T-cell immunity. Skin infections and deep-seated abscesses primarily reflect innate immune defects (such as chronic granulomatous disease); however, they may also appear in the autosomal dominant hyper-immunoglobulin E (IgE) syndrome. Finally, some PIDs increase the risk of cancer, notably but not exclusively lymphocytic cancers (e.g., lymphoma).

IX-5. **The answer is B.** *(Chap. 374)* This patient has axillary folliculitis, an infection of the hair follicles. Based on his history, including recurrent infections with the catalase-positive organism *Serratia marcescens*, he most likely has chronic granulomatous disease (CGD). CGDs are characterized by impaired phagocytic killing of microorganisms by neutrophils and macrophages. About 70% of cases are associated with X-linked recessive inheritance versus autosomal inheritance in the remaining 30%. CGD causes deep tissue bacterial and fungal abscesses in macrophage-rich organs such as the skin, lymph nodes, liver, and lungs. Recurrent skin infections, such as folliculitis, are common and can prompt an early diagnosis of CGD. The infectious agents are typically catalase-positive bacteria (such as *Staphylococcus aureus* and *Serratia marcescens*) but also include *Burkholderia cepacia*, pathogenic mycobacteria (in certain regions of the world), and fungi (mainly filamentous molds, such as *Aspergillus*). CGD is caused by defective production of reactive oxygen species (ROS) in the phagolysosome membrane following phagocytosis of microorganisms. Diagnosis of CGD is based on assays of ROS production in neutrophils and monocytes such as the dihydrorhodamine (DHR) fluorescence or nitroblue tetrazolium (NBT) assays. CGD is a granulomatous disease with macrophage-rich granulomas in the liver, spleen, and other organs. These are sterile granulomas that cause disease by obstruction (bladder, pylorus, etc.) or inflammation (colitis, restrictive lung disease). The treatment of bacterial infections is generally based on combination therapy with antibiotics that are able to penetrate into cells. The treatment of fungal infections requires aggressive, long-term use of antifungals. Inflammatory/granulomatous lesions are usually steroid sensitive; however, glucocorticoids often contribute to the spread of infections. The treatment of CGD mostly relies on preventing infections. It has been unambiguously demonstrated that prophylactic usage of trimethoprim/sulfamethoxazole is both well tolerated and highly effective in reducing the risk of bacterial infection. Daily administration of azole derivatives (notably itraconazole) also reduces the frequency of fungal complications. Human stem cell transplantation is an established curative approach for CGD; however, the risk-benefit ratio must be carefully assessed on a case-by-case basis. Gene therapy approaches are also being evaluated.

IX-6. **The answer is B.** *(Chap. 376)* The patient has classic symptoms of angioedema with rapid onset of facial swelling often involving the lips, frequently with preceding limb symptoms. Angioedema and urticaria are grouped by the underlying etiology. In this case, angiotensin-converting enzyme (ACE) inhibitor use is associated with increased levels of bradykinin, which in a predisposed individual can result in angioedema. Hereditary angioedema is associated with chronically depressed levels of C1 inhibitor, which is involved in the degradation of bradykinin. IgE-mediated angioedema occurs due to specific antigen sensitivity, and complement-mediated disease may be due to vasculitis, serum sickness, or reactions to blood products. Finally, nonimmunologic causes of angioedema include direct mast cell–releasing agents such as opiates and agents that alter arachidonic acid metabolism, most commonly nonsteroidal anti-inflammatory drugs (NSAIDs). IgE levels are not elevated in bradykinin-mediated angioedema. Because of the potentially life-threatening nature of disease, rechallenge with a second ACE inhibitor is not 1recommended.

IX-7. **The answer is D.** *(Chap. 376)* This patient presents with symptoms of cold urticaria, an IgE-dependent urticarial reaction to cold exposure. After exposure to cold, urticarial lesions appear in exposed areas and usually last for <2 hours. Histologic examination of the urticarial lesion would demonstrate mast cell degranulation with edema of the dermis and subcutaneous tissues. In experimental exposure to a cold challenge such as an ice water bath, elevated levels of histamine in venous blood may be demonstrated if assessed in the extremity exposed to a cold environment, whereas the histamine levels would be normal in a nonexposed extremity. The appearance of a linear wheal after a firm stroke is indicative of dermatographism. This condition can be seen in 1%–4% of the population and is often found in individuals with cold urticaria. In general, cold urticaria is a localized process without adverse consequences. However, vascular collapse may occur if an individual is submerged in cold water. Many individuals request treatment because they are embarrassed by their condition or are symptomatic from the recurrent urticaria and pruritus. Treatment with H_1 histamine receptor blockers is usually adequate for symptom control. Cyproheptadine or hydroxyzine can be added to therapy if H_1 antihistamines are inadequate. In this patient, there is a clear precipitant for developing urticaria—cold exposure. Thus, no other evaluation is necessary. In the evaluation and management of chronic urticaria, identification and elimination of precipitating factors are important. Possible etiologic factors include foods, pollens, molds, and medications. In this case, the urticaria predates the use of oral contraceptive medications; thus, stopping oral contraceptives would be unlikely to be helpful. Assessment of antithyroglobulin and antimicrosomal antibodies can be helpful in individuals with chronic urticaria in whom a cause is not otherwise identified. Deficiency of C1 or the presence of a C1 inhibitor presents as recurrent angioedema rather than urticaria.

IX-8. **The answer is E.** *(Chap. 376)* Allergic rhinitis is a common problem in the United States and North America. It is estimated that approximately one in five individuals experiences allergic rhinitis. The incidence is greatest in childhood and adolescence, and the symptoms tend to regress with aging. Complete remissions, however, are uncommon. Many individuals experience seasonal symptoms only. These symptoms are due to pollen production by weeds, grasses, and trees that are dependent on wind currents, rather than insects, for cross-pollination. The timing of the pollination events predicts seasonal severity of symptoms and varies little from year to year within a particular locale. Based on this pattern, one is able to predict which allergens are most likely responsible for a patient's symptoms. In the temperate regions of North America, trees pollinate in the spring, and ragweed pollinates in the fall. Grasses are responsible for seasonal allergic symptoms in the summer months. Mold allergens can have a variable pattern of symptoms, depending on climactic conditions that allow them to sporulate. Perennial rhinitis does not have a seasonal pattern and is more continually present. Allergens that cause perennial rhinitis include animal dander, dust, and cockroach-derived proteins.

IX-9. **The answer is D.** *(Chap. 376)* There is no convincing evidence that age, sex, race, or geographic location predisposes a human to anaphylaxis except through exposure to specific immunogens. According to most studies, atopy does not predispose individuals to anaphylaxis from penicillin therapy or venom of a stinging insect but is a risk factor for allergens in food or latex. Risk factors for a poor outcome, however, include older age, use of β-blockers, and the presence of preexisting asthma. Individuals differ in the time of appearance of symptoms and signs, but the hallmark of the anaphylactic reaction is the onset of some manifestation within seconds to minutes after introduction of the antigen. Early recognition of an anaphylactic reaction is mandatory, because death can occur within minutes to hours after the first symptoms.

Mild symptoms such as pruritus and urticaria can be controlled by administration of 0.3–0.5 mL of 1:1000 (1 mg/mL) epinephrine subcutaneously (SC) or intramuscularly (IM), with repeated doses as required at 5- to 20-minute intervals for a severe reaction. The failure to use epinephrine within the first 20 minutes of symptoms is a risk factor for poor outcome in studies of anaphylaxis to food. An intravenous (IV) infusion should be initiated to provide a route for administration of 2.5 mL epinephrine, diluted 1:10,000, at 5- to 10-minutes intervals, volume expanders such as normal saline, and vasopressor agents such as dopamine if intractable hypotension occurs. Replacement of intravascular volume due to postcapillary venular leakage may require several liters of saline. Epinephrine provides both α- and β-adrenergic effects, resulting in vasoconstriction, bronchial smooth muscle relaxation, and attenuation of enhanced venular permeability. Ancillary agents such as the antihistamine diphenhydramine, 50–100 mg IM or IV, and aminophylline, 0.25–0.5 g IV, are appropriate for urticaria-angioedema and bronchospasm, respectively. IV glucocorticoids (0.5–1 mg/kg of methylprednisolone) are not effective for the acute event but may alleviate later recurrence of bronchospasm, hypotension, or urticaria.

IX-10. The answer is E. *(Chap. 377e)* Derangements of normal processes may predispose to the development of autoimmunity. In general, these abnormal responses require both an exogenous trigger, such as infection (bacterial or viral) or cigarette smoking, and the presence of endogenous abnormalities in the cells of the immune system. One of the best examples of autoreactivity and autoimmune disease resulting from molecular mimicry is rheumatic fever, in which antibodies to the M protein of streptococci cross-react with myosin, laminin, and other matrix proteins as well as with neuronal antigens. Deposition of these autoantibodies in the heart initiates an inflammatory response, whereas their penetration into the brain can result in Sydenham chorea. Molecular mimicry between microbial proteins and host tissues has been reported in type 1 diabetes mellitus, rheumatoid arthritis, celiac disease, and multiple sclerosis.

TABLE IX-10 Mechanisms of Autoimmunity

- I. Exogenous
  - A. Molecular mimicry
  - B. Superantigenic stimulation
  - C. Microbial and tissue damage–associated adjuvanticity
- II. Endogenous
  - A. Altered antigen presentation
    1. Loss of immunologic privilege
    2. Presentation of novel or cryptic epitopes (epitope spreading)
    3. Alteration of self-antigen
    4. Enhanced function of antigen-presenting cells
       - a. Costimulatory molecule expression
       - b. Cytokine production
  - B. Increased T-cell help
    1. Cytokine production
    2. Costimulatory molecules
  - C. Increased B-cell function
    1. B-cell activating factor
    2. Costimulatory molecules
  - D. Apoptotic defects or defects in clearance of apoptotic material
  - E. Cytokine imbalance
  - F. Altered immunoregulation
  - G. Endocrine abnormalities

IX-11. The answer is D. *(Chap. 377e)* The mechanisms of tissue injury in autoimmune diseases can be divided into antibody-mediated and cell-mediated processes. Autoantibodies can interfere with normal physiologic functions of cells or soluble factors. Autoantibodies to hormone receptors can lead to stimulation of cells or to inhibition of cell function through interference with receptor signaling. For example, long-acting thyroid stimulators—autoantibodies that bind to the receptor for thyroid-stimulating hormone (TSH)—are present in Graves disease and function as agonists, causing the thyroid to respond as if there were an excess of TSH. In contrast, Hashimoto thyroiditis is due to antibody-dependent cellular cytotoxicity due to antibodies directed against thyroid peroxidase.

IX-12. The answer is C. *(Chap. 378)* Antinuclear antibodies are nearly ubiquitous in patients with systemic lupus erythematosus (SLE), with demonstration in 90% of affected patients. There are many other antibodies that can be demonstrated. The next most common antibodies are anti-dsDNA and anti-histone. Anti-dsDNA is very specific to SLE and may correlate with disease activity, nephritis, and vasculitis. Antiphospholipid antibodies can be demonstrated in about half of affected patients, whereas the remainder is present in less than half of SLE cases. Antierythrocyte antibodies are present in approximately 60% of SLE cases and can be measured by a direct Coombs test. In contrast, anti-La antibodies directed against the 47-kDa protein complexes to hY RNA is rare, present only in 10% of cases of SLE. It is associated with a *decreased* risk for nephritis.

IX-13. The answer is B. *(Chap. 378)* There are well-published, strict diagnostic criteria for SLE. They include four or more of the following criteria from the table below.

The patient described does not meet the arthritis criteria; her only criteria are oral ulcers and weakly positive ANA.

Malar rash	Fixed erythema, flat or raised, over the malar eminences
Discoid rash	Erythematous circular raised patches with adherent keratotic scaling
Photosensitivity	Exposure to ultraviolet light causes rash
Oral ulcers	Oral and nasopharyngeal ulcers observed by a physician
Arthritis	Nonerosive arthritis of two or more peripheral joints with tenderness, swelling, or effusion
Serositis	Pleuritis or pericarditis
Renal disorder	Proteinuria >0.5 g/d or 3+ or cellular casts
Neurologic disorder	Seizures, psychosis
Hematologic disorder	Hemolytic anemia or leukopenia, lymphopenia, thrombocytopenia
Immunologic disorder	Anti-dsDNA, anti-Sm, and/or antiphospholipid, low serum complement, positive direct Coombs
Antinuclear antibodies (ANA)	Abnormal titer of ANA

IX-14. The answer is A. *(Chap. 378)* The patient has Libman-Sacks endocarditis associated with her SLE. This results in fibrinous endocarditis and can lead to valvular insufficiencies, most often mitral or aortic, or embolism. It is not generally found with concomitant pericarditis, although this is another common cardiac manifestation of systemic lupus erythematosus. Although glucocorticoids and anti-inflammatory therapies have no proven benefit in this condition, they are often used in conjunction with supportive care. Because Libman-Sacks endocarditis is a culture-negative endocarditis and is not thought to be due to microbial infection, blood cultures will not be positive.

IX-15. The answer is D. *(Chap. 378)* SLE is a multisystem disease with diverse organ involvement and multiple different manifestations within an organ system. The most common system to be involved is the musculoskeletal system, with 95% of patients having involvement, most commonly as arthralgias or myalgias. Arthritis is also common and is one of the diagnostic criteria for SLE. Cutaneous and hematologic disease occurs in approximately 80%–85% of patients. Neurologic and cardiopulmonary disease affects approximately 60% of patients, whereas renal and gastrointestinal disease occurs in <50% of cases.

IX-16. The answer is C. *(Chap. 378)* This patient is presenting with acute lupus nephritis with evidence of hematuria, proteinuria, and an acute rise in creatinine. Together with infection, nephritis is the most common cause of mortality in the first decade after diagnosis of SLE and warrants prompt immunosuppressive therapy. It is important to assess for other potentially reversible causes of acute renal insufficiency, but this patient is not otherwise acutely ill and is taking no medications that would cause renal failure. The urinalysis shows evidence of active nephritis with hematuria and proteinuria. Even in the absence of red blood cell (RBC) casts, therapy should not be withheld to await biopsy results in someone with a known diagnosis of SLE with consistent clinical presentation and urinary findings. This patient also has other risk factors known to predict the development of lupus nephritis, including high titers of anti-dsDNA and African American race. The mainstay of treatment for any life-threatening or organ-threatening manifestation of SLE is high-dose systemic glucocorticoids. Addition of cytotoxic or other immunosuppressive agents (cyclophosphamide, azathioprine, mycophenolate mofetil) is recommended to treat serious complications of SLE, but their effects are delayed for 3–6 weeks after initiation of therapy, whereas the effects of glucocorticoids begin within 24 hours. Thus, these agents alone should not be used to treat acute serious manifestations of SLE. The choice of cytotoxic agent is at the discretion of the treating physician. Cyclophosphamide in combination with steroid therapy has been demonstrated to prevent development of end-stage renal disease better than steroids alone. Likewise, mycophenolate also prevents development of end-stage renal disease in combination with glucocorticoids, and some studies suggest that African Americans have a greater response to mycophenolate than to cyclophosphamide. Plasmapheresis is not indicated in the treatment of lupus nephritis but is useful in cases of severe hemolytic anemia or thrombotic thrombocytopenic purpura associated with SLE. Finally, this patient has no acute indication for hemodialysis and, with treatment, may recover renal function.

IX-17. The answer is A. *(Chap. 379)* The patient has multiple clinical manifestations of arterial thrombosis in her hand and brain and likely had placental insufficiency in the three prior pregnancies, which makes the possibility of antiphospholipid antibody syndrome likely. In addition, she has evidence of acute kidney injury, suggesting multisystem disease. Thrombocytopenia may be due to hemolytic anemia, but the absence of schistocytes makes it less likely that she has thrombotic thrombocytopenic purpura. Although magnetic resonance imaging (MRI) of her brain and extremity duplex may confirm the presence of thrombosis, these will not diagnose antiphospholipid antibody syndrome. An anticardiolipin antibody screening panel will look for evidence of antibodies directed against cardiolipin and β-2 glycoprotein I. Additional testing for lupus anticoagulant determined by clotting assays such as the Russel viper venom time, false-positive rapid plasma reagin (RPR), and the activated partial thromboplastin time (aPTT) may also be useful. ANA is likely to be positive given the common overlap with SLE, but is nonspecific.

IX-18. The answer is D. *(Chap. 379)* This patient has a typical presentation of antiphospholipid syndrome (APS) with a deep venous thrombosis, history of spontaneous abortion, and isolated elevated aPTT due to a lupus anticoagulant. Additional clinical features of APS involving the arterial or venous circulation include livedo reticularis (24%), pulmonary embolism (14%), stroke (20%), transient ischemic attack (10%), myocardial infarction (10%), migraine (20%), preeclampsia (10%), thrombocytopenia (30%), and autoimmune hemolytic anemia (10%). Laboratory criteria include demonstration of lupus anticoagulant (elevated aPTT that does not correct on mixing), in conjunction with the presence of anticardiolipin and/or anti-β-2 glycoprotein I on two occasions 3 month apart. After diagnosis of a thrombotic event due to APS, patients should receive warfarin for life with a goal international normalized ratio (INR) of 2.5–3.5 alone or in combination with daily aspirin. During pregnancy, patients should receive heparin plus aspirin. Patients who develop recurrent thrombosis while on effective anticoagulation may benefit from a 5-day infusion of IV γ-globulin or 4 weeks of rituximab therapy. The optimal therapy for patients with APS without a thrombotic event is not known; however, daily aspirin (80 mg) protects patients with SLE and antiphospholipid antibodies from thrombotic events. Warfarin for 3 months with INR goal of 2.0–3.0 is recommended therapy for deep vein thrombosis (DVT) with a known reversible precipitating event. Warfarin for 6–12 months with an INR goal of 2.0–3.0 is recommended therapy for first episode of idiopathic DVT.

IX-19. The answer is E. *(Chap. 379)* Patients with APS often possess antibodies recognizing *Treponema pallidum* PL/cholesterol complexes, which are detected as biologic false-positive serologic tests for syphilis (BFP-STS) and Venereal Disease Research Laboratory (VDRL) tests. If syphilis is suspected, a specific direct treponemal test, such as fluorescent treponemal antibody absorption (FTA-ABS) should be obtained.

IX-20. The answer is E. *(Chap. 380)* Once the disease process of rheumatoid arthritis is established, the most common joints of involvement are the wrists, metacarpophalangeal joints, and proximal interphalangeal joints. Distal interphalangeal joint involvement is rarely due to rheumatoid arthritis and more often due to coexisting osteoarthritis.

IX-21. The answer is C. *(Chap. 380)* There is potential involvement of multiple organ systems in rheumatoid arthritis (RA). The most common pulmonary complication is pleural effusion that is typically exudative and presents with chest pain and dyspnea. RA is associated with a form of diffuse interstitial lung disease that may present with dyspnea and bilateral interstitial infiltrates that may be so extensive as to develop into a honeycomb pattern. Pulmonary nodules associated with rheumatoid arthritis may be solitary or multiple. They often occur in conjunction with cutaneous nodules. Bronchiectasis and respiratory bronchiolitis may also be due to rheumatoid arthritis. Many of these manifestations respond to immunosuppressive therapy. Lobar infiltrate has not been described to be caused by RA and is more commonly caused by an acute infectious etiology, often as a complication of RA immunosuppressive therapy.

IX-22. The answer is A. *(Chap. 380)* Joint imaging is a critical tool for both diagnosis and monitoring of disease status in RA. Plain radiographs, because of their ready availability and ease of film comparison, are most commonly ordered. The earliest clinical sign of RA is juxta-articular osteopenia, although this may be difficult to appreciate on newer, digitized films. Other findings include soft tissue swelling, symmetric joint space loss, and subchondral erosions most frequently in the wrists, metacarpophalangeal and proximal interphalangeal joints, and metatarsophalangeal joint.

IX-23. The answer is E. *(Chap. 380)* Anemia is common in RA and parallels the degree of inflammation as measured by C-reactive protein or erythrocyte sedimentation rate (ESR). Felty syndrome, typically occurring in late-stage poorly controlled disease, is characterized by the triad of neutropenia, splenomegaly, and rheumatoid nodules. Rheumatoid vasculitis is not common and typically occurs in long-standing disease. It is associated with hypocomplementemia. The cutaneous signs are typical of vasculitic lesions with palpable purpura, digital infarcts, livedo reticularis, and ulcers. Clinical manifestations of pericarditis occur in 10% of patients with echocardiographic or autopsy findings in about half of those cases. Secondary Sjögren syndrome manifest as keratoconjunctivitis sicca or xerostomia occurs in approximately 10% of patients with RA. RA also appears to increase the risk of developing B-cell lymphoma by two- to fourfold compared with the general population. The risk of lymphoma appears to correlate with high levels of disease activity or the presence of Felty syndrome. Platelet counts in RA are typically elevated in association with the acute-phase response of inflammation. Immune thrombocytopenia is rare.

IX-24. The answer is D. *(Chap. 380)* The therapy of RA has changed dramatically in the past two decades with the development of drugs that modify the disease course of RA. Methotrexate is the disease-modifying antirheumatic drug (DMARD) of first choice for treatment of early RA. Other conventional DMARDs include hydroxychloroquine, sulfasalazine, and leflunomide. Leflunomide, an inhibitor of pyrimidine synthesis, is efficacious as a single agent or in combination with methotrexate. Hydroxychloroquine and sulfasalazine are typically reserved for mild disease. The biologic DMARDs have dramatically improved the treatment of RA in the past decade. There are currently five anti–tumor necrosis factor (TNF) agents, including infliximab, approved for use in patients with RA. Rituximab, an anti-CD20 antibody, is approved for refractory RA in combination with methotrexate. It is more efficacious in seropositive than seronegative patients.

Other biologics approved for use in RA include anakinra (interleukin [IL]-1 receptor antagonist), abatacept (CD28/CD80/86 antagonist), and tocilizumab (IL-6 antagonist). NSAIDs, including naproxen, were formerly used as core RA therapy. However, they are now used as adjunctive treatment for symptom management. They are not considered DMARDs.

IX-25. The answer is E. *(Chap. 381)* Felty syndrome is defined by the clinical triad of neutropenia, splenomegaly, and nodular RA and is seen in less than 1% of patients, although its incidence appears to be declining in the face of more aggressive treatment of the joint disease. It typically occurs in the late stages of severe RA and is more common in whites than other racial groups. T-cell large granular lymphocytic leukemia (T-LGL) may have a similar clinical presentation and often occurs in association with RA. T-LGL is characterized by a chronic, indolent clonal growth of LGL cells, leading to neutropenia and splenomegaly. As opposed to Felty syndrome, T-LGL may develop early in the course of RA. Leukopenia apart from these disorders is uncommon and most often due to drug therapy.

IX-26. The answer is C. *(Chap. 380)* Large cohort studies have shown a two- to fourfold increased risk of lymphoma in RA patients compared with the general population. The most common histopathologic type of lymphoma is a diffuse large B-cell lymphoma. The risk of developing lymphoma increases if the patient has high levels of disease activity or Felty syndrome.

IX-27. The answer is D. *(Chap. 381)* Acute rheumatic fever is almost universally due to group A streptococcal disease in present time, though virtually all streptococcal disease may be capable of precipitating rheumatic fever. Although skin infections may be associated with rheumatic fever, far and away the most common presentation is with preceding pharyngitis. There is a latent period of approximately 3 weeks from an episode of sore throat to presentation of acute rheumatic fever. The most common manifestations are fever and polyarthritis, with polyarthritis present in 60%–75% of cases. Carditis may also be present, although somewhat less frequently (50%–60% of cases). Chorea and indolent carditis may have a subacute presentation. Chorea is present in 2%–30% of affected individuals, whereas erythema marginatum and subcutaneous nodules are rare. Sixty percent of patients with acute rheumatic fever progress to rheumatic heart disease with the endocardium, pericardium, and myocardium all potentially involved. All patients with acute rheumatic fever should receive antibiotics sufficient to treat the precipitating group A streptococcal infection.

IX-28. The answer is D. *(Chap. 381)* This patient has a history suggestive of recurrent bouts of acute rheumatic fever (ARF) with evidence of mitral regurgitation, mitral stenosis, and aortic regurgitation on physical examination. This and the presence of atrial fibrillation imply severe rheumatic heart disease. Risk factors for this condition include poverty and crowded living conditions. As a result, ARF is considerably more common in the developing world. Daily aspirin is the treatment of choice for the migratory large-joint arthritis and fever that are common manifestations of ARF. Practitioners sometimes use steroids during acute bouts of carditis to quell inflammation, although this remains a controversial practice and has no role between flares of ARF. Secondary prophylaxis with either daily oral penicillin or, preferably, monthly IM injections is considered the best method to prevent further episodes of ARF and, therefore, prevent further valvular damage. Primary prophylaxis with penicillin on an as-needed basis is equally effective for preventing further bouts of carditis. However, most episodes of sore throat are too minor for patients to present to a physician. Therefore, secondary prophylaxis is considered preferable in patients who already have severe valvular disease. Doxycycline is not a first-line agent for group A *Streptococcus*, the pathogen that incites ARF.

IX-29. The answer is A. *(Chap. 381)* There is a latent period of approximately 3 weeks (1–5 weeks) between the precipitating group A streptococcal infection and the appearance of the clinical features of ARF. The exceptions are chorea and indolent carditis, which may follow prolonged latent periods lasting up to 6 months. Although many patients report a prior sore throat, the preceding group A streptococcal infection is commonly subclinical; in these cases, it can only be confirmed using streptococcal antibody testing. The most common clinical features are polyarthritis (present in 60%–75% of cases) and carditis (50%–60%). The prevalence of chorea in ARF varies substantially between populations, ranging from <2% to 30%. Erythema marginatum and subcutaneous nodules are now rare, being found in <5% of cases.

IX-30. The answer is A. *(Chap. 382)* The prognosis for patients with scleroderma renal disease is poor. In scleroderma renal crisis patients, prompt treatment with an ACE inhibitor may reverse acute renal failure. In recent studies, the initiation of ACE inhibitor therapy resulted in 61% of patients having some degree of renal recovery and not needing chronic dialysis support. The survival rate is estimated to be 80%–85% at 8 years. Among patients who needed dialysis, when treated with ACE inhibitors, over 50% were able to discontinue dialysis after 3–18 months. Therefore, ACE inhibitors should be used even if the patient requires dialysis support.

IX-31. The answer is C. *(Chap. 382)* Virtually every organ can be clinically affected with cutaneous systemic sclerosis (SSc). Most patients with SSc can be classified as either limited (lcSSc) or diffuse (dcSSc). Although stratification of SSc patients into diffuse and limited cutaneous subsets is useful, disease expression is far more complex, and several distinct endophenotypes exist within each subset. In general, pulmonary parenchymal involvement is more common in patients with dcSSc than lcSSc. See Figure IX-31.

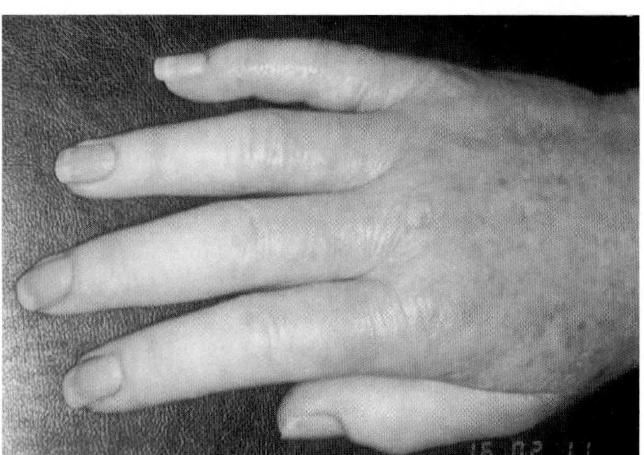

FIGURE IX-31

IX-32. The answer is E. *(Chap. 382)* Patients who have lcSSc coexisting with features of SLE, polymyositis, and rheumatoid arthritis may have mixed connective tissue disease (MCTD). This overlap syndrome is generally associated with the presence of high titers of autoantibodies to U1-RNP. Laboratory evaluation indicates features of inflammation with elevated ESR and hypergammaglobulinemia. Although anti–U1-RNP antibodies are detected in the serum in high titers, SSc-specific autoantibodies are not found. In contrast to SSc, patients with MCTD often show a good response to treatment with glucocorticoids, and the long-term prognosis is better than that of SSc. Anticentromere antibodies are typically associated with lcSSc.

IX-33. The answer is D. *(Chap. 383)* The patient presented with classic symptoms for Sjögren syndrome including dry mouth and eyes. This condition may be primary, as in this case, or secondary in association with another connective tissue disease such as scleroderma or rheumatoid arthritis. Many autoantibodies may be demonstrated in the serum of patients with Sjögren syndrome, including antibodies to Ro/SS-A or La/SS-B. Sialometry will demonstrate decreased production of saliva and MRI or magnetic resonance sialography of the major salivary glands may also demonstrate abnormalities. Ocular involvement with decreased tear production is demonstrated by the Schirmer I test. Scl-70 antibody is associated with scleroderma and should not be positive in primary Sjögren syndrome.

IX-34. The answer is D. *(Chap. 383)* Lymphoma is well known to develop specifically in the late stage of Sjögren syndrome. Common manifestations of this malignant condition include persistent parotid gland enlargement, purpura, leukopenia, cryoglobulinemia, and low C4 complement levels. Most of the lymphomas are extranodal, marginal zone B cell, and low grade. Low-grade lymphomas may be detected incidentally during a labial biopsy. Mortality is higher in patients with concurrent B symptoms (fevers, night sweats, and weight loss), a lymph node mass >7 cm, and a high or intermediate histologic grade.

IX-35. The answer is A. *(Chap. 383)* Although Sjogren syndrome most commonly affects the eyes and mouth, there are a number of common extraglandular sites of involvement. The most common is arthritis or arthralgias that complicate up to 60% of cases. Raynaud phenomenon is the second most common extraglandular site. Lung involvement and vasculitis are found in less than 20% of patients. Lymphoma, although a concerning and highly morbid complication, is relatively rare, affecting only 6% of Sjögren patients.

IX-36. The answer is B. *(Chap. 383)* Primary Sjögren syndrome is diagnosed if (1) the patient presents with eye and/or mouth dryness, (2) eye tests disclose keratoconjunctivitis sicca, (3) mouth evaluation reveals the classic manifestations of the syndrome, and/or (4) the patient's serum reacts with Ro/SS-A and/or La/SS-B autoantigens. Labial biopsy is needed when the diagnosis is uncertain or to rule out other conditions that may cause dry mouth or eyes or parotid gland enlargement. See Table IX-36 for the differential diagnosis of Sjögren syndrome.

TABLE IX-36 Differential Diagnosis of Sjögren Syndrome

HIV Infection and Sicca Syndrome	Sjögren Syndrome	Sarcoidosis
Predominant in young males	Predominant in middle-aged women	No age or sex preference
Lack of autoantibodies to Ro/SS-A and/or La/SS-B	Presence of autoantibodies	Lack of autoantibodies to Ro/SS-A and/or La/SS-B
Lymphoid infiltrates of salivary glands by CD8+ T lymphocytes	Lymphoid infiltrates of salivary glands by CD4+ T lymphocytes	Granulomas in salivary glands
Association with HLA-DR5	Association with HLA-DR3 and DRw52	Unknown
Positive serologic tests for HIV	Negative serologic tests for HIV	Negative serologic tests for HIV

IX-37. The answer is D. *(Chap. 384)* Ankylosing spondylitis is closely correlated with the presence of the histocompatibility antigen HLA-B27. In North American whites, the prevalence of B27 is 7%, but in patients with ankylosing spondylitis, it is 90%. Not all persons with B27 develop ankylosing spondylitis; the disease is only present in 1%–6% of B27-positive individuals.

IX-38. The answer is A. *(Chap. 384)* Although the most serious spine complication of ankylosing spondylitis is fracture, there are a number of important extra-articular manifestations. Anterior uveitis is the most common, occurring in 40% of patients with ankylosing spondylitis. Inflammatory bowel disease has been reported to be frequently present. Less common complications include aortic insufficiency, third-degree heart block, pulmonary nodules and upper lobe fibrosis, cardiac dysfunction, retroperitoneal fibrosis, prostatitis, and amyloidosis.

IX-39. The answer is B. *(Chap. 384)* NSAIDs are the first line of pharmacologic therapy for ankylosing spondylitis, for which this patient has a classic presentation. These agents have been shown to reduce pain and tenderness and increase mobility. There is even some evidence that they slow disease progression. Given their proven efficacy, tolerability, and safety, they remain first-line therapy. Anti–TNF-α agents have been reported to have dramatic effects in ankylosing spondylitis, with infliximab, etanercept, adalimumab, or golimumab having published reports of success. Because of their potential side effects, including serious infections, hypersensitivity reactions, and others, these agents should be reserved for patients failing therapy with NSAIDs.

IX-40. The answer is E. *(Chaps. 384 and 191)* Reactive arthritis refers to an acute, nonpurulent arthritis that occurs after an infection elsewhere in the body. Often presenting with lower joint inflammatory arthritis occurring 1–4 weeks after a diarrheal episode, reactive arthritis may also include uveitis or conjunctivitis, dactylitis, urogenital lesions, and characteristic mucocutaneous lesions such as keratoderma blennorrhagicum. The most common organisms associated with reactive arthritis are *Shigella* species, although *Yersinia*, *Chlamydia*, and, to a much lesser extent, *Salmonella* and *Campylobacter* have been described. Although more common in children residing in developing countries, over 400,000 annual cases of *Shigella* species infections occur in the United States. These infections mostly occur in children 4–11 years old. Most U.S. cases are due to *Shigella sonnei*, with *Shigella flexneri* the second most common cause.

IX-41. The answer is E. *(Chap. 384)* Whipple disease is a rare chronic bacterial infection of the gastrointestinal tract most commonly affecting middle-aged men. Arthritis is a common early manifestation of the disease, with arthritis predating gastrointestinal symptoms by 5 years or more. Large and small joints may be affected, and sacroiliitis is common. Arthritis is often migratory and lasts several days with spontaneous recovery. Synovial fluid is generally inflammatory, including polymorphonuclear cells. Radiographs rarely show joint erosions, although sacroiliitis may be demonstrated. Diagnosis is often made by polymerase chain reaction amplification of genetic material from *Tropheryma whipplei* in biopsied material, most commonly the gut.

IX-42. The answer is C. *(Chap. 384) Enthesopathy* or *enthesitis* is the term used to describe inflammation at the site of tendinous or ligamentous insertion into bone. This type of inflammation is seen most frequently in patients with seronegative spondyloarthropathies and various infections, especially viral infections. The other definitions apply to other terms used in the orthopedic and rheumatic examination. Subluxation is the alteration of joint alignment so that articulating surfaces incompletely approximate each other. Synovitis refers to inflammation at the site of tendinous or ligamentous insertion into bone. Inflammation of a saclike cavity near a joint that decreases friction is the definition of bursitis. Finally, crepitus is a palpable vibratory or crackling sensation elicited with joint motion.

IX-43. The answer is D. *(Chap. 384)* Nail changes in the fingers or toes occur in up to 90% of patients with psoriatic arthritis (PsA), compared with 40% of psoriatic patients without arthritis, and pustular psoriasis is said to be associated with more severe arthritis. Several articular features distinguish PsA from other joint disorders; such hallmark features include dactylitis and enthesitis. Dactylitis occurs in >30%; enthesitis and tenosynovitis are also common and are probably present in most patients, although often not appreciated on physical examination. Shortening of digits because of underlying osteolysis is particularly characteristic of PsA, and there is a much greater tendency than in RA for both fibrous and bony ankylosis of small joints. Rapid ankylosis of one or more proximal interphalangeal (PIP) joints early in the course of disease is not uncommon. Back and neck pain and stiffness are also common in PsA. Diarrhea is not a feature of PsA. See Figure IX-43.

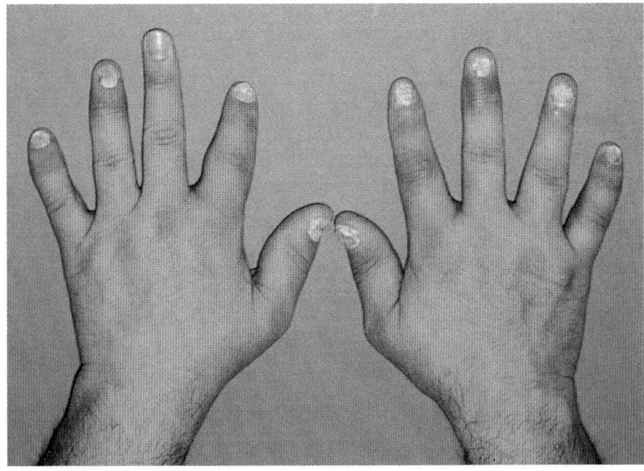

FIGURE IX-43

IX-44. The answer is A. *(Chap. 384)* Aortic insufficiency, sometimes leading to congestive heart failure, occurs in a small percentage of patients, occasionally early. Third-degree heart block may occur alone or together with aortic insufficiency. Subclinical pulmonary lesions and cardiac dysfunction may be relatively common.

IX-45. The answer is B. *(Chap. 385)* Although the molecular pathology of most vasculitic syndromes is poorly understood, the deposition of immune complexes is commonly thought to play an important role in vasculitis associated with Henoch-Schönlein purpura, cryoglobulinemic vasculitis associated with hepatitis C, serum sickness and cutaneous vasculitic syndromes, and polyarteritis nodosa–like vasculitis associated with hepatitis B. Granulomatosis with polyangiitis (previously Wegener granulomatosis), Churg-Strauss syndrome, and microscopic polyangiitis are thought to be due to production of antineutrophilic antibodies. Pathogenic T-lymphocyte responses are also implicated in granulomatosis with polyangiitis (previously Wegener), giant-cell arteritis, Takayasu arteritis, and Churg-Strauss syndrome.

IX-46. The answer is D. *(Chap. 385)* The patient presents with classic symptoms for granulomatosis with polyangiitis. The average age of diagnosis is 40 years, and there is a male predominance. Upper respiratory symptoms often predate lung or renal findings and may even present with septal perforation. The diagnosis is made by demonstration of necrotizing granulomatous vasculitis on biopsy. Pulmonary tissue offers the highest yield. Biopsy of the upper airway usually shows the granulomatous inflammation but infrequently shows vasculitis. Renal biopsy may show the presence of pauci-immune glomerulonephritis.

IX-47. The answer is C. *(Chap. 385)* The patient has a classic presentation for giant-cell arteritis with associated polymyalgia rheumatica including headache, jaw claudication, and visual disturbances. Her age makes this diagnosis highly likely as well. The diagnosis is confirmed by temporal artery biopsy; however, in the presence of visual symptoms, initiation of therapy should not be delayed pending a biopsy because the biopsy may be positive even after approximately 14 days of glucocorticoid therapy. Delay in therapy risks irreversible visual loss. Additionally, a dramatic response to therapy may lend further support to the diagnosis. The primary therapy is prednisone at 40–60 mg daily for 1 month with gradual tapering. Although ESR is nearly universally elevated, it is not specific for the diagnosis. Temporal artery ultrasound may be suggestive but is not diagnostic.

IX-48. The answer is C. *(Chap. 385)* The most common manifestations of cryoglobulinemic vasculitis are cutaneous vasculitis, arthritis, peripheral neuropathy, and glomerulonephritis.

The demonstration of circulating cryoprecipitates is a critical component of the diagnosis, and often rheumatoid factor can be found as well. Because hepatitis C infection is present in the vast majority of patients with cryoglobulinemic vasculitis, infection should be sought in all patients with this clinical syndrome.

IX-49. The answer is C. *(Chap. 385)* The most likely cause of the acute coronary syndrome in this patient is thrombosis of a coronary artery aneurysm in an individual with a past history of Kawasaki disease. Kawasaki disease is an acute multisystem disease that primarily presents in children <5 years of age. The clinical manifestations in childhood are nonsuppurative cervical lymphadenitis; desquamation of the fingertips; and erythema of the oral cavity, lips, and palms. Approximately 25% of cases are associated with coronary artery aneurysms that occur late in illness in the convalescent stage. Early treatment (within 7–10 days of onset) with IV immunoglobulin and high-dose aspirin decreases the risk of developing coronary aneurysms to about 5%. Even if coronary artery aneurysms develop, most regress over the course of the first year if the size is <6 mm. Aneurysms >8 mm, however, are unlikely to regress. Complications of persistent coronary artery aneurysms include rupture, thrombosis and recanalization, and stenosis at the outflow area. Dissection of the aortic root and coronary ostia is a common cause of death in Marfan syndrome and can also be seen with aortitis due to Takayasu arteritis. In this patient, there is no history of hypertension, limb ischemia, or systemic symptoms that would suggest an active vasculitis. In addition, there are no other ischemic symptoms that would be expected in Takayasu arteritis. Myocardial bridging overlying a coronary artery is seen frequently at autopsy but is an unusual cause of ischemia. The possibility of cocaine use as a cause of myocardial ischemia in a young individual must be considered, but given the clinical history, it is a less likely cause of ischemia in this case.

IX-50. The answer is E. *(Chap. 385)* Prior to initiation of azathioprine, thiopurine methyltransferase (TPMT), an enzyme involved in the metabolism of azathioprine, should be assayed because inadequate levels may result in severe cytopenia. The antineutrophil cytoplasmic antibody (ANCA) titer can be misleading and should not be used to assess disease activity. Many patients who achieve remission continue to have elevated titers for years. Results from a large prospective study found that increases in ANCA were not associated with relapse and that only 43% of patients relapsed within 1 year of an increase in ANCA levels. Thus, a rise in ANCA by itself is not a harbinger of immediate disease relapse and should not lead to reinstitution or increase in immunosuppressive therapy.

IX-51. The answer is C. *(Chap. 385)* Polyarteritis nodosa does not involve pulmonary arteries, although bronchial vessels may be involved; granulomas, significant eosinophilia, and an allergic diathesis are not observed. Vascular beds typically involved are listed in Table IX-51.

TABLE IX-51 Clinical Manifestations Related to Organ System Involvement in Polyarteritis Nodosa

Organ System	Percent Incidence	Clinical Manifestations
Renal	60	Renal failure, hypertension
Musculoskeletal	64	Arthritis, arthralgia, myalgia
Peripheral nervous system	51	Peripheral neuropathy, mononeuritis multiplex
Gastrointestinal tract	44	Abdominal pain, nausea and vomiting, bleeding, bowel infarction and perforation, cholecystitis, hepatic infarction, pancreatic infarction
Skin	43	Rash, purpura, nodules, cutaneous infarcts, livedo reticularis, Raynaud phenomenon
Cardiac	36	Congestive heart failure, myocardial infarction, pericarditis
Genitourinary	25	Testicular, ovarian, or epididymal pain
Central nervous system	23	Cerebral vascular accident, altered mental status, seizure

Source: From Cupps TR, Fauci AS: *The Vasculitides.* Philadelphia, PA: Saunders, 1981.

IX-52. **The answer is C.** *(Chap. 386e)* Granulomatosis with polyangiitis (Wegener) is a small-vessel vasculitis that involves the lung in >80% of cases. One-third of patients with radiographic abnormalities may be asymptomatic. It typically also involves the upper respiratory tract and the kidney. Surgical biopsies of radiographically abnormal pulmonary parenchyma have a diagnostic yield of approximately 90% in patients with granulomatosis with polyangiitis (Wegener). Biopsy may also differentiate vasculitis from infection or malignancy. The yield of bronchoscopic transbronchial biopsy is substantially lower than surgical biopsy. Cryoglobulinemic vasculitis and IgA vasculitis (Henoch-Schönlein) are small-vessel vasculitides that typically involve the skin and kidney. Polyarteritis nodosa is a medium-vessel vasculitis that typically involves the mesenteric vessels. Cutaneous vasculitis represents the most common vasculitic feature and can be seen in a broad spectrum of settings including infections, medications, malignancies, and connective tissue diseases.

IX-53. **The answer is A.** *(Chap. 386e)* In granulomatosis with polyangiitis (Wegener), 80% of patients may have pulmonary involvement during their disease course. The typical chest radiographic abnormalities are single or multiple nodular infiltrates that often cavitate (Figures IX-53A and IX-53B).

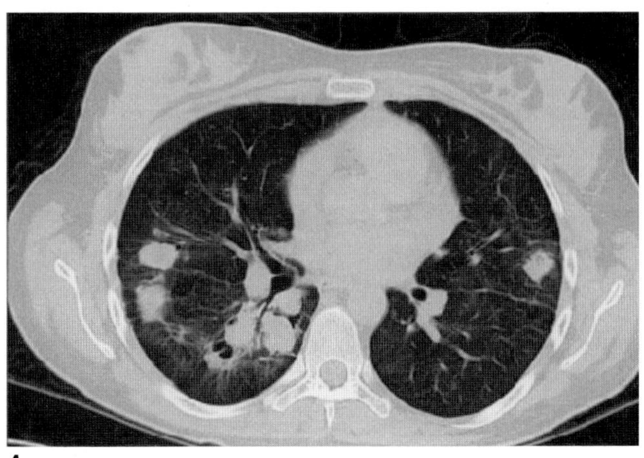

A

FIGURE IX-53A

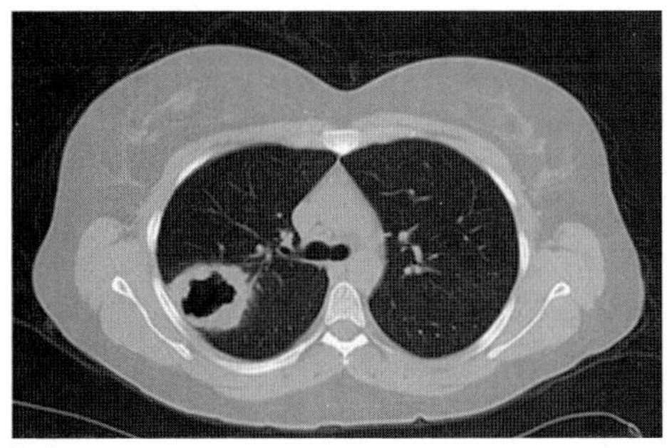

Left

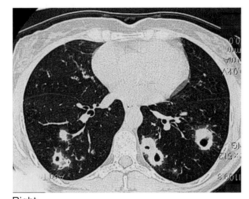

Right

B

FIGURE IX-53B

However, due to the frequent involvement of airways, tracheal or bronchial stenosis may occur. Ground glass infiltrates (Figure IX-53C) may occur due to capillaritis and subsequent pulmonary hemorrhage.

Microscopic polyangiitis and SLE are also causes of capillaritis. Patients with granulomatosis with polyangiitis on immunosuppressive therapy are at risk of opportunistic lung infections. Granulomatosis with polyangiitis typically will not cause bronchiectasis in the absence of a history of multiple respiratory infections. Bronchiectasis is more typical

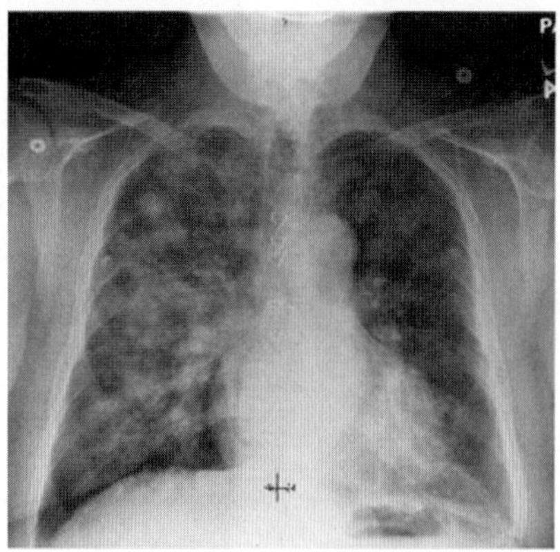

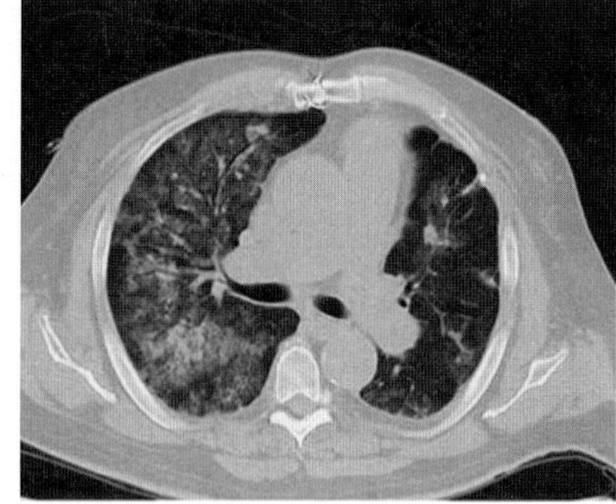

C

FIGURE IX-53C

of cystic fibrosis, ciliary dysfunction syndromes, obstructive lung disease, or congenital immunodeficiency.

IX-54. The answer is C. *(Chap. 387)* Recurrent oral ulceration is required for the diagnosis of Behçet disease. The ulcers may be single or multiple, are shallow based with a yellow necrotic base, and are painful. They are generally small, <10 mm in diameter. In addition, the diagnosis of Behçet disease requires two of the following: recurrent genital ulceration, eye lesions, skin lesions, and pathergy test. Nonspecific skin inflammatory reactivity to any scratches or intradermal saline injection (pathergy test) is common and specific.

IX-55. The answer is A. *(Chap. 387)* Behçet's disease is a multisystem disorder of uncertain cause that is marked by oral and genital ulcerations and ocular involvement. This disorder affects males and females equally and is more common in persons of Mediterranean, Middle Eastern, and Far Eastern descent. Approximately 50% of these persons have circulating autoantibodies to human oral mucosa. The clinical features are quite varied. The presence of recurrent aphthous ulcerations is essential for the diagnosis. Most of these patients have primarily oral ulcerations, although genital ulcerations are more specific for the diagnosis. The ulcers are generally painful, can be shallow or deep, and last for 1 or 2 weeks. Other skin involvement may occur, including folliculitis, erythema nodosum, and vasculitis. Eye involvement is the most dreaded complication because it may progress rapidly to blindness. It often presents as panuveitis, iritis, retinal vessel occlusion, or optic neuritis. This patient also presents with superficial venous thrombosis. Superficial and deep venous thromboses are present in one-fourth of these patients. Neurologic involvement occurs in up to 10%. Laboratory findings are nonspecific with elevations in the ESR and the white blood cell count. Bullous pemphigoid is a polymorphic autoimmune subepidermal blistering disease usually seen in the elderly. Initial lesions may consist of urticarial plaques; most patients eventually display tense blisters on either normal-appearing or erythematous skin. The lesions are usually distributed over the lower abdomen, groin, and flexor surface of the extremities; oral mucosal lesions are found in some patients. Discoid lupus erythematosus is the cutaneous form of SLE and is characterized by atrophic, depigmented plaques and patches surrounded by hyperpigmentation and erythema in association with scarring and alopecia.

IX-56. The answer is E. *(Chap. 387)* Superficial or deep peripheral vein thrombosis is seen in 30% of patients. Pulmonary emboli are a rare complication. The superior vena cava is obstructed occasionally, producing a dramatic clinical picture. Arterial involvement occurs in less than 5% of patients and presents with aortitis or peripheral arterial aneurysm and arterial thrombosis. Pulmonary artery vasculitis presenting with dyspnea, cough, chest pain, hemoptysis, and infiltrates on chest roentgenograms has been reported in 5% of patients and should be differentiated from thromboembolic disease because it warrants anti-inflammatory and not thrombolytic therapy. Neurologic involvement (5%–10%)

appears mainly in the parenchymal form (80%); it is associated with brainstem involvement and has a serious prognosis (central nervous system [CNS]-Behçet disease). IL-6 is persistently raised in cerebrospinal fluid of these patients. Cerebral venous thrombosis is most frequently observed in the superior sagittal and transverse sinuses and is associated with headache and increased intracranial pressure. MRI and/or proton magnetic resonance spectroscopy are very sensitive and should be employed if CNS-Behçet disease is suspected. Gastrointestinal involvement is seen more frequently in patients from Japan and consists of mucosal ulcerations of the gut, resembling Crohn disease. Epididymitis is seen in 5% of patients, whereas amyloidosis of AA type and glomerulonephritis are uncommon.

IX-57. The answer is B. *(Chap. 388)* When patients present with proximal muscle weakness and myositis, whether polymyositis, dermatomyositis, or inclusion body myositis, the diagnosis is confirmed by analysis of serum muscle enzymes, electromyography (EMG) findings, and muscle biopsy. The most sensitive serum enzyme is creatinine kinase (CK), which can be elevated as much as 50-fold in active disease. CK levels usually parallel disease activity, but can be normal in some patients with inclusion body myositis or dermatomyositis. CK is always elevated in active polymyositis and thus is considered most sensitive. Other enzymes may be elevated as well, including glutamic-oxaloacetic transaminase, glutamate pyruvate transaminase, lactate dehydrogenase, and aldolase.

IX-58. The answer is C. *(Chap. 388)* Various autoantibodies against nuclear antigens (e.g.m ANAs) and cytoplasmic antigens are found in up to 20% of patients with inflammatory myopathies. The antibodies to cytoplasmic antigens are directed against ribonucleoproteins involved in protein synthesis (antisynthetases) or translational transport (anti–signal-recognition particles). The antibody directed against the histidyl-transfer RNA synthetase, called anti-Jo-1, accounts for 75% of all the antisynthetases and is clinically useful because up to 80% of patients with this autoantibody will have interstitial lung disease. Patients with anti-Jo-1 may also have Raynaud phenomenon, nonerosive arthritis, and the MHC molecules DR3 and DRw52. Interstitial lung disease associated with anti-Jo-1 is often rapidly progressive and fatal, even if treated aggressively with cyclophosphamide or other immunosuppressants.

IX-59. The answer is A. *(Chap. 388)* Dermatomyositis is associated with malignancy in up to 15% of cases; thus, age-appropriate cancer screening is indicated when this diagnosis is made. Exhaustive cancer searches are not recommended, however. Dermatomyositis may be associated occasionally with scleroderma and mixed connective tissue disease, but less frequently with SLE, RA, or Sjögren syndrome, which are more closely associated with polymyositis or inclusion body myositis (IBM). Viruses may be associated with IBM and polymyositis but are not proven to be associated with dermatomyositis. Parasites and bacteria such as cestodes and nematodes are associated with polymyositis, but not other forms of inflammatory myopathy. Finally, thyroid-stimulating immunoglobulins are not known to be associated with dermatomyositis.

IX-60. The answer is A. *(Chap. 388)* Mild statin-induced myopathy is noninflammatory and usually resolves with discontinuation of therapy. In rare patients, however, muscle weakness continues to progress even after the statin is withdrawn; in these cases, a diagnostic muscle biopsy is indicated and search for antibodies to 3-hydroxy-3-methylglutarylcoenzyme A reductase (HMGCR) is suggested; if histologic evidence of polymyositis or necrotizing myositis is present, immunotherapy should be initiated. ANA may be present but is nonspecific in these cases. Anti-Jo-1 antibodies are associated with the antisynthetase syndromes where myositis is usually accompanied by interstitial lung disease and stereotypical skin changes. Antibodies against signal recognition particle (SRP) are not associated with statin-induced myopathy.

IX-61. The answer is E. *(Chap. 389)* Relapsing polychondritis most often presents with recurrent painful swelling of the ear. Although other cartilaginous sites may be involved such as the nose and the tracheobronchial tree, these are less frequent. Episodes of ear involvement may result in floppy ears. Typically the pinna is affected while the earlobe is spared because there is no cartilage in the lobe. Cogan syndrome is a rare vasculitic syndrome involving hearing loss, but cartilage inflammation is not a feature. Recurrent trauma or irritation is a consideration, but the history is not suggestive, and it would less likely be bilateral and accompanied by inflammatory findings and a relatively spared earlobe.

IX-62. The answer is E. *(Chap. 390)* Despite multiple investigations, the cause of sarcoidosis remains unknown. Currently, the most likely etiology is an infectious or noninfectious environmental agent that triggers an inflammatory response in a genetically susceptible host. Among the possible infectious agents, careful studies have shown a much higher incidence of *Propionibacterium acnes* in the lymph nodes of sarcoidosis patients compared to controls. An animal model has shown that *P acnes* can induce a granulomatous response in mice similar to sarcoidosis. Others have demonstrated the presence of a mycobacterial protein (*Mycobacterium tuberculosis* catalase-peroxidase [mKatG]) in the granulomas of some sarcoidosis patients. This protein is very resistant to degradation and may represent the persistent antigen in sarcoidosis. Immune response to this and other mycobacterial proteins has been documented by another laboratory. These studies suggest that a *Mycobacterium* similar to *M tuberculosis* could be responsible for sarcoidosis. The mechanism of exposure/infection with such agents has been the focus of other studies. Environmental exposures to insecticides and mold have been associated with an increased risk for disease. In addition, healthcare workers appear to have an increased risk. Also, sarcoidosis in a donor organ has occurred after transplantation into a sarcoidosis patient. Some authors have suggested that sarcoidosis is not due to a single agent but represents a particular host response to multiple agents. Some studies have been able to correlate the environmental exposures to genetic markers. These studies have supported the hypothesis that a genetically susceptible host is a key factor in the disease. Although helper T cells may be increased, particularly in the lung of patients with sarcoidosis, it is not a monoclonal or malignant expansion of cells.

IX-63. The answer is D. *(Chap. 390)* Lung involvement occurs in >90% of sarcoidosis patients and is by far the most common manifestation of sarcoidosis. Characteristic computed tomography (CT) features include peribronchial thickening and reticular nodular changes, which are predominantly subpleural. The peribronchial thickening seen on CT scan seems to explain the high yield of granulomas from bronchial biopsies performed for diagnosis. Usually the infiltrates in sarcoidosis are predominantly an upper lobe process. Approximately one-half of sarcoidosis patients present with obstructive disease, reflected by a reduced ratio of forced expiratory volume in 1 second to forced vital capacity. Cough is a common symptom. Airway involvement causing varying degrees of obstruction underlies the cough in most sarcoidosis patients. Pulmonary arterial hypertension is reported in at least 5% of sarcoidosis patients. Either direct vascular involvement or the consequence of fibrotic changes in the lung can lead to pulmonary arterial hypertension. In sarcoidosis patients with end-stage fibrosis awaiting lung transplant, 70% will have pulmonary arterial hypertension. This is a much higher incidence than that reported for other fibrotic lung diseases. In less advanced, but still symptomatic, patients, pulmonary arterial hypertension has been noted in up to 50% of the cases. Because sarcoidosis-associated pulmonary arterial hypertension may respond to therapy, evaluation for this should be considered in persistently dyspneic patients.

IX-64. The answer is D. *(Chap. 390)* Hypercalcemia and/or hypercalciuria occurs in about 10% of sarcoidosis patients. It is more common in whites than African Americans and in men. The mechanism of abnormal calcium metabolism is increased production of 1,25-dihydroxyvitamin D by the granuloma itself. The 1,25-dihydroxyvitamin D causes increased intestinal absorption of calcium, leading to hypercalcemia with a suppressed parathyroid hormone (PTH) level. Increased exogenous vitamin D from diet or sunlight exposure may exacerbate this problem. Serum calcium should be determined as part of the initial evaluation of all sarcoidosis patients, and a repeat determination may be useful during the summer months with increased sun exposure.

IX-65. The answer is C. *(Chap. 390)* The presence of cardiac involvement is influenced by race. Although over a quarter of Japanese sarcoidosis patients develop cardiac disease, only 5% of sarcoidosis patients in the United States and Europe develop symptomatic cardiac disease. However, there is no apparent racial predilection between whites and African Americans.

IX-66. The answer is E. *(Chap. 390)* Cardiac sarcoidosis classically presents as either congestive heart failure or cardiac arrhythmias, which results from infiltration of the heart muscle by granulomas. Valvular, coronary, or pericardial involvement with granulomatous disease has also been described. Diffuse granulomatous involvement of the heart muscle can lead to profound dysfunction with left ventricular ejection fractions below 10%. Even in this situation, improvement in the ejection fraction can occur with systemic therapy. Arrhythmias can also occur with diffuse infiltration or with more patchy cardiac involvement. If the atrioventricular node is infiltrated, heart block can occur, which can be detected by routine electrocardiography. Ventricular arrhythmias and sudden death due to ventricular tachycardia are common causes of death. Arrhythmias are best detected using 24-hour ambulatory monitoring, and electrophysiology studies may be negative. Other screening tests for cardiac disease include routine electrocardiography and echocardiography. The confirmation of cardiac sarcoidosis is usually performed with either MRI or positron emission tomography (PET) scanning.

IX-67. The answer is D. *(Chap. 391e)* This patient has IgG4-related disease (IgG4-RD). IgG4-RD is a fibroinflammatory condition characterized by a tendency to form tumefactive lesions. The clinical manifestations of this disease, however, are protean and continue to be defined. Pancreatic and retroperitoneal involvement is well described and may present as type 1 autoimmune pancreatitis, presenting as mild abdominal pain, weight loss, and acute, obstructive jaundice, mimicking adenocarcinoma of the pancreas (including a pancreatic mass). Imaging shows diffuse (termed *sausage-shaped pancreas*) or segmental pancreatic enlargement, with loss of normal lobularity; a mass often raises the suspicion of malignancy. The key histopathology characteristics of IgG4-RD are a dense lymphoplasmacytic infiltrate that is organized in a storiform pattern (resembling a basket weave), obliterative phlebitis, and a mild to moderate eosinophilic infiltrate. The inflammatory infiltrate is composed of an admixture of B and T lymphocytes. B cells are typically organized in germinal centers. Plasma cells staining for CD19, CD138, and IgG4 appear to radiate out from the germinal centers. Vital organ involvement must be treated aggressively, however, because IgG4-RD can lead to serious organ dysfunction and failure. Aggressive disease can lead quickly to end-stage liver disease, permanent impairment of pancreatic function, renal atrophy, aortic dissection or aneurysms, and destructive lesions in the sinuses and nasopharynx. Glucocorticoids are the first line of therapy. Treatment regimens, extrapolated from experience with the management of autoimmune pancreatitis, generally begin with 40 mg/d of prednisone, with tapering to discontinuation or maintenance doses of 5 mg/d within 2 or 3 months. The clinical response to glucocorticoids is usually swift and striking; however, longitudinal data indicate that disease flares occur in more than 90% of patients within 3 years. Conventional steroid-sparing agents such as azathioprine and mycophenolate mofetil have been used in some patients; however, evidence for their efficacy is lacking.

IX-68. The answer is A. *(Chap. 392)* Familial Mediterranean fever (FMF) is the prototype of a group of inherited diseases that are characterized by recurrent episodes of fever with serosal, synovial, or cutaneous inflammation. The FMF gene encodes a 781-amino acid, ~95-kDa protein denoted pyrin (or marenostrin) that is expressed in granulocytes, eosinophils, monocytes, dendritic cells, and synovial and peritoneal fibroblasts. Typical FMF episodes generally last 24–72 hours, with arthritic attacks tending to last somewhat longer. In some patients, the episodes occur with great regularity, but more often, the frequency of attacks varies over time, ranging from as often as once every few days to remissions lasting several years. Attacks are often unpredictable, although some patients relate them to physical exertion, emotional stress, or menses; pregnancy may be associated with remission.

If measured, fever is nearly always present throughout FMF attacks. Severe hyperpyrexia and even febrile seizures may be seen in infants, and fever is sometimes the only manifestation of FMF in young children. Over 90% of FMF patients experience abdominal attacks at some time. Episodes range in severity from dull, aching pain and distention with mild tenderness on direct palpation to severe generalized pain with absent bowel sounds, rigidity, rebound tenderness, and air-fluid levels on upright radiographs. CT scanning may demonstrate a small amount of fluid in the abdominal cavity. If such patients undergo exploratory laparotomy, a sterile, neutrophil-rich peritoneal exudate is present, sometimes with adhesions from previous episodes. Ascites is rare. Exercise-induced (nonfebrile) myalgia is common in FMF, and a small percentage of patients develop a protracted febrile myalgia that can last several weeks.

IX-69. The answer is A. *(Chap. 392)* The treatment of choice for FMF is daily oral colchicine, which decreases the frequency and intensity of attacks and prevents the development of amyloidosis in compliant patients. Intermittent dosing at the onset of attacks is not as effective as daily prophylaxis and is of unproven value in preventing amyloidosis. The usual adult dose of colchicine is 1.2–1.8 mg/d, which causes substantial reduction in symptoms in two-thirds of patients and some improvement in >90%. Children may require lower doses, although not proportionately to body weight.

IX-70. The answer is E. *(Chap. 394)* Osteoarthritis (OA) affects certain joints, yet spares others. Commonly, affected joints include the cervical and lumbosacral spine, hip, knee, and first metatarsal phalangeal joint (MTP). In the hands, the distal and proximal interphalangeal joints and the base of the thumb are often affected. Usually spared are the wrist, elbow, and ankle. Human joints were designed, in an evolutionary sense, for brachiating apes, animals that still walked on four limbs. We thus develop OA in joints that were ill designed for human tasks such as pincer grip (OA in the thumb base) and walking upright (OA in knees and hips). Some joints, like the ankles, may be spared because their articular cartilage may be uniquely resistant to loading stresses. See Figure IX-70.

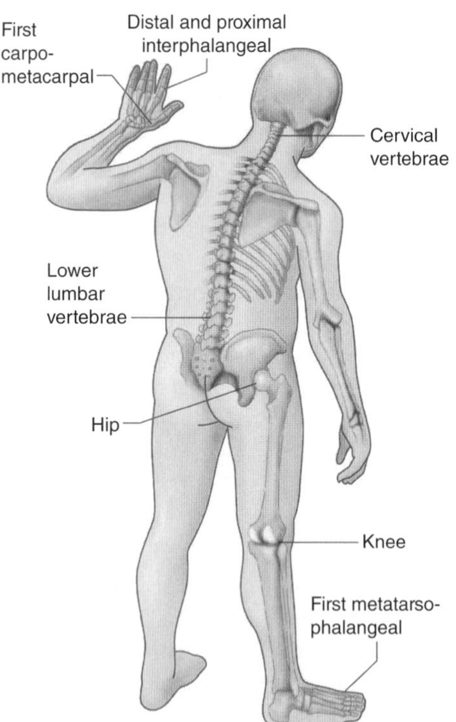

FIGURE IX-70

IX-71. The answer is D. *(Chap. 394)* Examination of the synovial fluid is often helpful in suspected osteoarthritis, particularly if inflammatory disease is possible. If the synovial fluid white blood cell count is >1000/μL, inflammatory arthritis, gout, or pseudogout is likely, with the latter two being also identified by the presence of crystals. Because cartilage is aneural, cartilage loss in a joint is not accompanied by pain. Thus, pain in OA likely arises from structures outside the cartilage. Innervated structures in the joint include the synovium, ligaments, joint capsule, muscles, and subchondral bone. Most of these are not visualized by the x-ray, and the severity of radiographic changes in OA correlates poorly with pain severity. OA is the most common type of arthritis. Its high prevalence, especially in the elderly, and the high rate of disability related to disease make it a leading cause of disability in the elderly. Although MRI may reveal the extent of pathology in an osteoarthritic joint, it is not indicated as part of the diagnostic workup.

IX-72. The answer is C. *(Chap. 394)* Recent guidelines recommend against the use of glucosamine or chondroitin for OA. Large publicly supported trials have failed to show that, compared with placebo, these compounds relieve pain in persons with disease. Glucocorticoid injections are efficacious in OA, but response is variable, with some patients having little relief of pain, whereas others experience pain relief lasting several months. Glucocorticoid injections are useful to get patients over acute flares of pain and may be especially indicated if the patient has coexistent OA and crystal deposition disease, especially from calcium pyrophosphate dihydrate crystals. Acetaminophen (paracetamol) is the initial analgesic of choice for patients with OA in knees, hips, or hands. For some patients, it is adequate to control symptoms, in which case more toxic drugs such as NSAIDs can be avoided. Doses up to 1 g three times daily can be used. NSAIDs are the most popular drugs to treat osteoarthritic pain. They can be administered either topically or orally. In clinical trials, oral NSAIDs produced approximately 30% greater improvement in pain than high-dose acetaminophen. Ultimately, when the patient with knee or hip OA has failed medical treatment modalities and remains in pain, with limitations of physical function that compromise the quality of life, the patient should be referred for total knee or hip arthroplasty. These are highly efficacious operations that relieve pain and improve function in the vast majority of patients, although rates of success are higher for hip than knee replacement.

IX-73. The answer is E. *(Chap. 395)* Figure IX-73B illustrates extracellular and intracellular monosodium urate crystals, as seen in a fresh preparation of synovial fluid. This is gout. Most patients with gout are overproducers of uric acid. Hyaline cartilage degeneration is typical of osteoarthritis, which usually has a bland synovial aspirate. Antibodies to ANA are typical of lupus, rare in an elderly man, and not associated with crystalline fluid. Bacterial joint infection would have a purulent synovial fluid. Increased production of inorganic pyrophosphate is a cause of calcium pyrophosphate deposition disease (CPPD; pseudogout), another crystalline arthropathy. CPPD crystals are shown in Figure IX-73B.

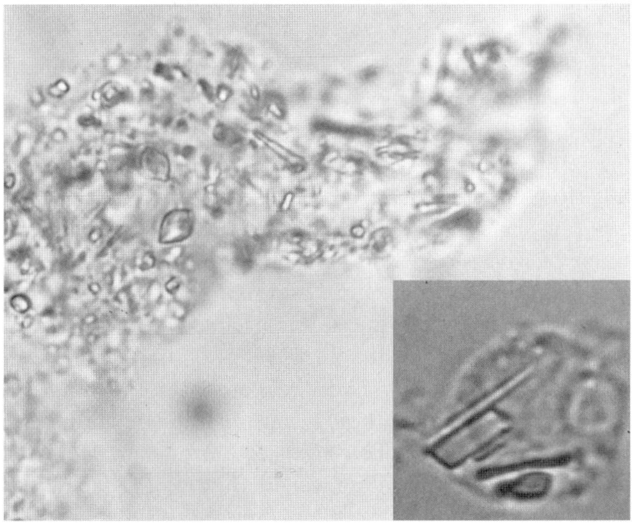

FIGURE IX-73B

IX-74. The answer is C. *(Chap. 395)* The xanthine oxidase inhibitor allopurinol is by far the most commonly used hypouricemic agent and is the best drug to lower serum urate in overproducers, urate stone formers, and patients with renal disease. It can be given in a single morning dose, usually 100 mg initially and increasing up to 800 mg if needed. In patients with chronic renal disease, the initial allopurinol dose should be lower and adjusted depending on the serum creatinine concentration; for example, with a creatinine clearance of 10 mL/min, one generally would use 100 mg every other day. Doses can be increased gradually to reach the target urate level of <6 mg/dL. Toxicity of allopurinol has been recognized increasingly in patients who use thiazide diuretics, in patients allergic to penicillin and ampicillin, and in Asians expressing HLA-B*5801. Colchicine is commonly used with allopurinol in the treatment of gout. Allopurinol and azathioprine should not be coprescribed because azathioprine can greatly increase blood levels of allopurinol and lead to toxicity.

IX-75. The answer is C. *(Chap. 396)* This patient presents with a characteristic history for fibromyalgia, a diffuse pain syndrome associated with increased sensitivity to evoked pain. The underlying pathophysiology of pain in fibromyalgia is felt to be related to altered pain processing in the central nervous system. Epidemiologically, women are affected nine times more frequently than men. The worldwide prevalence of fibromyalgia is 2%–3%, but in primary care practices, it is as high as 5%–10%. The disorder is even more common in patients with degenerative or inflammatory rheumatic disorders, with a prevalence of 20% or higher. The most common presenting complaint is diffuse pain that is difficult to localize. Pain is both above and below the waist and affects the extremities as well as the axial skeleton. However, it does not localize to a specific joint. The pain is noted to be severe in intensity and difficult to ignore and interferes with daily functioning. Although this patient demonstrates pain at several tender points, the American College of Rheumatology no longer includes tender point assessment in the diagnostic criteria for fibromyalgia. Rather, the new criteria focus on clinical symptoms of widespread pain and neuropsychological symptoms that have been present for at least 3 months. Some of the neuropsychological conditions that are frequently observed in fibromyalgia include sleep disturbance, impaired cognitive functioning, fatigue, stiffness, anxiety, and depression. The lifetime prevalence of mood disorders in patients with fibromyalgia is 80%. Sleep disturbances can include difficulty falling asleep, difficulty staying asleep, or nonrestorative sleep, among others.

IX-76. The answer is D. *(Chap. 396)* Fibromyalgia is a common disorder affecting 2%–5% of the population. It presents as a diffuse pain syndrome with associated neuropsychological symptoms including depression, anxiety, fatigue, cognitive dysfunction, and disturbed sleep. Treatment for fibromyalgia should include a combination of nonpharmacologic and pharmacologic approaches. Patient education regarding the disease is important to provide a framework for understanding symptoms. The focus of treatment should not be on eliminating pain, but rather improving function and quality of life. Physical conditioning is an important part of improving function and should include a multifaceted exercise program with aerobic exercise, strength training, and exercises that incorporate relaxation techniques such as yoga or tai chi. Cognitive behavioral therapy can be useful in improving sleep disturbance and also for decreasing illness behaviors. Pharmacologic therapy in fibromyalgia is targeted at the afferent and efferent pain pathways. The two most common categories of medications for fibromyalgia are antidepressants and anticonvulsants. Amitriptyline, duloxetine, and milnacipran have all been used with some efficacy in fibromyalgia. Duloxetine and milnacipran are approved by the U.S. Food and Drug Administration (FDA) for the treatment of fibromyalgia. The anticonvulsants that are predominantly used in fibromyalgia are those that are ligands of the α-2-δ subunit of voltage-gated calcium channels. These include gabapentin and pregabalin, which is also FDA approved for treatment of fibromyalgia. Anti-inflammatory medications and glucocorticoids are not effective in fibromyalgia. However, if there is a comorbid triggering condition such as RA, appropriate therapy directed at the underlying disorder is critical to controlling symptoms of fibromyalgia as well. Opioid analgesics such as oxycodone should be avoided. They have no efficacy in treating fibromyalgia and may induce hyperalgesia that can worsen both pain and function.

IX-77. The answer is A. *(Chap. 396)* Fibromyalgia is characterized by chronic widespread musculoskeletal pain, stiffness, paresthesia, disturbed sleep, and easy fatigability. It occurs in a 9:1 female-to-male ratio. It is not confined to any particular region, ethnicity, or climate. Although the pathogenesis is not clear, there are associations with disturbed sleep and abnormal pain perception. Fibromyalgia is diagnosed by the presence of widespread pain, a history of widespread musculoskeletal pain that has been present for >3 months, and presence of neuropsychological dysfunction (fatigue, waking unrefreshed, or cognitive symptoms). In the prior diagnostic criteria, it was required to demonstrate pain on palpation at 11 of 18 tender point sites. However, this was abandoned in the updated criteria because it was felt that strict application of a threshold of pain could lead to underdiagnosis of the disorder. Besides pain on palpation, the neurologic and musculoskeletal examinations are normal in patients with fibromyalgia. Psychiatric illnesses, particularly depression and anxiety disorders, are common comorbidities in these patients but do not help satisfy any diagnostic criteria.

IX-78. The answer is A. *(Chap. 397)* The finding shown in Figure IX-78 is characteristic of clubbing. Clubbing occurs in the distal portions of the digits and is characterized by widening of the fingertips, convexity of the nail contour, and loss of the normal 15-degree angle between the proximal nail and cuticle. Clinically, it can be sometimes difficult to ascertain whether clubbing is present. One approach to the diagnosis of clubbing is to measure the diameter of the finger at the base of the nail and at the tip of the finger in all 10 fingers. For each finger, a ratio between the base of the nail and the tip of the finger is determined. If the sum of all 10 fingers is greater than 1, then clubbing is felt to be present. A simpler approach is to have an individual place the dorsal surfaces of the distal fourth digits from each hand together. In a normal individual, there should be a diamond-shaped space between the digits. When an individual has clubbing, this space is obliterated. Clubbing most commonly occurs in advanced lung disease, especially bronchiectasis, cystic fibrosis, and interstitial lung diseases like sarcoidosis or idiopathic pulmonary fibrosis. Clubbing was originally described in individuals with empyema and can occur in chronic lung infections, including lung abscess, tuberculosis, or fungal infections. Pulmonary vascular lesions and lung cancer also are associated with clubbing. However, chronic obstructive pulmonary disease does not cause clubbing. However, the causes of clubbing are not limited to the pulmonary system alone. Clubbing can be a benign familial condition and is also associated with a variety of other disorders, including cyanotic congenital heart disease, subacute bacterial endocarditis, Crohn disease, ulcerative colitis, celiac disease, and cancer of the esophagus, liver, small bowel, and large bowel. In untreated hyperthyroidism, clubbing can occur in association with periostitis in a condition called thyroid acropachy. Although these numerous clinical associations have been described for many centuries, the cause of clubbing remains unknown.

IX-79. The answer is C. *(Chap. 397)* Symptoms of hemochromatosis usually begin between the ages of 40 and 60 but can appear earlier. Arthropathy, which occurs in 20%–40% of patients, usually begins after the age of 50 and may be the first clinical feature of hemochromatosis. The arthropathy is an osteoarthritis-like disorder affecting the small joints of the hands and later the larger joints, such as knees, ankles, shoulders, and hips. The second and third metacarpophalangeal joints of both hands are often the first and most prominent joints affected; this clinical picture may provide an important clue to the possibility of hemochromatosis because these joints are not predominantly affected by "routine" osteoarthritis. Patients experience some morning stiffness and pain with use of involved joints. The affected joints are enlarged and mildly tender. Radiographs show narrowing of the joint space, subchondral sclerosis, subchondral cysts, and juxta-articular proliferation of bone. Hooklike osteophytes are seen in up to 20% of patients; although they are regarded as a characteristic feature of hemochromatosis, they can also occur in osteoarthritis and are not disease specific. Bony erosions are typical of rheumatoid arthritis, not hemochromatosis. The synovial fluid is noninflammatory. In approximately half of patients, there is evidence of calcium pyrophosphate deposition disease, and some patients experience episodes of acute pseudogout late in the course of disease *(Chap. 395)*. The treatment of hemochromatosis is repeated phlebotomy. Unfortunately, this treatment has little effect on established arthritis, which, along with chondrocalcinosis, may progress.

Symptom-based treatment of the arthritis consists of administration of acetaminophen and NSAIDs, as tolerated. Acute pseudogout attacks are treated with high doses of an NSAID or a short course of glucocorticoids. Hip or knee total joint replacement has been successful in advanced disease.

IX-80. The answer is E. *(Chap. 398)* Trochanteric bursitis is a common cause of hip pain and results from inflammation within the bursa that surrounds the insertion of the gluteus medius onto the greater trochanter of the femur. Bursae lie throughout the body with the purpose of facilitating movement of tendons and muscles over bony prominences. Bursitis has many causes, including overuse, trauma, systemic disease, or infection. Trochanteric bursitis typically presents with acute or subacute hip pain with a varying quality. The pain localizes to the lateral aspect of the hip and upper thigh. Direct palpation over the posterior aspect of the greater trochanter reproduces the pain, and often sleeping on the affected side is painful. Pain is also elicited with external rotation and resisted abduction of the hip. Treatment of trochanteric bursitis includes use of NSAIDs and avoidance of overuse. If the pain persists, steroid injection into the affected bursa may be beneficial.

Other causes of hip pain include osteoarthritis, avascular necrosis, meralgia paresthetica, septic arthritis, occult hip fracture, and referred pain from lumbar spine disease. In patients with true disorders of the hip joint such as osteoarthritis, avascular necrosis, and occult hip fracture, the pain is most commonly localized to the groin area. Meralgia paresthetica (lateral femoral nerve entrapment syndrome) causes a neuropathic pain in the upper outer thigh with symptoms ranging from tingling sensations to a burning pain. When degenerative spinal disease is the cause of referred hip pain, there is typically back pain as well. In addition, palpation over the lateral joint would not reproduce the pain. Iliotibial band syndrome causes lateral knee pain but not hip pain.

IX-81. The answer is B. *(Chap. 398)* The iliotibial band is comprised of thick connective tissue that runs along the outer thigh from the ilium to the fibula. When this band becomes tightened or inflamed, pain most commonly occurs where the band passes over the lateral femoral condyle of the knee, leading to a burning or aching pain in this area that can radiate toward the outer thigh. This overuse injury is most often seen in runners and can be caused by improperly fitted shoes, running on uneven surfaces, and excessive running. It is also more common in individuals with a varus alignment of the knee (bowlegged). Treatment of iliotibial band syndrome involves rest, NSAIDs, physical therapy, and addressing risk factors such as poorly fitted shoes or uneven running surface. Glucocorticoid injection at the lateral femoral condyle may alleviate pain, but running must strictly be avoided for 2 weeks following injection. In refractory cases, surgical release of the iliotibial band may be beneficial.

IX-82. The answer is A. *(Chap. 398)* Adhesive capsulitis is characterized by pain and restricted motion of the shoulder. Usually this occurs in the absence of intrinsic shoulder disease, including osteoarthritis and avascular necrosis. It is, however, more common in patients who have had bursitis or tendinitis previously as well as patients with other systemic illnesses, such as chronic pulmonary disease, ischemic heart disease, and diabetes mellitus. The etiology is not clear, but adhesive capsulitis appears to develop in the setting of prolonged immobility. Reflex sympathetic dystrophy may also occur in the setting of adhesive capsulitis. Clinically, this disorder is more commonly seen in females over age 50. Pain and stiffness develop over the course of months to years. On physical examination, the affected joint is tender to palpation, with a restricted range of motion. The gold standard for diagnosis is arthrography with limitation of the amount of injectable contrast to less than 15 mL. In most patients, adhesive capsulitis will regress spontaneously within 1 to 3 years. NSAIDs, glucocorticoid injections, physical therapy, and early mobilization of the arm are useful therapies.

IX-83. The answer is B. *(Chap. 398)* Inflammation of the abductor pollicis longus and the extensor pollicis brevis at the radial styloid process tendon sheath is known as De Quervain tenosynovitis. Repetitive twisting of the wrist can lead to this condition. Pain occurs when grasping with the thumb and can extend radially along the wrist to the radial styloid process.

Mothers often develop this tenosynovitis by holding their babies with the thumb outstretched. The Finkelstein sign is positive in De Quervain tenosynovitis. It is positive if the patient develops pain by placing the thumb in the palm, closing the fingers around the thumb, and deviating the wrist in the ulnar direction. Management of De Quervain tenosynovitis includes NSAIDs and splinting. Glucocorticoid injections can be effective. A Phalen maneuver is used to diagnose carpal tunnel syndrome and does not elicit pain. The wrists are flexed for 60 seconds to compress the median nerve to elicit numbness, burning, or tingling. Gouty arthritis will present with an acutely inflamed joint with crystal-laden fluid. Rheumatoid arthritis is a systemic illness with characteristic joint synovitis and radiographic features.

IX-84. **The answer is C.** *(Chap. 398)* Ms. Rumpulo has plantar fasciitis, a diagnosis that often can be made clinically. It is a common cause of foot pain in adults, with the peak incidence occurring in people between the ages of 40 and 60 years. The pain originates at or near the site of the plantar fascia attachment to the medial tuberosity of the calcaneus. Several factors that increase the risk of developing plantar fasciitis include obesity, pes planus (flat foot or absence of the foot arch when standing), pes cavus (high-arched foot), limited dorsiflexion of the ankle, prolonged standing, walking on hard surfaces, and faulty shoes. In runners, excessive running and a change to a harder running surface may precipitate plantar fasciitis. Smoking and oral contraceptives are not specific risk factors. Patients experience severe pain with the first steps on arising in the morning or following inactivity during the day. The pain usually lessens with weight-bearing activity during the day, only to worsen with continued activity. Pain is made worse on walking barefoot or up stairs. On examination, maximal tenderness is elicited on palpation over the inferior heel corresponding to the site of attachment of the plantar fascia. Imaging studies may be indicated when the diagnosis is not clear. Plain radiographs may show heel spurs, which are of little diagnostic significance. Ultrasonography in plantar fasciitis can demonstrate thickening of the fascia and diffuse hypoechogenicity, indicating edema at the attachment of the plantar fascia to the calcaneus. MRI is a sensitive method for detecting plantar fasciitis, but it is usually not required for establishing the diagnosis. The differential diagnosis of inferior heel pain includes calcaneal stress fractures, the spondyloarthritides, rheumatoid arthritis, gout, neoplastic or infiltrative bone processes, and nerve compression/entrapment syndromes.

Resolution of plantar fasciitis symptoms occurs within 12 months in more than 80% of patients. Initial treatment consists of ice, heat, massage, and stretching. Orthotics providing medial arch support can be effective. A short course of NSAIDs can be given to patients when the benefits outweigh the risks. Local glucocorticoid injections have also been shown to be efficacious but may carry an increased risk for plantar fascia rupture. Plantar fasciotomy is reserved for those patients who have failed to improve after at least 6–12 months of conservative treatment.

SECTION X

Endocrinology and Metabolism

QUESTIONS

DIRECTIONS: Choose the one best response to each question.

X-1. All of the following hormones is produced by the anterior pituitary EXCEPT:

A. Adrenocorticotropic hormone
B. Growth hormone
C. Oxytocin
D. Prolactin
E. Thyroid-stimulating hormone

X-2. A 45-year-old man reports to his primary care physician that his wife has noted coarsening of his facial features over several years. In addition, he reports low libido and decreased energy. Physical examination shows frontal bossing and enlarged hands. An MRI confirms that he has a pituitary mass. Which of the following screening tests should be ordered to diagnose the cause of the mass?

A. 24-Hour urinary free cortisol
B. Adrenocorticotropic hormone (ACTH) assay
C. Growth hormone level
D. Serum insulin-like growth factor-1 (IGF-1) level
E. Serum prolactin level

X-3. Which of the following statements regarding the anatomy of the pituitary gland is true?

A. Growth hormone is derived from the precursor proopiomelanocortin (POMC).
B. Prolactin-secreting cells form the majority of cells in the anterior pituitary.
C. The anterior pituitary secretes hormones directly synthesized in neuroendocrine cells in the hypothalamus.
D. The pituitary gland forms from the Rathke pouch embryonically.
E. The posterior pituitary has dual arterial blood supply.

X-4. A 58-year-old man undergoes severe head trauma and develops pituitary insufficiency. After recovery, he is placed on thyroid hormone, testosterone, glucocorticoids, and vasopressin. On a routine visit, he questions his primary care physician regarding potential growth hormone deficiency. All of the following are potential signs or symptoms of growth hormone deficiency EXCEPT:

A. Abnormal lipid profile
B. Atherosclerosis
C. Increased bone mineral density
D. Increased waist-to-hip ratio
E. Left ventricular dysfunction

X-5. A 75-year-old man presents with development of abdominal obesity, proximal myopathy, and skin hyperpigmentation. His laboratory evaluation shows a hypokalemic metabolic alkalosis. Cushing syndrome is suspected. Which of the following statements regarding this syndrome is true?

A. Basal ACTH level is likely to be low.
B. Circulating corticotropin-releasing hormone is likely to be elevated.
C. Pituitary magnetic resonance imaging (MRI) will visualize all ACTH-secreting tumors.
D. Referral for urgent performance of inferior petrosal venous sampling is indicated.
E. Serum potassium level <3.3 mmol/L is suggestive of ectopic ACTH production.

X-6. Which of the following is common in patients with Kallmann syndrome?

A. Anosmia
B. A white forelock
C. Precocious (early) puberty in females
D. Syndactyly in males
E. Hyperphagic obesity

X-7. A 22-year-old woman who is otherwise healthy undergoes an uneventful vaginal delivery of a full-term infant. One day postpartum, she complains of visual changes and severe headache. Two hours after these complaints, she is found unresponsive and profoundly hypotensive. She is intubated and placed on mechanical ventilation. Her blood pressure is 68/28 mmHg, regular heart rate is 148 bpm, her oxygen saturation is 95% on fraction of inspired oxygen (FiO_2) of 0.40. Physical exam is unremarkable. Her laboratory tests are notable for glucose of 49 mg/dL, with normal hematocrit and white blood cell count. Which of the following is most likely to reverse her hypotension?

A. Activated drotrecogin alfa
B. Hydrocortisone
C. Piperacillin/tazobactam
D. Thyroxine (T_4)
E. Transfusion of packed red blood cells

X-8. You are caring for Mr. Gelston, a 19-year-old man who had a brain tumor when young and underwent cranial radiation. You note that he has short stature and has not yet gone through puberty. You suspect that he has pituitary insufficiency due to radiation. Which of the following is true regarding acquired hypopituitarism due to radiation?

A. At a dose of 50 Gy of radiation, only 5% of patients will manifest hypopituitarism.
B. The majority of patients who develop hypopituitarism after cranial radiation, do so within a year of treatment.
C. Growth hormone is the most common hormonal deficiency.
D. There is no correlation between radiation dose and likelihood of developing hypopituitarism.
E. Older adults are at highest risk from radiation-induced hypopituitarism.

X-9. A 23-year-old college student is followed in the student health center for medical management of panhypopituitarism after resection of craniopharyngioma as a child. She reports moderate compliance with her medications but feels generally well. Thyroid-stimulating hormone (TSH) is checked and is below the limits of detection of the assay. Which of the following is the next most appropriate action?

A. Decrease levothyroxine dose to half of current dose
B. Do nothing
C. Order free T_4 level
D. Order MRI of her brain
E. Order thyroid uptake scan

X-10. A patient visited a local emergency department 1 week ago with a headache. She received a head MRI, which did not reveal a cause for her symptoms, but the final report states "An empty sella is noted. Advise clinical correlation." The patient was discharged from the emergency department with instructions to follow up with her primary care physician as soon as possible. Her headache has resolved, and the patient has no complaints. However, she comes to your office 1 day later very concerned about this unexpected MRI finding. What should be the next step in her management?

A. Diagnose her with subclinical panhypopituitarism, and initiate low-dose hormone replacement.
B. Reassure her and follow laboratory results closely.
C. Reassure her and repeat MRI in 6 months.
D. This may represent early endocrine malignancy, so whole-body positron emission tomography (PET)/computed tomography (CT) is indicated.
E. This MRI finding likely represents the presence of a benign adenoma, so she should be referred to neurosurgery for resection.

X-11. Pituitary adenomas typically expand in which direction?

A. Anteriorly
B. Inferiorly
C. Laterally
D. Posteriorly
E. Superiorly

X-12. On MRI of the pituitary, which of the following findings is abnormal in an adult?

A. A slightly concave upper aspect of the pituitary
B. Brighter T1 intensity of the posterior pituitary
C. Heterogeneous anterior pituitary tissue
D. Pituitary height of 8–12 mm
E. Tissue that is lower intensity than the nearby brain tissue on T1 images and enhances on T2 images

X-13. Mr. Jones has a pituitary adenoma on imaging that has extended directly superiorly and is compressing his optic chiasm. Which of the following visual field deficits is most likely present?

A. Bilateral inferior visual field deficits
B. Bilateral superior visual field deficits
C. Bitemporal hemianopia
D. Central scotomas bilaterally
E. Right homonymous hemianopia

X-14. All of the following features are present in Carney syndrome EXCEPT:

A. Acromegaly
B. Adrenal adenomas
C. Atrial myxomas
D. Hypertrophic cardiomyopathy
E. Spotty skin pigmentation

X-15. Which of the following is the most common cause of preventable mental deficiency in the world?

A. Beriberi disease
B. Cretinism
C. Folate deficiency
D. Scurvy
E. Vitamin A deficiency

X-16. All of the following are associated with increased levels of total T_4 in the plasma with a normal free T_4 EXCEPT:

A. Cirrhosis
B. Pregnancy
C. Euthyroid sick syndrome
D. Familial dysalbuminemic hyperthyroxinemia
E. Familial excess thyroid binding globulin

X-17. Which of the following is the most common cause of hypothyroidism worldwide?

A. Graves disease
B. Hashimoto thyroiditis
C. Iatrogenic hypothyroidism
D. Iodine deficiency
E. Radiation exposure

X-18. A 75-year-old woman is diagnosed with hypothyroidism. She has longstanding coronary artery disease and is wondering about the potential consequences for her cardiovascular system. Which of the following statements is true regarding the interaction of hypothyroidism and the cardiovascular system?

A. A reduced stroke volume is found with hypothyroidism.
B. Blood flow is diverted toward the skin in hypothyroidism.
C. Myocardial contractility is increased with hypothyroidism.
D. Pericardial effusions are a rare manifestation of hypothyroidism.
E. Reduced peripheral resistance is found in hypothyroidism and may be accompanied by hypotension.

X-19. A 38-year-old mother of three presents to her primary care office with complaints of fatigue. She feels that her energy level has been low for the past 3 months. She was previously healthy and taking no medications. She does report that she has gained about 10 lb and has severe constipation, for which she has been taking a number of laxatives. A TSH is elevated at 25 mU/L. Free T_4 is low. She is wondering why she has hypothyroidism. Which of the following tests is most likely to diagnose the etiology?

A. Antithyroid peroxidase antibody
B. Antithyroglobulin antibody
C. Radioiodine uptake scan
D. Serum thyroglobulin level
E. Thyroid ultrasound

X-20. A 54-year-old woman with longstanding hypothyroidism is seen in her primary care physician's office for a routine evaluation. She reports feeling fatigued and somewhat constipated. Since her last visit, her other medical conditions, which include hypercholesterolemia and systemic hypertension, have been stable. She was diagnosed with uterine fibroids and started on iron recently. Her other medications include levothyroxine, atorvastatin, and hydrochlorothiazide. A TSH is checked, and it is elevated to 15 mU/L. Which of the following is the most likely reason for her elevated TSH?

A. Celiac disease
B. Colon cancer
C. Medication noncompliance
D. Poor absorption of levothyroxine due to ferrous sulfate
E. TSH-secreting pituitary adenoma

X-21. An 87-year-old woman is admitted to the intensive care unit with depressed level of consciousness, hypothermia, sinus bradycardia, hypotension, and hypoglycemia. She was previously healthy with the exception of hypothyroidism and systemic hypertension. Her family recently checked in on her and found that she was not taking any of her medications because of financial difficulties. There is no evidence of infection on exam, urine microscopy, or chest radiograph. Her serum chemistries are notable for mild hyponatremia and a glucose of 48 mg/dL. A TSH is >100 mU/L. All of the following statements regarding this condition are true EXCEPT:

A. External warming is a critical feature of therapy in patients with a temperature <34°C.
B. Hypotonic intravenous solutions should be avoided.
C. Intravenous (IV) levothyroxine should be administered with IV glucocorticoids.
D. Sedation should be avoided if possible.
E. This condition occurs almost exclusively in the elderly and often is precipitated by an unrelated medical illness.

X-22. A 29-year-old woman is evaluated for anxiety, palpitations, and diarrhea and found to have Graves disease. Before she begins therapy for her thyroid condition, she has an episode of acute chest pain and presents to the emergency department. Although a CT angiogram is ordered, the radiologist calls to notify the treating physician that this is potentially dangerous. Which of the following best explains the radiologist's recommendation?

A. Iodinated contrast exposure in patients with Graves disease may exacerbate hyperthyroidism.
B. Pulmonary embolism is exceedingly rare in Graves disease.
C. Radiation exposure in patients with hyperthyroidism is associated with increased risk of subsequent malignancy.
D. Tachycardia with Graves disease limits the image quality of CT angiography and will not allow accurate assessment of pulmonary embolism.
E. The radiologist was mistaken; CT angiography is safe in Graves disease.

X-23. A patient has neurosurgery for a pituitary tumor that requires resection of the gland. Which of the following functions of the adrenal gland will be preserved in this patient immediately postoperatively?

A. Morning peak of plasma cortisol level
B. Release of cortisol in response to stress
C. Sodium retention in response to hypovolemia
D. None of the above

X-24. Which of the following is the most common cause of Cushing syndrome?

A. ACTH-producing pituitary adenoma
B. Adrenocortical adenoma
C. Adrenocortical carcinoma
D. Ectopic ACTH secretion
E. McCune-Albright syndrome

X-25. All of the following are features of Conn syndrome EXCEPT:

A. Alkalosis
B. Hyperkalemia
C. Muscle cramps
D. Normal serum sodium
E. Severe systemic hypertension

X-26. All of the following statements regarding asymptomatic adrenal masses (incidentalomas) are true EXCEPT:

A. All patients with incidentalomas should be screened for pheochromocytoma.
B. Fine-needle aspiration may distinguish between benign and malignant primary adrenal tumors.
C. In patients with a history of malignancy, the likelihood that the adrenal mass is a metastasis is approximately 50%.
D. The majority of adrenal incidentalomas are nonsecretory.
E. The vast majority of adrenal incidentalomas are benign.

X-27. You are designing an experiment to determine the effect of psychosocial stress exposure on peak daily cortisol secretion. When should you measure cortisol to ensure that you are most likely assessing peak cortisol levels?

A. Midnight (12:00 AM)
B. 4:00 AM
C. 8:30 AM
D. Noon (12:00 PM)
E. 8:30 PM

X-28. Mr. McTrap is admitted to the hospital after a car accident. His medical history is unknown, and on presentation, he is obtunded and can provide no history. CT scan reveals a splenic laceration, and he is emergently taken to the operating room for splenectomy, which proceeds without complication. At the completion of the operation, all bleeding has stopped, and he returns to the intensive care unit. However, he remains deeply hypotensive with a blood pressure of 70/50 mmHg with an increase only to 82/52 mmHg after a bolus of 2 L of normal saline IV. He is afebrile with a normal white blood cell count. Repeat CT scan of the chest, abdomen, and pelvis shows no hemorrhage. Jugular venous pressure is not visible above the clavicle. He has a round face and is obese, and you note the following on physical exam (see Figure X-28).

He has no hand hyperpigmentation. What is the next most appropriate step?

A. Return to the operating room for exploratory laparotomy
B. Administer hydrocortisone 100 mg IV
C. Administer vancomycin and piperacillin/tazobactam
D. Insert intra-aortic balloon pump for counterpulsation
E. Perform MRI of the spine

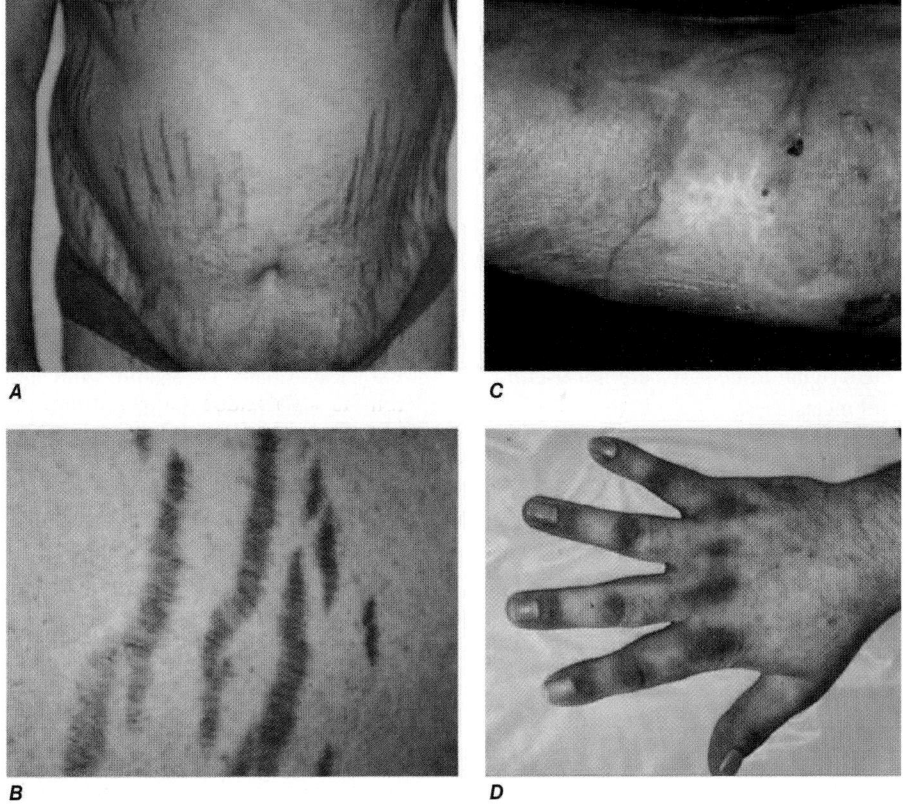

FIGURE X-28

X-29. A 43-year-old man with episodic, severe hypertension is referred for evaluation of possible secondary causes of hypertension. He reports feeling well generally, except for episodes of anxiety, palpitations, and tachycardia with elevation in his blood pressure during these episodes. Exercise often brings on these events. The patient also has mild depression and is presently taking sertraline, labetalol, amlodipine, and lisinopril to control his blood pressure. Urine 24-hour total metanephrines are ordered and show an elevation of 1.5 times the upper limit of normal. Which of the following is the next most appropriate step?

A. Hold labetalol for 1 week and repeat testing
B. Hold sertraline for 1 week and repeat testing
C. Refer immediately for surgical evaluation
D. Measure 24-hour urine vanillylmandelic acid level
E. Obtain MRI of the abdomen

X-30. A 45-year-old man is diagnosed with pheochromocytoma after presentation with confusion, marked hypertension to 250/140 mmHg, tachycardia, headaches, and flushing. His fractionated plasma metanephrines show a normetanephrine level of 560 pg/mL and a metanephrine level of 198 pg/mL (normal values: normetanephrine, 18–111 pg/mL; metanephrine, 12–60 pg/mL). CT scanning of the abdomen with IV contrast demonstrates a 3-cm mass in the right adrenal gland. A brain MRI with gadolinium shows edema of the white matter near the parieto-occipital junction consistent with reversible posterior leukoencephalopathy. You are asked to consult regarding management. Which of the following statements is true regarding management of pheochromocytoma in this individual?

A. β-Blockade is absolutely contraindicated for tachycardia even after adequate α-blockade has been attained.
B. Immediate surgical removal of the mass is indicated, because the patient presented with hypertensive crisis with encephalopathy.
C. Salt and fluid intake should be restricted to prevent further exacerbation of the patient's hypertension.
D. Treatment with phenoxybenzamine should be started at a high dose (20–30 mg three times daily) to rapidly control blood pressure, and surgery can be undertaken within 24–48 hours.
E. IV phentolamine is indicated for treatment of the hypertensive crisis. Phenoxybenzamine should be started at a low dose and titrated to the maximum-tolerated dose over 2–3 weeks. Surgery should not be planned until the blood pressure is consistently below 160/100 mmHg.

X-31. Mr. Robinson returns for a follow-up after a long hospital stay for hypertension when he was diagnosed with a pheochromocytoma and ultimately underwent a left adrenalectomy. He reports feeling well since then, and his hypertension is well controlled. He is curious about whether his pheochromocytoma was considered malignant. What should you tell him?

A. Approximately 50% of pheochromocytomas are malignant.
B. Cellular atypia and invasion of blood vessels on pathology define malignancy for pheochromocytoma.
C. ^{23}I-metaiodobenzylguanidine scans are not useful in locating distant metastases.
D. The absence of distant metastases rules out malignant disease.

X-32. An 18-year-old woman is evaluated at her primary care physician's office for a routine physical. She is presently healthy. Her family history is notable for a father and two aunts with multiple endocrine neoplasia type 1 (MEN1), and the patient has undergone genetic testing and carries the *MEN1* gene. Which of the following is the first and most common presentation for individuals with this genetic mutation?

A. Amenorrhea
B. Hypercalcemia
C. Hypoglycemia
D. Peptic ulcer disease
E. Uncontrolled systemic hypertension

X-33. You are seeing Mr. Avendaw in clinic today. He is a 35-year-old man who last year had a partial thyroidectomy for medullary thyroid carcinoma. You note that he was recently in the hospital and diagnosed with a pheochromocytoma, and after 2 weeks of intensive medical therapy, he underwent unilateral adrenalectomy. He is recovering nicely. You are reviewing his chart before the visit, when you note that on the pathology from his thyroid surgery last year, a single parathyroid gland was removed that was shown to be a parathyroid tumor. When you meet with Mr. Avendaw, you will tell him which of the following?

A. "Family and genetic screening for similar cancers is not useful because the mutations causing these cancers are certainly unrelated and spontaneously arise."
B. "I suspect you have a syndrome called multiple endocrine neoplasia type 1."
C. "I suspect you have a syndrome called multiple endocrine neoplasia type 2."
D. "The partial thyroidectomy was an appropriate treatment for this condition."
E. "These tumors were likely caused by a mutation in the *Menin* gene."

X-34. Johnny Stewart, a 4-year-old boy, presents to the hospital with hypotension, lethargy, and hyponatremia. You also note that his potassium is elevated to 5.7 mEq/dL. He is afebrile and has a normal complete blood count. However, you note extensive oral thrush. On review of his chart, you note that he has had multiple treatment courses for thrush and cutaneous candidal infections. Human immunodeficiency virus (HIV) antibody tests have been negative. Also, you note that at 1 year of age, he had an episode of tetany prompting an emergent presentation to the hospital, where he was found to be hypocalcemic. Ultimately, he was diagnosed with hypoparathyroidism. Given his current presentation, which of the following is the most appropriate course of treatment?

A. IV calcium
B. IV hydrocortisone
C. Kayexalate, IV insulin, and albuterol to treat presumed hyperkalemic periodic paralysis
D. Ketoconazole
E. Urgent echocardiogram for suspected cardiac tamponade

X-35. Mr. David presents to the emergency department with numbness and weakness in his legs and feet. On exam, you find that he is numb to the knees and has marked weakness in ankle dorsiflexion and plantar flexion. Two years ago, he developed diabetes, and last year, he was admitted when found to be profoundly hypothyroid. On examination, he has hepatosplenomegaly and appears to have a dark tan despite having no sun exposure recently. Which of the following tests will likely help make his diagnosis?

A. Anti–nuclear antibody titer measurement
B. Anti–thymoglobulin antibody titer measurement
C. Blood cultures
D. Serum protein electrophoresis
E. Skin biopsy searching for intravascular clonal T cells

X-36. A 37-year-old man is evaluated for infertility. He and his wife have been attempting to conceive a child for the past 2 years without success. He initially saw an infertility specialist but was referred to endocrinology after sperm analysis showed no sperm. He is otherwise healthy and only takes a multivitamin. On physical examination, his vital signs are normal. He is tall and has small testes, gynecomastia, and minimal facial and axillary hair. Chromosomal analysis confirms Klinefelter syndrome. Which of the following statements is true?

A. Androgen supplementation is of little use in this condition.
B. He is not at increased risk for breast tumors.
C. Increased plasma concentrations of estrogen are present.
D. Most cases are diagnosed before puberty.
E. Plasma concentrations of follicle-stimulating hormone (FSH) and luteinizing hormone (LH) are decreased in this condition.

X-37. A 17-year-old teenager is evaluated in your office for primary amenorrhea. She does not feel as if she has entered puberty because she has never had a menstrual period and has sparse axillary and pubic hair growth. On examination, she is noted to be 150 cm tall. She has a low hairline and slight webbing of her neck. Her FSH level is

75 mIU/mL, LH is 20 mIU/mL, and estradiol level is 2 pg/mL. You suspect Turner syndrome. All of the following tests are indicated in this individual EXCEPT:

A. Buccal smear for nuclear heterochromatin (Barr body)
B. Echocardiogram
C. Karyotype analysis
D. Renal ultrasound
E. TSH

X-38. An infant is born with ambiguous genitalia. Although amniocentesis analysis during pregnancy showed a 46, XX genotype, this infant has phallic-appearing genitalia and partially fused labia. You cannot palpate testes. Aside from a standard blood test, which biochemical screen is indicated?

A. Flow cytometry of the peripheral blood
B. Serum cortisol levels
C. Serum 17-hydroxyprogesterone levels
D. Serum TSH
E. Serum prolactin levels

X-39. A 58-year-old man is seen in his primary care physician's office for evaluation of bilateral breast enlargement. This has been present for several months and is accompanied by mild pain in both breasts. He reports no other symptoms. His other medical conditions include coronary artery disease with a history of congestive heart failure, atrial fibrillation, obesity, and type 2 diabetes mellitus. His current medications include lisinopril, spironolactone, furosemide, insulin, and digoxin. He denies illicit drug use and has fathered three children. Examination confirms bilateral breast enlargement with palpable glandular tissue that measures 2 cm bilaterally. Which of the following statements regarding his gynecomastia is true?

A. He should be referred for mammography to rule out breast cancer.
B. His gynecomastia is most likely due to obesity, with adipose tissue present in the breast.
C. Serum testosterone, LH, and FSH should be measured to evaluate for androgen insensitivity.
D. Spironolactone should be discontinued, and he should be followed for regression.
E. Liver function testing should be performed to screen for cirrhosis.

X-40. All the following drugs may interfere with testicular function EXCEPT:

A. Cyclophosphamide
B. Ketoconazole
C. Metoprolol
D. Prednisone
E. Spironolactone

X-41. Clinical signs and findings of the presence of ovulation include all of the following EXCEPT:

A. Detection of urinary LH surge
B. Estrogen peak during secretory phase of menstrual cycle
C. Increase in basal body temperature >0.5°F in second half of menstrual cycle
D. Presence of mittelschmerz
E. Progesterone level >5 ng/mL 7 days before expected menses

X-42. In the developmental progression from childhood through puberty to menopause, all of the following statements regarding levels of FSH and LH are true EXCEPT:

A. FSH is suppressed from birth to 20 months of age.
B. LH is increased during the neonatal year (birth to 20 months).
C. LH and FSH levels are reduced during childhood before puberty.
D. At the onset of puberty, pulsatile gonadotropin-releasing hormone (GnRH) drives pituitary FSH and LH levels.
E. LH and FSH levels rise sharply after menopause.

X-43. Which of the following occurs first in the majority of girls with normal pubertal development?

A. Achieving peak height velocity
B. Menarche
C. Breast development
D. Development of pubic hair
E. Development of axillary hair.

X-44. The Women's Health Initiative study investigated hormonal therapy in postmenopausal women. The study was stopped early due to increased risk of which of the following diseases in the estrogen-only arm?

A. Deep venous thrombosis
B. Endometrial cancer
C. Myocardial infarction
D. Osteoporosis
E. Stroke

X-45. All of the following are traditional contraindications for oral hormone replacement therapy in postmenopausal women EXCEPT:

A. Active liver disease
B. Blood clotting disorder
C. Breast cancer
D. Coronary heart disease risk over ensuing 10 years of 5%–10%
E. Unexplained vaginal bleeding

X-46. A couple that has been married for 5 years have been attempting to conceive a child for the last 12 months. Despite regular intercourse, they have not achieved pregnancy. They are both 32 years of age and have no medical problems. Neither partner is taking medications. Which of the following is the most common cause of infertility?

A. Endometriosis
B. Male causes
C. Ovulatory dysfunction
D. Tubal defect
E. Unexplained

X-47. A couple seeks advice regarding infertility. The female partner is 35 years old. She has never been pregnant and was taking oral contraceptive pills from age 20 until age 34. It is now 16 months since she discontinued her oral contraceptives. She is having menstrual cycles approximately once every 35 days, but occasionally will go as long as 60 days between cycles. Most months, she develops breast tenderness about 2–3 weeks after the start of her menstrual cycle. When she was in college, she was treated for *Neisseria gonorrhoeae* that was diagnosed when she presented to the student health center with a fever and pelvic pain. She otherwise has no medical history. She works about 60 hours weekly as a corporate attorney and exercises daily. She drinks coffee daily and alcohol at social occasions only. Her body mass index (BMI) is 19.8 kg/m^2. Her husband, who is 39 years old, accompanies her to the evaluation. He also has never had children. He was married previously from the ages of 24–28. He and his prior wife attempted to conceive for about 15 months but were unsuccessful. At that time, he was smoking marijuana on a daily basis and attributed their lack of success to his drug use. He has now been completely free of drugs for 9 years. He suffers from hypertension and is treated with lisinopril 10 mg daily. He is not obese (BMI 23.7 kg/m^2). They request evaluation for their infertility and request help with conception. Which of the following statements is true regarding their infertility and likelihood of success in conception?

A. Determination of ovulation is not necessary in the female partner because most of her cycles occur regularly and she develops breast tenderness midcycle, indicating ovulation.
B. Lisinopril should be discontinued immediately because of the risk of birth defects associated with its use.
C. The female partner should be assessed for tubal patency by a hysterosalpingogram. If significant scarring is found, in vitro fertilization should be strongly considered to decrease the risk of ectopic pregnancy.
D. The prolonged use of oral contraceptives for >10 years has increased the risk of anovulation and infertility.
E. The use of marijuana by the male partner is directly toxic to sperm motility, and this is the likely cause of their infertility.

X-48. Which of the following forms of contraception has a theoretical efficacy of >90%?

A. Condoms
B. Intrauterine devices
C. Oral contraceptives
D. Spermicides
E. All of the above

X-49. A 30-year-old man, the father of three children, has had progressive breast enlargement during the last 6 months. He does not use any drugs. Laboratory evaluation reveals that both LH and testosterone are low. Further evaluation of this patient should include which of the following?

A. 24-Hour urine collection for the measurement of 17-ketosteroids
B. Blood sampling for serum glutamic oxaloacetic transaminase (SGOT) and serum alkaline phosphatase and bilirubin levels
C. Breast biopsy
D. Karyotype analysis to exclude Klinefelter syndrome
E. Measurement of estradiol and human chorionic gonadotropin (hCG) levels

X-50. You are seeing a 36-year-old woman in clinic as her family practitioner. In her history, she reports no illness and is taking no medications. She does mention that she and her husband have been trying to conceive a child for the past 7 months but have been unsuccessful. Which of the following would be an appropriate response?

A. "You have likely entered menopause and cannot have a child."
B. "We do not recommend evaluation by a fertility specialist until you and her husband have tried for at least 12 months."
C. "I will refer you to an expert in fertility issues."
D. "Most causes of infertility are related to the male. I suggest you have him evaluated."
E. "Advancing age does not reduce a woman's chance of becoming pregnant until she reaches menopause."

X-51. Which of the following ethnic populations in the United States has the highest risk of diabetes mellitus?

A. Ashkenazi Jews
B. Asian American
C. Hispanic
D. Non-Hispanic black
E. Non-Hispanic white

X-52. Which of the following defines normal glucose tolerance?

A. Fasting plasma glucose <100 mg/dL
B. Fasting plasma glucose <126 mg/dL following an oral glucose challenge
C. Fasting plasma glucose <100 mg/dL, plasma glucose <140 mg/dL following an oral glucose challenge, and hemoglobin A1C <5.6%
D. Hemoglobin A1C <5.6% and fasting plasma glucose <140 mg/dL
E. Hemoglobin A1C <6.0%

X-53. A 37-year-old obese woman presents to clinic for routine health evaluation. She reports that over the last year she has had two yeast infections treated with over-the-counter remedies and she frequently feels thirsty. She reports waking up at night to urinate. Which of the following studies is the most appropriate first test in evaluating the patient for diabetes mellitus?

A. Hemoglobin A1C
B. Oral glucose tolerance test
C. Plasma C-peptide level
D. Plasma insulin level
E. Random plasma glucose level

X-54. A 27-year-old woman with mild obesity is seen by her primary care physician for increased thirst and polyuria. Diabetes mellitus is suspected, and a random plasma glucose of 211 mg/d confirms this diagnosis. Which of the following tests will strongly indicate that she has type 1 diabetes mellitus?

A. Anti-GAD-65 antibody
B. Peroxisome proliferator-activated receptor γ-2 polymorphism testing
C. Plasma insulin level
D. Testing for human leukocyte antigen (HLA) DR3
E. There is no laboratory test to detect type 1 diabetes mellitus.

X-55. You have admitted an 18-year-old patient to the adult medical intensive care unit for diabetic ketoacidosis (DKA). The patient was not known previously to be diabetic, but her mother notes that she had been "going to the bathroom a lot" recently and that "she had been really thirsty." The patient's BMI is 44 kg/m^2. There is no family history of diabetes. You successfully treat the patient for her DKA and note that serum anti-GAD antibodies and anti–islet cell antibodies (ICA) sent on admission are not detected. The patient and her mother want to know what "type" of diabetes she has. You should tell them which of the following?

A. "Due to the young age of onset, you likely have type 1 diabetes."
B. "Due to your presentation with diabetic ketoacidosis, you likely have type 1 diabetes."
C. "I suspect you have maturity-onset diabetes of the young."
D. "You likely have type 2 diabetes mellitus."
E. "I suspect your diabetes was triggered by a virus."

X-56. A patient is evaluated in the emergency department for complications of diabetes mellitus due to an episode of life stressors. All of the following laboratory tests are consistent with the diagnosis of DKA EXCEPT:

A. Arterial pH of 7.1
B. Glucose of 550 mg/dL
C. Markedly positive plasma ketones
D. Normal serum potassium
E. Plasma osmolality of 380 mOsm/mL

X-57. Pick the correct combination of onset of action and duration of action for the following insulins.

		Onset	Duration
A.	Aspart	1 hr	6 hr
B.	Detemir	2 hr	12 hr
C.	Lispro	0.5 hr	2 hr
D.	NPH	2 hr	14 hr
E.	Regular	0.25 hr	8 hr

X-58. A 54-year-old woman is diagnosed with type 2 diabetes mellitus after a routine follow-up for impaired fasting glucose showed that her hemoglobin A1C is now 7.6%. She has attempted to lose weight and exercise with no improvement in her hemoglobin A1C, and drug therapy is now recommended. She has mild systemic hypertension that is well controlled and no other medical conditions. Which of the following is the most appropriate first-line therapy?

A. Acarbose
B. Exenatide
C. Glyburide
D. Metformin
E. Sitagliptin

X-59. A 21-year-old woman with a history of type 1 diabetes mellitus is brought to the emergency department with nausea, vomiting, lethargy, and dehydration. Her mother notes that she stopped taking insulin 1 day before presentation. She is lethargic, has dry mucous membranes, and is obtunded. Blood pressure is 80/40 mmHg, and heart rate is 112 bpm. Heart sounds are normal. Lungs are clear. The abdomen is soft, and there is no organomegaly. She is responsive and oriented × 3 but diffusely weak. Serum sodium is 126 mEq/L, potassium is 4.3 mEq/L, magnesium is 1.2 mEq/L, blood urea nitrogen is 76 mg/dL, creatinine is 2.2 mg/dL, bicarbonate is 10 mEq/L, and chloride is 88 mEq/L. Serum glucose is 720 mg/dL. All the following are appropriate management steps EXCEPT:

A. 3% sodium solution
B. Arterial blood gas
C. IV insulin
D. IV potassium
E. IV fluids

X-60. You are seeing a 28-year-old woman with longstanding type 1 diabetes on insulin. She tells you that she and her husband have decided to try to conceive. Which of the following is true regarding reproductive issues and diabetes?

A. Women with diabetes have a reduced reproductive capacity.
B. Insulin crosses the placenta and may affect the fetus adversely.
C. The patient should expect her insulin requirements to increase during pregnancy.
D. High maternal serum glucose increases the risk of fetal abnormalities.
E. The most crucial period of glycemic control is in the third trimester to avoid fetal malformations.

X-61. Which of the following regarding care of the hospitalized diabetic patient is true?

A. General anesthesia leads to insulin sensitization and higher risk for hypoglycemia.
B. A greater degree of hyperglycemia during hospitalization has not been associated with worse infectious outcomes.
C. In clinical trials, strict glycemic control (goal, 81–108 mg/dL) is superior to moderate glycemic control (goal, 140 mg/dL).
D. The initiation of total parenteral nutrition is associated with increased insulin requirements.
E. In critically ill patients, subcutaneous insulin is invariably preferred over IV insulin.

X-62. In Figure X-62, what is the primary finding seen in this patient's fundus?

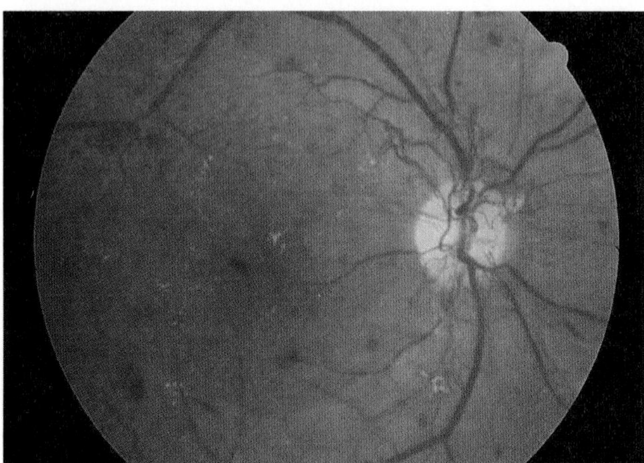

FIGURE X-62

A. Arteriovenous nicking
B. Microaneurysms
C. Neovascularization
D. Papilledema

X-63. Which of the following patients should be treated with either an angiotensin-converting enzyme (ACE) inhibitor or angiotensin receptor blocker?

A. A 24-year-old woman with type 1 diabetes with two positive spot microalbuminuria tests 1 week apart
B. A 32-year-old woman with type 1 diabetes with a blood glucose of 328 mg/dL and a positive spot microalbuminuria test
C. A 48-year-old man with type 2 diabetes with a positive spot microalbuminuria test 1 week after starting a new exercise program
D. A 56-year-old man with type 2 diabetes with two positive spot microalbuminuria tests 3 months apart
E. A 62-year-old man with type 2 diabetes and hypertension with a positive spot microalbuminuria test and a blood pressure on day of testing of 190/118 mmHg

X-64. A 58-year-old woman with type 2 diabetes mellitus is evaluated by her primary care provider for a tingling sensation in her hands and feet. She has had type 2 diabetes for 15 years with intermittently poor control. Her most recent hemoglobin A1C was 7.9%. She is currently managed with insulin detemir 40 units daily and metformin 1000 mg daily. On neurologic examination, there is loss of deep tendon reflexes at the ankles bilaterally. Deep tendon reflexes are 2+ at the knees, biceps, and triceps. Sensation is decreased to pinprick and light touch bilaterally to the ankle and wrists. She also has difficulty ascertaining if the great toe is being held in the up or down position when her eyes are closed. She finds it difficult to sleep at night sometimes due to the pain in her legs. She is diagnosed with distal sensory polyneuropathy due to her diabetes. Which of the following medications has been approved by the U.S. Food and Drug Administration for the treatment of pain associated with diabetic neuropathy?

A. Duloxetine
B. Gabapentin
C. Pregabalin
D. A and C only
E. All of the above

X-65. Plasma glucose is normally tightly regulated in the body, with fasting levels between 70 and 110 mg/dL. When the blood glucose falls below 80–85 mg/dL, which of the following physiologic changes is the first to occur?

A. Decrease in growth hormone
B. Decrease in insulin secretion
C. Increase in cortisol
D. Increase in epinephrine
E. Increase in glucagon

X-66. A 25-year-old healthcare worker is seen for evaluation of recurrent hypoglycemia. She has had several episodes at work over the past year in which she feels shaky, anxious, and sweaty; she measures her fingerstick glucose, and it is 40–55 mg/dL. This has been confirmed with a plasma glucose level during one episode of 50 mg/dL. She then drinks orange juice and feels better. These episodes have not happened outside the work environment. Aside from oral contraceptives, she takes no medications and is otherwise healthy. Which of the following tests is most likely to demonstrate the underlying cause of her hypoglycemia?

A. Measurement of IGF-1
B. Measurement of fasting insulin and glucose levels
C. Measurement of fasting insulin, glucose, and C-peptide levels
D. Measurement of insulin, glucose, and C-peptide levels during an symptomatic episode
E. Measurement of plasma cortisol

X-67. All of the following statements regarding hypoglycemia in diabetes mellitus are true EXCEPT:

A. Individuals with type 2 diabetes mellitus experience less hypoglycemia than those with type 1 diabetes mellitus.
B. From 2%–4% of deaths in type 1 diabetes mellitus are directly attributable to hypoglycemia.
C. Recurrent episodes of hypoglycemia predispose to the development of autonomic failure with defective glucose counterregulation and hypoglycemia unawareness.
D. The average person with type 1 diabetes mellitus has two episodes of symptomatic hypoglycemia weekly.
E. Thiazolidinediones and metformin cause hypoglycemia more frequently than sulfonylureas.

X-68. An 18-year-old man presents with severe mid-abdominal pain radiating to his back. Physical examination reveals a temperature of 38.0°C, blood pressure of 95/55 mmHg, heart rate of 110 bpm, and respiratory rate of 18 breaths/min, with room air oxygen saturation 96%. His abdomen is diffusely tender with voluntary guarding and no rebound tenderness. There is enlargement of the liver and spleen. He also has eruptive xanthomas on his hands, feet, and legs. His lipase is 2300 U/L, and he has a fasting triglyceride level of 1019 mg/dL. After appropriate evaluation, he is presumed to have pancreatitis and lipoprotein lipase deficiency. He stabilizes without complication and is ready for discharge after 4 days. What do you recommend for treatment?

A. Dietary fat restriction 15 g/d
B. Fish oil supplementation
C. Gemfibrozil 600 mg twice a day (bid)
D. Nicotinic acid sustained-release 250 mg bid
E. Simvastatin 20 mg daily

X-69. A 32-year-old man is evaluated at a routine clinic visit for coronary risk factors. He reports no tobacco use, his systemic blood pressure is normal, and he does not have diabetes. He is otherwise healthy. His family history is notable for high cholesterol in his mother and maternal grandfather and grandmother. Physical examination shows tendon xanthomas. A fasting cholesterol is notable for a low-density lipoprotein (LDL) cholesterol level of 387 mg/dL. Which of the following is the most likely genetic disorder affecting this individual?

A. Apolipoprotein (apo) A-V deficiency
B. Familial defective apoB-100
C. Familial hepatic lipase deficiency
D. Familial hypercholesterolemia
E. Lipoprotein lipase deficiency

X-70. All of the following are potential causes of elevated LDL EXCEPT:

A. Anorexia nervosa
B. Cirrhosis
C. Hypothyroidism
D. Nephrotic syndrome
E. Thiazide diuretics

X-71. Your 60-year-old patient with a monoclonal gammopathy of unclear significance presents for a follow-up visit and to review recent laboratory data. His creatinine is newly elevated to 2.0 mg/dL, potassium is 3.7 mg/dL, calcium is 12.2 mg/dL, LDL is 202 mg/dL, and triglycerides are 209 mg/dL. On further questioning, he reports 3 months of swelling around the eyes and "foamy" urine. On examination, he has anasarca. Concerned for multiple myeloma and nephrotic syndrome, you order a urine protein/creatinine ratio, which returns at 14:1. Which treatment option would be most appropriate to treat his lipid abnormalities?

A. Cholesterol ester transfer protein inhibitor
B. Dietary management
C. 3-Hydroxy-3-methylglutaryl–coenzyme A (HMG-CoA) reductase inhibitors
D. Lipid apheresis
E. Niacin and fibrates

X-72. Metabolic syndrome was defined initially as a clinical entity by the World Health Organization in 1998 as a constellation of findings including central obesity, hypertriglyceridemia, low high-density lipoprotein (HDL), hyperglycemia, and hypertension. Which of the following statements regarding the epidemiology of metabolic syndrome is true?

A. After the age of 60, men are more likely to have metabolic syndrome than women.
B. Among patients with diabetes mellitus, presence of metabolic syndrome confers a higher risk of cardiovascular disease.
C. BMI is the strongest predictor of insulin resistance and diabetes risk in metabolic syndrome.
D. The highest recorded prevalence of metabolic syndrome in the United States is among Mexican American women.
E. The nationality at the lowest risk of metabolic syndrome is the Japanese population.

X-73. A 47-year-old Chinese man is seen for an annual examination. He generally has no complaints but lives a sedentary lifestyle. He works as an accountant and spends of his work days at a computer screen. He does not maintain a regular exercise routine. He admits his diet is poor. He is divorced and lives alone. He eats out or gets take out about 4 nights a week. On other days, he prefers quick meals that he can heat up in the microwave. His past medical history is significant for hypertension and obesity. He is being treated with hydrochlorothiazide 25 mg daily. He has no allergies. His blood pressure today is 148/92 mmHg. His waist circumference is 93 cm (36.6 in). He is 177.8 cm (70 in) tall and weighs 105 kg (225 lb). His BMI is 32.3 kg/m^2. On his annual fasting labs, his total cholesterol is 220 mg/dL, HDL is 28 mg/dL, triglycerides are 178 mg/dL, and LDL is 103 mg/dL. Fasting plasma glucose is 98 mg/dL. Which of the following is true regarding a diagnosis of metabolic syndrome in this patient?

A. He cannot have metabolic syndrome because his fasting plasma glucose level is normal.
B. He has metabolic syndrome because he meets three out of five diagnostic criteria: high triglyceride levels, low HDL level, and hypertension.
C. He has metabolic syndrome because he meets four out of five diagnostic criteria: high BMI, high triglyceride levels, low HDL level, and hypertension.
D. He has metabolic syndrome because he meets four out of five diagnostic criteria: large waist circumference, high triglyceride levels, low HDL level, and hypertension.
E. Metabolic syndrome cannot be diagnosed on a single evaluation. Repeat testing is indicated in 3–6 months

X-74. A 55-year-old man is admitted to the intensive care unit with 1 week of fever and cough. He was well until 1 week before admission, when he noted progressive shortness of breath, cough, and productive sputum. On the day of admission, the patient was noted by his wife to be lethargic. Emergency response medics found the patient unresponsive. He was intubated in the field and brought to the emergency department. His only medications are insulin glargine 20 units daily and insulin aspart with meals. The past medical history is notable for alcohol abuse and diabetes mellitus. His recent alcohol use has been at least 12 beers daily. Upon arrival to the hospital, his temperature is 38.9°C (102°F), blood pressure is 76/40 mmHg, and oxygen saturation is 86% on ventilator setting of assist-control, with a tidal volume of 420 mL, respiratory rate of 22 breaths/min, positive end-expiratory pressure of 5, and FiO_2 of 1.0. On examination, the patient is intubated on mechanical ventilation. Jugular venous pressure is normal. There are decreased breath sounds at the right lung base with egophony. Heart sounds are normal. The abdomen is soft. There is no peripheral edema. Chest radiography shows a right lower lobe infiltrate with a moderate pleural effusion. An electrocardiogram is normal. Sputum Gram stain shows gram-positive diplococci. White blood cell count is $23 \times 10^3/\mu L$, with 70% polymorphonuclear cells and 6% bands. Blood urea nitrogen is 80 mg/dL, and creatinine is 3.1 mg/dL. Plasma glucose is 425 mg/dL. He is started on broad-spectrum antibiotics, IV fluids, omeprazole, and an insulin drip. A nasogastric tube is inserted, and tube feedings are started. On hospital day 2, his creatinine has improved to 1.6 mg/dL. However, plasma phosphate is 1.0 mg/dL (0.3 mmol/L), and calcium is 8.8 mg/dL. All of following are causes of hypophosphatemia is this patient EXCEPT:

A. Acute kidney injury
B. Alcoholism
C. Insulin
D. Malnutrition
E. Sepsis

X-75. In the patient described in Question X-74, what it the most appropriate approach to correcting the hypophosphatemia?

A. Administer IV calcium gluconate 1 g followed by infusion of IV phosphate at a rate of 8 mmol/hr for 6 hours.
B. Administer IV phosphate alone at a rate of 2 mmol/hr for 6 hours.
C. Administer IV phosphate alone at a rate of 8 mmol/hr for 6 hours.
D. Continued close observation as redistribution of phosphate is expected to normalize levels over the course of the next 24–48 hours.
E. Initiate oral phosphate replacement at a dose of 1500 mg/d.

X-76. You are caring for a 72-year-old man who has been living in a nursing home for the past 3 years. He has severe chronic obstructive pulmonary disease and requires continuous oxygen at 3 L/min. He also previously had a stroke, which has left him with a right hemiparesis. His current medications include aspirin, losartan, hydrochlorothiazide, fluticasone/salmeterol, tiotropium, and albuterol. His BMI is 18.5 kg/m^2. You are concerned that he may have vitamin D deficiency. Which of the following is the best test to determine if vitamin D deficiency is present?

A. 1,25-Hydroxy-vitamin D
B. 25-Hydroxy-vitamin D
C. Alkaline phosphatase
D. Parathyroid hormone
E. Serum total and ionized calcium levels

X-77. A 72-year-old woman was hospitalized with a right hip fracture. After initial surgical repair, she is transferred to rehabilitation for further care. While there, she has a 25-hydroxyvitamin D level checked, and it returns at 18.3 ng/L. What do you recommend for treatment in this patient?

A. Vitamin D_3 800 units daily
B. Vitamin D_3 800 units daily plus calcium carbonate 1500 mg daily
C. Vitamin D_3 2000 units daily
D. Vitamin D_3 2000 units daily plus calcium carbonate 1500 mg daily
E. Vitamin D_3 50,000 units weekly for 4 weeks, then 800 units weekly, plus calcium 1500 mg daily

X-78. A 60-year-old woman is referred to your office for evaluation of hypercalcemia. A serum calcium level of 12.9 mg/dL was found incidentally on a chemistry panel that was drawn during a hospitalization for cholecystectomy. Despite fluid administration in the hospital, her serum calcium at discharge was 11.8 mg/dL. The patient is asymptomatic, and her parathyroid hormone level is 95 ng/L (reference value 10–65 ng/L). She is otherwise in good health and has had her recommended age-appropriate cancer screening. She denies constipation or bone pain and is now 8 weeks out from her surgical procedure. Today, her serum calcium level is 12.6 mg/dL, and phosphate is 2.3 mg/dL. Her hematocrit and all other chemistries, including creatinine, were normal. Which of the following would be an indication for surgery in this patient to definitively treat her underlying diagnosis?

A. Age >50
B. Elevated 24-hour urine calcium
C. Nephrolithiasis
D. Osteopenia on bone density testing
E. Serum calcium >1 mg/dL above normal

X-79. A 42-year-old man presents to the emergency department with acute-onset right-sided flank pain. He describes the pain as 10 out of 10 in severity and radiating to the groin. He has had one episode of hematuria. A noncontrast CT scan confirms the presence of a right-sided renal stone that is currently located in the distal ureter. He has a past medical history of pulmonary sarcoidosis that is not currently treated. This was diagnosed by bronchoscopic biopsy showing noncaseating granulomas. His chest radiograph shows bilateral hilar adenopathy. His serum calcium level is 12.6 mg/dL. What is the mechanism of hypercalcemia in this patient?

A. Increased activation of 25-hydroxyvitamin D to 1,25-hydroxyvitamin D by macrophages within granulomas
B. Increased activation of 25-hydroxyvitamin D to 1,25-hydroxyvitamin D by the kidney
C. Increased activation of vitamin D to 25-hydroxyvitamin D by macrophages within granulomas
D. Missed diagnosis of lymphoma with subsequent bone marrow invasion and resorption of bone through local destruction
E. Production of parathyroid hormone–related peptide by macrophages within granulomas

X-80. A 52-year-old man has end-stage kidney disease from longstanding hypertension and diabetes mellitus. He has been managed with hemodialysis for the past 8 years. Throughout this time, he has been poorly compliant with his medications and hemodialysis schedule, frequently missing one session weekly. He is now complaining of bone pain and dyspnea. His oxygen saturation is noted to be 92% on room air, and his chest radiograph shows hazy bilateral infiltrates. Chest CT shows ground-glass infiltrates bilaterally. His laboratory data include a calcium of 12.3 mg/dL, phosphate of 8.1 mg/dL, and parathyroid hormone of 110 pg/mL. Which of the following would be the best approach to the treatment of the patient's current clinical condition?

A. Calcitriol 0.5 μg IV with hemodialysis with sevelamer three times daily
B. Calcitriol 0.5 μg orally daily with sevelamer 1600 mg three times daily
C. More aggressive hemodialysis to achieve optimal fluid and electrolyte balance
D. Parathyroidectomy
E. Sevelamer 1600 mg three times daily

X-81. A 54-year-old woman undergoes total thyroidectomy for follicular carcinoma of the thyroid. About 6 hours after surgery, the patient complains of tingling around her mouth. She subsequently develops a pins-and-needles sensation in the fingers and toes. The nurse calls the physician to the bedside to evaluate the patient after she has severe hand cramps when her blood pressure is taken. Upon evaluation, the patient is still complaining of intermittent cramping of her hands. Since surgery, she has received morphine sulfate for pain and metoclopramide for nausea. She has had no change in her vital signs and is afebrile. Tapping on the inferior portion of the zygomatic arch 2 cm anterior to the ear produces twitching at the corner of the mouth. An electrocardiogram shows a QT interval of 575 msec. What is the next step in evaluation and treatment of this patient?

A. Administration of benztropine
B. Administration of calcium gluconate
C. Administration of magnesium sulphate
D. Measurement of calcium, magnesium, phosphate, and potassium levels
E. Measurement of forced vital capacity

X-82. A 68-year-old woman with stage IIIB squamous cell carcinoma of the lung is admitted to the hospital because of altered mental status and dehydration. Upon admission, she is found to have a calcium level of 19.6 mg/dL and phosphate level of 1.8 mg/dL. Concomitant measurement of parathyroid hormone was 0.1 pg/mL (normal 10–65 pg/mL), and a screen for parathyroid hormone–related peptide was positive. Over the first 24 hours, the patient receives 4 L of normal saline with furosemide diuresis. The next morning, the patient's calcium is 17.6 mg/dL and phosphate is 2.2 mg/dL. She continues to have delirium. What is the best approach for ongoing treatment of this patient's hypercalcemia?

A. Continue therapy with large-volume fluid administration and forced diuresis with furosemide
B. Continue therapy with large-volume fluid administration, but stop furosemide and treat with hydrochlorothiazide
C. Initiate therapy with calcitonin alone
D. Initiate therapy with pamidronate alone
E. Initiate therapy with calcitonin and pamidronate

X-83. Which of the following statements regarding the epidemiology of osteoporosis and bone fractures is correct?

A. For every 5-year age increase after age 70, the incidence of hip fractures increases by 25%.
B. Fractures of the distal radius increase in frequency before age 50 and plateau by age 60, with only a modest age-related increase.
C. Most women meet the diagnostic criteria for osteoporosis between the ages of 60 and 70.
D. The risk of hip fracture is equal when white women are compared to black women.
E. Women outnumber men with osteoporosis at a ratio of about 10 to 1.

X-84. A 50-year-old woman presents to your office to inquire about her risk of fracture related to osteoporosis. She has a positive family history of osteoporosis in her mother, but her mother never experienced any hip or vertebral fractures. The patient herself has also not experienced any fractures. She is white and has a 20-pack-year history of tobacco use, quitting 10 years prior. At the age of 37, she had a total hysterectomy with bilateral salpingo-oophorectomy for endometriosis. She is lactose intolerant and does not consume dairy products. She currently takes calcium carbonate 500 mg daily. Her weight is 115 lb, and her height is 66 in (BMI 18.6 kg/m^2). All of the following are risk factors for an osteoporotic fracture in this woman EXCEPT:

A. Early menopause
B. Female sex
C. History of cigarette smoking
D. Low body weight
E. Low calcium intake

X-85. A 54-year-old woman is referred to the endocrinology clinic for evaluation of osteoporosis after a recent examination for back pain revealed a compression fracture of the T4 vertebral body. She is perimenopausal with irregular menstrual periods and frequent hot flashes. She does not smoke. She otherwise is well and healthy. Her weight is 70 kg, and height is 168 cm. She has lost 5 cm from her maximum height. A bone mineral density scan shows a T-score of –3.5 standard deviation (SD) and a Z-score of –2.5 SD. All of the following tests are indicated for the evaluation of osteoporosis in this patient EXCEPT:

A. 24-Hour urine calcium
B. FSH and LH levels
C. Serum calcium
D. TSH
E. Vitamin D levels (25-hydroxyvitamin D)

X-86. A 45-year-old white woman seeks advice from her primary care physician regarding her risk for osteoporosis and the need for bone density screening. She is a lifelong nonsmoker and drinks alcohol only socially. She has a history of moderate-persistent asthma since adolescence. She is currently on fluticasone, 44 mg/puff twice daily, with good control currently. She last required oral prednisone therapy about 6 months ago when she had influenza that was complicated by an asthma flare. She took prednisone for a total of 14 days. She has had three pregnancies and two live births at ages 39 and 41. She currently has irregular periods occurring approximately every 42 days. Her FSH level is 25 mIU/L and 17β-estradiol level is 115 pg/mL on day 12 of her menstrual cycle. Her mother and maternal aunt both have been diagnosed with osteoporosis. Her mother also has rheumatoid arthritis and requires prednisone therapy, 5 mg daily. Her mother developed a compression fracture of the lumbar spine at age 68. On physical examination, the patient appears well and healthy. Her height is 168 cm. Her weight is 66.4 kg. The chest, cardiac, abdominal, muscular, and neurologic examinations are normal. What do you tell the patient about the need for bone density screening?

A. Because she is currently perimenopausal, she should have a bone density screen every other year until she completes menopause and then have bone densitometry measured yearly thereafter.
B. Because of her family history, she should initiate bone density screening yearly beginning now.
C. Bone densitometry screening is not recommended until after completion of menopause.
D. Delayed childbearing until the fourth and fifth decade decreases her risk of developing osteoporosis, so bone densitometry is not recommended.
E. Her use of low-dose inhaled glucocorticoids increases her risk of osteoporosis threefold, and she should undergo yearly bone density screening.

X-87 to X-91. Match the following medications used for osteoporosis to the mechanism of action:

87. Calcitonin:

88. Denosumab:

89. Raloxifene:

90. Teriparatide:

91. Zoledronic acid

A. Recombinant parathyroid hormone (1-34hPTH) with direct stimulation of osteoblast activity
B. Polypeptide hormone that suppresses osteoclast activity through a specific receptor for the hormone
C. Bisphosphonate drug given on an annual basis that impairs osteoclast function and reduces osteoclast number
D. Selective estrogen receptor modulator
E. Human monoclonal antibody to RANKL, a protein necessary for osteoclast maturation

X-92. A 38-year-old woman with cystic fibrosis and vitamin D deficiency has a T-score of –2.8 in the lumbar spine and hip. She is initiated on treatment with alendronate 70 mg weekly, cholecalciferol 5000 units daily, and calcium carbonate 1500 mg daily. When should the bone densitometry testing be repeated to assess the response to therapy?

A. 1 year
B. 3 years
C. 5 years
D. 10 yeears
E. It does not need to be repeated. MRI should be performed instead.

X-93. A 19-year-old woman is evaluated by her primary care physician for recurrent long bone fractures. She has fractured her femur twice and her humerus three times. She has not had an abnormal number of falls and reports also having easy bruising. Aside from these repeated orthopedic injuries, she is otherwise healthy. Physical examination shows mildly disfigured bones, small, amber-yellowish teeth, and bluish-colored sclera. Osteogenesis imperfecta is suspected. Which of the following statements is true regarding this condition?

A. A mutation in type 1 procollagen likely is present in this patient.
B. Bone biopsy is needed for definitive diagnosis.
C. Bisphosphonates have shown long-term success in preventing long bone fractures in this condition.
D. Fractures in females tend to increase after puberty.
E. Increased bone mineral density may be demonstrated on x-ray absorptiometry.

X-94. A 20-year-old man is evaluated during a routine physical examination prior to playing for a college basketball team. He was recruited to play on the team and offered a scholarship after being noticed for his skills on a junior national team abroad. He is originally from Nigeria and has come to the United States only for his education. His medical history is significant for prior treatment for tuberculosis at the age of 13. He takes no medications and has no allergies. His father died of sudden cardiac death at the age of 46. No autopsy was performed. Other family members in his father's family have died at young ages from cardiac conditions. His mother is healthy. His height is 79 in (200.6 cm). His weight is 198 lb (89.8 kg). His BMI is 22.3 kg/m^2. You note that his torso is short relative to his limbs. His arm span measures 83 in. He also has pectus excavatum and arachnodactyly. A high-arched palate is present. He wears glasses for severe myopia and has had ectopia lentis on the right. On cardiovascular examination, a II/VI blowing diastolic murmur is noted in the third left intercostal space. He is anxious to begin practicing with the basketball team. What do you advise at this time?

A. He is not safe for further competitive basketball or other strenuous physical activities.
B. He is safe to resume physical activity without further evaluation.
C. He may continue to practice with the team while further evaluation with an echocardiogram, slit-lamp examination, and genetic testing is performed.
D. He should be placed on a β-blocker and then can resume physical activity.

X-95. A 40-year-old man is evaluated as part of an executive physical examination. He has read about different screening procedures on the Internet and is interested in being screened for hemochromatosis. He is otherwise healthy and takes only a daily multivitamin. His father died of cirrhosis at the age of 56 and also drank alcohol heavily. There is no other liver disease in his family. Which of the following tests is the most appropriate first step to screen for this disorder?

A. Genetic testing for C282Y mutation
B. *HFE* activity assay
C. Liver MRI
D. Screening for hemochromatosis is not cost effective and not advised
E. Transferrin saturation and serum ferritin

X-96. A 55-year-old white male with a history of diabetes presents to your office with complaints of generalized weakness, weight loss, nonspecific diffuse abdominal pain, and erectile dysfunction. The patient has a past history of hypercholesterolemia and takes atorvastatin. The examination is significant for hepatomegaly without tenderness, testicular atrophy, and gynecomastia. Skin examination shows a diffuse slate-gray hue slightly more pronounced on the face and neck. Joint examination shows mild swelling of the second and third metacarpophalangeal joints on the right hand. Which of the following studies is most likely to lead to the correct diagnosis?

A. Anti–smooth muscle antibody
B. Ceruloplasmin
C. Hepatic ultrasound with Doppler imaging
D. Hepatitis B surface antibody
E. *HFE* gene mutation screen

X-97. A 28-year-old man is admitted to the intensive care unit with fulminant hepatic failure and hemolysis. On further questioning, his family reports that he has been diagnosed with depression for 5 years and had a prior episode of acute hepatitis 2 years ago that resolved. At that time, his aspartate aminotransferase peaked at 1200 U/L and alanine aminotransferase peaked at 1900 U/L. He had only mild jaundice, with a total bilirubin of 7.2 g/dL. No cause of the hepatitis was found despite a workup that included viral and autoimmune causes. His liver function returned to normal. He is taking an antidepressant and occasional ibuprofen, but no other medications. Physical examination is notable for ascites and altered mental status with dystonia. Abdominal CT scan shows no biliary obstruction but a cirrhotic liver. Which of the following findings would be most likely to confirm the underlying diagnosis?

A. 24-Hour urine level of iron
B. Brain MRI showing damage to the basal ganglia
C. Genotype for *HFE* mutation
D. Schistocytes on peripheral blood smear
E. Slit-lamp ocular examination showing Kayser-Fleischer rings

X-98. Which of the following is the most appropriate initial treatment for the patient described in Question X-97?

A. Cholestyramine
B. D-Penicillamine
C. Liver transplantation
D. Trientine
E. Zinc

X-99. A 22-year-old woman presents to the emergency department for abdominal pain that she rates a 10 out of 10 in severity. Her current episode began about 5 hours ago. She describes it as diffuse and constant with a mild crampy quality. She has mild nausea and has vomited once. She feels that her abdomen is distended. Over the past 6 years, she has presented to the emergency department five times with similar symptoms and has been frustrated because nothing has been found. She reports that she was generally treated with IV fluids, antiemetics, and IV narcotics. She expresses that she was treated like a drug user because laboratory studies, urinalysis, and abdominal CT with IV and oral contrast were negative. Her symptoms have always resolved without intervention or hospitalization within 24–48 hours. She has had milder episodes approximately four to five times yearly and has avoided coming in for evaluation due to her prior bad experiences with healthcare. When she has pain, she has significant anxiety and insomnia. She has had two episodes of auditory hallucinations during an acute pain attack, which she attributed to the severity of the pain. She is currently in her senior year of college studying mechanical engineering and is an honors student. She has no past medical history. She stopped taking oral contraceptives due to her perception that it caused her episodes of abdominal pain to worsen. Her mother has had a few mild episodes of similar abdominal pain that she thinks has been due to endometriosis. Her mother has not sought specific evaluation. On examination, vital signs are heart rate of 120 bpm, temperature of 37.2°C, blood pressure of 138/88 mmHg, respiratory rate of 18 breaths/min, and arterial oxygen saturation (SaO_2) of 99% on room air. She appears in mild distress due to pain. Examination of the head, eyes, ears, nose, and throat is unremarkable. Chest is clear. Cardiovascular exam shows only a regular tachycardia without murmur. Abdominal examination shows hypoactive bowel sounds with mild distention. There is no localizing tenderness. Abdominal x-rays show an ileus. A urinalysis and toxicology screen are negative. Her complete blood count and comprehensive metabolic panel are normal with the exception of mild hyponatremia (sodium 132 mmol/L). Which of the following is the next most appropriate step in her evaluation?

A. Endoscopy and colonoscopy
B. Plasma HMB synthase mutation analysis
C. Measurement of urine porphyrobilinogen and 5-aminolevulinic acid during attack
D. Measurement of urine porphyrins
E. Prescription for lubiprostone

X-100. A 39-year-old man comes to clinic complaining of blistering skin lesions on the backs of his hands and arms that are painful. They are often precipitated by sunlight and heal with scarring. He also notices that they often occur after drinking alcohol heavily. His hands and forearms have numerous hypopigmented scars that he says are from previous episodes. The skin over the back of his hands appears thick and coarse. Otherwise his review of systems and physical examination are normal. The lesions on his hands are shown in Figure X-100. Testing confirms your suspected diagnosis. Which of the following treatments will most likely lead to long-term improvement for this patient?

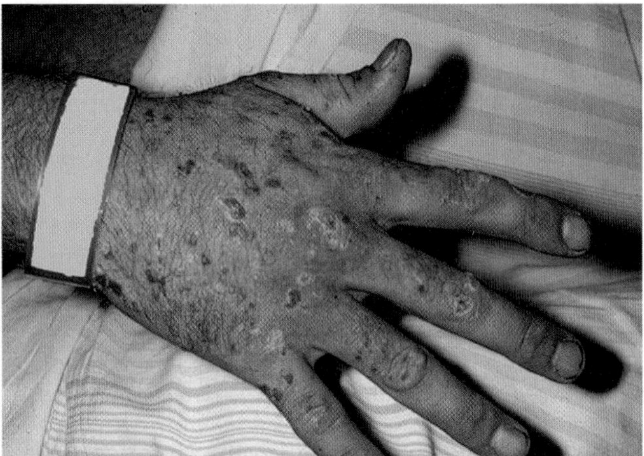

FIGURE X-100 Courtesy of Dr. Karl E. Anderson; with permission.

A. Avoidance of sun exposure and IV hemin for treatment of acute lesions
B. Hydroxychloroquine 200 mg twice daily
C. Phlebotomy of 450 mL of blood every 1–2 weeks
D. Prednisone 0.5 mg/kg orally daily
E. Triamcinolone 0.5% topically twice daily

ANSWERS

X-1. **The answer is C.** *(Chap. 401e)* Hormones produced by the anterior pituitary include adrenocorticotropic hormone (ACTH), thyroid-stimulating hormone (TSH), luteinizing hormone (LH), follicle-stimulating hormone (FSH), prolactin, and growth hormone. The posterior pituitary produces vasopressin and oxytocin. The anterior and posterior pituitary have a separate vascular supply, and the posterior pituitary is directly innervated by the hypothalamic neurons via the pituitary stalk, thus making it susceptible to shear stress–associated dysfunction. Hypothalamic control of anterior pituitary function is through secreted hormones; thus, it is less susceptible to traumatic injury.

X-2. **The answer is D.** *(Chap. 401e)* Functional pituitary adenoma presentations include acromegaly, as in this patient; prolactinomas; or Cushing syndrome. Hypersecretion of growth hormone underlies this syndrome in patients with pituitary masses, although ectopic production of growth hormone, particularly by tumors, has been reported. Because growth hormone is secreted in a highly pulsatile fashion, obtaining random serum levels is not reliable. Thus, the downstream mediator of systemic effects of growth hormone, insulin-like growth factor-1 (IGF-1), is measured to screen for growth hormone excess. IGF-1 is made by the liver in response to growth hormone stimulation. An oral glucose tolerance test with growth hormone obtained at 0, 30, and 60 minutes may also be used to screen for acromegaly because normal persons should suppress growth hormone to this challenge. Serum prolactin level is useful to screen for prolactinomas, and 24-hour urinary free cortisol and ACTH assay are useful screens for Cushing disease.

X-3. **The answer is D.** *(Chap. 401e)* The pituitary gland does form from the Rathke pouch embryonically. As shown in Figure X-3, blood supply of the pituitary gland comes from the superior and inferior hypophyseal arteries. The hypothalamic pituitary portal plexus provides the major blood source for the anterior pituitary, allowing reliable transmission

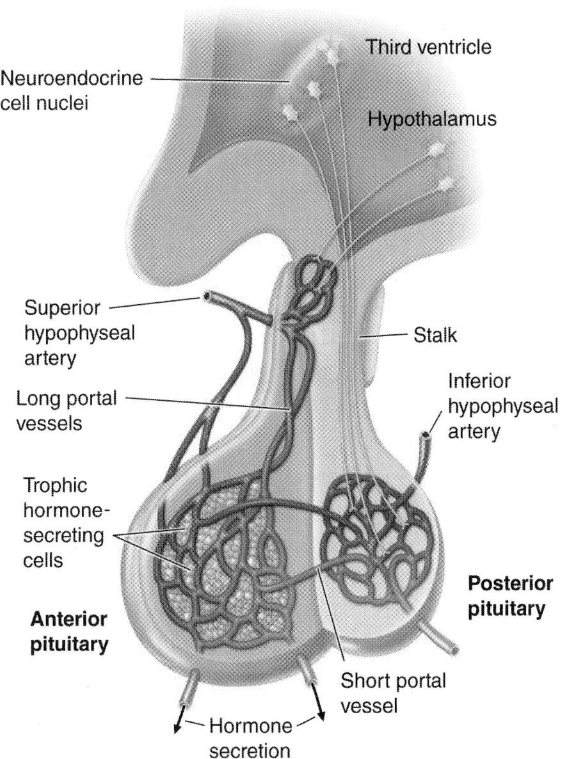

FIGURE X-3

of hypothalamic peptide pulses without significant systemic dilution; consequently, pituitary cells are exposed to releasing or inhibiting factors and, in turn, release their hormones as discrete pulses into the systemic circulation. The posterior pituitary is supplied by the inferior hypophyseal arteries. In contrast to the anterior pituitary, the posterior lobe is directly innervated by hypothalamic neurons (supraopticohypophyseal and tuberohypophyseal nerve tracts) via the pituitary stalk. Thus, posterior pituitary production of vasopressin (antidiuretic hormone) and oxytocin is particularly sensitive to neuronal damage by lesions that affect the pituitary stalk or hypothalamus. ACTH is derived from proopiomelanocortin, and prolactin is secreted in the posterior pituitary.

X-4. **The answer is C.** *(Chap. 401e)* Adult growth hormone deficiency is usually caused by hypothalamic or pituitary damage. Because growth hormone is no longer important for achieving stature, the presentation is different from childhood growth hormone deficiency. Although growth hormone has direct tissue effects, it primarily acts through increasing secretion of IGF-1, which in turn stimulates lipolysis, increases circulating fatty acids, reduces omental fat mass, and enhances lean body mass. Thus, deficiency of growth hormone causes the opposite effects. In addition, hypertension, left ventricular dysfunction, and increased plasma fibrinogen levels may also be present with deficient growth hormone. Reduced, not increased, bone mineral density may also occur in adults with growth hormone deficiency.

X-5. **The answer is E.** *(Chap. 401e)* The patient has a clinical presentation consistent with Cushing syndrome. Although many cases of inappropriate elevation of ACTH are due to pituitary tumors, a substantial proportion are due to ectopic ACTH secretion. Clues to this diagnosis include a rapid onset of hypercortisolism features associated with skin hyperpigmentation and severe myopathy. Additionally, hypertension, hypokalemic metabolic alkalosis, glucose intolerance, and edema are more prominent in ectopic ACTH secretion than in pituitary tumors. Serum potassium <3.3 mmol/L is present in 70% of patients with ectopic ACTH, but <10% of patients with pituitary-dependent Cushing syndrome. ACTH levels will be high, because this is the underlying cause of both types of Cushing syndrome. Corticotropin-releasing hormone is rarely the cause of Cushing syndrome. Unfortunately, magnetic resonance imaging (MRI) of the pituitary gland will not visualize lesions <2 mm; thus occasionally, sampling of the inferior petrosal veins is required, but this is not yet indicated in this patient at this point in the evaluation.

X-6. **The answer is A.** *(Chap. 402)* Kallmann syndrome results from defective hypothalamic gonadotropin-releasing hormone (GnRH) synthesis and is associated with anosmia or hyposmia due to olfactory bulb agenesis or hypoplasia. Classically, the syndrome may also be associated with color blindness, optic atrophy, nerve deafness, cleft palate, renal abnormalities, cryptorchidism, and neurologic abnormalities such as mirror movements. Associated clinical features, in addition to GnRH deficiency, vary depending on the genetic cause. GnRH deficiency prevents progression through puberty. Males present with delayed puberty and pronounced hypogonadal features, including micropenis, which are probably the result of low testosterone levels during infancy. Females present with primary amenorrhea and failure of secondary sexual development. A white forelock is typical of Waardenburg syndrome, whereas hyperphagic obesity is common in Prader-Willi syndrome.

X-7. **The answer is B.** *(Chap. 402)* This patient has evidence of Sheehan syndrome after giving birth. In this syndrome, the postpartum hyperplastic pituitary is at increased risk for hemorrhage and/or infarction. This leads to bilateral visual changes, headache, and meningeal signs. Ophthalmoplegia may be observed. In severe cases, cardiovascular collapse and altered levels of consciousness may be observed. Laboratory evaluation commonly shows hypoglycemia. Pituitary computed tomography (CT) or MRI may show signs of sellar hemorrhage if present. Involvement of all pituitary hormones may be seen, although the most acute findings are often hypoglycemia and hypotension from failure of ACTH. The hypoglycemia and hypotension present in this patient suggest failure of the glucocorticoid system; thus treatment with a corticosteroid is indicated. There is no evidence of sepsis;

thus antibiotics and drotrecogin alfa are not indicated. With a normal hematocrit and no reported evidence of massive hemorrhage, packed red cell transfusion is unlikely to be helpful. Although TSH production is undoubtedly low in this patient, the most immediate concern is replacement of glucocorticoid.

X-8. **The answer is C.** *(Chap. 402)* Cranial irradiation may result in long-term hypothalamic and pituitary dysfunction, especially in children and adolescents, because they are more susceptible to damage after whole-brain or head and neck therapeutic irradiation. The development of hormonal abnormalities correlates strongly with irradiation dosage and the time interval after completion of radiotherapy. Up to two-thirds of patients ultimately develop hormone insufficiency after a median dose of 50 Gy (5000 rad) directed at the skull base. The development of hypopituitarism occurs over 5–15 years and usually reflects hypothalamic damage rather than primary destruction of pituitary cells. Although the pattern of hormone loss is variable, growth hormone deficiency is most common, followed by gonadotropin and ACTH deficiency. When deficiency of one or more hormones is documented, the possibility of diminished reserve of other hormones is likely. Accordingly, anterior pituitary function should be continually evaluated over the long term in previously irradiated patients, and replacement therapy should be instituted when appropriate.

X-9. **The answer is C.** *(Chap. 402)* The patient has panhypopituitarism and is unable to make TSH; thus her plasma TSH level will always be low, regardless of the adequacy of her thyroxine (T_4) replacement. A free T_4 level will allow determination of whether her plasma level is in the normal range of thyroid hormone. This, coupled with her symptoms, will aid in determination of proper levothyroxine dosing. There is no evidence of recurrent disease clinically; thus MRI is not useful. She is unlikely to have primary thyroid disease, and T_4 level is unknown presently, so thyroid uptake scan is not indicated at this time.

X-10. **The answer is B.** *(Chap. 402)* The identification of an empty sella is often an incidental MRI finding. Typically, these patients will have normal pituitary function and should be reassured. It is likely that the surrounding rim of pituitary tissue is functioning normally. An empty sella may signal the insidious onset of hypopituitarism, and laboratory results should be followed closely. Unless her clinical situation changes, repeat MRI is not indicated. Endocrine malignancy is unlikely, and surgery is not part of the management of an empty sella.

X-11. **The answer is E.** *(Chap. 403)* The dorsal sellar diaphragm presents the least resistance to soft tissue expansion from the sella; consequently, pituitary adenomas frequently extend in a suprasellar direction. Bony invasion may occur as well.

X-12. **The answer is E.** *(Chap. 403)* Pituitary gland height ranges from 6 mm in children to 8 mm in adults; during pregnancy and puberty, the height may reach 10–12 mm. The upper aspect of the adult pituitary is flat or slightly concave, but in adolescent and pregnant individuals, this surface may be convex, reflecting physiologic pituitary enlargement. The stalk should be midline and vertical. Anterior pituitary gland soft tissue consistency is slightly heterogeneous on MRI, and signal intensity resembles that of brain matter on T1-weighted imaging. Adenoma density is usually lower than that of surrounding normal tissue on T1-weighted imaging, and the signal intensity increases with T2-weighted images. The high phospholipid content of the posterior pituitary results in a pituitary "bright spot."

X-13. **The answer is C.** *(Chap. 403)* Because optic tracts may be contiguous to an expanding pituitary mass, reproducible visual field assessment using perimetry techniques should be performed on all patients with sellar mass lesions that impinge the optic chiasm. Bitemporal hemianopia, often more pronounced superiorly, is observed classically. It occurs because nasal ganglion cell fibers, which cross in the optic chiasm, are especially vulnerable to compression of the ventral optic chiasm. Occasionally, homonymous hemianopia occurs as a result of postchiasmal compression, or monocular temporal field loss occurs as a result of prechiasmal compression.

X-14. **The answer is D.** *(Chap. 403)* Carney syndrome is characterized by spotty skin pigmentation, myxomas, and endocrine tumors, including testicular, adrenal, and pituitary adenomas. Acromegaly occurs in about 20% of these patients. A subset of patients have mutations in the R1α regulatory subunit of protein kinase A (*PRKAR1A*).

X-15. **The answer is B.** *(Chap. 405)* Nutritional and maternal iodine deficiencies are common in many parts of the developing world and, when severe, can result in cretinism. Cretinism is characterized by mental and growth retardation but is preventable by administration of iodine and/or thyroid hormone early in life. Concomitant selenium deficiency can contribute to the neurologic manifestations. Iodine supplementation of bread, salt, and other foods has markedly decreased the rates of this disease. Beriberi disease is a nervous system ailment caused by a thiamine deficiency in the diet. Scurvy is due to vitamin C deficiency. Folate deficiency in pregnant women is associated with an increased risk of preterm labor and a number of congenital malformations, most notably involving the neural tube. Folate supplementation can lower the risk of spina bifida, anencephaly, congenital heart disease, cleft lips, and limb deformities. Vitamin A deficiency is a common cause of blindness in the developing world.

X-16. **The answer is C.** *(Chap. 405)* A number of conditions are associated with normal thyroid function but hyperthyroxinemia. Although some of these are associated with clinical hyperthyroidism, many have simply elevated levels of total T_4 and normal conversion to triiodothyronine (T_3) and, thus, are clinically normal. Anything that increases liver production of thyroid-binding globulin will produce elevated total T_4 levels and normal free T_4 and T_3 levels. In this category are pregnancy, estrogen-containing oral contraceptives, cirrhosis, and familial excess thyroid-binding globulin production. Familial dysalbuminemic hyperthyroxinemia results in an albumin mutation and increased T_4 with normal free T_4 and T_3 levels. Euthyroid sick syndrome occurs during acute medical and psychiatric illness. In this syndrome, there is transiently increased unbound T_4 and decreased TSH. Total T_4 and T_3 may be decreased, particularly later in the course of disease.

X-17. **The answer is D.** *(Chap. 405)* Iodine deficiency remains the most common cause of hypothyroidism worldwide. It is present at relatively high levels even in the developed world, including Europe. In areas of iodine sufficiency, autoimmune disease (Hashimoto thyroiditis) and iatrogenic hypothyroidism (treatment of hyperthyroidism) are the most common causes.

X-18. **The answer is C.** *(Chap. 405)* There are a number of important effects of thyroid hormone (or its absence) on the cardiovascular system. Importantly, hypothyroidism is associated with bradycardia, reduced myocardial contractility, and thus reduced stroke volume. Increased peripheral resistance may be accompanied by systemic hypertension, particularly diastolic in hypothyroidism. Pericardial effusions are found in up to 30% of patients with hypothyroidism, although they rarely cause decreased cardiac function. Finally, in hypothyroid patients, blood flow is directed away from the skin, thus producing cool extremities.

X-19. **The answer is A.** *(Chap. 405)* The most common cause of hypothyroidism in the United States is autoimmune thyroiditis, because the United States is an iodine-replete area. Although earlier in the disease, a radioiodine uptake scan may have shown diffusely increased uptake from lymphocytic infiltration, at this point in the disease, when the infiltrate is "burned out," there is likely to be little found on the scan. Likewise, a thyroid ultrasound would only be useful for presumed multinodular goiter. Antithyroid peroxidase antibodies are commonly found in patients with autoimmune thyroiditis, whereas antithyroglobulin antibodies are found less commonly. Antithyroglobulin antibodies are also found in other thyroid disorders (Graves disease, thyrotoxicosis) as well as systemic autoimmune diseases (systemic lupus erythematosus). Thyroglobulin is released from the thyroid in all types of thyrotoxicosis with the exception of factitious disease. This patient, however, was hypothyroid, and thus serum thyroglobulin levels are unlikely to be helpful.

X-20. The answer is D. *(Chap. 405)* An increase in TSH in a patient with hypothyroidism that was previously stable with medication for many years suggests either a failure of taking the medication, difficulty with absorption from bowel disease, or medication interaction or drug–drug interaction affecting clearance. In patients with normal body weight taking >200 μg of levothyroxine per day, an elevated TSH strongly suggests noncompliance. Such patients should be encouraged to take two tablets at one time on the day they remember to attempt to reach the weekly target dose; the long drug half-life makes this practice safe. Other causes of increased thyroxine requirements include malabsorption, such as with celiac disease or small bowel surgery, estrogen therapy, and drugs that interfere with T_4 absorption (e.g., ferrous sulfate, cholestyramine) or clearance (e.g., lovastatin, amiodarone, carbamazepine, phenytoin).

X-21. The answer is A. *(Chap. 405)* The patient has myxedema coma. This condition of profound hypothyroidism most commonly occurs in the elderly, and often a precipitating condition may be identified such as myocardial infarction or infection. Clinical manifestations include altered level of consciousness, bradycardia, and hypothermia. Management includes repletion of thyroid hormone through IV levothyroxine, but also supplementation of glucocorticoids because there is impaired adrenal reserve in severe hypothyroidism. Care must be taken with rewarming because it may precipitate cardiovascular collapse. Therefore, external warming is indicated only if the temperature is <30°C. Hypertonic saline and glucose may be used if hyponatremia or hypoglycemia is severe; however, hypotonic solutions should be avoided because they may worsen fluid retention. Because metabolism of many substances is markedly reduced, sedation should be avoided or minimized. Similarly, blood levels of drugs should be monitored when available.

X-22. The answer is A. *(Chap. 405)* Patients with Graves disease produce thyroid-stimulating immunoglobulins. They subsequently produce higher levels of T_4 compared with the normal population. As a result, many patients with Graves disease are mildly iodine deficient, and T_4 production is somewhat limited by the availability of iodine. Exposure to iodinated contrast thus reverses iodine deficiency and may precipitate worsening hyperthyroidism. Additionally, the reversal of mild iodine deficiency may make iodine-125 therapy for Graves disease less successful because thyroid iodine uptake is lessened in the iodine-replete state.

X-23. The answer is C. *(Chap. 406)* The adrenal gland has three major functions: glucocorticoid synthesis, aldosterone synthesis, and androgen precursor synthesis. Glucocorticoid synthesis is controlled by the pituitary secretion of ACTH. The primary stimulus for aldosterone synthesis is the renin-angiotensin-aldosterone system, which is independent of the pituitary. Thus, morning cortisol secretion and release of cortisol in response to stress are regulated by the pituitary gland, whereas regulation of sodium retention and potassium excretion by aldosterone is independent of the pituitary and would be preserved in this patient.

X-24. The answer is A. *(Chap. 406)* Cushing syndrome is a constellation of features that result from chronic exposure to elevated levels of cortisol from any etiology. Although the most common etiology is an ACTH-producing pituitary adenoma, which accounts for 75% of Cushing syndrome, 15% of cases are due to ectopic ACTH syndromes such as bronchial or pancreatic tumors, small-cell lung cancer, and other causes. ACTH-independent Cushing syndrome is much rarer. Adrenocortical adenoma underlies 5%–10% of cases, and adrenocortical carcinoma is present in 1% of Cushing cases. McCune-Albright syndrome is a genetic cause of bone abnormalities, skin lesions (café-au-lait), and premature puberty, particularly in girls. Interestingly, it is caused by a sporadic in utero mutation, not an inherited disorder, and thus will not be passed on to progeny.

X-25. The answer is B. *(Chap. 406)* Conn syndrome refers to an aldosterone-producing adrenal adenoma. Although it accounts for 40% of hyperaldosterone states, bilateral micronodular adrenal hyperplasia is more common. Other causes of hyperaldosteronism are substantially rarer, accounting for <1% of disease. The hallmark of Conn syndrome is hypertension with hypokalemia. Because aldosterone stimulates sodium retention and potassium excretion, all patients should be hypokalemic at presentation. Serum sodium is usually normal because of concurrent fluid retention. Hypokalemia may be associated with muscle weakness, proximal myopathy, or even paralysis. Hypokalemia may be exacerbated by thiazide diuretics. Additional features include metabolic alkalosis that may contribute to muscle cramps and tetany.

X-26. **The answer is B.** *(Chap. 406)* Incidental adrenal masses are often discovered during radiographic testing for another condition and are found in approximately 6% of adults at autopsy. Fifty percent of patients with a history of malignancy and a newly discovered adrenal mass will actually have an adrenal metastasis. Fine-needle aspiration of a suspected metastatic malignancy will often be diagnostic. In the absence of a suspected nonadrenal malignancy, most adrenal incidentalomas are benign. Primary adrenal malignancies are uncommon (<0.01%), and fine-needle aspiration is not useful to distinguish between benign and malignant primary adrenal tumors. Although 90% of these masses are nonsecretory, patients with an incidentaloma should be screened for pheochromocytoma and hypercortisolism with plasma free metanephrines and an overnight dexamethasone suppression test, respectively. When radiographic features suggest a benign neoplasm (<3 cm), scanning should be repeated in 3–6 months. When masses are >6 cm, surgical removal (if more likely primary adrenal malignancy) or fine-needle aspiration (if more likely metastatic malignancy) is preferred.

X-27. **The answer is C.** *(Chap. 406)* The release of corticotropin-releasing hormone, and subsequently ACTH, occurs in a pulsatile fashion that follows a circadian rhythm under the control of the hypothalamus, specifically its suprachiasmatic nucleus (SCN), with additional regulation by a complex network of cell-specific clock genes. Reflecting the pattern of ACTH secretion, adrenal cortisol secretion exhibits a distinct circadian rhythm; it starts to rise in the early morning hours prior to awakening, with peak levels in the morning and low levels in the evening (Figure X-27).

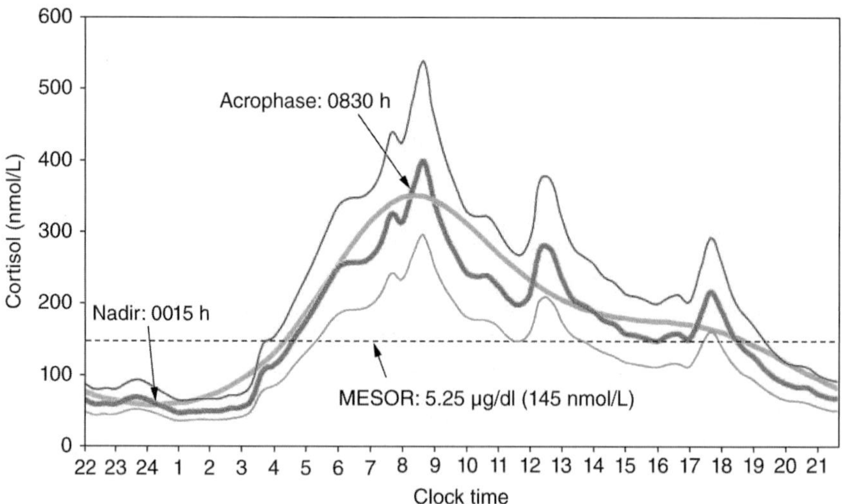

FIGURE X-27 Modified after Debono M, Ghobadi C, Rostami-Hodjegan A, et al: Modified-release hydrocortisone to provide circadian cortisol profiles. *J Clin Endocrinol Metab* 94:1548, 2009.

X-28. **The answer is B.** *(Chap. 406)* This patient is obese and has abdominal stria and a round (or moon) facies, which are all signs of glucocorticoid excess. Often, this is due to exogenous (corticosteroid) administration, although it could also be due to endogenous production (Cushing syndrome). A physiologic stressor, such as trauma or infection, may trigger adrenal crisis. Importantly (although not present in this case), hyperthyroidism can also trigger adrenal crisis via increased glucocorticoid inactivation. Thus, glucocorticoids must always be provided first in the setting of concomitant thyroid and adrenal insufficiency. Acute adrenal insufficiency requires immediate initiation of rehydration, usually carried out by saline infusion at initial rates of 1 L/hr with continuous cardiac monitoring. Glucocorticoid replacement should be initiated by bolus injection of 100 mg of hydrocortisone, followed by the administration of 100–200 mg of hydrocortisone over 24 hours, either by continuous infusion or by bolus intravenous (IV) or intramuscular injections. Mineralocorticoid replacement can be initiated once the daily hydrocortisone dose has been reduced to <50 mg because, at higher doses, hydrocortisone provides sufficient stimulation of mineralocorticoid receptors.

X-29. **The answer is A.** *(Chap. 407)* When the diagnosis of pheochromocytoma is entertained, the first step is measurement of catecholamines and/or metanephrines. This can be achieved by urinary tests for vanillylmandelic acid, catecholamines, fractionated metanephrines, or total metanephrines. Testing for total metanephrines has a high sensitivity and, therefore, is frequently used. A value of three times the upper limit of normal is highly suggestive of pheochromocytoma. Borderline elevations, as this patient had, are likely to be false positives. The next most appropriate step is to remove potentially confounding dietary or drug exposures, if possible, and repeat the test. Likely culprit drugs include levodopa, sympathomimetics, diuretics, tricyclic antidepressants, and α- and β-blockers (labetalol in this case). Sertraline is a selective serotonin reuptake inhibitor antidepressant, not a tricyclic. Alternatively, a clonidine suppression test may be ordered.

X-30. **The answer is E.** *(Chap. 407)* Complete removal of the pheochromocytoma is the only therapy that leads to a long-term cure, although 90% of tumors are benign. However, preoperative control of hypertension is necessary to prevent surgical complications and lower mortality. This patient is presenting with encephalopathy in a hypertensive crisis. The hypertension should be managed initially with IV medications to lower the mean arterial pressure by approximately 20% over the initial 24-hour period. Medications that can be used for hypertensive crisis in pheochromocytoma include nitroprusside, nicardipine, and phentolamine. Once the acute hypertensive crisis has resolved, transition to oral α-adrenergic blockers is indicated. Phenoxybenzamine is the most commonly used drug and is started at low doses (5–10 mg three times daily) and titrated to the maximum-tolerated dose (usually 20–30 mg daily). Once α-blockers have been initiated, β-blockade can be safely used and is particularly indicated for ongoing tachycardia. Liberal salt and fluid intake helps expand plasma volume and treat orthostatic hypotension. Once blood pressure is maintained below 160/100 mmHg with moderate orthostasis, it is safe to proceed to surgery. If blood pressure remains elevated despite treatment with α-blockade, the addition of calcium channel blockers, angiotensin receptor blockers, or angiotensin-converting enzyme inhibitors should be considered. Diuretics should be avoided because they will exacerbate orthostasis.

X-31. **The answer is D.** *(Chap. 407)* The diagnosis of malignant pheochromocytoma is problematic. The typical histologic criteria of cellular atypia, presence of mitoses, and invasion of vessels or adjacent tissues are insufficient for the diagnosis of malignancy in pheochromocytoma. Thus, the term malignant pheochromocytoma is restricted to tumors with distant metastases, most commonly found by nuclear medicine imaging in lungs, bone, or liver—locations suggesting a vascular pathway of spread.

X-32. **The answer is B.** *(Chap. 408)* Multiple endocrine neoplasia (MEN) syndrome is defined as a disorder with neoplasms affecting two or more hormonal tissues in several members of the family. The most common of these is MEN type 1 (MEN1), which is caused by the gene coding the nuclear protein called Menin. MEN1 is associated with tumors or hyperplasia of the parathyroid, pancreas, pituitary, adrenal cortex, and foregut and/or subcutaneous or visceral lipomas. The most common and earliest manifestation is hyperparathyroidism with symptomatic hypercalcemia. This most commonly occurs in the late teenage years, and 93%–100% of mutation carriers develop this complication. Gastrinomas, insulinomas, and prolactinomas are less common and tend to occur in the 20s, 30s, and 40s. Pheochromocytoma may occur in MEN1 but is more commonly found in MEN type 2A (MEN2A) or von Hippel-Lindau syndrome.

X-33. The answer is C. *(Chap. 408)* MEN type 2 (MEN2), also called Sipple syndrome, is characterized by the association of medullary thyroid carcinoma (MTC), pheochromocytomas, and parathyroid tumors. In MEN2A (the most common variant), MTC is associated with pheochromocytomas in 50% of patients (may be bilateral) and with parathyroid tumors in 20% of patients. MEN1, which is also referred to as Wermer syndrome, is characterized by the triad of tumors involving the parathyroids, pancreatic islets, and anterior pituitary. MEN1 syndrome is caused by a mutation in the Menin (or *MEN1*) gene. MEN2 is caused by a mutation in the *RET* gene. Family and genetic screening both have high value in this syndrome (MEN2) because prophylactic thyroidectomy, with life-long thyroxine replacement, has dramatically improved outcomes in patients with MEN2 and MEN3, such that approximately 90% of young patients with *RET* mutations who had a prophylactic thyroidectomy have no evidence of persistent or recurrent MTC at 7 years after surgery. Partial thyroidectomy is inappropriate for this patient; in patients with clinically evident MTC, a total thyroidectomy with bilateral central resection is recommended.

X-34. The answer is B. *(Chap. 409)* This patient almost certainly is hypotensive, hyponatremic, and hyperkalemic from primary adrenal insufficiency. Given the concomitant presence of hypoparathyroidism and mucocutaneous candidiasis, he likely suffers from autoimmune polyendocrine syndrome (APS) type 1. Mucocutaneous candidiasis, hypoparathyroidism, and Addison disease form the three major components of this disorder. It is an autosomal recessive disorder caused by mutations in the *AIRE* gene (autoimmune regulator gene) found on chromosome 21. APS type 1 develops very early in life, often in infancy. Chronic mucocutaneous candidiasis without signs of systemic disease is often the first manifestation. Hypoparathyroidism usually develops next, followed by adrenal insufficiency. Regarding the treatment of adrenal crisis, several issues merit mention. Adrenal insufficiency can be masked by primary hypothyroidism by prolonging the half-life of cortisol. Therefore, the caveat is that replacement therapy with thyroid hormone can precipitate an adrenal crisis in an undiagnosed individual. Hence, all patients with hypothyroidism and the possibility of APS should be screened for adrenal insufficiency to allow treatment with glucocorticoids prior to the initiation of thyroid hormone replacement. Treatment of mucocutaneous candidiasis with ketoconazole in an individual with subclinical adrenal insufficiency may also precipitate adrenal crisis. This patient may have concurrent hypocalcemia that merits treatment in conjunction with the adrenal insufficiency.

X-35. The answer is D. *(Chap. 409)* This patient likely has POEMS (polyneuropathy, organomegaly, endocrinopathy, M-protein, and skin changes). Patients usually present with a progressive sensorimotor polyneuropathy, diabetes mellitus (50%), primary gonadal failure (70%), and a plasma cell dyscrasia with sclerotic bony lesions. Associated findings can be hepatosplenomegaly, lymphadenopathy, and hyperpigmentation. Patients often present in the fifth and sixth decades of life and have a median survival after diagnosis of less than 3 years. The detection of an M-protein on serum electrophoresis would make POEMS the most likely diagnosis.

X-36. The answer is C. *(Chap. 410)* Klinefelter syndrome is a chromosomal disorder with 47, XXY. Because the primary feature of this disorder is gonadal failure, low testosterone is present, and thus, increased LH and FSH are produced in an attempt to increase testosterone production in the feedback loop of sex hormones. Increased estrogen production is often present because of chronic Leydig cell stimulation by LH and aromatization of androstenedione by adipose tissue. The lower testosterone-to-estrogen ratio results in mild feminization with gynecomastia. Features of low testosterone are small testes and eunuchoid proportions with long legs and incomplete virilization. Biopsy of the testes, although rarely performed, shows hyalinization of the seminiferous tubules and azoospermia. Although severe cases are diagnosed prepubertally as a result of small testes and impaired androgenization, approximately 75% of cases are not diagnosed, and the frequency in the general population is 1 in 1000. Patients with Klinefelter syndrome are at increased risk of breast tumors, thromboembolic disease, learning difficulties, obesity, diabetes mellitus, and varicose veins.

X-37. **The answer is A.** *(Chap. 410)* Turner syndrome most frequently results from a 45,X karyotype, but mosaicism (45,X/46,XX) also can result in this disorder. Clinically, Turner syndrome manifests as short stature and primary amenorrhea if presenting in young adulthood. In addition, chronic lymphedema of the hands and feet, nuchal folds, a low hairline, and high-arched palate are also common features. To diagnose Turner syndrome, karyotype analysis should be performed. A Barr body results from inactivation of one of the X chromosomes in women and is not seen in males. In Turner syndrome, the Barr body should be absent, but only 50% of individuals with Turner syndrome have the 45,X karyotype. Thus, the diagnosis could be missed in those with mosaicism or other structural abnormalities of the X chromosome. Multiple comorbid conditions are found in individuals with Turner syndrome, and appropriate screening is recommended. Congenital heart defects affect 30% of women with Turner syndrome, including bicuspid aortic valve, coarctation of the aorta, and aortic root dilatation. An echocardiogram should be performed, and the individual should be assessed with blood pressures in the arms and legs. Hypertension can also be associated with structural abnormalities of the kidney and urinary tract, most commonly horseshoe kidney. A renal ultrasound is also recommended. Autoimmune thyroid disease affects 15%–30% of women with Turner syndrome and should be assessed by screening TSH. Other comorbidities that may occur include sensorineural hearing loss, elevated liver function enzymes, osteoporosis, and celiac disease.

X-38. **The answer is C.** *(Chap. 410)* This infant likely has congenital adrenal hyperplasia (CAH). The classic form of 21-hydroxylase deficiency (21-OHD) is the most common cause of CAH. It has an incidence between 1 in 10,000 and 1 in 15,000 and is the most common cause of androgenization in chromosomal 46,XX females. Affected individuals are homozygous or compound heterozygous for severe mutations in the enzyme 21-hydroxylase (*CYP21A2*). This mutation causes a block in adrenal glucocorticoid and mineralocorticoid synthesis, increasing 17-hydroxyprogesterone and shunting steroid precursors into the androgen synthesis pathway. Glucocorticoid insufficiency causes a compensatory elevation of ACTH, resulting in adrenal hyperplasia and additional synthesis of steroid precursors proximal to the enzymatic block. Increased androgen synthesis in utero causes androgenization of the 46,XX fetus in the first trimester. Ambiguous genitalia are seen at birth, with varying degrees of clitoral enlargement and labial fusion. The salt-wasting form of 21-OHD results from severe combined glucocorticoid and mineralocorticoid deficiency. A salt-wasting crisis usually manifests between 5 and 21 days of life and is a potentially life-threatening event that requires urgent fluid resuscitation and steroid treatment. Thus, a diagnosis of 21-OHD should be considered in any baby with atypical genitalia with bilateral nonpalpable gonads.

X-39. **The answer is D.** *(Chap. 411)* Gynecomastia is a relatively common complaint in men and may be caused by either obesity with adipose tissue expansion in the breast or by an increased estrogen-to-androgen ratio in which there is true glandular enlargement, as in this case. If the breast is unilaterally enlarged or if it is hard or fixed to underlying tissue, mammography is indicated. Alternatively, if cirrhosis or a causative drug is present, these may be adequate explanations, particularly when gynecomastia develops later in life in previously fertile men. If the breast tissue is >4 cm or there is evidence of very small testes and no causative drugs or liver disease, a search for alterations in serum testosterone, LH, FSH, estradiol, and human chorionic gonadotropin (hCG levels) should be undertaken. An androgen deficiency or resistance syndrome may be present, or an hCG-secreting tumor may be found. In this case, spironolactone is the likely culprit, and it may be stopped or switched to eplerenone and gynecomastia reassessed.

X-40. **The answer is C.** *(Chap. 411)* Many drugs may interfere with testicular function through a variety of mechanisms. Cyclophosphamide damages the seminiferous tubules in a dose- and time-dependent fashion and causes azoospermia within a few weeks of initiation.

This effect is reversible in approximately half of these patients. Ketoconazole inhibits testosterone synthesis. Spironolactone causes a blockade of androgen action which may also cause gynecomastia. Glucocorticoids lead to hypogonadism predominantly through inhibition of hypothalamic-pituitary function. Sexual dysfunction has been described as a side effect of therapy with β-blockers. However, there is no evidence of an effect on testicular function. Most reports of sexual dysfunction were in patients receiving older β-blockers such as propranolol and timolol.

X-41. **The answer is B.** *(Chap. 412)* Women who have regular monthly bleeding cycles that do not vary by >4 days generally have ovulatory cycles, but several other indicators suggest that ovulation is likely. These include the presence of mittelschmerz, which is described as midcycle pelvic discomfort that is thought to be caused by rapid expansion of the dominant follicle at the time of ovulation or premenstrual symptoms such as breast tenderness, bloating, and food cravings. Additional objective parameters suggest the presence of ovulation including a progesterone level >5 ng/mL 7 days before expected menses, an increase in basal body temperature >0.5°F in the second half of the menstrual cycle, and detection of urinary LH surge. Estrogen levels are elevated at the time of ovulation and during the secretory phase of the menstrual cycle but are not useful in detection of ovulation.

X-42. **The answer is A.** *(Chap. 412)* After birth and the loss of placenta-derived steroids, gonadotropin levels rise. FSH levels are much higher in girls than in boys. This rise in FSH results in ovarian activation (evident on ultrasound) and increased inhibin B and estradiol levels. Studies that have identified mutations in *TAC3*, which encodes neurokinin B, and its receptor, *TAC3R*, in patients with GnRH deficiency indicate that both are involved in control of GnRH secretion and may be particularly important at this early stage of development. By 12–20 months of age, the reproductive axis is again suppressed, and a period of relative quiescence persists until puberty. At the onset of puberty, pulsatile GnRH secretion induces pituitary gonadotropin production. In the early stages of puberty, LH and FSH secretion are apparent only during sleep, but as puberty develops, pulsatile gonadotropin secretion occurs throughout the day and night. Gonadotropin levels are cyclic during the reproductive years and increase dramatically with the loss of negative feedback that accompanies menopause (Figure X-42).

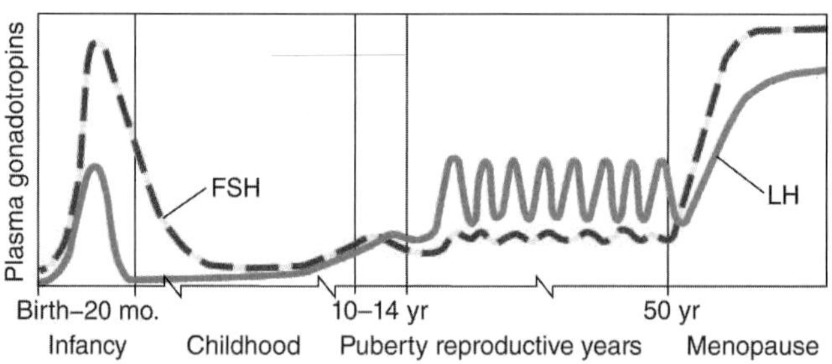

FIGURE X-42

X-43. **The answer is C.** *(Chap. 412)* The first menstrual period (menarche) occurs relatively late in the series of developmental milestones that characterize normal pubertal development. Menarche is preceded by the appearance of pubic and then axillary hair (adrenarche) as a result of maturation of the zona reticularis in the adrenal gland and increased adrenal androgen secretion, particularly dehydroepiandrosterone (DHEA). The triggers for adrenarche remain unknown but may involve increases in body mass index, as well as in utero and neonatal factors. Menarche is also preceded by breast development (thelarche). The breast is exquisitely sensitive to the very low levels of estrogen that result from peripheral conversion of adrenal androgens and the low levels of estrogen secreted from the ovary early in pubertal maturation. Breast development precedes the appearance of pubic and axillary hair in approximately 60% of girls. The interval between the onset of breast development and menarche is approximately 2 years. There has been a gradual decline in the age of menarche over the past century, attributed in large part to improvement in nutrition, and there is a relationship between adiposity and earlier sexual maturation in girls.

X-44. **The answer is E.** *(Chap. 413)* The Women's Health Initiative was the largest study of hormone therapy to date, including 27,000 postmenopausal women age 50 to 79 years who were followed for an average of 5–7 years. It was presumed that hormone replacement in this group of women would decrease cardiovascular risk. However, the trial was stopped early because of an unfavorable risk-benefit ratio in the estrogen-progestin arm and an increased risk of stroke that was not offset by lower coronary heart disease in the estrogen-only arm. Endometrial cancer risk was higher in patients with an intact uterus who were taking estrogen only. Use of progesterone eliminated this risk. Unopposed estrogen was associated with an increased risk of stroke that far outweighed the decreased risk of coronary heart disease. Estrogen-progestin together was associated with an increased risk of coronary heart disease. Osteoporosis risk was decreased in both the estrogen and estrogen-progestin groups. Venous thromboembolism risk was higher in both treatment groups as well. These therapies do reduce important menopausal symptoms such as hot flashes and vaginal drying. This seminal study caused a dramatic reevaluation of the use of estrogen and progesterone in postmenopausal women to reduce cardiovascular risk. In addition, it reiterated the importance of well-designed clinical studies to test accepted dogma.

X-45. **The answer is D.** *(Chap. 413)* Traditional contraindications for oral hormone replacement therapy are unexplained vaginal bleeding; active liver disease; history of venous thromboembolism due to pregnancy, oral contraceptive use, or an unknown etiology; blood clotting disorder; history of breast or endometrial cancer; and diabetes. Ten-year risk of coronary heart disease, based on the Framingham Coronary Heart Disease Risk Score, indicating a risk of 5%–10% is not a traditional contraindication for oral hormone replacement therapy.

X-46. **The answer is C.** *(Chap. 414)* Infertility, defined as the inability to conceive after 12 months of unprotected intercourse, is a common problem in the United States, with an estimated 15% of couples affected. Initial evaluation should include an evaluation of current menstrual history, counseling regarding the appropriate timing of intercourse, and education regarding modifiable risk factors such as drug use, alcohol intake, smoking, caffeine, and obesity. Male factors are at the root of approximately 25% of cases of infertility, unexplained infertility is found in 17% of cases, and female causes underlie 58% of infertility cases. Among the female causes, the most common is amenorrhea/ovulatory dysfunction, which is present in 46% of cases. This is most frequently due to hypothalamic or pituitary causes or polycystic ovary syndrome. Tubal defects and endometriosis are less common.

X-47. **The answer is C.** *(Chap. 414)* Evaluation of infertility should include evaluation of common male and female factors that could be contributing. Abnormalities of menstrual function are the most common cause of female infertility, and initial evaluation of infertility should include evaluation of ovulation and assessment of tubal and uterine patency. The female partner reports an episode of gonococcal infection with symptoms of pelvic inflammatory disease, which would increase her risk of infertility due to tubal scarring and occlusion. A hysterosalpingogram is indicated. If there is evidence of tubal abnormalities, many experts recommend in vitro fertilization for conception because these women are at increased risk of ectopic pregnancy if conception occurs. The female partner reports some irregularity of her menses, suggesting anovulatory cycles, and thus, evidence of ovulation should be determined by assessing hormonal levels. There is no evidence that prolonged use of oral contraceptives affects fertility adversely (Farrow A, et al: *Hum Reprod* 17:2754, 2002). Angiotensin-converting enzyme inhibitors, including lisinopril, are known teratogens when taken by women but have no effect on chromosomal abnormalities in men. Recent marijuana use may be associated with increased risk of infertility, and in vitro studies of human sperm exposed to a cannabinoid derivative showed decreased motility (Whan LB, et al: *Fertil Steril* 85:653, 2006). However, no studies have shown long-term decreased fertility in men who previously used marijuana.

X-48. **The answer is E.** *(Chap. 414)* All of the choices have a theoretical efficacy in preventing pregnancy of >90%. However, the actual effectiveness can vary widely. Spermicides have the greatest failure rate (21%). Barrier methods (e.g., condoms, cervical cap, diaphragm) have an actual efficacy between 82% and 88%. Oral contraceptives and intrauterine devices perform similarly, with 97% efficacy in preventing pregnancy in clinical practice.

X-49. **The answer is E.** *(Chap. 414)* Pathologic gynecomastia develops when the effective ratio of testosterone to estrogen is decreased due to diminished testosterone production (as in primary testicular failure) or increased estrogen production. The latter may arise from direct estradiol secretion by a testis stimulated by LH or hCG or from an increase in peripheral aromatization of precursor steroids, most notably androstenedione. Elevated androstenedione levels may result from increased secretion by an adrenal tumor (leading to an elevated level of urinary 17-ketosteroids) or decreased hepatic clearance in patients with chronic liver disease. A variety of drugs, including diethylstilbestrol, heroin, digitalis, spironolactone, cimetidine, isoniazid, and tricyclic antidepressants, also can cause gynecomastia. In this patient, the history of paternity and the otherwise normal physical examination indicate that a karyotype is unnecessary, and the bilateral breast enlargement essentially excludes the presence of carcinoma and thus the need for biopsy. The presence of low LH and testosterone levels suggests either estrogen or hCG production. Because of the normal testicular examination, a primary testicular tumor is not suspected. Carcinoma of the lung and germ cell tumors both can produce hCG, causing gynecomastia.

X-50. **The answer is C.** *(Chap. 414)* The spectrum of infertility ranges from reduced conception rates or the need for medical intervention to irreversible causes of infertility. Infertility can be attributed primarily to male factors in 25% of couples and female factors in 58% of couples and is unexplained in about 17% of couples. Not uncommonly, both male and female factors contribute to infertility. Decreases in the ability to conceive as a function of age in women have led to recommendations that women >34 years old who are not at increased risk of infertility seek attention after 6 months, rather than 12 months as suggested for younger women, and receive an expedited workup and approach to treatment.

X-51. **The answer is D.** *(Chap. 417)* The risk of both type 1 and type 2 diabetes mellitus is rising in all populations, but the risk of type 2 diabetes is rising at a substantially faster rate. In the United States, the age-adjusted prevalence of diabetes mellitus is 7.1% in non-Hispanic whites, 7.5% in Asian Americans, 11.8% in Hispanics, and 12.6% in non-Hispanic blacks. Comparable data are not available for individuals belonging to American Indian, Alaska Native, or Pacific Islander populations, but the prevalence is thought to be even higher than in the non-Hispanic black population.

X-52. **The answer is C.** *(Chap. 417)* Glucose tolerance is classified into three categories: normal glucose tolerance, impaired glucose homeostasis, and diabetes mellitus. Normal glucose tolerance is defined by the following: fasting plasma glucose <100 mg/dL, plasma glucose <140 mg/dL following an oral glucose challenge, and hemoglobin A1C <5.6%. Abnormal glucose homeostasis is defined as a fasting plasma glucose of 100–125 mmol/dL or a plasma glucose of 140–199 following an oral glucose tolerance test or hemoglobin A1C of 5.7%–6.4%. Actual diabetes mellitus is defined by either a fasting plasma glucose >126 mg/dL, glucose of 200 mg/dL after an oral glucose tolerance test, or hemoglobin A1C ≥6.5%.

X-53. **The answer is E.** *(Chap. 417)* Because the patient has symptoms, she is not being screened for diabetes mellitus. For screening, the fasting plasma glucose or hemoglobin A1C is recommended. Because the patient has symptoms, a random plasma glucose of >200 mg/dL is adequate to diagnose diabetes mellitus. Other criteria include fasting plasma glucose >126 mg/dL, hemoglobin A1C >6.4%, or 2-hour plasma glucose >200 mg/dL during an oral glucose tolerance test. C-peptide is a useful tool to determine if the normal cleavage of insulin from its precursor is occurring. A normal C-peptide level with hypoglycemia suggests surreptitious insulin use, and a low C-peptide level with hyperglycemia suggests pancreatic failure.

X-54. The answer is A. *(Chap. 417)* Type 1 diabetes mellitus often has a more severe presentation with diabetic ketoacidosis and often presents in younger individuals compared with type 2 diabetes; however, there are some cases where the distinction of type 1 from type 2 diabetes is not straightforward. Human leukocyte antigen (HLA) DR3 localization preferences exist for type 1 diabetes; several haplotypes are present in 40% of children with type 1 diabetes mellitus, but this is still the minority. Immunologic destruction of the β cell is the primary cause of disease in type 1 diabetes, and islet cell antibodies are commonly present. GAD, insulin, IA/ICA-512, and ZnT-8 are the most common targets. Commercially available assays for GAD-65 autoantibodies are widely available and can demonstrate antibodies in >85% of individuals with recent-onset type 1 diabetes. These autoantibodies are infrequently present in type 2 diabetes mellitus (5%–10%). There may be some residual insulin in the plasma in early type 1 diabetes; thus, this will not distinguish the two conditions reliably. Polymorphisms of the peroxisome proliferator-activated receptor γ-2 have been described in type 2 diabetes mellitus but cannot distinguish the two conditions.

X-55. The answer is D. *(Chap. 417)* Individuals with type 2 diabetes mellitus (T2DM) often exhibit the following features: (1) develop diabetes after the age of 30 years; (2) are usually obese (80% are obese, but elderly individuals may be lean); (3) may not require insulin therapy initially; and (4) may have associated conditions such as insulin resistance, hypertension, cardiovascular disease, dyslipidemia, or polycystic ovary syndrome. In T2DM, insulin resistance is often associated with abdominal obesity (as opposed to hip and thigh obesity) and hypertriglyceridemia. Although most individuals diagnosed with T2DM are older, the age of diagnosis is declining, and there is a marked increase among overweight children and adolescents. The age of the patient should not be the sole basis for determining the type of diabetes present. Some individuals with phenotypic T2DM present with diabetic ketoacidosis but lack autoimmune markers and may be later treated with oral glucose-lowering agents rather than insulin (this clinical picture is sometimes referred to as ketosis-prone T2DM). Monogenic forms of diabetes (maturity-onset diabetes of the young) should be considered in those with diabetes onset at <30 years of age, an autosomal pattern of diabetes inheritance (which this patient lacks), and the lack of nearly complete insulin deficiency.

X-56. The answer is E. *(Chap. 418)* Diabetic ketoacidosis and hyperglycemic hyperosmolar state exist on a spectrum with diabetic ketoacidosis more common in patients with type 1 diabetes mellitus, but does occur with some frequency in patients with T2DM. Both conditions include hyperglycemia, dehydration, absolute or relative insulin deficiency, and acid-base abnormalities. Ketosis is more common in diabetic ketoacidosis. In diabetic ketoacidosis, glucose normally ranges from 250–600 mg/dL, whereas it is frequently 600–1200 mg/dL in hyperglycemic hyperosmolar state. Sodium is often mildly depressed in ketoacidosis and is preserved in hyperosmolar state. Potassium is normal to elevated in diabetic ketoacidosis and normal in hyperglycemic hyperosmolar patients. Magnesium, chloride, and phosphate are normal in both conditions. Creatinine may be slightly elevated in diabetic ketoacidosis but is often moderately elevated in hyperglycemic hyperosmolar state. Plasma ketones may be slightly positive in hyperosmolar patients, but are always strongly positive in diabetic ketoacidosis. Because hyperosmolarity is the hallmark of hyperglycemic hyperosmolar patients, they have an osmolarity of 330–380 mOsm/mL, whereas patients with diabetic ketoacidosis typically have a slightly elevated plasma osmolarity ranging from 300–320 mOsm/mL. Serum bicarbonate is markedly depressed in diabetic ketoacidosis and normal or slightly depressed in hyperosmolar state. Arterial pH is depressed at <7.3 in ketoacidosis and >7.3 in hyperosmolar state. Finally, the anion gap is wide in diabetic ketoacidosis and normal to slightly elevated in hyperglycemic hyperosmolar state.

X-57. The answer is D. *(Chap. 418)* Insulin preparations can be divided into short-acting and long-acting insulins. The short-acting insulins include regular and new preparations including aspart, glulisine, and lispro. Regular insulin has an onset of action of 0.5–1 hour and is effective for 4–6 hours. The other three short-acting insulins have an onset of action of <0.25 hour and are effective for 3–4 hours. Long-acting insulins include detemir, glargine, and NPH. Detemir and glargine have an onset of action of 1–4 hours and last up to 24 hours, whereas NPH has an onset of action of 1–4 hours and is effective for 10–16 hours.

These insulins have a number of combination preparations that take advantage of the different durations of onset and action to provide optimal efficacy and compliance.

X-58. **The answer is D.** *(Chap. 418)* First-line oral therapy for patients with T2DM is metformin. It is contraindicated in patients with a glomerular filtration rate <60 mL/min, any form of acidosis, congestive heart failure, liver disease, or severe hypoxemia, but is well tolerated in most individuals. Insulin secretagogues, biguanides, α-glucosidase inhibitors, thiazolidinediones, GLP-1 agonists, dipeptidyl peptidase-4 (DPP-IV) inhibitors, and insulin have all been approved as monotherapy for T2DM. Because of extensive clinical experience, favorable side effect profile, and relatively low cost, metformin is the recommended first-line agent. It has additional benefits of promotion of mild weight loss, lower insulin levels, and mild improvements in lipid profile. Sulfonylureas such as glyburide, GLP-1 agonists such as exenatide, and insulin DPP-IV inhibitors such as sitagliptin may be appropriate as combination therapy but are not considered first-line therapy for most patients.

X-59. **The answer is A.** *(Chap. 418)* Diabetic ketoacidosis is an acute complication of diabetes mellitus. It results from a relative or absolute deficiency of insulin combined with a counterregulatory hormone excess. In particular, a decrease in the ratio of insulin to glucagons promotes gluconeogenesis, glycogenolysis, and the formation of ketone bodies in the liver. Ketosis results from an increase in the release of free fatty acids from adipocytes, with a resultant shift toward ketone body synthesis in the liver. This is mediated by the relationship between insulin and the enzyme carnitine palmitoyltransferase I. At physiologic pH, ketone bodies exist as ketoacids, which are neutralized by bicarbonate. As bicarbonate stores are depleted, acidosis develops. Clinically, these patients have nausea, vomiting, and abdominal pain. They are dehydrated and may be hypotensive. Lethargy and severe central nervous system depression may occur. The treatment centers on replacement of the body's insulin, which will result in cessation of the formation of ketoacids and improvement of the acidotic state. Assessment of the level of acidosis may be done with an arterial blood gas. These patients have an anion gap acidosis and often a concomitant metabolic alkalosis resulting from volume depletion. Volume resuscitation with intravenous fluids is critical. Many electrolyte abnormalities may occur. Total-body sodium, potassium, and magnesium are depleted in these patients. As a result of the acidosis, intracellular potassium may shift out of cells and cause a normal or even elevated potassium level. However, with improvement in the acidosis, the serum potassium rapidly falls. Therefore, potassium repletion is critical despite the presence of a "normal" level. Because of the osmolar effects of glucose, fluid is drawn into the intravascular space. This results in a drop in the measured serum sodium. There is a drop of 1.6 mEq/L in serum sodium for each rise of 100 mg/dL in serum glucose. In this case, the serum sodium will improve with hydration alone. The use of 3% saline is not indicated because the patient has no neurologic deficits, and the expectation is for rapid resolution with IV fluids alone.

X-60. **The answer is D.** *(Chap. 418)* Reproductive capacity in either men or women with diabetes mellitus appears to be normal. Menstrual cycles may be associated with alterations in glycemic control in women with diabetes. Pregnancy is associated with marked insulin resistance; the increased insulin requirements often precipitate diabetes and lead to the diagnosis of gestational diabetes mellitus. Glucose, which at high levels is a teratogen to the developing fetus, readily crosses the placenta, but insulin does not. Thus, hyperglycemia from the maternal circulation may stimulate insulin secretion in the fetus. The anabolic and growth effects of insulin may result in macrosomia. Pregnancy in individuals with known diabetes requires meticulous planning and adherence to strict treatment regimens. Intensive diabetes management and normalization of the hemoglobin A1C are essential for individuals with existing diabetes who are planning pregnancy. The most crucial period of glycemic control is soon after fertilization. The risk of fetal malformations is increased 4–10 times in individuals with uncontrolled diabetes at the time of conception, and normal plasma glucose during the preconception period and throughout the periods of organ development in the fetus should be the goal.

X-61. **The answer is D.** *(Chap. 418)* Virtually all medical and surgical subspecialties are involved in the care of hospitalized patients with diabetes. Hyperglycemia, whether in a patient with known diabetes or in someone without known diabetes, appears to be a predictor of poor outcome in hospitalized patients. General anesthesia, surgery, infection, or concurrent illness raises the levels of counterregulatory hormones (cortisol, growth hormone, catecholamines, and glucagon) and cytokines that may lead to transient insulin resistance and hyperglycemia. In a number of cross-sectional studies of patients with diabetes, a greater degree of hyperglycemia was associated with worse cardiac, neurologic, and infectious outcomes. In some studies, patients who do not have preexisting diabetes but who develop modest blood glucose elevations during their hospitalization appear to benefit from achieving near-normoglycemia using insulin treatment. However, a large randomized clinical trial (Normoglycemia in Intensive Care Evaluation Survival Using Glucose Algorithm Regulation [NICESUGAR]) of individuals in the intensive care unit (ICU; most of whom were receiving mechanical ventilation) found an increased mortality rate and a greater number of episodes of severe hypoglycemia with very strict glycemic control (target blood glucose of 4.5–6 mmol/L or 81–108 mg/dL) compared to individuals with a more moderate glycemic goal (mean blood glucose of 8 mmol/L or 144 mg/dL). Total parenteral nutrition (TPN) greatly increases insulin requirements. In addition, individuals not previously known to have diabetes may become hyperglycemic during TPN and require insulin treatment. Insulin infusions are preferred in the ICU or in a clinically unstable setting. The absorption of subcutaneous insulin may be variable in such situations. Insulin infusions can also effectively control plasma glucose in the perioperative period and when the patient is unable to take anything by mouth.

X-62. **The answer is C.** *(Chap. 419)* Diabetic retinopathy is the leading cause of blindness in individuals between the ages of 20 and 74 in the United States. Individuals with diabetes are 25 times more likely to go legally blind than individuals without diabetes. Diabetic retinopathy is classified into two stages: nonproliferative and proliferative. Nonproliferative retinopathy typically appears late in the first decade or early in the second decade of the disease. Characteristic findings include cotton wool spots, blot hemorrhages, and retinal vascular microaneurysms. Mild proliferative retinopathy may progress to more extensive disease, characterized by changes in venous vessel caliber, intraretinal microvascular abnormalities, and more numerous microaneurysms and hemorrhages. Pathophysiologically, there is loss of retinal pericytes, increased retinal vascular permeability, alterations in retinal blood flow, and abnormal retinal microvasculature. Severe nonproliferative diabetic retinopathy creates retinal hypoxemia and establishes the environment for development of proliferative retinopathy. Neovascularization, as shown in this patient's fundus, is the hallmark of proliferative retinopathy. Neovascular vessels appear at the optic disc. The most effective therapy for the treatment of diabetic retinopathy is prevention with intensive glycemic and blood pressure control. However, in established diabetic retinopathy, improved glycemic control leads to transient worsening of the disease. When proliferative retinopathy and neovascularization are present, retinal laser photocoagulation is required.

X-63. **The answer is D.** *(Chap. 419)* Diabetes mellitus is the most common cause of chronic kidney disease, end-stage renal disease, and chronic kidney disease requiring renal replacement therapy. In the first 5 years after diabetes onset, glomerular hyperfiltration and increased glomerular filtration rate are seen. The glomerular basement membrane subsequently thickens, with concomitant mesangial volume and glomerular hypertrophy. Typically within 5–10 years, many individuals will begin to excrete small amounts of albumin in their urine. It is recommended to screen for albumin excretion annually with a 24-hour collection or spot albumin-to-creatinine ratio. Microalbuminuria is defined as >30–299 g/d in a 24-hour collection or 30–299 g/mg creatinine in a spot collection. However, interpretation may be clouded by conditions known to transiently increase albumin excretion including urinary tract infection, hematuria, heart failure, febrile illness, severe hyperglycemia (option B), severe hypertension (option E), pregnancy, and vigorous exercise (option C). If testing is positive, it should be repeated within 3–6 months, and treatment should begin at that time. This makes option A too soon for repeat testing and option D the most appropriate answer to the question. Although direct comparisons have not been done, experts believe that angiotensin-converting enzyme (ACE) inhibitors and angiotensin receptor blockers are equivalent in the treatment of albuminuria and diabetic nephropathy.

X-64. The answer is D. *(Chap. 419)* Diabetic neuropathy occurs in as many as 50% of individuals with longstanding type 1 and type 2 diabetes and can manifests as polyneuropathy, mononeuropathy, and/or autonomic neuropathy. Like other complications of diabetes, the likelihood of developing neuropathy depends on the duration of the disease and the degree of glycemic control. The most common form of neuropathy is distal symmetric polyneuropathy, which typically presents as distal sensory loss and pain. However, as many as 50% of individuals will have no symptoms at all. Alternatively, hyperesthesia, paresthesia, and dysesthesia may also occur. Clinically, patients often complain of a pins-and-needles sensation in the distal extremities. Other symptoms include burning, numbness, or a sharp pain. Both the hands and feet may be affected, but usually, it starts in the lower extremities. Pain is worse at rest and at night. An acute form of diabetic neuropathy may worsen in the setting of improved glycemic control. As the neuropathy progresses, the pain may subside with worsening numbness and sensory deficit. Physical examination shows sensory loss to light touch and pinprick with loss of ankle deep tendon reflexes and abnormal position sense. Treatment of diabetic neuropathy is difficult. Improved glycemic control may improve nerve conduction velocity, but symptoms of neuropathy may not improve. Other neurotoxins, such as alcohol, smoking, and vitamin deficiencies, that could worsen neuropathy should be avoided. Multiple agents have been used to attempt to treat painful neuropathy, but the results of treatment are less than ideal. Only two agents—duloxetine and pregabalin—have been approved by the U.S. Food and Drug Administration for the treatment of diabetic neuropathy. Other agents that are sometimes used off-label include amitriptyline, gabapentin, valproate, and opioids.

X-65. The answer is B. *(Chap. 420)* Maintenance of euglycemia involves a number of systems to lower elevated blood glucose, but also to restore normal levels when hypoglycemia is present or impending. This is particularly important for neurologic functioning because the brain cannot synthesize glucose and has only a few minutes' supply stored as glycogen. In a nondiabetic individual, the normal fasting plasma glucose level is normally tightly controlled between 70 and 110 mg/dL. When the plasma glucose begins to fall below about 80–85 mg/dL, the first line of defense to protect against development of hypoglycemia is to decrease insulin secretion. When this occurs, hepatic glycogenolysis and gluconeogenesis increase. In addition, lowered insulin levels leads to decreased peripheral glucose utilization. If the glucose continues to fall to about 65–70 mg/dL, other protective mechanisms are employed. The second line of defense against hypoglycemia is glucagon secretion, which further stimulates hepatic gluconeogenesis. Epinephrine may also be secreted, although it is not normally critical unless glucagon is deficient. Cortisol and growth hormone are secreted later in the pathway when hypoglycemia is prolonged greater than 4 hours. These hormones have no role in acute hypoglycemia.

X-66. The answer is D. *(Chap. 420)* The patient presents with recurrent episodes of hypoglycemia that meet the Whipple triad of symptoms: (1) symptoms of hypoglycemia; (2) low plasma glucose concentration measured with a precise method (not a glucose monitor); and (3) relief of symptoms with raising the plasma glucose level. The differential starts with measuring insulin levels during hypoglycemia. The levels must be obtained during an episode to be interpretable. If insulin is elevated, it suggests either endogenous hyperproduction from an insulin-secreting tumor or exogenous administration causing factitious hypoglycemia. Because C-peptide is cleaved from native proinsulin to make the secreted product, it will be high in the case of endogenous hyperinsulinemia and will be low during an episode of factitious hypoglycemia. Surreptitious ingestion of sulfonylurea could cause hypoglycemia along with high insulin and C-peptide levels since the drug stimulates pancreatic insulin secretion. In this case, a sulfonylurea drug screen would be indicated. Red flags in this case that point to surreptitious insulin use include the patient being a healthcare worker and the presence of symptoms only at work. Other groups in which this is common are relatives of patients with diabetes and patients with a history of other factitious disorders. It is possible that the patient has an insulin-secreting β cell tumor, but this is much less likely, and symptoms would be present during times other than work. Evaluation is aimed at demonstrating that pancreatic insulin secretion is suppressed during the episode of hypoglycemia. Although a failure of counterregulatory hormones can produce hypoglycemia, this is a rare cause of hypoglycemia, and evaluation should be aimed at this only after surreptitious use is ruled out.

X-67. **The answer is E.** *(Chap. 420)* The most common cause of hypoglycemia is related to the treatment of diabetes mellitus. Individuals with type 1 diabetes mellitus (T1DM) have more symptomatic hypoglycemia than individuals with T2DM. On average, those with T1DM experience two episodes of symptomatic hypoglycemia weekly; and at least once yearly, individuals with T1DM will have a severe episode of hypoglycemia that is at least temporarily disabling. It is estimated that 6%–10% of individuals with T1DM will die from hypoglycemia. In addition, recurrent episodes of hypoglycemia in T1DM contribute to the development of hypoglycemia-associated autonomic failure. Clinically, this is manifested as hypoglycemia unawareness and defective glucose counterregulation, with lack of glucagon and epinephrine secretion as glucose levels fall. Individuals with T2DM are less likely to develop hypoglycemia. However, once an individual with T2DM requires insulin, the likelihood of symptomatic hypoglycemia increases, and although the incidence of hypoglycemia is overall lower in T2DM, the absolute number of individuals with T2DM with hypoglycemia episodes is far greater than those with T1DM given the higher prevalence of T2DM. Medications that are associated with hypoglycemia in T2DM are insulin and insulin secretagogues, such as sulfonylureas. Metformin, thiazolidinediones, α-glucosidase inhibitors, glucagon-like peptide-1 receptor agonists, and DPP-IV inhibitors should not cause hypoglycemia. However, when these medications are combined with another class of medications known to cause hypoglycemia, they do increase the risk of hypoglycemic episodes.

X-68. **The answer is A.** *(Chap. 421)* Lipoprotein lipase (LPL) deficiency is a very rare autosomal recessive disorder that results in elevated fasting triglyceride levels because the absence of LPL results in the inability of chylomicrons to undergo hydrolysis of triglycerides. Thus, circulating levels of chylomicrons, very-low-density lipoprotein (VLDL), and triglycerides are high. Fasting triglyceride levels are typically >1000 mg/dL. LPL deficiency has an incidence of approximately 1 in 1,000,000 in the population. The disease typically presents in childhood or young adulthood with recurrent episodes of pancreatitis. Ophthalmologic examination may show lipemia retinalis with an opalescent appearance to the retinal blood vessels. Eruptive xanthomas are small, yellowish-white papules and may appear on the back, buttocks, and extensor surfaces of the arms and legs. Hepatosplenomegaly occurs because of uptake of the circulating chylomicrons by the reticuloendothelial system. Primary treatment of the disorder is to restrict dietary fat to 15 g/d or less. If dietary fat restriction alone is not sufficient to control the triglyceride level, fish oil has been useful in some patients.

X-69. **The answer is D.** *(Chap. 421)* Familial hypercholesterolemia (FH) is the most common inherited cause of hypercholesterolemia and may be one of the most common single-gene disorders in humans. The incidence of the mutation that causes FH is estimated to be as common as 1 in 250 to 1 in 500 individuals in the population. FH is also known as autosomal dominant hypercholesterolemia, type 1, and is caused by loss-of-function mutations in the gene encoding the low-density lipoprotein (LDL) receptor. More than 1600 mutations in the gene have been reported. In the presence of a single mutation (heterozygous FH), there is a decrease of LDL receptors in the liver with a resulting decrease in clearance of LDL from the circulation, and plasma levels of LDL cholesterol typically range from 200–400 mg/dL. In the presence of two mutations (homozygous FH), LDL receptors are markedly reduced or absent. In these patients, the LDL cholesterol levels are markedly elevated to 400 to >1000 mg/dL. Many individuals with homozygous FH present with cutaneous xanthomas in childhood and early cardiovascular disease in late childhood or young adulthood. Although heterozygous patients have hypercholesterolemia from birth, disease recognition is usually not until adulthood when patients are found to have tendon xanthomas or coronary artery disease. In patients with heterozygous disease, there is generally a family history on at least one side of the family. Familial defective apolipoprotein (apo) B-100 has a similar presentation but is less common (1/1000). ApoA-V deficiency presents with xanthomas, but also pancreatitis and hepatosplenomegaly with elevated chylomicrons and VLDL. Familial hepatic lipase deficiency and lipoprotein lipase deficiency are associated with increased chylomicrons, not LDL cholesterol, and present with eruptive xanthomas, hepatosplenomegaly, and pancreatitis. These conditions occur rarely (<1/1,000,000).

X-70. The answer is B. *(Chap. 421)* There are many secondary forms of elevated LDL that warrant consideration in a patient found to have abnormal LDL. These include hypothyroidism, nephrotic syndrome, cholestasis, acute intermittent porphyria, anorexia nervosa, hepatoma, and drugs such as thiazides, cyclosporine, and carbamazepine. Cirrhosis is associated with reduced LDL because of inadequate production. Malabsorption, malnutrition, Gaucher disease, chronic infectious disease, hyperthyroidism, and niacin toxicity are all similarly associated with reduced LDL.

X-71. The answer is C. *(Chap. 421)* This patient has nephrotic syndrome, which is likely a result of multiple myeloma. The hyperlipidemia of nephrotic syndrome appears to be due to a combination of increased hepatic production and decreased clearance of VLDL, with increased LDL production. It is usually mixed but can manifest as hypercholesterolemia or hypertriglyceridemia. Effective treatment of the underlying renal disease normalizes the lipid profile. Of the choices presented, 3-hydroxy-3-methylglutaryl–coenzyme A (HMG-CoA) reductase inhibitors would be the most effective to reduce this patient's LDL. Dietary management is an important component of lifestyle modification but seldom results in a >10% fall in LDL. Niacin and fibrates would be indicated if the triglycerides were higher, but the LDL is the more important lipid abnormality to address at this time. Lipid apheresis is reserved for patients who cannot tolerate the lipid-lowering drugs or who have a genetic lipid disorder refractory to medication. Cholesterol ester transfer protein inhibitors have been shown to raise high-density lipoprotein (HDL) levels, and their role in the treatment of lipoproteinemias is still under investigation.

X-72. The answer is B. *(Chap. 422)* Metabolic syndrome is a common disorder that features central obesity, hypertriglyceridemia, low levels of HDL cholesterol, hyperglycemia, and hypertension. The prevalence of the disease varies around the world, reflecting the age, ethnicity, and varying diagnostic criteria applied. The highest prevalence of metabolic syndrome worldwide occurs in the Native American populations in the United States, with nearly 60% of women age 45–49 and 45% of men age 45–49 being affected. In the United States, African American men are less commonly affected, whereas Mexican American women are more commonly affected. In France, the disease prevalence is generally the lowest in the world, with <10% of individuals between 30 and 60 years of age affected, although after age 60, the prevalence rises to 17.5%. Risk factors that confer increasing likelihood of developing metabolic syndrome included overweight/obesity, aging, sedentary lifestyle, diabetes mellitus, cardiovascular disease, and lipodystrophy. Central obesity is both a risk factor and a feature central to defining the presence of the disease. Central obesity as measured by waist circumference, not body mass index, is most strongly associated with insulin resistance and risk of diabetes mellitus and cardiovascular disease. The precise waist circumference at which the risk increases may vary between men and women and across different ethnicities. For instance, in Japanese women, the waist circumference that is used for diagnosis of metabolic syndrome is 90 cm compared to 85 cm for men. However, in individuals of Europoid descent, women are diagnosed with metabolic syndrome at a waist circumference ≥80 cm, whereas men are diagnosed at a waist circumference ≥94 cm. Aging is also associated with increased risk of metabolic syndrome. Metabolic syndrome affects about half of the population older than age 50, and after age 60, women are more affected than men. Physical inactivity is a predictor of cardiovascular events and death in individuals with metabolic syndrome. Spending more than 4 hours a day watching television or videos or using a computer confers a twofold greater risk of metabolic syndrome. Insulin resistance is felt to be the pathophysiologic hallmark of the metabolic syndrome, and about 75% of individuals with T2DM or impaired glucose tolerance have metabolic syndrome. When these diseases coexist in an individual, there is a higher prevalence of cardiovascular disease than with T2DM or glucose tolerance alone.

X-73. The answer is D. *(Chap. 422)* The most recent criteria for the diagnosis of metabolic syndrome is called the Harmonizing Definition and was published in 2009. This definition brought together multiple international medical societies to create a unifying definition, including the International Diabetes Federation; the National Heart, Lung, and Blood Institute; the American Heart Association; the World Heart Federation; the International Atherosclerosis Society; and the International Association for the Study of Obesity. When compared to prior guidelines, the most important change was to recognize that the waist circumference that confers the risk of metabolic syndrome is different across ethnic groups. The harmonizing definition creates three different waist circumference groupings by gender and ethnic group (Table X-73).

TABLE X-73 NCEP:ATPIII[a] 2001 and Harmonizing Definition Criteria for the Metabolic Syndrome

<table>
<tr><th>NCEP:ATPIII 2001</th><th>Harmonizing Definition[b]</th></tr>
<tr><td>
Three or more of the following:
• Central obesity: waist circumference >102 cm (male), >88 cm (female)
• Hypertriglyceridemia: triglyceride level ≥150 mg/dL or specific medication
• Low HDL[c] cholesterol: <40 mg/dL and <50 mg/dL for men and women, respectively, or specific medication
• Hypertension: blood pressure ≥130 mmHg systolic or ≥85 mmHg diastolic or specific medication
• Fasting plasma glucose level ≥100 mg/dL or specific medication or previously diagnosed type 2 diabetes
</td><td>
Three of the following:
• Waist circumference (cm)
<table>
<tr><th>Men</th><th>Women</th><th>Ethnicity</th></tr>
<tr><td>≥94</td><td>≥80</td><td>Europid, sub-Saharan African, Eastern and Middle Eastern</td></tr>
<tr><td>≥90</td><td>≥80</td><td>South Asian, Chinese, and ethnic South and Central American</td></tr>
<tr><td>≥85</td><td>≥90</td><td>Japanese</td></tr>
</table>
• Fasting triglyceride level >150 mg/dL or specific medication
• HDL cholesterol level <40 and <50 mg/dL for men and women, respectively, or specific medication
• Blood pressure >130 mmHg systolic or >85 mmHg diastolic or previous diagnosis or specific medication
• Fasting plasma glucose level ≥100 mg/dL (alternative indication: drug treatment of elevated glucose levels)
</td></tr>
</table>

[a]National Cholesterol Education Program and Adult Treatment Panel III.
[b]In this analysis, the following thresholds for waist circumference were used: white men, ≥94 cm; African American men, ≥94 cm; Mexican American men, ≥90 cm; white women, ≥80 cm; African American women, ≥80 cm; Mexican American women, ≥80 cm. For participants whose designation was "other race—including multiracial," thresholds that were once based on Europid cutoffs (≥94 cm for men and ≥80 cm for women) and on South Asian cutoffs (≥90 cm for men and ≥80 cm for women) were used. For participants who were considered "other Hispanic," the International Diabetes Federation thresholds for ethnic South and Central Americans were used.
[c]High-density lipoprotein.

Furthermore, when compared with the National Cholesterol Education Program and Adult Treatment Panel III 2001 classification, the waist circumference that is considered abnormal is lower by at least 8 cm in both men and women. The remainder of the diagnostic criteria for metabolic syndrome remain the same when compared to prior guidelines:

- Fasting triglycerides >150 mg/dL or specific medication
- HDL cholesterol <40 mg/dL in men or <50 mg/dL in women or specific medication
- Blood pressure >130 mmHg systolic or >85 mmHg diastolic or specific medication or previous diagnosis
- Fasting plasma glucose >100 mg/dL or drug treatment of elevated glucose level

This individual meets diagnostic criteria with elevated waist circumference (>90 cm in Chinese man), elevated triglyceride level, low HDL level, and hypertension.

X-74. and X-75. The answers are A and C, respectively. *(Chap. 423)* Hypophosphatemia results from one of three mechanisms: inadequate intestinal phosphate absorption, excessive renal phosphate excretion, and rapid redistribution of phosphate from the extracellular space into bone or soft tissue. Inadequate intestinal absorption is rare because antacids containing aluminum hydroxide are no longer commonly prescribed. Malnutrition from fasting or starvation may result in depletion of phosphate. This is also commonly seen in alcoholism. In hospitalized patients, redistribution is the main cause. Insulin promotes phosphate entry into cells along with glucose. When nutrition is initiated, refeeding further increases redistribution of phosphate into cells and is more pronounced when IV glucose is used alone. Sepsis may cause destruction of cells and metabolic acidosis, resulting in a net shift of phosphate from the extracellular space into cells. Renal failure is associated with hyperphosphatemia, not hypophosphatemia, and initial prerenal azotemia, such as in this presentation, can obscure underlying phosphate depletion. The approach to treating hypophosphatemia should take into account several factors, including the likelihood (and magnitude) of underlying phosphate depletion, renal function, serum calcium levels, and the concurrent administration of parenteral glucose. In addition, the treating physician should assess the patient for complications of hypophosphatemia, which can include neuromuscular weakness, cardiac dysfunction, hemolysis, and platelet dysfunction. Severe hypophosphatemia generally occurs when the serum concentration falls below 2 mg/dL (<0.75 mmol/L). This becomes particularly dangerous when there is underlying chronic phosphate depletion. However, there is no simple formula to determine the body's phosphate needs from measurement of the serum phosphate levels because most phosphate is intracellular. It is generally recommended to use oral phosphate repletion when the serum phosphate levels are greater than 1.5–2.5 mg/dL (0.5–0.8 mmol/L). The dose of oral phosphate is 750–2000 mg daily of elemental phosphate given in divided doses. More severe hypophosphatemia, as in the case presented, requires IV repletion. IV phosphate repletion is given as neutral mixtures of sodium and potassium phosphate salts at doses of 0.2–0.8 mmol/kg given over 6 hours. Table X-75 outlines the total dose and recommended infusion rates for a range of phosphate levels. In this patient with a level of 1.0 mg/dL, the recommended infusion rate is 8 mmol/hr over 6 hours for a total dose of 48 mmol. Until the underlying hypophosphatemia is corrected, one should measure phosphate and calcium levels every 6 hours. The infusion should be stopped if the calcium phosphate product rises to higher than 50 to decrease the risk of heterotopic calcification. Alternatively, if hypocalcemia is present coincident with the hypophosphatemia, it is important to correct the calcium prior to administering phosphate.

TABLE X-75 Intravenous Therapy for Hypophosphatemia

Consider			
Likely severity of underlying phosphate depletion			
Concurrent parenteral glucose administration			
Presence of neuromuscular, cardiopulmonary, or hematologic complications of hypophosphatemia			
Renal function (reduce dose by 50% if serum creatinine >220 μmol/L [>2.5 mg/dL])			
Serum calcium level (correct hypocalcemia first; reduce dose by 50% in hypercalcemia)			
Guidelines			
Serum Phosphorus, mmol/L (mg/dL)	**Rate of Infusion, mmol/hr**	**Duration, hr**	**Total Administered, mmol**
<0.8 (<2.5)	2	6	12
<0.5 (<1.5)	4	6	24
<0.3 (<1)	8	6	48

Note: Rates shown are calculated for a 70-kg person; levels of serum calcium and phosphorus must be measured every 6–12 hours during therapy; infusions can be repeated to achieve stable serum phosphorus levels >0.8 mmol/L (>2.5 mg/dL); most formulations available in the United States provide 3 mmol/mL of sodium or potassium phosphate.

X-76. The answer is B. *(Chap. 423)* Vitamin D deficiency is highly prevalent in the United States and is most common in older individuals who are hospitalized or institutionalized. Vitamin D deficiency can occur as a result of inadequate dietary intake, decreased production in the skin, decreased intestinal absorption, accelerated losses, or impaired vitamin D activation in the liver or kidney. Clinically, vitamin D deficiency in older individuals is most often silent. Often practitioners fail to consider vitamin D deficiency until a patient has been diagnosed with osteoporosis or suffered a fracture. However, some individuals can experience diffuse muscle and bone pain. When assessing vitamin D levels, the appropriate test is 25-hydroxyvitamin D [25(OH)D] levels. The Institute of Medicine has defined vitamin D sufficiency as a level of 25(OH)D >50 nmol/L (>20 ng/L). However, in the elderly and in some disease states, higher levels may be required to maximize intestinal calcium absorption. Levels less than 37 nmol/L (15 ng/mL) are associated with a rise in parathyroid hormone levels and a fall in bone density. Vitamin D deficiency may also lead to decreased intestinal absorption of calcium with resultant hypocalcemia and secondary hyperparathyroidism. As a result, there is higher bone turnover, which can be associated with an increase in alkaline phosphatase levels. In addition, elevated parathyroid hormone (PTH) stimulates renal conversion of 25(OH)D to 1,25-hydroxyvitamin D [1,25(OH)D], the activated form of vitamin D. Thus, even in the face of severe vitamin D deficiency, the activated 1,25(OH)D levels may be normal and do not accurately reflect vitamin D stores. Thus, 1,25(OH)D should not be used to make a diagnosis of vitamin D deficiency. Although vitamin D deficiency may be associated with abnormalities in PTH, alkaline phosphatase, and calcium levels, these biochemical abnormalities are seen in many other diseases and are neither sensitive nor specific for the diagnosis of vitamin D deficiency.

X-77. The answer is D. *(Chap. 423)* Vitamin D deficiency is common in all areas of the United States and has resulted from decreased solar exposure with deficient production of vitamin D in the skin, lack of dietary intake, accelerated losses of vitamin D, impaired vitamin D activation, or resistance to the biologic effects of $1,25(OH)_2D$, the activated form of vitamin D. Vitamin D stores are best assessed by measuring 25(OH)D. Levels less than 20 ng/L (<50 nmol/L) should be repleted. The recommended daily intake in the absence of vitamin D deficiency is 800 IU of vitamin D, typically administered as vitamin D_3 or cholecalciferol, daily. However, higher doses of vitamin D are required when vitamin D deficiency is present to return vitamin D levels to normal. In most individuals, supplementation with vitamin D_3 at 2000 IU daily along with calcium supplementation would be recommended. In severe cases of vitamin D deficiency, high-dose repletion may be required. This is given as ergocalciferol (vitamin D) 50,000 IU weekly for 3 to 12 weeks before decreasing to the maintenance daily dose of cholecalciferol 800 IU daily.

X-78. The answer is E. *(Chap. 424)* Primary hyperparathyroidism is the most common cause of hypercalcemia and is the most likely cause in an adult who is asymptomatic. Primary hyperparathyroidism results from autonomous secretion of PTH that is no longer regulated by serum calcium levels, usually related to development of parathyroid adenomas. Most patients are asymptomatic or have minimal symptoms at the time of diagnosis. When present, symptoms include recurrent nephrolithiasis, peptic ulcers, dehydration, constipation, and altered mental status. Distinctive bone manifestations include osteitis fibrosa cystica, which histologically results from an increase in the giant multinucleated osteoclasts in scalloped areas on the surface of the bone and a replacement of the normal cellular and marrow elements by fibrous tissue. On x-ray, this will appear as resorption of the phalangeal tufts and replacement of the usually sharp cortical outline of the bone in the digits by an irregular outline. Historically, this finding was present on presentation in 10%–25% of cases but is rare today due to earlier diagnosis of disease. Laboratory studies show elevated serum calcium with decreased serum phosphate. Diagnosis can be confirmed with measurement of PTH levels. The optimal management of asymptomatic primary hyperparathyroidism has been debated because surgical removal of autonomous adenomas is generally curative. However, it is unclear whether all patients need to be treated surgically. The most recent recommendations suggest that the more aggressive surgical approach be considered in most patients due to concerns of subtle neuropsychiatric symptoms, long-term skeletal effects, and potential for cardiovascular deterioration. The current guidelines recommend surgery for individuals less than 50 years in age or with creatinine clearance <60 mL/min, osteoporosis on bone density scanning, or serum calcium >1 mg/mL above normal. There is no indication for surgery based on 24-hour urine calcium levels or presence of nephrolithiasis. Likewise, presence of cardiovascular disease is not in the guidelines for recommendation of surgical intervention.

X-79. The answer is A. *(Chap. 424)* Granulomatous disorders including sarcoidosis, tuberculosis, and fungal infections can be associated with hypercalcemia caused by increased conversion of 25(OH)D to 1,25(OH)D by macrophages within the granulomas. This process bypasses the normal feedback mechanisms, and elevated levels of both 25(OH)D and 1,25(OH)D can be seen. This does not normally occur because 1,25(OH)D levels are normally tightly controlled through feedback mechanisms on renal 1-α-hydroxylase, the primary producer of activated vitamin D in normal circumstances. In addition, the normal feedback provided by PTH concentrations is also bypassed and the PTH level may be low.

X-80. The answer is D. *(Chap. 424)* This patient demonstrates evidence of tertiary hyperparathyroidism, with inappropriate elevations in PTH despite increases in calcium and phosphate. In addition, the patient is demonstrating clinical evidence of disease including bony pain and ectopic calcification. Tertiary hyperparathyroidism most commonly develops in individuals with longstanding renal failure who have been nonadherent to therapy. In this patient scenario, the hypoxemia and ground-glass infiltrates on chest CT represent ectopic calcification of the lungs. This can be difficult to identify with typical imaging, and a technetium-99 bone scan will show increased uptake in the lungs. Treatment of tertiary hyperparathyroidism with severe clinical manifestations requires parathyroidectomy. Pathologically, these individuals demonstrate the emergence of monoclonal growth in one or more previously hyperplastic parathyroid glands with subsequent autonomous parathyroid function.

X-81. The answer is B. *(Chap. 424)* Hypocalcemia can be a life-threatening consequence of thyroidectomy if the parathyroid glands are inadvertently removed during the surgery, because the four parathyroid glands are located immediately posterior to the thyroid gland. This currently occurs infrequently because the parathyroid glands are better able to be identified both before and during surgery. However, hypoparathyroidism may occur even if the parathyroid glands are not removed by thyroidectomy due to devascularization or trauma to the parathyroid glands. Hypocalcemia following removal of the parathyroid glands may begin any time during the first 24–72 hours, and monitoring of serial calcium levels is recommended for the first 72 hours. The earliest symptoms of hypocalcemia are typically circumoral paresthesias and paresthesias with a "pins-and-needles" sensation in the fingers and toes. The development of carpal spasms upon inflation of the blood pressure cuff is a classic sign of hypocalcemia and is known as Trousseau sign. Chvostek sign is the other classic sign of hypocalcemia and is elicited by tapping the facial nerve in the preauricular area causing spasm of the facial muscles. A prolongation of the QT interval on the electrocardiogram suggests life-threatening hypocalcemia that may progress to fatal arrhythmia, and treatment should not be delayed while waiting for serum testing to occur in a patient with a known cause of hypocalcemia. Immediate treatment with IV calcium should be initiated. Maintenance therapy with calcitriol and vitamin D is necessary for ongoing treatment of acquired hypoparathyroidism. Alternatively, surgeons may implant parathyroid tissue into the soft tissue of the forearm, if it is thought that the parathyroid glands will be removed. Hypomagnesemia can cause hypocalcemia by suppressing PTH release despite the presence of hypocalcemia. However, in this patient, hypomagnesemia is not suspected after thyroidectomy, and magnesium administration is not indicated. Benztropine is a centrally acting anticholinergic medication that is used in the treatment of dystonic reactions that can occur after taking centrally acting antiemetic medications with dopaminergic activity, such as metoclopramide or Compazine. Dystonic reactions involve focal spasms of the face, neck, and extremities. Although this patient has taken medications that can cause a dystonic reaction, the spasms that she is experiencing are more consistent with tetanic contractions of hypocalcemia than dystonic reaction. Finally, measurement of forced vital capacity is most commonly used as a measurement of disease severity in myasthenia gravis or Guillain-Barré syndrome. Muscle weakness is a typical presenting feature, but not paresthesias.

X-82. **The answer is E.** *(Chap. 424)* Malignancy can cause hypercalcemia by several different mechanisms, including metastasis to bone, cytokine stimulation of bone turnover, and production of a protein structurally similar to PTH by the tumor. This protein is called PTH-related peptide (PTHrp) and acts at the same receptors as PTH. Squamous cell carcinoma of the lung is the most common tumor associated with the production of PTHrp. Serum calcium levels can become quite high in malignancy because of unregulated production of PTHrp that is outside of the negative feedback control that normally results in the setting of hypercalcemia. PTH hormone levels should be quite low or undetectable in this setting. When hypercalcemia is severe (>15 mg/dL), symptoms frequently include dehydration and altered mental status. The electrocardiogram may show a shortened QTc interval. Initial therapy includes large-volume fluid administration to reverse the dehydration that results from hypercalciuria. In addition, furosemide is also added to promote further calciuria. If the calcium remains elevated, as in this patient, additional measures should be undertaken to decrease the serum calcium. Calcitonin has a rapid onset of action, with a decrease in serum calcium seen within hours. However, tachyphylaxis develops, and the duration of benefit is limited. Pamidronate is a bisphosphonate that is useful for the hypercalcemia of malignancy. It decreases serum calcium by preventing bone resorption and release of calcium from the bone. After IV administration, the onset of action of pamidronate is 1–2 days, with a duration of action of several weeks. Thus, in this patient with ongoing severe symptomatic hypercalcemia, addition of both calcitonin and pamidronate is the best treatment. The patient should continue to receive IV fluids and furosemide. The addition of a thiazide diuretic is contraindicated because thiazides cause increased calcium resorption in the kidney and would worsen hypercalcemia.

X-83. **The answer is B.** *(Chap. 425)* Osteoporosis refers to a chronic condition characterized by decreased bone strength and frequently manifests as vertebral and hip fractures. In the United States, about 8 million women have osteoporosis compared to about 2 million men, for a ratio in women to men of 4 to 1. An additional 48 million individuals are estimated to have osteopenia. The risk of osteoporosis increases with advancing age and rapidly worsens following menopause in women. Most women meet the diagnostic criteria for osteoporosis between the ages of 70 and 80. White women have an increased risk for osteoporosis when compared to African American women. The epidemiology for bone fractures follows the epidemiology for osteoporosis. Fractures of the distal radius (Colles fracture) increase up to age 50 and plateau by age 60, and there is only a modest increase in risk thereafter. This is contrasted with the risk of hip fractures. Incidence rates for hip fractures double every 5 years after the age of 70. This change in fracture pattern is not entirely due to osteoporosis but is also related to the fact that fewer falls in the elderly occur onto an outstretched arm and are more likely to occur directly on the hip. Black women experience hip fractures at approximately half the rate as white women. The mortality rate in the year following a hip fracture is 5%–20%. Vertebral fractures are also common manifestations of osteoporosis. Although most are found incidentally on chest radiograph, severe cases can lead to height loss, pulmonary restriction, and respiratory morbidity.

X-84. **The answer is C.** *(Chap. 425)* There are multiple risks for osteoporotic bone fractures that can be either modifiable or nonmodifiable. These are outlined in Table X-84. Nonmodifiable risk factors include a previous history of fracture as an adult, female sex, white race, dementia, advanced age, and history of fracture (but not osteoporosis) in a first-degree relative. Risk factors that are potentially modifiable include low calcium intake, alcoholism, impaired eyesight, recurrent falls, inadequate physical activity, poor health, and estrogen deficiency, including menopause prior to age 45 or prolonged premenstrual amenorrhea. Excessive thinness and low body weight are also risk factors for osteoporosis, although the osteoporosis guidelines do not clearly delineate what is considered excessive thinness. Current cigarette smoking is a risk factor for osteoporosis-related fracture, whereas a prior history of cigarette use is not.

TABLE X-84 Conditions, Diseases, and Medications That Contribute to Osteoporosis and Fractures

Lifestyle Factors		
Alcohol abuse	High salt intake	Falling
Low calcium intake	Inadequate physical activity	Excessive thinness
Vitamin D insufficiency	Immobilization	Prior fractures
Excess vitamin A	Smoking (active or passive)	
Genetic Factors		
Cystic fibrosis	Homocystinuria	Osteogenesis imperfecta
Ehlers-Danlos syndrome	Hypophosphatasia	Parental history of hip fracture
Gaucher disease	Idiopathic hypercalciuria	Porphyria
Glycogen storage diseases	Marfan syndrome	Riley-Day syndrome
Hemochromatosis	Menkes steely hair syndrome	
Hypogonadal States		
Androgen insensitivity	Hyperprolactinemia	Athletic amenorrhea Panhypopituitarism
Anorexia nervosa and bulimia	Premature menopause Premature ovarian failure	
Turner and Klinefelter syndromes		
Endocrine Disorders		
Adrenal insufficiency	Cushing syndrome	Central adiposity
Diabetes mellitus (types 1 and 2)	Hyperparathyroidism	Thyrotoxicosis
Gastrointestinal Disorders		
Celiac disease	Inflammatory bowel disease	Primary biliary cirrhosis
Gastric bypass	Malabsorption	
Gastrointestinal surgery	Pancreatic disease	
Hematologic Disorders		
Multiple myeloma	Monoclonal gammopathies	Sickle cell disease
Hemophilia	Leukemia and lymphomas	Systemic mastocytosis
Thalassemia		
Rheumatologic and Autoimmune Diseases		
Ankylosing spondylitis	Lupus	Rheumatoid arthritis
Other rheumatic and autoimmune diseases		
Central Nervous System Disorders		
Epilepsy	Parkinson disease	Stroke
Multiple sclerosis	Spinal cord injury	
Miscellaneous Conditions and Diseases		
AIDS/HIV Alcoholism Amyloidosis Chronic metabolic acidosis Chronic obstructive pulmonary disease	Congestive heart failure Depression End-stage renal disease Hypercalciuria Idiopathic scoliosis Muscular dystrophy	Posttransplantation bone disease Sarcoidosis Weight loss
Medications		
Aluminum (in antacids) Anticoagulants (heparin) Anticonvulsants Aromatase inhibitors Barbiturates Cancer chemotherapeutic drugs Cyclosporine A and tacrolimus Depo-medroxyprogesterone (premenopausal contraception)	Glucocorticoids (≥5 mg/d prednisone or equivalent for ≥3 months) Gonadotropin-releasing hormone antagonists and agonists Lithium Methotrexate Proton pump inhibitors Selective serotonin reuptake inhibitors	Tamoxifen (premenopausal use) Thiazolidinediones (such as pioglitazone and rosiglitazone) Thyroid hormones (in excess) Parenteral nutrition

Source: From the 2014 National Osteoporosis Foundation Clinician's Guide to the Prevention and Treatment of Osteoporosis. © National Osteoporosis Foundation.

X-85. **The answer is B.** *(Chap. 425)* Osteoporosis is a common disease affecting 8 million women and 2 million men in the United States. It is most common in postmenopausal women, but the incidence is also increasing in men. Estrogen loss probably causes bone loss by activation of bone remodeling sites and exaggeration of the imbalance between bone formation and resorption. Osteoporosis is diagnosed by bone mineral density scan. Dual-energy x-ray absorptiometry (DXA) is the most accurate test for measuring bone mineral density. Clinical determinations of bone density are most commonly measured at the lumbar spine and hip. In the DXA technique, two x-ray energies are used to measure the area of the mineralized tissues, and results are compared to gender- and race-matched normative values. The T-score compares an individual's results to a young population, whereas the Z-score compares the individual's results to an age-matched population. Osteoporosis is diagnosed when the T-score is −2.5 standard deviations (SD) in the lumbar spine, femoral neck, or total hip. An evaluation for secondary causes of osteoporosis should be considered in individuals presenting with osteoporotic fractures at a young age and those who have very low Z-scores. Initial evaluation should include serum and 24-hour urine calcium levels, renal function panel, hepatic function panel, serum phosphorous level, and vitamin D levels. Other endocrine abnormalities including hyperthyroidism and hyperparathyroidism should be evaluated, and urinary cortisol levels should be checked if there is a clinical suspicion for Cushing syndrome. FSH and LH levels would be elevated but are not useful in this individual because she presents with a known perimenopausal state.

X-86. **The answer is C.** *(Chap. 425)* Determination of when to initiate screening for osteoporosis with bone densitometry testing can be complicated by multiple factors. In general, most women do not require screening for osteoporosis until after completion of menopause unless there have been unexplained fractures or other risk factors that would suggest osteoporosis. There is no benefit to initiating screening for osteoporosis in the perimenopausal period. Indeed, most expert recommendations do not recommend routine screening for osteoporosis until age 65 or older unless risk factors are present. Risk factors for osteoporosis include advanced age, current cigarette smoking, low body weight (<57.7 kg), family history of hip fracture, and long-term glucocorticoid use. Inhaled glucocorticoids may cause increased loss of bone density, but because this patient is on a low dose of inhaled fluticasone and is not estrogen deficient, bone mineral densitometry cannot be recommended at this time. The risk of osteoporosis related to inhaled glucocorticoids is not well defined, but most studies suggest that the risk is relatively low. Delaying childbearing until the fourth and fifth decades does increase the risk of osteoporosis but does not cause early onset of osteoporosis prior to completion of menopause. The patient's family history of osteoporosis likewise is not an indication for early screening for osteoporosis.

X-87, X-88, X-89, X-90, and X-91. **The answers are B, E, D, A, and C, respectively.** *(Chap. 425)* In the past 20 years, multiple pharmacologic options have become available for the treatment of osteoporosis. Prior to the 1990s, estrogen, either alone or in combination with a progestin, was the primary treatment for osteoporosis. Since that time, many new agents have been introduced, although estrogen is effective at preventing bone loss and reducing bone turnover and yields small increases in bone mass of the spine, hip, and total body. The selective estrogen receptor modulator (SERM) raloxifene binds to the estrogen receptor and is approved for the prevention and treatment of osteoporosis as well as the prevention of breast cancer. Tamoxifen is another well-known SERM, but it is only approved for the treatment and prevention of breast cancer. Both drugs have a favorable effect on bone turnover and bone mass. Raloxifene has been demonstrated in clinical trials to reduce the occurrence of vertebral fracture by 30%–50%, although the effect on nonvertebral fracture is not known. Bisphosphonates are the most widely used category of medications for the prevention and treatment of osteoporosis. Alendronate, risedronate, ibandronate, and zoledronic acid are approved medications in this class. Bisphosphonates act to impair osteoclast function and reduce osteoclast number by inducing apoptosis. Zoledronic acid is retained in the bone for a very long time and is dosed intravenously only once yearly. Exogenous administration of calcitonin, a polypeptide hormone produced by the thyroid gland, is sometimes administered as a nasal spray in the treatment of osteoporosis. It acts to suppress osteoclast activity by direct action on the osteoclast calcitonin receptor. In clinical studies, the effect on bone mass and vertebral fracture risk was small, and there was no effect on nonvertebral fractures. Denosumab is a fully human monoclonal antibody to RANKL, the final common effector of osteoclast formation, activity, and survival. When denosumab binds to RANKL, osteoclast maturation is significantly impaired. It is administered by subcutaneous injection twice yearly and has been demonstrated to decrease fracture risk in the spine, hip, and forearm over a 3-year period by 20%–70%. Teriparatide is a recombinant PTH (1-34hPTH) that is approved for the treatment of osteoporosis. It is administered by daily subcutaneous injection and has been shown to decrease both vertebral and nonvertebral fracture risk. Because teriparatide is an analogue of PTH, the drug acts like PTH with direct actions on osteoblast to stimulate new bone formation, which is unique among the treatments for osteoporosis.

X-92. The answer is B. *(Chap. 425)* This individual with cystic fibrosis has malabsorption of vitamin D and chronic inflammation, placing her at increased risk of osteoporosis. Upon diagnosis of osteoporosis with a T-score less than –2.5, the patient was appropriately initiated on therapy with a bisphosphonate, vitamin D_3, and calcium. The appropriate interval for following osteoporosis with bone densitometry after initiating treatment is not clearly established because most treatments yield only small or moderate bone mass increments. Thus, the changes need to be greater than approximately 4% in the spine and approximately 6% in the hip to be considered significant in any given individual. Medications take several years to produce significant changes in bone mineral density (BMD); therefore, bone densitometry should be repeated at intervals of >2 years. Only further declines in BMD should prompt a change in regimen.

X-93. The answer is A. *(Chap. 427)* Osteogenesis imperfecta (OI) is a heritable disorder of connective tissue in which there is a severe decrease of bone mass that makes bone brittle and prone to fracture due to a deficiency or abnormality in type I procollagen. The disease is often inherited in an autosomal dominant fashion. There are several subtypes of OI that are currently based on the clinical phenotype of the disease. There is debate about whether the disease should be reclassified based on genetic abnormalities, but at present, the classification based on clinical presentation remains the standard. Type 1 OI has a varied clinical presentation, but generally has the mildest bone disease with minimal or no apparent skeletal deformities. The disease may not present until adulthood in those with type 1 OI. However, type 2 OI produces very brittle bones and typically is lethal in utero or shortly after birth. Other types of OI have variable bone disease that can yield bone deformity with frequent fractures or kyphoscoliosis or result in only mild disease. Another common clinical feature of type 1 OI includes blue sclera, which is thought to be due to the thinness of the collagen fibers of the sclerae, allowing the choroid layers to be seen. Additionally, the teeth may have an amber or yellowish brown color due to a deficiency of dentin that is rich in type I collagen. The deciduous teeth are often smaller than normal, whereas the permanent teeth may be bell-shaped and restricted at the base. Hearing loss is common beginning in the second decade of life and affects >50% of individuals over the age of 30. Fractures tend to decrease after puberty in both sexes but may increase in women at the time of pregnancy and after menopause. Diagnosis of OI is usually based on clinical criteria in an individual with fractures and other typical clinical features. Given the autosomal dominant nature of inheritance, a family history of disease may be present. Decreased bone mineral density is demonstrated in a variety of imaging techniques including x-ray absorptiometry and plain radiographs. Bone biopsy is not required for diagnosis and may cause morbidity. Treatment of the disease is primarily aimed at treating complications. Fractures typically are only slightly displaced with little soft tissue swelling. Minimal support and traction are required. Although bisphosphonates are well tolerated and often used for moderate to severe disease, where they may decrease bony pain and fracture risk, their long-term effects and safety in osteogenesis imperfecta are unknown.

X-94. The answer is A. *(Chap. 427, http://www.marfan.org/dx/home)* This patient presents with evidence of Marfan syndrome (MFS), an autosomal disorder most commonly associated with mutations in the fibrillin-1 gene. MFS is one of the most common heritable connective tissue disorders, with an incidence of 1 in 3000–5000 and is found in most racial and ethnic groups. The diagnosis of MFS is based on the revised Ghent criteria, which include major and minor criteria for evaluation. In the most recent revision, there has been stronger emphasis on the cardiovascular and ocular manifestations of MFS. In the absence of family history, the presence of aortic root aneurysm and ectopia lentis is sufficient to make the diagnosis. The diagnosis can also be made with a combination of systemic manifestations and the presence of aortic root dilation or ectopia lentis. Some of the systemic manifestations that this patient exhibits include the presence of long limbs and tall stature. The ratio of the upper segment to the lower segment of the body is usually 2 standard deviations below mean for age, race, and sex, and the arm span is usually >1.05 times the height. Arachnodactyly with long, slender fingers and hands is present. Other skeletal deformities include pectus excavatum, pectus carinatum, scoliosis, kyphosis, pes planus, and high-arched palate. A calculator is available at http://www.marfan.org/dx/score to allow one to easily calculate the number of systemic symptoms an individual has on presentation. In individuals with a family history of MFS, the presence of ectopia lentis, aortic root dilation, or a positive systemic score would be adequate for diagnosis. In this clinical scenario, the patient has a strong likelihood of having MFS and should be advised to refrain from engaging in strenuous physical activity or contact sports immediately, although further workup with echocardiogram and slit-lamp examination will be required. Although there is no definitive family diagnosis, the sudden death of the patient's father is likely to represent an aortic aneurysm rupture. In the most recent diagnostic criteria, an echocardiogram would be required for definitive diagnosis to evaluate for aortic root dilation. However, because this patient has several clinical features and a murmur concerning for aortic regurgitation, an echocardiogram would not be required before acting in the best interest of the man's health and removing him from further physical activity. Cardiovascular abnormalities may include mitral valve prolapse with or without mitral regurgitation and aortic root dilation. Dilation of the aortic root and the sinuses of Valsalva are characteristic of MFS and are an ominous sign of the disease. The dilation can occur at any age and place the patient at risk for aortic regurgitation, aortic dissection, and aneurysmal rupture. Dilation can be accelerated by physical and emotional stress and pregnancy. Individuals may require surgical repair of the dilated aortic root, and routine follow-up echocardiography is required to ensure that further dilation is not occurring. Use of β-blockers and, more recently, angiotensin II receptor blockers has been demonstrated to reduce the rate or delay the onset of aortic dilation. Physical activity guidelines have been published that suggest that all patients with MFS should avoid strenuous physical activity and contact sports. However, regular exercise that is low impact and low intensity should be encouraged.

X-95. The answer is E. *(Chap. 428)* Hereditary hemochromatosis is a common genetic condition. One out of 10 individuals of northern European ancestry will be a heterozygous carrier for the most common mutation, *HFE*, and 0.3%–0.5% of the population are homozygous for this mutation. However, disease expression in individuals who are homozygous for the *HFE* gene varies widely and is modified by a variety of environmental and clinical factors including alcohol intake, dietary iron intake, blood loss from pregnancy and menstruation, and blood donation. It is estimated that about 30% of men who are homozygous for the *HFE* gene will develop symptomatic iron overload, with about 6% progressing to hepatic cirrhosis. In women, clinical disease is less prevalent, with only 1% progressing to cirrhosis. Clinical manifestations include iron overload (as measured biochemically) initially without symptoms, and then iron overload with symptoms. Initial symptoms often include lethargy, arthralgia, change in skin color, loss of libido, and diabetes mellitus. Cirrhosis, cardiac arrhythmias, and infiltrative cardiomyopathy are later manifestations. Because the clinical manifestations of the disease can be prevented with iron chelation and the mutation is so common, some have advocated for screening the population for evidence of iron overload. Although routine screening remains controversial, recent studies indicate that it is highly effective for primary care physicians to screen subjects using transferrin saturation and serum ferritin levels. This will detect anemia and iron deficiency as well. Liver biopsy or MRI may demonstrate later findings of increased iron deposition and/or cirrhosis, but these are more costly, possibly invasive, or risky and not recommended for screening. Genetic testing is also not recommended as a first step, although it is indicated if evidence of iron overload is found on serum iron studies. No *HFE* activity assay is currently available.

X-96. The answer is E. *(Chap. 428)* This patient presents with the classic finding of diffuse organ iron infiltration due to hemochromatosis. The iron accumulation in the pancreas, testes, liver, joints, and skin explains his findings. Hemochromatosis is a common disorder of iron storage in which inappropriate increases in intestinal iron absorption result in excessive deposition in multiple organs, but predominantly in the liver. There are two forms: hereditary hemochromatosis, in which the majority of cases are associated with mutations of the *HFE* gene, and secondary iron overload, which usually is associated with iron-loading anemias such as thalassemia and sideroblastic anemia. In this case, without a history of prior hematologic disease, the most likely diagnosis is hereditary hemochromatosis. Serum ferritin testing and plasma iron studies can be very suggestive of the diagnosis, with the ferritin often >500 μg/L and transferrin saturation of 50%–100%. However, these tests are not conclusive, and further testing is still required for the diagnosis. Although liver biopsy and evaluation for iron deposition or a hepatic iron index [(μg/g dry weight)/56 × age >2] provide the definitive diagnosis, genetic testing is widely available today is recommended for diagnostic evaluation because of the high prevalence of *HFE* gene mutations associated with hereditary hemochromatosis. If the genetic testing is inconclusive, an invasive liver biopsy evaluation may be indicated. Anti–smooth muscle antibody testing is useful for the evaluation of autoimmune hepatitis and is indicated in any case of cryptogenic cirrhosis. Plasma ceruloplasmin is the initial study in the evaluation of Wilson disease, which is also a cause of occult liver disease. However, Wilson disease would not be likely to be associated with pancreatic, joint, and skin findings. If chronic hepatitis B is suspected, a viral load or surface antigen test would be indicated. Hepatitis B surface antibody is useful to demonstrate resolved hepatitis B or prior vaccination. Hepatic ultrasound is useful in the evaluation of acute and chronic liver disease to demonstrate portal flow or vascular occlusion; it may be useful in the physiologic evaluation of this patient but would have little diagnostic value.

X-97. and X-98. The answers are E and D, respectively. *(Chap. 429)* This patient presents with liver disease, hemolysis, and psychiatric illness, which suggests the presence of Wilson disease. Wilson disease is an autosomal recessive disorder caused by mutations in the *ATP7B* gene, a copper-transporting ATP-ase. As a result of this mutation, patients store abnormally high levels of copper in their liver initially, but later, copper is stored in other organs such as the brain. Although liver dysfunction is a hallmark of the disease, it may have several presentations, such as acute hepatitis, cirrhosis, or hepatic decompensation, as in this patient. Hemolysis may complicate acute decompensation because of massive release of copper from the liver into the blood, leading to hemolysis. Accumulation of copper in the basal ganglia results in Parkinson-like syndromes. Up to 50% of patients with Wilson disease will have Kayser-Fleischer rings on ocular slit-lamp examination. These brownish rings surrounding the cornea are due to copper deposition within the cornea and are diagnostic when found. Twenty-four-hour urinary copper levels are universally elevated in this disease and are the primary diagnostic modality when Kayser-Fleischer rings are absent. Liver biopsy can also be used to confirm increased copper content. Although MRI will show basal ganglia damage, it is not specific for Wilson disease. *HFE* mutation is present in hemochromatosis, which this patient does not have. Urine iron levels are not indicated.

Therapy for Wilson disease is dependent on the degree of disease at the time of presentation. Patients with mild hepatitis may be treated with zinc, which blocks intestinal absorption of copper, results in a negative copper balance, and induces hepatic metallothionein synthesis, which sequesters additional toxic copper. Trientine serves as a copper chelator and is used for more severe liver dysfunction or neurologic or psychiatric disease. In acutely decompensated liver failure, zinc should not be administered for at least 1 hour following trientine because the zinc could be chelated instead of copper if administered simultaneously. Liver transplantation is appropriate for patients who have experienced treatment failed with initial therapy.

X-99. The answer is C. *(Chap. 430)* This patient has a classic presentation for acute intermittent porphyria (AIP), an inherited disorder of heme biosynthesis. There are many different types of porphyrias, which are classified as either hepatic or erythropoietic depending on the primary site of overproduction and accumulation of their respective porphyrin precursors or porphyrins. AIP is classified as a hepatic porphyria and is typically inherited in an autosomal dominant fashion, although clinical expression of the disease is variable. It is most common in Scandinavia and Great Britain, with an estimated frequency of approximately

1 in 20,000. The genetic defect in AIP occurs in the enzyme hydroxymethylbilane (HMB) synthase, and over 300 mutations in this enzyme have been described. The disease typically presents with attacks of acute abdominal pain and neurologic symptoms that occur after puberty. Often, a precipitating cause of symptomatic episodes can be identified such as steroid hormone use, oral contraceptive use, systemic illness, reduced caloric intake, or use of many other medications (Table X-99A) This diagnosis should be considered in any individual with recurrent abdominal pain, especially when accompanied by neuropsychiatric complaints. The abdominal symptoms are often more prominent and nonspecific. These include severe nonlocalizing abdominal pain, abdominal distention, constipation or diarrhea, and vomiting. However, the physical examination shows no localizing findings, and workup fails to show any abnormalities with the exception of mild ileus. Other common findings on examination include tachycardia and hypertension due to increased sympathetic activation. Fever and leukocytosis are rare. Neuropsychiatric findings are considered a part of the diagnostic features and can be quite variable. A peripheral motor neuropathy that is associated with motor weakness and absent reflexes may occur. Sensory changes are less prominent. Psychiatric features may include depression, anxiety, insomnia, and hallucinations. The initial diagnostic test of choice for an acute porphyria is to perform a spot urine for presence of urinary porphyrin precursors (urinary porphyrobilinogen and 5-aminolevulinic acid) during an attack. Urinary porphyrobilinogen (PBG) is almost always elevated during an attack of AIP or one of the other acute porphyrias but not in any other medical condition, making it sensitive and specific for diagnosis of an acute porphyria (Table X-99B). A 24-hour collection is not required and may only delay diagnosis. If the urinary PBG is elevated, then second-line testing is measurement of red blood cell HMB synthase levels and urinary, plasma, and fecal porphyrins. Urinary porphyrin levels are not recommended as a screening test, however, because they are not sensitive markers. Other conditions, including chronic liver disease, can cause elevations in urinary porphyrins. If the diagnosis of AIP is made, genetic analysis for mutations in the HMB synthase gene should be performed, but this is not the test of choice for initial screening and diagnosis. The porphobilinogen level will drop in the recovery phase and may be normal between attacks. Therapy for acute attack is with carbohydrate loading, narcotic pain control, anxiolysis, and IV hemin, which repletes the end product in heme synthesis.

TABLE X-99A Unsafe Drugs in Porphyria

Documented Porphyrinogenic	Probably Porphyrinogenic	Possibly Porphyrinogenic	
Carbamazepine	Altretamine	Aceclofenac	Parecoxib
Carisoprodol	Aminophylline	Acitretin	Pentifylline
Chloramphenicol	Amiodarone	Acrivastine	Pentoxyverine
Clindamycin	Amitriptyline	Alfuzosin	Phenylpropanolamine + cinnarizine
Dextropropoxyphene	Amlodipine	Anastrozole	Pizotifen
Dihydralazine	Amprenavir	Auranofin	Polidocanol
Dihydroergotamine	Aprepitant	Azelastine	Polyestradiol
Drospirenone + estrogen	Atorvastatin	Benztropine	Phosphate
Dydrogesterone	Azathioprine	Benzydamine	Potassium canrenoate
Etonogestrel	Bosentan	Betaxolol	Pravastatin
Fosphenytoin sodium	Bromocriptine	Bicalutamide	Prednisolone
Hydralazine	Buspirone	Biperiden	Prilocaine
Hydroxyzine	Busulfan	Bupropion	Proguanil
Indinavir	Butylscopolamine	Carvedilol	Propafenone
Ketamine	Cabergoline	Chlorambucil	Pseudoephedrine + dexbrompheniramine
Ketoconazole	Ceftriaxone + lidocaine	Chlorcyclizine + guaifenesin	Quillaia extract
Lidocaine	Cerivastatin	Chloroquine	Quinagolide
Lynestrenol	Cetirizine	Chlorprothixene	Quinine
Lynestrenol + estrogen	Cholinetheophyllinate	Chlorzoxazone	Quinupristin + Dalfopristin
Mecillinam	Clarithromycin	Chorionic	Reboxetine

(*continued*)

TABLE X-99A Unsafe Drugs in Porphyria (Continued)

Documented Porphyrinogenic	Probably Porphyrinogenic	Possibly Porphyrinogenic	
Medroxyprogesterone	Clemastine	Gonadotropin	Repaglinide
Megestrol	Clonidine	Ciclosporin	Rizatriptan
Methylergometrine	Cyclizine	Cisapride	Rofecoxib
Methyldopa	Cyproterone	Citalopram	Ropinirole
Mifepristone	Danazol	Clomethiazole	Ropivacaine
Nicotinic acid/meclozine/ hydroxyzine	Delavirdine	Clomiphene	Roxithromycin
	Desogestrel + estrogen	Clomipramine	Sertraline
Nitrofurantoin	Diazepam	Clopidogrel	Sevoflurane
Norethisterone	Dienogest + estrogen	Clotrimazole	Sibutramine
Norgestimate + estrogen	Diclofenac	Cortisone	Sildenafil
Orphenadrine	Diltiazem	Cyclandelate	Sirolimus
Phenobarbital	Diphenhydramine	Cyclophosphamide	Sodium aurothiomalate
Phenytoin	Disopyramide	Cyproheptadine	Sodium oleate + chlorocymol
Pivampicillin	Disulfiram	Dacarbazine	Stavudine
Pivmecillinam	Drospirenone + estrogen	Daunorubicin	Sulindac
Primidone	Dydrogesterone	Desogestrel	Sumatriptan
Rifampicin	Ergoloid mesylate	Dichlorobenzyl alcohol	Tacrolimus
Ritonavir	Erythromycin	Dithranol	Tadalafil
Spironolactone	Estramustine	Docetaxel	Tegafur + uracil
Sulfadiazine + trimethoprim	Ethosuximide	Donepezil	Telmisartan
Tamoxifen	Etoposide	Doxycycline	Thioridazine
Testosterone, injection	Exemestane	Ebastine	Thioguanine
Thiopental	Felbamate	Econazole	Tolfenamic acid
Trimethoprim	Felodipine	Efavirenz	Tolterodine
Valproic acid	Fluconazole	Escitalopram	Torsemide
Venlafaxine	Flunitrazepam	Esomeprazole	Triamcinolone
Vinblastine	Fluvastatin	Estradiol/tablets	Trihexyphenidyl
Vincristine	Glibenclamide	Estriol/tablets	Trimipramine
Vindesine	Halothane	Estriol/vaginal crème, tablet	Valerian
Vinorelbine	Hyoscyamine		Venlafaxine
Xylometazoline	Ifosfamide	Estrogen, conjugate	Vinblastine
Zaleplon	Imipramine	Finasteride	Vincristine
Ziprasidone	Irinotecan	Flecainide	Vindesine
Zolmitriptan	Isoniazid	Flucloxacillin	Vinorelbine
Zolpidem	Isradipine	Fluoxetine	Xylometazoline
Zuclopenthixol	Itraconazole	Flupentixol	Zaleplon
	Lamivudine + zidovudine	Flutamide	Ziprasidone
	Lansoprazole	Fluvoxamine	Zolmitriptan
	Lercanidipine	Follitropin alfa and beta	Zolpidem
	Levonorgestrel	Galantamine	Zuclopenthixol
	Lidocaine	Glimepiride	
	Lopinavir	Glipizide	
	Lutropin alfa	Gonadorelin	
	Lymecycline	Gramicidin	
	Meclozine	Guaifenesin	
	Medroxyprogesterone + estrogen	Hydrocortisone	
	Metoclopramide	Hydroxycarbamide	
	Metronidazole	Hydroxychloroquine	
	Metyrapone	Ibutilide	
	Moxonidine	Imatinib	

(*continued*)

TABLE X-99A Unsafe Drugs in Porphyria (Continued)

Documented Porphyrinogenic	Probably Porphyrinogenic	Possibly Porphyrinogenic
	Nandrolone	Indomethacin
	Nefazodone	Ketobemidone + DDBA
	Nelfinavir	Ketoconazole
	Nevirapine	Ketorolac
	Nifedipine	Lamotrigine
	Nimodipine	Letrozole
	Nitrazepam	Levodopa + benserazide
	Norethisterone	Levonorgestrel intra-uterine
	Nortriptyline	Levosimendan
	Oxcarbazepine	Lidocaine
	Oxytetracycline	Linezolid
	Paclitaxel	Lofepramine
	Paroxetine	Lomustine
	Phenazone + caffeine	Malathion
	Pioglitazone	Maprotiline
	Probenecid	Mebendazole
	Progesterone, vaginal gel	Mefloquine
	Quinidine	Melperone
	Rabeprazole	Melphalan
	Raloxifene	Mepenzolate
	Rifabutin	Mepivacaine
	Riluzole	Mercaptopurine
	Risperidone	Methadone
	Rosiglitazone	Methylprednisolone
	Saquinavir	Methixene
	Selegiline	Metolazone
	Simvastatin	Metronidazole
	Sulfasalazine	Mexiletine
	Telithromycin	Mianserin
	Terbinafine	Midazolam
	Terfenadine	Minoxidil
	Testosterone, transdermal patch	Mirtazapine
	Tetracycline	Mitomycin
	Theophylline	Mitoxantrone
	Thiamazole	Moclobemide
	Tibolone	Montelukast
	Ticlopidine	Morphine + scopolamine
	Tinidazole	Multivitamins
	Thiotepa	Mupirocin
	Topiramate	Nabumetone
	Topotecan	Nafarelin
	Toremifene	Naltrexone
	Tramadol	Nateglinide
	Trimegestone + estrogen	Nilutamide
	Verapamil	Noscapine
	Voriconazole	Omeprazole
	Zidovudine (AZT)	Oxybutynin
		Oxycodone
		Pantoprazole
		Papaverine

Note: Based on list in "Patient's and Doctor's Guide to Medication in Acute Porphyria," Swedish Porphyria Association and Porphyria Centre Sweden. Also see the website Drug Database for Acute Porphyrias (www.drugs-porphyria.org) for a searchable list of safe and unsafe drugs.

TABLE X-99B Diagnosis of Acute and Cutaneous Porphyrias

Symptoms	First-Line Test: Abnormality	Possible Porphyria	Second-Line Testing if First-Line Testing Is Positive: to include urine (U), plasma (P), and fecal (F) porphyrins; for acute porphyrias, add red blood cell (RBC) HMB synthase; for blistering skin lesions, add P and RBC porphyrins	Confirmatory Test: Enzyme Assay and/or Mutation Analysis
Neurovisceral	**Spot U:** ↑↑ ALA and normal PBG	ADP	**U porphyrins:** ↑↑, mostly COPRO III **P & F porphyrins:** normal or slightly ↑ **RBC HMB synthase:** normal	Rule out other causes of elevated ALA; ↓↓ RBC ALA dehydratase activity (<10%); ALA dehydratase mutation analysis
	Spot U: ↑↑ PBG	AIP	**U porphyrins:** ↑↑, mostly URO and COPRO **P & F porphyrins:** normal or slightly ↑ **RBC HMB synthase:** usually ↓	HMB synthase mutation analysis
	"	HCP	**U porphyrins:** ↑↑, mostly COPRO III **P porphyrins:** normal or slightly ↑ (↑ if skin lesions present) **F porphyrins:** ↑↑, mostly COPRO III	Measure RBC HMB synthase: normal activity COPRO oxidase mutation analysis
	"	VP	**U porphyrins:** ↑↑, mostly COPRO III **P porphyrins:** ↑↑(characteristic fluorescence peak at neutral pH) **F porphyrins:** ↑↑, mostly COPRO and PROTOO	Measure RBC HMB synthase: normal activity PROTO oxidase mutation analysis
Blistering skin lesions	**P:** ↑ porphyrins	PCT and HEP	**U porphyrins:** ↑↑, mostly URO and heptacarboxylate porphyrin **P porphyrins:** ↑↑ **F porphyrins:** ↑↑, including increased isocoproporphyrin **RBC porphyrins:** ↑↑ zinc PROTO in HEP[a]	RBC URO decarboxylase activity: half-normal in familial PCT (~20% of all PCT cases); substantially deficient in HEP URO decarboxylase mutation analysis: mutation(s) present in familial PCT (heterozygous) and HEP (homozygous)
	"	HCP and VP	See HCP and VP above. Also, U ALA and PBG: may be ↑	
	"	CEP	**RBC and U porphyrins:** ↑↑, mostly URO I and COPRO I **F porphyrins:** ↑↑; mostly COPRO I	↓↓ RBC URO synthase activity (<15%) on URO synthase mutation analysis
Nonblistering photosensitivity	**P:** porphyrins usually ↑	EPP	**RBC porphyrins:** ↓↓, mostly free PROTO **U porphyrins:** normal **F porphyrins:** normal or ↓, mostly PROTO	*FECH* mutation analysis
	P: porphyrins usually ↑	XLP	**RBC porphyrins:** ↑↑, approximately equal free and zinc PROTO **U porphyrins:** normal **F porphyrins:** normal or ↑, mostly PROTO	*ALAS2* mutation analysis

[a]Nonspecific increases in zinc protoporphyrins are common in other porphyrias.

Abbreviations: ADP, 5-ALA dehydratase-deficient porphyria; AIP, acute intermittent porphyria; ALA, 5-aminolevulinic acid; CEP, congenital erythropoietic porphyria; COPRO I, coproporphyrin I; COPRO III, coproporphyrin III; EPP, erythropoietic protoporphyria; F, fecal; HCP, hereditary coporphyria; HEP, hepatoerythropoietic porphyria; ISOCOPRO, isocoproporphyrin; P, plasma; PBG, porphobilinogen; PCT, porphyria cutanea tarda; PROTO, protoporphyrin IX; RBC, erythrocytes; U, urine; URO I, uroporphyrin I; URO III, uroporphyrin III; VP, variegate porphyria; XLP, X-linked protoporphyria.

Source: Based on KE Anderson et al: Ann Intern Med 142:439, 2005.

X-100. The answer is C. *(Chap. 430)* This patient has porphyria cutanea tarda (PCT), the most common porphyria. Although PCT can be inherited, it most commonly occurs sporadically and is associated with a defect in hepatic uroporphyrinogen (URO) decarboxylase. For clinical symptoms to be present, the patient needs to have less than 20% of normal enzyme activity, and PCT occurs when an individual develops an inhibitor of URO decarboxylase in the liver. The majority of PCT patients have no mutations in URO decarboxylase. The major clinical feature of PCT is blistering skin lesions predominantly affecting the back of the hands that also may involve the forearms, face, legs, and feet. The lesions start as blisters that rupture and crust over, leaving scarring. Chronically, the areas most involved can develop thickened skin similar to systemic sclerosis. Precipitating factors for development of lesions include hepatitis C, human immunodeficiency virus, excess alcohol, elevated iron levels, and estrogens. Diagnosis of PCT is made by measuring porphyrin levels, which would demonstrate elevated plasma, urine, and fecal porphyrins. Liver levels of porphyrins are also high. Urinary 5-aminolevunilinic acid level may be slightly elevated, but the urinary porphyrobilinogen level is normal. In addition to avoiding precipitating factors, treatment of PCT is primarily through phlebotomy every 1–2 weeks to achieve a low-normal ferritin level. With this approach, a complete remission can almost always be achieved, typically after only five to six phlebotomies. After remission, continued phlebotomy may not be required, but plasma porphyrin levels should continue to be followed every 6–12 months to assess for recurrence. An alternative effective treatment is use of the antimalarial drugs chloroquine or hydroxychloroquine. These drugs complex with the excess porphyrins and promote their excretions. Doses typically are lower in PCT because standard doses may actually worsen symptoms transiently. Recent studies have shown that hydroxychloroquine may be as safe and effective as phlebotomy, although phlebotomy remains the standard of care at this time. None of the other treatments, including hemin, are used in the treatment of PCT.

SECTION XI

Neurologic Disorders

QUESTIONS

DIRECTIONS: Choose the one best response to each question.

XI-1. A 78-year-old man with a history of prostate cancer presents to the emergency department with weakness affecting his right arm and leg and left face. The weakness began abruptly earlier during the day and is associated with numbness and paresthesias. On physical examination, strength is 4/5 in the right leg and arm. The upper and lower facial muscles fail to move on the left. Babinski sign is positive. Sensation is decreased in the right extremities and on the left face. Based on this information, what is the most likely site of the lesion causing the patient's symptoms?

A. Brainstem
B. Cerebrum
C. Cervical spinal cord
D. Multiple spinal cord levels
E. Neuromuscular junction

XI-2. During a neurologic examination, you ask a patient to stand with both arms fully extended and parallel to the ground with his eyes closed for 10 seconds. What is the name of this test?

A. Babinski sign
B. Dysdiadochokinesis
C. Lhermitte symptom
D. Pronator drift
E. Romberg sign

XI-3. The test described in Question XI-2 is considered positive if there is flexion at the elbows or forearms or if there is pronation of the forearms. A positive test is a sign of which of the following?

A. Abnormal sensation
B. Early dementia
C. Localized brainstem disease
D. Potential weakness
E. Underlying cerebellar dysfunction

XI-4 through XI-8. For each of the following clinical findings on neurologic examination, identify the most likely anatomic location:

4. Anal sphincter dysfunction

5. Bilateral ptosis and diplopia

6. Diminished sensation bilaterally at the ankles and feet in a patient with diabetes

7. Left homonymous hemianopia

8. Right lateral extraocular muscle paresis

A. Brainstem
B. Cerebrum
C. Neuromuscular junction
D. Peripheral nerve
E. Spinal cord

XI-9. A 54-year-old woman presents to the emergency department complaining of the abrupt onset of what she describes as the worst headache of her life. You are concerned about the possibility of subarachnoid hemorrhage. What is the most appropriate initial test for diagnosis?

A. Cerebral angiography
B. Computed tomography (CT) of the head with intravenous contrast
C. CT of the head without intravenous contrast
D. Lumbar puncture
E. Transcranial Doppler ultrasound

XI-10. A 74-year-old woman has a recent diagnosis of small-cell lung cancer. She is now complaining of headaches, and her family has noticed confusion as well. Metastatic disease to the brain is suspected. A mass lesion on magnetic resonance imaging (MRI) is demonstrated in the right parietal lobe. Which MRI technique would best identify the extent of the edema surrounding the lesion?

A. Magnetic resonance angiography
B. Fluid-attenuated inversion recovery (FLAIR)
C. T1-weighted
D. T2-weighted
E. B and D

XI-11. Which of the following is a possible complication of administration of gadolinium to a patient with chronic kidney disease?

A. Acute renal failure
B. Hyperthyroidism
C. Hypocalcemia
D. Lactic acidosis
E. Nephrogenic systemic sclerosis

XI-12. A 45-year-old woman is admitted to the emergency department after a first episode of witnessed generalized tonic-clonic seizure. She is administered lorazepam 2 mg with cessation of seizure activity. All of the following are likely possible causes of her seizure EXCEPT:

A. Alcohol withdrawal
B. Autoantibodies
C. Brain tumor
D. Genetic disorder
E. Hyperglycemia

XI-13. A 48-year-old woman is evaluated for seizure-like episodes. She has a history of major depression and borderline personality disorder. She is currently taking escitalopram 10 mg daily. She smokes one pack of cigarettes daily and drinks one to two glasses of wine daily. You are called to the bedside during an episode. You observe her head turning vigorously side to side with large-amplitude limb shaking and upward thrusting of the pelvis. You are concerned about psychogenic seizures. Which of the following findings could assist in this diagnosis?

A. A normal creatine kinase level within 30 minutes of the episode
B. A normal prolactin level within 30 minutes of the episode
C. An elevated creatine kinase within 30 minutes of the episode
D. An elevated prolactin level within 30 minutes of the episode
E. Decreased arousability in the period immediately following the episode

XI-14. A 56-year-old man with glioblastoma multiforme in the right parietal lobe experiences his first generalized tonic-clonic seizure. What is the best course of action for this patient?

A. Initiate therapy with ethosuximide
B. Initiate therapy with lamotrigine
C. Initiate therapy with phenytoin
D. Observe for additional seizures and initiate therapy only if additional seizures occur
E. Refer for electroencephalogram (EEG) and treat only if an epileptogenic focus is identified

XI-15. A 24-year-old man presents to your office requesting to be taken off of his antiepileptic drugs. He was in an automobile accident at the age of 12, resulting in significant head trauma. He was in a medically induced coma for 6 weeks and had intracranial edema with generalized tonic-clonic seizures at that time. These persisted for several years afterward. His last seizure that he is aware of occurred at the age of 18 and was generalized. He continues to take valproic acid 1000 mg bid. On physical examination, he demonstrates normal cognition and affect. He has ongoing focal weakness involving his left lower extremity with spasticity. You refer him for a sleep-deprived EEG, which shows no evidence of focal abnormalities. Which of the following factors is of greatest concern regarding his risk of recurrent seizures?

A. Focal defect on neurologic examination
B. Generalized seizure disorder
C. Head trauma
D. Seizure within the past 7 years

XI-16. A 38-year-old man with a history of seizure disorder presents with generalized convulsive status epilepticus. He had been having persistent seizure activity for 20 minutes when emergency medical services were activated. He was given paralytic agents in the field to allow for intubation as well as lorazepam 8 mg intravenously (IV). Upon arrival in the emergency department 20 minutes later, the neuromuscular blockade has worn off and generalized seizure activity is again apparent. His initial temperature is 39.2°C with blood pressure of 182/92 mmHg, heart rate of 158 bpm, respiratory rate of 38 breaths/min, and SaO_2 of 95% on mechanical ventilation with an assist control mode with a set rate of 15, tidal volume of 420 mL, positive end-expiratory pressure of 5 cmH_2O, and FiO_2 of 0.6. What is the next step in the management of this patient?

A. Additional dosing of neuromuscular blockers
B. Isoflurane anesthesia
C. Fosphenytoin 20 mg/kg IV
D. Pentobarbital 5 mg/kg bolus followed by an infusion at 1 mg/kg/hr
E. Propofol 2 mg/kg bolus followed by an infusion at 2 mg/kg/hr

XI-17. A 68-year-old man presents to the emergency department with right-sided face, arm, and leg weakness that began abruptly 1 hour prior to arrival. The patient is accompanied by his wife. He exhibits Broca aphasia and dysarthria. Physical examination confirms a dense hemiparesis of the right face, arm, and leg with decreased sensation. In addition, there is a gaze preference to the left. The patient's initial blood pressure on presentation to the emergency department is 195/115 mmHg. Multiple follow-up blood pressures have been sustained between 160–170/100–110 mmHg without treatment. An emergent noncontrast head CT shows no evidence of intracranial hemorrhage or edema with only mild loss of gray-white matter differentiation. On further review of the patient's medical history, he had a prior embolic stroke affecting the posterior circulation 12 months ago. He also has a history of colon cancer that was diagnosed 3 months ago when he presented with a lower gastrointestinal (GI) bleed requiring transfusion of 4 units of packed red blood cells. He successfully underwent left hemicolectomy of a stage I adenocarcinoma. In the postoperative period, he developed a deep venous thrombosis of the superficial femoral vein on the right. He is currently being treated with warfarin at 5 mg daily. His last international normalized ratio (INR) was therapeutic at 2.2. It was checked 4 days ago. Which of the following factors is a contraindication to use of IV recombinant tissue plasminogen activator in this patient?

A. GI bleeding within the past 3 months
B. Initial blood pressure elevation >180/110 mmHg
C. Major surgery within the past 3 months
D. Prior embolic stroke
E. Use of warfarin with elevated INR

XI-18. A 54-year-old woman is seen in your office for a new patient visit. She is very concerned about her risk of stroke and wants to do whatever she can to prevent it. Her mother died following a stroke related to untreated hypertension at the age of 62. The patient has hypertension and diabetes mellitus. She currently is taking hydrochlorothiazide 25 mg daily and metformin 500 mg twice daily. She smokes one pack of cigarettes daily. Her blood pressure today is 158/92 mmHg. Fasting lipids show a total cholesterol of 232 mg/dL, triglyceride level of 168 mg/dL, high-density lipoprotein of 32 mg/dL, and low-density lipoprotein of 166 mg/dL. The hemoglobin A1C is 7.5%. What advice is LEAST helpful in primary prevention of stroke in this individual?

A. Add aspirin 81 mg daily as an antiplatelet agent
B. Add atorvastatin 10 mg daily to lower cholesterol
C. Add lisinopril 20 mg daily to decrease blood pressure to a target blood pressure of 130/80 mmHg
D. Increase metformin to 1000 mg twice daily and change diet to obtain a goal hemoglobin A1C level of less than 7%
E. Recommend smoking cessation and offer counseling and nicotine replacement

XI-19. A 76-year-old man was seen in the emergency department for left-sided arm weakness that rapidly improved over the course of 4 hours. He has a past medical history positive for hypertension, dyslipidemia, and coronary artery disease. He previously has undergone coronary angioplasty with stenting to both his left anterior descending artery and right coronary artery on two occasions. He is currently being treated with aspirin 81 mg daily, metoprolol 100 mg bid, benazepril 20 mg daily, rosuvastatin 10 mg daily, and clopidogrel 75 mg daily. Evaluation demonstrates a 75% occlusion of the right internal carotid artery. The patient is considering whether he would like to undergo carotid endarterectomy. What information is needed for him to make an informed decision about the risks and benefits of the surgery for him?

A. Perioperative mortality rate for the surgeon performing his surgery
B. Perioperative stroke rate for the surgeon performing his surgery
C. Risk of stroke in the next 90 days
D. Risk of stroke in the next year
E. The surgeon cannot schedule his surgery for 6 weeks

XI-20. A 48-year-old man presents to the emergency department with stupor. He was feeling well until 30 minutes ago when he complained of headache and right-sided weakness. He has a history of hypertension and cocaine use. He is prescribed hydrochlorothiazide 25 mg daily, but it is unknown whether he is taking his medication. On presentation, he is drowsy and minimally responsive to questioning. His blood pressure is 242/148 mmHg, heart rate is 124 bpm, respiratory rate is 24 breaths/min, SaO2 is 98% on room air, and temperature is 37.0°C. He is not moving his right arm and leg. He does withdraw to pain. His noncontrast head CT is shown in Figure XI-20. What is the diagnosis?

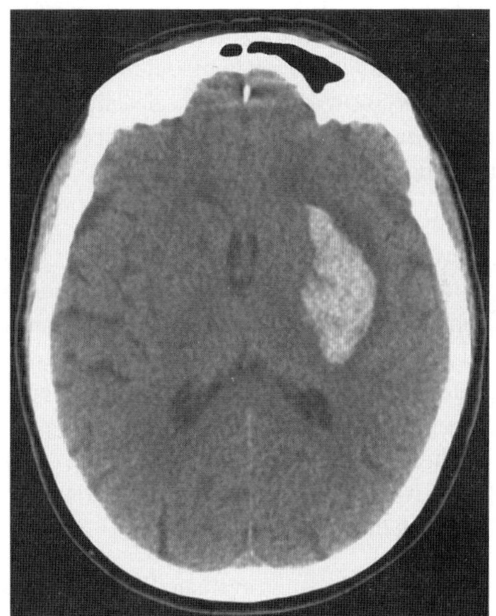

FIGURE XI-20

A. Brain mass
B. Epidural hematoma
C. Intracranial hemorrhage
D. Ischemic stroke in the left middle cerebral artery territory
E. Subdural hematoma

XI-21. A 26-year-old woman has throbbing right-sided headaches that are centered around her right eye. They are worse with movement and aggravated by loud noises. There are no premonitory warning features. Triggers for the headaches include lack of sleep, stress, and red wine. A mild attack can be treated by ibuprofen, but nonsteroidal anti-inflammatory drugs have no effect on more severe pain. Which of the following best characterizes what is understood about the pathogenesis of the patient's headache syndrome?

A. Diffuse muscular contraction of the neck and scalp
B. Disinhibition of the central pacemaker neurons in the posterior hypothalamic region
C. Dysfunction of monoaminergic sensory control systems in brainstem and hypothalamus
D. Focal cerebral vasodilation in the region of the brain that is the focus of the pain
E. Vascular compression of the trigeminal nerve as it enters the pons

XI-22. A 34-year-old woman is evaluated for migraine headaches. She has had migraines since her early 20s, and they are worse with recovery from sleep loss, menstrual cycles, stress, and certain foods that she tries to avoid. She describes the pain as left occipital in nature, throbbing, and severe. She has photophobia with episodes and occasionally vomits. With an acute episode, she takes rizatriptan 10 mg. It works within 1–2 hours in about 75% of attacks. However, recently, she has been having about six episodes per month. She has missed some days of work due to attacks. She would like to escalate her therapy and is asking for your advice. What is your advice about medications for migraine prevention?

A. Methysergide and phenelzine are first-line medications for this indication.
B. No drugs have a Food and Drug Administration–approved indication for migraine prevention.
C. Preventive therapy would not be recommended unless she has more than seven attacks per month.
D. The probability of success with use of a preventive medication is 90%.
E. There is a lag of 2–12 weeks after starting a new medication before an effect is seen.

XI-23. A 42-year-old man is evaluated for severe headaches that have occurred several times over the past 5–7 years. He describes the headaches as occurring behind his left eye and coming on suddenly. The headaches have a stabbing quality and are associated tearing of his eye and nasal congestion. He says the pain is a "12" out of 10 when it occurs, and he finds that he can't even sit still due to pain. The headaches last about 20 minutes and then subside. He says that the headaches seem to occur at the same time every day, around 5 AM, but he can go months without having any headache at all. He has a difficult time identifying a trigger for the headaches. What is the most likely cause of his headaches?

A. Cluster headache
B. Migraine
C. Paroxysmal hemicrania
D. Short-lasting unilateral neuralgiform headaches with conjunctival injection and tearing (SUNCT)
E. Tension headache

XI-24. A 72-year-old woman is evaluated for memory problems. She and her husband first noticed some mild problems about 2 or 3 years ago, but attributed her symptoms to "old age." They decided to seek an evaluation when she became lost while returning home from the grocery store last week. She had driven back and forth from this same store weekly for the past 20 years, and this incident frightened them both. She does not know what happened and had to call her husband for help. She has shown no changes to her personality. Her medical history is significant for hypertension and stage II breast cancer treated 10 years ago. She is taking ramipril 5 mg bid. She smoked one pack of tobacco daily from the age of 20 until she was 64. She drinks a glass of wine nightly. She retired from her position as an accountant at the age of 60. On examination, she appears well-groomed and pleasant. Her blood pressure is 158/90 mmHg, and heart rate is 82 bpm. Her neurologic examination is normal without focal defect. Gait is normal. No rigidity is present. Neuropsychological testing shows impairment 1.5 standard deviations below the norm. What would be the most likely pathologic finding in the brain?

A. Deposition of amyloid within cerebral blood vessels
B. Loss of cortical serotonergic innervation with atrophy of the frontal, insular, and/or temporal cortex
C. Neuritic plaques and neurofibrillary tangles in the medial temporal lobes
D. Presence of intraneuronal cytoplasmic inclusions that stain with periodic acid–Schiff and ubiquitin in the substantia nigra, amygdala, cingulate gyrus, and neocortex

XI-25. A 78-year-old man has been diagnosed with mild cognitive impairment after complaining of decreased memory. He asks you to prescribe something that will decrease his likelihood to progress to Alzheimer disease. What treatment do you recommend?

A. Brain training exercises
B. Donepezil
C. Gingko biloba
D. Memantine
E. No treatment at this time has been demonstrated to delay the progression of mild cognitive impairment to Alzheimer disease.

XI-26. A 62-year-old man presents with memory and behavior problems. Until 1 year ago, he had worked as a senior account manager at a local bank, but he had to retire after he had an angry outburst with a client and was inappropriate with a female colleague in a departmental meeting. His family reports that this behavior was entirely out of character for him, and since then, he is increasingly brusque and easily angered. He also has been overly sexual and has said many inappropriate things within the hearing of his teenaged grandchildren. At the same time, it has been noted that his memory has been worsening. He has an MBA degree, but his wife has recently began managing the money after he could no longer be relied on to do this. The financial records were highly disorganized when she began to look into them. The patient also recently had a near-miss accident while driving the wrong way down a one-way street. On examination, he is gruff and says that he doesn't want to do "this damn thing." He needs to "get the hell out of here." He is quite rude and insults his wife several times. He has a positive glabellar reflex. Mini Mental State Examination score is 20/30. There is no rigidity. Gait is normal. Deep tendon reflexes are 3+ and symmetric. Strength is 5/5 throughout, and there are no sensory deficits. Cerebellar function is normal. What is the most likely diagnosis?

A. Alzheimer disease
B. Dementia with Lewy bodies
C. Frontotemporal dementia
D. Progressive supranuclear palsy
E. Vascular dementia

XI-27. Which of the following statements regarding Parkinson disease is true?

A. Cigarette smoking reduces the risk of developing the disease.
B. Older age at presentation is more likely to be associated to genetic predisposition.
C. Parkinson disease has been identified as a monogenetic disorder related to mutations in the α-synuclein protein.
D. The typical age of onset of symptoms is about 70 years.
E. The hallmark pathologic feature of Parkinson disease is presence of neurofibrillary tangle and tau protein in the substantia nigra pars compacta.

XI-28. A 64-year-old man presents with symptoms of tremor and a generalized feeling of slowing down. His tremor bothers him most on his left side. His past medical history is significant for depression, hypertension, and hyperlipidemia. He is taking fluoxetine 40 mg daily, lisinopril 40 mg daily, and atorvastatin 20 mg daily. On physical examination, he has a resting tremor with presence of cogwheel rigidity. When observing his gait, you note slow, shuffling steps with difficulty maneuvering to turn around. His facial features show decreased range of emotion and appear somewhat flat. Eye movements are full. Mental status examination shows normal mentation. You suspect Parkinson disease. What is your first choice of therapy?

A. Defer therapy until further diagnostic studies are performed
B. Levodopa-carbidopa
C. Rotigotine
D. Selegiline
E. Either B or C can be used
F. Any of the above can be used

XI-29. Which of the following patients with Parkinson disease is the best candidate for deep brain stimulation?

A. A 64-year-old woman on levodopa-carbidopa who continues to experience episodes of freezing while walking
B. A 68-year-old man with recurrent falls due to orthostatic hypotension
C. A 70-year-old woman with severe tremor unresponsive to dopaminergic therapy
D. A 71-year-old man with worsening symptoms of dementia
E. All of the above patients will respond to deep brain stimulation.

XI-30. A 54-year-old man presents complaining of weakness. He has a difficult time pinpointing an onset. He believes he first noticed weakness in his right foot and leg about 6 months ago. He reports that he frequently trips over his toes and drags his foot. He also gets frequent cramps when he stretches in bed in the mornings. The weakness is progressing to involve both legs now. On examination, you note tongue fasciculations. Deep tendon reflexes are 3+ at the knees and ankles. Strength is 4– at the extensors and flexors of the right foot and 4+ at the left foot. Hand grip strength is also 4+. Which of the following is the suspected pathologic cause of this patient's symptoms?

A. Degeneration of the corticospinal tracts
B. Demyelinating plaques
C. Loss of anterior horn cells in the spinal cord
D. Loss of large pyramidal cells in the precentral gyrus
E. Lymphocytic infiltrate of spinal roots and nerves
F. A and C

XI-31. A 62-year-old woman is evaluated for symptoms of "slowing down." She used to be very active and ran 2–4 miles at least 3 days per week. For the past 6 months, she has not been able to complete even 1 mile, and her husband feels she has been moving more slowly and with a shuffling gait. She reports no tremor. She frequently feels lightheaded upon standing and has been evaluated in the emergency department twice for falls that occurred soon after standing. After one fall, she did require sutures for a scalp laceration. She has also been experiencing significant constipation requiring daily treatment with polyethylene glycol and bisacodyl suppositories. On physical examination, she has a blood pressure of 122/78 mmHg and a heart rate of 72 bpm while seated. Upon standing, her blood pressure falls to 92/60 mmHg with a heart rate of 102 bpm. She does report dizziness with the maneuver. She has bradykinesia and walks with a shuffling gait. Cranial nerves are intact with full eye movements. Deep tendon reflexes are 2+ and symmetric. There is rigidity with passive motion of the forearms. She has no tremor. Mental status examination is normal. What is the most likely diagnosis?

A. Diffuse Lewy body disease
B. Multiple system atrophy
C. Parkinson disease
D. Postural orthostatic tachycardia syndrome
E. Progressive supranuclear palsy

XI-32. A 58-year-old woman is seen for complaints of very sharp pain lasting about 1 minute over her right cheek and lips. These pain episodes occur in clusters with intense pain during the episode. When an episode occurs, it is present both day and night and can recur over a period of about a week. Paroxysms of pain can be elicited by washing her face. On physical examination, there is no sensory or motor loss in the right face. There are no masses. Touching the right face does bring about an episode of pain for the patient. What is the next best step in management of this patient?

A. Initiate treatment with carbamazepine 100 mg with a goal dose of 200 mg qid
B. Perform an MRI/magnetic resonance angiography (MRA) of the brain
C. Refer patient for a temporal artery biopsy
D. Refer patient for electromyography and nerve conduction study
E. Refer patient for microvascular decompression surgery

XI-33. A 65-year-old woman with a prior history of stage IIB carcinoma of the right breast presents with a 1-week history of sharp mid-back pain. She reports that it becomes worse with movement and coughing. She has not slept well because the pain awakens her. On the day of presentation, she developed weakness in her lower extremities such that she is not able to bear weight. She has had incontinence of the bladder. On examination, the patient has tenderness to palpation over the lower thoracic spine. The strength in the lower extremities is 3 out of 5 with decreased deep tendons reflexes. Anal sphincter tone is decreased. Sensation to light touch and pinprick also demonstrates a decrease in perception to the level of T8. Metastatic disease to the spine is demonstrated in multiple thoracic and lumbar vertebral bodies with cord compression at T8 on T1-weighted MRI. What is the next best step in the management of this patient?

A. Administer dexamethasone 10 mg IV every 6 hours
B. Consult neurosurgery for surgical decompression
C. Consult medical oncology for additional chemotherapy
D. Consult radiation oncology for urgent radiotherapy
E. A and D
F. A, C, and D
G. A, B, C, and D

XI-34. A 32-year-old African American man presents to the emergency department with progressive lower extremity weakness that has been present for the past month. It has now progressed to the point that he is unable to bear weight. He also has been experiencing loss of sensation and aching pains in his mid-back and a sensation of incomplete voiding with mild urinary incontinence. Today, he also had incontinence of stool. His past medical history is significant for a stab wound to the left chest 9 months prior. He required surgical repair. A CT scan was negative at that time for any lymph node abnormalities. He is on no medications and does not smoke or drink alcohol. Physical examination confirms lower extremity paresis with strength of only 3/5 and decreased deep tendon reflexes. Sensation to light tough and pinprick is absent in the lower extremities. He develops sensory perception at the umbilicus. An MRI shows multilevel enhancement of the spinal cord consistent with edema. It has a predominance in the mid-thoracic spinal cord. Gadolinium administration shows enhancement in a nodular fashion of the surface of the cord. Lumbar puncture is performed. There are 32 white blood cells (WBC)/μL in the first tube and 24 WBC/μL in the fourth tube. These are 90% lymphocytes. The cerebrospinal fluid protein level is 75 mg/dL. The glucose level is normal. A chest radiograph demonstrates enlargement of the hilar lymph nodes without pulmonary infiltrates. On chest CT, bilateral hilar, subcarinal, and precarinal lymphadenopathy is observed with the largest lymph node measuring 2 × 1.8 cm. Serum calcium is 12.5 mg/dL. A biopsy of the hilar lymph nodes is planned. What is the most likely finding on biopsy?

A. Abundant atypical lymphocytes that demonstrate clonality on flow cytometry
B. Caseating granulomatous inflammation
C. Noncaseating granulomatous inflammation
D. Nonspecific chronic inflammatory changes
E. Sheets of small, round cells with dark nuclei, scant cytoplasm, and salt-and-pepper chromatin with indistinct nucleoli; frequent mitotic figures are also seen

XI-35. A 32-year-old woman presents for neurologic evaluation after experiencing a severe burn on the palm of her right hand. She had placed her hand onto the hot surface of a smooth electric range. She did not feel the burn when it occurred, and only when she picked her hand up did she notice the burn. After that, it was discovered that the patient unknowingly has bilateral loss of pain and temperature sensation in both hands. However, she does have touch and vibratory sense. Mapping of her loss of sensation shows decreased pain sensation in the nape of her neck, shoulders, and upper arms as well in a cape-like distribution. Deep tendon reflexes are absent at the biceps and triceps, and there is visible muscle wasting of the right biceps and shoulder musculature. What is the most likely diagnosis?

A. Arteriovenous malformation of the spine
B. Neoplastic spinal cord compression
C. Subacute combined degeneration
D. Syringomyelia
E. Transverse myelitis

XI-36. A 31-year-old white woman is evaluated for symptoms of blurred vision and weakness. She is not really sure how long the symptoms have been occurring. She has had intermittent blurring of her vision for the past 2 months, although it has been more persistent for the past 2 weeks. She states that she also notes that colors seem less vivid and that her symptoms are worse in the right eye. Three months ago, she did notice some sharp pains in the right eye that were worse when she looked around. They subsided after about a week, and since then, her vision has worsened. At the same time, she feels as though she is stiff in her legs and also feels that her left leg is weak. She sometimes feels as if her left leg will give out on her if she stands on it for a prolonged period. Her past medical history is significant for type 1 diabetes mellitus for which she uses an insulin pump. She has smoked one pack of cigarettes daily since the age of 18. On physical examination, there is spasticity in both of her lower extremities with passive motion. Deep tendon reflexes are 3+ bilaterally with strength at the quadriceps on the right at 4/5. All other strength in the lower extremity is 5/5 bilaterally. Sensation to light touch and pinprick is decreased in the lower extremities. A dilated funduscopic examination shows swelling of the optic disc. Which of the following findings is most likely to be demonstrated?

A. Elevated protein levels in the cerebrospinal fluid to more than 100 mg/dL
B. Hyperintensity on T1-weight images consistent with a mass lesion in the occipital lobe with hydrocephalus
C. Hyperintensity on T2-weighted MRI images in multiple areas of the brain, brainstem, and spinal cord
D. Marked increased in transmission of somatosensory evoked potentials of lower limbs
E. Presence of 15 polymorphonuclear cells/μL in the cerebrospinal fluid

XI-37. In the patient in Question XI-36, the expected finding is demonstrated on testing. On further historical review, the patient reports that she had one prior episode of blurred vision that resolved spontaneously about 8 months ago. She never sought treatment for it, although it lasted for about 2 weeks. You make the correct diagnosis. All of the following are epidemiologic risks factors for her disease EXCEPT:

A. Age between 20 and 40
B. Cigarette smoking
C. Female sex
D. History of an autoimmune disorder (type 1 diabetes mellitus)
E. White race

XI-38. A 38-year-old woman has relapsing/remitting multiple sclerosis. She has experienced two attacks of disease previously that have left her with residual lower extremity weakness. She was initially treated with glucocorticoids with some improvement in her symptoms. However, she is currently only able to walk with a rolling walker about 100 m. A prior antibody test shows that she is positive for reactivity to the JC virus. You are planning to start a disease-modifying therapy. Which of the following is LEAST appropriate for this individual?

A. Dimethyl fumarate (DMF)
B. Interferon-β-1a
C. Fingolimod
D. Natalizumab
E. Teriflunomide

XI-39. You are evaluating a 42-year-old woman for complaints of muscle weakness and tingling in her lower extremities. You suspect a peripheral neuropathy. All of the following questions are important for the history and physical examination EXCEPT:

A. Are there any important comorbid conditions?
B. Is there evidence of upper motor neuron involvement?
C. What does the electromyogram and nerve conduction study demonstrate?
D. What is the distribution of the weakness?
E. Which systems are involved—motor, sensory, autonomic, or combination?

XI-40. A 24-year-old man presents for evaluation of foot drop. He has noted that for the last several months, he has had difficulty picking his feet up to walk up stairs and over thresholds. His right leg is more affected than his left leg. He has not noted any sensory changes. His father and paternal aunt each have had some weakness in their lower extremities. However, his father is currently 50 years of age and only began to develop some weakness in the past 2 years. His paternal aunt has always had a limp for as long as he can recall. He does not remember his grandparents having any symptoms, although his paternal grandfather died in a car accident at the age of 46 prior to his birth. The patient's examination is notable for distal leg weakness with reduced sensation to light touch in both lower extremities. Knee and ankle jerk reflexes are unobtainable. Calves are reduced in size bilaterally. Upper extremity examination is normal. Which of the following is the most likely diagnosis?

A. Charcot-Marie-Tooth syndrome
B. Fabry disease
C. Guillain-Barré syndrome
D. Hereditary neuralgic amyotrophy
E. Hereditary sensory and autonomic neuropathy

XI-41. A 57-year-old immigrant from Vietnam is evaluated by his primary care giver for dysesthesias that have been present in his hands and feet for the past several weeks. He also reports some difficulty walking. His past medical history is notable for hypertriglyceridemia, tobacco abuse, and a recently discovered positive purified protein derivative (PPD) with sputum that is smear-negative for *Mycobacterium tuberculosis*. His medications include niacin, aspirin, and isoniazid. Which of the following is likely to reverse his symptoms?

A. Cobalamin
B. Levothyroxine
C. Neurontin
D. Pregabalin
E. Pyridoxine

XI-42. A 52-year-old woman with long-standing poorly controlled type 2 diabetes mellitus is evaluated for a sensation of numbness in her fingers and toes, as if she is wearing gloves and socks all the time. She also reports tingling and burning in the same location, but no weakness. Her symptoms have been intermittently present for the last several months. After a thorough evaluation, nerve biopsy is obtained and demonstrates axonal degeneration, endothelial hyperplasia, and perivascular inflammation. Which of the following statements regarding this condition is true?

A. Autonomic neuropathy is rarely seen in combination with sensory neuropathy.
B. The presence of retinopathy or nephropathy does not portend increased risk for diabetic neuropathy.
C. This is the most common cause of peripheral neuropathy in developed countries.
D. Tight glucose control will reverse her neuropathy.
E. None of the above is true.

XI-43. A 52-year-old man presents to the emergency department complaining of weakness that has developed over the past 2 days. He first noticed that he had generalized fatigue and felt like he was having a hard time moving his feet. Over the past 24 hours, the weakness has progressed to the point that he can barely stand with assistance. He was brought into the emergency department in a wheelchair. He is beginning to feel that it is difficult to lift his arms. He also complains of a sharp pain in his shoulders and along his spine. Both his hands and feet are tingling. On physical examination, his initial blood pressure is 138/82 mmHg. On repeat 1 hour later, it is 92/50 mmHg. His heart rate is 108 bpm, respiratory rate is 24 breaths/min, temperature is 37.0°C, and SaO_2 is 96% on room air. He appears anxious and weak. Deep tendon reflexes are absent at the knee, ankle, and wrist. The brachioradialis reflex is 1+. Strength throughout the lower extremities is diminished as the patient is unable to lift either leg against gravity. In the arms, strength is 4/5 in the deltoids, biceps, and triceps. However, he is unable to maintain a grip, and wrist flexion and extension are 3/5. Which of the following features would most commonly accompany this patient's history?

A. A diagnosis of "walking pneumonia" that was treated with azithromycin 2 weeks prior to presentation
B. An acute diarrheal illness 2 weeks prior to presentation
C. Presence of a massive mediastinal lymphadenopathy on chest radiograph
D. Presence of a monoclonal gammopathy of unknown significance on laboratory testing
E. Recent immunization with the H1N1 vaccine

XI-44. You make the correct diagnosis for the patient in Question XI-43 and transfer him to the intensive care unit for close monitoring. Forced vital capacity on admission is 1.5 L (20 mL/kg), and maximum negative inspiratory force is 30 cmH_2O. You are very concerned about impending respiratory failure. Cerebrospinal fluid analysis shows a protein level of 100 mg/dL. There is 1 WBC in the first tube and none in the fourth tube. What is the next step in the management of this patient?

A. Azithromycin
B. IV immunoglobulin
C. Oseltamivir
D. Prednisone
E. Pyridostigmine

XI-45. A 34-year-old woman is seen for complaints of weakness for the past month. She notes this to be particularly worse in the late afternoon and evening. Initially, she attributed the weakness to stress from her job, but she feels that the weakness is worsening despite taking several days off work. She also is now noticing some occasional double vision, and her husband has noticed that her voice sounds weak. The patient denies pain. On physical examination, you note the appearance of mild ptosis and a nasal, breathy tone to her voice. Which of the following tests would be most sensitive and specific for making a diagnosis in this patient?

A. Acetylcholine receptor (AChR) antibodies
B. Edrophonium test
C. Muscle-specific kinase (MuSK) antibodies
D. Repetitive nerve stimulation test
E. Voltage-gated calcium channel antibodies

XI-46. A 26-year-old woman is diagnosed with myasthenia gravis in the setting of complaints of diplopia, dysphagia, and weakness with fatigability. Acetylcholine receptor antibodies are positive. She is initially treated with pyridostigmine 60 mg three times daily with improvement. She is further evaluated for concomitant conditions. A CT scan of the neck reveals a "thymic shadow" but no evidence of thymoma. She is not found to have hyperthyroidism or any other autoimmune disorder. Her forced vital capacity after treatment with pyridostigmine is 2.9 L (73% predicted). What is the next best approach for treatment of this patient?

A. Continue pyridostigmine at current dose only
B. Continue pyridostigmine at current dose and add mycophenolate mofetil 1 g twice daily
C. Continue pyridostigmine at current dose and add prednisone 20 mg daily
D. Refer for treatment with plasmapheresis
E. Refer for thymectomy

XI-47. A 56-year-old man with facial and ocular weakness has just been diagnosed with myasthenia gravis. All of the following tests are necessary before instituting therapy EXCEPT:

A. CT of mediastinum
B. Lumbar puncture
C. Pulmonary function tests
D. Purified protein derivative skin test
E. Thyroid-stimulating hormone

XI-48. All of the following lipid-lowering agents are associated with muscle toxicity EXCEPT:

A. Atorvastatin
B. Ezetimibe
C. Gemfibrozil
D. Niacin
E. All of the above are associated with muscle toxicity.

XI-49. All of the following endocrine conditions are associated with myopathy EXCEPT:

A. Hypothyroidism
B. Hyperparathyroidism
C. Hyperthyroidism
D. Acromegaly
E. All of the above are associated with myopathy.

XI-50. A 34-year-old woman seeks evaluation for weakness. She has noted tripping when walking, particularly in her left foot, for the past 2 years. She also has recently begun to drop things, once allowing a full cup of coffee to spill onto her legs. The patient also feels as if the appearance of her face has changed over the course of many years, stating that she feels as if her face is becoming more hollow and elongated although she hasn't lost any weight recently. She has not seen a physician in many years and has no past medical history. Her only medications are a multivitamin and calcium with vitamin D. Her family history is significant for similar symptoms of weakness in her brother who is 2 years older. Her mother, who is 58 years old, was diagnosed with mild weakness after her brother was evaluated but is not symptomatic. On physical examination, the patient's face appears long and narrow with wasting of the temporalis and masseter muscles. Her speech is mildly dysarthric, and the palate is high and arched. Strength is 4/5 in the intrinsic muscles of the hand, wrist extensors, and ankle dorsiflexors. After testing handgrip strength, you notice that there is a delayed relaxation of the muscles of the hand. What is the most likely diagnosis?

A. Acid maltase deficiency (Pompe disease)
B. Becker muscular dystrophy
C. Duchenne muscular dystrophy
D. Myotonic dystrophy
E. Nemaline myopathy

XI-51. A 33-year-old woman seeks an additional medical opinion after seeing multiple physicians in the past 3 years. She describes unrelenting fatigue that has lasted for approximately 2 years to the point where she no longer exercises and is in danger of losing her job as a copy editor. Her sleep is typically unsettled, and no matter how much she sleeps, she reports never feeling refreshed. She dates the onset of the fatigue to an episode of serologically confirmed mononucleosis 3 years prior. Her husband agrees that "she has never recovered from that episode." She has tried antidepressants and various supplements with no benefit. Her past medical history is unremarkable other than having anorexia and depression as a teenager. She says she is fully recovered from that since college. Her physical examination is unremarkable other than a resting heart rate of 95 bpm. She has a normal body mass index (BMI). Which of the following is an exclusion to the diagnosis of chronic fatigue syndrome?

A. History of anorexia and depression
B. History of mononucleosis
C. Normal BMI
D. Resting heart rate >90 bpm
E. None of the above

XI-52. In the patient described in Question XI-51, which of the following has been shown to improve symptoms?

A. Acyclovir
B. Cognitive behavioral therapy
C. Gabapentin
D. Psychoanalysis
E. Venlafaxine

XI-53. A 34-year-old woman seeks evaluation because of insomnia. She reports difficulty both falling and staying asleep because she cannot calm her mind. When questioned, she says she has always been a worrier. You are considering a diagnosis of generalized anxiety disorder. All of the following characteristics are common in this disorder EXCEPT:

A. She has episodic palpitations and shortness of breath lasting 10–30 minutes associated with feelings of impending doom.
B. She particularly worries about her job as a data analyst at a major telecommunications company, and she frequently avoids social outings because she "freezes" in social situations.
C. She reports concomitant feelings of hopelessness and sadness and worries about death.
D. She reports drinking four glasses of wine or more nightly to calm herself prior to bed.
E. Symptoms began during her teenage years.

XI-54. You are paged by the clinic staff covering the sleep laboratory. A 24-year-old man has walked into the sleep laboratory asking if a sleep study will help him understand where the voices in his head are coming from. The staff says he appears somewhat agitated and is talking to himself. You arrive at the sleep laboratory to find a disheveled-appearing young man pacing in the lobby. When you attempt to speak with him, he says that he has been hearing an angry voice telling him that he is a worthless pig. It gets loudest whenever he is lying in bed. Sometimes it tells him he is a demon and to hurt himself. He says these voices are being sent into his brain by an alien satellite and thinks a sleep study will help show the abnormal brain waves that are not his since the voices are worse at night. His speech is pressured, and he speaks rapidly, pacing the entire time. He refuses to go to the emergency department for help. You call 911 because it is obvious that the patient is having active hallucinations. The man is unwilling to provide any medical history or even his last name. He is admitted involuntarily to a psychiatric facility and diagnosed with acute psychosis and eventually schizophrenia, as this was his first episode of psychosis. He is treated appropriately with antipsychotics. Which of the following statements regarding his prognosis is true?

A. Antipsychotics are effective in treating 95% of patients with a first episode of psychosis.
B. Full remission from an episode of psychosis typically takes 3–6 months.
C. If medications are discontinued, the relapse rate is 60% at 6 months.
D. More than 25% of schizophrenia patients commit suicide.
E. Prognosis depends on severity of symptoms at initial presentation.

XI-55. A 26-year-old woman presents to the emergency department complaining of shortness of breath and chest pain. These symptoms began abruptly while at a shopping mall and became progressively worse over 10 minutes, prompting her to call 911. Over this same period, the patient describes feeling her heart pounding, and she states that she felt like she was dying. She feels lightheaded and dizzy. It is currently about 20 minutes since the onset of symptoms, and the severity has abated, although she is not back to her baseline. She denies any immediate precipitating cause, although she has been under increased stress because her mother has been hospitalized recently with advanced breast cancer. She has never had any episode like this previously. She does not take any medications and has no medical history. She denies tobacco, alcohol, or drug use. On initial examination, she appears somewhat anxious and diaphoretic. Her initial vital signs show a heart rate of 108 bpm, blood pressure of 122/68 mmHg, and respiratory rate of 20 breaths/min. She is afebrile. Her examination is normal. Her arterial blood gas shows a pH of 7.52, $PaCO_2$ of 28 mmHg, and PaO_2 of 116 mmHg. The electrocardiogram (ECG) shows sinus tachycardia. A D-dimer is normal. What is the next best step in the management of this patient?

A. Initiate therapy with alprazolam 0.5 mg as needed
B. Initiate therapy with fluoxetine 20 mg daily
C. Perform a CT pulmonary angiogram
D. Reassure the patient and suggest medical and/or psychological therapy if symptoms recur on a frequent basis
E. Refer for cognitive behavioral therapy

XI-56. All of the following antidepressant medications are correctly paired with their class of medication EXCEPT:

A. Duloxetine—Selective serotonin reuptake inhibitor
B. Fluoxetine—Selective serotonin reuptake inhibitor
C. Nortriptyline—Tricyclic antidepressant
D. Phenelzine—Monoamine oxidase inhibitor
E. Venlafaxine—Mixed norepinephrine/serotonin reuptake inhibitor and receptor blocker

XI-57. A 42-year-old woman seeks your advice regarding symptoms concerning for posttraumatic stress disorder. She was the victim of a home invasion 6 months previously where she was robbed and beaten by a man at gunpoint. She thought she was going to die and was hospitalized with multiple blunt force injuries including a broken nose and zygomatic arch. She now states that she is unable to be alone in her home and frequently awakens with dreams of the event. She is irritable with her husband and children and cries frequently. She has worsening insomnia and often stays awake most of the night watching out her window because she is afraid her assailant will return. She has begun drinking a bottle of wine nightly to help her fall asleep, although she notes that this has worsened her nightmares in the early morning hours. You concur that posttraumatic stress disorder is likely. What treatment do you recommend for this patient?

A. Avoidance of alcohol
B. Cognitive behavioral therapy
C. Paroxetine 20 mg daily
D. Trazodone 50 mg nightly
E. All of the above

XI-58. A 36-year-old man is being treated with venlafaxine 150 mg twice daily for major depression. He has currently been on the medication for 4 months. After 2 months, his symptoms were inadequately controlled, necessitating an increase in the dose of venlafaxine from 75 mg twice daily. He has had one prior episode of major depression when he was 25. At that time, he was treated with fluoxetine 80 mg daily for 12 months, but found the sexual side effects difficult to tolerate. He asks when he can safely discontinue his medication. What is your advice to the patient?

A. He should continue on the medication indefinitely because his depression is likely to recur.
B. The current medication should be continued for a minimum of 6–9 months following control of his symptoms.
C. The medication can be discontinued safely if he establishes a relationship with a psychotherapist who will monitor his progress and symptoms.
D. The medication can be discontinued safely now because his symptoms are well controlled.
E. The medication should be switched to fluoxetine to complete 12 months of therapy because this was previously effective for him.

XI-59. You are seeing a 28-year-old man in your primary care clinic. He reports drinking alcohol on most days. Typically, he drinks 3–4 beers daily, but on weekends, he will drink as many as 8–12 beers per night. He has not missed work due to his drinking, although he does state that he has been hungover at work at least twice in the past month. He also has blacked out from binge drinking at least once in the past 6 months. However, he does not feel that he has any problem with alcohol. He states he never drinks and drives and has not ever felt guilt related to his drinking. You suspect he may be minimizing his level of alcohol consumption. Which of the following laboratory tests has the greatest sensitivity and specificity in identifying heavy alcohol consumption?

A. Aspartate aminotransferase (AST) elevated >2× alanine aminotransferase (ALT)
B. Carbohydrate-deficient transferrin (CDT) >20 U/L or >2.6%
C. γ-Glutamyl transferase >35 U/L
D. Mean corpuscular volume (MCV) >91 μm^3
E. A and D
F. B and C

XI-60. Which of the following will lead to a faster rate of absorption of alcohol from the gut into the blood?

A. Coadministration with a carbonated beverage
B. Concentration of alcohol of more than 20% by volume
C. Concurrent intake of a high-carbohydrate meal
D. Concurrent intake of a high-fat meal
E. Concurrent intake of a high-protein meal

XI-61. Which of the following statements best reflects the effect of alcohol on neurotransmitters in the brain?

A. Decreases dopamine activity
B. Decreases serotonin activity
C. Increases γ-aminobutyric acid activity
D. Stimulates muscarinic acetylcholine receptors
E. Stimulates *N*-methyl-D-aspartate excitatory glutamate receptors

XI-62. In an individual without any prior history of alcohol intake, what serum concentration of ethanol (in g/dL) would likely result in death?

A. 0.02
B. 0.08
C. 0.28
D. 0.40
E. 0.60

XI-63. All of the following statements regarding the epidemiology and genetics of alcoholism are true EXCEPT:

A. Approximately 60% of the risk for alcohol abuse disorders is attributed to genetics.
B. At least 20% of all patients seen in primary care offices have an alcohol use disorder.
C. Children of alcoholics have a 10-fold higher risk of alcohol abuse and dependence even if adopted early in life and raised by nonalcoholics.
D. Presence of a mutation of aldehyde dehydrogenase that results in intense flushing with alcohol consumption confers a decreased risk of alcohol dependence.
E. The lifetime risk of alcohol dependence in most Western countries is about 10%–15% for men and 5%–8% for women.

XI-64. A 42-year-old man with alcohol dependence is admitted to the hospital for acute pancreatitis. Upon admission, he has an abdominal CT that shows pancreatic edema without necrosis or hemorrhage. He is treated with IV dextrose-containing fluids, multivitamins, thiamine 50 mg daily, pain control, and bowel rest. He typically drinks 24 12-ounce beers daily. Forty-eight hours after admission, you are called because the patient is febrile and combative with the nursing staff. His vital signs demonstrate a heart rate of 132 bpm, blood pressure of 184/96 mmHg, respiratory rate of 32 breaths/min, temperature of 38.7°C, and oxygen saturation of 94% on room air. He is agitated, diaphoretic, and pacing his room. He is oriented to person only. His neurologic examination appears nonfocal, although he does not cooperate. He is tremulous. What is the next step in the management of this patient?

A. Administration of a bolus of 1 L of normal saline and thiamine 100 mg IV
B. Administration of diazepam 10–20 mg IV followed by bolus doses of 5–10 mg as needed until the patient is calm but arousable
C. Perform an emergent head CT
D. Perform two peripheral blood cultures and begin treatment with imipenem 1 g IV every 8 hours
E. Place the patient in four-point restraints and treat with haloperidol 5 mg IV

XI-65. A 48-year-old woman is recovering from alcohol dependence and requests medication to help prevent relapse. She has a medical history of stroke occurring during a hypertensive crisis. Which of the following medications could be considered?

A. Acamprosate
B. Disulfiram
C. Naltrexone
D. A and C
E. A, B, or C

XI-66. Which of the following statements about cigarette smoking is true?

A. Approximately 75% of cigarette smokers will die prematurely due to cigarette smoking unless they are able to quit.
B. Approximately 90% of peripheral vascular disease in nondiabetic individuals is attributable to cigarette smoking.
C. Cigarette smoking causes small airway inflammation and alveolar destruction sufficient to cause clinical symptoms in about 40% of smokers.
D. More than one-half of smokers have attempted to quit in the past year, and of these, 25% remain quit for 6 months or more.
E. Two of every five deaths in the United States can be attributed to cigarette use.

XI-67. A 42-year-old woman presents for a yearly office visit. She is in general good health and takes no medications. Her BMI is 32 kg/m^2. She was previously treated for depression with sertraline 100 mg daily for 12 months. She last took the medication 6 months ago. She is feeling mentally healthy now. She has smoked since the age of 21 and smokes one pack of cigarettes daily. You advise her to quit smoking. She tells you she has been thinking about this a lot lately since her father died at the age of 74 from complications of lung cancer and was a smoker. He died 2 years ago this month. She previously has tried on her own, both "cold turkey" and using nicotine patches. She was unable to sustain abstinence longer than 1 month. The only time she had sustained abstinence was when she was pregnant 18 years ago, but she quickly started again after delivery. What do you recommend for this patient?

A. Close follow-up with ongoing counseling
B. Nicotine replacement therapy with patches or nasal inhaler
C. Varenicline orally
D. A and B only
E. A combined with either B or C is an acceptable option.

XI-68. A 32-year-old man is seen in your office to discuss smoking cessation. He has been smoking since the age of 16 years. He typically smokes 1.5 to 2 packs of cigarettes each day. At the age of 21, he was hospitalized in a psychiatric facility for severe depression with psychotic features. He was originally treated with venlafaxine and quetiapine. After 6 months, the quetiapine was tapered off without recurrence of the psychosis. His depression has waxed and waned over time, but generally has been well controlled. He has had no suicide attempts and denies suicidal ideations. He has had multiple quit attempts in the past with nicotine replacement therapy but has failed each attempt. He says he would like to try varenicline and asks your opinion about its safety given his psychiatric history. What advice do you give him?

A. Varenicline has been recommended by the U.S. Food and Drug Administration for further monitoring and supervision because it is unclear how frequently severe psychiatric responses occur.
B. A recent publication did not demonstrate an increased risk of suicide or psychosis with varenicline use even though varenicline was used more frequently in individuals with a preexisting psychiatric diagnosis.
C. Alternative therapies such as bupropion and/or nicotine replacement therapy should be considered.
D. All of the above

XI-69. You are counseling your patient on the need to quit smoking cigarettes. She has been smoking for over two decades and wants to quit in order to avoid the harmful physical effects of smoking. Wanting to take "baby steps," she has switched to low-tar, low-nicotine cigarettes. Which of the following statements is true about the potential benefit of switching to these low-yield cigarettes?

A. Fewer smoking–drug interactions are found among smokers of low-yield cigarettes.
B. Most smokers inhale the same amount of nicotine and tar even if they switch to low-yield cigarettes.
C. Smokers of low-yield cigarettes tend to inhale less deeply and smoker fewer cigarettes daily.
D. Smoking low-yield cigarettes decreases the harmful cardiovascular effects of cigarette smoking.
E. Smoking low-yield cigarettes is a reasonable alternative to complete smoking cessation for chronic smokers.

ANSWERS

XI-1. **The answer is A.** *(Chap. 437)* This patient is presenting with symptoms of metastatic neurologic disease, and a careful neurologic examination can localize the site of disease in most patients. The patient has "crossed" weakness and sensory abnormalities, which localizes the lesion to the brainstem. In this setting, the limbs exhibit weakness and sensory symptoms opposite from the facial symptoms. Moreover, the facial weakness localizes to lower motor neuron as it involves both the upper and lower facial muscles. If the upper facial muscles had preserved movement, this might suggest multiple areas of metastatic disease in both the cerebrum and spinal cord.

XI-2 and XI-3. **The answers are D and D, respectively.** *(Chap. 437)* The ability to perform a thorough neurologic examination is an important skill for all internists to master. A careful neurologic examination can localize the site of the lesion and is important in directing further workup. The components of the neurologic examination include mental status, cranial nerves, motor function, sensory function, gait, and coordination. The motor examination is further characterized by appearance, tone, strength, and reflexes. Pronator drift is a useful tool for determining if upper extremity weakness is present. In this test, an individual is asked to stand with both arms fully extended and parallel to the floor while closing his or her eyes. If the arms flex at the elbows or fingers or there is pronation of the forearm, this is considered a positive test. Other tests of motor strength include tests of maximal effort in a specific muscle or muscle group. Most commonly, this type of strength testing is graded from 0 (no movement) to 5 (full power) with varying degree of weakness noted against resistance. However, many individuals find it more practical to use qualitative grading of strength, such as paralysis, severe weakness, moderate weakness, mild weakness, or full strength. Babinski sign is a sign of upper motor neuron disease above the level of the S1 vertebra and is characterized by paradoxical extension of the great toe with fanning and extension of the other toes as well. Dysdiadochokinesis refers to the inability to perform rapid alternating movements and is a sign of cerebellar disease. Lhermitte symptom causes electric shock–like sensations in the extremities associated with neck flexion. It has many causes including cervical spondylosis and multiple sclerosis. Romberg sign is performed with an individual standing with feet together and arms at the side. An individual is then asked to close his or her eyes. If the individual begins to sway or fall, this is considered a positive test and is a sign of abnormal proprioception.

XI-4 to XI-8. **The answers are E, C, D, B, and A, respectively.** The clinical data obtained from the history and examination are interpreted to arrive at a possible anatomic localization that best explains the clinical findings, helps to narrow the list of diagnostic possibilities, and helps to select the laboratory tests most likely to be informative (Table XI-8).

TABLE XI-8 **Global Disability-Adjusted Life-Years (DALYs) and Number of Annual Deaths for Selected Neurologic Disorders in 2010**

Disorder	DALYs	Deaths
Low back and neck pain	116,704,000	—
Cerebrovascular diseases	102,232,000	5,874,000
Meningitis and encephalitis	26,540,000	541,000
Migraine	22,362,000	—
Epilepsy	17,429,000	177,000
Dementia	11,349,000	485,000
Parkinson disease	1,918,000	111,000
% of total DALYs or deaths for all causes that are neurologic	**12.0%**	**13.6%**
% change of DALYs for neurologic disorders between 2000 and 2010	**51.6%**	**114.3%**

Source: R Lozano et al: Lancet 380:2095, 2012.

XI-9. The answer is C. *(Chap. 440e)* Appropriate and timely evaluation is needed to determine whether a subarachnoid hemorrhage is present because it can be rapidly fatal if undetected. The procedure of choice for initial diagnosis is a computed tomography (CT) of the head without intravenous (IV) contrast. On the CT, blood in the subarachnoid space would appear whiter compared to the surrounding brain tissue. The head CT is most sensitive when it is performed shortly after the onset of symptoms, but sensitivity declines over several hours. It can also demonstrate significant mass effect and midline shift, factors that increase the severity of the underlying hemorrhage. In the situation where the head CT is negative but clinical suspicion is high, a lumbar puncture can be performed. This may demonstrate increased numbers of red blood cells that do not clear with successive aliquots of cerebrospinal fluid (CSF). If the lumbar puncture is performed more than 12 hours after a small subarachnoid hemorrhage, then the red blood cells may begin to decompose, leading to xanthochromia—a yellow to pink coloration of CSF that can be measure spectrographically. A basic head CT with IV contrast is rarely useful in subarachnoid hemorrhage because the brightness of the contrast material may make it difficult to identify blood in the subarachnoid space. However, a CT angiography that is performed with IV contrast can be useful in identifying the aneurismal vessel leading to the bleeding. Classic angiography is a more direct way to visualize the anatomy of the cranial vasculature and is now often combined with interventional procedures to coil a bleeding vessel. Transcranial Doppler ultrasound is a test that measures the velocity of blood flow through the cranial vasculature. It is used in some centers following subarachnoid hemorrhage to assess for the development of vasospasm, which can worsen ischemia leading to increased damage to brain tissue following subarachnoid hemorrhage.

XI-10. The answer is E. *(Chap. 440e)* Magnetic resonance imaging (MRI) is generated from the interaction between the hydrogen protons in biologic tissues, the magnetic field, and the radiofrequency (Rf) of waves generated by the coil placed next to the body part of interest. The Rf pulses transiently excite the protons of the body with a subsequent return to the equilibrium energy state, a process known as relaxation. During relaxation, the protons release Rf energy creating an echo that is then transformed via Fourier analysis to generate the MRI. The two relaxation rates that influence the signal intensity of the image are T1 and T2. T1 refers to the time in milliseconds that it takes for 63% of protons to return to their baseline state. T2 relaxation is the time for 63% of protons to become dephased due to interactions among nearby protons. The intensity of the signal is also influenced by the interval between Rf pulses (TR) and the time between the Rf pulse and the signal reception (TE). T1-weighted images are produced by keeping both TR and TE relatively short, whereas T2-weighted images require long TR and TE times. Fat and subacute hemorrhage have relatively short TR and TE times and thus appear more bright on T1-weighted images. Conversely, structures with more water such as CSF or edema have long T1 and T2 relaxation times, resulting in higher signal intensity on T2-weighted images. T2 images are also more sensitive for detecting demyelination, infarction, and chronic hemorrhage.

Fluid-attenuated inversion recovery (FLAIR) is a type of T2-weighted image that suppresses the high-intensity signal of CSF. As a result, images created by the FLAIR technique are more sensitive to detecting water-containing lesions or edema than the standard spin images.

Magnetic resonance angiography refers to several different techniques that are useful for assessing vascular structures but does not provide details of the underlying brain parenchyma.

XI-11. The answer is E. *(Chap. 440e)* For many years, MRI was considered the modality of choice for patients with renal insufficiency because it does not lead to acute renal failure. However, gadolinium was recently linked to a rare disorder called nephrogenic systemic fibrosis. This newly described disorder results in widespread fibrosis in skin, skeletal muscle, bone, lungs, pleura, pericardium, myocardium, and many other tissues. Histologically, thickened collagen bundles are seen in the deep dermis of the skins with increased numbers of fibrocytes and elastic fibers. There is no known medical treatment for nephrogenic systemic fibrosis, although improvement may be seen following kidney transplantation. It has only recently been linked to the receipt of gadolinium-containing contrast agents with a typical onset between 5 and 75 days following administration of the contrast. The incidence of nephrogenic systemic fibrosis following administration of gadolinium in individuals with a glomerular filtration rate of <30 mL/min may be as high as 4%, and thus, gadolinium is absolutely contraindicated in individuals with severe renal dysfunction.

Pseudohypocalcemia can occur following administration of gadolinium in individuals with renal dysfunction, but not true hypocalcemia. This occurs because of an interaction of the contrast dye with standard colorimetric assays for serum calcium that are commonly used. If ionized calcium is measured, it would be normal, often in the face of very low levels of serum calcium.

The other reported complications can be seen following administration of iodinated contrast that is used for CT imaging. The most common complication of CT imaging outside of allergic reactions is the development of worsening renal function or acute renal failure. This risk can be minimized if the patient is adequately hydrated. Lactic acidosis is a rare but dreaded side effect of iodinated contrast that has been linked to the coadministration of metformin in diabetic patients. Typically a patient is asked to hold metformin for 48 hours before and after a CT scan. The reason for the development of lactic acidosis is actually related to development of renal insufficiency and a subsequent buildup of lactic acid. In very rare instances, administration of iodinated contrast can unmask hyperthyroidism.

XI-12. The answer is D. *(Chap. 445)* Age of presentation is an important consideration when an individual presents with a new onset of seizure because certain causes of seizures are more likely to present within certain age ranges (Table XI-12), ranging from the neonatal period throughout older adulthood (age >35 years). In individuals >35 years old, the most likely causes of new-onset seizures include alcohol withdrawal, cerebrovascular disease, brain

TABLE XI-12 Causes of Seizures

Neonates (<1 month)	Perinatal hypoxia and ischemia Intracranial hemorrhage and trauma CNS infection Metabolic disturbances (hypoglycemia, hypocalcemia, hypomagnesemia, pyridoxine deficiency) Drug withdrawal Developmental disorders Genetic disorders
Infants and children (>1 month and <12 years)	Febrile seizures Genetic disorders (metabolic, degenerative, primary epilepsy syndromes) CNS infection Developmental disorders Trauma
Adolescents (12–18 years)	Trauma Genetic disorders Infection Illicit drug use Brain tumor
Young adults (18–35 years)	Trauma Alcohol withdrawal Illicit drug use Brain tumor Autoantibodies
Older adults (>35 years)	Cerebrovascular disease Brain tumor Alcohol withdrawal Metabolic disorders (uremia, hepatic failure, electrolyte abnormalities, hypoglycemia, hyperglycemia) Alzheimer disease and other degenerative CNS diseases Autoantibodies

Abbreviation: CNS, central nervous system.

tumor, autoantibodies, Alzheimer disease or other neurodegenerative disease, and a range of metabolic disorders. These disorders can include either hyper- or hypoglycemia, uremia, hepatic failure, and a host of electrolyte abnormalities or acid-base disorders. Inherited disorders of ion channels have been implicated in a variety of rare epilepsy syndromes. These genetic disorders typically present in childhood and rarely after the age of 18.

XI-13. **The answer is B.** *(Chap. 445)* Psychogenic seizures are nonepileptic behaviors that resemble seizures and may be conversion reactions that occur under psychological distress. Psychogenic seizures may occur in individuals with underlying seizure disorder and may be difficult to distinguish. Clinical features prominent in psychogenic seizures include side-to-side turning of the head, asymmetric and large-amplitude movements of the limbs, twitching of all four extremities without loss of consciousness, and pelvic thrusting. Psychogenic seizures also often last longer than epileptic seizures and may wax and wane over minutes to hours. Video electroencephalogram (EEG) monitoring can be quite helpful in this situation as EEG monitoring during the episode is normal. In addition, there is no postictal period. Measurement of prolactin levels may also help to distinguish generalized and some focal seizures from psychogenic seizures because prolactin levels rise in these disorders but remain normal in psychogenic seizures. Serum creatine kinase may rise following a seizure, but this is not sensitive for detection of seizure disorder.

XI-14. **The answer is B.** *(Chap. 445)* Determination of when to initiate epileptic drug therapy can be difficult in clinical practice given the variability in presentation of seizure disorders and the large number of antiepileptic drugs available. In general, antiepileptic drugs should be initiated when an individual presents with either recurrent seizures of unknown etiology or known cause that cannot be reversed. In individuals with a single seizure and a clear cause such as a brain tumor, infection, or trauma, these individuals should also be treated. Currently, lamotrigine and valproic acid are considered the best initial therapies for individuals with generalized seizures. Although used with good efficacy for many years, phenytoin is no longer first-line therapy for generalized seizures due to its long-term side effect profile including gingival hyperplasia. Ethosuximide is generally only used for absence seizures.

XI-15. **The answer is A.** *(Chap. 445)* Overall, 70% of children and 60% of adults will be able to successfully discontinue antiepileptic drugs without recurrence of seizures. However, the data regarding the time frame to attempt weaning of antiepileptic drugs are scarce. Once the determination to discontinue antiepileptic drugs has been made, the dosage of medication is typically decreased over a 2–3 month period, gradually weaning to off. If a recurrence of seizure were to happen, it is most likely during the first 3 months after discontinuation of therapy. Four factors predict the greatest likelihood of remaining seizure-free upon discontinuation of antiepileptic drugs: (1) complete control of seizures for 1–5 years; (2) single seizure type—focal or generalized; (3) normal EEG; and (4) normal neurologic examination, including intelligence. Given that this patient continues to have an abnormal neurologic examination following closed head trauma, he would have a greater likelihood to have a poorer outcome after withdrawal of his seizure medication.

XI-16. **The answer is C.** *(Chap. 445)* Status epilepticus is a medical emergency that can result in severe metabolic derangements, hyperthermia, cardiorespiratory collapse, and irreversible neuronal injury. Prompt recognition and appropriate treatment are necessary to prevent long-term sequelae of this neuronal injury. Status epilepticus is defined as continuous seizures or repetitive discrete seizures with impaired consciousness in the interictal period. Status epilepticus has many subtypes, with the most common subtype leading to presentation and critical care admission being generalized convulsive status epilepticus (GCSE). The duration of seizure activity that leads to a diagnosis of GCSE is typically defined as 15–30 minutes, but practically, if intervention with anticonvulsant medication is required to stop the seizure activity, then one must be concerned about GCSE. Likewise, if a seizure is of sufficient duration to cause significant metabolic or cardiorespiratory consequence, GCSE must be considered. Once GCSE is diagnosed, initial treatment should include basic cardiopulmonary support, including maintaining an appropriate airway, establishing venous access, and obtaining samples of laboratory analysis to identify contributing laboratory abnormalities. It is important to understand that suppression of convulsive activity through the use of paralytic agents does not suppress the epileptic activity in the central nervous system and does not prevent ongoing neuronal injury and death. Thus, when these agents are used for rapid-sequence intubation, the treating team should also continue treatment for GCSE through appropriate use of IV benzodiazepines initially followed by loading doses of either IV phenytoin or fosphenytoin, valproic acid, or levetiracetam. In many cases, continuous EEG monitoring may be required to determine when the seizure activity has ceased. If the seizure activity fails to break with these agents, further therapy with propofol or pentobarbital may be required. In more severe cases, inhaled anesthetics may be required. In addition, it is important to treat any underlying infection or metabolic derangements.

XI-17. **The answer is E.** *(Chap. 446)* This patient is presenting with symptoms of an acute ischemic stroke affecting the middle cerebral artery territory. All patients older than age 18 should be evaluated promptly upon arrival to determine if they are candidates for administration of recombinant tissue plasminogen activator (rtPA). A large trial showed a significant improvement in patients with only minimal disability (32% on placebo vs. 44% on rtPA) and a nonsignificant reduction in mortality (21% on placebo vs. 17% on rtPA) when IV rtPA was administered within 3 hours of the onset of symptoms. However, rtPA was associated with a significant increase in the risk of symptomatic intracranial hemorrhage (6.4% on rtPA vs. 0.6% on placebo). A more recent trial has confirmed this benefit and that rtPA is both cost-effective and cost-saving. Carefully choosing the correct patients for administration of rtPA is key to best achieve benefits while minimizing risk of adverse events. Thrombolytic administration should be considered in all patients ≥18 years old with a clinical diagnosis of stroke presenting with symptom onset of ≤4.5 hours. A noncontrast head CT should be performed promptly to ensure there is no intracranial hemorrhage or edema of more than one-third of the middle cerebral artery territory. If a patient meets these criteria, then a careful assessment for possible contraindications should be undertaken. Hypertension is common in acute stroke. A sustained blood pressure >185/110 mmHg despite treatment is a contraindication to administration of rtPA. However, a single blood pressure reading higher than this value would not prevent treatment with thrombolytics. Individuals with rapidly improving symptoms more indicative of a transient ischemic attack or mild cerebrovascular accident should not be treated with rtPA because the risk outweighs the potential benefits. At the opposite end of the spectrum, individuals presenting with stupor or coma should not be treated with thrombolytics. Findings on past medical history that would be contraindications to the use of rTPA include prior stroke or head injury within 3 months, any prior history of intracranial hemorrhage, major surgery in the preceding 14 days, gastrointestinal (GI) bleeding in the preceding 21 days, and recent myocardial infarction. Individuals with platelets <100,000, hematocrit <25%, use of heparin within 48 hours, prolonged activated partial thromboplastin time, or elevated international normalized ratio should also not receive rtPA.

XI-18. **The answer is D.** *(Chap. 446)* Multiple atherosclerotic risk factors contribute to the risk for stroke. Among these are hypertension, diabetes mellitus, dyslipidemia, cigarette smoking, and atrial fibrillation. Primary prevention of stroke is largely targeted at these modifiable risk factors. Untreated or undertreated hypertension is the most significant risk factor for stroke. All hypertension should be treated to a goal blood pressure of <140–150/90 mmHg. Data are strongest for thiazide diuretics and angiotensin-converting enzyme inhibitors for secondary prevention of stroke. This patient also has an elevated total cholesterol, elevated triglycerides, low high-density lipoprotein (HDL), and high low-density lipoprotein (LDL). Therefore, she should be treated with a statin for primary stroke prevention. However, even in the absence of elevated LDL or low HDL, there is evidence that statins can be useful for stroke prevention, decreasing the incidence of stroke by 51%. Tobacco smoking should be discouraged in all patients, and the patient should be given assistance in quitting smoking. The use of antiplatelet agents for primary prevention of stroke is somewhat controversial. The most recent guidelines for primary stroke prevention recommend aspirin for individuals who are at high risk for stroke. In those with diabetes, additional risk factors for stroke must also be present. This patient also has the risk factors of hypertension, smoking, and dyslipidemia. Although diabetes is a risk factor for stroke, no trial has ever demonstrated that improving glucose control decreases stroke risk.

XI-19. **The answer is B.** *(Chap. 446)* The choice to perform a carotid endarterectomy for a carotid stenosis depends on many factors, including the degree of stenosis and whether the patient is symptomatic. In general, carotid endarterectomy has been demonstrated to have the greatest benefit in those who are symptomatic and have stenosis of ≥70%. In individuals with asymptomatic carotid artery stenosis, the risk of stroke is ~2% per year, and the potential benefits of the procedure may be outweighed by the risks. A more measured approached with risk factor modification may be more prudent. In symptomatic individuals such as the patient in this case, several trials have attempted to address the value of carotid endarterectomy. There is a significant absolute risk reduction favoring surgery of 17%. In the symptomatic patient, the annual risk of stroke is ~13%. A recent meta-analysis showed that carotid endarterectomy is most beneficial when performed within 2 weeks of symptoms onset and has greater benefits in men and those ≥75 years old. However, the procedure should be performed only in institutions familiar with the procedure. The benefit of the procedure is questionable for any surgeon whose perioperative stroke rate is ≥6%.

XI-20. **The answer is C.** *(Chap. 446)* The noncontrast head CT shows blood within the left putamen in this patient presenting with marked hypertension and abrupt onset of right hemiparesis. This is consistent with intracranial hemorrhage. On a noncontrast head CT, blood is demonstrated as a hyperdense white area, and this is an emergent finding. Most patients have symptoms that begin abruptly and acutely worsen over the first 30–90 minutes. Diminished level of consciousness is common, and signs of increased intracranial pressure may occur. Intracranial hemorrhage is associated with a 40% mortality rate. The patient should be admitted to a neurologic intensive care unit, if available, and monitored. Any coagulopathy should be corrected. The goal for blood pressure management at this level of blood pressure is unclear. A recent clinical trial enrolled patients with blood pressure between 150 and 220 mmHg and demonstrated improved outcomes with lowering of blood pressure to 140 mmHg over 6 hours. However, it is not known how individuals with higher blood pressures would respond. The patient should be carefully monitored for development of increased intracranial pressure and treated appropriately. Intracranial pressure monitoring is sometimes required with a goal cerebral perfusion pressure of >60 mmHg.

XI-21. **The answer is C.** *(Chap. 447)* The patient describes a typical history for migraine headaches, the second most common cause of headache and most common cause of headache-related disability worldwide. Migraine affects approximately 15% of women and 6% of men in any given year. Diagnostic criteria for migraine have been simplified recently. To diagnose migraine, an individual should complain of repeated attacks of headache lasting from 4–72 hours, with a normal physical examination, and no other clear cause. The headache should be associated with two of the following four features: unilateral pain, throbbing pain, aggravation by movement, and moderate to severe intensity. In addition, the individual should complain of either nausea/vomiting or phonophobia and photophobia. Most individuals with migraine headaches can identify triggers associated with an attack. Common triggers include lack of sleep or excessive sleep, stress, hormonal fluctuations, alcohol, and barometric pressures changes. The pathophysiology that underlies migraine is increasingly understood as a dysfunction of the monoaminergic sensory control systems located in the brainstem and hypothalamus. Activation of cells in the trigeminal nucleus leads to release of vasoactive neuropeptides at vascular terminations of the trigeminal nerve and within the trigeminal nucleus. These neurons also project centrally, crossing the midline, to project to ventrobasal and posterior nuclei of the posterior thalamus. The primary vasoactive peptide that has been implicated is calcitonin gene-related peptide (CGRP). A new class of medication called gepants is being developed to act as an antagonist at the CGRP receptor and has been demonstrated to be effective against migraine in early clinical trials. The most common medications used for acute relief of severe migraine pain are the triptans, potent agonists of the 5-hydroxytryptamine (serotonin) receptor, implicating serotonin in pathogenesis of migraine as well. It is thought that serotonin is necessary for nociceptive signaling in the trigeminovascular system and that triptans arrest this pathway. Finally, dopamine may also play a role in pathogenesis of migraine because migraine symptoms can be induced by dopamine stimulation, and individuals with migraine have been demonstrated to have hypersensitivity to dopamine agonists at doses that do not affect non–migraine-affected persons. In the past, the "vascular theory" of migraine was frequently espoused, with the cause of migraine thought to be related to abnormal cerebral vasodilation. This theory has been discounted as the pathogenesis has become more widely understood.

XI-22. **The answer is E.** *(Chap. 447)* Patients who have increasing frequency of migraines or attacks that are poorly responsive to abortive treatment should be considered for preventive therapy. The typical patient considered for preventive therapy has four or more attacks per month. The U.S. Food and Drug Administration (FDA)-approved medications for migraine prevention include propranolol, timolol, sodium valproate, topiramate, and methysergide (not currently available). In addition, many medications are commonly used for migraine prevention off-label including amitriptyline, nortriptyline, flunarizine, phenelzine, gabapentin, and cyproheptadine. When considering which medication to choose in a particular patient, one must carefully consider the potential side effects that may limit use. The appropriate dose for migraine prevention may also be unclear as the dosing for these drugs was determined for an indication other than migraine. Patients should be started on a low dose and titrated upward to limit side effects. The efficacy in decreasing migraine attacks is 50%–75%. However, the treatment effect is delayed 2–12 weeks. Once efficacy is achieved, the drug is continued for 6 months before tapering downward. Many patients exhibit fewer and milder attacks after cessation of medications, indicating that these drugs may potentially alter the natural history of migraine.

XI-23. **The answer is A.** *(Chap. 447)* Cluster headache is a rare disorder affecting only about 0.1% of the population. This episodic headache disorder is characterized by severe unilateral headache of relatively short duration that occurs over 8–10 weeks a year, followed by prolonged pain-free intervals that average a little less than a year. As opposed to migraine, men are more likely to have cluster headache, but cluster headache does share some features common to migraine including the unilateral nature of the pain and the stabbing or throbbing characteristics of the pain. In addition, a patient with cluster headache may also complain of nausea, photophobia, or phonophobia during the attack. In contrast, however, patients with cluster headache tend to move about during at attack. A cluster headache is accompanied by ipsilateral symptoms of cranial parasympathetic activation including lacrimation, rhinorrhea or nasal congestion, and ptosis. The headache in cluster headache is explosive in onset and associated with intense pain. During a cluster attack, the headaches can occur as infrequently as every other day to several times daily. The duration of pain is variable, between 15 and 180 minutes. Cluster headache falls within a category of trigeminal autonomic cephalgias, along with paroxysmal hemicranias, short-lasting unilateral neuralgiform headaches with conjunctival injection and tearing (SUNCT), and short-lasting unilateral neuralgiform headaches with cranial autonomic symptoms (SUNA). It can be differentiated from these based on historical factors. In paroxysmal hemicrania, the attacks are more frequent, occurring between 1 and 20 times per day, and last 2–30 minutes. Males and females are equally affected. In contrast to cluster headache, indomethacin provides very effective prophylactic treatment. SUNCT and SUNA are rare disorders that are easily distinguished from cluster headache. A patient with one of these disorders will have 3–200 episodes of unilateral pain daily, but the duration is less than 5 minutes. Migraine headache is a unilateral throbbing headache associated with phonophobia, photophobia, and nausea and vomiting. It is more common in women than men and is not associated with the symptoms of tearing or nasal congestion. Tension headache is the most common cause of headache and does not typically cause debilitating pain. The pain of a tension headache is described as band-like.

XI-24. **The answer is C.** *(Chap. 448)* Significant memory loss affects about 10% of all individuals greater than 70 years of age, and in more than half, the cause is Alzheimer disease (AD). AD is the leading cause of dementia and typically presents as slowly progressive memory loss that develops over many years. Early in the disease, the memory loss often goes unrecognized or is attributed to the effects of aging. Memory deficits are typically not noticeable to the patient or spouse until the deficits fall to 1.5 standard deviations below normal on standardized memory tests. When this occurs, the term mild cognitive impairment (MCI) is applied. Among those diagnosed with MCI, about 50% progress to AD over 4 years. Many neurologists have begun to replace MCI with the term "early symptomatic AD." As the cognitive disease progresses, patients will lose their ability to maintain their higher order daily activities such as driving, shopping, housekeeping, and maintaining finances. Most patients are aware of the loss of these abilities in early stages of the disease. In middle stages of the disease, the patient loses the ability to work and is easily lost and confused. Language is increasingly impaired in both comprehension and fluency. Motor apraxia also becomes noticeable. In advanced stages of the disease, patients may remain ambulatory but often wander aimlessly. There is a loss of judgment and reasoning. The patient may have delusions and may not recognize caregivers. The pathologic hallmark of AD is the presence of neuritic plaques containing amyloid beta and neurofibrillary tangles (option C) containing hyperphosphorylated tau filament. The earliest and most severe degeneration is seen in the medial temporal lobe, lateral temporal cortex, and nuclear basalis of Meynert. Amyloid deposition in cerebral blood vessels (option A) can be seen in AD but is not the pathologic hallmark of AD. It is also seen in a condition called cerebral amyloid angiopathy, which predisposes individuals to cerebral hemorrhage. Frontotemporal lobar degeneration spectrum disorders are a heterogeneous group of disorders including Pick disease, progressive supranuclear palsy, and corticobasal syndrome that share a common gross pathologic hallmark of focal atrophy of the frontal, insular, and/or temporal cortex (option B) with a concomitant loss of serotonergic innervation in many patients. Lewy bodies are intracytoplasmic inclusions that stain positive with periodic acid–Schiff (PAS) and ubiquitin (option D) that are found throughout specific brainstem nuclei, substantia nigra, amygdala, cingulate gyrus, and neocortex. Lewy bodies are seen in dementia syndromes with parkinsonian features.

XI-25. The answer is E. *(Chap. 448)* MCI refers to a condition of impaired memory that is 1.5 standard deviations below normal on standardized memory tests. Over 4 years, about 50% of individuals with MCI will progress to AD. However, no treatment currently has been demonstrated to slow the decline in memory or delay the progression to AD. Donepezil, rivastigmine, and galantamine are anticholinesterase inhibitors that are FDA approved for use in patients diagnosed with AD. Memantine is also approved for use in moderate to severe AD and blocks N-methyl-D-aspartate (NMDA)–glutamate receptors. These medications have modest effects on caregiver ratings of patient functioning and slight decrease in rate of decline in cognitive test scores over periods of up to 3 years. However, these medications have significant side effects including nausea, diarrhea, altered sleep with vivid dreams, and muscle cramps. Interventions that have been attempted and failed to show benefit have included hormone replacement therapy in postmenopausal women and gingko biloba. Many potential therapies are being investigated to ascertain benefit including vaccination against amyloid beta and statin use in early AD. Despite the popularity in the media, "brain training" has not been shown to slow decline in cognitive function.

XI-26. The answer is C. *(Chap. 448)* Frontotemporal dementia (FTD) refers to a group of clinical syndromes that demonstrate frontotemporal lobe degeneration (FTLD) on pathologic examination. FTD typically presents in the fifth to seventh decades of life and is nearly as predominant as Alzheimer disease in this age group. Three distinct clinical syndromes are described: behavioral variant FTD, semantic primary progressive aphasia, and nonfluent/agrammatic primary progressive aphasia. These syndromes have clinical and MRI findings that allow the clinician to determine the primary diagnosis, although patients may evolve to have prominent features of another syndrome. This patient has behavioral variant FTD, the most common of the FTD syndromes. Individuals with behavioral variant FTD demonstrate social and emotional dysfunction with a variety of symptoms including apathy, disinhibition, compulsivity, loss of empathy, and overeating. In addition, there are typically deficits in executive control. Upper motor neuron disease is often seen as well. The MRI shows atrophy of anterior cingulate and frontoinsular areas. In the semantic primary progressive aphasia variant of FTD, patients slowly lose the ability to decode word, object, person-specific, and emotion meaning, and the MRI shows prominent atrophy in the temporopolar area that is greater on the left. The nonfluent/agrammatic primary progressive aphasia variant of FTD demonstrates profound inability to produce words and motor speech impairment. The MRI shows dominant frontal opercular and dorsal insula degeneration.

XI-27. **The answer is A.** *(Chap. 449)* Parkinson disease (PD) is the second most common neurodegenerative disorder after Alzheimer disease, affecting approximately 1 million individuals in the United States. PD affects men and women equally, with a typical age of symptom onset around age 60. The frequency of PD increases with age but can present as early as the third decade of life. Most cases of PD occur sporadically, although genetic factors play a role in some individuals. These individuals are more likely to present at a younger age. There is no single gene found to be associated with PD. The most likely genes to be altered in PD patients include *α-synuclein*, *PINK1/Parkin*, and *LRRK2*, but many others have been identified. Other epidemiologic risk factors for PD include exposure to pesticides, rural living, and drinking well water. Cigarette smoking and caffeine are associated with reduced risk of PD. Pathologically, the characteristic finding in PD is degeneration of the dopaminergic neurons in the substantia nigra pars compacta. Lewy bodies, which are intracytoplasmic inclusions containing primarily α-synuclein, may also be seen.

XI-28. **The answer is E.** *(Chap. 449)* This patient exhibits classic features of PD, a diagnosis made based on clinical presentation. Historically, PD could be diagnosed if the patient had two out of three of the following: bradykinesia, tremor, and rigidity. However, given the significant overlap of these symptoms with atypical or secondary Parkinson syndrome, the diagnosis of PD was incorrect in about 24% of cases. More recently, it has been determined that a more predictive trio of features is rest tremor, asymmetry, and positive response to levodopa. Imaging of the brain may show reduced uptake of striatal dopaminergic markers in the posterior putamen with sparing of the caudate nucleus on positron emission tomography (PET) or single-photon emission computed tomography (SPECT) imaging. However, imaging is not required for a diagnosis of PD and is typically only performed under research settings or if there are features that would cause one to suspect an atypical Parkinson syndrome. This patient does not have features that would lead one to suspect atypical parkinsonism (Table XI-28). He also has no medications or other clinical conditions that would lead to secondary parkinsonism. The most common causes of secondary parkinsonism include stroke, tumor, infection, exposure to toxins such as carbon monoxide, and particularly medications. The medications most likely to cause secondary parkinsonism are neuroleptic agents, including metoclopramide and chlorpromazine. Treatment of PD is typically with either levodopa-carbidopa or a dopamine agonist. Levodopa has a long history of use in PD dating to the 1960s. Levodopa is administered in combination with carbidopa to prevent peripheral conversion to dopamine and thus prevent side effects, especially nausea and vomiting. In Europe, levodopa is combined with benserazide to prevent this conversion. Levodopa is the most effective symptomatic treatment of PD. It improves motor features, quality of life, and life span as well as improving productive years of life with increased independence and employability. However, the majority of patients treated with levodopa develop motor complications with "on/off" periods, referring to fluctuations in motor responsiveness to the drug. In addition, patients may develop involuntary movements as well. Further, the duration of benefit of levodopa subsides over time to where it approaches the short half-life of the drug. Nondopaminergic features, including falling, freezing, and autonomic dysfunction, are also not treated with levodopa. Many providers now prefer dopamine agonists as first-line therapy. These drugs include pramipexole, ropinirole, and rotigotine as non–ergot derivatives. Although these agents do not show comparable efficacy compared to levodopa, they are associated with fewer motor complications. It should be noted that even with use of the dopamine agonists, eventual treatment with levodopa is required in most patients. Selegiline is a monoamine oxidase inhibitor (MAOI). Although MAOIs can be used as monotherapy in early disease, there is a risk of serotonin syndrome when used with selective serotonin reuptake inhibitor (SSRI) agents such as fluoxetine. The risk is low overall, but because this patient is untreated, there are other better options for his care.

TABLE XI-28 Features Suggesting an Atypical or Secondary Cause of Parkinsonism

Symptoms/Signs	Alternative Diagnosis to Consider
History	
Early speech and gait impairment (lack of tremor, lack of motor asymmetry)	Atypical parkinsonism
Exposure to neuroleptics	Drug-induced parkinsonism
Onset prior to age 40	Genetic form of PD
Liver disease	Wilson disease, non-Wilsonian hepatolenticular degeneration
Early hallucinations and dementia with later development of PD features	Dementia with Lewy bodies
Diplopia, impaired downgaze	PSP
Poor or no response to an adequate trial of levodopa	Atypical or secondary parkinsonism
Physical Exam	
Dementia as first or early feature	Dementia with Lewy bodies
Prominent orthostatic hypotension	MSA-p
Prominent cerebellar signs	MSA-c
Slow saccades with impaired downgaze	PSP
High-frequency (6–10 Hz) symmetric postural tremor with a prominent kinetic component	Essential tremor

Abbreviations: MSA-c, multiple system atrophy–cerebellar type; MSA-p, multiple system atrophy–Parkinson type; PD, Parkinson disease; PSP, progressive supranuclear palsy.

XI-29. **The answer is C.** *(Chap. 449)* Deep brain stimulation (DBS) is the most common surgical therapy performed for PD. In this surgery, an electrode is placed into a target area, typically the subthalamic nucleus or globus pallidus pars interna. The electrode is connected to a stimulator usually placed in the chest wall. The precise mechanism by which DBS works is not known, but it is thought to act by disrupting the abnormal signal associated with PD and motor symptoms. Once in place, DBS can be adjusted on many variables, including voltage, frequency, and pulse duration. The primary indication for DBS is severe tremor or levodopa-induced motor complications that cannot be controlled with medications. It does not improve features that fail to respond to levodopa, including falling, freezing, and dementia.

XI-30. **The answer is F.** *(Chap. 452)* Amyotrophic lateral sclerosis (ALS) is a common motor neuron disease with an incidence of 1–3 per 100,000 population and prevalence of 3–5 per 100,000 population. ALS is responsible for about 1 in 1000 deaths in North America and Western Europe. This progressive disease has no treatment and leads to disability and death due to respiratory failure within 3–5 years after diagnosis. The pathologic hallmark of ALS is loss or death of both upper and lower motor neurons. The upper motor neuron loss can be demonstrated by degeneration of the corticospinal tracts typically originating in layer five of the motor cortex and descending downward via the pyramidal tract to synapse with the lower motor neurons both directly and indirectly via interneurons. The lower motor neuron disease is manifested by death of anterior horn cells in the spinal cord and brainstem, which can lead to bulbar symptoms. Clinically, this leads to the classic findings of both upper and lower motor neuron disease in ALS. The most common presenting symptom in ALS is asymmetric weakness of insidious onset, which is most prominent in the lower extremities. Muscle wasting and atrophy may be prominent. A detailed history can elicit cramping with volitional movements, such as stretching, that is most common in the early morning hours. Fasciculations may be identified. When the muscles of the hands are involved, extensor weakness is more common than flexor weakness. Bulbar symptoms include difficulty with chewing, swallowing, and movements of the face and tongue. Upper motor neuron symptoms may lead to spasticity with increased deep tendon reflexes. However, even in late stages of the disease, sensory and cognitive functions are preserved. At present, the treatment for ALS is largely supportive. Riluzole has been approved for treatment of ALS as it may confer a modest increase in survival, although its true benefits are not clearly known. Its mechanism of action may be to reduce excitotoxicity by decreasing glutamate release. Supportive therapy may include use of cough assist devices, invasive or noninvasive ventilatory support, and gastrostomy feeding in addition to a variety of orthopedic assistive devices.

XI-31. **The answer is B.** *(Chap. 454)* The patient is presenting with parkinsonism with symptoms of orthostatic hypotension and constipation indicating concomitant autonomic dysfunction. Because the patient exhibits no dementia and has no tremor, the most likely diagnosis would be multiple system atrophy (MSA). This rare disorder has a prevalence of about 2–5 per 100,000 and is commonly grouped within a category of disorders of atypical parkinsonism that includes progressive supranuclear palsy, corticobasal ganglionic degeneration, and frontotemporal dementia. MSA is typically diagnosed in the sixth decade of life and is slightly more common in men. MSA is characterized by degeneration of the substantia nigra pars compacta, striatum, cerebellum, and inferior olivary nuclei. Glial cytoplasmic inclusions that stain positive for α-synuclein are also a defining feature. The diagnosis of MSA should be suspected in individuals presenting with parkinsonian symptoms in combination with prominent cerebellar and/or autonomic complaints. In most patients, either cerebellar or parkinsonian symptoms predominate, leading to a subclassification as MSA-c or MSA-p, respectively. Autonomic symptoms occur in all patients. The most frequent autonomic symptoms include prominent orthostatic hypotension, severe constipation, neurogenic bladder, impotence in men, rapid eye movement (REM) behavior disorder, and laryngeal stridor. Diagnosis is made by clinical features. Treatment with dopaminergic agents is typically ineffective. Management is primarily symptomatic and focused on managing the concomitant autonomic features. Orthostatic hypotension often requires fludrocortisone. If that approach fails, other agents including midodrine, ephedrine, pseudoephedrine, or phenylephrine may be used. Conservative treatment of the gastrointestinal and urinary symptoms include frequent small meals, stool softeners, bulking agents, and intermittent bladder catheterization. The median time to death after diagnosis is 10 years. Risk factors for decreased survival include female gender, urinary dysfunction, older age at onset, and parkinsonian variant of the disease.

XI-32. **The answer is A.** *(Chap. 455)* Trigeminal neuralgia is a relatively common disorder with an annual incidence of 4–8 cases per 100,000 population. It is more common in women and typically presents in middle-aged or elderly individuals. It presents as sharp, and sometimes excruciating, paroxysms of pain in the lips, gums, cheek, or chin. The pain typically lasts from just a few seconds to no more than a few minutes. The painful sensations recur frequently in clusters and can occur day or night. Episodes of pain can last for several weeks at a time. Pain can occur spontaneously, but is often elicited by light touch or movements of the affected areas, including chewing, speaking, or smiling. On physical examination, there are no objective signs of sensory or motor loss. Trigeminal neuralgia is caused by ectopic generation of action potentials by pain-sensitive afferent fibers in the fifth cranial nerve. Compression of the trigeminal nerve root by a blood vessel is believed to be the most common cause of trigeminal neuralgia. Demyelination near the entry of the fifth nerve root has also been implicated. Diagnosis of trigeminal neuralgia is made based on clinical features, and laboratory or radiologic examination is not required. There is no role for electromyography (EMG) or nerve conduction studies in the evaluation of the disease. The initial treatment is typically with carbamazepine, which has been demonstrated to be effective in 50%–75% of cases. The initial dose is 100 mg in two to three divided doses daily. The medication is titrated upward to achieve pain relief. Most patients require a dose of 200 mg qid or greater, although doses >1200 mg daily confer no added benefit. For patients who do not tolerate carbamazepine, other antiseizure medications have been used to control the symptoms. These include oxcarbazepine, lamotrigine, and Dilantin. In cases that are refractory to medical therapy, microvascular surgical decompression can be considered and has a >70% success rate in relieving pain. Gamma knife radiosurgery may also be used. Radiofrequency thermal rhizotomy is used less frequently. Despite an initial success rate of >95%, up to one-third of individuals will have recurrence of symptoms, and the procedure is associated with an increased risk of complications including facial numbness and jaw weakness. The differential diagnosis of trigeminal neuralgia includes temporal arteritis, migraine or cluster headaches, and multiple sclerosis.

Temporal arteritis may present with superficial facial pain. One typically also has symptoms including jaw claudication, diffuse myalgias, and potential visual symptoms. Testing of erythrocyte sedimentation rate and performance of temporal artery biopsy are appropriate if this diagnosis is suspected. Migraine and cluster headaches present with a deeper sensation of pain. Although the pain is often throbbing in nature, it lacks the stabbing quality of trigeminal neuralgia. Multiple sclerosis can present with trigeminal neuralgia, but most patients have other symptoms of the disease as well, including weakness or visual symptoms. Multiple sclerosis may be more likely if a patient presents with bilateral trigeminal neuralgia or at a young age, and an MRI would be appropriate at that time.

XI-33. **The answer is F.** *(Chap. 456)* This patient presents with spinal cord compression, which represents an urgent need for treatment. Spinal cord compression can occur with any tumor but is most common with tumors of the breast, lung, prostate, and kidney and lymphoma and myeloma. The thoracic spinal column is the most commonly affected area for most tumors. However, metastases from prostate or ovarian cancer invade locally into the spinal column. Thus, they more commonly affect the sacral and lumbar vertebrae. Pain is typically the initial symptom of vertebral metastases. The pain can be dull and aching or sharp and radiating. The pain is usually worsened by movement, cough, and sneezing and at night. When cord compression occurs, the patient will develop weakness, sensory abnormalities, and bowel or bladder dysfunction. When spinal cord compression is suspected, imaging should be obtained promptly. Diagnosis typically is made with MRI, which also allows one to differentiate between metastasis, epidural abscess, epidural hemorrhage, or other lesions. On T1-weighted MRI, the vertebral metastases will appear hypodense relative to normal bone marrow. With gadolinium administration, the MRI may pseudo-normalize as uptake of the contrast causes the lesions to appear at the same density as the bone marrow. Plain radiographs of the spine and radionuclide bone scans will not identify 10%–20% of metastatic lesions. Management of cord compression should include glucocorticoids, local radiotherapy, and treatment of the underlying malignancy. Glucocorticoids decrease cord edema, and dexamethasone is the most commonly used medication. Up to 40 mg daily of dexamethasone is frequently used. Prompt treatment with radiotherapy to the area of cord compression is essential to decrease morbidity associated with the finding. A good response to therapy is expected for individuals who are ambulatory at the time of presentation. If motor deficits persist for longer than 12 hours, however, these will not improve. Treatment would be expected to prevent new weakness. Finally, specific therapy for the underlying tumor type is important. Surgical decompression of cord compression is generally not a preferred therapy. If there is only a single metastasis to the spine, it can sometimes be considered as a therapy. Otherwise, surgical therapy is typically limited to individuals who fail to respond to the maximum-tolerated dose of radiotherapy.

XI-34. **The answer is C.** *(Chap. 456)* Sarcoidosis is an important cause of acute or subacute myelopathy. It most often presents with slowly progressive weakness or a relapsing-remitting course. The patient affected with sarcoid myelopathy typically has concomitant sensory loss with weakness. A distinct cord level may be demonstrated. The MRI often shows diffuse edema of the spinal cord with gadolinium enhancement in active lesions. Nodular enhancement of the adjacent surface of the spinal cord is frequently seen, and the disease may affect many levels of the spinal cord. A lumbar puncture shows a lymphocyte-predominant cell count with mildly elevated CSF protein. Because sarcoidosis is often a multisystem disease, examination for evidence of disease outside of the spinal cord should be performed, including a chest radiograph, slit-lamp eye examination, serum calcium levels, and electrocardiogram. If there is evidence of abnormalities in other body systems, then definitive diagnosis can be made with a biopsy demonstrating noncaseating granulomas on pathologic examination. Patients are treated initially with high-dose glucocorticoids to decrease swelling and stimulate regression of the granulomatous lesions. Many patients will also require alternative immunosuppression including azathioprine, mycophenolate mofetil, or infliximab. Presence of caseating granulomas typically signifies an infectious process, most commonly tuberculosis or fungal infection. Atypical lymphocytes with clonality on flow cytometry are found in various types of lymphoma. A biopsy with small round cells that often resemble lymphocytes and that demonstrate scant cytoplasm, indistinct nucleoli, and mitotic figures is typical of small-cell lung carcinoma. Nonspecific chronic inflammation is nondiagnostic, and further workup would be required.

XI-35. **The answer is D.** *(Chap. 456)* Syringomyelia is a development disorder of the spinal cord that results in enlargement of the central cavity of the spinal cord. More than half of all cases are associated with a concomitant Chiari I malformation of the brainstem with protrusion of the cerebellar tonsils through the foramen magnum and into the cervical spinal canal. Although controversial, one theory for the pathogenesis of syringomyelia is impaired CSF flow with secondary enlargement of the central spinal cord, and the common coexistence with Chiari malformations may provide support of this theory. Symptoms of syringomyelia develop gradually, often beginning in late adolescence or early adulthood. The symptoms progress irregularly and may even arrest for a prolonged period. The presentation of syringomyelia includes both sensory loss and muscle wasting and weakness. The sensory disturbance is dissociative, with loss of pain and temperature sensation but preservation of vibration and touch. Patients may present with injuries or burns that occur when the patient is unaware of a painful sensation in the affected limb. The distribution of sensory loss is classically described as cape-like, affecting the nape of the neck, shoulders, upper arms, and hands. Patients are areflexic in the upper limbs. Symptoms may be asymmetric. As the cavity enlarges, it can further lead to spasticity and weakness in the lower extremities as well. There are no definitive treatment options for the disease. If a Chiari malformation is also present, surgical decompression may be required. Surgeons have attempted direct decompression of the spinal canal with varied results.

XI-36 and XI-37. **The answers are C and D, respectively.** *(Chap. 458)* This patient presents with visual disturbance and weakness affecting the lower extremities with a past history of prior visual disturbance. This suggests a diagnosis of multiple sclerosis (MS), an autoimmune demyelinating disorder of the central nervous system. This disease affects about 350,000 individuals in the United States and has a variable clinical course, with some individuals experiencing limited symptoms and others becoming very incapacitated due to the disease. MS is three times more common in women, with a typical age of onset between 20 and 40 years of age. MS is more common in white individuals that those of African or Asian descent. In addition, geographic variations in disease prevalence have also been demonstrated, with higher prevalence in the temperate zone areas of northern North America, northern Europe, and southern Australia and New Zealand. In contrast, the tropics have a prevalence that is 10 to 20 times less. Other well-established risk factors for development of MS include vitamin D deficiency, exposure to Epstein-Barr virus after early childhood, and cigarette smoking. Despite the fact that this is an autoimmune disorder, there has not been an associated between MS and other autoimmune disorders. The clinical manifestations of MS are varied. The disease can present with an abrupt onset of symptoms or may develop gradually. The most common initial presenting symptoms include sensory loss, optic neuritis, weakness, paresthesias, and diplopia. Weakness of the limbs may be asymmetric and manifest as loss of strength, speed, dexterity, or endurance. Symptoms are upper neuron in origin and have associated spasticity, hyperreflexia, and Babinski sign most commonly. However, if there is a spinal cord lesion, lower motor neuron signs and loss of reflexes may also be seen. The spasticity that is present may lead to spontaneous or movement-induced muscle spasms and affects up to 30% of patients with MS. Optic neuritis presents with blurred vision, dimness, or decreased color perception in the central visual fields. Visual symptoms typically only affect one eye. Periorbital pain often precedes or accompanies visual loss. Funduscopic examination may be normal or show optic disc swelling. Other common symptoms that occur with MS include bladder dysfunction, ataxia, constipation, chronic pain, fatigue, and depression. A diagnosis of MS can be difficult to confirm in some individuals. There is no definitive test for MS. The diagnostic criteria require two or more episodes of symptoms and two or more signs of dysfunction in noncontiguous white matter tracts. MRI characteristically shows multiple hyperintense T2-weighted lesions that can be present in the brain, brainstem, and spinal cord. More than 90% of lesions seen on MRI, however, are asymptomatic. Approximately one-third of lesions that appear hyperintense on T2-weighted images will be hypointense on T1-weighted images. These "black holes" may be a marker of irreversible demyelination and axonal loss. Evoked potentials are no longer commonly used in MS and are most useful in studying pathways that are not exhibiting clinical symptoms. Evoked potentials are not specific to MS, although a marked delay in latency of transmission suggests demyelination. The CSF may show an increased number of mononuclear cells, although CSF protein is typically normal. Oligoclonal bands help to assess the intrathecal production of immunoglobulin (Ig) G. The presence of two or more discrete oligoclonal bands in the CSF that are not present in serum is found in more than 75% of MS patients. If a patient has a pleocytosis of >75 cells/μL, presence of polymorphonuclear cells, or protein concentration >100 mg/dL, an alternative diagnosis should be sought.

XI-38. **The answer is D.** *(Chap. 458)* Over the past two decades, 10 disease-modifying agents for the treatment of MS have been approved. Due to these multiple options, it is preferred that a patient with MS be referred to a treatment center with experience in the disease. The disease-modifying drugs approved for MS include interferon-β-1a, interferon-β-1b, glatiramer acetate, natalizumab, fingolimod, dimethyl fumarate, teriflunomide, mitoxantrone, and alemtuzumab. Given this patient's poor functional status, her disease should be treated as moderate disease. Generally, in those with moderate disease, the preferred agents are dimethyl fumarate, fingolimod, teriflunomide, and natalizumab, with interferon-β-1a and -1b treatment being reserved for individuals with milder disease. However, natalizumab is not recommended in this patient due to the presence of antibody to JC virus. About half of the population is antibody positive for JC virus, indicating past exposure typically with an asymptomatic infection. JC virus is implicated in the development of progressive multifocal leukoencephalopathy. This life-threatening condition has occurred in 0.3% of all patients treated with natalizumab and in about 0.6% of patients who are positive for JC virus antibody. The risk is lower in the first year of treatment and increases thereafter. Thus, natalizumab should not be used in this patient unless she has failed alternative therapies or if the disease course has been particularly aggressive. If natalizumab is ultimately chosen for a patient who is JC virus antibody positive, it should not be used for any longer than 1 year. In patients who are JC virus antibody negative, it is recommended to follow the patient for development of antibody approximately every 6 months.

XI-39. **The answer is C.** *(Chap. 459)* When evaluating a patient with peripheral neuropathy, the clinician should consider the history and physical examination carefully to determine the location of the lesion, which will then further identify the cause and appropriate treatment. However, in as many as 50% of patients presenting with peripheral neuropathy, no cause is ever found, and these patients generally have a predominate sensory polyneuropathy. Seven keys questions in the history and physical examination can assist with the identification of the site of the lesion and the cause (Table XI-39). The first determination the clinician should make is which systems are involved—sensory, motor, autonomic, or some combination of these. An isolated motor neuropathy without sensory involvement should lead to diagnostic possibilities that include myopathy, motor neuropathy, or disorder of the neuromuscular junction. Autonomic symptoms can accompany a diabetic neuropathy and can also be seen in amyloid polyneuropathy. Another important determination is the distribution of the weakness (proximal vs. distal, symmetric vs. asymmetric). A third determination is the nature of the sensory involvement. Small-fiber neuropathy often has a burning or stabbing quality along with temperature loss, whereas a large-fiber sensory neuropathy will show loss of vibratory sense and proprioception. One should also consider whether upper motor neuron symptoms are also present, which occurs with vitamin B_{12} deficiency most commonly, but also occurs with other causes of combined system degeneration such as human immunodeficiency virus (HIV) and copper deficiency. The temporal evolution of symptoms further provides the clinician with clues as to the cause of the disease. Most neuropathies have an insidious onset over weeks to months. Acute development of symptoms points to causes such as Guillain-Barré syndrome vasculitis or Lyme disease. Asking about symptoms in other family members will help to establish whether a hereditary neuropathy is present. Finally, it is important to obtain a full medical history to assess whether any associated conditions could be contributing to the neuropathy. Once a full history and physical examination is completed, a clinician will often order EMG and nerve conduction studies to complete the work up. Autonomic studies may also be helpful in selected patients.

TABLE XI-39 Approach to Neuropathic Disorders: Seven Key Questions

1. What systems are involved?
- Motor, sensory, autonomic, or combinations

2. What is the distribution of weakness?
- Only distal versus proximal and distal
- Focal/asymmetric versus symmetric

3. What is the nature of the sensory involvement?
- Temperature loss or burning or stabbing pain (e.g., small fiber)
- Vibratory or proprioceptive loss (e.g., large fiber)

4. Is there evidence of upper motor neuron involvement?
- Without sensory loss
- With sensory loss

5. What is the temporal evolution?
- Acute (days to 4 weeks)
- Subacute (4–8 weeks)
- Chronic (>8 weeks)
- Monophasic, progressive, or relapsing-remitting

6. Is there evidence for a hereditary neuropathy?
- Family history of neuropathy
- Lack of sensory symptoms despite sensory signs

7. Are there any associated medical conditions?
- Cancer, diabetes mellitus, connective tissue disease or other autoimmune diseases, infection (e.g., HIV, Lyme disease, leprosy)
- Medications including over-the-counter drugs that may cause a toxic neuropathy
- Preceding events, drugs, toxins

XI-40. The answer is A. *(Chap. 459)* Charcot-Marie-Tooth (CMT) syndrome is the most common type of hereditary neuropathy. CMT is comprised of several similar but genetically distinct conditions with different associated mutations. CMT1 is the most common syndrome and is an inherited demyelinating sensorimotor neuropathy. CMT1 most often affects patients in the first to third decades of life with distal leg weakness (ie, foot drop). There are several subtypes of CMT1, most of which are inherited in an autosomal dominant fashion. However, the penetrance is variable, and some affected family members may remain asymptomatic even late in life. The most common genetic defect in CMT1 (*CMT1A*) is a 1.5-megabase duplication in the gene for peripheral myelin production (*PMP-22*) on chromosome 17. This results in a patient having three copies of the gene rather than two. Although patients generally do not complain of sensory symptoms, these can be elicited often on physical examination. Muscle stretch reflexes are unobtainable or reduced throughout, and muscles below the knee are often atrophied, which makes legs appear to have so-called inverted champagne bottle appearance. There are no medical therapies for CMT, but patients are generally referred for physical and occupational therapy. Bracing and other orthotic devices are frequently used. Hereditary neuralgic amyotrophy is an autosomal dominant disorder characterized by recurrent attacks of pain, weakness, and sensory loss in the distribution of the brachial plexus that often begins in childhood. Hereditary sensory and autonomic neuropathy is a rare group of hereditary neuropathies in which sensory and autonomic dysfunction predominates over muscle weakness. This would not fit the clinical pattern described here. Guillain-Barré syndrome generally presents acutely with rapid development of ascending paralysis. The prolonged symptom period and distribution described here are not typical for Guillain-Barré syndrome. Fabry disease is an X-linked disorder in which men are more commonly affected then women. Patients have angiokeratomas, which are reddish-purple lesions usually found around the umbilicus, scrotum, and inguinal region. Burning pain in the hands and feet often is found in late childhood or early adult life. Patients also have premature atherosclerosis from the underlying mutation in the α-galactosidase gene with accumulation of ceramide in nerves and blood vessels.

XI-41. The answer is E. *(Chap. 459)* One of the most common side effects of isoniazid treatment is peripheral neuropathy. The elderly, malnourished patients, and "slow acetylators" are at increased risk for developing the neuropathy. Isoniazid inhibits pyridoxal phosphokinase, resulting in pyridoxine (vitamin B_6) deficiency and the neuropathy. Prophylactic administration of pyridoxine can prevent the neuropathy from developing. Symptoms are generally dysesthesias and sensory ataxia. Impaired large-fiber sensory modalities are found on examination. Cobalamin (vitamin B_{12}) is not reduced in this condition and unaffected by isoniazid. Neurontin and pregabalin may alleviate symptoms but will not reverse the neuropathy. There is no indication that hypothyroidism is present.

XI-42. The answer is C. *(Chap. 459)* Diabetes mellitus is the most common cause of peripheral neuropathy in developed countries and is associated with several different types of polyneuropathy including distal symmetric sensory or sensorimotor polyneuropathy, autonomic neuropathy, diabetic neuropathic cachexia, polyradicular neuropathies, cranial neuropathies, and other mononeuropathies. Risk factors for development of neuropathy include long-standing and poorly controlled diabetes and the presence of retinopathy or nephropathy. The patient here appears to have diabetic distal symmetric sensory and sensorimotor polyneuropathy (DSPN), which is the most common form of diabetic neuropathy. DSPN presents with sensory loss beginning in the toes and gradually progressives over time up the legs and into the fingers and arms. Symptoms also may include tingling, burning, and deep aching pains. Nerve biopsy, although rarely indicated, often shows axonal degeneration, endothelial hyperplasia, and occasionally perivascular inflammation. Tight glucose control prevents development of disease but does not reverse established disease. Diabetic autonomic neuropathy is often seen in combination with DSPN and manifests by abnormal sweating, dysfunctional thermoregulation, dry eyes and mouth, postural hypotension, gastrointestinal abnormalities including gastroparesis, and genitourinary dysfunction.

XI-43 and XI-44. The answers are B and B, respectively. *(Chap. 460)* Guillain-Barré syndrome (GBS) is an acute demyelinating polyneuropathy that can be severe and life-threatening if not immediately recognized and treated. Each year, there are about 5000–6000 cases in the United States, with an incidence of about 1–4 cases per 100,000 population annually. Men are slightly more commonly affected than women, and GBS is more commonly diagnosed in adulthood. The typical presentation is a rapid ascending paralysis that may be first noticed as weak or "rubbery" legs. The weakness can evolve over hours to a few days, with the legs being more affected than the arms. Tingling dysesthesias are also frequently present, although sensory neuropathy is always present. Facial paresis occurs in about 50% of patients, and other lower cranial nerves may also be affected. Pain is a frequent complaint, with pain in the neck, shoulders, back, and diffusely over the spine. In addition, vague sensation of deep aching pain in the weakened muscles may also be present. Up to 30% of patients will require mechanical ventilation due to weakness of the respiratory muscles. Moreover, bulbar involvement increases the risk of aspiration and subsequent pneumonia. Deep tendon reflexes are decreased or disappear entirely within the first few days of onset. Cutaneous sensory deficits are usually only mild if present at all. Bladder dysfunction only rarely occurs and is transient. Persistent or severe bladder dysfunction should stimulate a workup for other causes. Autonomic symptoms are common. Blood pressure may be quite labile with marked postural changes. Cardiac dysrhythmias may also occur and require continuous monitoring. Typically within 4 weeks of onset or sooner, there is a plateau in symptoms with no further progression. Diagnosis of GBS relies upon a high degree of clinical suspicion because there is no one test that is diagnostic for the disorder. Typical CSF findings include a high CSF protein without pleocytosis. The presence of a high CSF white blood cell count should prompt a search for an alternative diagnosis. Early in the disease process, electrodiagnostic testing may be normal or only show mild findings of demyelination. Approximately 70% of GBS cases occur within 1–3 weeks of an antecedent infectious illness. Most commonly, the illness is respiratory or gastrointestinal in nature. About 20%–30% of all cases in North America, Europe, and Australia are preceded by infection or reinfection with *Campylobacter jejuni*. A similar proportion of individuals will have had an infection with a human herpes virus, most often cytomegalovirus or Epstein-Barr virus. Less frequently, HIV, hepatitis E, or *Mycoplasma pneumoniae* may be implicated. Recent immunizations are a rare cause of GBS, with a risk of <1 per million.

When a case of GBS is suspected, clinical vigilance and prompt treatment are required. Admission to intensive care is often required to monitor for development of respiratory failure or cardiac arrhythmias. If treatment is delayed longer than 2 weeks after initial symptoms or during the plateau stage, it may not be effective. Either high-dose IV immunoglobulin (IVIg) or plasmapheresis should be begun as soon as possible. IVIg is given as a daily infusion for 5 days. Plasmapheresis should be performed four to five times over the first week. Functionally significant recovery may begin to be evident after the first week but may take several weeks. Lack of noticeable improvement following either IVIg or plasmapheresis is not an indication to switch to the alternative therapy as they are equally effective in treatment. Glucocorticoids have not been shown to be effective in GBS and should not be used. Approximately 85% of patients with GBS achieve full functional recovery after several months to a year. However, some physical examination findings such as areflexia may persist. The mortality rate is <5%, and death is most often due to respiratory complications. Although macrolides have activity against *Campylobacter* species, most cases of diarrhea resolve spontaneously, and treatment has no effect on the course of GBS. Pyridostigmine may increase strength in patients with myasthenia gravis but will have no effect on strength in patients with GBS.

XI-45. The answer is A. *(Chap. 461)* Myasthenia gravis (MG) is a relatively common neuromuscular disorder that is caused by antibody-mediated autoimmune destruction of acetylcholine receptors at the neuromuscular junction. MG has a prevalence of about 2–7 in 10,000 individuals and affects women more commonly than men at a ratio of 3:2. The age of presentation in women is generally in the 20s to 30s, whereas men more commonly present in their 50s and 60s. The key features of MG are weakness and fatigability of muscles. The weakness increases with repeated use and is typically more prominent late in the day. The distribution of muscle weakness often follows a typical pattern, with cranial muscles being affected early in the course of disease. Common clinical features include diplopia, ptosis, inability to smile fully, weakness with chewing, dysarthria, and dysphagia. Aspiration of liquids may also occur. In the majority of patients, the weakness becomes generalized, affecting proximal muscles greater than distal muscles. Deep tendon reflexes are preserved, and the disease may be asymmetric. The diagnosis is suspected after the appearance of the characteristic symptoms and signs. The diagnosis should be confirmed with further testing because treatment may involve surgery and the prolonged use of immunosuppressive agents. The most sensitive test for the diagnosis of MG is the presence of antibodies to the acetylcholine receptor (AChR). These antibodies are present in about 85% of patients with MG. The presence of AChR antibodies in a patient with typical signs and symptoms is diagnostic. If AChR antibodies are negative, additional testing for muscle-specific kinase (MuSK) antibodies will be positive in another 40% of individuals. However, if the disease is limited to the ocular muscles alone, both of these tests are likely to be negative. Use of repetitive nerve stimulation characteristically shows decrements of >10%–15% in action potential amplitude with successive electric shocks delivered at two to three per second. Patients should be tested with repetitive stimulation in a proximal muscle group or in muscles that have been demonstrated to be weakened in the disease. Edrophonium is an acetylcholinesterase inhibitor that allows acetylcholine to interact repeatedly with the limited number of AChRs, producing improvement in the strength of myasthenic muscles. An objective end point must be chosen when performing the edrophonium test to determine if there is an improvement in muscle strength after administration. At this time, edrophonium is only used in individuals with suspected MG with negative antibody testing as well as negative electrodiagnostic testing. False-positive tests may occur in patients with other neurologic diseases, such as amyotrophic lateral sclerosis. Antibodies to voltage-gated calcium channels are found in patients with Lambert-Eaton syndrome, another neuromuscular disorder associated with complaints of weakness. In this disorder, however, individuals develop improved responses with repetitive nerve stimulation. Clinically, Lambert-Eaton syndrome can also be distinguished from MG because Lambert-Eaton syndrome typically has prominent autonomic changes as well as depressed deep tendon reflexes.

XI-46. The answer is E. *(Chap. 461)* The treatment of MG may include a variety of modalities including anticholinesterase medications, immunosuppression, IVIg or plasmapheresis, or surgical intervention. Initial treatment of symptoms with anticholinesterase medications such as pyridostigmine yields partial improvement in most patients. However, few patients achieve complete relief with this class of medications alone. In addition, dose-limiting side effects such as diarrhea, abdominal cramping, and excessive salivation are frequent. Thymectomy should be considered in all patients with MG. When considering thymectomy, there are two separate issues to be considered. If the patient has evidence of thymoma, thymectomy is necessary because local spread may occur. However, presence of a thymic shadow on CT scan is not indicative of thymoma and is common in young adulthood. In individuals without evidence of thymoma, thymectomy should still be considered an important therapeutic option. Even in the absence of tumor, up to 85% of individuals will experience improvement in disease after thymectomy, with ~35% achieving drug-free remission. Current literature suggests that individuals who undergo thymectomy are 1.7 times more likely to improve and 2 times more likely to achieve remission than those who do not undergo thymectomy. It is now consensus that individuals between the ages of puberty and 55 with generalized MG should be referred for thymectomy if surgically appropriate candidates. In the absence of thymectomy, addition of immunosuppressants in the form of glucocorticoids or other steroid-sparing agents will yield further benefits and often control the disease. Prednisone at a dose of 15–25 mg daily is the initial choice in most patients and should be increased for residual symptoms. Other immunomodulatory agents with proven effectiveness in MG include mycophenolate mofetil, azathioprine, cyclosporine, and tacrolimus. In addition, rituximab may be considered in refractory cases. In acute presentations with myasthenic crisis, IVIg or plasmapheresis is used concomitantly with immunosuppressants. Anticholinesterase drugs are typically withheld during a myasthenic crisis because overdosage of these drugs can worsen weakness.

XI-47. **The answer is B.** *(Chap. 461)* Except for lumbar puncture, all of the options listed are indicated at this time. Thymic abnormalities are present in 75% of patients with MG. A CT or MRI of the mediastinum may show enlargement or neoplastic changes in the thymus and is recommended upon diagnosis. Hyperthyroidism occurs in 3%–8% of patients with MG and may aggravate weakness. Testing for rheumatoid factor and antinuclear antibodies should also be obtained because of the association of MG with other autoimmune diseases. Due to side effects of immunosuppressive therapy, a thorough evaluation should be undertaken to rule out latent or chronic infections such as tuberculosis. Measurements of ventilatory function are valuable as a baseline because of the frequency and seriousness of respiratory impairment in patients with MG, and they can be used as an objective measure of response to therapy.

XI-48. **The answer is E.** *(Chap. 462e)* All classes of lipid-lowering agents have been implicated in muscle toxicity including fibrates, HMG-CoA reductase inhibitors, niacin, and ezetimibe. Myalgia, malaise, and muscle tenderness are the most common manifestations, and muscle pain may be exacerbated by exercise. Proximal weakness may be found on examination. In severe cases, rhabdomyolysis and myoglobinuria may occur, although most cases are more mild. Concomitant use of statins with fibrates and cyclosporine are more likely to cause adverse muscle reactions. Elevated serum creatine kinase (CK) is often identified, and muscle weakness is evidenced by myopathic EMG studies and myonecrosis on muscle biopsy. Severe myalgias, muscle weakness, significant elevations in CK (>3× upper limit of normal), and myoglobinuria are indications for stopping. After cessation, improvement generally occurs in up to several weeks.

XI-49. **The answer is E.** *(Chap. 462e)* A number of endocrinologic conditions are associated with myopathy. Both hypo- and hyperthyroidism are associated with proximal muscle weakness. Hypothyroidism is associated with an elevated CK frequently, even with minimal clinical evidence of muscle disease. Thyrotoxic patients may have fasciculations in addition to proximal myopathy, but in contrast to hypothyroid patients, CK is not generally elevated. Hyperparathyroidism is associated with muscle weakness, generally proximal. Muscle wasting and brisk reflexes are also generally present. Serum CK levels may be normal or slightly elevated. Serum calcium and phosphate levels show no correlation with clinical weakness. Hypoparathyroid patients also often have myopathy due to hypocalcemia. Patients with acromegaly usually have mild proximal weakness without atrophy. The duration of acromegaly, not the serum growth hormone levels, correlates with the degree of myopathy. Diabetes mellitus is a rare cause of myopathy, generally due to ischemic infarction of muscle, and not a primary myopathy. Finally, vitamin D deficiency is associated with muscle weakness, as are glucocorticoid excess states (e.g., Cushing disease).

XI-50. **The answer is D.** *(Chap. 462e)* There are two recognized clinical forms of myotonic dystrophy, both of which are characterized by autosomal dominant inheritance. Myotonic dystrophy type 1 (DM1) is the most common form and the most likely disorder in this patient. Characteristic clinical features of this disorder include a "hatchet-faced" appearance, due to wasting of the facial muscles, and weakness of the neck muscles. In contrast to the muscular dystrophies (Becker and Duchenne), distal limb muscle weakness is more common in DM1. Palatal, pharyngeal, and tongue involvement are also common and produce the dysarthric voice that is frequently heard. The failure of relaxation after a forced hand grip is characteristic of myotonia. Myotonia can also be elicited by percussion of the thenar eminence. In most individuals, myotonia is present by age 5, but clinical symptoms of weakness that lead to diagnosis may not be present until adulthood. Cardiac conduction abnormalities and heart failure are also common in myotonic dystrophy. Diagnosis can often be made by clinical features alone in an individual with classic symptoms and a positive family history. An EMG would confirm myotonia. Genetic testing for DM1 would show a characteristic trinucleotide repeat on chromosome 19. Genetic anticipation occurs with an increasing number of repeats and worsening clinical disease over successive generations. Myotonic dystrophy type 2 (DM2) causes proximal muscle weakness primarily and is also known by the name proximal myotonic myopathy. Other features of the disease overlap with DM1. Acid maltase deficiency (glucosidase deficiency, or Pompe disease) has three recognized forms, only one of which has onset in adulthood. In the adult-onset form, respiratory muscle weakness is prominent and often is the presenting symptom. As stated previously, Becker and Duchenne muscular dystrophies present with primarily proximal muscle weakness and are X-linked recessive disorders. Becker muscular dystrophy presents at a later age than Duchenne muscular dystrophy and has a more prolonged course. Otherwise, features are similar to one another. Nemaline myopathy is a heterogeneous disorder marked by the threadlike appearance of muscle fibers on biopsy. Nemaline myopathy usually presents in childhood and has a striking facial appearance similar to myotonic dystrophy with a long, narrow face. This disease is inherited in an autosomal dominant fashion.

XI-51. **The answer is E.** *(Chap. 464e)* Chronic fatigue syndrome (CFS) is a disorder characterized by persistent and unexplained fatigue resulting in severe impairment in daily functioning. Besides intense fatigue, most patients with CFS report concomitant symptoms such as pain, cognitive dysfunction, and unrefreshing sleep. Additional symptoms can include headache, sore throat, tender lymph nodes, muscle aches, joint aches, feverishness, difficulty sleeping, psychiatric problems, allergies, and abdominal cramps. Criteria for the diagnosis of CFS have been developed by the U.S. Centers for Disease Control and Prevention (Table XI-51). CFS is seen worldwide, with adult prevalence rates varying between 0.2% and 0.4%. In the United States, the prevalence is higher among women (~75% of cases), members of minority groups (African and Native Americans), and individuals with lower levels of education and occupational status. The mean age of onset is between 29 and 35 years. Many patients probably go undiagnosed and/or do not seek help. There are numerous hypotheses about the etiology of CFS; there is no definitively identified cause. Physical inactivity and trauma in childhood tend to increase the risk of CFS in adults. Neuroendocrine dysfunction may be associated with childhood trauma, reflecting a biological correlate of vulnerability. Psychiatric illness and physical hyperactivity in adulthood raise the risk of CFS in later life. Twin studies suggest a familial predisposition to CFS, but no causative genes have been identified. Physical or psychological stress may elicit the onset of CFS. Most patients report an infection (usually a flulike illness or infectious mononucleosis) as the trigger of their fatigue. Relatively high percentages of CFS cases occur after Q fever and Lyme disease.

TABLE XI-51 **Diagnostic Criteria for Chronic Fatigue Syndrome**

Characteristic Persistent or Relapsing Unexplained Chronic Fatigue
Fatigue lasts for at least 6 months.
Fatigue is of new or definite onset.
Fatigue is not the result of an organic disease or of continuing exertion.
Fatigue is not alleviated by rest.
Fatigue results in a substantial reduction in previous occupational, educational, social, and personal activities.
Four or more of the following symptoms are concurrently present for 6 months: impaired memory or concentration, sore throat, tender cervical or axillary lymph nodes, muscle pain, pain in several joints, new headaches, unrefreshing sleep, or malaise after exertion.
Exclusion Criteria
Medical condition explaining fatigue
Major depressive disorder (psychotic features) or bipolar disorder
Schizophrenia, dementia, or delusional disorder
Anorexia nervosa, bulimia nervosa
Alcohol or substance abuse
Severe obesity (body mass index >40)

XI-52. **The answer is B.** *(Chap. 464e)* Cognitive behavioral therapy (CBT) and graded exercise therapy (GET) have been found to be the only beneficial interventions in CFS. Some patient groups argue against these approaches because of the implication that CFS is a purely mental disorder. CBT is a psychotherapeutic approach directed at changing unhealthy disease-perpetuating patterns of thoughts and behaviors. It includes educating the patient about the etiologic model, setting goals, restoring fixed bedtimes and wake-up times, challenging and changing fatigue and activity-related concerns, reducing a focus on symptoms, spreading activities evenly throughout the day, gradually increasing physical activity, planning a return to work, and resuming other activities. The intervention, which typically consists of 12–14 sessions spread over 6 months, helps CFS patients gain control over their symptoms. GET targets deconditioning and exercise intolerance and usually involves a home exercise program that continues for 3–5 months. Walking or cycling is systematically increased, with set goals for maximal heart rates. CBT and GET appear to improve fatigue primarily by changing the patient's perception of the fatigue and also by reducing the focus on symptoms. In general, CBT studies tend to yield better improvement rates than GET trials. Not all patients benefit from CBT or GET. Predictors of poor outcome are medical (including psychiatric) comorbidities, current disability claims, and severe pain. CBT offered in an early stage of the illness reduces the burden of CFS for the patient as well as for society in terms of decreased medical and disability-related costs. Full recovery from untreated CFS is rare: the median annual recovery rate is 5% (range, 0%–31%), and the median improvement rate is 39% (range, 8%–63%). Patients with an underlying psychiatric disorder and those who continue to attribute their symptoms to an undiagnosed medical condition have poorer outcomes. The other listed therapies have been tried in patients with CFS with no proven lasting benefit.

XI-53. **The answer is A.** *(Chap. 466)* Generalized anxiety disorder (GAD) has a lifetime prevalence of about 5%–6% and presents with persistent, excessive, and/or unrealistic worry occurring on most days that persists for at least 6 months. The worry typically pervades most aspects of life and is to a degree that it is uncontrollable and causes impairment in social, work, or interpersonal functioning. Associated physical symptoms include tension, restlessness, impaired concentration, insomnia, autonomic arousal, and feeling of being "on edge." Typical onset of symptoms is before the age of 20, although patients may not seek treatment for many years. A history of childhood fears may be present. More than 80% of patients with GAD have a concomitant mood disorder such as major depression or dysthymia or social phobia, but panic attacks (e.g., 10–30 minute episodes including palpitations, shortness of breath, and feelings of impending doom) generally do not occur. Comorbid substance abuse, most often with alcohol or sedative/hypnotics, is also common, perhaps as an attempt to self-treat anxiety. Treatment of GAD is most effective when psychotherapy is combined with medications, although complete relief of symptoms is rare. Initial intervention with benzodiazepines is often required for a period of 4–6 weeks. Other medications that are FDA-approved for the treatment of GAD are escitalopram, paroxetine, and venlafaxine, although other SSRIs have been demonstrated in clinical trials to be effective as well, typically at doses comparable to the effective dose for major depression. Buspirone is another anxiolytic agent that is nonsedating, does not produce tolerance or dependence, and has no abuse potential. However, it generally has mild effects and takes several weeks to produce results. It has demonstrated best results in individuals with dementia or head injury who develop agitation and/or anxiety. Anticonvulsants with GABAergic properties such as gabapentin, oxcarbazepine, tiagabine, pregabalin, and divalproex also may have efficacy against anxiety.

XI-54. **The answer is C.** *(Chap. 466)* There are an estimated 300,000 episodes of acute schizophrenia in the United States annually. This disorder has a high degree of morbidity, with many individuals failing to achieve their premorbid level of functioning after an episode of acute schizophrenia. Symptoms of schizophrenia are heterogeneous with perturbations in language, thinking, perception, social activity, affect, and volition. The most typical age of onset is late adolescence and young adulthood. Onset is insidious as individuals progressively experience social withdrawal and perceptual distortion and often progress to experience frank delusions and hallucinations. As individuals age, the positive symptoms of delusions and hallucinations tend to recede, and the negative symptoms of anhedonia, decreased emotional expression, and loss of function become more predominant. In a first episode, antipsychotic agents are effective about 70% of the time. Symptoms may improve within hours or days of dosing, but full remission often takes 6–8 weeks. If medications are discontinued, relapse will occur in 60% of patients within 6 months. The long-term prognosis of most individuals with schizophrenia is somewhat grim. Prognosis of schizophrenia depends not on symptom severity at initial diagnosis but on the response to antipsychotic medication. A permanent remission rarely occurs. About 10% of schizophrenic patients commit suicide.

XI-55. **The answer is D.** *(Chap. 466)* This patient is experiencing her first episode of a panic attack and does not meet criteria for panic disorder. In this situation, no specific treatment is required. The patient should be reassured that she does not have any evidence of a serious medical disorder in a manner that is empathetic and supportive. Panic disorder is a frequently occurring mental disorder with a lifetime prevalence of about 2%–3%. Panic attacks begin abruptly, most commonly without an immediate precipitating cause, and peak in severity over 10 minutes. The first episode of panic attack is most often outside the home. The symptoms usually subside spontaneously over the course of an hour. Panic attacks are often accompanied by intense fear and a variety of physical symptoms, including palpitations, dizziness, sweating, shortness of breath, chest pain, and a feeling of impending doom or death. Gastrointestinal distress, paresthesias, and syncope may occur. Panic disorder could be diagnosed if the patient developed recurrent attacks lasting at least 1 month or exhibited excessive worry or change in behavior related to these attacks. If the patient subsequently develops panic disorder, a variety of treatment options can be pursued. The goals of therapy for panic attacks are to decrease the frequency of attacks and severity of symptoms during the attack. Antidepressant medications are the cornerstone of therapy with SSRIs being the most frequently used class of medication. The dose of medication for panic disorder is typically lower than the antidepressant dose. For fluoxetine, this would be 5–10 mg daily. Because these medications take 2–6 weeks to become effective, they are often combined with benzodiazepines early in the course of treatment to alleviate anticipatory anxiety and provide immediate relief of panic symptoms. Alprazolam and clonazepam are common agents used for panic disorder, although alprazolam may have more associated dependence with need for escalating doses of medications. In combination with pharmacologic therapy, psychotherapy and education are also useful for the treatment of panic disorder. The therapy often includes breathing techniques, cognitive behavioral therapy, and even homework assignments.

XI-56. **The answer is A.** *(Chap. 466)* There are an increasing number of antidepressant medications available in a variety of classes. SSRIs are the most commonly used antidepressant drugs. This class of medications includes fluoxetine, sertraline, paroxetine, fluvoxamine, citalopram, and escitalopram. These medications are taken once daily and have side effects including sexual dysfunction, headache, and insomnia. Tricyclic antidepressants were commonly used in past decades for treatment of depression. However, overdoses can be lethal, and anticholinergic side effects including dry mouth, constipation, and urinary retention can limit the dose. Medications in the tricyclic class of antidepressants include amitriptyline, nortriptyline, imipramine, desipramine, doxepin, and clomipramine. Mixed norepinephrine/serotonin reuptake inhibitors and receptor blockers are a newer class of medications. These medications are increasing in use because they are quite effective and do not have the same frequency of sexual dysfunction. Medications in this class includes venlafaxine, desvenlafaxine, duloxetine, and mirtazapine. Monoamine oxidase inhibitors were once a common antidepressant class of medication, but these medications are now only rarely used because of a wide range of drug and food interactions that can lead to hypertensive crises. Examples of medication in this class include phenelzine, tranylcypromine, and isocarboxazid. A final class of antidepressants, called simply mixed-action, and includes trazodone, bupropion, and nefazodone.

XI-57. **The answer is E.** *(Chap. 466)* Posttraumatic stress disorder (PTSD) was only added as a discrete disorder in 1980. The diagnostic criteria for PTSD are long and require that an individual experiences an event where there was an actual or perceived threat of death or serious injury and that the individual's reaction included intense fear or helplessness. Following the event, the individual continues to reexperience the event and avoids stimuli associated with the trauma. In association with this, there is also often a generalized withdrawal and decrease in responsiveness. At the same time, the patient exhibits an increase in arousal that is often exhibited by insomnia, irritability, hypervigilance, and difficulty concentrating. Treatment of PTSD is almost always multifactorial, including both pharmacotherapy and psychotherapy. It is not uncommon for an individual with PTSD to develop dependence on drugs or alcohol as an attempt to control the symptoms, and any substance abuse issues need to be treated simultaneously as well. This patient's treatment would include avoidance of alcohol and intensive substance abuse treatment, as needed. Treatment with antidepressant medications can decrease anxiety and avoidance behaviors. Trazodone is often given at night for its sedating properties. Psychotherapeutic strategies include cognitive behavioral therapy to overcome avoidance behaviors.

XI-58. **The answer is B.** *(Chap. 466)* Fifteen percent of the population will experience at least one episode of major depression over the course of a lifetime, and most episodes of major depression are treated by primary care practitioners. Treatment can be with any of a number of medications across a variety of classes. Despite the popularity of newer antidepressants, there is no evidence that these medications are more efficacious than older drugs like tricyclic antidepressants. Indeed, 60%–70% of patients will respond to any drug chosen if given in a sufficient dose for 6–8 weeks. However, up to 40% of patients treated at primary care offices discontinue treatment if there has not been a response within 1 month. Once a patient has been on treatment for ~2 months, the response should be evaluated, and if there has been an insufficient response, a dose increase should be considered. In this patient, a dose increase yielded control of depressive symptoms at 4 months. Once control of symptoms has been achieved, the drug should be continued for an additional 6–9 months to prevent relapse. If a patient experiences any additional episodes of major depression, he will likely require indefinite maintenance treatment because it is recommended that anyone with more than two episodes of major depression continue treatment indefinitely.

XI-59. **The answer is F.** *(Chap. 467)* About 20% of all patients have an alcohol use disorder, even in affluent locales. Patients should be screened for an alcohol use disorder by asking specific questions regarding alcohol consumption, although many patients may minimize their alcohol use. The patient in the scenario presented reports daily alcohol consumption and some symptoms of an alcohol use disorder, including blackouts from drinking and frequent hangovers while working. Laboratory tests may be helpful in this situation as they can be elevated in individuals who regularly consume six or more drinks daily. The two tests with the greatest sensitivity and specificity (≥60%) are γ-glutamyl transferase (GGT) >35 U/L and carbohydrate-deficient transferrin (CDT). Using both of these tests combined is more likely to be accurate than using either test alone. Other blood tests that may be useful include high-normal MCV >91 μm^3 and serum uric acid >7 mg/dL. Elevations in AST or ALT are neither sensitive nor specific.

XI-60. The answer is A. *(Chap. 467)* Alcohol is primarily absorbed through the proximal small intestine, but small amounts can also be absorbed in the mouth, esophagus, stomach, and large intestines as well. Several factors can increase the rate of absorption. One factor that increases absorption is rapid gastric emptying, which can be induced by concurrent consumption of carbonated beverages. Another factor that increases absorption from the gut to the blood is the ingestion of alcohol in the absence of other calorie sources such as proteins, fat, or carbohydrates. A final factor that can increase absorption is to drink alcohol that is diluted to a modest concentration (~20% or less). At high alcohol concentrations, absorption is decreased, although high blood levels may be achieved because the amount of alcohol ingested is high.

XI-61. The answer is C. *(Chap. 467)* Alcohol has effects on many neurotransmitters in the brain. The predominant effect of alcohol lies in its ability to cause release of γ-aminobutyric acid (GABA), and it acts primarily at the $GABA_A$ receptors. GABA is the primary inhibitory neurotransmitter in the brain and is associated with the sedative effects of alcohol. Many other drugs affect the GABA system including benzodiazepines, nonbenzodiazepine sleep aids such as zolpidem, anticonvulsants, and muscle relaxants. The euphoric effects of alcohol consumption are related to increases in dopamine, which is common to all pleasurable activities. The effects on dopamine are thought to be important in alcohol craving and relapse. In addition, alcohol alters opioid receptors and can lead to a release of β-endorphins during acute ingestion. In addition to these effects, alcohol also inhibits postsynaptic NMDA excitatory glutamate receptors. Glutamate is the primary excitatory neurotransmitter of the brain, and its inhibition further contributes to the sedative effects of alcohol. Additional important effects on neurotransmitters include increased serotonin activity and decreased nicotinic acetylcholine receptors.

XI-62. The answer is D. *(Chap. 467)* The acute effects of any drug depend on many factors including amount consumed and absorbed, presence of other drugs, and past experience with the drug. In an individual who is naïve to alcohol, levels as low as 0.02 g/dL can lead to a decrease in inhibitions and a slight feeling of intoxication. In the United States, "legal" intoxication occurs at a blood alcohol level of 0.08 g/dL in most states. At this level, decreases in cognitive and motor abilities are seen. Once an alcohol level of 0.20 g/dL is achieved, an individual is obviously impaired with slurred speech, poor judgment, and impaired coordination. Light coma and depression of respiratory rate, blood pressure, and pulse occur at levels around 0.30 g/dL, and death is likely to occur at levels of 0.40 g/dL. However, in individuals who drink heavily, tolerance begins to develop to alcohol. After a period of 1–2 weeks of daily alcohol consumption, liver metabolism of alcohol increases by as much as 30%, but disappears quite quickly with abstinence. Cellular or pharmacodynamic tolerance also occurs and refers to the neurochemical changes that allow an individual to maintain more normal physiologic function despite the presence of alcohol.

XI-63. The answer is C. *(Chap. 467)* In the most recent fifth edition of *Diagnostic and Statistical Manual of Mental Disorders*, the term *alcohol use disorder* replaced the two terms used to describe problem areas with alcohol use: alcohol abuse and alcohol dependence. Under the new terminology, alcohol use disorder is defined as repeated alcohol-related difficulties in at least 2 of 11 life areas that cluster together in the same 12-month period, and this disorder combines many of the criteria of dependence and abuse into a single diagnosis. The diagnosis of alcohol use disorder is further characterized as mild, moderate, or severe based on how many criteria a person fulfills. Examples of these criteria include failure to fulfill obligations, drinking in hazardous situations, tolerance, withdrawal, craving, and inability to control drinking behaviors. The lifetime risk of an alcohol use disorder in most Western countries is about 10%–15% in men and 5%–8% in women. However, there may be higher rates in Ireland, France, and Scandinavian countries. In addition, native cultures appear to be especially susceptible to problems with alcohol use. This has been seen in Native Americans, Maoris, and the aboriginal tribes of Australia. About 60% of the risk for alcohol use disorders is attributed to genetic influences. Children of alcoholics do have a higher risk of an alcohol use disorder; however, this risk is about 4 times higher, not 10 times higher. This risk is conferred even when the children are adopted early and raised by nonalcoholics. Identical twins also exhibit a higher risk of concurrent alcoholism when compared to fraternal twins. The genetic factors that appear to be most strongly linked to alcohol use disorders include genes that are linked to impulsivity, schizophrenia, and bipolar disorder. In addition, genes that affect alcohol metabolism or sensitivity to alcohol also contribute to the genetics of alcoholism. A mutation in aldehyde dehydrogenase that is more common in individuals of Asian descent results in intense flushing when alcohol is consumed and confers a decreased risk of alcohol dependence. Conversely, genetic variants that lead to a low sensitivity to alcohol increase the risk of a subsequent alcohol use disorder as higher doses of alcohol are required to achieve the same effects. It is estimated that 20% of all patients have at least mild alcohol use disorder. The age at first drink is similar between alcoholics and nonalcoholics. However, alcoholics report a slightly earlier onset of regular drinking and drunkenness. In most individuals with alcoholism, the course of the disease is one of remissions and relapse, but most individuals do require treatment to be able to sustain abstinence. The chance of spontaneous remission is about 20%. If drinking continues without remission, the lifespan will decrease by about 10 years, with leading causes of death including heart disease, cancer, suicide, and accidents.

XI-64. **The answer is B.** *(Chap. 467)* Individuals with alcohol dependence are susceptible to alcohol withdrawal when alcohol intake is stopped abruptly. The individual in this case scenario is likely alcohol dependent given his large amount of alcohol intake on a daily basis. Symptoms of alcohol withdrawal can range from mild tremulousness to hallucinations, seizures, or development of delirium tremens. Other clinical features of alcohol withdrawal include anxiety, insomnia, and autonomic nervous system overactivity manifested as tachycardia, tachypnea, elevated blood pressure, and fever. This patient exhibits symptoms of the more severe delirium tremens, with mental confusion, agitation, and fluctuating levels of consciousness. Although minor symptoms of alcohol withdrawal may begin as soon as 5–10 hours after cessation of alcohol intake, the symptoms do not peak for 48–72 hours, putting this patient in the appropriate time frame for alcohol withdrawal. The best approach to the alcohol-dependent patient who abruptly stops all alcohol intake is a prophylactic approach, and the patient should be screened early for symptoms of alcohol withdrawal. Tools such as the Revised Clinical Institute for Withdrawal Assessment for Alcohol (CIWA-Ar) may help clinicians and nurses screen for early development of symptoms and allow intervention before symptoms escalate. In this setting, most experts recommend use of oral long-acting benzodiazepines such as chlordiazepoxide or diazepam beginning on the first day. However, in this case, the patient received no such treatment and is now experiencing severe alcohol withdrawal and delirium tremens. IV medications that have a rapid onset of action and can be titrated for more aggressive symptom management are often employed in this setting. Thus, use of IV lorazepam or diazepam is preferred in this patient. Following an initial bolus, repeated doses can be used in short intervals until the patient is calm but arousable. In some instances, a continuous infusion may be required, although bolus dosing is preferred. In the most severe cases, propofol or barbiturates may be required, although the patient would most likely need to be intubated for airway protection with use of these medications. The other options listed are not appropriate for initial management of this patient. IV fluids and thiamine had been administered since hospital admission. Administration of glucose-containing fluids without thiamine in the alcohol-dependent patient can precipitate Wernicke encephalopathy, which would present with ophthalmoparesis, ataxia, and encephalopathy. Given the patient's fever, an infectious etiology can be considered, and it would be appropriate to perform blood cultures in this patient. However, given the clear symptoms of alcohol withdrawal and lack of necrotizing pancreatitis on abdominal CT, empiric treatment with antibiotics is not required. Likewise, without focal neurologic findings, a head CT would be a low-yield diagnostic procedure that would be difficult to perform in the patient's current agitated condition and would only delay appropriate therapy. Finally, restraints are best avoided if the patient's safety can be ensured through appropriate use of benzodiazepines because restraints are only likely to make the patient's agitation worse and may lead to iatrogenic harm. Haloperidol may have some sedative effect on the patient but could lead to torsades de pointes arrhythmia because this patient is at risk for electrolyte deficiencies from his alcoholism and pancreatitis.

XI-65. The answer is D. *(Chap. 467)* In individuals recovering from alcoholism, several medications may have a modest benefit in increasing abstinence rates. The two medications with the best risk-benefit ratio are acamprosate and naltrexone. Acamprosate inhibits NMDA receptors, decreasing symptoms of prolonged alcohol withdrawal. Naltrexone is an opioid antagonist that can be administered orally or as a monthly injection. It is thought to act by decreasing activity in the dopamine-rich ventral tegmental area of the brainstem and subsequently decreasing the pleasurable feelings associated with alcohol consumption. There is some research to suggest that the use of these medications in combination may be more effective than either one alone. Disulfiram is an aldehyde dehydrogenase inhibitor that has been used for many years in the treatment of alcoholism. However, it is no longer a commonly used drug due to its many side effects and risks associated with treatment. The primary mechanism by which it acts is to create negative effects of vomiting and autonomic nervous system hyperactivity when alcohol is consumed concurrently with use of the medication. Because it inhibits an enzyme that is part of the normal metabolism of alcohol, it allows the buildup of acetaldehyde, which creates these unpleasant symptoms. As a result of the autonomic side effects, it is contraindicated in individuals with hypertension, a history of stroke, heart disease, or diabetes mellitus.

XI-66. The answer is B. *(Chap. 470)* Although declining in prevalence, cigarette smoking and use of other nicotine-containing products remain a significant contributor to premature death in the United States and account for about one out of every five deaths in the United States, for a total of 400,000 deaths annually. Approximately 40% of cigarette smokers will die prematurely due to the habit unless they are able to quit. The primary causes of premature death related to cigarette smoking are cardiovascular diseases, including both myocardial infarction and stroke; chronic obstructive pulmonary disease (COPD); and myriad cancers including lung, oral, esophageal, urogenital, and pancreatic cancer. Cigarette smoking promotes both large- and small-vessel vascular disease. Approximately 90% of peripheral vascular disease in the nondiabetic population can be attributed to cigarette smoking. In addition, 50% of aortic aneurysms, 20%–30% of coronary artery diseases, and 10% of ischemic and hemorrhagic strokes are caused by cigarette smoking. Moreover, if additional cardiac risk factors are present, the incremental risk added by cigarette smoking is multiplicative. As mentioned earlier, cigarette smoking increases the risk of many different cancers, not just those of the respiratory tract. The digestive tract appears to be particularly susceptible to the effects of cigarette smoking because cigarette smoking has been linked to esophageal, stomach, pancreatic, liver, and colorectal cancer. Urogenital cancers are also increased in cigarette smokers, with increases in both kidney and bladder cancer. In women, cervical cancer is also increased among smokers. Interestingly, however, uterine cancer may be decreased among postmenopausal woman who smoke. Cigarette smoking is responsible for 90% of COPD. Cigarette smoking induces chronic inflammation in the small airways, although most smokers do not develop symptomatic respiratory disease. Chronic inflammation, narrowing of the small airways, and destruction of the alveoli lead to symptoms of COPD and emphysema in 15%–25% of smokers. In any given year, more than half of smokers would like to quit smoking. However, only 6% quit for 6 months, and less than 3% remain abstinent at 3 years. Most individuals have to make multiple attempts to quit before being successful, and they are more likely to be successful if advised to quit by a physician. Other triggers for smoking cessation include an acute illness, the cost of cigarettes, media campaigns, and workplace smoking restrictions.

XI-67. The answer is E. *(Chap. 470)* Smoking cessation is more likely to be successful when an individual is advised to quit by a physician and has a supervised smoking cessation plan.

At every medical visit, all patients should be asked whether they smoke, how much they smoke, and whether they are interested in quitting. Even patients who state that are not interested in quitting should receive a clear message from their provider that smoking is an important health hazard and be offered assistance with quitting in the future. For those interested in quitting, negotiating a quit date is an important step in the process, and close follow-up with office contact near the quit date is an important part of the process. In addition, sometimes a more intensive counseling approach may be necessary. Current recommendations are to offer pharmacologic therapy with either nicotine replacement therapy (NRT) or varenicline. A variety of NRTs are available, including transdermal patches, nasal inhaler, gum, oral inhaler, or lozenge, with success rates of 1.5–2.7 times greater than no intervention. Varenicline is an oral partial agonist of the nicotinic acetylcholine receptor that has a published success rate of 2.7 times greater than no intervention. There has been some concern regarding use of varenicline in individuals with severe psychiatric illness, including suicidal ideation, but this individual does not meet this level of concern. With planned close follow-up, varenicline should be considered an available option for this patient.

XI-68. **The answer is D.** *(Chap. 470)* Varenicline is a partial agonist of the nicotinic acetylcholine receptor and has been demonstrated to be more effective than placebo in promoting smoking cessation. Severe psychiatric symptoms including suicidal ideation have been reported, prompting a warning by the FDA. In addition, closer therapeutic supervision has been recommended, but at this time, the true frequency of these responses remains unclear. A recent publication retrospectively reviewed the use of varenicline in over 69,000 individuals in Sweden. When compared to the general population, there was no increased risk of suicide or psychosis in individuals prescribed varenicline even though these individuals were twice as likely to have had a prior psychiatric diagnosis (Thomas KH et al. *BMJ* 347:f5704, 2013). However, the FDA is currently continuing its surveillance of the drug until more data are available. Alternative agents such as bupropion in combination with nicotine replacement therapy should be considered.

XI-69. **The answer is B.** *(Chap. 470)* Smokers regulate their blood levels of nicotine by adjusting the frequency and intensity of their tobacco use. Smokers can compensate for the lower levels of nicotine in low-yield cigarettes by smoking more cigarettes or by adjusting their smoking technique with a deeper inhalation and breathhold. Therefore, smoking low-yield cigarettes is not a reasonable alternative to smoking cessation. Moreover, there is no difference in the harmful physical effects of smoking or in the potential for drug interactions. Finally, although not definitively proven, there is some thought that the rise in adenocarcinoma of the lung over the past 50 years is associated with introduction of the low-tar cigarette and the resultant change in smoking behavior associated with this introduction.